Clinical Gynecologic Endocrinology and Infertility

Fifth Edition

Clinical Gynecologic Endocrinology and Infertility

Fifth Edition

Leon Speroff
Robert H. Glass
Nathan G. Kase

**Illustration and Page Design
by Lisa Million**

SANS TACHE

Williams & Wilkins

BALTIMORE • PHILADELPHIA • HONG KONG
LONDON • MUNICH • SYDNEY • TOKYO

A WAVERLY COMPANY

Editor: Charles Mitchell
Project Manager: Victoria Rybicki Vaughn

Copyright © 1994
Williams & Wilkins
428 East Preston Street
Baltimore, Maryland 21202, USA

Accurate indications, adverse reactions, and dosage schedules for drugs are provided in this book, but it is possible that they may change. The reader is urged to review the package information data of the manufacturers of the medications mentioned.

Printed in the United States of America

First Edition 1973

Library of Congress Cataloging in Publication Data

Speroff, Leon, 1935–
    Clinical gynecologic endocrinology & infertility / Leon Speroff,
Robert H. Glass, Nathan G. Kase ; illustration and page design by
Lisa Million. —5th ed.
        p.   cm.
    Includes bibliographical references and index.
    ISBN 0-683-07899-2
    1. Endocrine gynecology. 2. Infertility—Endocrine aspects.
I. Glass, Robert H., 1932–   . II. Kase, Nathan G., 1930–   .
III. Title.
    [DNLM: 1. Genital Diseases, Female. 2. Endocrine Diseases.
3. Infertility, Female. WP 505 S749c 1994]
RG159.S62 1994
618.1—dc20
DNLM/DLC
for Library of Congress   94-6960
                                                                 CIP

94 95 96 97 98
1 2 3 4 5 6 7 8 9 10

Preface

We are pleased to present the 5th edition of our book; 5 editions over a span of approximately 20 years. We hope that our efforts have contributed to the improved and informed care of women.

Over these 20 years, our objective has been to provide both useful information and practical clinical management. Our text is an expression and formulation of our collective professional activities as teachers, investigators, and most importantly, as clinicians in the field of reproductive endocrinology and infertility.

The basic form of the book is unchanged, but the increase in weight and size testify to the massive expansion of knowledge since the first editon. We now provide sufficient information so that the book can serve as a resource for basic data (anatomical, physiological, and biochemical) that we all have trouble remembering. However, we believe we have held true to our objective: to provide both factual knowledge and systematic approaches to clinical problems.

As always, this book is dedicated to the improvement of patient care, and we hope that it will aid all readers in accomplishing that goal. We would like to express our gratitude to the scholars, epidemiologists, laboratory investigators, and clinical researchers who have contributed the facts that are the substance of our formulations. Most importantly, we thank our patients, who, in the final analysis, are the most informative teachers.

Leon Speroff, M.D.
Portland, Oregon

Robert H. Glass, M.D.
San Francisco, California

Nathan G. Kase, M.D.
New York, New York

P.S. Perhaps some would be interested in the history of the cover colors of our 5 editions. The 1st edition, when we were all at Yale, was supposed to be Yale blue, but the printer erred and it turned out to be light blue. The 2nd edition was in green and yellow, the colors of the University of Oregon. The cover and endpapers of the 3rd edition featured the colors of the Cleveland Browns. The 4th edition was a nostalgic return to Yale blue. The colors of the present edition represent the Portland Trail Blazers. Go Blazers!

Contents

The International System of Units (SI Units); methods and interpretations of laboratory assays that are useful in reproductive endocrine diagnosis.

Part I

Reproductive Physiology

1 Molecular Biology for Clinicians

GCAGCCGTATTTCTACTGCGACGAGGAG
GAGAACTT**SPEROFF**CTACCAGCAGCAG
AGCGAGCTGGC**GLASS**AGCCCCGGCGC
CCAGGGATATCTGGAA**KASE**GAAATTCGA
GCTGCTGCCGCCCTGTCCCTAGCCGCG

The above DNA sequence is obviously a mutant. But the fact that we can recognize this cryptogram as a nucleotide sequence, and diagnose a mutant change, illustrates the incredible progress made in the understanding of human biology. Molecular biology is the subspecialty of science devoted to understanding the structure and function of the genome, the full complement of DNA (desoxyribonucleic acid), the macromolecule which contains all the hereditary information.

The Austrian monk, Gregor Mendel, studied his garden of peas for much of his life at his monastery, and was the first to express the principles of heredity in the 1860s. He described dominant and recessive traits, and the "laws" of transmission governing the homozygous and heterozygous inheritance of these traits. Mendel's theories remained unknown until 1900, when they were discovered. Unfortunately, Mendel died 16 years before recognition of his work.

The pairing and splitting of chromosomes at cell division was proposed in 1903, but it was not until 1946 that Edward Tatum and Joshua Lederberg at Yale University demonstrated in bacteria that DNA carried hereditary information. James Watson and Francis Crick, working at the Cavendish Laboratories in Cambridge, proposed in 1953, the structure of DNA by creating a model based upon the parameters provided by Maurice Wilkins and Rosalind Franklin obtained with x-ray crystallography. Crick, Watson, and Wilkins received the Nobel Prize in 1962; Franklin died in 1958, and Nobel prizes are not awarded posthumously.

DNA replication involves many enzyme systems. DNA polymerase was isolated in 1958, and RNA polymerase in 1960. In 1978, Werner Arber, Hamilton Smith, and Daniel Nathans received the Nobel prize for their discovery, in the 1960s, of the enzymes for joining or cutting DNA. The use of ligase and restriction endonuclease enzymes permitted the production of recombinant DNA molecules, first accomplished by Paul Berg at Stanford University in 1972.

E.M. Southern of Edinburgh University developed in 1975 the technique to transfer (to blot) DNA from agarose gels onto nitrocellulose filters, enabling DNA fragments to be joined with radiolabeled RNA probes and thus isolated. The cloning of genes or DNA fragments followed the breakthrough discovery that plasmids carrying foreign DNA molecules could be inserted into bacteria, leading to the replication of the foreign DNA.

We have entered the age of molecular biology. It won't be long before endocrine problems will be explained, diagnosed, and treated at the molecular level. Soon the traditional hormone assays will be a medical practice of the past. The power of molecular biology will touch us all, and the many contributions of molecular biology will be perceived throughout this book. But unfortunately, molecular biology has its own language, a language that is almost unintelligible to the uninitiated. We offer this chapter as a guide for the new molecular medicine.

To begin a clinical book with a chapter on molecular biology and a chapter on biochemistry only serves to emphasize that competent clinical judgment is founded upon a groundwork of basic knowledge. On the other hand, clinical practice does not require a technical and sophisticated proficiency in a basic science. The purpose of these first two chapters, therefore, is not to present an intensive course in a basic science, but rather to present a selective review of the most important principles and information necessary for the development of the physiological and clinical concepts to follow. It is further intended that certain details, which we all have difficulty remembering, will be available in these chapters for reference.

The Chromosomes

We are *eukaryotes,* organisms with cells having a true nucleus bounded by a nuclear membrane, with multiplication by mitosis. Bacteria are *prokaryotes,* organisms without a true nucleus, with reproduction by cell division. With the exception of DNA within mitochondria, all of our DNA is packaged in a nucleus surrounded by a nuclear membrane. Mitochondria are believed to be descendants of primitive bacteria engulfed by our ancestors, and they still contain some important genes.

Chromosomes are packages of genetic material, consisting of a DNA molecule (which contains many genes) to which are attached large numbers of proteins that maintain chromosome structure and play a role in gene expression. Human somatic cells contain 46 chromosomes, 22 pairs of autosomes and one pair of sex chromosomes. All somatic cells are diploid — 23 pairs of chromosomes. Only gametes are haploid with 22 autosome chromosomes and one sex chromosome. The chromosomes vary in size, and all contain a pinched portion called a centromere, which divides the chromosome into two arms, the shorter p arm and the longer q arm. The two members of any pair of autosomes are homologous, one homologue derived from each parent. The number of chromosomes does not indicate the level of evolutionary sophistication and complexity; the dog has 78 chromosomes and the carp has 104!

A single gene is a unit of DNA within a chromosome that can be activated to transcribe a specific RNA. The location of a gene on a particular chromosome is designated its locus. Because there are 22 pairs of autosomes, most genes exist in two pairs. The pairs are homozygous when similar and heterozygous when dissimilar.

The usual human karyotype is an arrangement of the chromosomes into pairs, usually after proteolytic treatment and Giemsa staining to produce characteristic banding patterns allowing a blueprint useful for location. The staining characteristics divide each arm into regions, and each region into bands that are numbered from the centromere outwards. A given point on a chromosome is designated by the following order: chromosome number, arm symbol (p for short arm, q for long arm), region number, band number. Example: 7q31.1 is the location for the cystic fibrosis gene.

Mitosis

All eukaryotes, from yeast to humans, undergo similar cell division and multiplication. The process of nuclear division in all somatic cells is called mitosis, during which each chromosome divides into two. For normal growth and development, the entire genomic information must be faithfully reproduced in every cell.

Mitosis consists of the following stages.

Interphase
During this phase, all normal cell activity occurs except active division. It is during this stage that the inactive X chromosome (the Barr body or the sex chromatin) can be seen in female cells.

Prophase
As division begins, the chromosomes condense, and the two chromatids become visible. The nuclear membrane disappears. The centriole is an organelle outside the nucleus that forms the spindles for cell division; the centriole duplicates itself and the two centrioles migrate to opposite poles of the cell.

Metaphase
The chromosomes migrate to the center of the cell, forming a line designated the equatorial plate. The chromosomes are now maximally condensed. The spindle, microtubules of protein that radiate from the centrioles and attach to the centromeres, is formed.

Anaphase
Division occurs in the longitudinal plane of the centromeres. The two new chromatids move to opposite sides of the cell drawn by contraction of the spindles.

Telophase
Division of the cytoplasm begins in the equatorial plane, ending with the formation of two complete cell membranes. The two groups of chromosomes are surrounded by nuclear membranes forming new nuclei. Each strand of DNA serves as a template, and the DNA content of the cell doubles.

Meiosis

Meiosis is the cell division that forms the gametes, each with a haploid number of chromosomes. Meiosis has two purposes: reduction of the chromosome number and recombination to transmit genetic information. In Meiosis I, homologous chromosomes pair and split apart. Meiosis II is similar to mitosis as the already divided chromosomes split and segregate into new cells.

The First Meiotic Division (Meiosis I)
Prophase:
Leptotene: Condensation of the chromosomes.

Zygotene: Pairing of homologous chromosomes (synapsis).

Pachytene: Each pair of chromosomes thickens to form four strands. This is the stage when crossing-over or recombination can occur (exchange of homologous segments between two of the four strands). Chiasmata are the places of contact where cross-overs occur (and can be visualized).

Diplotene: Longitudinal separation of each chromosome.

Metaphase, Anaphase, and Telophase of Meiosis I:
The nuclear membrane disappears and the chromosomes move to the center of the cell. One member of each pair goes to each pole, and the cells divide. Meiosis I is often referred to as reduction division because each new product now has the haploid chromosome number. It is during the first meiotic division that mendelian inheritance occurs. Cross-overs, which occur prior to metaphase, result in new combinations of genetic material, both favorable and unfavorable.

The Second Meiotic Division (Meiosis II)
The second division follows the first without DNA replication. In the oocyte, meiosis II occurs after fertilization. The end result is the production of 4 haploid cells.

The Structure and Function of DNA

DNA is the material of the gene responsible for coding the genetic message as transmitted through specific proteins. Thus, it is the most important molecule of life and the fundamental mechanism for evolution. Genes are segments of DNA which code for specific proteins, together with flanking and intervening sequences that serve controlling and regulating functions. Each molecule of DNA has a deoxyribose backbone, identical repeating groups of deoxyribose sugar linked through phosphodiester bonds. Each deoxyribose is attached in order (giving individuality and specificity) to one of 4 nucleic acids, the nuclear bases:

A purine — adenine or guanine.
A pyrimidine — thymine or cytosine.

A nucleotide is the basic building block of DNA. It consists of 3 major components: the deoxyribose sugar, a phosphate group, and a nucleic acid base. The phosphate-sugar linkages are asymmetric; the phosphorous is linked to the 5-carbon of one sugar and to the 3-carbon of the following sugar. Thus, one end is the 5' (5 prime) end and the other the 3' (3 prime) end. By convention, DNA and its nuclear acid sequences are written from left to right, from the 5' end to the 3' end, the direction of the transcription process. The 5' end leads to the formation of the amino end of the protein; the 3' end forms the carboxy end of the protein.

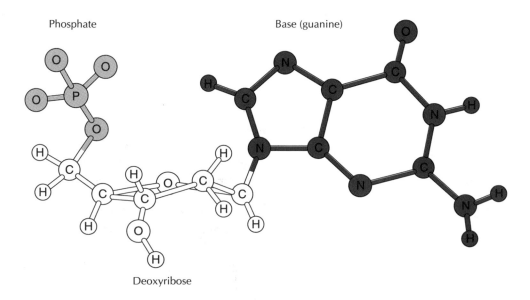

Phosphate   Base (guanine)

Deoxyribose

6

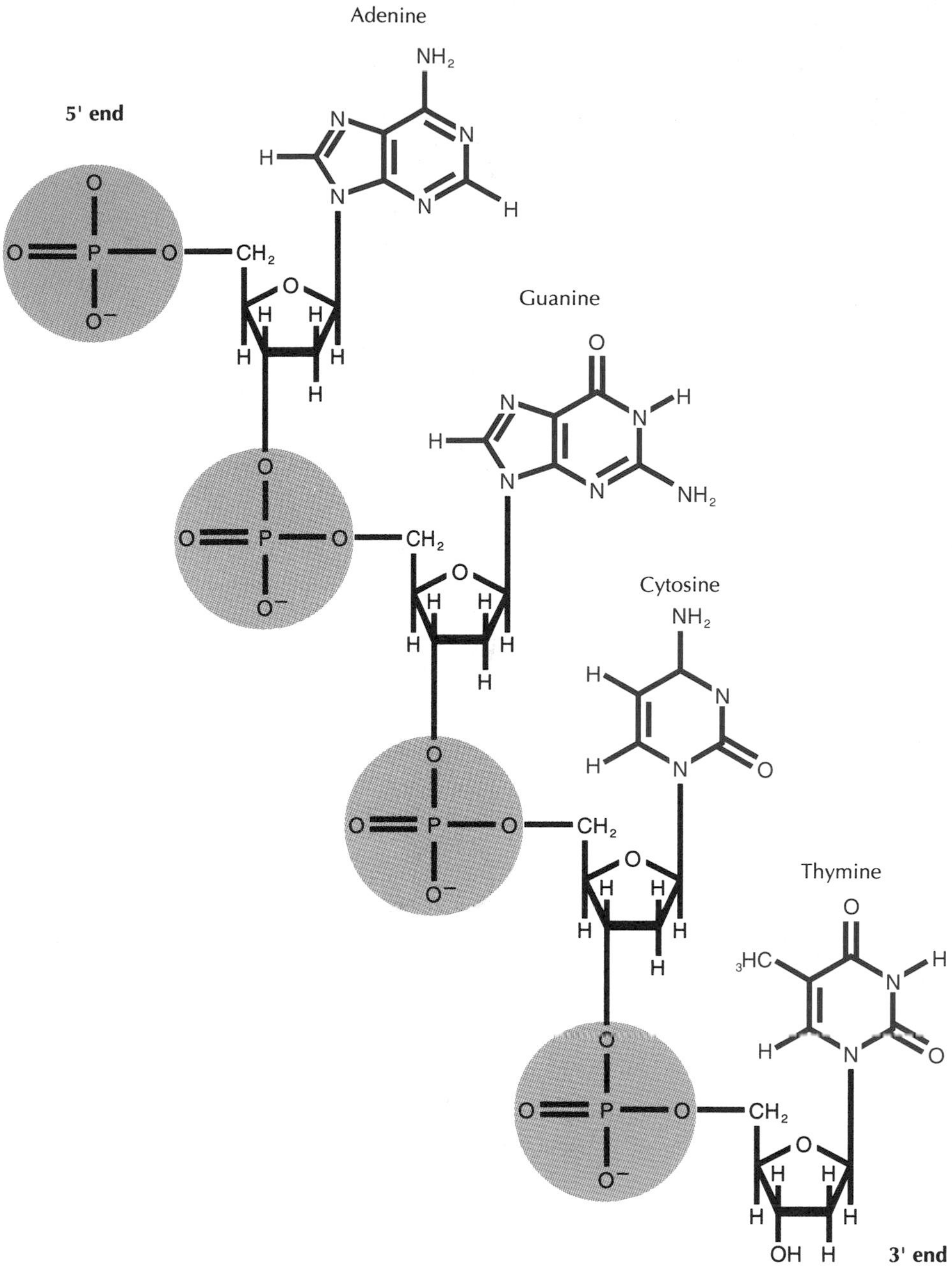

Adenine

Guanine

Cytosine

Thymine

5' end

3' end

DNA consists of two deoxyribose strands in a double helix with the nucleic acids on the inside and the nuclear bases paired by hydrogen bonding, adenine with thymine and cytosine with guanine. RNA differs from DNA in that it is single stranded, its sugar moiety is ribose, and it substitutes uracil for thymine.

How can a cell's DNA, which stretched out measures nearly 2 meters long, fit into a cell? Watson and Crick figured this out when they proposed a tightly coiled two-stranded helix, the double helix. Like the cm is a measure of length, the base pair (bp) is the unit of measure for DNA. The base pair is either adenine-guanine or cytosine-thymine, the nucleic acid of one chain paired with the facing nucleic acid of the other chain. A fragment of DNA is therefore measured by the number of base pairs: e.g., a 4,800-bp fragment (a 4.8-kb fragment). It is estimated that we have 3 billion bp of DNA, only a small portion of which actually codes out for proteins.

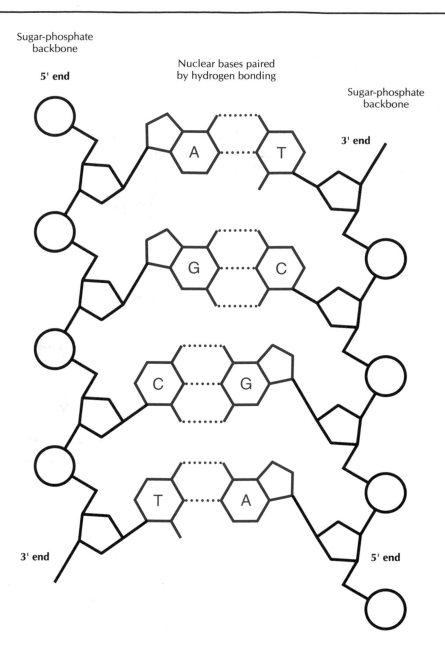

Sugar-phosphate backbone

5' end

Nuclear bases paired by hydrogen bonding

Sugar-phosphate backbone

3' end

3' end

5' end

DNA does not exist within the cell as a naked molecule. The nucleotide chains wind about a core of proteins (histones) to form a nucleosome. The nucleosomes become condensed into many bands, the bands that are recognized in karyotype preparations. This condensation is another important mechanism for packing the long DNA structure into a cell. A variety of other proteins is associated with DNA, important for both structure and function.

The process of DNA replication begins with a separation of the double-stranded DNA helix, initiated at multiple steps by enzyme action. As the original DNA unwinds into template strands, DNA polymerase catalyzes the synthesis of new duplicate strands, which reform a double helix with each of the original strands (this is called replication). Each daughter molecule, therefore, contains one of the parental strands. It is estimated that the original DNA molecule present in the fertilized zygote must be copied approximately 10^{15} times during the course of a human lifetime. Rapidity and accuracy are essential. By combining precision with error-correction systems, errors that affect the function of the gene's protein are surprisingly rare.

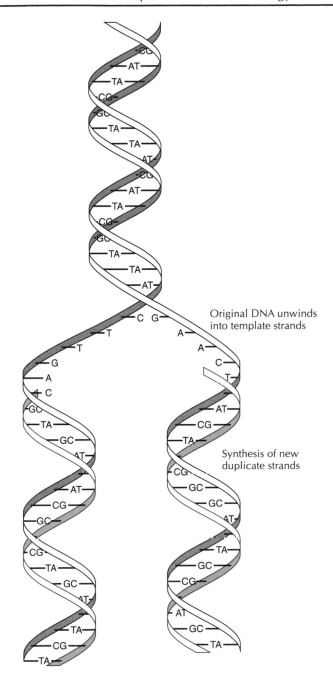

Original DNA unwinds
into template strands

Synthesis of new
duplicate strands

The ***homeobox*** is a DNA sequence, highly conserved throughout evolution, that encodes a series of 60 amino acids, called a homeodomain. Homeodomain protein products function as transcription factors by binding to DNA. The homeobox influences specific tissue functions that are critical for growth and development of the embryo.

The Human Genome

There are 3 billion base pairs in each haploid genome; in the double stranded helix DNA, there are 6 billion nucleotides; and there are an estimated 100,000 to 300,000 genes. Although enormously complex at first glance, the entire genetic language is written with only four letters: A, C, G, and T (U in RNA). Furthermore, the language is limited to only 3 letter words, codons. Finally the entire genetic message is fragmented into the 23 pairs of chromosomes. With four nucleotides, reading groups of three, there are 64 possible combinations. Essentially all living organisms use this code. The genome changes only by new combinations derived from parents or by mutation.

The 20 Amino Acids in Proteins

Amino Acid	Three-Letter Abbreviation	Single-Letter Code
Glycine	Gly	G
Alanine	Ala	A
Valine	Val	V
Isoleucine	Ile	I
Leucine	Leu	L
Serine	Ser	S
Threonine	Thr	T
Proline	Pro	P
Aspartic acid	Asp	D
Glutamic acid	Glu	E
Lysine	Lys	K
Arginine	Arg	R
Asparagine	Asn	N
Glutamine	Gln	Q
Cysteine	Cys	C
Methionine	Met	M
Tryptophan	Trp	W
Phenylalanine	Phe	F
Tyrosine	Tyr	Y
Histidine	His	H

The mRNA Genetic Code

First Position (5' end)	Second Position				Third Position (3' end)
	U	C	A	G	
U	Phe	Ser	Tyr	Cys	U
	Phe	Ser	Tyr	Cys	C
	Leu	Ser	Stop	Stop	A
	Leu	Ser	Stop	Trp	G
C	Leu	Pro	His	Arg	U
	Leu	Pro	His	Arg	C
	Leu	Pro	Gln	Arg	A
	Leu	Pro	Gln	Arg	G
A	Ile	Thr	Asn	Ser	U
	Ile	Thr	Asn	Ser	C
	Ile	Thr	Lys	Arg	A
	Met	Thr	Lys	Arg	G
G	Val	Ala	Asp	Gly	U
	Val	Ala	Asp	Gly	C
	Val	Ala	Glu	Gly	A
	Val	Ala	Glu	Gly	G

Reading across the first row of the table, the codon UUU specifies Phenylalanine, the codon UCU specifies Serine, the codon UAU specifies Tyrosine, and the codon UGU specifies Cysteine. UAA, UAG, and UGA are stop codons.

Gene Structure and Function

The linear arrangement of many genes forms a chromosome. A gene is composed of a segment of DNA containing exons separated by introns, the coding and noncoding codons of nucleotides, respectively. Intron-exon patterns tend to be conserved during evolution. The alpha- and beta-globin genes are believed to have arisen 500 million years ago, with the introns in the same location as they are today.

Exon
The segment of a gene that yields a messenger RNA product that codes for a specific protein.

Intron
The segment of a gene not represented in mature RNA and, therefore, noncoding for protein.

Codon
A sequence of 3 bases in RNA or DNA that codes for a specific amino acid; the triplet codon.

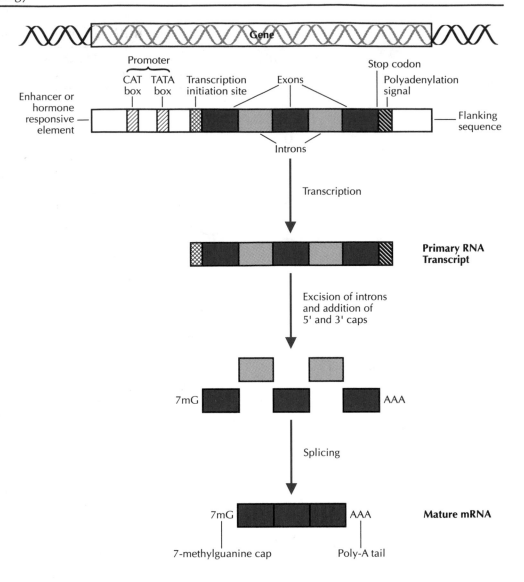

With some exceptions, essentially one gene yields one protein. As noted above, the introns are not translated into protein products. Only the DNA sequences in the exons (the part that "exits" the nucleus) are transcribed into messenger RNA and then translated into proteins. Genes also include flanking sequences important for gene transcription. The area that will initiate DNA action (e.g., DNA binding to the hormone-receptor complex) is called an ***enhancer*** region. The actual area where transcription begins is the ***promoter*** region. Only a few relatively short nucleotide sequences are promoters, such as the T-A-T-A-A sequence, or TATA box, and the C-C-A-A-T sequence, or CAT box. The promoter sites are usually near the start of the coding region of the gene. Enhancer sites are larger than promoter sites and can be located anywhere, even far from the gene, but usually are in the 5' flanking end. At the 3' end, a coding sequence is usually present for the polyadenine tail common for most messenger RNA molecules.

The enhancer sites bind proteins that serve as signals to regulate gene expression by either increasing or repressing the binding of RNA polymerase in the promoter region. This is one method of creating unique cellular functions. For example, a hormone target tissue can respond to the hormone because it contains a specific receptor protein that upon binding to the hormone will bind to a DNA enhancer site. Specific proteins (called transcription factors) bind to enhancer sites and activate transcription. The regulation of gene transcription usually involves DNA sequences in the 5' flanking upstream region of a gene.

Three codons (UAG, UAA, UGA) are called *stop codons,* because they specify a stop to translation of RNA into protein (like a period at the end of a sentence). By contrast, an *open reading frame* is a long series of base pairs between two stop codons; therefore, an open reading frame encodes the amino acid sequence of the protein product. Finding and identifying an open reading frame is an important step in analyzing DNA sequences because such a long sequence is usually encountered only in an active gene.

Gene expression is composed of the following steps: transcription of DNA to RNA, RNA processing to produce functional messenger RNA by splicing out introns, translation of messenger RNA on a ribosome to a peptide chain, and protein structural processing to the functional form.

Transcription

Transcription is the synthesis of single-stranded messenger RNA from a gene (double-stranded DNA). The amino acid sequence of the protein is coded in the DNA by codons; a single amino acid is coded by each codon, a triplet of 3 nucleic acid bases. RNA polymerase constructs the messenger RNA by reading the DNA strand that is complementary to the RNA; thus, the RNA is an exact copy of the other DNA strand, which is also called the complementary strand of the DNA molecule (remember, an important difference is that thymine in DNA is replaced by uracil in RNA).

Molecular complementarity is both a difficult and a simple concept to grasp. The simple aspect is the concept of one thing being like another. The difficult part is the necessity to understand and visualize that the complementary molecule is not identical to its template, but more like: where the template goes in, the complementary molecule goes out. Thus, the strands of the double helix are not identical. Each DNA strand has a complementary structure, in a sense, one positive template and one negative template, each specifying the other. Each strand, therefore, serves as a template for its complementary DNA (in the process of replication) or complementary RNA (in the process of transcription). Thus, messenger RNA is synthesized from the negative template, the "antisense" strand, so that it will have the same structure as the positive template, the "sense" strand. Molecular biologists have to think in three dimensions!

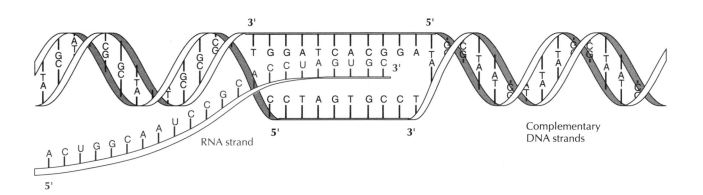

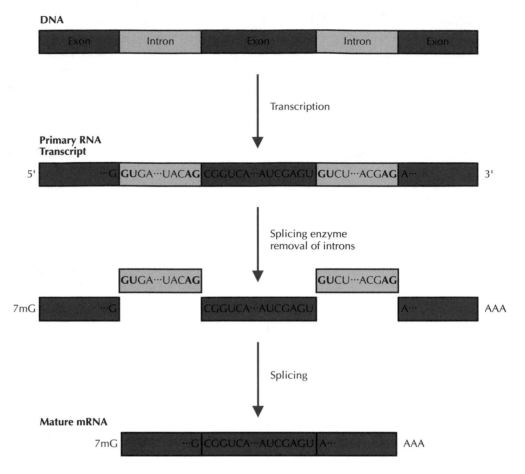

Transcription is initiated at the upstream start site, the 5' untranslated flanking region where the two strands of the double helix come apart. The process continues downstream, copying one of the strands until a specific codon is reached which provides a stop message. RNA synthesis continues with the addition of a long chain of adenines, the poly-A tail; this is the 3' untranslated region that is believed to stabilize RNA by preventing degradation. After transcription from a gene, the RNA moves into the cytoplasm where the intron regions are excised, and the exons are joined together *(RNA splicing)* to produce a complete, mature RNA molecule. The start and end of each exon and intron have sequences which when copied onto the RNA signal an enzyme to remove the intervening parts. Almost all introns begin with G-U and end with A-G (G-T and A-G in the DNA intron). Introns are of varying lengths; a single intron can be longer than the final RNA product. The mature RNA molecule has an addition at one end ("capping," by the addition of a modified nucleotide, 7-methyl guanosine) to protect against RNAases and at the other end, a polyadenine tail (the poly-A tail) is added (in addition to a stabilizing factor, perhaps a signal to direct exit from the nucleus). Both ends are untranslated in the ribosomes.

Translation

The messenger RNA travels from the chromosome on which it was synthesized to a ribosome in the cytoplasm, where it directs the assembly of amino acids into proteins (translation). Amino acids are brought into the process by specific transfer RNA molecules. The specific sequence of 3 bases at one end of the transfer RNA is complementary to the codon coding for the specific amino acid. Binding of this area to the messenger RNA codon places the specific amino acid at the other end into the proper sequence for the protein. The amino acids are placed one at a time as the transfer RNA molecules read the RNA template beginning at the amino acid end (the 5' end) and finishing at the carboxy end (the 3' end). The process begins at the first AUG triplet and

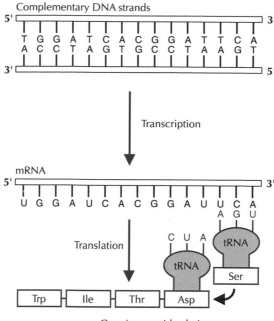

Complementary DNA strands

mRNA

Transcription

Translation

Growing peptide chain

continues until a stop codon (UAA, UAG, or UGA) is reached, whereupon the messenger RNA falls off the ribosome and degenerates. The specific linear sequence of amino acids is specified by the genetic coding; in turn, this sequence determines the 3-dimensional form of the protein, the folded structure necessary for function.

The final expression of a gene may not end with the translation process. Further (posttranslational) processing of proteins occurs, such as glycosylation (the gonadotropins) or proteolytic cleavage (conversion of proopiomelanocortin to ACTH).

Mutations

Any change in DNA sequence constitutes a mutation. Substitution refers to a change in a single nucleic acid base. A substitution in a codon can result in the incorporation of the wrong amino acid into a protein, leading to a change or loss in function. Insertion or deletion of amino acids into the final protein product can result from improper RNA splicing. Because of great redundancy in the genetic code (many triplet codons code out for the same amino acid, and there are only 20 amino acids), not all substitutions produce an effect. A clinical example of a single base substitution (point mutation) is the sickle mutation, where thymine is substituted for adenine in the beta-globin gene. If homologous regions of DNA are misaligned, unequal crossover can occur, resulting in deletions and insertions (additions). Deletions and insertions can involve single bases, up to entire exons, or genes or several genes. Recombination or exchange of genetic material usually occurs in meiosis. Even a change at the junction of a coding and noncoding region can lead to abnormal mRNA.

Chromosomal Abnormalities	**Numerical Abnormalities**

Numerical Abnormalities

Numerical abnormalities usually are due to nondisjunction, a failure of separation at anaphase, either during mitotic division or during meiosis. *Aneuploidy* is a chromosome number that is not an exact multiple of the haploid number, e.g., monosomy (45,X Turner syndrome) or trisomy (trisomy 13 Patau syndrome, trisomy 18 Edward syndrome, trisomy 21 Down syndrome, 47,XXY Klinefelter syndrome). *Mosaicism* indicates one or more cell lines with a different karyotype, usually arising from nondisjunction during early mitosis (failure of two paired chromosomes to separate). *Polyploidy,* multiples of the haploid number of chromosomes, is a significant cause of spontaneous abortion.

Structural Abnormalities

Structural abnormalities are usually due to chromosomal breaks induced by radiation, drugs, or viruses. The resulting abnormality depends upon the rearrangement of the broken pieces. Thus in a *translocation* there is interchange of material between two or more nonhomologous chromosomes. A balanced translocation is associated with neither gain nor loss of genetic material, and such an individual is a translocation carrier.

Single Gene Defects

Single gene defects are due to mutations in specific genes. These mutations are transmitted according to mendelian inheritance: autosomal dominant, autosomal recessive, X-linked recessive, and rarely X-linked dominant.

Autosomal Dominance. Transmission is not linked to the sex of an individual, and homozygous and heterozygous children are affected (only one allele need be abnormal). With two heterozygous parents, each child has a 75% risk of being affected. With one heterozygous parent, each child has a 50% risk of being affected. The effect is subject to variable expression. Examples of autosomal dominant conditions include Huntington disease, neurofibromatosis, and Marfan syndrome.

Autosomal Recessive. These conditions are phenotypically expressed only in homozygotes (both alleles must be abnormal). With heterozygote parents, each child has a 25% risk of being affected, a 50% chance of being a carrier. Examples of autosomal recessive conditions are cystic fibrosis, sickle cell disease, and adrenal hyperplasia due to a deficiency in 21-hydroxylase.

X-Linked Recessive Inheritance. An affected father can transmit the condition only to daughters. Only homozygous females are affected when the condition is recessive. Red-green color blindness and hemophilia A are examples.

Genomic Imprinting

Genomic imprinting indicates persisting influences on genome function by the male and female parental contributions. For example, placental development is controlled mostly by paternally derived genes. Thus a hydatidiform mole has a normal karyotype, but all of its chromosomes are derived from the father. Experiments in nature and animal experiments indicate that the maternal contribution to the genome is more important for embryonic development. In certain autosomal recessive conditions, the expression, severity, and age of onset will be influenced by the gender of the parent providing the mutant gene or chromosome.

Techniques of Molecular Biology

An enyzme that breaks the phosphodiester bonds and cuts the DNA molecule into fragments is an endonuclease; a ***restriction enzyme*** (restriction endonuclease) will cut only at sites with specific nucleic acid sequences. Restriction enzymes were discovered in bacteria where they form a defense mechanism to cut (and thus inactivate) any foreign DNA (from invading viruses) introduced into the bacterial cell. As part of this protection mechanism, bacteria also contain methylases that methylate recognition sites in native DNA, directing the action of the restriction enzyme to the nonmethylated foreign DNA. Different bacteria have different restriction enzymes with specific action sites. Restriction enzymes are available that cut DNA into pieces ranging from many small fragments to a few large pieces, depending upon the number of nucleotides in the recognition sequence. They are named for the organism and strain from which they are derived.

DNA polymerase is an enzyme that brings single nucelotides into a DNA molecule. A DNA polymerase can form DNA only in the presence of a DNA template; the synthesized DNA will be complementary to the template. RNA polymerase can make RNA also only in the presence of a DNA template.

A ***DNAase*** can remove nucleotides. By combining DNAase treatment with DNA polymerase action, radiolabeled nucleotides can be introduced into a DNA molecule, producing a ***DNA probe.*** A DNA probe can be compared to the antibody used in immunoassays. The antibody is specific and recognizes the hormone against which it is formed. The DNA probe specifically detects a sequence of DNA.

Reverse transcriptase is DNA polymerase that is RNA dependent. It is called reverse transcriptase because the flow of information is from RNA to DNA, the reverse of the usual direction of flow. This enzyme permits the copying of essentially any RNA molecule into single-stranded DNA; such DNA is called ***complementary DNA*** because it is a mirror image of the messenger RNA. Complementary DNA probes are limited by their reading only the exons (remember that introns are excised from RNA), and thus these probes read only large areas.

DNA and RNA are charged molecules and, therefore, will migrate in an electrical field. Fragments can be analyzed by gel (agarose or polyacrilamide) electrophoresis, the largest fragments migrating the slowest. By convention, the gels are read from top to bottom, with the smallest fragments at the bottom.

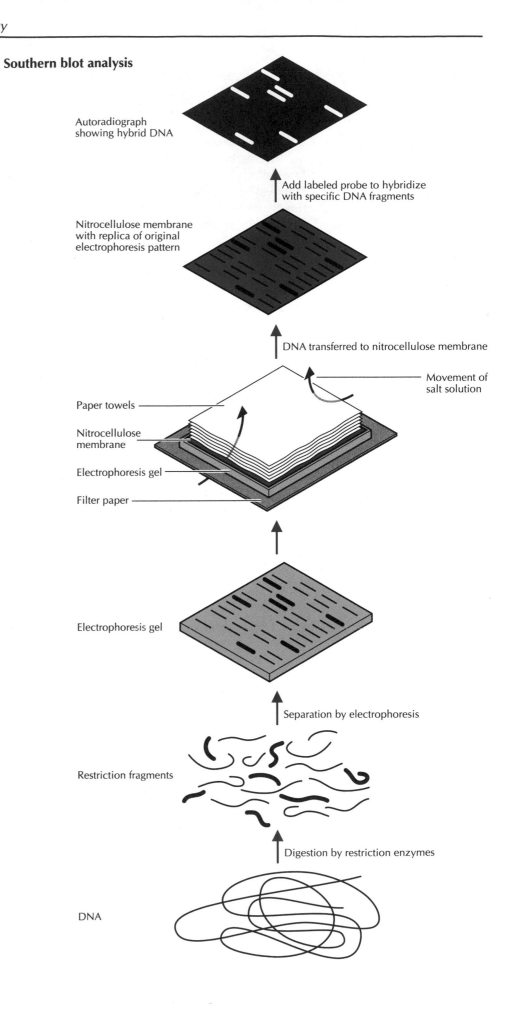

Southern blot analysis

Autoradiograph showing hybrid DNA

Add labeled probe to hybridize with specific DNA fragments

Nitrocellulose membrane with replica of original electrophoresis pattern

DNA transferred to nitrocellulose membrane

Movement of salt solution

Paper towels

Nitrocellulose membrane

Electrophoresis gel

Filter paper

Electrophoresis gel

Separation by electrophoresis

Restriction fragments

Digestion by restriction enzymes

DNA

Southern Blot Analysis

DNA is first denatured to separate the two strands, then digested by restriction enzymes to produce smaller fragments. The Southern blot method, named after E.M. Southern, determines the fragment sizes. The fragments are separated by electrophoresis. The electrophoresis gel is placed over a thick piece of filter paper with its ends dipped in a high salt solution. A special membrane (nitrocellulose) is placed over the gel and over this is placed a stack of paper towels compressed by a weight. The salt solution rises by wick action into the filter paper; it moves by capillary action through the gel carrying the DNA with it. The DNA is carried to the nitrocellulose membrane to which it binds. The salt solution keeps moving and is absorbed by the paper towels. The nitrocellulose membrane thus creates a replica of the original electrophoresis pattern. The DNA is fixed to the membrane either by high temperature baking or by ultraviolet light. Specific labeled probes than can be introduced for hybridization. *Hybridization* means that a specific probe anneals to its complementary sequence. The fragments with this sequence are then identified by autoradiography.

Northern blotting refers to RNA processing, Northern because RNA is the opposite image of DNA. Extracted RNA is separated by electrophoresis and transferred to a cellulose membrane as in Southern blotting for hybridization with probes (complementary DNA). Northern blotting would be used, for example, to determine whether hormone stimulation of a specific protein in a tissue is mediated by messenger RNA, i.e., gene expression.

Electrophoresis to separate proteins is called *Western blotting,* and antibodies are used for the hybridization identification process. Like Northern blotting, Western blotting tests gene expression, not just the presence of a gene. Northern and Western represent intentional witticisms (a rare event in science) in response to Southern blotting. Hybridization without electrophoresis by placing a drop of the cell extract directly on filter paper is called *dot or slot blotting.*

Hybridization

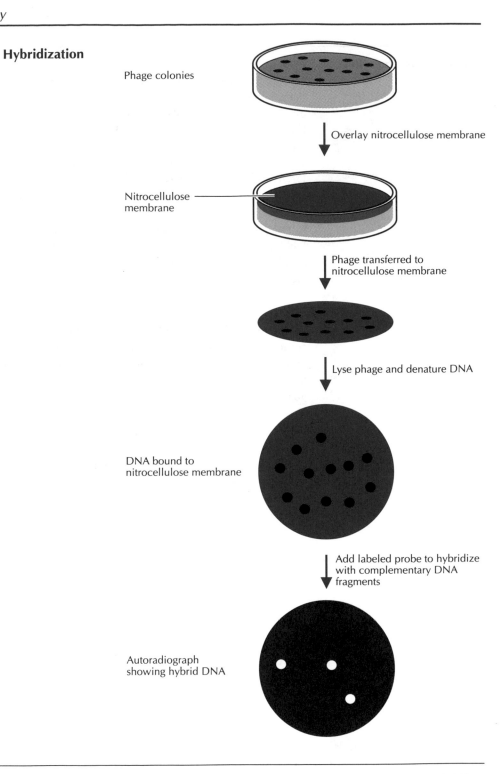

Phage colonies

Overlay nitrocellulose membrane

Nitrocellulose membrane

Phage transferred to nitrocellulose membrane

Lyse phage and denature DNA

DNA bound to nitrocellulose membrane

Add labeled probe to hybridize with complementary DNA fragments

Autoradiograph showing hybrid DNA

Hybridization   When two complementary strands of DNA reassociate, the process is called hybridization. Hybridization allows a specific area of the DNA to be studied using a radiolabeled DNA probe that is specific (a complementary sequence). The nitrocellulose membrane produced after Southern blotting is first treated to block nonspecific binding sites. The membrane is then treated (hybridized) with the labeled probe. The location of bound probe is then identified by autoradiography (for radiolabeled probes) or by colorimetric methods. The sequence of the probe therefore determines the sequence at the site of binding. Whenever two products are complementary, hybridization occurs. Thus, complementary DNA can be hybridized to its template messenger RNA. In situ hybridization is the technique where labeled DNA or RNA probes are placed directly on a slide of tissue or cells.

Polymerase Chain Reaction (PCR)

The polymerase chain reaction (PCR) is a technique to amplify (relatively quickly) small fragments or areas of DNA into quantities large enough to be analyzed with electrophoresis and blotting methods. This technique produces enormous numbers of copies of a specific DNA sequence without resorting to cloning. The sequence to be amplified must be known. Specific markers (synthesized short sequences of DNA corresponding to each end of the sequence to be studied) are selected that will delineate the region of DNA to be amplified. These flanking sequences are called primers. The DNA sample, the primers, and an excess of free single nucleotides are incubated with a DNA polymerase.

The first step involves separating DNA into its single strands by denaturation with heat (92°C), then the temperature is lowered (40°C), causing the primers to stick (anneal) to their complementary regions on the DNA. The temperature is raised to 62°C, and DNA polymerase then synthesizes a new strand beginning and ending at the primers, forming a new double-stranded DNA. Repeating the cycle many times (by alternating the reaction temperature) amplifies the amount of DNA available for study (more than 1 million-fold); the increase occurs exponentially. Thus, DNA can be analyzed from a single cell, and genes can be visualized by blotting without labeled probes.

Because the process requires alternate heating and cooling, a DNA polymerase resistant to heat is an advantage in that periodic replenishment is not necessary. This problem was solved with the discovery of DNA polymerase (Taq polymerase) in a microorganism (*Thermus aquaticus*) that lives in hot springs and was found in Yellowstone National Park geysers. This high temperature polymerase allows automation of the process.

The technique of polymerase chain reaction has made possible the study of incredibly small amounts of DNA. Most impressive is the amplification of small amounts of degraded DNA from extinct and rare species preserved in museums. DNA from fossils has been amplified and sequenced (e.g., from an 18 million year old magnolia plant).

Part I Reproductive Physiology

Cloning DNA

Cloning means isolating a gene and making copies of it. A DNA library is a collection of DNA molecules derived from cloning methods. A complementary DNA library is the DNA counterpart of all of the messenger RNA isolated from a particular cell or tissue. By starting with messenger RNA, the search for the gene of interest can be focused (instead of searching the entire genome). Such a library is made using reverse transcriptase. The DNA molecules then can be inserted into an appropriate vector (described below) and replicate molecules can be produced. Using probes, the complementary DNA can be selected that matches the gene of interest (keeping in mind that complementary DNA only includes the exons of a gene). Cloning the DNA simply means the production of many identical copies of a specified fragment of DNA. Cloning can also be performed using the polymerase chain reaction. As indicated above, complementary DNA cloning focuses on the DNA counterpart of messenger RNA; genomic DNA cloning, using a restriction endonuclease, copies the DNA in genes. Cloning can be also used to make multiple copies of probes or unknown DNA fragments.

Identification of specific DNA by hybridization with known oligonucleotide sequences

Known amino acid sequence   Met — Tyr — Lys — Asp — Trp — Gln — Cys

Possible cDNA sequence   ATG TAT AAA GAT TGG CAA TGT
                                TAC AAG GAC   CAG TGC

Bacterial colonies with various cDNA segments

Synthesize labeled DNA oligonucleotides for possible cDNA sequences

Correct oligonucleotide hybridized to the cDNA

Autoradiography showing hybrid DNA

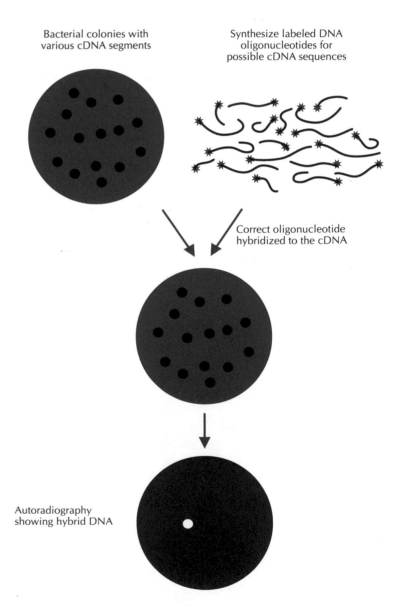

22

If the amino acid sequence is unknown, one can work backward. Knowing the specific protein product, antibodies can be produced against the protein. When complementary DNA is inserted into certain vectors, production of the protein can be identified with the antibodies; thus the DNA fragment will be isolated.

A vector is an entity in which foreign DNA can be inserted. The vector plus the foreign DNA are inserted into a host cell; the host cell produces both the vector and the foreign DNA. The first vectors were bacterial plasmids, circular DNA molecules (minichromosomes) that coexist in the cytoplasm with the bacterial chromosomal DNA. Most noteworthy, they carry genes that code for antibiotic resistance. This enables the bacterial cells that contain the plasmid to be selected by appropriate antibiotic treatment. Plasmid vectors have also been developed that allow selection by color. A variety of bacterial strains have been developed, each for a specific use.

Disruption of the plasmid DNA with restriction enzymes, followed by incorporation of foreign DNA with DNA ligase, produces plasmid DNA molecules (recombinant DNA containing the foreign DNA) which can be replicated. Plasmid vectors can incorporate foreign DNA fragments up to 10 kb in size. Digestion of recovered plasmids with restriction enzymes releases the desired DNA fragment, which can then be recovered by electrophoresis.

Other vectors exist. Bacteriophages (or phages) are viruses that infect and replicate within bacteria. Phage vectors can incorporate larger DNA inserts, up to 20 kb. Cloning DNA with phage vectors follows the same basic design as with plasmids. Larger fragments of foreign DNA are cloned with cosmid vectors, artificially produced combinations of phage and plasmid vectors. Very large fragments, up to 1,000 kb, can be cloned using yeast artificial chromosomes. This method can work with whole genes.

Basic Steps for Cloning.
1. Choose a DNA source: either genomic DNA or complementary DNA.

2. Fragment the DNA by restriction endonucleases.

3. Insert the fragments into vectors.

4. Introduce the vectors into bacteria.

5. Collect the cloned DNA propagated in the bacteria to form a library.

6. Screen the library for the desired sequence. Possible methods include the use of complementary nucleotide probes for fragments that hybridize or the detection of a specific protein produced with antibodies to the protein or by assaying the function of the protein.

Identification of specific DNA by detecting a known protein product

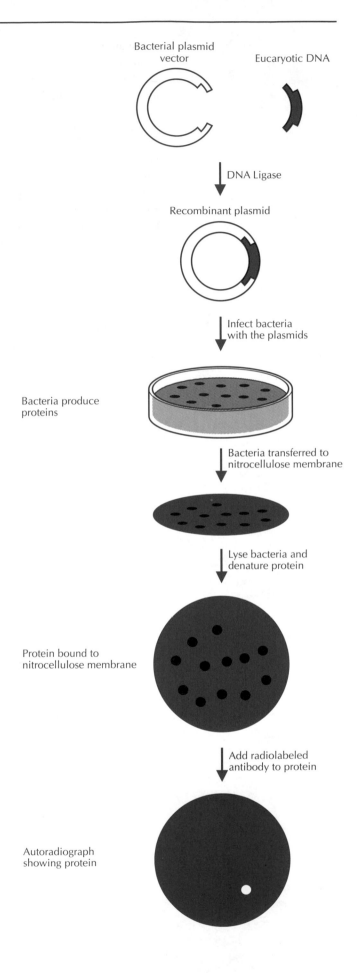

The Identification of Genes

To clone an entire gene whose protein product is known, a complementary DNA library is produced. The specific DNA fragment is identified by linking it to the protein. Once identified, the total gene can be screened using the identified complementary DNA, indicating the introns and exons. Another strategy is to synthesize an oligonucleotide probe, basing the sequence upon the known amino acid sequence in the protein product (from the peptide sequence, the DNA sequence that codes for that protein can be predicted). This method can be used with just a relatively small piece of the peptide. As more and more genes are cloned, the codon frequency for particular amino acids is being established. Complementary DNA can be cloned without producing a library by using the polymerase chain reaction to amplify complementary DNA made from messenger RNA by reverse transcriptase. Overlapping sequences of the genome can be cloned, using a piece of DNA from each succeeding product, to work across a chromosome in a systematic manner to search for a gene; this is called *chromosome walking.*

The entire sequencing process can be performed by a computer, even searching for open reading fames. Once the sequence of a DNA fragment has been identified, the computer can utilize DNA and protein data bases to predict sequence, recognition site, protein translation, and homology with known sequences. The scientist can then select restriction fragment sizes for cloning. Once a gene has been analyzed, it has to be compared to the gene in the disease state. If a mutation is of large size, this can be detected by Southern blotting. Minor alterations require comparisons in DNA sequences, which is possible by using polymerase chain amplification to produce specific gene sequences in amounts readily studied.

A gene can be localized to a specific chromosome when its protein product is unknown by studies involving chromosome rearrangements and linkage analysis. Specific diseases are associated with karyotypic changes. Thus, the specific chromosome can be targeted for gene localization. Linkage analysis utilizes restriction fragment length polymorphisms.

Restriction Fragment Length Polymorphism (RFLP)

Southern blotting reveals specific patterns of bands that reflect the varying lengths of the DNA fragments produced by restriction enzyme action. A specific site can exhibit a mutation by having a different pattern (a different length of the DNA fragment on Southern blotting). This is called a restriction fragment length polymorphism (RFLP), usually a benign variation. A polymorphism will be governed by the mendelian regulations of inheritance, and if by chance, a polymorphism is identified in a patient with a specific disease, the transmission of the disease can be studied. The RFLP, which is linked to the disease by chance, can be used to study the inheritance of a disease when the genes are unknown. This method of study requires DNA from at least one affected individual and a sufficient number of family members to trace the length polymorphism.

Minisatellites are a form of RFLPs. Minisatellites are noncoding areas of DNA that repeat in variable numbers, so-called variable number tandem repeats. These areas can be followed by DNA probes, providing a "fingerprint" for specific individuals. This uniqueness is applied in forensic medicine. Microsattelites, as the name implies, are smaller than minisatellites. Usually microsatellites consist of repetitions of only two nucleotides.

The Human Genome Project

The goal of the international human genome project is to sequence the 3 billion base pairs of the human genome, enough information to occupy 10,000 conventional floppy disks. Using the standard thin-layer vertical gel electrophoresis followed by autoradiographs of gel blots, it would require tens of millions of gels to accomplish this project. Shared data and computer analysis are necessary, and high speed automated sequencing technology must be utilized. Each lab will determine its small part of the sequence and then have to figure out where it fits in the big picture. When the computer finds an open reading frame, the probable amino acid sequence and the function can be predicted for the gene's protein. By the end of 1992, 92% of the autosomal length of the genome and 95% of the X chromosome were estimated to be included in a genetic linkage map constructed by an American/French collaborative mapping group. This map serves as a foundation for locating disease sites and for integrating the genetic sequencing with biologic functions.

The chromosomal locations of genes responsible for hormone production are rapidly being mapped. From the cloned DNA sequences, the amino acid sequences can be predicted. Hormones then can be synthesized in large and pure amounts, and hybridization probes will be available to study endocrine gene structure and function. And of course, inherited disorders will be subject to characterization and, eventually, gene therapy.

The future will see preventive medicine by prediction. By knowing an individual's genetic constitution, appropriate and intensive screening can be directed to predisposed conditions. This kind of knowledge will also require social and political considerations. It is not farfetched to envision marriages and children avoided because of a bad match of genetic predispositions. Society will have to develop guidelines regarding the use of this information: by individuals, by employers, by insurance companies, by the government. Scientific progress must be matched by public and professional education to appropriately manage this knowledge.

Clinical Applications

Polymerase chain reaction carried out by automatic machinery allows speedy DNA diagnosis with material amplified from a single cell. This is an important advantage in prenatal genetic analysis and in preimplantation sexing and diagnosis. PCR makes it possible to perform DNA diagnosis from a single cell removed from embryos fertilized in vitro.

At least one type of growth hormone deficiency is inherited in an autosomal recessive pattern. The cloning of growth hormone DNA complementary to its messenger RNA permitted localization of the growth hormone gene. The growth hormone gene is in a cluster that also includes the gene for human placental lactogen. This cluster of genes contains multiple units of DNA that are homologous and prone to recombination, which leads to deletion on one chromosome and duplication on another. Similar mechanisms operate for other protein products governed by genes in clusters, such as the globins.

Congenital adrenal hyperplasia is an autosomal recessive disorder with a deficiency in an enzyme necessary for adrenal steroidogenesis, most commonly the 21-hydroxylase enzyme. The 21-hydroxylase gene has been localized to the short arm of chromosome 6. Molecular analysis indicates that the genetic defect involves the structural gene for cytochrome P450c21-hydroxylase.

The commercial production of proteins from cloned genes inserted into bacteria is rapidly increasing. The production of insulin (the first) and growth hormone are good examples. Glycosylation does not occur in bacterial systems, and therefore the commercial production of recombinant glycoproteins requires a mammalian cell line for the process. This has been accomplished, and recombinant gonadotropins are now available. The gene for gonadotropin releasing hormone (GnRH) on the short arm of chromosome 8 has been isolated and cloned. Molecular technology was important in the characterization of inhibin, the ovarian follicular hormone that inhibits follicle-stimulating hormone (FSH) secretion. The inhibin gene has been sequenced and found to be homologous to the gene for antimüllerian hormone. The alpha-subunit common to gonadotropins, thyroid-stimulating hormone (TSH), and human chorionic gonadotropin (HCG) has been traced to a gene which has been isolated, sequenced, and localized on chromosome 6.

The beta-subunit gene for FSH is on chromosome 11p. The similar biologic action of luteinizing hormone (LH) and HCG is understandable when it is appreciated that they originated from a common ancestral gene. The beta-subunits for LH and HCG are derived from a family of genes on chromosome 19q. It is believed that a cluster of genes indicates an origin from a single primordial gene. The differences between LH and HCG can be attributed to different promoter regions. A different translational stop signal in the HCG gene permits the addition of extra glycosylation sites and thus a longer half-life.

The Y chromosome carries a genetic locus responsible for differentiation of the testes, called the testis determining factor. The theory that this is a male-specific histocompatibility antigen (the H-Y antigen) has been abandoned. Using material from intersex patients, maps of the Y chromosome have placed the testis determinant genes on the short arm. Certain intersex disorders, therefore, result from an exchange of X and Y DNA when the short arms of the X and Y chromosomes pair and crossover during meiosis. The exact locus (or loci) of the ovarian determinants on the X chromosomes has not yet been identified.

Because of the importance of X-linked disease, the X chromosome is one of the most studied of all human chromosomes. By 1993, about 40% of the 160 million base pairs of the X chromosome DNA had been cloned; in addition, 26 inherited disease genes had been cloned, and more than 50 other genes had been localized by linkage analysis.

Insertion of a foreign gene into an embryo results in a transgenic animal. The inserted foreign gene will be present in many tissues, and if the animal is fertile, it will be inherited. There are many applications for transgenic animals. Transgenic animals provide animal models for inherited diseases and malignant tumors and provide a means to carry out experiments in gene therapy. The transfer of new or altered genes is an important method to study gene function. Transgenic plants can even be developed to produce new pharmaceuticals, and the introduction of genes conferring resistance to insects may solve the problem of insecticide contamination.

The human genome contains many genes with the potential to cause cancer. Other genes have the ability to block malignant growth. Cancer is a genetic disease in that tumors can be said to be clonal; all the cells are genetically related. Oncogenes, discovered in tumor viruses, are genes that transform cells from normal to abnormal growth by encoding proteins that activate DNA replication. There are many oncogenes and many different pathways of action, all of which result in uncontrolled growth. The mutations that activate these genes either lead to protein activity independent of incoming signals or to activity at the wrong place at the wrong time. The bottom line is the turning on (by an altered oncogene) of persistent growth. There are also anti-oncogenes in normal cells, growth suppressing genes that must be inactivated before tumors can grow. Inherited susceptibility for cancer can also result from a mutation in tumor suppresser genes. Whereas activation of an oncogene is a dominant effect, tumor suppresser mutations are recessive and can be carried and transmitted, but are not active as long as pairing occurs with a normal anti-oncogene. Cancer, therefore, is a genetic disease, but regulation of normal growth involves a complex system that takes a long time to overcome. During this time period, the technology of recombinant DNA may be able to achieve diagnosis sufficiently early to yield cures. Knowing the specific oncogene involved in a given tumor also offers therapeutic possibilities. For example, an antimetabolite can be attached to antibody for an oncogene, targeting the cancer cells.

Molecular biology is changing both diagnosis and therapy. Viral and bacterial DNA can be identified. The automated PCR process can produce electrophoretic patterns that can also be read automatically. With this technique, a single human papillomavirus DNA molecule can be detected among 10,000 or more human cells.

Faulty endogenous protein production can be corrected by replacing the problematic mechanism. There are two strategies: foreign cells that produce the missing protein could be introduced, or the faulty gene could be replaced (or more accurately, adding a complementary corrected DNA). Thus, recessive single-gene disorders are potentially amenable to gene therapy, as are acquired diseases such as cancer and infections.

Specific guidelines for gene therapy have been developed requiring several levels of review. One class of human therapy is the use of retroviral vectors to transfer marker genes into cultured human cells that are returned to patients of origin. For example, this allows tracking of tumor-infiltrating lymphocytes, donor hepatocytes, or killer T cells that are specific for the human immunodeficiency virus. These transferred genes can also be crafted to provide a function in patients with single-gene inherited disorders. Another class of therapy involves the transfer of genes which encode for factors that destroy tumor cells, such as tumor necrosis factor or interleukin. Retroviral vectors are viruses that have been altered so that no viral proteins can be made by cells infected by the vectors. Thus, viral replication and spread are prevented, but gene transfer into replicating cells can take place. Other transfer methods being developed include the use of adenovirus vectors and specifically targeted plasmid DNA.

References

1. **Caskey CT,** Molecular medicine, JAMA 269:1986, 1993.

2. **Collins F, Galas D,** A new five-year plan for the U.S. human genome project, Science 262:43, 1993.

3. **Mandel J-L, Monaco AP, Nelson DL, Schlessinger D, Willard H**, Genome analysis and the human X chromosome, Science 258:103, 1992.

4. **Miller AD,** Human gene therapy comes of age, Nature 357:455, 1992.

5. **NIH/CEPH Collaborative Mapping Group,** A comprehensive genetic linkage map of the human genome, Science 258:67, 1992.

6. **Ross DW,** *Introduction to Molecular Medicine,* Springer-Verlag, New York, 1992.

7. **Watson JD,** The human genome project: past, present and future, Science 248:44, 1990.

8. **Watson JD, Gilman M, Witkowski J, Zoller M,** *Recombinant DNA,* second edition, Scientific American Books, New York, 1992.

2 Hormone Biosynthesis, Metabolism, and Mechanism of Action

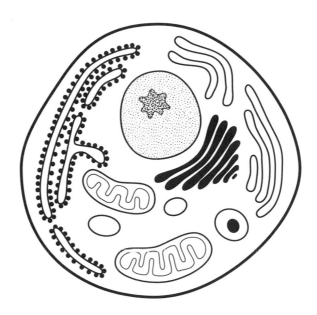

The classical definition of a hormone is a substance that travels from a special tissue, where it is released into the bloodstream, to distant responsive cells where the hormone exerts its characteristic effects. What was once thought of as a simple voyage is now appreciated as an odyssey which becomes more complex as new facets of the journey are unraveled in research laboratories throughout the world. Indeed, the notion that hormones are products only of special tissues has been challenged.

Complex hormones and hormone receptors have been discovered in primitive, unicellular organisms, suggesting that endocrine glands are a late development of evolution. The widespread capability of cells to make hormones explains the puzzling discoveries of hormones in strange places, such as gastrointestinal hormones in the brain, reproductive hormones in intestinal secretions, and the ability of cancers to unexpectedly make hormones. Hormones and neurotransmitters were and are a means of communication. Only when animals evolved into complex organisms did special glands develop to produce hormones which could be used in a more sophisticated fashion. Furthermore, hormones must have appeared even before plants and animals diverged because there are many plant substances similar to hormones and hormone receptors. Therefore it is not surprising that every cell should contain genes necessary for hormonal expression, and cancer cells, because of their dedifferentiation, can uncover gene expression and, in inappropriate locations and at inappropriate times, make hormones.

Hormones, therefore, are substances that provide a means of communication. The classic endocrine hormones travel through the bloodstream to distant sites, but cellular communication is also necessary at local sites. Two words which are now encountered relatively frequently are paracrine and autocrine, depicting a more immediate form of communication.

Paracrine Communication
Intercellular communication involving the local diffusion of regulating substances from a cell to nearby (contiguous) cells.

Autocrine Communication
Intracellular communication whereby a single cell produces regulating substances that in turn act upon receptors on or within the same cell.

Intracrine Communication
This form of intracellular communication occurs when unsecreted substances bind to intracellular receptors.

Let us follow an estradiol molecule throughout its career and in so doing gain an overview of how hormones are formed, how hormones work, and how hormones are metabolized. Estradiol begins its lifespan with its synthesis in a cell specially suited for this task. For this biosynthesis to take place, the proper enzyme capability must be present along with the proper precursors. In the human female the principal sources of estradiol are the granulosa cells of the developing follicle and the corpus luteum. These cells possess the ability to turn on steroidogenesis in response to specific stimuli. The stimulating agents are the gonadotropins, follicle-stimulating hormone (FSH) and luteinizing hormone (LH). The initial step in the process that will give rise to estradiol is the transmission of the message from the stimulating agents to the steroid-producing mechanisms within the cells.

Messages that stimulate steroidogenesis must be transmitted through the cell membrane. This is necessary because gonadotropins, being large glycopeptides, do not ordinarily enter cells but must communicate with the cell by joining with specific receptors on the cell membrane. In so doing they activate a sequence of communication. A considerable amount of investigation has been devoted to determining the methods by which this communication takes place. E. M. Sutherland received the Nobel Prize in 1971 for proposing the concept of a second messenger.

Gonadotropin, the first messenger, activates an enzyme in the cell membrane called adenylate cyclase. This enzyme transmits the message by catalyzing the production of a second messenger within the cell, cyclic adenosine 3'5'-monophosphate (cyclic AMP). The message passes from gonadotropin to cyclic AMP, much like a baton in a relay race.

Cyclic AMP, the second messenger, initiates the process of steroidogenesis, leading to the synthesis and secretion of the hormone estradiol. This notion of message transmission has grown more and more complex with the appreciation of new physiologic concepts such as the heterogeneity of peptide hormones, the up- and down-regulation of cell membrane receptors, the regulation of adenylate cyclase activity, and the important roles for autocrine and paracrine regulating factors.

Secretion of estradiol into the bloodstream directly follows its synthesis. Once in the bloodstream, estradiol exists in two forms, bound and free. A majority of the hormone is bound to protein carriers, albumin and sex steroid hormone binding globulin. The purpose of this binding is not totally clear. The biologic activity of a hormone may be limited by binding in the blood, thereby avoiding extreme or sudden reactions. In addition, binding may prevent unduly rapid metabolism, allowing the hormone to exist for the length of time necessary to ensure a biologic effect. This reservoir-like mechanism avoids peaks and valleys in hormone levels and allows a more steady state of hormone action.

The biologic and metabolic effects of a hormone are determined by a cell's ability to receive and retain the hormone. The estradiol that is not bound to a protein, but floats freely in the bloodstream, readily enters cells by rapid diffusion. For estradiol to produce its effect, however, it must be grasped by a receptor within the cell. Only those cells which contain estradiol-specific receptors will respond to estradiol. The job of the receptor is to aid in the transmission of the hormone's message to nuclear gene transcription. The result is production of messenger RNA leading to protein synthesis and a cellular response characteristic of the hormone.

Once estradiol has accomplished its mission, it is probably released back into the bloodstream. It is possible that estradiol can perform its duty several times before being cleared from the circulation by metabolism. On the other hand, many molecules will be metabolized without ever having the chance to produce an effect. Unlike estradiol, other hormones, such as testosterone, are metabolized and altered within the cell in which an effect is produced. In the latter case, a steroid is released into the bloodstream as an inactive compound. Clearance of steroids from the blood varies according to the structure of the molecules.

Cells that are capable of clearing estradiol from the circulation accomplish this by biochemical means (conversion to estrone and estriol, moderately effective and very weak estrogens, respectively) and conjugation to products which are water soluble and excreted in the urine and bile (sulfo- and glucuro-conjugates).

Thus, a steroid hormone has a varied career packed into a short lifetime. We are now ready to review the important segments of this lifespan in greater detail.

Nomenclature

All steroid hormones are of basically similar structure with relatively minor chemical differences leading to striking alterations in biochemical activity. The basic structure is the perhydrocyclopentanephenanthrene molecule. It is composed of three 6-carbon rings and one 5-carbon ring. One ring is benzene, two rings naphthalene, and three rings phenanthrene; add a cyclopentane (5-carbon ring) and you have the perhydrocyclopenta-nephenanthrene structure of the steroid nucleus.

The sex steroids are divided into 3 main groups according to the number of carbon atoms they possess. The 21-carbon series includes the corticoids and the progestins, and the basic structure is the **pregnane** nucleus. The 19-carbon series includes all the androgens and is based on the **androstane** nucleus, whereas the estrogens are 18-carbon steroids based on the **estrane** nucleus.

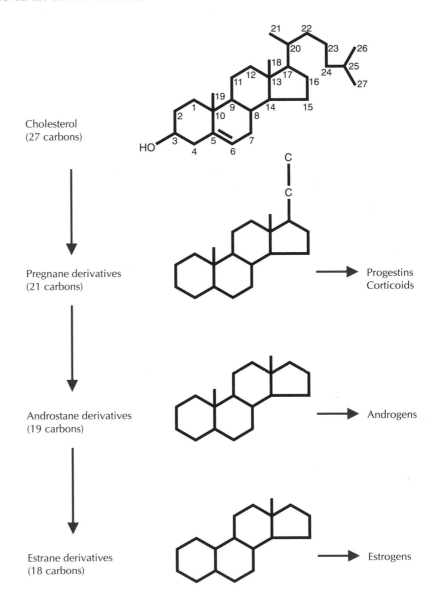

Cholesterol
(27 carbons)

Pregnane derivatives
(21 carbons)   → Progestins
                       Corticoids

Androstane derivatives
(19 carbons)   → Androgens

Estrane derivatives
(18 carbons)   → Estrogens

There are 6 centers of asymmetry on the basic ring structure, and there are 64 possible isomers. Almost all naturally occurring and active steroids are nearly flat, and substituents below and above the plane of the ring are designated alpha (α) (dotted line) and beta (β)(solid line), respectively. Changes in the position of only one substituent can lead to inactive isomers. For example, 17-epitestosterone is considerably weaker than testosterone, the only difference being a hydroxyl group in the α position at C-17 rather than in the β position.

Progesterone

Top View

Side View

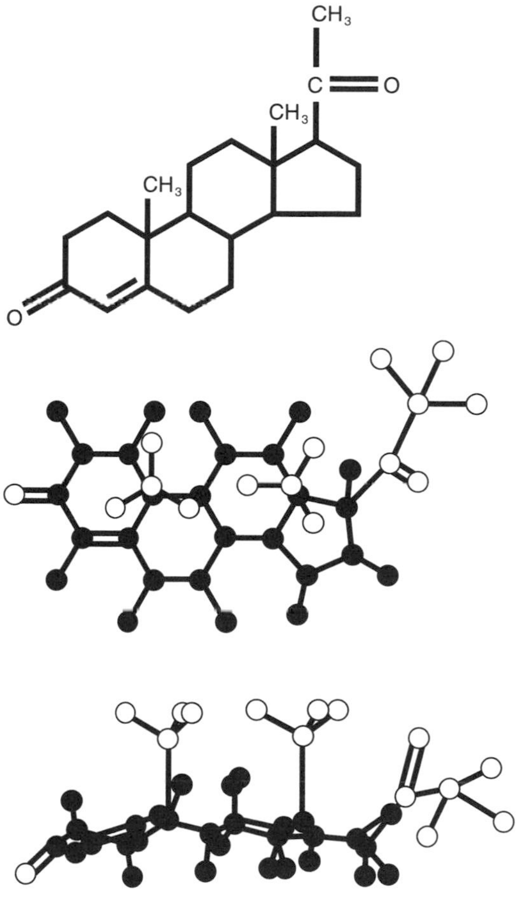

The convention of naming steroids uses the number of carbon atoms to designate the basic name (e.g., pregnane, androstane, or estrane). The basic name is preceded by numbers which indicate the position of double bonds and the name is altered as follows to indicate 1, 2, or 3 double bonds: -ene, -diene, and -triene. Following the basic name, hydroxyl groups are indicated by the number of the carbon attachment, and 1, 2, or 3 hydroxyl groups are designated -ol, -diol, or -triol. Ketone groups are listed last with numbers of carbon attachments, and 1, 2, or 3 groups designated -one, -dione, or -trione. Special designations include: dehydro, elimination of 2 hydrogens; deoxy, elimination of oxygen; nor, elimination of carbon; delta or Δ, location of double bond.

Estrone
1,3,5(10)-Estratriene-3β-ol-17-one

Testosterone
4-Androstene-17β-ol-3-one

Progesterone
4-Pregnene-3,20-dione

Lipoproteins and Cholesterol

Cholesterol is the basic building block in steroidogenesis. All steroid-producing organs except the placenta can synthesize cholesterol from acetate. Progestins, androgens, and estrogens, therefore, can be synthesized in situ in the various ovarian tissue compartments from the 2-carbon acetate molecule via cholesterol as the common steroid precursor. However, in situ synthesis cannot meet the demand, and therefore the major resource is blood cholesterol which enters the ovarian cells and can be inserted into the biosynthetic pathway or stored in esterified form for later use. The cellular entry of cholesterol is mediated via a cell membrane receptor for low-density lipoprotein (LDL), the bloodstream carrier for cholesterol.

Lipoproteins are large molecules that facilitate the transport of nonpolar fats in a polar solvent, the blood plasma. There are 5 major categories of lipoproteins according to their charge and density (flotation during ultracentrifugation). They are derived from each other in the following cascade of decreasing size and increasing density.

Chylomicrons
Large, cholesterol (10%) and triglyceride (90%) carrying particles formed in the intestine after a fatty meal.

Very Low-Density Lipoproteins (VLDL)
Also carry cholesterol, but mostly triglyceride; more dense than chylomicrons.

Intermediate-Density Lipoproteins (IDL)
Formed (for a transient existence) with the removal of some of the triglyceride from the interior of VLDL particles.

Low-Density Lipoproteins (LDL)
The end products of VLDL catabolism, formed after further removal of triglyceride leaving approximately 50% cholesterol; the major carriers (2/3) of cholesterol in the plasma and thus a strong relationship exists between elevated LDL levels and cardiovascular disease.

High-Density Lipoproteins (HDL)
The smallest and most dense of the lipoproteins with the highest protein and phospholipid content; HDL levels are inversely associated with atherosclerosis (high levels are protective). HDL can be further separated into a lighter fraction (HDL_2) and a denser fraction (HDL_3). HDL_2 is strongly associated with cardiovascular disease.

The lipoproteins contain 4 ingredients: 1) cholesterol in two forms: free cholesterol on the surface of the spherical lipoprotein molecule and esterified cholesterol in the molecule's interior; 2) triglycerides in the interior of the sphere; 3) phospholipid, and 4) protein: electrically charged substances on the surface of the sphere and responsible for miscibility with plasma and water. The surface proteins, called *apoproteins,* constitute the sites which bind to the lipoprotein receptor molecules on the cell surfaces. The principal surface protein of LDL is apoprotein B, and apoprotein A-1 is the principal apoprotein of HDL.

Lipids for peripheral tissues are provided by the secretion of VLDL by the liver. Triglycerides are liberated from VLDL by lipoprotein lipase located in the capillary endothelial cells as well as a lipase enzyme located on the endothelial cells in liver sinusoids. In this process, the surface components (free cholesterol, phospholipids, and apolipoproteins) are transferred to HDL. Finally the VLDL is converted to LDL, which plays the important role of transporting cholesterol to cells throughout the body. The hepatic lipase enzyme is sensitive to sex steroid changes: suppression by estrogen and stimulation by androgens.

LDL is removed from the blood by cellular receptors that recognize one of the surface apoproteins. The lipoprotein bound to the cell membrane receptor is internalized and degraded. Intracellular levels of cholesterol are partly regulated by the up- and down-regulation of cell membrane LDL receptors. When these LDL receptors are saturated or deficient, LDL is taken up by "scavenger" cells (most likely derived from macrophages) in other tissues, notably the arterial intima. Thus, these cells can become the nidus for atherosclerotic plaques.

HDL is secreted by the liver and intestine or is a product of the degradation of VDL. Cholesteryl ester molecules move to form a core in a small spherical particle, the HDL_3 particle. These particles accept additional free cholesterol, perhaps mediated by receptors which recognize apoprotein A-1. With uptake of cholesterol, the particle size increases to form HDL_2, the fraction that reflects changes in diet and hormones. HDL_3 levels remain relatively stable.

The protein moieties of the lipoprotein particles are strongly related to the risk of cardiovascular disease, and genetic abnormalities in their synthesis or structure can result in atherogenic conditions. The lipoproteins are a major reason for the disparity in atherosclerosis risk between men and women. Throughout adulthood, the blood HDL-cholesterol level is about 10 mg/dL higher in women, and this difference continues through the postmenopausal years. Total and LDL-cholesterol levels are lower in premenopausal women than in men, but after menopause they rise rapidly.

The protective nature of HDL is due to its ability to pick up free cholesterol from cells or other circulating lipoproteins. This lipid-rich HDL is known as HDL_3, which is then converted to the larger, less dense particle, HDL_2. Thus, HDL converts lipid-rich scavenger cells (macrophages residing in arterial walls) back to their low-lipid state and carries the excess cholesterol to sites (mainly liver) where it can be metabolized. Another method by which HDL removes cholesterol from the body focuses on the uptake of free cholesterol from cell membranes. The free cholesterol is esterified and moves to the core of the HDL particle. Thus HDL can remove cholesterol by delivering cholesterol to sites for utilization (steroid-producing cells) or metabolism and excretion (liver).

Understanding the role of the cell surface receptors for the homeostasis of cholesterol (discussed later in this chapter), the work of the 1985 Nobel Laureates, M.S. Brown and J.L. Goldstein, revolutionized our concepts of cholesterol, lipoprotein metabolism, and hormone action at the cell membrane.[1] In their Nobel lecture, Brown and Goldstein paid tribute to cholesterol as the most highly decorated small molecule in biology.

For good cardiovascular health, the blood concentration of cholesterol must be kept low, and its escape from the bloodstream must be prevented. The problem of cholesterol transport is solved by esterifying the cholesterol and packaging the ester within the cores of plasma lipoproteins. The delivery of cholesterol to cells is in turn solved by lipoprotein receptors. After binding the lipoprotein with its package of esterified cholesterol, the complex is delivered into the cell by receptor-mediated endocytosis, where the lysosomes liberate cholesterol for use by the cell.

Major protection against atherosclerosis depends upon the high affinity of the receptor for LDL and the ability of the receptor to recycle multiple times, thus allowing large amounts of cholesterol to be delivered while maintaining a healthy low blood level of LDL. Cells can control their uptake of cholesterol by increasing or decreasing the number of LDL receptors according to the intracellular cholesterol levels. Thus, a high cholesterol diet influences the liver to reduce the number of LDL receptors on its cells, causing an elevated blood level of LDL.

There are 3 important clinical points:

1. Atherosclerotic disease is related to increased LDL- and decreased HDL-cholesterol concentrations.

2. Lowering LDL levels and raising HDL levels can reduce the incidence of atherosclerotic disease.

3. Atherosclerosis is not a disease limited to aging people. It begins in early childhood, and its manifestation later in life can be influenced by health care behavior during younger years.

All adults should have a screening measurement of total cholesterol and the lipoproteins. Familial hypercholesterolemia is not always associated with a family history of premature cardiovascular disease. Dietary efforts to lower cholesterol and change the LDL:HDL ratio should be directed to any individual with a cholesterol level over 200 mg/dL. Brown and Goldstein postulate that the LDL receptor evolved under dietary conditions of a lower fat intake, and that the high fat, high cholesterol modern diet suppresses the production of LDL receptors, thereby allowing cholesterol to rise to levels associated with cardiovascular disease.

Steroidogenesis

The overall steroid biosynthesis pathway shown in the figure is based primarily on the pioneering work of K. J. Ryan and his coworkers. These pathways follow the fundamental pattern displayed by all steroid-producing endocrine organs. As a result, it should be no surprise that the normal human ovary produces all 3 classes of sex steroids: estrogens, progestins, and androgens. The importance of ovarian androgens is appreciated, not only as obligate precursors to estrogens, but also as clinically important secretory products. The ovary differs from the testis in its fundamental complement of critical enzymes and, hence, its distribution of secretory products. The ovary is distinguished from the adrenal gland in that it is deficient in 21-hydroxylase and 11β-hydroxylase reactions. Glucocorticoids and mineralocorticoids, therefore, are not produced in normal ovarian tissue.

During steroidogenesis, the number of carbon atoms in cholesterol or any other steroid molecule can be reduced but never increased. The following reactions can take place.

1. Cleavage of a side chain (desmolase reaction).

2. Conversion of hydroxyl groups into ketones or ketones into hydroxyl groups (dehydrogenase reactions).

3. Addition of OH group (hydroxylation reaction).

4. Creation of double bonds (removal of hydrogen).

5. Addition of hydrogen to reduce double bonds (saturation).

The traditional view of steroidogenesis was that each step was mediated by many enzymes, with differences from tissue to tissue. A fundamental simplicity to the system emerged when complementary DNAs and genes were cloned.[2]

Steroidogenic enzymes are members of the cytochrome P450 group of oxidases. Cytochrome P450 is a generic term for a family of oxidative enzymes, termed 450 because of a pigment (450) absorbance shift when reduced. P450 enzymes can metabolize many substrates; e.g., in the liver, P450 enzymes metabolize toxins and environmental

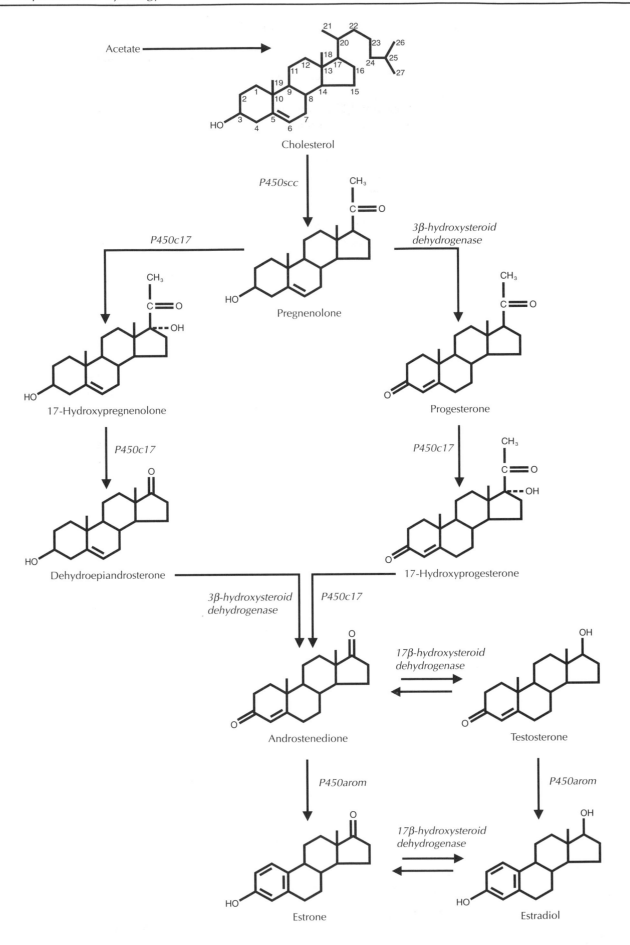

Enzyme	Cellular Location	Reactions
P450scc	Mitochondria	Cholesterol side chain cleavage
P450c11	Mitochondria	11-hydroxylase 18-hydroxylase 19-methyloxidase
P450c17	Endoplasmic reticulum	17-hydroxylase, 17,20-lyase
P450c21	Endoplasmic reticulum	21-hydroxylase
P450arom	Endoplasmic reticulum	Aromatase

pollutants. The following distinct P450 enzymes are identified with steroidogenesis: P450scc is the cholesterol side chain cleavage enzyme; P450c11 mediates 11-hydroxylase, 18-hydroxylase, and 19-methyloxidase; P450c17 mediates 17-hydroxylase and 17,20-lyase; P450c21 mediates the 21-hydroxylase; and P450arom mediates aromatization of androgens to estrogens. Marked differences in the exon-intron organization of the P450 genes are compatible with an ancient origin; thus, the superfamily of P450 genes diverged more than 1.5 billion years ago.

The structural knowledge of the P450 enzymes that has been derived from amino acid and nucleotide sequencing studies demonstrated that all the steps between cholesterol and pregnenolone were mediated by a single protein, P450scc, bound to the inner mitochondrial membrane. Cloning data indicate the presence of a single, unique P450scc gene on chromosome 15. These experiments indicated that multiple steps did not require multiple enzymes. Differing activity may reflect posttranslational modifications. These genes contain tissue specific promoter sequences which is at least one reason that regulatory mechanisms can differ in different tissues (e.g., placenta and ovary).

Genetic lesions in P450scc are very rare, usually resulting in death due to the inability to synthesize steroid hormones. Southern blot studies of survivers indicate no gross deletions in their P450scc genes, suggesting small deletions or point mutations causing this autosomal recessive lethal defect.

Conversion of cholesterol to pregnenolone involves hydroxylation at the carbon 20 and 22 positions, with subsequent cleavage of the side chain. Conversion of cholesterol to pregnenolone by P450scc takes place within the mitochondria. It is a rate-limiting step in the steroid pathway and is one of the principal effects of tropic hormone stimulation, which also causes the uptake of the cholesterol substrate for this step. This stimulation is marked by the accumulation of messenger RNA for growth factors, especially insulin-like growth factor, the probable mediator of tissue hyperplasia in response to the tropic hormones.

It is important to note that once pregnenolone is formed further steroid synthesis in the ovary can proceed by one of 2 pathways, either via Δ^5-3β-hydroxysteroids or via the Δ^4-3-ketone pathway. The first (the Δ^5 pathway) proceeds by way of pregnenolone and dehydroepiandrosterone (DHA) and the second (the Δ^4 pathway) via progesterone and 17α-hydroxyprogesterone.

The conversion of pregnenolone to progesterone involves two steps: the 3β-hydroxysteroid dehydrogenase and Δ^{4-5} isomerase reactions which convert the 3-hydroxyl group to a ketone and transfer the double bond from the 5–6 position to the 4–5 position. A single polypeptide catalyzes both the dehydrogenation and isomerization reactions, encoded by two separate genes on chromosome 1. Once the Δ^{4-5} ketone is formed, progesterone is hydroxylated at the 17 position to form 17α-hydroxyprogesterone. 17α-Hydroxyprogesterone is the immediate precursor of the C-19 (19 carbons) series of androgens in this pathway. By peroxide formation at C-20, followed by epoxidation of the C-17, C-20 carbons, the side chain is split off forming androstenedione. The 17-ketone may be reduced to a 17β-hydroxyl to form testosterone by the 17β-hydroxysteroid dehydrogenase reaction. Both C-19 steroids (androstenedione and testosterone) are rapidly converted to corresponding C-18 phenolic steroid estrogens (estrone and estradiol) by microsomal reactions in a process referred to as aromatization. This process includes hydroxylation of the angular 19-methyl group, followed by oxidation, loss of the 19-carbon as formaldehyde, and ring A aromatization (dehydrogenation).

As an alternative, pregnenolone can be directly converted to the Δ^5-3β-hydroxy C-19 steroid, DHA, by 17α-hydroxylation followed by cleavage of the side chain. With formation of the Δ^4-3-ketone, DHA is converted into androstenedione. It is thought that conversion of each of the Δ^5 compounds to their corresponding Δ^4 compounds can occur at any step; however, the principal pathways are via progesterone and DHA. Regardless of the precursor source, C-19 Δ^4-3-ketone substrates proceed to estrogens as noted above.

The four reactions involved in converting pregnenolone and progesterone to their 17-hydroxylated products are mediated by a single enzyme, P450c17, bound to smooth endoplasmic reticulum, regulated by a gene on chromosome 10. 17-Hydroxylase and 17,20 lyase were traditionally regarded as separate enzymes. These two different functions of a single enzyme, P450c17, are not genetic or structural but represent the effect of local influencing factors.

Characterization of the P450c21 protein and gene cloning indicate that there is only one 21-hydroxylase enzyme, the P450c21 in the smooth endoplasmic reticulum. Two human P450c21 genes (the A and B genes) have been cloned (on chromosome 6p), and the evidence indicates that only one (the B gene) is active. The molecular genetics of 21-hydroxylase deficiency indicate that the syndrome can be due to gene conversions of material in the active B gene to resemble material in the inactive A gene, as well as deletions in the P450c21B gene. A conversion is similar to a cross-over in genetic effect. However, rather than appearing as a deletion or addition, the gene changes, but the number of gene copies does not change.

Aromatization is mediated by P450arom found in the endoplasmic reticulum. The human genome has one P450arom gene, located on chromosome 15q21.1. Aromatization in different tissues with different substrates is the result of the single P450arom enzyme encoded by the single gene.[3] Aromatase transcription is regulated by several promotor sites that respond to cytokines, cyclic nucelotides, gonadotropins, glucocorticoids, and growth factors. Very specific inhibitors of P450arom are being developed which would allow intense blockage of estrogen production, with potential clinical applications that include the treatment of breast cancer and dysfunctional uterine bleeding.[4]

The 17β-hydroxysteroid dehydrogenase and 5α-reductase reactions are due to non-P450 enzymes. The 17β-hydroxysteroid dehydrogenase is bound to the endoplasmic reticulum and the 5α-reductase to the nuclear membrane. The 17β-hydroxysteroid dehydrogenase enzyme converts estrone to estradiol, androstenedione to testosterone, and DHEA to androstenediol, and vice-versa.

The Two Cell System

The two cell system is a logical explanation of the events involved in ovarian follicular steroidogenesis.[5] This explanation brings together information on the site of specific steroid production, along with the appearance and importance of hormone receptors. The following facts are important:

1. FSH receptors are present on the granulosa cells.

2. FSH receptors are induced by FSH itself.

3. LH receptors are present on the theca cells and initially absent on the granulosa cells, but, as the follicle grows, FSH induces the appearance of LH receptors on the granulosa cells.

4. FSH induces aromatase enzyme activity in granulosa cells.

5. The above actions are modulated by autocrine/paracrine factors secreted by the theca and granulosa cells.

These facts combine into the two cell system to explain the sequence of events in ovarian follicular growth and steroidogenesis. The initial change from a primordial follicle is independent of hormones, and the stimulus governing this initial step in growth is unknown. Continued growth, however, depends upon FSH stimulation. As the granulosa responds to FSH, growth is associated with an increase in FSH receptors, a specific effect of FSH itself, but an action which is enhanced very significantly by the autocrine/ paracrine peptides. The theca cells are characterized by steroidogenic activity in response to LH, specifically resulting in androgen production. Aromatization of androgens to estrogens is a distinct activity within the granulosa layer induced by FSH. Androgens produced in the theca layer, therefore, must diffuse into the granulosa layer. In the granulosa layer they are converted to estrogens, and the increasing level of estradiol in the peripheral circulation reflects release of the estrogen back toward the theca layer and into blood vessels.

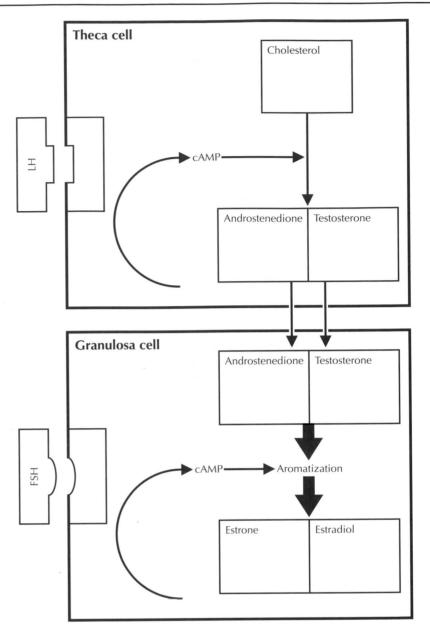

The theca and granulosa cells secrete peptides that operate as both autocrine and paracrine factors.[6] Insulin-like growth factor-I is secreted by the theca and enhances the LH stimulation of androgen production in the theca cells as well as FSH-mediated aromatization in the granulosa. Theca production of transforming growth factor can promote the growth of granulosa cells and FSH induction of LH receptors on the granulosa. The regulation of FSH receptors on granulosa cells is relatively complex. Although FSH increases the activity of its own receptor gene in a cyclic AMP-mediated mechanism, this action is influenced by inhibitory agents such as epidermal growth factor, fibroblast growth factor, and even a gonadotropin releasing hormone (GnRH)-like protein.[7,8] Inhibin and activin are produced in the granulosa in response to FSH. Activin augments FSH activities, and inhibin enhances LH stimulation of androgen synthesis in the theca to serve as substrate for aromatization to estrogen in the granulosa.

After ovulation the dominance of the luteinized granulosa layer is dependent upon preovulatory induction of an adequate number of LH receptors, and therefore, dependent upon adequate FSH action. Prior to ovulation the granulosa layer is characterized by aromatization activity and conversion of the theca androgens to estrogens, an FSH-mediated activity. After ovulation the granulosa layer secretes progesterone and estrogens directly into the bloodstream, an LH-mediated activity.

Granulosa and theca cells each have an androgen aromatase system that can be demonstrated in vitro. However, in vivo, the activity of the granulosa layer in the follicular phase is several hundred times greater than the activity of the theca layer, and therefore the granulosa is the main biosynthetic source of estrogen in the growing follicle. The rate of aromatization in the granulosa layer is directly related to the androgen substrate made available by the theca cells. Hence, estrogen secretion by the follicle prior to ovulation is the result of combined LH and FSH stimulation of the 2 cell types, the theca and the granulosa. After ovulation, it is believed the 2 cell types continue to function as a two cell system; luteal cells derived from theca produce androgens for aromatization into estrogens by luteal cells derived from granulosa.

Blood Transport of Steroids

While circulating in the blood a majority of the principal sex steroids, estradiol and testosterone, is bound to a β-globulin, a protein carrier, known as sex hormone binding globulin (SHBG). Another 10–40% is loosely bound to albumin, leaving only about 1% unbound and free. A very small percentage also binds to corticosteroid binding globulin. Hyperthyroidism, pregnancy, and estrogen administration all increase SHBG levels, whereas corticoids, androgens, progestins, and growth hormone decrease SHBG.

	Free (Unbound)	Albumin-Bound	SHBG-Bound
Estrogen	1%	30%	69%
Testosterone	1%	30%	69%
DHA	4%	88%	8%
Androstenedione	7%	85%	8%
Dihydrotestosterone	1%	71%	28%

From Mendel[9]

The circulating level of SHBG is inversely related to weight, and thus significant weight gain can decrease SHBG and produce important changes in the unbound levels of the sex steroids.[10] Another important mechanism for a reduction in circulating SHBG levels is insulin resistance and hyperinsulinemia (independent of age and weight).[11] Thus, increased insulin levels in the circulation lower SHBG levels, and this may be the major mechanism that mediates the impact of increased body weight on SHBG. This relationship between the levels of insulin and SHBG is so strong that SHBG concentrations are a marker for hyperinsulinemic insulin resistance, and a low level of SHBG is a predictor for the development of type II diabetes mellitus.[12]

SHBG is a glycoprotein that contains a single binding site for androgens and estrogens even though it is composed of two monomers. Its gene has been localized to the short arm of chromosome 17.[13] Transcortin, also called corticosteroid binding globulin, is a plasma glycoprotein that binds cortisol, progesterone, deoxycorticosterone, corticosterone, and some of the other minor corticoid compounds. Normally about 75% of circulating cortisol is bound to transcortin, 15% is loosely bound to albumin, and 10% is unbound or free. Binding in the circulation follows the law of mass action: the amount of the free, unbound hormone is in equilibrium with the bound hormone. Thus, the total binding capacity of SHBG will influence the amount that is free and unbound.

The biologic effects of the major sex steroids are largely determined by the unbound portion, known as the <u>free hormone</u>. In other words, the active hormone is unbound and free while the bound hormone is relatively inactive. This concept is not without controversy. The hormone-protein complex may be involved in an active uptake process at the target cell plasma membrane.[14] The albumin-bound fraction of steroids may also be available for cellular action because this binding is of low affinity. Routine assays determine the total hormone concentration, bound plus free, and special steps are required to measure the active free level of testosterone, estradiol, and cortisol.

Estrogen Metabolism

<u>Androgens are the common precursors of estrogens.</u> 17β-Hydroxysteroid dehydrogenase activity converts androstenedione to testosterone which is not a major secretory product of the normal ovary. It is rapidly demethylated at the C-19 position and <u>aromatized to estradiol, the major estrogen secreted by the human ovary.</u> Estradiol also arises to a major degree from androstenedione via estrone, and estrone itself is secreted in significant daily amounts. <u>Estriol is the peripheral metabolite of estrone and estradiol and not a secretory product of the ovary.</u> The formation of estriol is typical of general metabolic "detoxification," conversion of biologically active material to less active forms.

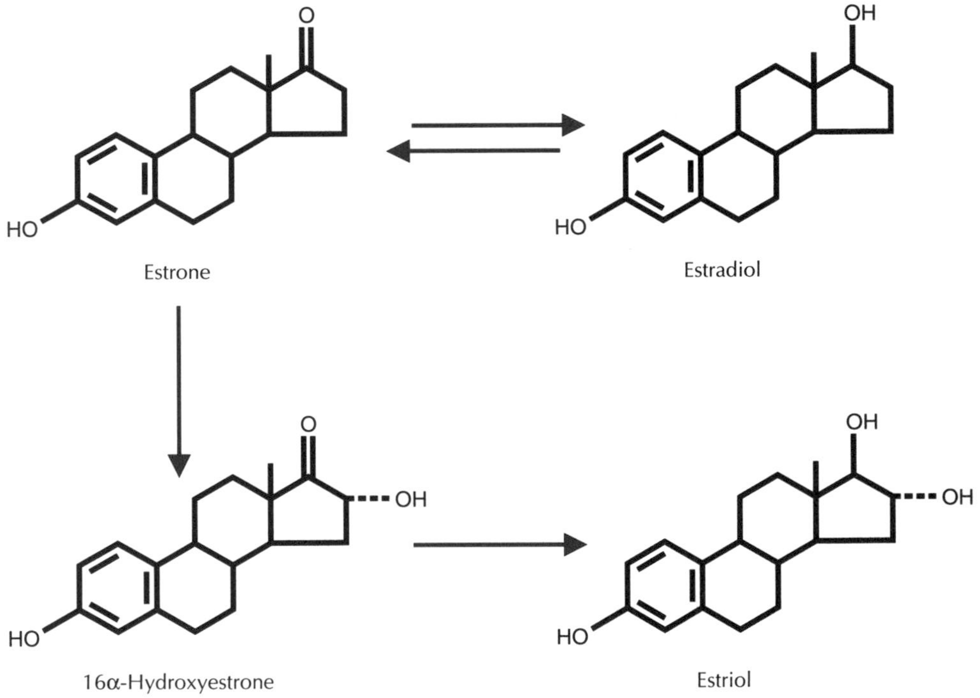

Estrone

Estradiol

16α-Hydroxyestrone

Estriol

The conversion of steroids in peripheral tissues is not always a form of inactivation. Free androgens are peripherally converted to free estrogens, for example, in skin and adipose cells. The location of the adipose cells influences their activity. Women with central obesity (the abdominal area) have more androgens.[15] The work of Siiteri and MacDonald[16] demonstrated that enough estrogen can be derived from circulating androgens to produce bleeding in the postmenopausal woman. <u>In the female the adrenal gland remains the major source of circulating androgens, in particular androstenedione.</u> In the male, almost all of the circulating estrogens are derived from peripheral conversion of androgens.

It can be seen, therefore, that the pattern of circulating steroids in the female is influenced by the activity of various processes outside the ovary. Because of the peripheral contribution to steroid levels, the term *secretion rate* is reserved for direct organ secretion, whereas ***production rate*** includes organ secretion plus peripheral contribution via conversion of precursors. The ***metabolic clearance rate (MCR)*** equals the volume of blood that is cleared of the hormone per unit of time. The ***blood production rate (PR)*** then equals the metabolic clearance rate multiplied by the concentration of the hormone in the blood.

MCR = Liters/Day
PR = MCR x Concentration
PR = Liters/Day x Amount/Liter = Amount/Day

In the normal nonpregnant female, estradiol is produced at the rate of 100–300 µg/day. The production of androstenedione is about 3 mg/day, and the peripheral conversion (about 1%) of androstenedione to estrone accounts for about 20–30% of the estrone produced per day. Since androstenedione is secreted in milligram amounts, even a small percent conversion to estrogen results in a significant contribution to estrogens which exist and function in microgram amounts. Thus, the circulating estrogens in the female are the sum of direct ovarian secretion of estradiol and estrone, plus peripheral conversion of C-19 precursors.

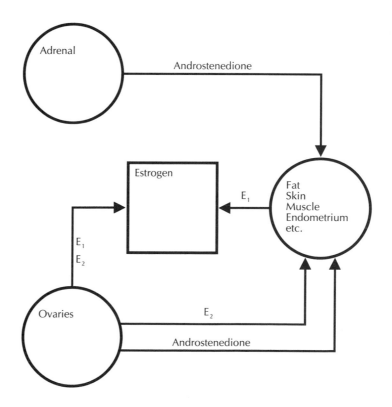

Premenopausal Peripheral Conversion

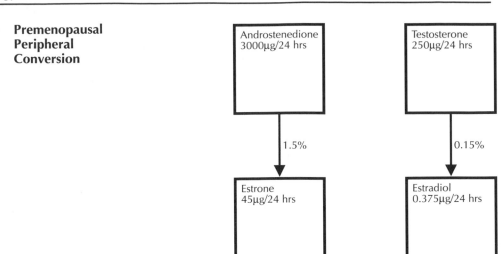

Androstenedione 3000μg/24 hrs		Testosterone 250μg/24 hrs
↓ 1.5%		↓ 0.15%
Estrone 45μg/24 hrs		Estradiol 0.375μg/24 hrs

Progesterone Metabolism

Peripheral conversion of steroids to progesterone is not seen in the nonpregnant female, rather the production rate is a combination of secretion from the adrenal and the ovaries. Including the small contribution from the adrenal, the blood production rate of progesterone in the preovulatory phase is less than 1 mg/day. During the luteal phase, production increases to 20–30 mg/day. The metabolic fate of progesterone, as expressed by its many excretion products, is more complex than estrogen. About 10–20% of progesterone is excreted as pregnanediol.

Pregnanediol glucuronide is present in the urine in concentrations less than 1 mg/day until ovulation. Postovulation pregnanediol excretion reaches a peak of 3–6 mg/day, which is maintained until 2 days prior to menses. The assay of pregnanediol in the urine now has little use, except in home test kits that allow women to self test for ovulation.

Progesterone

17-Hydroxyprogesterone

Pregnanediol

Pregnanetriol

In the preovulatory phase in adult females, in all prepubertal females, and in the normal male, the blood levels of progesterone are at the lower limits of immunoassay sensitivity: less than 100 ng/dL (320 nmol/L). After ovulation, i.e., during the luteal phase, progesterone ranges from 500 to 2,000 ng/dL. In congenital adrenal hyperplasia, progesterone blood levels can be as high as 50 times above normal.

Pregnanetriol is the chief urinary metabolite of 17α-hydroxyprogesterone and has clinical significance in the adrenogenital syndrome, where an enzyme defect results in accumulation of 17α-hydroxyprogesterone and increased excretion of pregnanetriol. The plasma or serum assay of 17α-hydroxyprogesterone is a more sensitive and accurate index of this enzyme deficiency than measurement of pregnanetriol. Normally the blood level of 17α-hydroxyprogesterone is less than 100 ng/dL (3 nmol/L), although after ovulation and during the luteal phase of a normal menstrual cycle, a peak of 200 ng/dL (6 nmol/L) can be reached. In syndromes of adrenal hyperplasia, values can be 10–400 times normal.

Androgen Metabolism

The major androgen products of the ovary are dehydroepiandrosterone (DHA) and androstenedione (and only a little testosterone) which are secreted mainly by stromal tissue derived from theca cells. With excessive accumulation of stromal tissue or in the presence of an androgen-producing tumor, testosterone becomes a significant secretory product. Occasionally, a nonfunctioning tumor can induce stromal proliferation and increased androgen production. The normal accumulation of stromal tissue at midcycle results in a rise in circulating levels of androstenedione and testosterone at the time of ovulation.

The adrenal cortex produces 3 groups of steroid hormones, the glucocorticoids, the mineralocorticoids, and the sex steroids. The adrenal sex steroids represent intermediate by-products in the synthesis of glucocorticoids and mineralocorticoids, and excessive secretion of the sex steroids occurs only with neoplastic cells or in association with enzyme deficiencies. Under normal circumstances, adrenal gland production of the sex steroids is less significant than gonadal production of androgens and estrogens. About one-half of the daily production of DHA and androstenedione comes from the adrenal gland; the other half of androstenedione is secreted by the ovary, but the other half of DHA is split almost equally between the ovary and peripheral tissues. The production rate of testosterone in the normal female is 0.2–0.3 mg/day, and approximately 50% arises from peripheral conversion of androstenedione (and a small amount from DHA) to testosterone, whereas 25% is secreted by the ovary and 25% by the adrenal. The major androgens are excreted in the urine as 17-ketosteroids.

There is no circadian cycle of the major sex steroids in the female. However, short-term variations in the blood levels due to episodic secretion require multiple sampling for absolutely accurate assessment. *Although frequent sampling is necessary for a high degree of accuracy, a random sample is sufficient for clinical purposes to determine whether a level is within a normal range.*

The testosterone binding capacity is decreased by androgens; hence, the binding capacity in men is lower than that in normal women. The binding globulin level in women with increased androgen production is also depressed. Androgenic effects are dependent upon the unbound fraction which can move freely from the vascular compartment into the target cells. Routine assays determine the total hormone concentration, bound plus free. Thus, a total testosterone concentration may be in the normal range in a woman who is hirsute or even virilized, but, since the binding globulin level is depressed by the androgen effects, the percent free and active testosterone is elevated. The need for a specific assay for the free portion of testosterone can be questioned since the very presence of hirsutism or virilism indicates increased androgen effects. In the face of hirsutism, one can reliably interpret a normal testosterone level as compatible with decreased binding capacity and increased active free testosterone.

Both total and unbound testosterone are normal in only a few women with hirsutism. In these cases, the hirsutism, heretofore regarded as idiopathic, most likely results from excessive intracellular androgen effects (specifically increased intracellular conversion of testosterone to dihydrotestosterone).

Reduction of the Δ^4 unsaturation (an irreversible pathway) in testosterone is very significant, producing derivatives very different in their spatial configuration and activity. The 5β derivatives are not androgenic, and this is not an important pathway; however, the 5α derivative (a very active pathway) is extremely potent. Indeed, dihydro-testosterone (DHT), the 5α derivative, is the principal androgenic hormone in a variety of target tissues and is formed within the target tissue itself.

In men, the majority of circulating DHT is derived from testosterone that enters a target cell and is converted by means of 5α-reductase to DHT. In women, because the production rate of androstenedione is greater than testosterone, blood DHT is primarily derived from androstenedione and partly from dehydroepiandrosterone.[17,18] Thus in women, the skin production of DHT may be predominantly influenced by androstenedione. DHT is by definition an autocrine and paracrine hormone, formed and acting within target tissues.[19]

The blood DHT is only about one-tenth the level of circulating testosterone, and it is clear that testosterone is the major circulating androgen. In tissues sensitive to DHT (which includes hair follicles), only DHT enters the nucleus to provide the androgen message. DHT also can perform androgenic actions within cells that do not possess the ability to convert testosterone to DHT. DHT is further reduced by a 3α-keto-reductase to androstanediol, which is relatively inactive. The metabolite of androstanediol, 3α-androstanediol glucuronide, is the major metabolite of DHT and can be measured in the plasma, indicating the level of activity of target tissue conversion of testosterone to DHT.

Not all androgen-sensitive tissues require the prior conversion of testosterone to DHT. In the process of masculine differentiation, the development of the wolffian duct structures (epididymis, the vas deferens, and the seminal vesicle) is dependent upon testosterone as the intracellular mediator, whereas development of the urogenital sinus and urogenital tubercle into the male external genitalia, urethra, and prostate requires the conversion of testosterone to DHT.[20] Muscle development is under the direct control of testosterone.

Excretion of Steroids

Active steroids and metabolites are excreted as sulfo- and glucuro-conjugates. Conjugation of a steroid generally reduces or eliminates the activity of a steroid. This is not completely true, however, since hydrolysis of the ester linkage can occur in target tissues and restore the active form. Furthermore, estrogen conjugates can have biologic activity, and it is known that sulfated conjugates are actively secreted and may serve as precursors. Ordinarily, however, conjugation by liver and intestinal mucosa is a step in deactivation preliminary to, and essential for, excretion into urine and bile.

Glucosiduronate

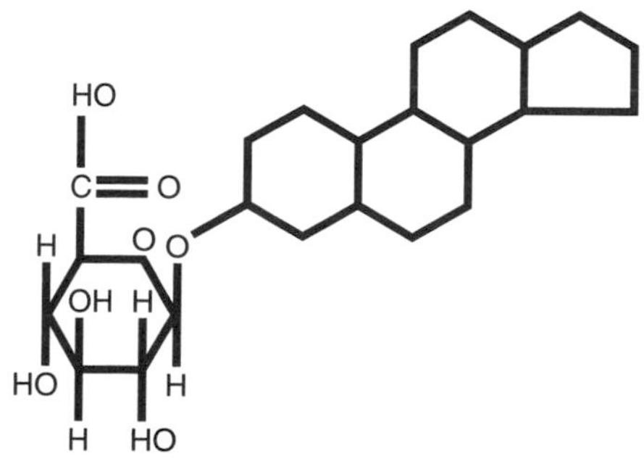

Sulfate

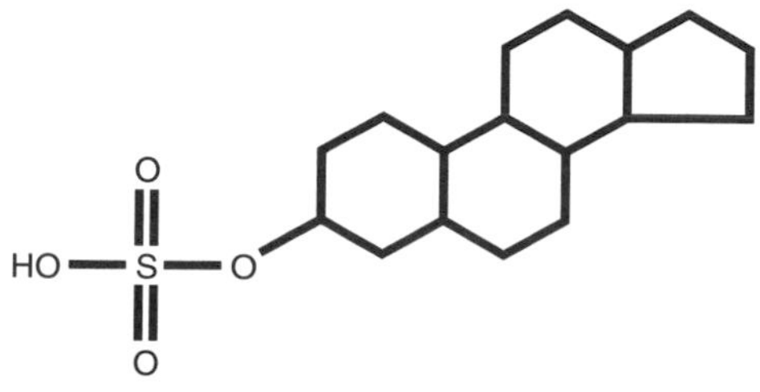

Cellular Mechanism of Action

Hormones circulate in extremely low concentrations and, in order to respond with specific and effective actions, target cells require the presence of special mechanisms. There are 2 major types of hormone action at target tissues. One mediates the action of tropic hormones (peptide and glycoprotein hormones) with receptors at the cell membrane level. In contrast, the smaller steroid hormones enter cells readily, and the basic mechanism of action involves specific receptor molecules within the cells. It is the affinity and specificity of the receptors together with the large concentration of receptors in cells that allow a small amount of hormone to produce a biologic response.

The many different types of receptors can be organized into the following basic categories.

Intracellular Receptors

Receptors in the nucleus lead to transcription activation. Examples include the receptors for steroid and thyroid hormones.

G Protein Coupled Receptors

These receptors are composed of a single polypeptide chain that spans the cell membrane. Binding to a specific hormone leads to interaction with G proteins that in turn activate second messengers. Examples include receptors for tropic hormones, prostaglandins, light, and odors. The second messengers include the adenylate cyclase enzyme, the phospholipase system, and calcium ion changes.

Ion Gate Channels

These cell surface receptors are composed of multiple units, that after binding, open ion channels. The influx of ions changes the electrical activity of the cells. The best example of this type is the acetylcholine receptor.

Receptors with Intrinsic Enzyme Activity

These transmembrane receptors have an intracellular component with tyrosine or serine kinase activity. Binding leads to receptor autophosphorylation and activity. Examples include the receptors for insulin and growth factors (tyrosine kinase) and the receptors for activin and inhibin (serine kinase).

Other Receptors

Receptors that do not fit the above categories include the receptors for LDL, prolactin, growth hormone, and some of the growth factors.

Mechanism of Action for Steroid Hormones

The specificity of the reaction of tissues to sex steroid hormones is due to the presence of intracellular receptor proteins.[21] Different types of tissues, such as liver, kidney, and uterus, respond in a similar manner. The mechanism includes: 1) diffusion across the cell membrane, 2) transfer across the nuclear membrane to the nucleus and binding to receptor protein, 3) interaction of a hormone-receptor complex with nuclear DNA, 4) synthesis of messenger RNA (mRNA), 5) transport of the mRNA to the ribosomes, and finally, 6) protein synthesis in the cytoplasm that results in specific cellular activity. Each of the major classes of the sex steroid hormones, including estrogens, progestins, and androgens, has been demonstrated to act according to this general mechanism. Glucocorticoid and mineralocorticoid receptors, when in the unbound state, reside in the cytoplasm and move into the nucleus after hormone-receptor binding.

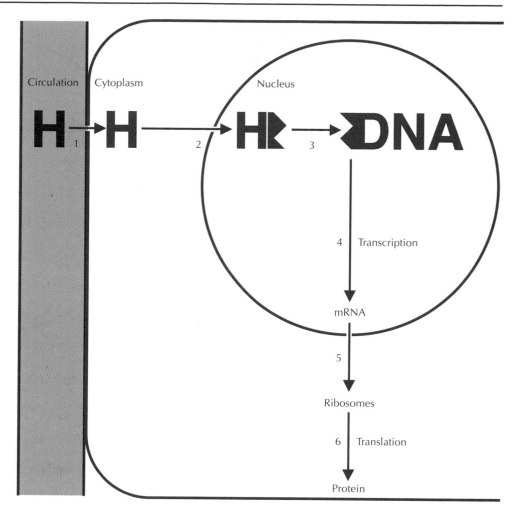

Steroid hormones are rapidly transported across the cell membrane by simple diffusion. The factors responsible for this transfer are unknown, but the concentration of free (unbound) hormone in the bloodstream seems to be an important and influential determinant of cellular function. Once in the cell, the sex steroid hormones bind to their individual receptors within the nucleus.[22–24] During this process, ***transformation or activation*** of the receptor occurs. Transformation refers to a conformational change of the hormone-receptor complex revealing or producing a binding site that is necessary in order for the complex to bind to the chromatin. In the unbound state, the receptor is associated with heat shock proteins that stabilize and protect the receptor and maintain the DNA binding region in an inactive state. Activation of the receptor is driven by hormone binding that causes a dissociation of the receptor-heat shock protein complex.

The hormone-receptor complex binds to specific DNA sites (***hormone responsive elements***) that are located upstream of the gene. The specific binding of the hormone-receptor complex with DNA results in RNA polymerase initiation of transcription. Transcription leads to translation, mRNA-mediated protein synthesis on the ribosomes. The principal action of steroid hormones is the regulation of intracellular protein synthesis by means of the receptor mechanism.

Biologic activity is maintained only while the nuclear site is occupied with the hormone-receptor complex. The dissociation rate of the hormone and its receptor as well as the half-life of the nuclear chromatin-bound complex are factors in the biologic response because the hormone response elements are abundant and, under normal conditions, are occupied only to a small extent.[25] Thus, an important clinical principle is the following: duration of exposure to a hormone is more important than dose. One reason only small

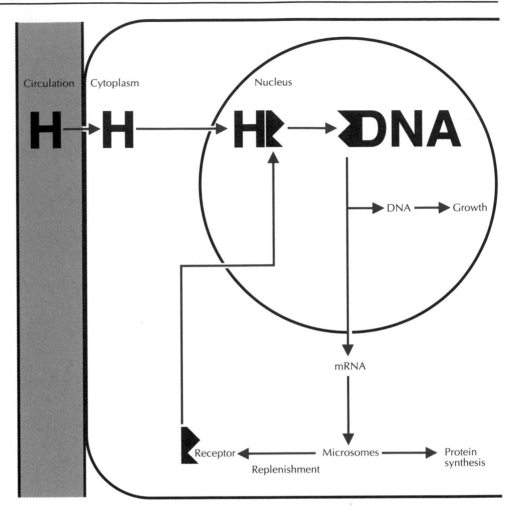

Circulation Cytoplasm Nucleus

DNA → Growth

mRNA

Receptor ← Microsomes → Protein synthesis

Replenishment

amounts of estrogen need be present in the circulation is the long half-life of the estrogen hormone-receptor complex. Indeed, a major factor in the potency differences among the various estrogens (estradiol, estrone, estriol) is the length of time the estrogen-receptor complex occupies the nucleus. The higher rate of dissociation with the weak estrogen (estriol) can be compensated for by continuous application to allow prolonged nuclear binding and activity. Cortisol and progesterone must circulate in large concentrations because their receptor complexes have short half-lives in the nucleus.

An important action of estrogen is the modification of its own and other steroid hormone activity by affecting receptor concentration. Estrogen increases target tissue responsiveness to itself and to progestins and androgens by increasing the concentration of its own receptor and that of the intracellular progestin and androgen receptors. This process is called *replenishment*. Progesterone and clomiphene, on the other hand, limit tissue response to estrogen by blocking the replenishment mechanism, thus decreasing over time the concentration of estrogen receptors. Replenishment is very responsive to the available amount of steroid and receptors. Small amounts of receptor depletion and small amounts of steroid in the blood activate the mechanism.

Replenishment, the synthesis of the sex steroid receptors, obviously takes place in the cytoplasm, but it must be quickly followed by transportation into the nucleus. There is an incredible nuclear traffic.[26] The nuclear membrane contains 3,000 to 4,000 pores. A cell synthesizing DNA imports about one million histone molecules from the cytoplasm every 3 minutes. If the cell is growing rapidly, about 3 newly assembled ribosomes will be transported every minute in the other direction. The typical cell can synthesize 10,000 to 20,000 different proteins. How do they know where to go? The answer is that these proteins have localization signals. In the case of steroid hormone receptor proteins, the signal sequences are in the hinge region.

Steroid hormone receptors exit continuously from the nucleus to the cytoplasm and are actively transported back to the nucleus. This is a constant shuttle; constant diffusion into the cytoplasm is balanced by the active transport into the nucleus. This raises the possibility that some diseases are due to poor traffic control. This can be true of some acquired diseases as well, e.g., Reye's syndrome, an acquired disorder of mitochondrial enzyme function.

The fate of the hormone-receptor complex after gene activation is referred to as hormone-receptor *processing.* In the case of estrogen receptors, processing involves the conversion of high affinity estrogen receptor sites to a rapidly dissociating form followed by loss of binding capacity which is completed in about 6 hours.[27] The rapid turnover of estrogen receptors has clinical significance. The continuous presence of estrogen is an important factor for continuing response.

The best example of the importance of these factors is the difference between estradiol and estriol. Estriol has only 20–30% affinity for the estrogen receptor compared to estradiol; therefore, it is rapidly cleared from a cell. But if the effective concentration is kept equivalent to that of estradiol, it can produce a similar biologic response.[28] In pregnancy, where the concentration of estriol is very great, it can be an important hormone, not just a metabolite.

The depletion of estrogen receptors in target tissues by progestational agents is the fundamental reason for adding progestins to estrogen treatment programs. The progestins accelerate the turnover of pre-existing receptors, and this is followed by inhibition of estrogen-induced receptor synthesis. Using monoclonal antibody immuno-cytochemistry, this action has been pinpointed to the interruption of transcription in estrogen-regulated genes.[29] The mechanism is different for androgen antiestrogen effects. Androgens do not involve depletion of estrogen receptors but in some way decrease estrogen-induced RNA activity in the cytoplasm.[30]

The Receptor Superfamily

Recombinant DNA techniques have permitted the study of the gene sequences that code for the synthesis of nuclear receptors. Steroid hormone receptors share a common structure with the receptors for thyroid hormone, 1,25-dihydroxy vitamin D_3, and retinoic acid; thus these receptors are called a superfamily.[31] Each receptor contains characteristic domains that are similar and interchangeable. Therefore, it is not surprising that the specific hormones can interact with more than one receptor in this family. Analysis of these receptors suggests a complex evolutionary history during which gene duplication and swapping between domains of different origins occurred.[32]

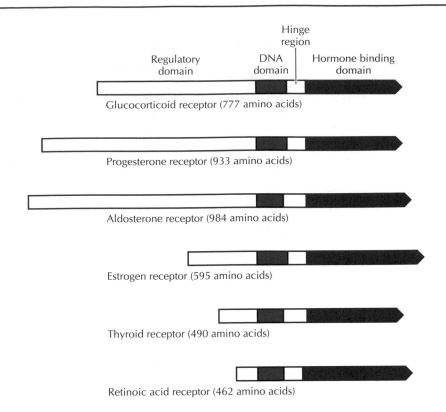

There are three domains and a "hinge" region in the superfamily receptor molecule.

1. The Regulatory Domain

The amino acid terminal is the immunoactive domain. It contains several phosphorylation sites and is involved in activation of the hormone-receptor complex (and thus influences gene transcription). This domain binds other protein factors.

2. The DNA-Binding Domain

The middle domain binds to DNA and consists of 66–68 amino acids with 9 cysteines in fixed positions. This domain is essential for activation of transcription. Hormone binding induces a conformational change which allows binding to the hormone responsive elements in the target gene. This domain is very similar for each member of the steroid and thyroid receptor superfamily; however, the genetic message is specific for the hormone which binds to the hormone binding domain, and this domain controls which gene will be regulated by the receptor.

3. The Hormone Binding Domain

The carboxy end is the hormone binding domain, consisting of about 250 amino acids. This domain is not essential for activation of transcription; thus, the hormone binding domain (in its unbound state) appears to normally prevent the function of the DNA binding domain and transcription activation. Hormone binding (with its conformational change) removes this inhibition. This domain also contributes to DNA localization and binding.

The Hinge Region

The region between the DNA binding domain and the hormone binding domain contains a signal area that is important for the movement of the receptor to the nucleus following synthesis in the cytoplasm.

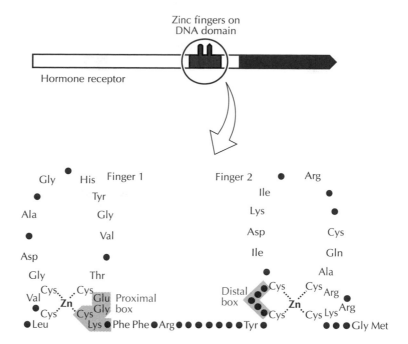

The similar amino acid sequence of the DNA binding domains indicates evolutionary conservation of homologous segments. An important part of the conformational pattern consists of multiple cysteine-repeating units found in two structures, each held in a finger-like shape by a zinc ion, the so-called zinc fingers.[33] The zinc fingers on the various hormone receptors are not identical. These fingers of amino acids are thought to interact with similar complementary patterns in the DNA. Directed changes (experimental mutations) indicate that conservation of the cysteine residues is necessary for binding activity, as is the utilization of zinc.

The DNA binding domain is specific for an enhancer site (called the hormone responsive element) in the gene promoter, located in the 5' flanking region. The activity of the hormone responsive element requires the presence of the hormone-receptor complex. Thus this region is the part of the gene to which the DNA binding domain of the receptor binds. There are four different hormone responsive elements, one for glucocorticoids/progesterone/androgen, one for estrogen, one for vitamin D_3, and one for thyroid/retinoic acid.[34,35] These sites significantly differ only in the number of intervening nucleotides.[36]

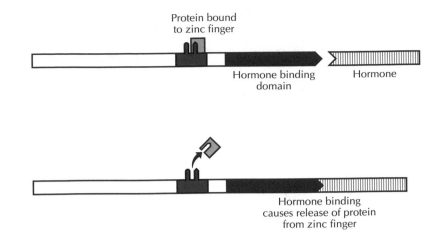

Protein bound
to zinc finger

Hormone binding
domain

Hormone

Hormone binding
causes release of protein
from zinc finger

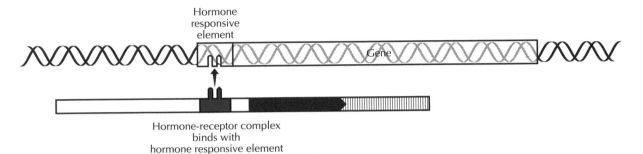

Hormone
responsive
element

Gene

Hormone-receptor complex
binds with
hormone responsive element
in the gene

Binding of the hormone-receptor complex to its hormone responsive element leads to many changes, one of which is a conformational alteration in the DNA.[37] Although the hormone responsive element for glucocorticoids, progesterone, and androgens mediates all of these hormonal responses, there are subtle differences in the binding sites, and there are additional sequences outside of the DNA binding sites that influence the activation by the three different hormones.[38] The cloning of complementary DNAs for steroid receptors has revealed a large number of similar structures of unknown function. It is believed that the protein products of these sequences are involved in the regulation of transcription initiation that occurs at the TATA box. *Estrogen, progesterone, and glucocorticoid receptors bind to their response elements as dimers, one molecule of hormone to each of the two units in the dimer.* This interaction produces greater stabilization and greater affinity for the hormone response element sequences. Even though receptors can bind to each other's sites because of their similarity, transcription activation occurs only when the right hormone binds to the right receptor, presumably because of proper turning on of the right regulators.

Multiple regions of the receptors are involved in the activation of transcription. The estrogen, progesterone, and glucocorticoid receptors contain two specific areas, known as TAF-1 and TAF-2 (transcription activation functions) which allow promotor-induced specific operation of transcription.[39] Phosphorylation of specific sites is an important method of regulation, as well as phosphorylation of other transcription factors.[40] Studies have indicated that the receptors interact with other transcription factors in synergistic ways to influence transcription. One example of a modulator, active in all of the genes of the receptor superfamily, is vitamin B_6.[41]

The specificity of receptor binding to its hormone responsive element is determined by the zinc finger region, especially the first finger. The specific message can be changed by changing the amino acids in the base of the fingers. Substitutions of amino acids in the finger tips leads to loss of function. Functional specificity is localized to the second zinc finger in an area designated the d (distal) box.[42] Different responses are due to the different genetic expression of each target cell (the unique activity of each cell's genetic constitution allows individual behavior).

Receptor activation is a complex series of events: separation of the receptor from inhibiting proteins, conformational change, and phosphorylation. Phosphorylation can be regulated by cell membrane receptors and ligand binding, thus establishing a method for cell membrane bound ligands to communicate with steroid receptor genes. One of the aspects of activation, for example with the estrogen receptor, is an increase in affinity for estrogen. This is an action of estrogen, and it is greatest with estradiol and least with estriol. This action of estradiol, the ability of binding at one site to affect another site, is called ***cooperativity***. An increase in affinity is called positive cooperativity. The biologic advantage of positive cooperativity is that this increases the receptor's ability to respond to small changes in the concentration of the hormone. One of the antiestrogen actions of clomiphene is its property of negative cooperativity, the inhibition of the transition from a low affinity to a high affinity state. The relatively long duration of action exhibited by estradiol is due to the high affinity state achieved by the receptor. Another form of cooperativity is the synergism observed when several hormone-receptor complexes interact with hormone responsive elements.[43]

Receptor activation also involves interactions with other proteins. In the unactivated state, steroid receptors are associated with other proteins; one group is the so-called heat shock proteins. One of the purposes of the heat shock proteins is to maintain the receptor in a high affinity conformation. Upon binding, the heat shock proteins are released from their attachments in the steroid-binding domain, contributing to the change in form that enables the DNA-binding domain to associate with the target gene.

The Progesterone Receptor
The progesterone receptor is induced by estrogens at the transcriptional level and decreased by progestins at both the transcriptional and translational levels (probably through receptor phosphorylation).[44] Estrogen exerts its influence on the progesterone receptor gene by means of an estrogen responsive element in the 5' flanking region.

The progesterone receptor gene encodes a collection of messenger RNAs that direct the synthesis of several structurally related receptor proteins, with two major forms, designated the A and B receptors.[45] The two forms are each associated with a different estrogen responsive element. Each form is associated with additional proteins, which are important for folding of the polypeptide into a structure that allows hormone binding and receptor activity.[46]

Progesterone is unique in the steroid superfamily in having two forms of its receptor. Therefore, progestational agents can elicit a variety of responses determined by target tissue production and activity of the two receptor forms with dimerization as A:A and B:B (homodimers) or A:B (heterodimer).

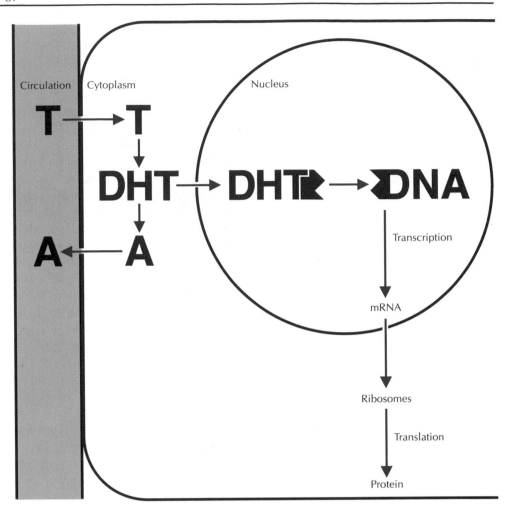

The Androgen Receptor

The cellular mechanism is more complex for androgens. Androgens can work in any one of three ways.

1. By intracellular conversion of testosterone to dihydrotestosterone (DHT).

2. By testosterone itself.

3. By intracellular conversion of testosterone to estradiol (aromatization).

Tissues that exclusively operate via the testosterone pathway are the derivatives of the wolffian duct, whereas hair follicles and derivatives of the urogenital sinus and urogenital tubercle require the conversion of testosterone to DHT. The hypothalamus actively converts androgens to estrogens; hence, aromatization may be necessary for certain androgen feedback messages in the brain.

In those cells that respond only to DHT, only DHT will be found within the nucleus activating messenger RNA production. Because testosterone and DHT bind to the same high affinity androgen receptor, why is it necessary to have the DHT mechanism? One explanation is that this is a mechanism for amplifying androgen action, because the androgen receptor preferentially will bind DHT (greater affinity). The antiandrogens, including cyproterone acetate and spironolactone, bind to the androgen receptor with about 20% of the affinity of testosterone.[47] This weak affinity is characteristic of binding without activation of the biologic response.

The amino acid sequence of the androgen receptor in the DNA-binding domain resembles that of the receptors for progesterone, mineralocorticoids, and glucocorticoids but most closely that of the progesterone receptor.[48] Androgens and progestins can crossreact for their receptors but do so only when present in pharmacologic concentrations. Progestins not only compete for androgen receptors but also compete for the metabolic utilization of the 5α-reductase enzyme. The dihydroprogesterone which is produced in turn also competes with testosterone and DHT for the androgen receptor. A progestin, therefore, can act both as an antiandrogen and as an antiestrogen. Androgen-responsive gene expression can also be modifed by estrogen; it has been known for years that androgens and estrogens can counteract each other's biologic responses. These responses of target tissues are determined by gene interactions with the hormone-receptor complexes, androgen with its receptor and estrogen with its receptor. The ultimate biologic response reflects the balance of actions of the different hormones with their respective receptors, modified by various transcription regulators.[49]

The syndrome of testicular feminization (androgen insensitivity) represents a congenital abnormality in the androgen intracellular receptor. The androgen receptor gene is localized on the human X chromosome, the only steroid hormone receptor to be located on the X chromosome.[50] Thus testicular feminization is an X-linked disorder. Molecular studies of patients with testicular feminization have indicated a deletion of amino acids from the steroid binding domain due to nucleotide alterations in the gene which encodes the androgen receptor.[51] What was once a confusing picture is now easily understood as a progressive increase in androgen receptor action. At one end, there is a complete absence of androgen binding — complete testicular feminization. In the middle is a spectrum of clinical presentations representing varying degrees of abnormal receptors and binding. While at the other end, it has been suggested that about 25% of infertile men with normal genitalia and normal family histories have azoospermia due to a receptor disorder.[52]

Mechanism of Action for Tropic Hormones

Tropic hormones include the releasing hormones originating in the hypothalamus and a variety of peptides and glycoproteins released by the anterior pituitary gland. The specificity of the tropic hormone depends upon the presence of a receptor in the cell membrane of the target tissue. Tropic hormones do not enter the cell to stimulate physiologic events but unite with a receptor on the surface of the cell.

The receptor protein in the cell membrane can either act as the active agent and, after binding, operate as an ion channel or function as an enzyme. Alternatively, the receptor protein is coupled to an active agent, an intracellular messenger. The major intracellular messenger molecules are cyclic AMP, inositol 1,4,5-triphosphate (IP$_3$), 1,2-diacyl-glycerol (1,2,-DG), calcium ion, and cyclic GMP.

Receptors from this membrane family are also found in the membranes of lysosomes, endoplasmic reticulum, Golgi complex, and in nuclei. The regulation of these intracellular organelle receptors differs from those of the cell surface membranes.

The Cyclic AMP Mechanism

Cyclic AMP is the intracellular messenger for FSH, LH, human chorionic gonadotropin (HCG), thyroid-stimulating hormone (TSH), and ACTH. Union of a tropic hormone with its cell membrane receptor activates the adenylate cyclase enzyme within the membrane wall leading to the conversion of adenosine 5'-triphosphate (ATP) within the cell to cyclic AMP.[53] Specificity of action and/or intensity of stimulation can be altered by changes in the structure or concentration of the receptor at the cell wall binding site. In addition to changes in biologic activity due to target cell alterations, changes in the molecular structure of the tropic hormone can interfere with cellular binding and physiologic activity.

The cell's mechanism for sensing the low concentrations of circulating tropic hormone is to have an extremely large number of receptors but to require only a very small percentage (as little as 1%) to be occupied by the tropic hormone. The cyclic AMP released is specifically bound to a cytoplasm receptor protein, and this cyclic AMP-receptor protein complex activates a protein kinase. The protein kinase is thought to be present in an inactive form as a tetramer containing 2 regulatory subunits and 2 catalytic subunits. Binding of cyclic AMP to the regulatory units releases the catalytic units, with the regulatory units remaining as a dimer. The catalytic units catalyze the phosphorylation of cellular proteins such as enzymes and mitochondrial, microsomal, and chromatin proteins. The physiologic event follows this cyclic AMP-mediated energy-producing event. Cyclic AMP is then degraded by the enzyme phosphodiesterase into the inactive compound, 5'-AMP.

Most noteworthy, DNA contains responsive elements that bind proteins phosphorylated by the catalytic units, thus leading to activation of gene transcription. The *cyclic AMP responsive element (CRE)* functions as an enhancer element upstream from the start of transcription.[54] A large family of transcription factors interact with the CRE, creating an important regulatory unit for gene transcription. Cyclic AMP activates a specific transcription factor, cyclic AMP regulatory element binding protein (CREB); the binding of CREB to CRE activates many genes. This system can also involve DNA sequences upstream from the CRE site.

Because LH can stimulate steroidogenesis without apparent changes in cyclic AMP (at low hormone concentrations), it is possible that an independent pathway exists; i.e., a mechanism independent of cyclic AMP. Mechanisms independent of cyclic AMP could include ion flow, calcium distribution, and changes in phospholipid metabolism.

The cyclic AMP system can be regarded as an example of evolutionary conservation. Rather than developing new regulatory systems, certain critical regulators have been preserved from bacteria to mammals. How is it that a single intracellular mediator can regulate different events? This is accomplished by turning on different biochemical events governed by the different gene expression in individual cells.

The cyclic AMP system provides a method for amplification of the faint hormonal signal swimming in the sea of the bloodstream. Each cyclase molecule produces a lot of cyclic AMP; the protein kinases activate a large number of molecules that in turn lead to an even greater number of products. This is an important part of the sensitivity of the endocrine system. This is a major reason why only a small percentage of the cell membrane receptors need be occupied in order to generate a response.

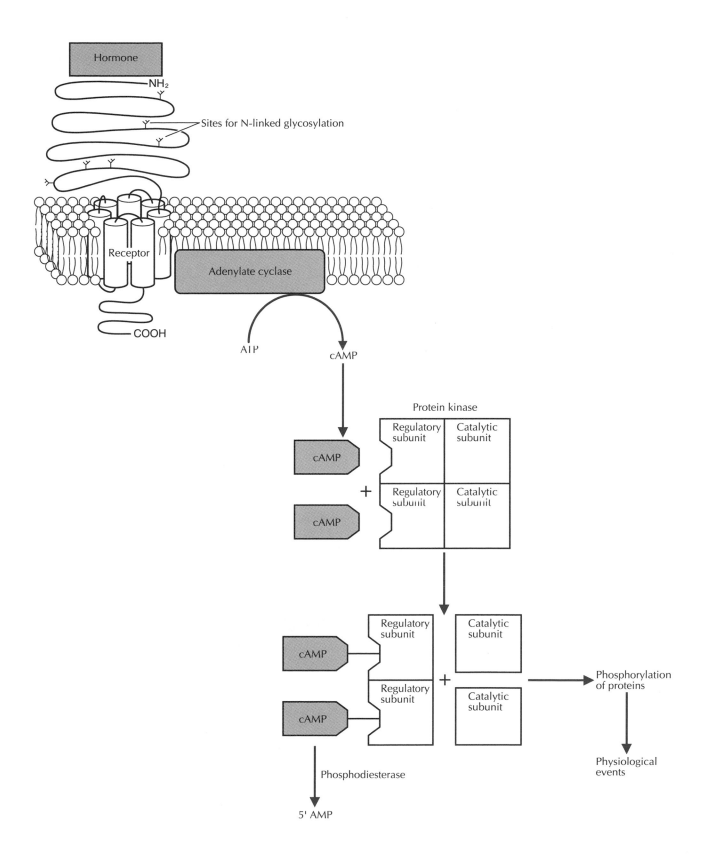

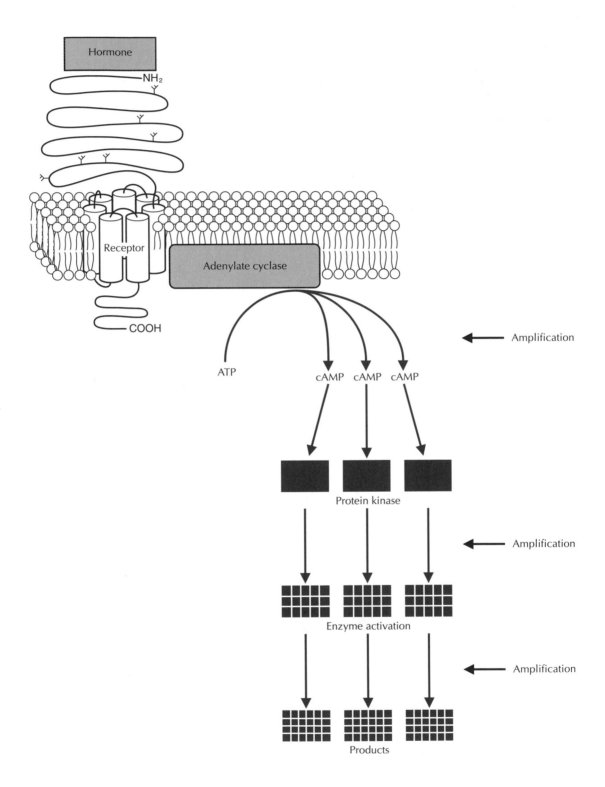

Prostaglandins stimulate adenylate cyclase activity and cyclic AMP accumulation. Despite the effect on adenylate cyclase, prostaglandins appear to be synthesized after the action of cyclic AMP. This implies that tropic hormone stimulation of cyclic AMP occurs first; cyclic AMP then activates prostaglandin synthesis and, finally, intracellular prostaglandin moves to the cell wall to facilitate the response to the tropic hormone. In addition to actions mediated by cyclic AMP, prostaglandins can also operate through changes in intracellular concentrations of calcium.[55]

Prostaglandins and cyclic GMP (cyclic guanosine 3'5'-monophosphate) may participate in an intracellular negative feedback mechanism governing the degree of, or direction of, cellular activity (e.g., the extent of steroidogenesis or shutting off of steroidogenesis after a peak of activity is reached). In other words, the level of cellular function may be determined by the interaction among prostaglandins, cyclic AMP, and cyclic GMP.

There are differences among the tropic hormones. Oxytocin, insulin, growth hormone, prolactin, and human placental lactogen (HPL) do not utilize the adenylate cyclase mechanism. Receptors for prolactin, growth hormone, and a number of cytokines (including erythropoietin and interleukins) belong to a single transmembrane domain receptor family.[56] Studies of this receptor family indicate that prolactin operates through various signal transduction mechanisms, including ion channels and nuclear kinase activation.

Gonadotropin releasing hormone (GnRH) is calcium dependent in its mechanism of action and utilizes IP$_3$ and 1,2-DG as second messengers to stimulate protein kinase activity.[57] These responses require a G protein and are associated with cyclical release of calcium ions from intracellular stores and the opening of cell membrane channels to allow entry of extracellular calcium.

The Calcium Messenger System

The intracellular calcium concentration is a regulator of both cyclic AMP and cyclic GMP levels.[58] Activation of the surface receptor either opens a channel in the cell membrane that lets calcium ions into the cell, or calcium is released from internal stores (the latter is especially the case in muscle). This calcium flux is an important intracellular mediator of response to hormones, functioning itself as a second messenger in the nervous system and in muscle.

The calcium messenger system is linked to hormone-receptor function by means of a specific enzyme, phospholipase C, that catalyzes the hydrolysis of polyphosphatidylinositols, specific phospholipids in the cell membrane. Activation of this enzyme by hormone binding to its receptor leads to the generation of 2 intracellular messengers, inositol trisphosphate (IP$_3$) and diacylglycerol (1,2-DG), which initiate the function of the 2 parts of the calcium system. The first part is a calcium activated protein kinase responsible for sustained cellular responses, and the second part involves a regulator called calmodulin responsible for acute responses. These responses are secondary to alterations in enzyme activity and in transcription factors.

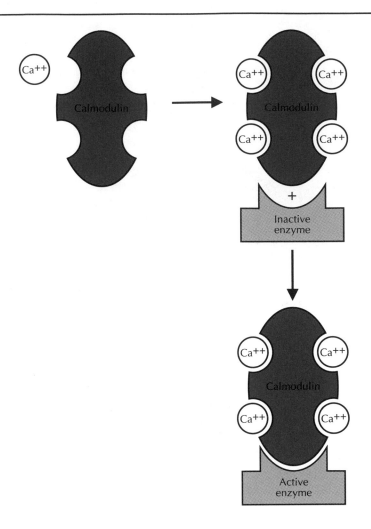

Calmodulin has been identified in all animal and plant cells that have been examined. Therefore, it is a very ancient protein. It is a single polypeptide chain of 148 amino acid residues whose sequence and structural and functional properties are similar to those of troponin C, the substance that binds calcium during muscle contractions, facilitating the interaction between actin and myosin. The calmodulin molecule has 4 calcium binding sites, and binding with calcium gives a helical conformation which is necessary for biologic activity. A typical animal cell contains more than 10 million molecules of calmodulin, constituting about 1% of the total cell protein. As a calcium regulatory protein, it serves as an intracellular calcium receptor and modifies calcium transport, enzyme activity, the calcium regulation of cyclic nucleotide and glycogen metabolism, and such processes as secretion and cell motility. Thus, calmodulin serves a role analogous to that of troponin C, mediating calcium's actions in noncontractile tissues, and cyclic AMP works together with calcium and calmodulin in the regulation of intracellular metabolic activity.

Kinase Receptors

The cell membrane receptors of insulin, insulin-like growth factor-I, epidermal growth factor, platelet derived growth factor, and fibroblast growth factor are tyrosine kinases. All tyrosine kinase receptors have a similar structure: an extracellular domain for ligand binding, a single transmembrane domain, and a cytoplasmic domain. The unique amino acid sequences determine a 3-dimensional conformation that provides ligand specificity. The transmembrane domains are not highly conserved (thus differing in make-up). The cytoplasmic domains respond to ligand binding by undergoing conformational changes and autophosphorylation. The structure of the receptors for insulin and insulin-like growth factor-I is more complicated, with two alpha- and two beta-subunits, forming two transmembrane domains connected extracellularly by disulfide bridges. The receptors for the important autocrine/paracrine factors, activin and inhibin, function as serine-specific protein kinases.

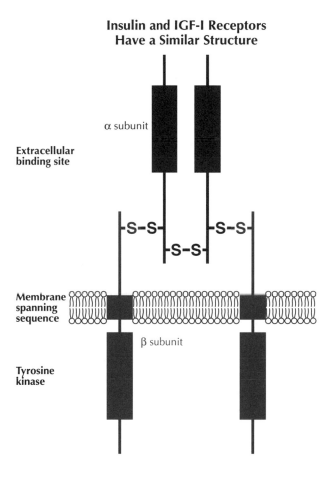

Insulin and IGF-I Receptors Have a Similar Structure

Kinase activation requires distinctive sequences; thus there is considerable homology among the kinase receptors in the cytoplasmic domain. Many of the substrates for these kinases are the enzymes and proteins in other messenger systems, e.g., the calcium messenger system. Thus, the kinase receptors can cross talk with other receptor regulated systems that involve the G proteins.

Autocrine and Paracrine Regulation Factors

Growth factors are polypeptides that modulate activity either in the cells in which they are produced or in nearby cells; hence, they are autocrine and paracrine regulators. Regulation factors of this type (yet another biologic family) are produced by local gene expression and protein translation, and they operate by binding to cell membrane receptors. The receptors usually contain an intracellular component with tyrosine kinase activity which is energized by a binding-induced conformational change that induces autophosphorylation. However, some factors work through the other second messenger systems, such as cyclic AMP or IP3. Growth factors are involved in a variety of tissue functions, including mitogenesis, tissue and cellular differentiation, chemotactic actions, and angiogenesis.

In addition to the growth factors, various immune factors, especially cytokines, modulate ovarian steroidogenesis.[59] These factors, including interleukin-1, tumor necrosis factor, and interferon, are found in human follicular fluid and, in general, inhibit gonadotropin stimulation of steroidogenesis.

The following growth factors are those which have been best studied in reproductive physiology:

Transforming growth factor-beta —	TGF-β
Fibroblast growth factor	— FGF
Epidermal growth factor	— EGF
Insulin-like growth factor-I	— IGF-I
Insulin-like growth factor-II	— IGF-II

For mitogenesis to occur, cells may require exposure to a sequence of growth factors, with important limitations in duration and concentrations.[60] Growth factors are important for the direction of embryonic and fetal growth and development. In cellular differentiation, growth factors can operate in a cooperative, competititve, or synergistic fashion with other hormones. For example, IGF-I plus FSH, but not IGF-I alone, increases the number of LH receptors, progesterone synthesis, and aromatase activity in granulosa cells.[61]

TGF-β belongs to a large family of proteins that includes inhibin, activin, and antimüllerian hormone. It can either stimulate or inhibit growth and differentiation, depending on the target cell and the presence or absence of other growth factors. In the ovary, TGF-β promotes granulosa cell differentiation by enhancing the actions of FSH (especially in expression of FSH and LH receptors) and antagonizing the down-regulation of FSH receptors. TGF-β and the insulin-like growth factors are required for the maintenance of normal bone mass. EGF is a structural analog of TGF-α and is involved in mitogenesis. In the ovary, EGF, secreted by theca cells, is important for granulosa cell proliferation, an action opposed by TGF-β which is also secreted by the theca cells. The most potent mitogens are the two forms of FGF. Additional roles for FGF, secreted by the granulosa, include modulation of enzyme activity involved in the physical act of ovulation and angiogenic function during the development of the corpus luteum.

The Insulin-Like Growth Factors

The insulin-like growth factors (also called somatomedins) are single chain polypeptides that resemble insulin in structure and function. These factors are widespread and are involved in growth and differentiation in response to growth hormone, and as local regulators of cell metabolism. IGF-II is more prominent during embryogenesis, while IGF-I is more active postnatally. Only the liver produces more IGF-I than the ovary. Both IGF-I and IGF-II are secreted by granulosa cells. IGF-I amplifies the action of gonadotropins and coordinates the functions of theca and granulosa cells. IGF-I receptors on the granulosa are increased by FSH and LH and augmented by estrogen. In the theca, IGF-I increases steroidogenesis. In the granulosa, IGF-I is important for the formation and increase in numbers of FSH and LH receptors, steroidogenesis, the secretion of inhibin, and oocyte maturation. Granulosa cells also contain receptors for insulin, and insulin can bind to the IGF receptors. The IGF-I receptor is a heterotetramer with two alpha- and two beta-subunits in a structure similar to that of the insulin receptor. Insulin can bind to the alpha-subunit ligand binding domain and activate the beta-subunit which is a protein kinase. Thus, insulin can modulate ovarian cellular functions. The biologic potency and availability of the insulin-like growth factors are further modulated by a collection of IGF-binding proteins which bind circulating insulin-like growth factors and also alter cellular responsiveness. IGF-binding protein-3, for example, is secreted, bound, and processed by cells, affecting both the function of the binding protein and IGF activity.[62]

Regulation of Tropic Hormones

Modulation of the peptide hormone mechanism is an important biologic system for enhancing or reducing target tissue response. This regulation of tropic hormone action currently has 3 major components

1. Heterogeneity of the hormone.
2. Up- and down-regulation of receptors.
3. Regulation of adenylate cyclase.

Heterogeneity

The glycoproteins, such as FSH and LH, are not single proteins but should be viewed as a family of heterogeneous forms of varying immunologic and biologic activity. The various forms (isoforms) arise in various ways, including different DNA promoter actions, alterations in RNA splicing, point mutations, and post-translational carbohydrate changes.[63] The impact of the variations is to alter structure and metabolic clearance, thus affecting binding and activity. The isoforms have different molecular weights, circulating half-lives, and biologic activities. Throughout the menstrual cycle, the amazing number of at least 20–30 isoforms of both FSH and LH are present in the bloodstream.[64] *The overall activity of a glycoprotein, therefore, is due to the effects of the mixture of forms which reach and bind to the target tissue.*

The nonglycosylated subunit precursors of glycoprotein hormones are synthesized in the endoplasmic reticulum, followed by glycosylation. The glycosylated subunits combine and then are transported to the Golgi apparatus for further processing of the carbohydrate component. The units combine to form a compact heterodimer. The protein moiety binds to specific target tissue receptors, while the carbohydrate moiety plays a critical role in coupling the hormone-receptor complex to adenylate cyclase (perhaps by determining the necessary conformational structure).[65]

The preciseness of the chemical make-up of the tropic hormones is an essential element in determining the ability of the hormone to mate with its receptor. The glycopeptides (FSH, LH, TSH, and HCG) are dimers composed of two glycosylated polypeptide subunits, the α- and β-subunits. The α- and β-subunits are tightly bound in a noncovalent association. The three-dimensional structure of the subunits is maintained by internal disulfide bonds. All of the glycopeptides of the human species (FSH, LH, TSH, and HCG) share a common α-chain, an identical structure containing 92 amino acids. The β-chains (or the β-subunits) differ in both amino acid and carbohydrate content, conferring the specificity inherent in the relationship between hormones and their receptors. Therefore, the specific biologic activity of a glycopeptide hormone is determined by the β-subunit; hypogonadism has been reported due to single amino acid substitution in the LH beta-subunit.[66]

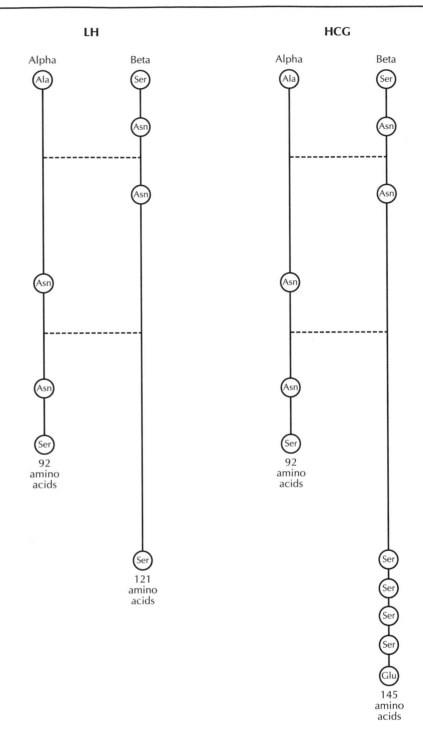

β-HCG is the largest β-subunit, containing a larger carbohydrate moiety and 145 amino acid residues, including a unique carboxyl terminal tail piece of 24 amino acid groups. It is this unique part of the HCG structure which allows the production of highly specific antibodies and the utilization of highly specific immunologic assays. The extended sequence in the carboxy-terminal region of β-HCG contains 4 sites for glycosylation, the reason why HCG is glycosylated to a greater extent than LH.

These differences in structure are associated with a different promoter and transcriptional site that is located upstream in the HCG beta-subunit gene compared to the site in the LH beta-subunit gene. The HCG beta-subunit site does not contain a hormone response element, allowing HCG secretion to escape feedback regulation by the sex steroids, in contrast to FSH and LH.

The rate-limiting step in the synthesis of gonadotropins and TSH is the availability of β-subunits, since excess α-units can be found in blood and in tissue. Furthermore, the three dimensional structure of the β-subunit, accomplished by folding the subunit by the formation of the disulfide bonds, is an important conformational step that is essential for assembly with the α-subunit.[67] This conformational change is not completed until the subunits are fully united to produce the final whole hormone.

The half-life of α-HCG is 6–8 minutes, that of whole HCG from the placenta about 12 hours. All human tissues appear to make HCG a whole molecule, but the placenta is different in having the ability to glycosylate the protein, thus reducing its rate of metabolism and giving it biologic activity through a long half-life. The carbohydrate components of the glycoproteins are comprised of fructose, galactose, mannose, galactosamine, glucosamine, and sialic acid. Whereas the other sugars are necessary for hormonal function, sialic acid is the critical determinant of biologic half-life. Removal of sialic acid residues in HCG, FSH, and LH leads to very rapid elimination from the circulation.

FSH consists of the α-subunit of 92 amino acids and a β-subunit of 110 amino acids. It has four carbohydrate side chains, two on each subunit. The β-subunit of LH consists of 121 amino acids. LH has 3 carbohydrate side chains with a single glycosylation site (with less than half of the sialic acid in FSH). The initial half-life of LH is approximately 20 minutes, compared to the initial half-life of FSH of 3–4 hours.

Genes for tropic hormones contain promoter and enhancer or inhibitor regions located in the 5' flanking regions upstream from the transcription site. These sites respond to second messengers (cyclic AMP) as well as steroids and other yet unknown regulators. The protein cores of the two subunits are the products of distinct genes.[68] Using recombinant DNA technology, it has been demonstrated that there is a single human gene for the expression of the α-subunit. The gene for the α-subunit shared by FSH, LH, HCG, and TSH is located on chromosome 6q21.1–23. A single promoter site regulates transcription of the α-gene in both placenta and pituitary. The gene for the FSH beta-subunit is on chromosome 11.

The genes that encode for the beta-subunits of LH, HCG, and TSH are located in a cluster on chromosome 19q13.3. There are 6 genes for the β-subunit of HCG, and only one for β-LH.[69,70] Transcription for the 6 HCG genes, each with different promoter activity, varies, and it is not certain why HCG requires multigenic expression (perhaps this is necessary to reach the extremely high level of production in early pregnancy).[71] It is thought that β-HCG evolved relatively recently from β-LH, and the unique amino acid terminal extension of β-HCG arose by reading a gene similar to β-LH; the DNA sequences of the β-HCG genes and the β-LH gene are 96% identical.[70,72] Only primates and horses have been demonstrated to have genes for the β-subunit of chorionic gonadotropin. In contrast to human chorionic gonadotropin, equine chorionic gonadotropin exerts both LH and FSH activities in many mammalian species because it contains peptide sequences in its beta-subunit which are homologous to those in the pituitary gonadotropins of other species. The equine β-chorionic gonadotropin gene is identical to the equine β-LH gene, and while the primate β-HCG gene evolved from an ancestral β-LH gene, the horse chorionic gonadotropin gene evolved in a different way.

Variations in Carbohydrate

The glycopeptide hormones can be found in the pituitary existing in a variety of forms, differing in their carbohydrate make-up. Removal of carbohydrate residues from the FSH molecule produces forms of FSH with antagonistic properties. Treatment of women with a GnRH antagonist yields circulating levels of deglycosylated FSH that bind to gonadal receptors but exert no biological activity.[73] Thus, the pituitary can secrete forms of the glycopeptide hormones which can function as naturally occurring antihormones. The isoform mixture is influenced both quantitatively and qualitatively by GnRH and the feedback of the steroid hormones.

Certain clinical conditions may be associated with alterations in the usual chemical structure of the glycopeptides, resulting in an interference with the ability to bind to receptors and stimulate biological activity. In addition to deglycosylation and the formation of antihormones, gonadotropins can be produced with an increased carbohydrate content. A low estrogen environment in the pituitary gland, for example, favors the production of so-called big gonadotropins, gonadotropins with an increased carbohydrate component and, as a result, decreased biological activity. Immunoassay in these situations may not reveal the biologic situation; an immunoassay sees only a certain set of molecules but not all. Therefore, immunologic results do not always indicate the biologic situation.

Bioactive levels of FSH are very low in women receiving oral contraceptives and during the luteal and late follicular phases. The highest values are during the midcycle surge and in postmenopausal women (including women with premature ovarian failure). The levels of bioactive FSH parallel those of immunoactive FSH with a constant ratio throughout the cycle. The greater bioactivity of FSH at midcycle is associated with less sialyated, shorter-lived isoforms. This is an effect of both GnRH and estrogen.

The carbohydrate component, therefore, affects target tissue response in two ways: 1) metabolic clearance and half-life and 2) biologic activity. The latter action focuses on two functions for the hormone-receptor complex: binding and activation. One structural domain is important for binding and another for triggering the biologic response. Carbohydrate residues, especially the sialic acid residues, are less important in binding. Indeed, experimental data indicate that the carbohydrate chains have no role in the binding of gonadotropins to their receptors.[74] Nevertheless, removal of the carbohydrate moiety of either subunit diminishes gonadotropic activity. Therefore, the carbohydrate component affects the biologic activity of the hormone-receptor complex after binding. Specific studies indicate that the carbohydrate component plays a critical role in activation (coupling) of the adenylate cyclase system.[75-77]

While the β-subunit specifies the biologic activity of an individual glycoprotein, the combination of the α- and β-subunits is necessary for full hormonal expression. Furthermore, the α-subunit also plays an important role in accomplishing normal receptor binding and activation.[78,79] Neither subunit alone can effectively bind to the receptor with high affinity or exert biologic effect. In other words, binding and activation occur only when the hormone is in the combined α-β form.

Heterogeneity of Prolactin

In most mammalian species, prolactin consists of 197–199 amino acids, similar in structure to growth hormone and placental lactogen. All three hormones are believed to have originated in a common ancestral protein about 60–70 million years ago. Simultaneous measurements of prolactin by both bioassay and immunoassay reveal discrepancies. At first differences in prolactin were observed based on size, leading to the use of terms such as little, big, and the wonderfully sophisticated term, big big prolactin. Further chemical studies have revealed structural modifications which include

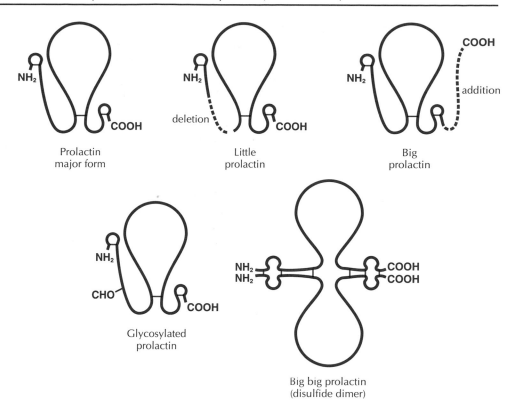

glycosylation, phosphorylation, and variations in binding and charge. This heterogeneity is the result of many influences at many levels: transcription, translation, and peripheral metabolism.[80]

Prolactin is encoded by a single gene, producing a molecule that in its major form is maintained in 3 loops by disulfide bonds. Both smaller and larger forms have been identified. Little prolactin probably represents a splicing variant resulting from the deletion of amino acids. Big prolactin can result from the failure to remove introns; it has little biologic activity and does not cross react with antibodies to the major form of prolactin. The so-called big big variants of prolactin are due to separate molecules of prolactin binding to each other, either noncovalently or by interchain disulfide bonding. Some of the apparently larger forms of prolactin are prolactin molecules complexed to binding proteins.

Other variations exist. Enzymatic cleavage of the prolactin molecule yields fragments that may be capable of biologic activity. Prolactin that has been glycosylated continues to exert activity. However, the nonglycosylated form of prolactin is the predominant form of prolactin secreted into the circulation.[81] Posttranslational modification of prolactin also occurs and includes phosphorylation, deamidation, and sulfation.

At any one point of time, the bioactivity (e.g., galactorrhea) and the immunoactivity (circulating level by immunoassay) of prolactin represent the cumulative effect of the family of structural variants. Remember, immunoassays do not always reflect the biologic situation (e.g., a normal prolactin level in a women with galactorrhea).

Up- and Down-Regulation   Positive or negative modulation of receptors by homologous hormones is known as up- and down-regulation. Little is known regarding the mechanism of up-regulation; however, hormones such as prolactin and GnRH can increase the cell membrane concentration of their own receptors.

Theoretically, deactivation of the hormone-receptor complex could be accomplished by dissociation of the complex or loss of receptors from the cell, either by shedding (externally) or by internalization of the receptors into the cell. It is the process of ***internalization*** which is the major biologic mechanism by which polypeptide hormones down-regulate their own receptors and thus limit hormonal activity. As a general rule, an excess concentration of a tropic hormone such as LH or GnRH will stimulate the process of internalization, leading to a loss of receptors in the cell membrane and a decrease in biological response. We now understand that the principal reason for the episodic (pulsatile) secretion of hormones is to avoid down-regulation and to maintain, if not up-regulate, its receptors. The pulse frequency is a key factor, therefore, in regulating receptor number; however further effects on target tissue response also occur at sites distal to receptors.[82]

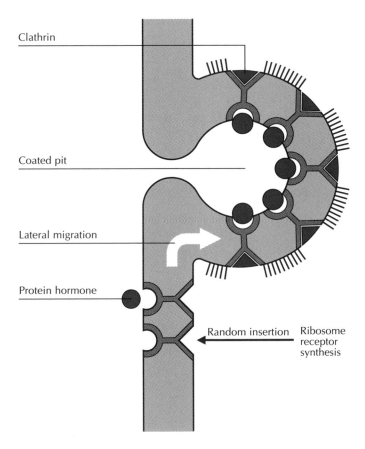

Clathrin

Coated pit

Lateral migration

Protein hormone

Random insertion   Ribosome receptor synthesis

It is believed that receptors are randomly inserted into the cell membrane after intra-cellular synthesis. The receptor may be viewed as having 3 important segments, an external binding site that is specific for a polypeptide hormone, the transmembrane region, and an internal site that plays a role in the process of internalization. When the receptor is bound to a polypeptide hormone and when high concentrations of the hormone are present in the circulation, the hormone-receptor complex moves through the cell membrane in a process called lateral migration. Lateral migration carries the complex to a specialized region of the cell membrane, ***the coated pit.*** Each cell in target tissues contains from 500 to 1,500 coated pits. Lateral migration thus concentrates hormone-receptor complexes in the coated pit (***clustering***), allowing increased internal-ization of the complex via the special mechanism of receptor-mediated endocytosis.[83] The time course for this process (minutes rather than seconds) is too slow to explain the immediate hormone-induced responses, but other cellular events may be mediated by this mechanism which circumvents the intracellular messenger, cyclic AMP.

The coated pit is a lipid vesicle hanging on a basket of specific proteins, called ***clathrins*** (from the Latin "clathra" meaning "lattice"). The unit is a network of hexagons and pentagons, thus looking like a soccer ball. The internal margin of the pit has a brush border, hence the name coated pit. The clathrin protein network serves to localize the hormone-receptor complexes by binding to the internal binding site on the receptor.

Clathrin protein network

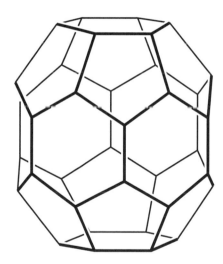

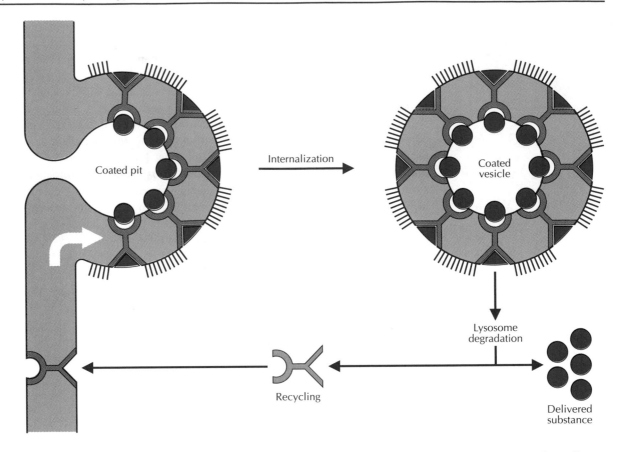

When fully occupied, the coated pit invaginates, pinches off, and enters the cell as a coated vesicle also called a receptosome. The coated vesicle is delivered to the lysosomes where the structure then undergoes degradation, releasing the substance (e.g., a polypeptide hormone) and the receptor. The receptor may be recycled; i.e., it may be reinserted into the cell membrane and used again. On the other hand, the receptor and the hormone may be metabolized, thus decreasing that hormone's biologic activity. The internalized hormones may also mediate biologic response by influencing cellular organelles such as the Golgi apparatus, the endoplasmic reticulum, and even the nucleus. For example, nuclear membranes from human ovaries bind HCG and LH and there follows an enzyme response that is involved in the transfer of mRNA from nucleus to the cytoplasm.[84]

Besides down-regulation of polypeptide hormone receptors, the process of internalization can be utilized for other cellular metabolic events, including the transfer into the cell of vital substances such as iron or vitamins. Hence, cell membrane receptors can be separated into 2 classes.[85]

The Class I receptors are randomly distributed in the cell membrane and transmit information to modify cell behavior. For these receptors, internalization is a method for down-regulation by degradation in lysosomes. Because of this degradation, recycling is usually not a feature of this class of receptors. Hormones that utilize this category of receptors include FSH, LH, HCG, GnRH, TSH, TRH, and insulin. For these hormones, the coated pit can be viewed as a trap to immobilize hormone-receptor complexes. The fate of the hormone, however, can vary from tissue to tissue. In some target tissues, HCG is internalized and the HCG-receptor complex is transferred intact from the coated vesicle into the lysosomes for dissociation and degradation. In other tissues, especially the placenta, it is thought that the HCG-receptor complex is recycled back to the cell surface as a means of transporting HCG across the placenta into both maternal and fetal circulations.[86]

The Class II receptors are located in the coated pits, and binding leads to internalization (thus providing the cell with required factors), the removal of noxious agents from the biologic fluid bathing the cell, or the transfer of substances through the cell (transendocytosis). These receptors are spared from degradation and can be recycled. Examples of this category include low-density lipoproteins (LDL) which supply cholesterol to steroid-producing cells, cobalamin and transferrin, which supply vitamin B_{12} and iron, respectively, and the transfer of immunoglobulins across the placenta to provide fetal immunity.

A closer look at LDL and its receptor is informative. The low-density lipoprotein particle is a sphere. It contains in its center about 1,500 molecules of cholesterol which are attached as esters to fatty acids. This core is contained by a bilayer lipid membrane. Protein binding proteins (the apoproteins) project on the surface of this membrane, and it is these proteins that the receptor must recognize.

Remember, this is an important story, because all cells that produce steroids must use cholesterol as the basic building block. Such cells do not contain and cannot synthesize enough cholesterol and therefore must bring cholesterol into the cell from the bloodstream. LDL is the principal messenger delivering the cholesterol. Experimental evidence, however, indicates that HDL-cholesterol as well as LDL can provide cholesterol to steroid producing cells.[87]

Different cell surface receptors and proteins contain similar structural parts.[88] For example, the receptor for LDL contains a region that is homologous to the precursor of epidermal growth factor and another region that is homologous to a component of complement. The LDL receptor is a "mosaic protein." There are regions of proteins derived from the exons of different gene families. This is an example of a protein that evolved as a new combination of pre-existing functional units of other proteins.

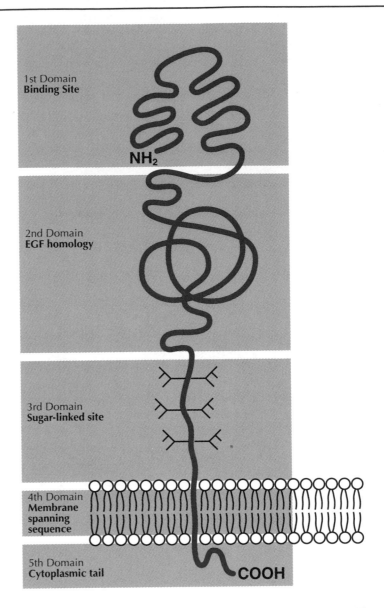

The LDL receptor is synthesized as a precursor of 860 amino acids. The precursor includes 22 amino acids which constitute a hydrophobic signal sequence that is cleaved prior to its insertion into the cell surface. This signal sequence presumably directs the protein where to go in the cell. This leaves an 839 amino acid protein that has 5 recognizable domains.

1. NH_2-terminal of 292 amino acids, composed of a sequence of 40 amino acids repeated with some variation some 7 times. This domain is the binding site for LDL and is located on the external surface of the cell membrane.

2. Approximately 400 amino acids homologous to epidermal growth factor precursor.

3. The sugar-linked site.

4. 22 Hydrophobic amino acids that cross the cell membrane. Deletion of the transmembrane signal sequence (found in a naturally occurring mutation) results in an LDL receptor that is secreted from the cell instead of being inserted into the membrane.

5. Cytoplasmic tail of 50 amino acids that is located internally and serves to cluster LDL receptors in coated pits.

When the coated pit is fully occupied with LDL, a coated vesicle is delivered into the cell in the process called endocytosis. The vesicle moves to the Golgi system and then is routed by an unknown mechanism (although a similar coated pit system in the Golgi appears to be involved) to the lysosomes where the structure undergoes degradation, releasing cholesterol esters and the receptor. The receptor may be recycled or degraded. The intracellular level of free cholesterol influences the following important activities: the rate-limiting enzyme for cholesterol synthesis, the reesterification of excess cholesterol for storage as lipid droplets, and the synthesis of LDL receptors. The cholesterol derived from the LDL transport process can have any one of the following fates: utilization in the mitochondria for steroidogenesis, reesterification for storage, use in membrane structures, or excretion (by the HDL mechanism).[89]

Synthesis and insertion of new LDL receptors are a function of LH in the gonads and ACTH in the adrenal. This process is relatively fast. It has been calculated that the coated pit system turns over an amount of cell surface equivalent to the total amount of plasma membrane every 30–90 minutes.[89] The LDL receptor makes one round trip every 10 minutes during its 20-hour lifespan for a total of several hundred trips.[1] A genetic defect in receptors for LDL can lead to a failure in internalization and hyperlipidemia.

Autoantibodies to membrane receptors can compete with a hormone for binding to the receptor and result in specific diseases, e.g., myasthenia gravis with antibodies to acetylcholine receptors, Graves' disease with antibodies to TSH receptors, and asthma with antibodies to adrenergic receptors.

Regulation of Adenylate Cyclase

The biologic activity of polypeptide or glycoprotein hormones (such as FSH or LH) can be altered by the heterogeneity of the molecules, up- and down-regulation of the receptors, and, finally, by modulation of the activity of the enzyme, adenylate cyclase.

The G Protein System

Adenylate cyclase is composed of 3 protein units: the receptor, a guanyl nucleotide regulatory unit, and a catalytic unit.[90] The regulatory unit is a coupling protein, regulated by guanine nucleotides (specifically GTP), and therefore it is called GTP binding protein or G protein for short.[91] The catalytic unit is the enzyme itself which converts ATP to cyclic AMP. The receptor and the nucleotide regulatory unit are structurally linked, but inactive until the hormone binds to the receptor. Upon binding, the complex of hormone, receptor, and nucleotide regulatory unit is activated leading to an uptake of guanosine 5'-triphosphate (GTP) by the regulatory unit. The activation and uptake of GTP result in an active enzyme which can convert ATP to cyclic AMP. This result can be viewed as the outcome of the regulatory unit *coupling* with the catalytic unit, forming an intact complete enzyme. Enzyme activity is then terminated by hydrolysis of the GTP to guanosine 5'-diphosphate (GDP) returning the enzyme to its inactive state. Quick action and acute control of adenylate cyclase are assured because the G protein is a GTPase that self activates upon binding of GTP.

The G protein has been purified. From the amino acid sequence, complementary DNA clones have been produced. These studies have indicated that a family of G proteins exists that couples receptors to active proteins, playing roles in signal transduction, intracellular transport, and exocytosis. The ability of the hormone-receptor complex to work through a common messenger (cyclic AMP) and produce contrasting actions (stimulation and inhibition) is thought to be due to the presence of both stimulatory nucleotide regulatory G proteins and inhibitory nucleotide regulatory G proteins.[92]

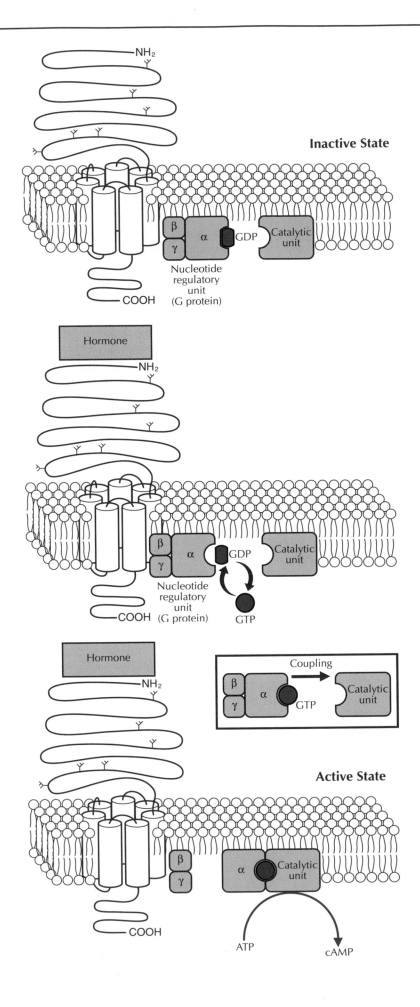

Inactive State

Hormone

Active State

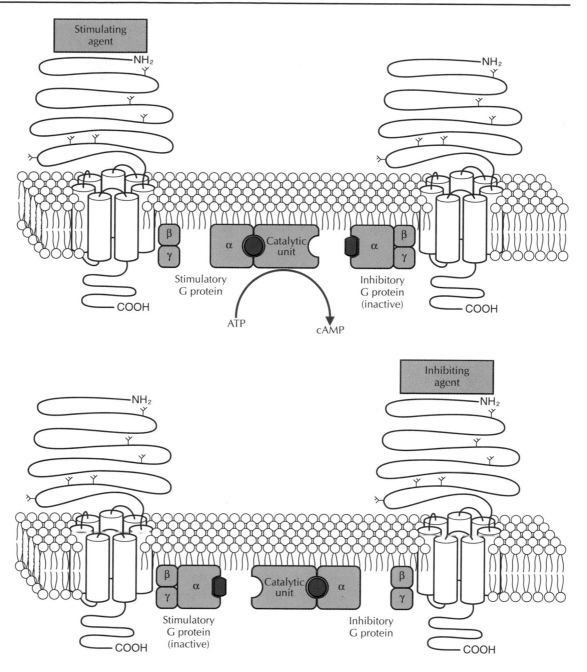

Thus, stimulating agents bind to their receptors and interact with G$_{\text{stimulatory}}$ protein while inhibiting agents interact with G$_{\text{inhibitory}}$ protein that prohibits cyclic AMP synthesis.

The G proteins are composed of α-, β-, and γ-subunits, each the product of a distinct gene. The β- and γ-subunits are similar, but each G protein has an unique α-subunit. In the inactive state GDP is bound to the α-subunit. Hormone-receptor interaction and binding changes the α-subunit conformation. GTP replaces GDP on the α-subunit, freeing the β- and γ-subunits which allows the GTP-α-subunit to bind to the catalytic unit of adenylate cyclase, forming the active enzyme. The GTP-α-subunit can also activate other messengers, such as ion channels. Intrinsic GTPase activity quickly hydrolyzes the GTP-α to GDP-α, which leads to reassociation with the β- and γ-subunits, reforming the G protein complex for further activation. The functional specificity is due to the α-subunit which differs for each G protein, and therefore there are many different α-subunits encoded by different genes.

Another potential mechanism for influencing target tissue response is the regulation of the G protein subunits.[93] Diversity in G protein activity is accomplished by multiple forms with different subunits encoded by different genes and by alterations due to variations in exon splicing.

Mutations that alter the structure and activity of G proteins can result in disease. A subset of growth hormone-secreting pituitary tumors has been identified with mutations (forming an oncogene) in the G protein α-subunit. The McCune-Albright syndrome (sexual precocity, polyostotic fibrous dysplasia, cafe-au-lait skin pigmentation, and autonomous functioning of various endocrine glands) can be explained by unregulated activity of the adenylate cyclase system. G protein mutations have been identified in tissues from patients with this syndrome.[91] G protein mutations have also been found in some, but not most, adrenal and ovarian tumors. It is possible that alterations in G protein function may ultimately explain abnormalities in endocrine-metabolic functions, as well as oncogenic mutations.[92,93]

The G Protein Receptors

The receptors linked to G proteins are derived from a supergene family, presumably originating from a common ancestral gene. These receptors consist of a single polypeptide chain composed of alternating stretches of hydrophobic and hydrophilic amino acids. This structure allows the prediction of 7 transmembrane stretches with the amino terminus located extracellularly and the carboxy terminus intracellularly.[94]

The gonadotropin receptor contains a transmembrane region that has the structural features of a receptor that couples with G protein and a large extracellular domain.[95] Receptors that utilize the G proteins are inserted in membranes and consist of a long polypeptide chain that folds into seven helixes, the amino acid loops that connect the helixes extend either into the cytoplasm or into the extracellular space. The amino end extends outside the cell, and the carboxy end extends into the cell. The large extracellular segment is the site for specific gonadotropin recognition and binding. Binding changes the conformation (which is associated with phosphorylation), leading to interaction with the G proteins which in turn activate second messengers, either enzymes or ion channels.[96] These are ancient proteins; e.g., they are used by yeast to detect mating pheromones (perhaps this is why this protein is the basic structure for sight and smell in higher organisms; rhodopsin is a G protein located in the light-sensitive rod of the retina). Thus, the G receptors can be activated by hormones, neurotransmitters, odorants, and photons of light.

LH and HCG bind to a common receptor, encoded by a gene on chromosome 2. The LH/HCG receptor is highly conserved in mammals; the human receptor is very similar to that of rat and bovine receptors.[97] In the rat model, FSH, LH, and prolactin stimulate LH receptor formation, while EGF, FGF, and GnRH have an inhibitory action.[98] It is likely that expression of the LH/HCG receptor is regulated by many factors, including endocrine, paracrine, and autocrine mechanisms.

The receptor for FSH is very similar to the LH/HCG receptor, but it is structurally distinct.[99] Appropriately (for specificity) the extracellular segment contains the major sequence divergence. The FSH receptor is also regulated by its hormone environment, especially by FSH and estradiol. Other members of this family include receptors for TSH, catecholamines, vasopressin, angiotensin II, and dopamine.

This receptor complex can be the site of abnormal function. Cholera toxin is an enzyme that alters the G protein so that it no longer hydrolyzes its bound GTP. Once activated by a hormone-receptor complex, it remains irreversibly turned on, and in the gastrointestinal tract this turn on of cyclic AMP results in massive efflux of sodium and water into the gut. A genetic deficiency of the coupling protein has been reported to be responsible for the manifestations of at least certain types of pseudohypoparathyroidism. Finally, some manifestations of abnormal thyroid function are due to the ability of thyroid hormone to alter receptor coupling.

Coupling and Uncoupling

Another way to explain stimulating and inhibiting actions at the adenylate cyclase level focuses on the mechanism of coupling. LH stimulates steroidogenesis in the corpus luteum and works through the coupling of stimulatory regulatory units to the catalytic units of adenylate cyclase. Prostaglandin $F_{2\alpha}$ is directly luteolytic, inhibiting luteal steroidogenesis through a mechanism which follows binding to specific receptors. This luteolytic action may be exerted via an inhibitory regulatory unit which leads to uncoupling with the catalytic unit, thus interfering with gonadotropin action.

Desensitization

Increasing concentrations of tropic hormones, such as gonadotropins, are directly associated with desensitization of adenylate cyclase independently of the internalization of receptors. Desensitization is a rapid, acute change without loss of receptors in contrast to the slower process of internalization and true receptor loss. The desensitization process after prolonged agonist exposure involves receptor phosphorylation (which uncouples the receptor from the G protein).[100] The LH/HCG receptor, a member of the G protein family, undergoes desensitization/uncoupling in response to LH or HCG in a process that involves phosphorylation of the C-terminal cytoplasmic tail of the receptor.[101]

Summary of Down-Regulation

Down-regulation is a decrease in response in the presence of continuous stimulation. It involves the following 3 mechanisms:

1. Loss of receptors by internalization.

2. Densensitization by autophosphorylation of the cytoplasmic segment of the receptor.

3. Uncoupling of the regulatory and catalytic subunits of the adenylate cyclase enzyme.

Agonists and Antagonists

An agonist is a substance that stimulates a response. An antagonist completely inhibits the actions of an agonist. Agonistic activity follows receptor binding which leads to stimulation of the message associated with that receptor. Antagonistic activity follows receptor binding and is characterized by blockage of the receptor message or nontransmission of the message. Most compounds used in this fashion that bind to hormone nuclear receptors have a mix of agonist and antagonist responses, depending upon the tissue and hormonal milieu. Examples of antagonists include tamoxifen, RU486, and the histamine receptor antagonists.

Short Acting Antagonists

Short-acting antagonists such as estriol are actually a mixed combination of agonism and antagonism depending upon time. Short-term estrogen responses can be elicited because estriol binds to the nuclear receptor, but long-term responses do not occur because this binding is short-lived. Antagonism results when estriol competes with estradiol for receptors. However, if a constant presence of the weak hormone, estriol, can be maintained, then long-term occupation is possible, and a potent estrogen response can be produced.

Long-Acting Antagonists

Clomiphene and tamoxifen are mixed agonists and antagonists. The endometrium is very sensitive to the agonistic response, while the breast is more sensitive to the antagonistic behavior. The antagonistic action is the result of nuclear receptor binding with an alteration in the normal receptor-DNA processing and a failure to replenish hormone receptors resulting in eventual depletion.

Alteration of the GnRH molecule has produced both agonists and antagonists. GnRH is a decapeptide; antagonists have substitutions at multiple positions, while agonists have substitutions at the 6 or 10 positions. The GnRH agonist molecules first stimulate the pituitary gland to secrete gonadotropins, then because of the constant stimulation, down-regulation and desensitization of the cell membrane receptors occur, and gonadotropin secretion is literally turned off. The antagonist molecules bind to the cell membrane receptor and fail to transmit a message and thus are competitive inhibitors. Various GnRH agonists are used to treat endometriosis, uterine leiomyomas, precocious puberty, cancer of the prostate gland, ovarian hyperandrogenism, and the premenstrual syndrome.

Physiologic Antagonists

Strictly speaking, a progestin is not an estrogen antagonist. It modifies estrogen action by causing a depletion of estrogen receptors.[102] There is also evidence that a progestin can inhibit transcription activation by the estrogen receptor.[103] In addition progestins induce enzyme activity that converts the potent estradiol to the impotent estrone sulfate which is then secreted from the cell.[104] Androgens do block the actions of estrogen, but the mechanism is not entirely clear. Rather than a direct impact on estrogen receptor levels, the action is directed to gene activity subsequent to estrogen-receptor binding.[30] High levels of androgen can produce estrogen and progestational effects by binding to the estrogen and progesterone receptors.

The Antiestrogen: Tamoxifen

Tamoxifen is very similar to clomiphene (in structure and actions), both being nonsteroidal compounds structurally related to diethylstilbestrol. Tamoxifen, in binding to the estrogen receptor, competitively inhibits estrogen binding. In vitro, the estrogen binding affinity for its receptor is 100–1,000 times greater than that of tamoxifen. Thus, tamoxifen must be present in a concentration 100–1,000 times greater than estrogen to maintain inhibition of breast cancer cells.[105] In vitro studies demonstrate that this action is not cytocidal, but rather cytostatic (and thus its use must be long-term). The tamoxifen-estrogen receptor complex binds to DNA, but whether an agonistic, estrogenic message occurs because of gene transcription is probably determined by what promoter elements are present in specific cell types.

Tamoxifen also has actions not mediated by the estrogen receptor. It binds to calmodulin, microsomal binding sites, and stimulates certain enzymes. Thus, tamoxifen disrupts calcium transport across membranes and also modulates immunoregulatory mechanisms.

There have been many clinical trials with the adjuvant treatment of breast cancer with tamoxifen, and many are still on-going.[106] Overall the impact on breast cancer can be summarized as follows: disease-free survival is prolonged. There is an increased survival at 5 years of approximately 20%, most evident in women over age 50. Response rates in advanced breast cancer are 30–35%, most marked in patients with tumors that are positive for estrogen receptors, reaching 75% in tumors highly positive for estrogen receptors.

Serum protein changes reflect the estrogenic (agonistic) action of tamoxifen. This includes decreases in antithrombin III, cholesterol, and LDL-cholesterol, while HDL-cholesterol and sex hormone binding globulin (SHBG) levels increase (as do other binding globulins). The estrogenic activity of tamoxifen, 20 mg daily, is nearly as potent as 2 mg estradiol in lowering FSH levels in postmenopausal women, 26% vs. 34% with estradiol.[107] The estrogenic actions of tamoxifen include the stimulation of progesterone receptor synthesis, an estrogen-like maintenance of bone, and estrogenic effects on the vaginal mucosa and the endometrium. Tamoxifen increases the frequency of hepatic carcinoma in rats at very large doses. This is consistent with its estrogenic, agonistic action, but this effect is unlikely to be a clinical problem (and it has not been observed) at doses currently used. There has been concern that tamoxifen might be associated with thrombotic events; however, the decrease in antithrombin III observed with tamoxifen is still within the normal range, and the clinical trials have indicated no significant increase in thrombotic events.

All too often the antagonistic, antiestrogenic action of tamoxifen is featured, and the estrogenic, agonistic action is ignored. In the 1980s, it was reported that human endometrial cancer transplanted into mice would grow more rapidly during tamoxifen therapy, although the growth of breast cancer cells would be inhibited. This growth in response to tamoxifen can be duplicated in laboratory culture preparations of endometrial cancer cells.

There now have been many reports of endometrial hyperplasia, endometrial polyps, and endometrial cancer occurring in women receiving tamoxifen treatment.[108] In addition, tamoxifen has been associated with major flare-ups in endometriosis. The development of endometrial cancer in women receiving tamoxifen should not be so surprising. We know that duration of exposure to estrogen is more important than the dose of estrogen in influencing progression from proliferative endometrium through hyperplasia to cancer. It is logical to expect a tissue (endometrium) highly sensitive to estrogen to respond to the estrogenic, agonistic action of tamoxifen. Appropriate clinical surveillance of this effect is very important.

The menopause commonly brings women to clinicians for consultation and advice. With increasing success, we are impressing upon our patients and our colleagues the importance of cardiovascular disease and osteoporosis during the postmenopausal years. Prevention of these two conditions is an important part of preventive health care for older women. The interaction of tamoxifen with the risks for osteoporosis and cardiovascular disease is an important issue. Thus far, studies indicate that the estrogenic, agonistic actions of tamoxifen influence the cholesterol profile and bone density.[109,110] Tamoxifen is associated with an estrogen-like decrease in total cholesterol and LDL-cholesterol, with an increase in triglycerides and HDL-cholesterol (although some studies do not find a significant impact on HDL). Patients can be reassured that the antagonistic actions of tamoxifen do not prevail in regard to osteoporosis and cardiovascular disease. Whether the agonistic effect protects against clinical events and how it compares to the benefits of hormone therapy will require future epidemiologic studies.

The Antiprogestin: RU486   Both progesterone and RU486 form hormone responsive element-receptor complexes that are similar, but the RU486 complex has a slightly different conformational change (in the hormone binding domain) that prevents full gene activation.[111,112] The agonistic activity of this progestin antagonist is due to its ability to activate certain, but not all, of the transcription activation functions on the progesterone receptor. New antiprogestins are in development which bind to the progesterone receptor and prevent the subsequent binding of the receptor to gene response elements.

The search for inhibitors of progesterone binding began over 20 years ago, in the late 1960s, but it wasn't until the early 1980s that RU486, the first successful antiprogestin was produced by scientists at Roussel Uclaf, a pharmaceutical company in Paris. RU486 (the generic name is mifepristone) is a 19 nortestosterone derivative. The dimethyl (dimethylaminophenyl) side chain at carbon 11 is the principal factor in its anti-progesterone action. There are three major characteristics of its action which are important: a long half-life, high affinity for the progesterone receptor, and active metabolites.

The affinity of RU486 for the progesterone receptor is 5 times greater than that of the natural hormone. In the absence of progesterone, it can produce an agonistic (progesterone) effect. It does not bind to the estrogen receptor, but it can act as a weak antiandrogen because of its low affinity binding to the androgen receptor. RU486 also binds to the glucocorticoid receptor, but higher doses are required to produce effects. The binding affinity of RU486 and its metabolites for the glucocorticoid receptor is very, very high. The reason why it takes such a high dose to produce an effect is because the circulating level of cortisol is so high, 1,000-fold higher than progesterone. This allows titration of clinical effects by adjustments of dose.

RU486 is most noted for its abortifacient activity and the political controversy surrounding it. However, the combination of its agonistic and antagonistic actions can be exploited for many uses, including contraception, therapy of endometriosis, induction of labor, treatment of Cushing's syndrome, and, potentially, treatment of various cancers.

References

1. **Brown MS, Goldstein JL,** A receptor-mediated pathway for cholesterol homeostasis, Science 232:34, 1986.

2. **Miller WL**, Molecular biology of steroid hormone synthesis, Endocr Rev 9:295, 1988.

3. **Simpson E, Lauber M, Demeter M, Means G, Mahendroo M, Kilgore M, Mendelson C, Waterman M,** Regulation of expression of the genes encoding steroidogenic enzymes in the ovary, J Steroid Biochem Mol Biol 41:409, 1992.

4. **Iveson TJ, Smith IE, Ahern J, Smithers DA, Trunet PF, Dowsett M,** Phase I study of the oral non-steroidal aromatase inhibtor CGS 20267 in postmenopausal patients with advanced breast cancer, Cancer Res 53:266, 1993.

5. **Erickson GF,** An analysis of follicle development and ovum maturation, Seminars Reprod Endocrinol 4:233, 1986.

6. **Magoffin DA,** Regulation of differentiated functions in ovarian theca cells, Seminars Reprod Endocrinol 9:321, 1991.

7. **Tilly JL LaPolt PS, Hsueh AJ,** Hormonal regulation of follicle-stimulating hormone receptor messenger ribonucleic acid levels in cultured rat granulosa cells, Endocrinology 130:1296, 1992.

8. **LaPolt PS, Tilly JL, Aihara T, Nishimori K, Hsueh AJ,** Gonadotropin-induced up- and down-regulation of ovarian follicle-stimulating hormone (FSH) receptor gene expression in immature rats: effects of pregnant mare's serum gonadotropin, human chorionic gonadotropin, and recombinant FSH, Endocrinology 130:1289, 1992.

9. **Mendel CM,** The free hormone hypothesis: a physiologically based mathematical model, Endocrin Rev 10:232, 1989.

10. **Vermeulen A,** Physiology of the testosterone-binding globulin in man, Ann NY Acad Sci 538:103, 1988.

11. **Preziosi P, Barrett-Connor E, Papoz L, Roger M, Saint-Paul M, Nahoul K, Simon D,** Interrelation between plasma sex hormone-binding globulin and plasma insulin in healthy adult women: the Telecom Study, J Clin Endocrinol Metab 76:283, 1993.

12. **Lindstedt G, Lundberg P-A, Lapidus L, Lundgren H, Bengtsson C, Bjorntorp P,** Low sex hormone-binding globulin concentration as independent risk factor for development of NIDDM. 12-year follow-up of population study of women in Gothenburg, Sweden, Diabetes 40:123, 1991.

13. **Berube D, Seralini GE, Gagne R, Hammond GL,** Localization of the human sex hormone-binding globulin gene (SHBG) to the short arm of chromosome 17 (17p12-13), Cytogenet Cell Genet 54:65, 1990.

14. **Rosner W,** The functions of corticosteroid-binding globulin and sex hormone-binding globulin: recent advances, Endocr Rev 11:80, 1990.

15. **Kirschner MA, Samojlik E, Drejka M, Szmal E, Schneider G, Ertel N,** Androgen-estrogen metabolism in women with upper body versus lower body obesity, J Clin Endocrinol Metab 70:473, 1990.

16. **Siiteri PK, MacDonald PC,** Role of extraglandular estrogen in human endocrinology, in Geiger SR, Astwood EB, Greep RO, editors, *Handbook of Physiology, Section 7, Endocrinology,* American Physiological Society, Washington, DC, 1973, pp 615-629.

17. **Silva PD, Gentzschein EEK, Lobo RA,** Androstenedione may be a more important precursor of tissue dihydrotestosterone than testosterone in women, Fertil Steril 48:419, 1987.

18. **Rittmaster R, Thompson D,** Effect of leuprolide and dexamethasone on hair growth in hirsute women, J Clin Endocrinol Metab 70:1096, 1990.

19. **Horton R,** Dihydrotestosterone is a peripheral paracrine hormone, J Androl 13:23, 1992.

20. **Mooradian AD, Morley JE, Korenman SG,** Biological actions of androgens, Endocrin Rev 8:1, 1987.

21. **King RJB,** Structure and function of steroid receptors, J Endocrinol 114:341, 1987.

22. **King WJ, Greene GL,** Monoclonal antibodies localize oestrogen receptor in the nuclei of target cells, Nature 307:745, 1984.

23. **Welshons WV, Lieberman ME, Gorski J,** Nuclear localization of unoccupied oestrogen receptors, Nature 307:747, 1984.

24. **Press MF, Greene GL,** Localization of progesterone receptor with monoclonal antibodies to the human progestin receptor, Endocrinology 122:1165, 1988.

25. **Webb P, Lopez GN, Greene GL, Baxter JD, Kushner PJ,** The limits of the cellular capacity to mediate an estrogen response, Mol Endocrinol 6:157, 1992.

26. **Gerace L,** Molecular trafficking across the nuclear pore complex, Curr Opin Cell Biol 4:637, 1992.

27. **Strobl JS, Kasid A, Huff KK, Lippman ME,** Kinetic alterations in estrogen receptors assocated with estrogen receptor processing in human breast cancer cells, Endocrinology 115:1116, 1984.

28. **Katzenellenbogen BS,** Biology and receptor interactions of estriol and estriol derivatives in vitro and in vivo, J Steroid Biochem 20:1033, 1984.

29. **DeSombre ER, Kuivanen PC,** Progestin modulation of estrogen-dependent marker protein synthesis in the endometrium, Seminars Oncol 12:Suppl 1:6, 1985.

30. **Hung TT, Gibbons WE,** Evaluation of androgen antagonism of estrogen effect by dihydro-testosterone, J Steroid Biochem 19:1513, 1983.

31. **Evans RM,** The steroid and thyroid hormone receptor family, Science 240:889, 1988.

32. **Laudet V, Hanni C, Coll J, Catzeflis F, Stehelin D,** Evolution of the nuclear receptor gene superfamily, EMBO J 11:1003, 1992.

33. **Freedman LP,** Anatomy of the steroid receptor zinc finger region, Endocr Rev 13:129, 1992.

34. **Carson-Jurica MA, Schrader WT, O'Malley BW,** Steroid receptor family: structure and functions, Endocr Rev 11:201, 1990.

35. **O'Malley BW, Tsai M-J,** Molecular pathways of steroid receptor action, Biol Reprod 46:163, 1992.

36. **Beato M,** Gene regulation by steroid hormones, Cell 56:335, 1989.

37. **Nardulli AM, Shapiro DJ,** Binding of the estrogen receptor DNA-binding domain to the estrogen response element induces DNA bending, Mol Cell Biol 12:2037, 1992.

38. **Danielian PS, White R, Lees JA, Parker MG,** Identification of a conserved region required for homone dependent transcriptional activation by steroid hormone receptors, EMBO J 11:1025, 1992.

39. **Meyer M-E, Quirin-Stricker C, Lerouge T, Bocquel M-T, Gronemeyer H**, A limiting factor mediates the differential activation of promoters by the human progesterone receptor isoforms, J Biol Chem 267:10882, 1992.

40. **Orti E, Bodwell JE, Munck A,** Phosphorylation of steroid hormone receptors, Endocr Rev 13:105, 1992.

41. **Allgood VE, Cidlowski JA,** Vitamin B6 modulates transcriptional activation by multiple members of the steroid hormone receptor superfamily, J Biol Chem 267:3819, 1992.

42. **Umesono K, Evans RM,** Determinants of target gene specificity for steroid/thyroid hormone receptors, Cell 57:1139, 1989.

43. **Klinge CM, Bambara RA, Hilf R,** What differentiates antiestrogen-liganded vs estradiol-liganded estrogen receptor action? Oncol Res 4:137, 1992.

44. **Chauchereau A, Savouret J-F, Milgrom E,** Control of biosynthesis and post-transcriptional modification of the progesterone receptor, Biol Reprod 46:174, 1992.

45. **Kastner P, Bocquel M-T, Turcotte B, Garnier J-M, Horwitz KB, Chambon P, Gronemeyer H,** Transient expression of human and chicken progesterone receptors does not support alternative translational initiation from a single mRNA as the mechanism generating two receptor isoforms, J Biol Chem 265:12163, 1990.

46. **Rehberger P, Rexin M, Gehring U,** Heterotetrameric structure of the human progesterone receptor, Proc Natl Acad Sci USA 89:8001, 1992.

47. **Tindall DJ, Chang CH, Lobl TJ, Cunningham, GR,** Androgen antagonists in androgen target tissues, Pharmacol Ther 24:367, 1984.

48. **Jenster G, van der Korput JAGM, Trapman J, Brinkmann AO,** Functional domains of the human androgen receptor, J Steroid Biochem Mol Biol 41:671, 1992.

49. **Jaussi R, Watson G, Paigen K,** Modulation of androgen-responsive gene expression by estrogen, Mol Cell Endocrinol 86:187, 1992.

50. **Lubahn DB, Joseph DR, Sullivan PM, Willard HF, French FS, Wilson EM,** Cloning of human androgen receptor complementary DNA and localization to the X chromosome, Science 240:327, 1988.

51. **Brinkmann AO, Jenster G, Kuiper GGJM, Ris C, van Laar JH, van der Korput JAGM, Degenhart HJ, Trifiro MA, Pinsky L, Romalo G, Schweikert HU, Veldscholte J, Mulder E, Trapman J,** The human androgen receptor: structure/function relationship in normal and pathological situations, J Steroid Biochem Mol Biol 41:361, 1992.

52. **Griffin JE, Wilson JD,** Disorders of androgen receptor function, Ann NY Acad Sci 438:61, 1984.

53. **Taylor SS,** cAMP-dependent protein kinase: model for an enzyme family, J Biol Chem 264:8443, 1989.

54. **Roesler WJ, Vandenbark GR, Hanson RW,** Cyclic AMP and the induction of eukaryotic gene transcription, J Biol Chem 263:9063, 1988.

55. **Currie WD, Li W, Baimbridge KG, Yuen BH, Leung PC,** Cytosolic free calcium increased by prostaglandin F_{2alpha} (PGF_{2alpha}), gonadotropin-releasing hormone, and angiotensin II in rat granulosa cells and PGF_{2alpha} in human granulosa cells, Endocrinology 130:1837, 1992.

56. **Kelly PA, Djiane J, Edery M,** Different forms of the prolactin receptor: insights into the mechanism of prolactin action, Trends Endocrinol Metab 3:54, 1992.

57. **Tse A, Hille B,** GnRH-induced Ca^{2+} oscillations and rhythmic hyperpolarizations of pituitary gonadotropes, Science 255:462, 1992.

58. **Rasmussen H,** The calcium messenger system, New Engl J Med 314:1094,1164, 1986.

59. **Fukuoka M, Yasuda K, Emi N, Fujiwara H, Iwai M, Takakura K, Kanzaki H, Mori T,** Cytokine modulation of progesterone and estradiol secretion in cultures of luteinized human granulosa cells, J Clin Endocrinol Metab 75:254, 1992.

60. **Hill D,** Growth factors and their cellular actions, J Reprod Fertil 85:723, 1989.

61. **Giudice LC,** Insulin-like growth factors and ovarian follicular development, Endocr Rev 13:641, 1992.

62. **Conover CA,** Potentiation of insulin-like growth factor (IGF) action by IGF-binding protein-3: studies of underlying mechanism, Endocrinology 130:3191, 1992.

63. **Beitins IZ, Padmanabhan V,** Bioactive follicle-stimulating hormone, Trends Endocrinol Metab 2:145, 1991.

64. **Wide L, Bakos O,** More basic forms of both follicle-stimulating hormone and luteinzing hormone in serum at midcycle compared with the follicular or luteal phase, J Clin Endocrinol Metab 76:885, 1993.

65. **Kahl KD, Stone MP,** FSH isoforms, radioimmunoassays, bioassays, and their significance, J Androl 13:11, 1992.

66. **Weiss J, Axelrod L, Whitcomb RW, Harris PE, Crowley WF, Jameson JL,** Hypogonadism caused by a single amino acid substitution in the β subunit of luteinizing hormone, New Engl J Med 326:179, 1992.

67. **Huth JR, Mountjoy K, Perini F, Ruddon RW,** Intracellular folding pathway of human chorionic gonadotropin β subunit, J Biol Chem 267:8870, 1992.

68. **Gharib SD, Wierman ME, Shupnik MA, Chin WW,** Molecular biology of the pituitary gonadotropins, Endocr Rev 11:177, 1990.

69. **Jameson JL, Lindell CM,** Isolation and characterization of the human chorionic gonadotropin β subunit (CGβ) gene cluster: regulation of a transcriptionally active CGβ gene by cyclic AMP, Molec Cellular Biol 8:5100, 1988.

70. **Jameson JL, Hollenberg AN,** Regulation of chorionic gonadotropin gene expression, Endocr Rev 14:203, 1993.

71. **Bo M, Boime I,** Identification of the transcriptionally active genes of the chorionic gonadotropin β gene cluster in vivo, J Biol Chem 267:3179, 1992.

72. **Fiddes JC, Talmadge K,** Structure, expression, and evolution of the genes for the human glycoprotein hormones, Recent Prog Horm Res 40:43, 1984.

73. **Dahl KD, Bicsak TA, Hsueh AJW,** Naturally occurring antihormones: secretion of FSH antagonists by women treated with a GnRH analog, Science 239:72, 1988.

74. **Combarnous Y,** Molecular basis of the specificity of binding of glycoprotein hormones to their receptors, Endocrin Rev 13:670, 1992.

75. **Richardson MC, Masson GM, Sairam MR,** Inhibitory action of chemically deglycosylated human chorionic gonadotrophin on hormone-induced steroid production by dispersed cells from human corpus luteum, J Endocrinol 101:327, 1984.

76. **Sairam MR,** Role of carbohydrates in glycoprotein hormone signal transduction, FASEB J 3:1915, 1989.

77. **Galway AB, Hsueh AJ, Keene JL, Yamoto M, Fauser BC, Boime I,** In vitro and in vivo bioactivity of recombinant human follicle-stimulating hormone and partially deglycosylated variants secreted by transfected eukaryotic cell lines, Endocrinology 127:93, 1990.

78. **Hwang J, Menon KMJ,** Spatial relationships of the human chorionic gonadotropin (hCG) subunits in the assembly of the hCG-receptor complex in the luteinized rat ovary, Proc Natl Acad Sci USA 81:4667, 1984.

79. **Merz WE, Dorner M,** Studies on structure-function relationships of human choriogonadotropins with C-terminally shortened alpha subunits. I. Receptor binding and immunologic properties, Biochem Biophys Acta 844:62, 1985.

80. **Sinha YN,** Prolactin variants, Trends Endocrinol Metab 3:100, 1992.

81. **Brue T, Caruso E, Morange I, Hoffmann T, Evrin M, Gunz G, Benkirane M, Jaquet P,** Immunoradiometric analysis of circulating human glycosylated and nonglycosylated prolactin forms: spontaneous and stimulated secretions, J Clin Endocrinol Metab 75:1338, 1992.

82. **Katt JA, Duncan JA, Herbon L, Barkan A, Marshall JC,** The frequency of gonadotropin-releasing hormone stimulation determines the number of pituitary gonadotropin-releasing hormone receptors, Endocrinology 116:2113, 1985.

83. **Goldstein JL, Anderson RGW, Brown MS,** Coated pits, coated vesicles, and receptor-mediated endocytosis, Nature 279:679, 1979.

84. **Toledo A, Ramani N, Rao ChV,** Direct stimulation of nucleoside triphosphatase activity in human ovarian nuclear membranes by human chorionic gonadotropin, J Clin Endocrinol Metab 65:305, 1987.

85. **Kaplan J,** Polypeptide-binding membrane receptors: analysis and classification, Science 212:14, 1981.

86. **Ascoli M,** Lysosomal accumulation of the hormone-receptor complex during receptor-mediated endocytosis of human chorionic gonadotropin, J Cell Biol 99:1242, 1984.

87. **Parinaud J, Perret B, Ribbes H, Chap H, Pontonnier G, Douste-Blazy L,** High density lipoprotein and low density lipoprotein utilization by human granulosa cells for progesterone synthesis in serum-free culture: respective contributions of free and esterified cholesterol, J Clin Endocrinol Metab 64:409, 1987.

88. **Sudhof TC, Goldstein JL, Brown MS, Russell DW,** The LDL receptor gene: a mosaic of exons shared with different proteins, Science 228:815, 1985.

89. **Reinhart MP,** Intracellular sterol trafficking, Experientia 46:599, 1990.

90. **Gilman AG,** Guanine nucleotide-binding regulatory proteins and dual control of adenylate cyclase, J Clin Invest 73:1, 1984.

91. **Spiegel AM, Shenker A, Weinstein LS,** Receptor-effector coupling by G proteins: implications for normal and abnormal signal transduction, Endocr Rev 13:536, 1992.

92. **Birnbaumer L, Abramowitz J, Brown AM,** Receptor-effector coupling by G proteins, Biochem Biophys Acta 1031:163, 1990.

93. **Loganzo F Jr, Fletcher PW,** Follicle-stimulating hormone increases guanine nucleotide-binding regulatory protein subunit a_{i-3} mRNA but decreases a_{i-1} and a_{i-2} mRNA in Sertoli cells, Molec Endocrinol 6:1259, 1992.

94. **Dohlman HG, Thorner J, Caron MG, Lefkowitz RJ,** Model systems for the study of seven-transmembrane-segment receptors, Ann Rev Biochem 60:653, 1991.

95. **Segaloff DL, Ascoli M,** The lutropin/choriogonadotropin receptor. . .4 years later, Endocr Rev 14:324, 1993.

96. **Freissmuth M, Casey PJ, Gilman AG,** G proteins control diverse pathways of transmembrane signalling, FASEB J 3:2125, 1989.

97. **Alpaugh K, Indrapichate K, Abel JA, Rimerman R, Wimalasena J,** Purification and characterization of the human ovarian LH/hCG receptor and comparison of the properties of mammalian LH/hCG receptors, Biochem Pharmacol 40:2093, 1990.

98. **Piquette GN, LaPolt PS, Oikawa M, Hsueh AJ,** Regulation of luteinizing hormone receptor messenger ribonucleic acid levels by gonadotropins, growth factors, and gonadotropin-releasing hormone in cultured granulosa cells, Endocrinology 128:2449, 1991.

99. **Minegishi T, Nakamura K, Takakura Y, Ibuki Y, Igarashi M,** Cloning and sequencing of human FSH receptor cDNA, Biochem Biophys Res Commun 175:1125, 1991.

100. **Sibley DR, Benovic JL, Caron MG, Lefkowitz RJ,** Phosphorylation of cell surface receptors: a mechanism for regulating signal transduction pathways, Endocr Rev 9:38, 1988.

101. **Sanchez-Yague J, Rodriguez MC, Segaloff DL, Ascoli M,** Truncation of the cytoplasmic tail of the lutropin/choriogonadotropin receptor prevents agonist-induced uncoupling, J Biol Chem 267:7217, 1992.

102. **Leavitt WW, MacDonald RC, Okulicz WC,** Hormonal regulation of estrogen and progesterone receptor systems, Biochem Actions Horm 10:323, 1983.

103. **Kirkland JL, Murthy L, Stancel GM,** Progesterone inhibits the estrogen-induced expression of *c-fos* messenger ribonucleic acid in the uterus, Endocrinology 130:3223, 1992.

104. **Tseng L, Lui HC,** Stimulation of arylsulfotransferase activity by progestins in human endometrium in vitro, J Clin Endocrinol Metab 53:418, 1981.

105. **Jordan VC, Murphy CS,** Endocrine pharmacology of antiestrogens as antitumor agents, Endocr Rev 11:578, 1990.

106. **Early Breast Cancer Trialists' Collaborative Group,** Systemic treatment of early breast cancer by hormonal, cytotoxic, or immune therapy, Lancet 339:1,71, 1992.

107. **Helgason S, Wilking N, Carlstrom K, Damber MG, von Schoultz B,** A comparative study of the estrogenic effects of tamoxifen and 17β-estradiol in postmenopausal women, J Clin Endocrinol Metab 54:404, 1982.

108. **De Muylder X, Neven P, DeSome M, Van Belle Y, Vandearick G, De Muylder E,** Endometrial lesions in patients undergoing tamoxifen therapy, Int J Gynecol Obstet 36:127, 1991.

109. **Bagdade JD, Wolter J, Subbaiah PV, Ryan W,** Effects of tamoxifen treatment on plasma lipids and lipoprotein composition, J Clin Endocrinol Metab 70:1132, 1990.

110. **Love RR, Mazess RB, Barden HS, Epstein S, Newcomb PA, Jordan VC, Carbone PP, DeMets DL,** Effects of tamoxifen on bone mineral density in postmenopausal women with breast cancer, New Engl J Med 326:852, 1992.

111. **Spitz IM, Bardin CW,** Clinical pharmacology of RU 486 — an antiprogestin and anti-glucocorticoid, Contraception 48:403, 1993.

112. **Gronemeyer H, Benhamous B, Berry M, Bocquel MT, Gofflo D, Garcia T, Lerouge T, Metzger D, Meyer ME, Tora L, Vergezac A, Chambon P,** Mechanisms of antihormone action, J Steroid Biochem Mol Biol 41:217, 1992.

3 The Ovary — Embryology and Development

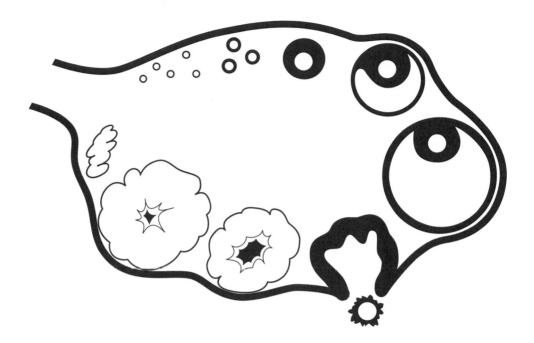

The great names of early medicine were Hippocrates, Soranus, and Galen. Although Aristotle (384–322 B.C.) referred to castration as a common agricultural practice, it was Soranus who provided the first anatomical description of the ovaries. Soranus of Ephesus (a Roman city on the coast of what is now Turkey) lived from 98 to 138 A.D. and has often been referred to as the greatest gynecologist of antiquity.[1] He studied in Alexandria and practiced in Rome. His great text was lost for centuries and was not published until 1838.

Galen was born in 130 A.D. in Pergamum, a Greek city in eastern Turkey, studied in Alexandria and became a famous practitioner and teacher of medicine in Rome. He lived 70 years and wrote about 400 treatises, 83 of which are still in existence. Galen preserved in his own writings (in Greek) Aristotle's descriptions of reproduction. He was a true scholar and was regarded as the ultimate authority on anatomy and physiology until the sixteenth century.[2] It was Galen who established bleeding as the appropriate treatment for almost every disorder. Although in retrospect Galen's conclusions and teachings contained many errors, how many other individuals have been able to satisfy the needs of scholars and physicians for hundreds of years?

After Galen, no further thoughts or advances were recorded for well over 1,000 years as the dark weight of the medieval ages descended upon Western civilization. During the medieval years, it was safe to copy Galen's works but literally dangerous to contribute anything original. Medieval scholars believed it was impossible to progress in knowledge beyond Galen. The doctrine according to Galen was not challenged until the introduction of printing made Galen's works available to scholars.

Although Leonardo da Vinci (1452–1519) drew accurately the anatomy of the uterus and the ovaries, the major advances in anatomical knowledge can be traced to the University of Padua, the famed Italian university where a succession of anatomists made important contributions.[3] It was Andreas Vesalius (1514–1564), who while still in his 20s, because of his own human dissections, realized that Galen described only animals. Appointed Professor of Surgery and Anatomy at the University of Padua at the age of 23, he published *The Fabric of the Human Body,* his authoritative, illustrated book on human anatomy, in 1543, at the age of 29. Vesalius was harshly attacked by the medical establishment, and one year after the publication of his book, he left Padua to become the court physician in Spain.

Vesalius was the first to describe ovarian follicles and probably the corpus luteum. Fallopius (1534–1562), remembered for his description of the fallopian tubes, was a pupil of Vesalius, and then a successful and popular teacher of anatomy at Padua. Fabricius (Girolamo Fabrici d'Acquapendente, 1533–1619), a pupil of Fallopius, succeeded Fallopius as chair of anatomy at Padua and made major contributions to embryology. During this period of time, the ovaries came to be recognized as structures, but their function remained a mystery.

William Harvey published the first original English book on reproductive anatomy and physiology in 1651, at the age of 69, 35 years after his discovery of the circulation of blood. He obtained his medical education at the University of Padua where he learned to describe accurately his own observations, a practice he was to continue and which culminated in his writings. Unfortunately, Harvey promoted and maintained the Aristotelian belief that the egg was a product of conception. This view was corrected by Bishop Niels Stensen of Denmark in 1667, and in 1672, at the age of 31, Reinier de Graaf published his great work on the female reproductive organs, *De Mulierum Organis.*

Ovarian follicles had been described by Vesalius and Fallopius, but the impact of his publication earned de Graaf eternal recognition as the ovarian follicle became known as the Graafian follicle, even though de Graaf believed that the whole follicle was the egg. de Graaf, however, was the first to accurately describe the corpus luteum. Malpighi, whose works were published posthumously in 1697, invented the name "corpus luteum."

With the discovery of mammalian spermatozoa by van Lecuwenhoek in 1677, it became possible to speculate that fertilization resulted from the combination of a spermatozoon and the Graafian follicle. It would be another 150 years before it was appreciated that the oocyte resides within the follicle, and that there is a relationship between the ovaries and menstruation. The process of fertilization was described by Newport in 1853–54, bringing to a close the era of descriptive anatomy of the ovary and marking the beginning of scientific explorations into physiology and endocrinology.

The Human Ovary

The physiologic responsibilities of the ovary are the periodic release of gametes (eggs) (oocytes) and the production of the steroid hormones, estradiol and progesterone. Both activities are integrated in the continuous repetitive process of follicle maturation, ovulation, and corpus luteum formation and regression. The ovary, therefore, cannot be viewed as a relatively static endocrine organ whose size and function expand and contract depending on the vigor of stimulating tropic hormones. Rather, the female gonad is a heterogeneous ever-changing tissue whose cyclicity is measured in weeks, rather than hours.

The ovary consists of three major portions, the outer cortex, the central medulla, and the rete ovarii (the hilum). The hilum is the point of attachment of the ovary to the mesovarium. It contains nerves and blood vessels, and hilus cells which have the potential to become active in steroidogenesis or to form tumors. These cells are very similar to the testosterone producing Leydig cells of the testes. The outermost portion of the cortex is called the tunica albuginea, topped on its surface by a single layer of cuboidal epithelium, the germinal epithelium. The oocytes, enclosed in complexes called follicles, are in the inner part of the cortex, embedded in stromal tissue. The stromal tissue is composed of connective tissue and interstitial cells which are derived from mesenchymal cells, and have the ability to respond to luteinizing hormone (LH) or human chorionic gonadotropin (HCG) with androgen production. The central medullary area of the ovary is derived largely from mesonephric cells.

The Fetal Ovary

During fetal life, the development of the human ovary can be traced through four stages.[4] These are 1) the indifferent gonad stage, 2) the stage of differentiation, 3) the period of oogonal multiplication and maturation, and finally 4) the stage of follicle formation.

The Indifferent Gonad Stage

At approximately 5 weeks of gestation, the paired gonads are structurally consolidated coelomic prominences overlying the mesonephros, forming the gonadal ridges. At this point, the gonad is morphologically indistinguishable as a primordial testis or ovary. The gonad is composed of primitive germ cells intermingled with coelomic surface epithelial cells and an inner core of medullary mesenchymal tissue. Just below this ridge lies the mesonephric duct. This indifferent stage lasts about 7–10 days. Together the mesonephros and the genital ridge are called the urogenital ridge, indicating the close association of the urinary and reproductive systems.

The origin of the gonadal somatic cells is still not certain. The earliest recognizable gonad contains besides the germ cells, somatic cells derived from at least 3 different tissues: coelomic epithelium, mesenchyme, and mesonephric tissue. In one model, the gonad is formed by the invasion of the "germinal epithelium" into the underlying mesenchyme. The germinal epithelium is simply that part of the coelomic epithelium which gives rise to gonadal tissue. The invading cells form the primary sex cords which contain the germ cells surrounded by somatic cells (the cells destined to form the tissue which holds the germ cells). In a newer model, the somatic cells of the gonad are believed to arise from the mesonephros and not the coelomic epithelium.[5]

The primordial germ cells originate within the primitive ectoderm, but the specific cells of origin cannot be distinguished. The germ cells are first identified in the primitive endoderm at the caudal end and in the adjacent yolk sac, and soon they also appear in the splanchnic mesoderm of the hindgut. The gonadal ridge is the one and only site where the germ cells can survive. By displacement because of growth of the embryo and also by active movement, the germ cells "migrate" to their gonadal sites between weeks 4 and 6 of gestation. The factors that initiate and guide the migration of the germ cells are not known. During this "movement," the germ cells begin their proliferation.

The germ cells are the direct precursors of sperm and ova, and by the 6th week, on completion of the indifferent state, these primordial germ cells have multiplied by mitosis to a total of 10,000. By the 6th week of gestation, the indifferent gonads contain the germ cells and supporting cells derived from the coelomic epithelium and the mesenchyme of the gonadal ridge.

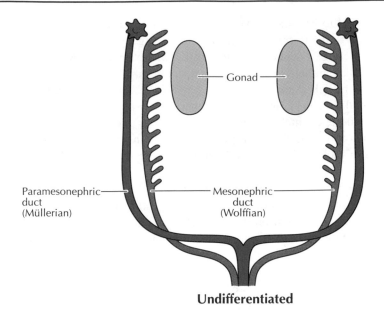

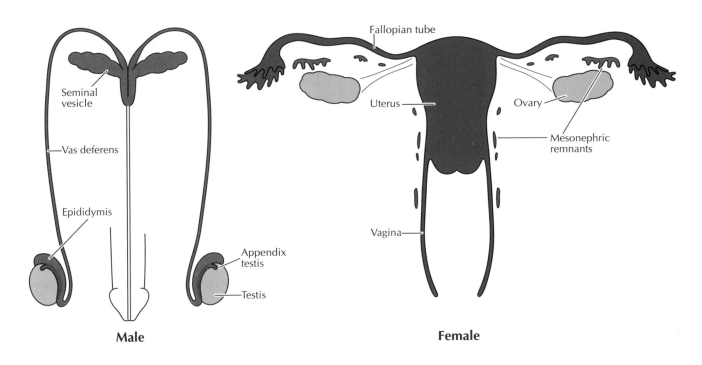

The Stage of Differentiation

If the indifferent gonad is destined to become a testis, differentiation along this line will take place at 6–9 weeks. The absence of testicular evolution (formation of medullary primary sex cords, primitive tubules, and incorporation of germ cells) gives implicit evidence of the existence of a primitive, albeit momentarily quiescent, ovary. In contrast to the male, female internal and external genitalia differentiation precedes gonadal maturation. These events are related to the genetic constitution and the territorial receptivity of the mesenchyme. If either factor is deficient or defective, improper development occurs. As has been noted, primitive germ cells are unable to survive in locations other than the gonadal ridge. If partial or imperfect gonadal tissue is formed, the resulting abnormal nonsteroidal and steroidal events have wide ranging morphologic, reproductive, and behavioral effects.

The Testes

The factor that determines whether the indifferent gonad will become a testis is called, appropriately, the testes-determining factor (TDF), a product of a gene located on the Y chromosome.[6] Currently, the best candidate for the testicular determining factor gene is located within a region named SRY, the sex-determining region on the Y chromosome.[7] The protein product of the TDF gene contains a DNA binding domain to activate gene transcription. The expression of the TDF gene is confined to the genital ridge during fetal life, but the gene is also active in the germ cells of the adult, perhaps playing a role in spermatogenesis.[6] The traditional view assigns active gene control and expression for testicular differentiation and a more passive, "default" mode of development for the ovary. However, any process of differentiation requires gene expression, and therefore ovarian development, too, must involve genes and gene products.

When the Y chromosome containing the testes determining region is present, the gonads develop into testes. The male phenotype is dependent upon the products (antimüllerian hormone and testosterone) of the fetal testes, while the female phenotype is the result of an absence of these fetal gonadal products.[8] Antimüllerian hormone (AMH), which inhibits the formation of the müllerian ducts, is secreted at the time of Sertoli cell differentiation, beginning at 7 weeks. After involution of the müllerian system, AMH continues to be secreted, but there is no known function. In the ovary, very small amounts of AMH mRNA are present early in life, and although there may be no role in female development, its production later in life by the granulosa cells raises the possibility of autocrine/paracrine actions in oocyte maturation and follicular development.[9]

The testis begins its differentiation in week 6–7 of gestation by the appearance of Sertoli cells that aggregate to form the testicular cords. The primordial germ cells are embedded in the testicular cords that will form the Sertoli cells and spermatogonia. The mature Sertoli cells are the site of production of ABP (androgen binding protein, important in maintaining the high local androgen environment necessary for spermatogenesis) and inhibin.

The Leydig cells differentiate (beginning week 8) from mesenchymal cells of the interstitial component surrounding the testicular cords. Thus secretion of AMH precedes steroidogenesis in Leydig cells. Shortly after the appearance of the Leydig cells, secretion of testosterone begins. Androgen secretion increases in conjunction with increasing Leydig cell numbers until a peak is reached at 15–18 weeks. At this time, Leydig cell regression begins, and at birth, only a few Leydig cells are present.

The cycle of fetal Leydig cells follows the rise and decline of fetal human chorionic gonadotropin (HCG) levels during pregnancy. This relationship and the presence of HCG receptors in the fetal testis indicate a regulatory role for HCG.[4] The pattern of HCG in the fetus parallels that of the mother, peaking at about 10 weeks and declining to a nadir at 20 weeks gestation, but the concentrations are only 5% of maternal concentrations.

Testosterone synthesis in human fetal testes begins at the 8th week of gestation, reaches a peak between 15–18 weeks, and then declines. Testicular function in the fetus can be correlated with the fetal hormonal patterns. While the initial testosterone production and sexual differentiation are in response to the fetal levels of HCG, further testosterone production and masculine differentiation appear to be maintained by the fetal pituitary gonadotropins. Decreased testosterone levels in late gestation probably reflect the decrease in gonadotropin levels. The fetal Leydig cells, by an unknown mechanism, avoid down-regulation and respond to high levels of HCG and LH by increased steroidogenesis and cell multiplication. This generation of cells is replaced by the adult generation of Leydig cells which becomes functional at puberty and responds to high levels of HCG and LH with down-regulation and decreased steroidogenesis.

Leydig cells, therefore, are composed of two distinct populations, one active during fetal life and one active during adult life. The regression of fetal Leydig cells and the appearance of morphologically distinct adult cells during the peripubertal period raise many questions: what is the relationship between these two types, what is the mechanism for the regression and for the new appearance, and what is the origin of the adult cells?

The fetal spermatogonia, derived from the primordial germ cells, are in the testicular cords, surrounded by the Sertoli cells. In contrast to the female, male germ cells do not start meiotic division before puberty.

The differentiation of the wolffian system begins with the increase in testicular testosterone production. The classic experiments by Jost indicate that this effect of testosterone is due to local action, probably explaining why male internal genitalia in true hermaphrodites are only on the side of the testis.[8] Not all androgen-sensitive tissues require the prior conversion of testosterone to dihydrotestosterone (DHT). In the process of masculine differentiation, the development of the wolffian duct structures (epididymis, the vas deferens, and the seminal vesicle) is dependent upon testosterone as the intracellular mediator, whereas development of the urogenital sinus and urogenital tubercle into the male external genitalia, urethra, and prostate requires the conversion of testosterone to DHT.[10] In the female, the loss of the wolffian system is due to the lack of locally produced testosterone.

The Stage of Oogonal Multiplication and Maturation

At 6–8 weeks, the first signs of ovarian differentiation are reflected in the rapid mitotic multiplication of germ cells, reaching 6–7 million oogonia by 16–20 weeks.[11,12] This represents the maximal oogonal content of the gonad. From this point in time germ cell content will irretrievably decrease until, some 50 years later, the store of oocytes will be finally exhausted.

By mitosis, the germ cells give rise to the oogonia. The oogonia are transformed to oocytes as they enter the first meiotic division and arrest in prophase. This process begins at 11–12 weeks, perhaps in response to a factor or factors produced by the rete ovarii.[13] Progression of meiosis to the diplotene stage is accomplished throughout the rest of pregnancy and completed by birth. Arrest of meiosis at the end of the first stage is probably maintained by inhibiting substances produced by granulosa cells. A single ovum is formed from the two meiotic divisions of the oocyte, one just before ovulation and the second at the time of sperm penetration. The excess genetic material is extruded as one polar body at each meiotic division.

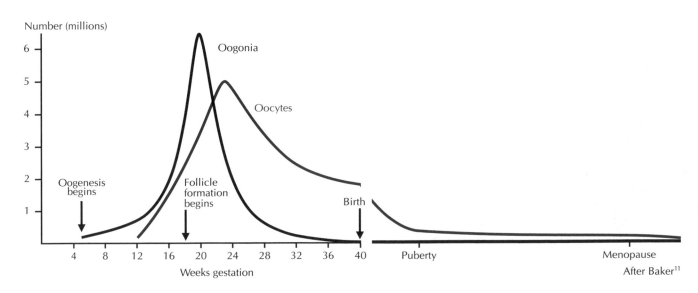

After Baker[11]

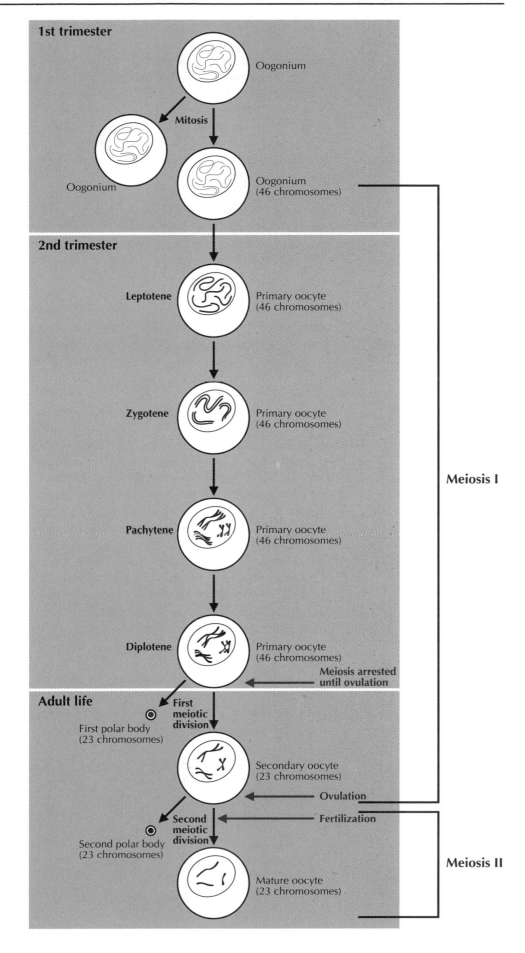

1st trimester

Oogonium

Mitosis

Oogonium

Oogonium
(46 chromosomes)

2nd trimester

Leptotene — Primary oocyte
(46 chromosomes)

Zygotene — Primary oocyte
(46 chromosomes)

Pachytene — Primary oocyte
(46 chromosomes)

Diplotene — Primary oocyte
(46 chromosomes)

Meiosis arrested
until ovulation

Adult life

First
meiotic
division

First polar body
(23 chromosomes)

Secondary oocyte
(23 chromosomes)

Ovulation

Second
meiotic
division

Fertilization

Second polar body
(23 chromosomes)

Mature oocyte
(23 chromosomes)

Meiosis I

Meiosis II

Loss of germ cells takes place throughout all of these events: during mitosis of germ cells, during the various stages of meiosis, and finally, after follicle formation. The massive loss of oocytes during the second half of pregnancy is the consequence of several mechanisms. Besides follicular growth and atresia, substantial numbers of oocytes regress during meiosis, and those follicles which fail to be enveloped by granulosa cells undergo degeneration. In addition, germ cells (in the cortical area) migrate to the surface of the gonad and become incorporated into the surface epithelium or are eliminated into the peritoneal cavity.[14,15] In contrast, once all oocytes are encased in follicles (shortly after birth), the loss of oocytes will be only through the process of follicular growth and atresia.

Chromosomal anomalies can accelerate germ cell loss. Individuals with Turner syndrome (45,X) experience normal migration and mitosis of germ cells, but the oogonia do not undergo meiosis, and rapid loss of oocytes leaves the gonad without follicles by birth, and it appears as a fibrous streak.

The Stage of Follicle Formation

At 14–20 weeks, the highly cellular cortex is gradually perforated by vascular channels originating in the deeper medullary areas. As the finger-like vascular projections enter the cortex, it takes on the appearance of secondary sex cords. As blood vessels invade and penetrate, they divide the previously solid cortical cell mass into smaller and smaller segments. Drawn in with the blood vessels are perivascular cells that are either mesenchymal or epithelial in origin. These cells surround the oocytes that have completed the first stage of meiosis. The resulting unit is the *primordial follicle — an oocyte arrested in prophase of meiosis enveloped by a single layer of granulosa cells, surrounded by a basement membrane.* Eventually all oocytes are covered in this fashion. Residual mesenchyme not utilized in primordial follicle formation is noted in the interstices between follicles, forming the primitive ovarian stroma. The granulosa cells differentiate from coelomic epithelial or mesenchymal precursors (their specific origin is still disputed). This process of primordial follicular development continues until all oocytes in the diplotene stage can be found in follicles, some time shortly after birth.

As soon as the oocyte is surrounded by the rosette of pregranulosa cells, the entire follicle can undergo variable degrees of maturation before arresting and becoming atretic. These events include in sequence: oocyte cytoplasmic enlargement, eccentric migration of the nucleus, and proliferation of several layers of granulosa cells by mitosis. As a result, a primary follicle is formed. Less frequently, but by no means rarely, further differentiation is expressed as more complete granulosa proliferation. Call-Exner body formation (coalescence to form an antrum) and occasionally a minor thecal layer system which differentiates from surrounding mesenchymal cells can be seen. Preantral follicles can be found in the 6th month of gestation, and antral follicles are present by the end of pregnancy, but not in large numbers. It is only during the last third of gestation that theca cells can be found surrounding follicles.[12]

Thus, even in fetal life the cycle of follicle formation, variable ripening, and atresia occurs. Although these steps are precisely those typical of adult reproductive life, full maturity, as expressed in ovulation, does not occur. Estrogen production does not occur until late in pregnancy when follicular development takes place, and even then steroidogenesis is not significant. Unlike the male, gonadal steroid production is not required for development of a normal phenotype. The development of the müllerian duct into the fallopian tubes, the uterus, and the upper third of the vagina is totally independent of the ovary.

The ovary at birth can contain cystic follicles of varying size, undoubtedly stimulated by the reactive gonadotropin surge accompanying the withdrawal of the neonatal hypothalamus and pituitary from the negative feedback of fetoplacental steroids. Ovarian cysts can also be occasionally detected in fetuses by ultrasonography.[16]

The anterior pituitary begins development between 4 and 5 weeks of fetal life. The median eminence is apparent by week 9, and the hypothalamic-pituitary portal circulation is functional by the 12th week of gestation. Pituitary levels of follicle-stimulating hormone (FSH) peak at 20–23 weeks, and circulating levels peak at 28 weeks. Levels are higher in female fetuses compared to males until the last 6 weeks of gestation. Ovaries in anencephalic fetuses (which lack gonadotropin releasing hormone [GnRH] and gonadotropin secretion) lack antral follicles and are smaller at term, but progression through meiosis and development of primordial follicles occur, apparently not dependent upon gonadotropins.[4] The ovary develops receptors for gonadotropins only in the second half of pregnancy. Thus the loss of oocytes during fetal life cannot be solely explained by the decline in gonadotropins. The follicular growth and development observed in the second half of pregnancy, however, is gonadotropin dependent.

The Neonatal Ovary

The total cortical content of germ cells falls to 1–2 million by birth as a result of prenatal oocyte depletion.[17] This huge depletion of germ cell mass (close to 4–5 million) has occurred over as short a time as 20 weeks. No similar rate of depletion will be seen again. Due to the fixed initial endowment of germ cells, the newborn female enters life, still far from reproductive potential, having lost 80% of her oocytes.

The ovary is approximately 1 cm in diameter and weighs about 250–350 mg at birth, although sizable cystic follicles can enlarge the total dimensions. Intriguingly, the gonad on the right side of the body in both males and females is larger, heavier, and greater in protein and DNA content than the gonad on the left side.[18] Compartmentalization of the gonad into cortex and a small residual medulla has been achieved. In the cortex almost all the oocytes are involved in primordial follicle units. Varying degrees of maturation in some units can be seen as in the prenatal state.

There is a sex difference in fetal gonadotropin levels. There are higher pituitary and circulating FSH and pituitary LH levels in female fetuses. The lower male levels are probably due to testicular testosterone and inhibin production. In infancy, the postnatal FSH rise is more marked and more sustained in females, while LH values are not as high. The FSH levels are greater than the levels reached during a normal adult menstrual cycle, decreasing to low levels usually by one year of age, sometimes later.[19] LH levels are in the range of lower adult levels. This early activity is accompanied by inhibin levels comparable to the low range observed during the follicular phase of the menstrual cycle. The most common cause of abdominal masses in fetuses and newborns is ovarian cysts, presumably a consequence of gonadotropin stimulation.[20]

Interference with the postnatal rise in gonadotropins in monkeys is associated with disturbances in normal hypothalamic-pituitary function at puberty.[21] After the postnatal rise, gonadotropin levels reach a nadir during early childhood (by about 6 months of age in males and 1–2 years in females) and then rise slightly between 4 and 10 years.

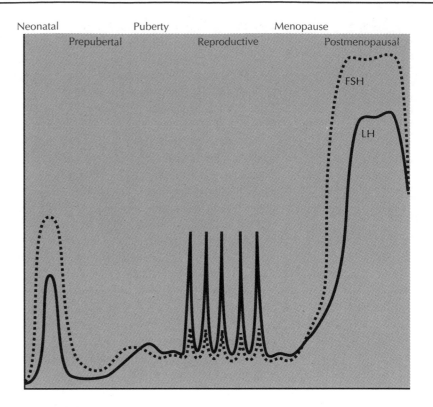

The Ovary in Childhood

The childhood period is characterized by low levels of gonadotropins in the pituitary and in the blood, little response of the pituitary to GnRH, and maximal hypothalamic suppression. The ovary, however, is not quiescent during childhood. Follicles begin to grow at all times and frequently reach the antral stage. Ultrasonography can commonly demonstrate ovarian follicular cysts during childhood, ranging in size from 2 to 15 mm.[16] These small unilocular ovarian cysts are not clinically significant.[22] The process of atresia with an increasing contribution of follicular remnants to the stromal compartment yields progressive ovarian enlargement during childhood, about a ten-fold increase in weight. Of course, the lack of gonadotropin support prevents full follicular development and function. There is no evidence that ovarian function is necessary until puberty. However, the oocytes during this time period are active, synthesizing mRNAs and protein.

The Adult Ovary

At the onset of puberty, the germ cell mass has been reduced to 300,000 units.[23] During the next 35–40 years of reproductive life, these units will be depleted further to a point at menopause where only a few hundred remain.[24] In the last 10–15 years before menopause, there appears to be an acceleration of follicular loss. This loss correlates with a subtle but real increase in FSH and decrease in inhibin.[25–27] The accelerated loss is probably secondary to the increase in FSH stimulation. Fewer follicles grow per cycle as a woman ages and cycles lengthen.[28–30] These changes, including the increase in FSH (which is probably due to the decrease in inhibin), all reflect the reduced quality and capability of aging follicles.

The loss of oocytes (and follicles) through atresia is a response to changes in many factors. Certainly gonadotropin stimulation and withdrawal are important, but ovarian steroids and autocrine/paracrine factors are also involved. The consequence of these unfavorable changes, atresia, is a process called *apoptosis*, programmed cell death. This process is heralded by alterations in mRNAs required for cell proteins that maintain follicle integrity.[31]

During the reproductive years, the typical cycle of follicle maturation, including ovulation and corpus luteum formation, will be realized. This results from the complex but well-defined sequence of hypothalamic-pituitary-gonadal interactions in which follicle and corpus luteum steroid hormones, pituitary gonadotropins, and autocrine/paracrine factors are integrated to yield ovulation. These important events are described in detail in Chapters 5 and 6. For the moment, our attention will be exclusively directed to a description of the events as the gonad is driven inexorably to final and complete exhaustion of its germ cell supply. The major feature of this reproductive period in the ovary's existence is the full maturational expression of some follicle units in ovulation and corpus luteum formation and the accompaniment of varying steroid output of estradiol and progesterone. For every follicle that ovulates, close to 1,000 will pursue abortive growth periods of variable length.

Follicular Growth

In the adult ovary, the stages of follicle development noted even in the prenatal period are repeated but to a more complete degree. Initially the oocyte enlarges and the granulosa cells proliferate markedly. A solid sphere of cells encasing the oocyte is formed. At this point the theca interna is noted in initial stages of formation. The zona pellucida begins to form. If gonadotropin increments are available, as can be seen early in a menstrual cycle, a further FSH-dependent stage of follicle maturation is seen. The number of follicles that mature is dependent on the amount of FSH available to the gonad and the sensitivity of the follicles to the gonadotropins.

The antrum first appears as a coalescence of numerous intragranulosa cavities called Call-Exner bodies, which were described by Emma Call and Siegmund Exner in Vienna in 1875. Emma Call was one of the first woman physicians in the United States.[32] After receiving her medical degree from the University of Michigan in 1873, she went to Vienna as Exner's postgraduate student. She returned to Boston and practiced as an obstetrician for more than 40 years. Emma Call was the first woman elected to the Massachusetts Medical Society (in 1884). Her description of the Call-Exner bodies was her only publication.

Whether Call-Exner bodies represent liquefaction or granulosa cell secretion is uncertain. At first the cavity is filled with a coagulum of cellular debris. Soon a liquor accumulates, which is essentially a transudation of blood filtered through the avascular granulosa from the thecal vessels. With antral formation, the theca interna develops more fully, expressed by increased cell mass, increased vascularity, and the formation of lipid-rich cytoplasmic vacuoles within the theca cells. As the follicle expands, the surrounding stroma is compressed and is called the theca externa.

At any point in this development, individual follicles become arrested and eventually regress in the process known as atresia. At first the granulosa component begins to disrupt. The antral cavity constituents are resorbed, and the cavity collapses and obliterates. The oocyte degenerates in situ. Finally, a ribbon-like scarred streak surrounded by theca is seen. Eventually this theca mass loses its lipid and becomes indistinguishable from the growing mass of stroma. Prior to regression, cystic follicles can be retained in the cortex for variable periods of time.

Ovulation

If gonadotropin stimulation is adequate, one of the several follicle units propelled to varying degrees of maturity will advance to ovulation. Morphologically these events include distension of the antrum by increments of antral fluid, and compression of the granulosa against the limiting membrane separating the avascular granulosa and the luteinized, vascularized theca interna. In addition, the antral fluid increment gradually pinches off the cumulus oophorous, the mound of granulosa enveloping the oocyte. The mechanisms of the thinning of the theca over the surface of the now protruding, distended follicle, the creation of an avascular area weakening the ovarian capsule, and the final acute distension of the antrum with rupture and extrusion of the oocyte in its cumulus, are multiple and complex. Repeated evaluation of intrafollicular pressures has failed to indict an explosive factor in this crucial event.

As demonstrated in a variety of animal experiments, the physical expulsion of the oocyte is dependent upon a preovulatory surge in prostaglandin synthesis within the follicle. Inhibition of this prostaglandin synthesis produces a corpus luteum with an entrapped oocyte. Both prostaglandins and the midcycle surge of gonadotropins are thought to increase the concentration and activity of local proteases, such as plasminogen conversion to plasmin. As a result of generalized tissue weakening (loss of intercellular gap junction integrity and disruption of elastic fibers), there is swift accumulation of antral fluid followed by rupture of the weakened tissue envelope surrounding the follicle.

Corpus Luteum

Shortly after ovulation profound alterations in cellular organization occur in the ruptured follicle that go well beyond simple repair. After tissue integrity and continuity are retrieved, the granulosa cells hypertrophy markedly, gradually filling in the cystic, sometimes hemorrhagic, cavity of the early corpus luteum. In addition, for the first time, the granulosa becomes markedly luteinized by incorporation of lipid-rich vacuoles within its cytoplasm. Both these properties had been the exclusive features of the theca prior to ovulation. For its part, the theca of the corpus luteum becomes less prominent, vestiges being noted eventually only in the interstices of the typical scalloping of the mature corpus luteum. As a result, a new yellow body is formed, now dominated by the enlarged, lipid-rich, fully vascularized granulosa. In the 14 days of its life, dependent on the low but important quantities of LH available in the luteal phase, this unit produces estradiol and progesterone. Failing a new enlarging source of LH-like human chorionic gonadotropin (HCG) from a successful implantation, the corpus luteum rapidly ages. Its vascularity and lipid content wane, and the sequence of scarification (albicantia) ensues.

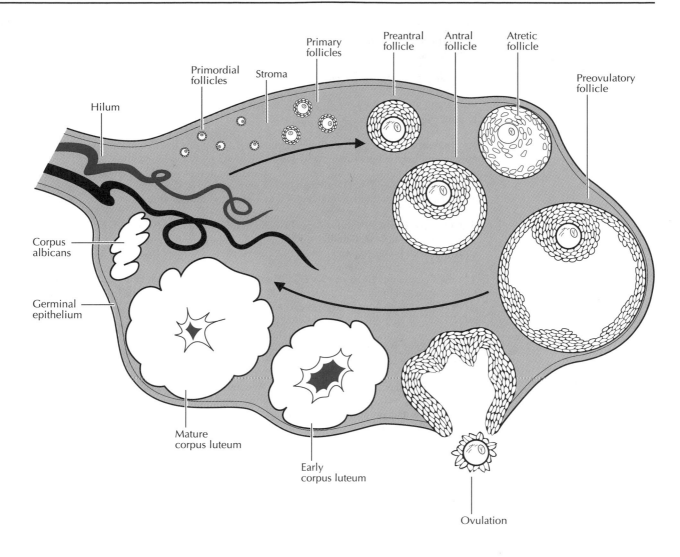

References

1. **Graham H,** *Eternal Eve, The History of Gynaecology & Obstetrics,* Doubleday & Company, Inc., Garden City, 1951.

2. **Magner LN,** *A History of Medicine,* Marcel Dekker, Inc., New York, 1992.

3. **Short RV,** The discovery of the ovaries, in Zuckerman S, Weir BJ, editors, *The Ovary,* Vol. 1, 2nd edition, Academic Press, New York, 1977, pp 1-67.

4. **Rabinovici J, Jaffe RB,** Development and regulation of growth and differentiated function in human and subhuman primate fetal gonads, Endocr Rev 11:532, 1990.

5. **Yoshinaga K, Hess DL, Hendrickx AG, Zamboni L,** The development of the sexually indifferent gonad in the prosimian, Galago *crassicaudatus crassicaudatus,* Am J Anat 181:89, 1988.

6. **Sinclair AH, Berta P, Palmer MS, Hawkins JR, Griffiths BL, Smith JJ, Foster JW, Frischauf A-M, Lovell-Badge R, Goodfellow PN,** A gene from the human sex-determining region encodes a protein with homology to a conserved DNA-binding motif, Nature 346:240, 1990.

7. **Tho SPT, Layman LC, Lanclos DK, Plouffe L Jr, Byrd JR, McDonough PG,** Absence of the testicular determining factor gene SRY in XX true hermaphrodites and presence of this locus in most subjects with gonadal dysgenesis caused by Y aneuploidy, Am J Obstet Gynecol 167:1794, 1992.

8. **Jost A, Vigier B, Prepin J, Perchellet JP,** Studies on sex differentiation in mammals, Recent Prog Horm Res 29:1, 1973.

9. **Kim JH, Seibel MM, MacLaughlin DT, Donahoe PK, Ransil BJ, Hametz PA, Richards CJ,** The inhibitory effects of müllerian-inhibiting substance on epidermal growth factor induced proliferation and progesterone production of human granulosa-luteal cells, J Clin Endocrinol Metab 75:911, 1992.

10. **Mooradian AD, Morley JE, Korenman SG,** Biological actions of androgens, Endocr Rev 8:1, 1987.

11. **Baker TG,** A quantitative and cytological study of germ cells in human ovaries, Proc R Soc Lond 158:417, 1963.

12. **Gondos B, Bhiraleus P, Hobel CJ,** Ultrastructural observations on germ cells in human fetal ovaries, Am J Obstet Gynecol 110:644, 1971.

13. **Gondos B, Westergaard L, Byskov A,** Initiation of oogenesis in the human fetal ovary: ultrastructural and squash preparation study, Am J Obstet Gynecol 155:189, 1986.

14. **Motta PM, Makabe S,** Germ cells in the ovarian surface during fetal development in humans. A three-dimensional microanatomical study by scanning and transmission electron microscopy, J Submicrosc Cytol Pathol 18:271, 1986.

15. **Speed RM,** The possible role of meiotic pairing anomalies in the atresia of human fetal ooctyes, Hum Genet 78:260, 1988.

16. **Cohen HL, Eisenberg P, Mandel F, Haller JO,** Ovarian cysts are common in premenarchal girls: a sonographic study of 101 children 2–12 years old, Am J Radiol 159:89, 1992.

17. **Himelstein-Braw R, Byskov AG, Peters H, Faber M,** Follicular atresia in the infant human ovary, J Reprod Fertil 46:55, 1976.

18. **Mittwoch U, Mahadevaiah S,** Comparison of development of human fetal gonads and kidneys, J Reprod Fertil 58:463, 1980.

19. **Burger HG, Famada Y, Bangah ML, McCloud PI, Warne GL,** Serum gonadotropin, sex steroid, and immunoreactive inhibin levels in the first two years of life, J Clin Endocrinol Metab 72:682, 1991.

20. **Hengster P, Menardi G,** Ovarian cysts in the newborn, Pediatr Surg Int 7:372, 1992.

21. **Mann DR, Akinbami MA, Gould KG, Tanner JM, Wallen K,** Neonatal treatment of male monkeys with a gonadotropin-releasing hormone agonist alters differentiation of central nervous system centers that regulate sexual and skeletal development, J Clin Endocrinol Metab 76:1319, 1993.

22. **Millar DM, Blake JM, Stringer DA, Hara H, Babiak C,** Prepubertal ovarian cyst formation: 5 years' experience, Obstet Gynecol 81:434, 1993.

23. **Block E,** Quantitative morphological investigations of the follicular system in women. Variations at different ages, Acta Anat 14:108, 1952.

24. **Richardson SJ, Senikas V, Nelson JF,** Follicular depletion during the menopausal transition — evidence for accelerated loss and ultimate exhaustion, J Clin Endocrinol Metab 65:1231, 1987.

25. **Metcalf MG, Livesay JH,** Gonadotropin excretion in fertile women: effect of age and the onset of the menopausal transition, J Endocrinol 105:357, 1985.

26. **Lee SJ, Lenton EA, Sexton L, Cooke ID,** The effect of age on the cyclical patterns of plasma LH, FSH, oestradiol and progesterone in women with regular menstrual cycles, Hum Reprod 3:851, 1988.

27. **Hughes EG, Robertson DM, Handelsman DJ, Hayward S, Healy DL, de Kretser DM,** Inhibin and estradiol responses to ovarian hyperstimulation: effects of age and predictive value for in vitro fertilization outcome, J Clin Endocrinol Metab 70:358, 1990.

28. **Lenton EA, Landgren B, Sexton L, Harper R,** Normal variation in the length of the follicular phase of the menstrual cycle: effect of chronological age, Br J Obstet Gynaecol 91:681, 1984.

29. **Cha KY, Koo JJ, Ko JJ, Choi DH, Han SY, Yoon TK,** Pregnancy after IVF of human follicular ooctyes collected from nonstimulated cycles, their culture in vitro and their transfer in a donor occyte program, Fertil Steril 55:109, 1991.

30. **Treloar AE, Boynton RE, Borghild GB, Brown BW,** Variation of the human menstrual cycle through reproductive life, Int J Fertil 12:77, 1967.

31. **Tilly JL, Kowalski KI, Schomberg DW, Hsueh AJ,** Apoptosis in atretic ovarian follicles is associated with selective decreases in messenger ribonucleic acid transcripts for gonadotropin receptors and cytochrome P450 aromatase, Endocrinology 131:1670, 1992.

32. **Speert H,** *Obstetric and Gynecologic Milestones,* The Macmillan Company, New York, 1958.

4 The Uterus

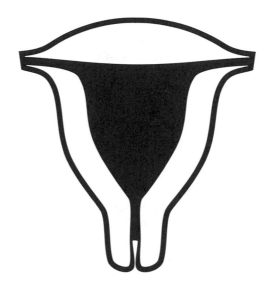

Anatomical knowledge of the uterus was slow to accumulate.[1,2] Papyrus writings from 2500 B.C. indicate that the ancient Egyptians made a distinction between the vagina and uterus. Because the dead had to be embalmed, dissection was precluded, but prolapse was recognized because it was important to return the uterus into its proper place prior to mummification. Next to the Egyptian papyri in antiquity were Hindu writings in which descriptions of the uterus, tubes, and vagina indicate knowledge gained from dissections. This was probably the earliest description of the fallopian tubes.

There is little information in Greek writings about female anatomy; however, Herophilus (4th century B.C.), the great anatomist in Alexandria and the originator of scholarly dissection, recorded the different positions of the uterus. Soranus of Ephesus (98–138 A.D.) accurately described the uterus (probably the first to do so), obviously from multiple dissections of cadavers. He recognized that the uterus is not essential for life, acknowledged the presence of leiomyomata, and treated prolapse with pessaries.

Herophilus and Soranus were uncertain regarding the function of the fallopian tubes, but Galen, Rufus, and Aetisu guessed correctly their function. Galen promoted the practice of bleeding for the treatment of almost every disorder. In his argument that nature prevented disease by discharging excess blood, Galen maintained that women were healthier because their superfluous blood was eliminated by menstruation.[3] The writings of Galen (130–200 A.D.) represented the knowledge of medicine for over 1,000 years until the end of the medieval dark ages. Galen's description of the uterus and tubes indicates that he had only seen the horned uteri of animals.

In the 16th century, Berengarius, Vesalius, Eustachius, and Fallopius made significant contributions to the anatomical study of the female genitalia. Berengarius (Giacomo Berengario da Carpi) was the first anatomist to work with an artist. His anatomical text, published in 1514, depicted dissected subjects as if they were still alive.

Gabriele Fallopio (or Fallopius) published his work, *Observationes Anatomicae,* in Venice in 1561, one year before his death from pleurisy at age 40. He provided the first descriptions of the clitoris and the hymen, and the first exact descriptions of the ovaries and the tubes. He named the vagina and the placenta and called the tubes the uteri tuba (the trumpet of the uterus), but soon they were known universally as the fallopian tubes. It was his professor and mentor at the University of Padua, however, Andreas Vesalius, who was the first to accurately reveal the presence of the endometrial cavity.

Development of the Müllerian System

The wolffian and müllerian ducts are discrete primordia that temporarily coexist in all embryos during the ambisexual period of development (up to 8 weeks). Thereafter, one type of duct system persists normally and gives rise to special ducts and glands, whereas the other disappears during the 3rd fetal month, except for nonfunctional vestiges.

Hormonal control of mammalian somatic sex differentiation was established by the classic experiments of Alfred Jost.[4] In Jost's landmark studies, the active role of male determining factors, as opposed to the constitutive nature of female differentiation, was defined as the directing feature of sex differentiation. This principle applies not only to the internal ducts but to the gonad, external genitalia, and perhaps even the brain. The critical factors in determining which of the duct structures stabilize or regress are the secretions from the testes: AMH (antimüllerian hormone, also known as müllerian inhibiting substance or müllerian inhibiting factor) and testosterone.

AMH is a member of the transforming growth factor-β family of glycoprotein differentiation factors that include inhibin and activin. The gene for AMH has been mapped to chromosome 19. AMH is synthesized by Sertoli cells soon after testicular differentiation and is responsible for the ipsilateral regression of the müllerian ducts by 8 weeks. Despite its presence in serum up to puberty, lack of regression of the uterus and tubes is the only consistent expression of AMH gene mutations. In the absence of AMH, the fetus will develop fallopian tubes, uterus, and upper vagina from the paramesonephric ducts (the müllerian ducts). This development requires the prior appearance of the mesonephric ducts, and for this reason, abnormalities in development of the tubes, uterus, and upper vagina are associated with abnormalities in the renal system.

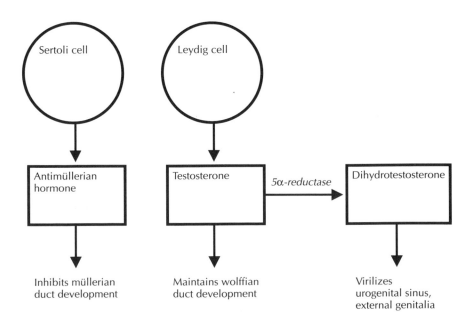

The internal genitalia possess the intrinsic tendency to feminize. In the absence of a Y chromosome and a functional testis, the lack of AMH allows retention of the müllerian system and development of fallopian tubes, uterus, and upper vagina. In the absence of testosterone, the wolffian system regresses. In the presence of a normal ovary or the absence of any gonad, müllerian duct development takes place.

The fallopian tubes, uterus, and the upper portion of the vagina are created by the fusion of the müllerian ducts by the 10th week of gestation. Under the epithelium lies mesenchymal tissue that will be the origin of the the uterine stroma and smooth muscle cells. By the 20th week of pregnancy, the uterine mucosa is fully differentiated into the endometrium.

The endometrium, derived from the mucosal lining of the fused müllerian ducts, may be one of the most complex tissues in the human body. It is always changing, responding to the cyclic patterns of estrogen and progesterone of the ovarian menstrual cycle, and to a complex interplay among its own autocrine/paracrine factors.[5]

The Histologic Changes in Endometrium during an Ovulatory Cycle

The sequence of endometrial changes associated with an ovulatory cycle has been carefully studied by Noyes in the human and Bartlemez and Markee in the subhuman primate.[6–8] From these data a description of menstrual physiology has developed based upon specific anatomic and functional changes within glandular, vascular, and stromal components of the endometrium.[9] These changes will be discussed in five phases: 1) the menstrual endometrium, 2) the proliferative phase, 3) the secretory phase, 4) preparation for implantation, and finally 5) the phase of endometrial breakdown. While these distinctions are not entirely arbitrary, it must be recalled that the entire process is an integrated evolutionary cycle of endometrial growth and regression, which is repeated some 300–400 times during the adult life of the human female.

The endometrium can be divided morphologically into an upper two-thirds "functionalis" layer and a lower one-third "basalis" layer. The purpose of the functionalis layer is to prepare for the implantation of the blastocyst and, therefore, it is the site of proliferation, secretion, and degeneration. The purpose of the basalis layer is to provide the regenerative endometrium following menstrual loss of the functionalis.

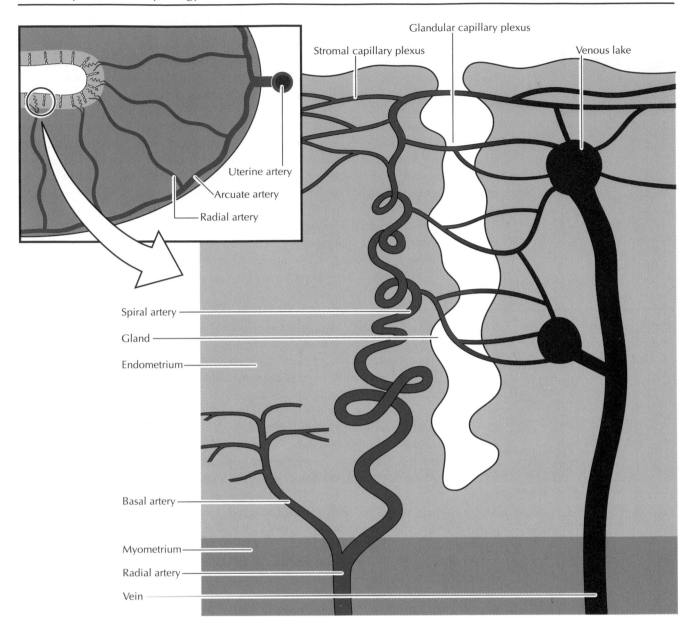

The Uterine Vasculature

The two uterine arteries which supply the uterus are branches of the internal iliac arteries. At the lower part of the uterus, the uterine artery separates into the vaginal artery and an ascending branch that divides into the arcuate arteries. The arcuate arteries run parallel to the uterine cavity and anastomose with each other, forming a vascular ring around the cavity. Small centrifugal branches (the radial arteries) leave the arcuate vessels, perpendicular to the endometrial cavity, to supply the myometrium. When these arteries enter the endometrium, small branches (the basal arteries) extend laterally to supply the basalis layer. These basal arteries do not demonstrate a response to hormonal changes. The radial arteries continue in the direction of the endometrial surface, now assuming a corkscrew appearance (and now called the spiral arteries), to supply the functionalis layer of the endometrium. It is the spiral artery (an end artery) segment which is very sensitive to hormonal changes. One reason the functionalis layer is more vulnerable to vascular permutations is that there are no anastomoses among the spiral arteries. The endometrial glands and the stromal tissue are supplied by capillaries that emerge from the spiral arteries at all levels of the endometrium. The capillaries drain into a venous plexus and eventually into the myometrial arcuate veins and into the uterine veins. This unique vascular architecture is important in allowing a repeated sequence of endometrial growth and desquamation.

The Menstrual Endometrium

The menstrual endometrium is a relatively thin but dense tissue. It is composed of the stable, nonfunctioning basalis component and a variable, but small, amount of residual stratum spongiosum. At menstruation, this latter tissue displays a variety of functional states including disarray and breakage of glands, fragmentation of vessels and stroma with persisting evidence of necrosis, white cell infiltration, and red cell interstitial diapedesis. Even as the remnants of menstrual shedding dominate the overall appearance of this tissue, evidence of repair in all tissue components can be detected. The menstrual endometrium is a transitional state bridging the more dramatic proliferative and exfoliative phases of the cycle. Its density implies that the shortness of height is not entirely due to desquamation. Collapse of the supporting matrix also contributes significantly to the shallowness. Reticular stains in rhesus endometrium confirm this "deflated" state. Nevertheless, as much as two-thirds of the functioning endometrium may be lost during menstruation. The more rapid the tissue loss, the shorter the duration of flow. Delayed or incomplete shedding is associated with heavier flow and greater blood loss.

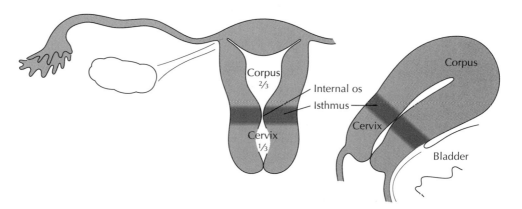

DNA synthesis is occurring in those areas of the basalis that have been completely denuded by day 2 3 of the menstrual cycle (the endometrium in the isthmic area, the narrow area between the cervix and the corpus, and the endometrium in the cornual recesses at the ostia of the tubes remain intact). The new surface epithelium emanates from the flanks of stumps of glands in the basalis layer left standing after menstrual desquamation.[10] Rapid reepithelialization follows the proliferation of the cells in the basalis layer and the surface epithelium in the isthmic and tubal ostial endometrium. This epithelial repair is supported by underlying fibroblasts. The stromal fibroblast layer forms a compact mass over which the resurfacing epithelium can "migrate." In addition, it is likely that the stromal layer contributes important autocrine/paracrine factors for growth and migration. Because hormone levels are at their nadir during this repair phase, the response may be due to injury rather than hormone mediated. However, the basalis layer is rich in its content of estrogen receptors. This "repair" is fast; by day 4 of the cycle, more than two-thirds of the cavity is covered with new epithelium.[10] By day 5–6, the entire cavity is reepithelialized, and stromal growth begins.

The Proliferative Phase

The proliferative phase is associated with ovarian follicle growth and increased estrogen secretion. Undoubtedly as a result of this steroidal action, reconstruction and growth of the endometrium are achieved. The glands are most notable in this response. At first they are narrow and tubular, lined by low columnar epithelium cells. Mitoses become prominent and pseudostratification is observed. As a result, the glandular epithelium extends peripherally and links one gland segment with its immediate neighbor. A continuous epithelial lining is formed facing the endometrial cavity. The stromal component evolves from its dense cellular menstrual condition through a brief period of edema to a final loose syncytial-like status. Coursing through the stroma, spiral vessels

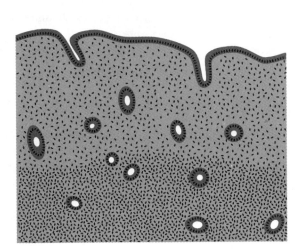

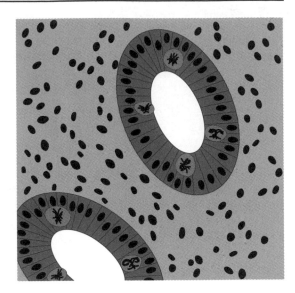

Early Proliferative

extend unbranched to a point immediately below the epithelial binding membrane. Here they form a loose capillary network. All of the tissue components (glands, stromal cells, and endothelial cells) demonstrate proliferation which peaks on days 8–10 of the cycle. This proliferation is marked by increased mitotic activity and increased nuclear DNA and cytoplasmic RNA synthesis. Intranuclear concentrations of estrogen and progesterone receptors reach a peak at midcycle prior to ovulation.

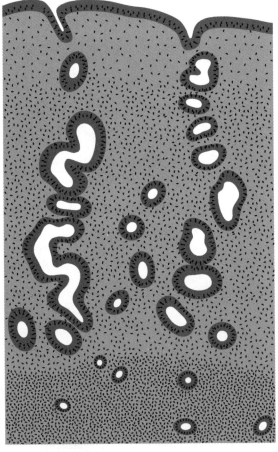

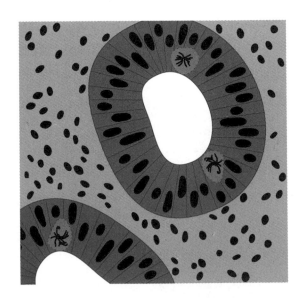

Late Proliferative

During proliferation, the endometrium grows from approximately 0.5 mm to 3.5–5.0 mm in height. This proliferation is mainly in the functionalis layer. Restoration of tissue constituents has been achieved by estrogen-induced new growth as well as incorporation of ions, water, and amino acids. The stromal ground substance has reexpanded from its menstrual collapse. Although true tissue growth has occurred, a major element in achievement of endometrial height is "reinflation" of the stroma.

A major feature of this estrogen dominant phase of endometrial growth is the increase in ciliated and microvillous cells. Ciliogenesis begins on days 7–8 of the cycle.[10] This response to estrogen is exaggerated in hyperplastic endometrium that is the result of hyperestrogenism. The concentration of these ciliated cells around gland openings and the ciliary beat pattern influence the mobilization and distribution of endometrial secretions during the secretory phase.

At all times, a large number of cells derived from bone marrow are present in the endometrium. These include lymphocytes and macrophages, diffusely distributed in the stroma.

The Secretory Phase

After ovulation, the endometrium now demonstrates a combined reaction to estrogen and progesterone activity. Most impressive is that total endometrial height is fixed at roughly its preovulatory extent (5–6 mm) despite continued availability of estrogen. This restraint or inhibition is believed to be induced by progesterone. This limitation of growth is associated with a decline in mitosis and DNA synthesis, significantly due to progesterone interference with estrogen receptor expression and progesterone stimulation of 17β-hydroxysteroid dehydrogenase and sulfotransferase, which convert estradiol to estrone sulfate (which is rapidly excreted from the cell).[11] In addition, estrogen stimulates many oncogenes that probably mediate estrogen-induced growth. Progesterone also antagonizes this action by suppressing the estrogen-mediated transcription of oncogene mRNA.[12]

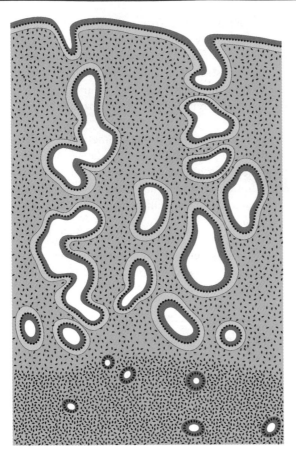

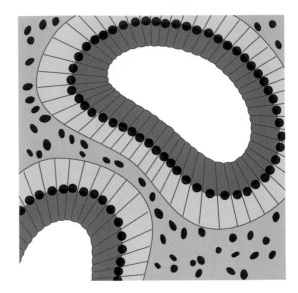

Early Secretory

Individual components of the tissue continue to display growth, but confinement in a fixed structure leads to progressive tortuosity of glands and intensified coiling of the spiral vessels. The secretory events within the glandular cells, with progression of vacuoles from intracellular to intraluminal appearance, are well-known and take place approximately over a 7-day postovulatory interval. At the conclusion of these events the glands appear exhausted, the tortuous lumina variably distended, and individual cell surfaces fragmented and lost (sawtooth appearance). Stroma is increasingly edematous, and spiral vessels are prominent and densely coiled.

The first histologic sign that ovulation has occurred is the appearance of subnuclear intracytoplasmic glycogen vacuoles in the glandular epithelium. Giant mitochondria and the "nucleolar channel system" appear in the gland cells. The nucleolar channel system is a unique appearance due to progesterone, presumably an infolding of the nuclear membranes. Individual components of the tissue continue to display growth, but confinement in a fixed structure leads to progressive tortuosity of glands and intensified coiling of the spiral vessels. These structural alterations are soon followed by active secretion of glycoproteins and peptides into the endometrial cavity. Transudation of plasma also contributes to the endometrial secretions. Important immunoglobulins are obtained from the circulation and delivered to the endometrial cavity by binding proteins produced by the epithelial cells. The peak secretory level is reached 7 days after the midcycle gonadotropin surge, coinciding with the time of blastocyst implantation.

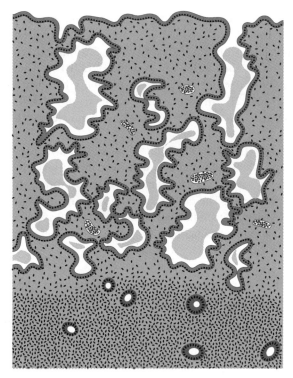

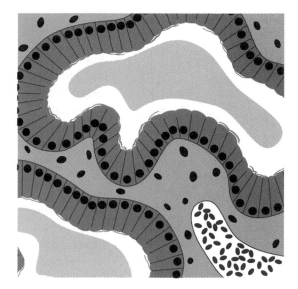

Late Secretory

The Implantation Phase

Significant changes occur within the endometrium from the 7th to the 13th day post-ovulation (days 21–27 of the cycle). At the onset of this period, the distended tortuous secretory glands have been most prominent with little intervening stroma. By 13 days postovulation, the endometrium has differentiated into three distinct zones. Something less than one-fourth of the tissue is the unchanged basalis fed by its straight vessels and surrounded by indifferent spindle-shaped stroma. The midportion of the endometrium (approximately 50% of the total) is the lace-like stratum spongiosum, composed of loose edematous stroma with tightly coiled but ubiquitous spiral vessels and exhausted dilated glandular ribbons. Overlying the spongiosum is the superficial layer of the endometrium (about 25% of the height) called the stratum compactum. Here the prominent histologic feature is the stromal cell, which has become large and polyhedral. In its cytoplasmic expansion one cell abuts the other, forming a compact, structurally sturdy layer. The necks of the glands traversing this segment are compressed and less prominent. The subepithelial capillaries and spiral vessels are engorged.

At the time of implantation, on days 21–22 of the cycle, the predominant morphologic feature is edema of the endometrial stroma. This change may be secondary to the estrogen and progesterone mediated increase in prostaglandin production by the endometrium. An increase in capillary permeability is a consequence of this local increase in prostaglandins. Receptors for the sex steroids are present in the muscular walls of the endometrial blood vessels and the enzyme system for prostaglandin synthesis is present in both the muscular walls and the endothelium of the endometrial arterioles. The vascular proliferation that leads to the coiling of the spiral vessels is a response to the sex steroids, the prostaglandins, and to autocrine/paracrine factors produced in response to estrogen and progesterone.

During the secretory phase, so-called K cells appear. These are probably granulocytes that have an immunoprotective role. They are located perivascularly and are believed to be derived from the blood.

The stromal cells of the endometrium respond to hormonal signals, synthesize prostaglandins, and, when transformed into decidual cells, produce an impressive array of substances, some of which are prolactin, relaxin, renin, insulin-like growth factors (IGFs), and insulin-like growth factor binding proteins (IGFBPs). The endometrial stromal cells, the progenitors of decidual cells, were originally believed to be derived from the bone marrow (from cells invading the endometrium), but they are now considered to emanate from the primitive uterine mesenchymal stem cells.[5]

The decidualization process begins in the luteal phase under the influence of progesterone. On cycle day 23, predecidual cells can be identified, initially surrounding blood vessels, characterized by cytonuclear enlargement, increased mitotic activity, and the formation of a basement membrane. The decidua becomes an important structural and biochemical tissue of pregnancy. Decidual cells control the invasive nature of the trophoblast, and the products of the decidua play important autocrine/paracrine roles in fetal and maternal tissues.

The Phase of Endometrial Breakdown

In the absence of fertilization, implantation, and the consequent lack of sustaining quantities of human chorionic gonadotropin from the trophoblast, the otherwise fixed lifespan of the corpus luteum is completed, and estrogen and progesterone levels wane. Predecidual transformation has formed the "compacta" layer in the upper part of the functionalis layer by day 25 (3 days before menstruation). In the first half of the secretory phase, acid phosphatase and potent lytic enzymes are confined to lysosomes. Their release is inhibited by progesterone stabilization of the lysosomal membranes. With the waning of estrogen and progesterone levels, the lysosomal membranes are not maintained, and the enzymes are released into the cytoplasm. These active enzymes will digest their cellular constraints, leading to the release of prostaglandins, extravasation of red blood cells, tissue necrosis, and vascular thrombosis. Endometrial tissue breakdown also involves a family of enzymes, matrix metalloproteinases, that degrade components of the extracellular matrix and basement membrane.[13]

The withdrawal of estrogen and progesterone initiates three endometrial events: vasomotor reactions, tissue loss, and menstruation. The most prominent immediate effect of this hormone withdrawal is a modest shrinking of the tissue height and remarkable spiral arteriole vasomotor responses. The following vascular sequence has been constructed from direct observations of rhesus endometrium. With shrinkage of height, blood flow

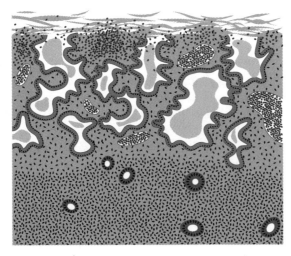
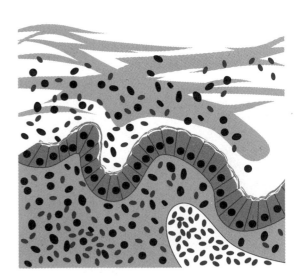

Menstruation

within the spiral vessels diminishes, venous drainage is decreased, and vasodilatation ensues. Thereafter, the spiral arterioles undergo rhythmic vasoconstriction and relaxation. Each successive spasm is more prolonged and profound, leading eventually to endometrial blanching. Within the 24 hours immediately preceding menstruation, these reactions lead to endometrial ischemia and stasis. White cells migrate through capillary walls, at first remaining adjacent to vessels, but then extending throughout the stroma. During arteriolar vasomotor changes, red blood cells escape into the interstitial space. Thrombin-platelet plugs also appear in superficial vessels. The prostaglandin content ($PGF_{2\alpha}$ and PGE_2) in the secretory endometrium reaches its highest levels at the time of menstruation. The vasoconstriction and myometrial contractions associated with the menstrual events are believed to be significantly mediated by the prostaglandins.

Eventually considerable leakage occurs as a result of diapedesis, and finally, interstitial hemorrhage occurs due to breaks in superficial arterioles and capillaries. As ischemia and weakening progress, the continuous binding membrane is fragmented and intercellular blood is extruded into the endometrial cavity. New thrombin-platelet plugs form intravascularly upstream at the shedding surface, limiting blood loss. Increased blood loss is a consequence of reduced platelet numbers and inadequate hemostatic plug formation. With further tissue disorganization, the endometrium shrinks further and coiled arterioles are buckled. Additional ischemic breakdown ensues with necrosis of cells and defects in vessels adding to the menstrual effluvium. A natural cleavage point exists between basalis and spongiosum, and, once breached, the loose, vascular, edematous stroma of the spongiosum desquamates and collapses. In the end, the typical deflated shallow dense menstrual endometrium results. Menstrual flow stops as a result of the combined effects of prolonged vasoconstriction, tissue collapse, vascular stasis, and estrogen-induced "healing." In contrast to postpartum bleeding, myometrial contractions are not important for control of menstrual bleeding. Resumption of estrogen secretion with its healing effects leads to clot formation over the decapitated stumps of endometrial vessels. Within 13 hours, the endometrial height shrinks from 4 mm to 1.25 mm.[9]

The basalis endometrium remains during menses, and repair takes place from this layer. This endometrium is protected from the lytic enzymes in the menstrual fluid by a mucinous layer of carbohydrate products that are discharged from the glandular and stromal cells.[14] The menstrual fluid is composed of the autolysed functionalis, inflammatory exudate, red blood cells, and proteolytic enzymes (at least one of which, plasmin, lyses fibrin clots as they form). The high fibrinolytic activity advances emptying of the uterus by liquefaction of tissue and fibrin. If the rate of flow is great, clotting can and does occur.

Normal Menses

Most women have menstrual cycles with an interval of 21 to 35 days (Chapter 6). Menarche is followed by approximately 5–7 years of increasing regularity as cycles shorten to reach the usual reproductive age pattern. In the forties, cycles begin to lengthen again. The perfect 28-day cycle is the most common mode, but only 15% of reproductive age cycles are 28 days in length. The usual duration of flow is 4–6 days, but many women flow as little as 2 days and as much as 8 days. The normal volume of menstrual blood loss is 30 mL; greater than 80 mL is abnormal (Chapter 16).

Dating the Endometrium

The postovulatory endometrium can be dated according to the histologic changes throughout a hypothetical 28-day menstrual cycle. These changes were described by Noyes, Hertig, and Rock in the lead article of the first volume of *Fertility and Sterility* in 1950.[6] Dating of the endometrium is most accurately accomplished with biopsy specimens obtained 2–3 days before the onset of menses. This method continues to be the most accepted way to diagnose an inadequate luteal phase (endometrium inadequate to sustain a pregnancy because of deficient progesterone secretion by the corpus luteum).

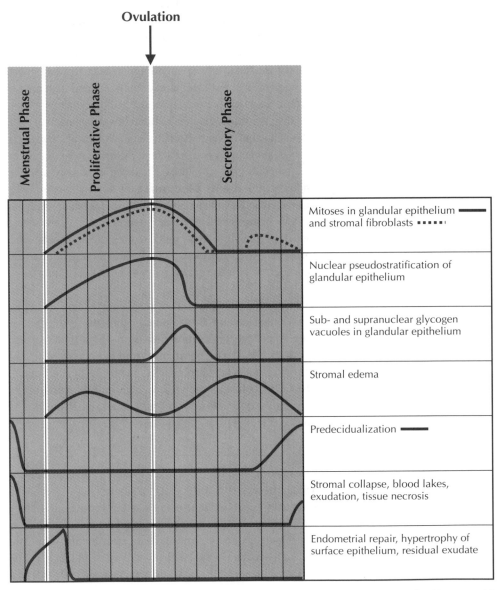

After Noyes, et al [6]

A Teleologic Theory of Endometrial-Menstrual Events

An unabashedly teleologic view of the events just described has been offered by Rock et al.[15] The basic premise of this thesis is that every endometrial cycle has, as its only goal, support of an early embryo. Failure to accomplish this objective is followed by orderly elimination of unutilized tissue and prompt renewal to achieve a more successful cycle.

The ovum must be fertilized within 12–24 hours of ovulation. Over the next 2 days, it remains unattached within the tubal lumen utilizing tubal fluids and residual cumulus cells to sustain nutrition and energy for early cellular cleavage. After this stay, the solid ball of cells (morula) that is the embryo leaves the tube and enters the uterine cavity. Here the embryo undergoes another 2–3 days of unattached but active existence. Fortunately, by this time endometrial gland secretions have filled the cavity and they bathe the embryo in nutrients. This is the first of many neatly synchronized events that mark the conceptus-endometrial relationship. By 6 days after ovulation the embryo (now a blastocyst) is ready to attach and implant. At this time it finds an endometrial lining of sufficient depth, vascularity, and nutritional richness to sustain the important events of early placentation to follow. Just below the epithelial lining, a rich capillary plexus has been formed and is available for creation of the trophoblast-maternal blood interface. Later, the surrounding zona compactum, occupying more and more of the endometrium, will provide a sturdy splint to retain endometrial architecture despite the invasive inroads of the burgeoning trophoblast.

Failure of the appearance of human chorionic gonadotropin, despite otherwise appropriate tissue reactions, leads to the vasomotor changes associated with estrogen-progesterone withdrawal and menstrual desquamation. However, not all the tissue is lost, and, in any event, a residual basalis is always available, making resumption of growth with estrogen a relatively rapid process. Indeed, even as menses persists, early regeneration can be seen. As soon as follicle maturation occurs (in as short a time as 10 days), the endometrium is ready once again to perform its reproductive function.

The Uterus is an Endocrine Organ

The uterus is dynamic. It not only responds and changes in a sensitive fashion to classic hormonal signals (the endocrine events of the menstrual cycle), but it is also composed of complex tissues, with important autocrine/paracrine functions that serve not only the uterus but the contiguous tissues of the fetoplacental unit during pregnancy.

Endometrial Products

The endometrium secretes many substances, the functions of which (and their interrelationships) represent a major investigative challenge. The endometrium plays an important role in suppressing the immune response within the pregnant uterus. The mechanisms controlling the immune response in decidual cells are not understood, but hormonal influence is undoubtedy important.

Because the growth factors are potent mitogens, it is not surprising that the follicular phase of the cycle, associated with proliferative activity of the endometrium, is also marked by dramatic alterations in growth factors. Estrogen stimulates gene expression for epidermal growth factor (EGF) (and its receptor) and insulin-like growth factor (IGF) production. In turn, EGF elicits estrogen-like actions by interacting with the estrogen receptor mechanism.[16] Thus, growth factors can cross-talk with steroid hormone receptors. EGF is present in endometrial stromal and epithelial cells during the follicular phase of the cycle and in the stromal cells during the luteal phase.[17] Transforming growth factor-α (TGF-α) and EGF work through the same receptor and are important mediators of estrogen-induced growth of the endometrium. The presence of the cytokine family, involved in inflammation, is also not surprising in a tissue that undergoes cyclic degeneration.

Lipids	Cytokines	Peptides
Prostaglandins	Interleukin-1α	Prolactin
Thromboxanes	Interleukin-1β	Relaxin
Leukotrienes	Interleukin-6	Renin
	Interferon-γ	Endorphin
	Colony-stimulating factor-1	Epidermal growth factor
		Insulin-like growth factors
		Fibroblast growth factor
		Platelet-derived growth factor
		Transforming growth factor
		IGFBPs
		Corticotropin releasing hormone
		Fibronectin
		Tumor necrosis factor
		Parathyroid hormone-like

The insulin-like growth factors are expressed in a pattern controlled by estrogen and progesterone. IGF-I is predominant in proliferative and early secretory endometrium, while IGF-II appears in the mid to late secretory phase and persists in early pregnancy decidua.[18] This suggests that IGF-I mediates estrogen-induced growth, and IGF-II is involved in differentiation in response to progesterone.

Human myometrial smooth muscle and endometrial stromal cells express mRNA for parathyroid hormone-like protein, the function of which is unknown.[19] Transforming growth factor-β (TGF-β) stimulates the production of the parathyroid hormone-like protein. The chorion laeve, villous trophoblast, and decidua are all sites of TGF-β production.[20] TGF-β can signal its own production; thus, TGF-β can be a messenger from fetal tissues to decidua.

Prostaglandins are produced by both epithelial and stromal cells, and the prostaglandin content in the endometrium reaches a peak level in late secretory endometrium. The predominant prostaglandin produced by endometrium is prostaglandin $F_{2\alpha}$, a potent stimulus for myometrial contractions.[21] Endometrial prostaglandin production decreases dramatically after implantation, suggesting the presence of an active mechanism for suppression.[22] The production of prostaglandins requires estrogen support, but the increased production by secretory endometrium suggests progesterone enhancement, and acute withdrawal of progesterone further promotes an increase.[21] Endometrial stromal cells produce prostacyclin and thromboxane in response to estrogen, a response that can be blocked by progestins.[23] The myometrium principally produces prostacyclin, utilizing precursors derived from the endometrium. However, receptors for all members of the prostaglandin family are present on human myometrial cells, and contraction of the myometrium is a major consequence of prostaglandin $F_{2\alpha}$.[24]

Thromboxane is synthesized by uterine tissues. Gene expression for the thromboxane synthase and for the thromboxane receptor can be identified in endometrial glands, stromal cells, myometrial smooth muscle, and uterine blood vessels.[25] Thromboxane A_2

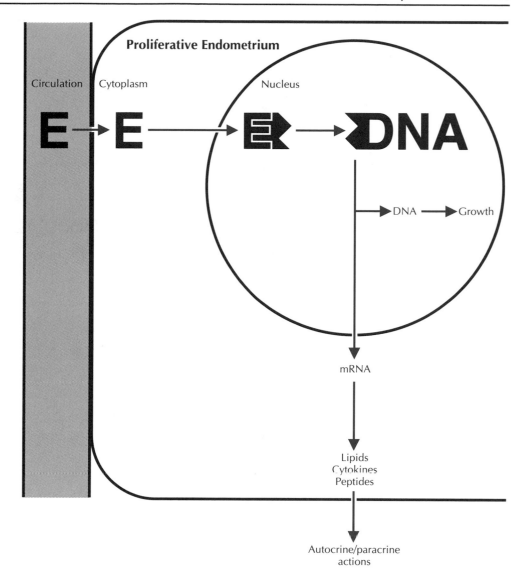

is a potent vasoconstrictor and stimulator of smooth muscle cells. Because of its rapid metabolism, it is limited to autocrine/paracrine activity.

Women with excessive menstrual bleeding have alterations in the normal rates of prostaglandin production. For this reason, effective reductions in menstrual blood loss can be achieved with treatment utilizing one of the nonsteroidal anti-inflammatory agents that inhibit prostaglandin synthesis. These agents are also effective treatment for prostaglandin-mediated dysmenorrhea.

Fibronectin is an extracellular matrix substance that is secreted by stromal cells and epithelial cells of the endometrium. Its secretion is suppressed by progesterone.[26] This suppression would reduce the action of fibronectin in binding heparin sulfate proteoglycans that are important in the attachment of the embryo.

Uteroglobin is a small protein expressed in endometrial epithelial cells.[27] The physiologic function of uteroglobin is uncertain. Uteroglobin, with high affinity, binds progestins and may play a role in immunosuppression. Uteroglobin gene expression is stimulated by estrogen, and this response is enhanced by progesterone. Human endometrium can secrete β-endorphin, yet another candidate for involvment in endometrial immunologic events, and its release is inhibited by both estrogens and

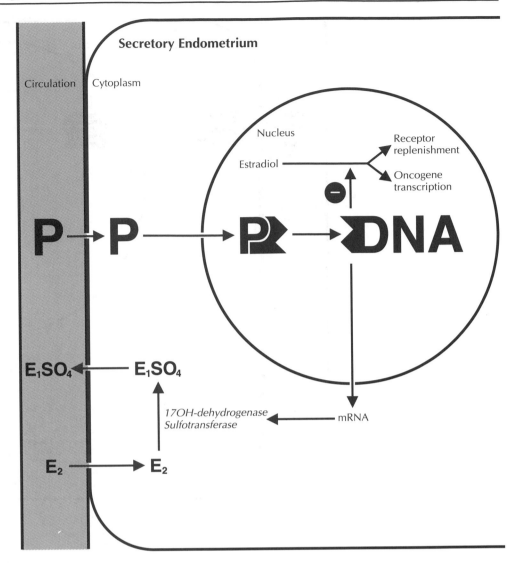

glucocorticoids.[28] Tumor necrosis factor-α (TNF-α) gene expression is present in endometrium, and its activity is increased during the proliferative phase, decreased early in the secretory phase, and increased again in the midsecretory phase.[29] TNF-α exerts multiple influences on cellular growth.

Endothelin-1 is a potent vasoconstrictor, but its vasoconstrictor activity is balanced by the fact that it promotes the synthesis of endothelium-derived relaxing factor and prostacyclin. Endothelin-1 is synthesized in endometrial stromal cells and the glandular epithelium, stimulated by both TGF-β and interleukin-1α.[30] Endothelin-1 may be at least one agent that is responsible for the vasoconstriction that shuts off menstrual bleeding. It is also a potent stimulator of myometrial contractions and can contribute to dysmenorrhea. Finally, endothelin-1 is also a mitogen and can promote the healing reepithelialization of the endometrium. Human decidual cells also synthesize and secrete endothelin-1, from where it may be transported into the amniotic fluid.[31]

Angiogenesis, the formation of new blood vessels, is an essential process in tissue growth and development. Angiogenesis is necessary for tumor growth, and in normal tissues, it is usually kept in check by regulating factors. The female reproductive tissues (specifically ovarian follicles, trophoblast, and the endometrium), however, must experience periodic and rapid growth and regression. In these tissues, angiogenesis is part of normal events. The endometrium is a major source for angiogenic factors during the menstrual cycle and during pregnancy.[32] Angiogenesis is also influenced by many of the growth factors, and other substances such as fibronectin and prostaglandins.

In all types of endometrial and myometrial cells, estrogen receptor expression reaches a maximum in the late follicular phase.[33,34] During the early luteal phase, estrogen receptor expression declines, followed by an increase in the mid and late luteal phases. These changes reflect the cyclic changes in estradiol (which increases estrogen receptor expression) and progesterone (which decreases estrogen receptor expression).

Progesterone receptor expression in endometrial glandular epithelium reaches a maximum in the late follicular and early luteal phases, then declines. Stromal cells in the endometrium show only minor fluctuations during the menstrual cycle. Decidualizing stromal cells exhibit strong progesterone receptor expression, although progesterone receptors are absent from decidual epithelial cells. Smooth muscle cells of the uterus demonstrate strong progesterone receptor expression throughout the menstrual cycle. Androgen receptor is present in endometrium at all stages of the menstrual cycle, in postmenopausal endometrium, and in the decidua of pregnancy.[35] Surprisingly, the androgen receptor concentration is constant throughout the cycle. Many of the events in uterine growth and function are regulated by the interplay between estrogen and progesterone. In general, progesterone antagonizes estrogen stimulation of proliferation and metabolism. This antagonism can be explained by the effects of progestins on the estrogen receptor (a decrease in levels) and on the enzymes that lead to excretion of estrogen from cells and by progesterone suppression of estrogen-mediated transcription of oncogenes.

The Decidua

The decidua is the specialized endometrium of pregnancy. The biochemical dialogue between the fetoplacental unit and the mother must pass back and forth through the decidua. The classic view of the decidua conformed to its designation as a thin line in anatomical diagrams, a minor, inactive structural component. We now know that the decidua is a vigorous, active tissue.

Decidual cells are derived from the stroma cells of the endometrium, under the stimulation of progesterone. Thus, they appear during the luteal phase and continue to proliferate during early pregnancy, eventually lining the entire uterus, including the implantation site. The decidual cell is characterized by the accumulation of glycogen and lipid droplets and the new expression of a host of substances, including prolactin, relaxin, renin, insulin-like growth factors (IGFs), and insulin-like growth factor binding proteins (IGFBPs). There is no evidence that these proteins are secreted into the circulation, therefore they serve as autocrine/paracrine agents.[36,37]

Riddick was the first to detect prolactin in the decidualizing endometrium of the late luteal phase.[38] The amino acid sequence and the chemical and biological properties of decidual prolactin are identical to those of pituitary prolactin. Decidual prolactin synthesis and release are controlled by the placenta, fetal membranes, and decidual factors. Dopamine, bromocriptine, and thyroid releasing hormone (TRH), in contrast to their action in the pituitary, have no effect on decidual synthesis and release of prolactin. A protein named decidual prolactin-releasing factor has been purified from the placenta, and an inhibiting protein, which blocks the stimulatory activity of the releasing factor, has been purified from decidua.[37] IGF-1, relaxin, and insulin all stimulate decidual prolactin synthesis and release, each through its own receptor. The same decidual cells produce both prolactin and relaxin.

Lipocortin-1 is a calcium and phospholipid binding protein, present in the placenta and decidua, that inhibits phospholipase A_2 and responds to glucocorticoids. Lipocortin-1 inhibits decidual prolactin release but in a mechanism independent of phospholipase action and independent of glucocorticoids. The prostaglandin system is not involved in decidual prolactin production, and corticoid steroids do not affect decidual prolactin release.[39]

There is good reason to believe that the amniotic fluid prolactin is derived from the decidua. In vitro experiments indicate that the passage of prolactin across the fetal membranes is in the direction of the amniotic cavity. The amniotic fluid concentration correlates with the decidual content, not maternal circulating levels. Amniotic fluid prolactin reaches peak levels in the first half of gestation (about 4,000 ng/mL [180 nmol/L]) when maternal plasma levels are approximately 50 ng/mL (2,220 pmol/L) and fetal levels about 10 ng/mL (440 pmol/L). Maternal circulating prolactin reaches maximal levels near term. Finally, amniotic fluid prolactin is unaffected by bromocriptine treatment (which reduces both fetal and maternal circulating levels to baseline levels).

It is believed that decidual prolactin regulates amniotic fluid volume and electrolyte concentrations. It can be demonstrated that prolactin regulates water and ion transport in lower animals, and prolactin binds to amniotic membranes. Disorders in human pregnancy associated with abnormal amniotic fluid volumes may be explained by this mechanism, especially idiopathic polyhydramnios (which is associated with a decrease in the number of prolactin receptors in the membranes). Prolactin may be involved in the regulation of surfactant synthesis in the fetus, and prolactin may inhibit uterine muscle contractility. Prolactin also suppresses the immune response and contributes to the prevention of immunologic rejection of the conceptus.

Fibroblast growth factor, derived from decidua, stimulates blood vessel growth in early pregnancy. Another factor, endothelial-cell-stimulating angiogenesis factor (a nonprotein mitogen), is also derived from decidua and contributes to the vascularization of the decidua during the first trimester of pregnancy.[40] The expression of corticotropin releasing hormone (CRH) has been demonstrated in human decidua, and many actions for decidual CRH are possible: activation of prostaglandins, stimulation of myometrial contractions, and a contribution to both maternal and fetal stress responses during pregnancy and labor.[41]

Prorenin (the inactive precursor of renin) is produced in decidua in response to IGF-1, insulin, endothelin, and relaxin.[42,43] The insulin-like growth factor binding proteins, IGFBP-1, -2, -3, and -4, are produced by endometrial stromal cells.[44] Although their exact function is unknown, it is likely that IGFBPs modulate the action of the IGFs. Large amounts of IGFBP-1 are present in amniotic fluid. The IGFBPs appear to be regulated by insulin, the IGFs, and relaxin.[45]

IGFBP-1 begins to appear in midluteal phase endometrium and reaches a level of major production in decidua by late in the first trimester of pregnancy. IGFBP-1, when first identified, was known as endometrial protein 12 and then as pregnancy-associated α-globulin. By the second trimester of pregnancy high levels of IGFBP-1 are present in the amniotic fluid, which then fall significantly during the third trimester. The decidual production of IGFBP-1 is correlated with the morphologic and histologic changes induced by progesterone. Binding of the insulin-like growth factors to the IGFBPs would limit further mitogenic activity in the endometrium in the secretory phase and during pregnancy.

The continuous stimulation of IGFBP-1 production by human endometrium can be maintained in women as long as they retain an intrauterine device that releases a progestin into the endometrial cavity.[46] In endometrial samples from these women, areas of endometrial atrophy correlate with intense staining for IGFBP-1. This makes a strong argument for the importance of insulin-like growth factors for endometrial growth and the potential for prevention of endometrial growth by providing IGFBP-1.

Anatomical Abnormalities of the Uterus

Congenital abnormalities of the müllerian ducts are relatively common and contribute to the problems of infertility, recurrent pregnancy loss, and poor outcome in pregnancy (encountered in approximately 25% of women with uterine anomalies).[47–50] The problems encountered in pregnancy include preterm labor, breech presentations, and complications that lead to interventions and greater perinatal mortality. Cervical cerclage is often indicated for prevention of preterm labor due to these anomalies. In addition, these abnormalities can produce the symptoms of dysmenorrhea and dyspareunia, and even amenorrhea. Because the embryologic origin of the ovaries is separate and distinct from that of the müllerian structures, patients with müllerian anomalies have normal ovaries and ovarian function.

Anomalies can originate in the failure of the müllerian ducts to fuse in the midline, to connect with the urogenital sinus, or to create the appropriate lumen in the upper vagina and uterus by resorption of the central vaginal cells and the septum between the fused müllerian ducts. Because fusion begins in the midline and extends caudally and cephalad, abnormal results can exist at either end. Formation of the uterine cavity begins at the lower pole and extends cephalad with dissolution of midline tissue; hence, incomplete resorbtion of tissue commonly yields persistence of midline uterine wall intruding into the cavity. The molecular pathophysiology of these abnormalities has been insufficiently studied; however, the association with other somatic anomalies and occasional reports of familial transmission suggest genetic linkages.

Vaginal outflow tract obstruction can be minimal with a transverse septum or complete due to agenesis. A septum is the result of a defect in the connection of the fused müllerian ducts to the urogenital sinus or a failure of canalization of the vagina. Vaginal agenesis is the result of a complete failure in canalization. These patients present with amenorrhea or pain due to accumulated menstrual effluvium. Surgical correction is frequently necessary to relieve the relative constriction (and obstruction) of the vaginal canal. An absent vagina is usually accompanied by an absent uterus and tubes, the classic müllerian agenesis of the Mayer-Rokitansky-Kuster-Hauser syndrome (discussed in Chapter 12).

Uterine anomalies can be organized into the following categories.[51]

Unicornuate Uterus

An abnormality that is unilateral obviously is due to a failure of development in one müllerian duct (probably a failure of one duct to migrate to the proper location). The altered uterine configuration is associated with an increase in obstetrical complications (abnormal presentations, intrauterine growth retardation, premature labor, and incompetent cervix). There may be a rudimentary horn present, and implantation in this horn is followed by a very high rate of pregnancy wastage or tubal pregnancies. A rudimentary horn can also be a cause of chronic pain, and surgical excision may be worthwhile.

Uterus Didelphus

Lack of fusion of the two müllerian ducts results in duplication of corpus and cervix. These patients usually have no difficulties with menstruation and coitus. Occasionally, one side is obstructed and symptomatic. Pregnancy is associated with an increased risk of malpresentations and premature labor.

The Bicornuate Uterus

Partial lack of fusion of the two müllerian ducts produces a single cervix with a varying degree of separation in the two uterine horns. This anomaly is relatively common, and pregnancy outcome has usually been reported to be near normal. Some, however, find a high rate of early abortion, preterm labor, and breech presentations.[50]

Classification of Müllerian Anomalies[51]

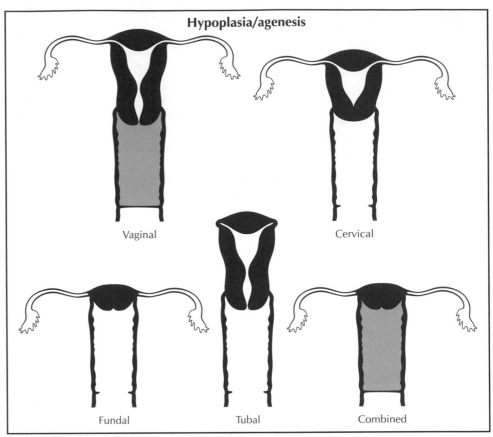

Hypoplasia/agenesis

Vaginal

Cervical

Fundal

Tubal

Combined

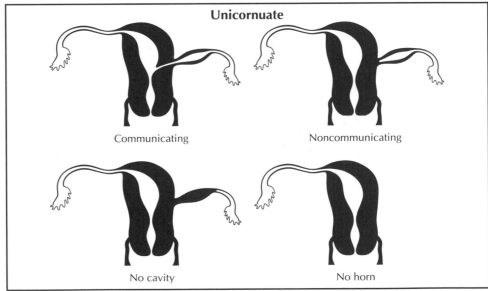

Unicornuate

Communicating

Noncommunicating

No cavity

No horn

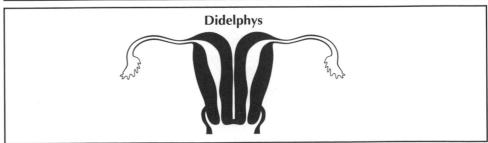

Didelphys

Classification of Müllerian Anomalies[51]

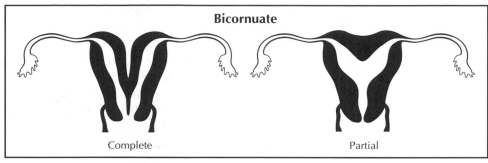

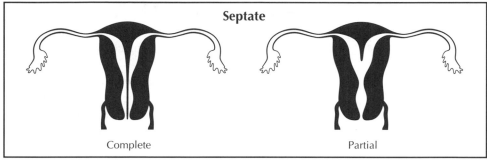

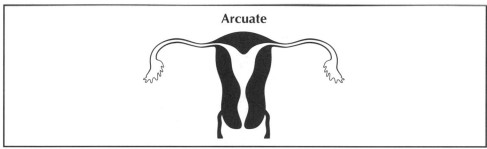

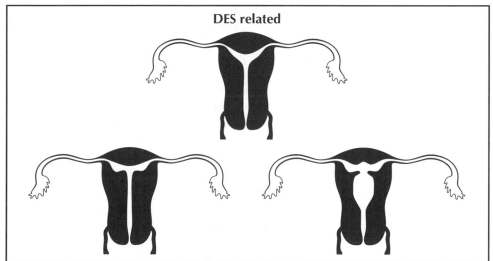

The Septate Uterus

Partial lack of resorption of the midline septum between the two müllerian ducts results in defects that range from a slight midline septum (the arcuate, heart-shaped cavity) to a significant midline division of the endometrial cavity. A total failure in resorption can leave a longitudinal vaginal septum (a double vagina). This defect is not a cause of infertility, but once pregnant, the greater the septum the greater the risk of recurrent spontaneous abortion. The complete septate uterus is associated with a high risk of preterm labor and breech presentation.[50] Outcomes are excellent with treatment by hysteroscopy.[52] Posttreatment abortion rates are approximately 10% in contrast to the 90% pretreatment rates. A longitudinal vaginal septum usually does not have to be excised (unless dyspareunia is a problem).

Very Rare Anomalies

Isolated agenesis of the cervix or the endometrium is incredibly rare. Absence of the cervix can lead to so much pain and obstruction that hysterectomy is the only solution.

The Diethylstilbestrol-Associated Anomaly

We are still encountering women whose mothers were treated with high doses of estrogen during their pregnancies. Exposure to these high levels of estrogen during müllerian development caused a variety of anomalies, ranging from the hypoplastic "T" shaped uterus to irregular cavities with adhesions. Women with uterine abnormalities usually also have cervical defects. In these individuals, the chance of term pregnancy is decreased because of higher risks of ectopic pregnancy, spontaneous abortion, and premature labor. An incompetent cervix is common. Poor outcome is correlated with an abnormal uterus on hysterosalpingography. No treatment is available beyond cervical cerclage.

Diagnosis. In the past full diagnosis has required surgical intervention, first laparotomy and then, more recently, laparoscopy. Today, vaginal ultrasonography and magnetic resonance imaging are highly accurate, and surgical intervention is usually not necessary.[53] Hysterosalpingography is relatively inaccurate, and decisions should not be based upon hysterosalpingography alone. Congenital anomalies of the müllerian ducts are frequently accompanied by abnormalities in the urinary tract. Renal agenesis is often present on the same side as a müllerian defect.

Leiomyomata (Uterine Fibroids)

Uterine leiomyomas are benign neoplasms that arise from uterine smooth muscle. It is hypothesized that leiomyomas originate from somatic mutations in myometrial cells, resulting in progressive loss of growth regulation.[54] The tumor grows as genetically abnormal clones of cells derived from a single progenitor cell (in which the original mutation took place). Studies indicate that leiomyomas are monoclonal. Different rates of growth can reflect the different cytogenetic abnormalities present in individual tumors. Multiple myomas within the same uterus are not clonally related; each myoma arises independently. The presence of multiple myomas (which have a higher recurrence rate than single myomas) argues in favor of a genetic predisposition for myoma formation; however, the familial inheritance of uterine myomas has not been well studied. It is not certain whether leiomyosarcomas arise independently or from leiomyomas.

If surgical specimens are serially sectioned, about 77% of women who come to hysterectomy will have myomas, many of which are occult.[55] Overall, about 17% of hysterectomies are performed for myomas in the U.S. (44% in women 45–54 years old).[56] The peak incidence for myomas requiring surgery occurs around age 45, approximately 8 cases per 1,000 women each year. In the U.S., approximately 10–15% of women require hysterectomy for myomas.

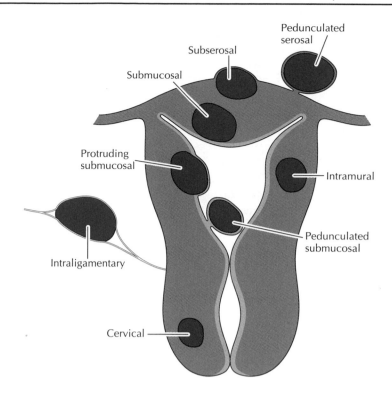

Myomas will be encountered in about 1% of pregnant women. The risk of myoma is decreased with increasing parity and with increasing age at last term birth. Women with at least two full term pregnancies have half the risk for myomas. Smoking decreases the risk (presumably by decreasing estrogen levels), and obesity increases the risk (presumably by increasing estrogen levels). Indeed, a lower risk for myomas is associated with factors that decrease estrogen levels, including leaness, smoking, and exercise. The use of oral contraceptives is not associated with an increased risk of uterine myomas.[57]

The hormone sensitivity of leiomyomas is indicated by the following clinical observations. Leiomyomas develop during the reproductive (hormonally active) years and regress after menopause. Occasionally, leiomyomas grow during pregnancy, and the hypogonadal state induced by treatment with gonadotropin releasing hormone (GnRH) agonists often causes shrinkage of myomas.

The environment within the leiomyoma is hyperestrogenic. The estradiol concentration is increased, and leiomyomas contain more estrogen receptors.[58,59] Endometrial hyperplasia is frequently observed at the margins of submucous myomas.[60] In the myometrium and in leiomyomas, peak mitotic activity occurs during the luteal phase, and mitotic activity is increased by the administration of high doses of progestational agents.[61,62] These facts indicate that progesterone stimulates mitotic activity in leiomyomas, but animal studies indicate both stimulation and inhibition of myometrial growth. Similarly, clinicians have reported both regression and growth with progestational treatment. Nevertheless, most of the evidence supports a growth-promoting role for progestins (the association with estrogen can be explained by the estrogen enhancement of progesterone receptor expression).[63] Treatment with RU486, the progesterone antagonist, is associated with a reduction in leiomyomata size.[64]

As in the normal uterus, the effects of estrogen and progestins on leiomyomata are mediated by growth factors. EGF receptors are present in leiomyomata, and GnRH agonist treatment (and hypogonadism) decreases EGF concentration in myomas (but not in normal myometrium).[65] IGF-I and IGF-II and their receptors are abundant in myometrium, and actively expressed in leiomyomas.[66] Leiomyomas express more IGF-II and less IGFBP-3 compared to myometrium, a situation which would enhance growth factor availability and activity in the tumor.[67] Like the endometrium and myometrium, leiomyomas secrete prolactin. Even hematopoiesis is possible in a leiomyoma.[68]

Reproductive Function and Leiomyomata

Leiomyomas are an infrequent cause of infertility, either by mechanical obstruction or distortion (and interference with implantation).[69] Most women with myomas are fertile. When a mechanical obstruction of fallopian tubes, cervical canal, or endometrial cavity is present and no other cause of infertility or recurrent abortion can be identified, myomectomy is usually followed by a prompt achievement of pregnancy in a high percentage of patients (usually within the first year).[70] Submucous myomas are best treated by hysteroscopic resection. Preoperative visualization is important, and mapping of myomas by magnetic resonance imaging (MRI) is superior to ultrasonography (which is relatively inaccurate).[71] It is difficult to distinguish between submucous myomas and endometrial polyps with ultrasonography.[72] Very large myomas (greater than 4–5 cm) and myomas that do not have greater than 50% protrusion into the cavity are not good candidates for hysteroscopic removal.

The recurrence rate after myomectomy is about 15%, with subsequent hysterectomy necessary in 1–5% of patients.[73] In a series with long follow-up, the recurrence rate over 10 years reached 27%.[74] Women who gave birth after myomectomy had a recurrence rate (over 10 years) of 16%, compared to a rate of 28% in those who did not give birth.

An increased incidence of spontaneous abortion because of myomas has not been definitively documented in the literature. Myomectomy for infertility or recurrent abortion requires a deliberate and careful decision after all factors have been considered. Intracavitory myomas, however, usually require surgery. Because of the rapid regrowth of myomas following cessation of GnRH agonist therapy, medical therapy for infertility is not recommended.

Most myomas do not grow during pregnancy.[75] When they do, most of the growth is in the first trimester, and most myomas regress in size after the pregnancy. The size of a myoma will not predict its course; large myomas will not necessarily grow more than a small one. So-called red degeneration of myomas is occasionally observed during pregnancy, a condition due to central hemorrhagic infarction of the myoma. Pain is the hallmark of this condition, occasionally associated with rebound tenderness, mild fever, leukocytosis, nausea, and vomiting. Usually pain is the only symptom and resolution follows rest and analgesic treatment.[76] Surgery should be a last resort. The larger the myoma, the greater the risk of premature labor.[77]

Medical Therapy of Leiomyomata

The goals of medical therapy for leiomyomas are to temporarily reduce symptoms and to reduce myoma size, and the therapy of choice is treatment with a GnRH agonist.[78]

The short half-life of GnRH is due to rapid cleavage of the bonds between amino acids 5–6, 6–7, and 9–10. By altering amino acids at these positions, analogues of GnRH can be synthesized with different properties. Substitution of amino acids at the 6 position or replacement of the C-terminal glycine-amide (inhibiting degradation) produces agonists. The GnRH agonists are administered either intramuscularly, subcutaneously, or by intranasal absorption. An initial agonistic action (the so-called flare effect) is associated with an increase in the circulating levels of follicle-stimulating hormone (FSH) and luteinizing hormone (LH). This response is greatest in the early follicular phase when GnRH and estradiol have combined to create a large reserve pool of gonadotropins. After 1–3 weeks, down-regulation and densensitization of the pituitary produce a hypo-gonadotropic, hypogonad state. The initial response is due to a loss of receptors, while the sustained response is due to desensitization, the uncoupling of the receptor from its effector system. Furthermore, postreceptor mechanisms lead to secretion of biologically inactive gonadotropins, which, however, can still be detected by immunoassay.

The GnRH analogues cannot escape destruction if administered orally. Higher doses administered subcutaneously can achieve nearly equal effects as observed with intravenous treatment; however, the smaller blood peaks are slower to develop and take longer to return to baseline. Other forms of administration include nasal spray, sustained release implants, and injections of biodegradable microspheres.

Treatment with GnRH Agonists

Summarizing the experience with GnRH agonist treatment of leiomyomata, the mean uterine size decreases 30–64% after 3–6 months of treatment.[78] Maximal response is usually achieved by 3 months. The reduction in size correlates with the estradiol level and with body weight. Menorrhagia, anemia, pelvic pressure, and urinary frequency all respond favorably to GnRH agonist treatment. A decrease in operative blood loss is significant when the uterus is the size of a 16 week pregnancy. Why is there a variation in response? When one considers the many factors involved in myoma growth (estrogen, progesterone, growth factors, receptors), it makes sense that not every myoma is the same. After cessation of GnRH agonist therapy, menses return in 4–10 weeks, and myoma and uterine size return to pretreatment levels in 3–4 months.

Preoperative GnRH agonist therapy offers several advantages for hysteroscopic removal of submucous tumors. In addition to a decrease in myoma size, endometrial atrophy will improve visualization, and decreased vascularity will reduce blood loss.

Leiomyomatosis Peritonealis Disseminata is a condition in which multiple small nodules of benign smooth muscle are found throughout the abdominal cavity, and occasionally in the pulmonary cavity. This condition appears to be sensitive to estrogen because it has been aggravated by postmenopausal estrogen treatment, and regression has been achieved with GnRH agonist treatment.[79]

Adenomyosis is the ectopic presence of endometrial glands within the myometrium. This diagnosis can be made by magnetic resonance imaging, and successful treatment with a GnRH agonist has been reported.[80,81]

Side Effects with GnRH Agonists

Hot flushes are experienced by more than 75% of patients, usually in 3–4 weeks after beginning treatment. Approximately 5–15% of patients will complain of headache, vaginal dryness, joint and muscle stiffness, and depression. About 30% of patients will continue to have irregular (although light) vaginal bleeding. It is useful to measure the circulating estradiol level. If the level is greater than 30 pg/mL (110 pmol/L), suppression is inadequate. On the other hand, Friedman and colleagues have suggested that maintaining the estradiol level in the early follicular phase range (30–50 pg/mL [110–180 pmol/L]) can protect against osteoporosis and reduce hot flushes, but not allow the growth of myomas.[82] The efficacy of this titration of response requires validation by clinical studies.

A small number (10%) of patients will experience a localized allergic reaction at the site of injection of depot forms of GnRH analogues. More serious reaction is rare, but immediate and delayed anaphylaxis can occur, requiring intense support and management.[83]

Bone loss occurs with GnRH therapy, but not in everyone, and it is reversible (although it is not certain if it is totally reversible in all patients). A significant vaginal hemorrhage 5–10 weeks after beginning treatment is encountered in about 2% of treated women, due to degeneration and necrosis of submucous myomas.[84] A disadvantage of agonist treatment is a delay in diagnosis of a leiomyosarcoma. Keep in mind that almost all leiomyosarcomas present as the largest or only uterine mass. Close monitoring is necessary and surgery is indicated when either enlargement or no shrinkage of myomas occurs during GnRH agonist treatment.[85] The use of Doppler ultrasonography or magnetic resonance imaging offer greater accuracy of evaluation.

Escape of suppression can result in an unexpected pregnancy. No adverse effects of fetal exposure to GnRH agonists have been reported, even when exposure has persisted throughout the early weeks of pregnancy.[86]

GnRH Agonists and Steroid Add-Back

Treatment with a GnRH agonist with steroid add-back has been explored to permit long-term therapy without bone loss.[78] Two strategies have been employed: simultaneous agonist and steroid add-back treatment or a sequential regimen in which the agonist is used alone for 3–6 months, followed by the combination of the agonist and steroid add-back. This long-term treatment is attractive for women who are perimenopausal, perhaps avoiding surgery. In addition, long-term treatment would be useful for women with coagulopathies, and in women with medical problems who need to postpone surgery.

Simultaneous treatment with agonist and medroxyprogesterone acetate (20 mg orally daily) effectively reduced hot flushing, but was less effective in reducing uterine volume.[78] A sequential program, adding a traditional postmenopausal hormone regimen (0.625 mg conjugated estrogens on days 1–25 and 10 mg medroxyprogesterone acetate on days 16–25) effectively reduced uterine volume and maintained the reduced volume for 2 years (and avoided any loss in bone density).[78] We recommend 3–6 months of GnRH agonist treatment followed by agonist treatment combined with a daily, continuous add-back of estrogen and progestin (0.625 mg conjugated estrogens or 1.0 mg estradiol and 2.5 mg medroxyprogesterone acetate or 0.35 mg norethindrone). In view of the sensitivity of leiomyomata tissue to progestational agents, it makes sense to keep the dose of progestin relatively low.

Summary of Clinical Advantages with GnRH Treatment

Reduction in menstrual blood loss.
Improvement in anemia prior to surgery.
Time for autologous blood donation.
Less operative blood loss.
Hysterectomy less likely.
More likely to allow laparoscopic technique.
Possible conversion from abdominal to vaginal hysterectomy.

References

1. **Graham H,** *Eternal Eve, The History of Gynaecology & Obstetrics,* Doubleday & Company, Inc., Garden City, 1951.

2. **Medvei VC,** *A History of Endocrinology,* MTP Press Limited, Lancaster, England, 1982.

3. **Magner LN,** *A History of Medicine,* Marcel Dekker, Inc., New York, 1992.

4. **Jost A, Vigier B, Prepin J, Perchellet JP,** Studies on sex differentiation in mammals, Recent Prog Horm Res 29:1, 1973.

5. **Ferenczy A, Bergeron C,** Histology of the human endometrium: from birth to senescence, in Bulletti C, Gurpide E, editors, *The Primate Endometrium,* The New York Academy of Sciences, New York, 1991, pp 6-27.

6. **Noyes RW, Hertig AW, Rock J,** Dating the endometrial biopsy, Fertil Steril 1:3, 1950.

7. **Bartlemez GW,** The phases of the menstrual cycle and their interpretation in terms of the pregnancy cycle, Am J Obstet Gynecol 74:931, 1957.

8. **Markee JE,** Morphological basis for menstrual bleeding, Bull NY Acad Med 24:253, 1948.

9. **Christiaens GCML, Sixma JJ, Haspels AA,** Hemostasis in menstrual endometrium: a review, Obstet Gynecol Survey 37:281, 1982.

10. **Ludwig H, Spornitz UM,** Microarchitecture of the human endometrium by scanning electron microscopy: menstrual desquamation and remodeling, in Bulletti C, Gurpide E, editors, *The Primate Endometrium,* The New York Academy of Sciences, New York, 1991, pp 28-46.

11. **Gurpide E, Gusberg S, Tseng L,** Estradiol binding and metabolism in human endometrial hyperplasia and adenocarcinoma, J Steroid Biochem 7:891, 1976.

12. **Kirkland JL, Murthy L, Stancel GM,** Progesterone inhibits the estrogen-induced expression of *c-fos* messenger ribonucleic acid in the uterus, Endocrinology 130:3223, 1992.

13. **Rodgers WH, Osteen KG, Matrisian LM, Navre M, Giudice LC, Gorstein F,** Expression and localization of matrilysin, a matrix metalloproteinase, in human endometrium during the reproductive cycle, Am J Obstet Gynecol 168:253, 1993.

14. **Wilborn WH, Flowers CE Jr,** Cellular mechanisms for endometrial conservation during menstrual bleeding, Seminars Reprod Endocrinol 2:307, 1984.

15. **Rock J, Garcia CR, Menkin M,** A theory of menstruation, Ann NY Acad Sci 75:830, 1959.

16. **Ignar-Trowbridge DM, Nelson KG, Bidwell MC, Curtis SW, Washburn TF, McLachlan JA, Korach KS,** Coupling of dual signaling pathways: epidermal growth factor action involves the estrogen receptor, Proc Natl Acad Sci USA 89:4658, 1992.

17. **Hofmann GE, Scott RT Jr, Bergh PA, Deligdisch L,** Immunohistochemical localization of epidermal growth factor in human endometrium, decidua, and placenta, J Clin Endocrinol Metab 73:882, 1991.

18. **Giudice LC, Dsupin BA, Jin IH, Vu TH, Hoffman AR,** Differential expression of messenger ribonucleic acids encoding insulin-like growth factors and their receptors in human uterine endometrium and decidua, J Clin Endocrinol Metab 76:1115, 1993.

19. **Casey ML, Mibe M, Erk A, MacDonald PC,** Transforming growth factor-β stimulation of parathyroid hormone-rleated protein expression in human uterine cells in culture: mRNA levels and protein secretion, J Clin Endocrinol Metab 74:950, 1992.

20. **Kauma S, Matt D, Strom S, Eierman D, Turner T,** Interleukin-1β, human leukocyte antigen HLA-DRα, and transforming growth factor-β expression in endometrium, placenta, and placental membranes, Am J Obstet Gynecol 163:1430, 1990.

21. **Eldering JA, Nay MG, Hoberg LM, Longcope C, McCracken JA,** Hormonal regulation of prostaglandin production by Rhesus monkey endometrium, J Clin Endocrinol Metab 71:596, 1990.

22. **Maathuis JB, Kelly RW,** Concentrations of prostaglandin $F_{2\alpha}$ and E_2 in the endometrium thorughout the human menstrual cycle after the administration of clomiphene or an oestrogen-progesterone pill and in early pregnancy, J Endocrinol 77:361, 1978.

23. **Levin JH, Stanczyk FZ, Lobo RA,** Estradiol stimulates the secretion of prostacylin and thromboxane from endometrial stromal cells in culture, Fertil Steril 58:530, 1992.

24. **Senior J, Sangha R, Baxter GS, Marshall K, Clayton JK,** In vitro characterization of prostanoid FP- DP- IP- and TP-receptors on the non-pregnant human myometrium, Br J Pharmacol 107:215, 1992.

25. **Swanson ML, Lei ZM, Swanson PH, Rao ChV, Narumiya S, Hirata M,** The expression of thromboxane A_2 synthase and thromboxane A_2 receptor gene in human uterus, Biol Reprod 47:105, 1992.

26. **Mularoni A, Mahfoudi A, Beck L, Coosemans V, Bride J, Nicollier M, Adessi GL,** Progesterone control of fibronectin secretion in guinea pig endometrium, Endocrinology 131:2127, 1992.

27. **Helftenbein G, Misseyanni A, Hagen G, Peter W, Slater EP, Wiehle RD, Suske G, Beato M,** Expression of the uteroglobin promoter in epithelial cell lines from endometrium, in Bulletti C, Gurpide E, editors, *The Primate Endometrium,* The New York Academy of Sciences, New York, 1991, pp 69-79.

28. **Makrigiannakis A, Margioris A, Markogiannakis E, Stournaras C, Gravanis A,** Steroid hormones regulate the release of immunoreactive β-endorphin from the Ishikawa human endometrial cell line, J Clin Endocrinol Metab 75:584, 1992.

29. **Hunt JS, Chen H-L, Hu X-L, Tabibzadeh S,** Tumor necrosis factor-α messenger ribonucleic acid and protein in human endometrium, Biol Reprod 47:141, 1992.

30. **Economos K, MacDonald PC, Casey ML,** Endothelin-1 gene expression and protein biosynthesis in human endometrium: potential modulator of endometrial blood flow, J Clin Endocrinol Metab 74:14, 1992.

31. **Kubota T, Kamada S, Hirata Y, Eguchi S, Imai T, Marumo F, Aso T,** Synthesis and release of endothelin-1 by human decidual cells, J Clin Endocrinol Metab 75:1230, 1992.

32. **Reynolds LP, Killilea SD, Redmer DA,** Angiogenesis in the female reproductive system, FASEB J 6:886, 1992.

33. **Lessey BA, Killiam AP, Metzger DA, Haney AF, Greene GL, McCarty KS,** Immunohistochemical analysis of uterine estrogen and progesterone receptors throughout the menstrual cycle, J Clin Endocrinol Metab 67:334, 1988.

34. **Snijders MPML, de Goeij AFPM, Debets-Te Baerts MJC, Rousch MJM, Koudstaal J, Bosman FT,** Immunocytochemical analysis of oestrogen receptors and progesterone receptors in the human uterus throughout the menstrual cycle and after the menopause, J Reprod Fertil 94:363, 1992.

35. **Horie K, Takakura K, Imai K, Liao S, Mori T,** Immunohistochemical localization of androgen receptor in the human endometrium, decidua, placenta and pathological conditions of the endometrium, Hum Reprod 7:1461, 1992.

36. **Handwerger S, Richards RG, Markoff E,** The physiology of decidual prolactin and other decidual protein hormones, Trends Endocrinol Metab 3:91, 1992.

37. **Handwerger S, Harman I, Golander A, Handwerger DA,** Prolactin release from perifused human decidual explants: effects of decidual prolactin-releasing factor (PRL-RF) and prolactin release-inhibitory factor (PRL-IF), Placenta 13:55, 1992.

38. **Maslar IA, Riddick DH,** Prolactin production by human endometrium during the normal menstrual cycle, Am J Obstet Gynecol 135:751, 1979.

39. **Pihoker C, Pheeney R, Handwerger S,** Lipocortin 1 inhibits the synthesis and release of prolactin from human decidual cells, Endocrinology 128:1123, 1991.

40. **Taylor CM, McLaughlin B, Weiss JB, Maroudas NG,** Concentrations of endothelial-cell-stimulating angiogenesis factor, a major component of human uterine angiogenesis factor, in human and bovine embryonic tissues and decidua, J Reprod Fertil 94:445, 1992.

136

41. **Petraglia F, Tabanelli S, Galassi MC, Garuti GC, Mancini AC, Genazzani AR, Gurpide E,** Human decidua and in vitro decidualized endometrial stromal cells at term contain immunoreactive corticotropoin-releasing factor (CRF) and CRF messenger ribonucleic acid, J Clin Endocrinol Metab 74:1427, 1992.

42. **Poisner AM, Thrailkill K, Poisner R, Handwerger S,** Cyclic AMP and protein kinase C as second messengers for prorenin relase from human decidual cells, Placenta 12:263, 1991.

43. **Chao H-S, Poisner A, Poisner R, Handwerger S,** Endothelins stimulate the synthesis and release of prorenin from human decidual cells, J Clin Endocrinol Metab 76:615, 1993.

44. **Giudice LC, Dsupin BA, Irwin JC,** Steroid and peptide regulation of insulin-like growth factor-binding proteins secreted by human endometrial stromal cells is dependent on stromal differentiation, J Clin Endocrinol Metab 75:1235, 1992.

45. **Tseng L, Gao J-G, Chen R, Zhu HH, Mazella J, Powell DR,** Effect of progestin, antiprogestin, and relaxin on the accumulation of prolactin and insulin-like growth factor-binding protein-1 messenger ribonucleic acid in human endometrial cells, Biol Reprod 47:441, 1992.

46. **Pekonen F, Nyman T, Lahteenmaki P, Haukkamaa M, Rutanen E-M,** Intrauterine progestin induces continuous insulin-like growth factor-binding protein-1 production in the human endometrium, J Clin Endocrinol Metab 75:660, 1992.

47. **Heinonen PK, Saarikoski S, Pystynen P,** Reproductive performance of women with uterine anomalies, Acta Obstet Gynecol Scand 61:157, 1982.

48. **Rock JA, Schlaff WD,** The obstetrical consequences of utero-vaginal anomalies, Fertil Steril 43:681, 1985.

49. **Golan A, Langer R, Bukovsky I, Caspi E,** Congenital anomalies of the müllerian system, Fertil Steril 51:747, 1989.

50. **Acien P,** Reproductive performance of women with uterine malformations, Hum Reprod 8:122, 1993.

51. **The American Fertility Society,** Classifications of adnexal adhesions, distal tubal occlusion, tubal occlusion secondary to tubal ligation, tubal pregnancies, müllerian anomalies and intrauterine adhesions, Fertil Steril 49:944, 1988.

52. **Daly DC, Maier D, Soto-Albors C,** Hysteroscopic metroplasty: six years experience, Obstet Gynecol 73:201, 1989.

53. **Pellerito JS, McCarthy SM, Doyle MB, Glickman MG, DeCherney AH,** Diagnosis of uterine anomalies: relative accuracy of MR imaging, endovaginal sonography, and hysterosalpingography, Genitourin Radiol 183:795, 1992.

54. **Barbieri RL, Andersen J,** Uterine leiomyomas: the somatic mutation theory, Seminars Reprod Endocrinol 10:301, 1992.

55. **Cramer SF, Patel D,** The frequency of uterine leiomyomas, Am J Clin Pathol 94:435, 1990.

56. **Cramer DW,** Epidemiology of myomas, Seminars Reprod Endocrinol 10:320, 1992.

57. **Parazzini F, Negri E, La Vecchia C, Fedele L, Rabaiotti M, Luchini L,** Oral contraceptive use and risk of uterine fibroids, Obstet Gynecol 79:430, 1992.

58. **Otubu JA, Buttram VC, Besch NF, Besch PK,** Unconjugated steroids in leiomyomas and tumor-bearing myometrium, Am J Obstet Gynecol 143:130, 1982.

59. **Rein MS, Friedman AJ, Stuart JM, MacLaughlin DT,** Fibroid and myometrial steroid receptors in women treated with the gonadotropin-releasing hormone agonist leuprolide acetate, Fertil Steril 53:1018, 1990.

60. **Deligdish L, Loewenthal M,** Endometrial changes associated with myomata of the uterus, J Clin Pathol 23:676, 1970.

61. **Kawaguchi K, Fujii S, Konishi I, Nanbu Y, Nonogaki H, Mori T,** Mitotic activity in uterine leiomyomas during the menstrual cycle, Am J Obstet Gynecol 160:637, 1989.

137

62. **Tiltman AJ,** The effect of progestins on the mitotic activity of uterine fibromyomas, Int J Gynecol Pathol 4:89, 1985.

63. **Brandon DD, Bethea CL, Strawn EY, Novy MJ, Burry KA, Harrington MS, Erickson TE, Warner C, Keenan EJ, Clinton GM,** Progesterone receptor messenger ribonucleic acid and protein are overexpressed in human uterine leiomyomas, Am J Obstet Gynecol 169:78, 1993.

64. **Murphy AA, Kettell LM, Morales AJ, Roberts VJ, Yen SSC,** Regression of uterine leiomyomata in response to the antiprogesterone RU 486, J Clin Endocrinol Metab 76:513, 1993.

65. **Lumsden MA, West CP, Bramley T, Rumgay L, Baird DT,** The binding of epidermal growth factor to the human uterus and leiiomyomata in women rendered hypoestrogenic by continuous administration of an LHRH agonist, Br J Obstet Gynaecol 95:1299, 1988.

66. **Gloudemans T, Prinsen I, Van Unnik JAM, Lips CJ, Den Otter W, Sussenbach JS,** Insulin-like growth factor gene expression in human smooth muscle tumors, Cancer Res 50:6689, 1990.

67. **Vollenhoven BJ, Herington AC, Healy DL,** Messenger ribonucleic acid expression of the insulin-like growth factors and their binding proteins in uterine fibroids and myometrium, J Clin Endocrinol Metab 76:1106, 1993.

68. **Schmid CH, Beham A, Kratochvil P,** Haematopoiesis in a degenerating uterine leiomyoma, Arch Gynecol Obstet 248:81, 1990.

69. **Buttram VC, Reiter RC,** Uterine leiomyomata: etiology, symptomatology and management, Fertil Steril 36:433, 1981.

70. **Verkauf BS,** Myomectomy for fertility enhancement and preservation, Fertil Steril 58:1, 1992.

71. **Zawin M, McCarthy S, Scoutt LM, Comite F,** High-field MRI and US evaluation of the pelvis in women with leiomyomas, Mag Reson Imaging 8:371, 1990.

72. **Fedele L, Bianchi S, Dorta M, Brioschi D, Zanottie F, Vercellini P,** Transvaginal ultrasonography versus hysteroscopy in the diagnosis of uterine submucous myomas, Obstet Gynecol 77:745, 1991.

73. **Malone LJ,** Myomectomy: recurrence after removal of solitary and multiple myomas, Obstet Gynecol 34:200, 1969.

74. **Candiani GB, Fedele L, Parazzini F, Villa L,** Risk of recurrence after myomectomy, Br J Obstet Gynaecol 98:385, 1991.

75. **Rossi G, Diamond MP,** Myomas, reproductive function, and pregnancy, Seminars Reprod Endocrinol 10:332, 1992.

76. **Katz VL, Dotters DJ, Droegemueller W,** Complications of uterine leiomyomas in pregnancy, Obstet Gynecol 73:593, 1989.

77. **Rice JP, Kay HH, Mahony BS,** The clinical significance of uterine leiomyomas in pregnancy, Am J Obstet Gynecol 160:1212, 1989.

78. **Stewart EA, Friedman AJ,** Steroidal treatment of myomas: preoperative and long-term medical therapy, Seminars Reprod Endocrinol 10:344, 1992.

79. **Hales HA, Peterson CM, Jones KP, Quinn JD,** Leiomyomatosis peritonealis disseminata treated with a gonadotropin-releasing hormone agonist, Am J Obstet Gynecol 167:515, 1992.

80. **Hirata JD, Moghissi KS, Ginsburg KA,** Pregnancy after medical therapy of adenomyosis with a gonadotropin-releasing hormone agonist, Fertil Steril 59:444, 1993.

81. **Nelson JR, Corson SL,** Long-term management of adenomyosis with a gonadotropin-releasing hormone agonist: a case report, Fertil Steril 59:441, 1993.

82. **Friedman AJ, Lobel SM, Rein MS, Barbieri RL,** Efficacy and safety considerations in women with uterine leiomyomas treated with gonadotropin-releasing hormone agonists: the estrogen threshold hypothesis. Am J Obstet Gynecol 163:1114, 1990.

83. **Letterie GS, Stevenson D, Shah A,** Recurrent anaphylaxis to a depot form of GnRH analogue, Obstet Gynecol 78:943, 1991.

84. **Friedman AJ,** Vaginal hemorrhage associated with degeneratiing submucous leiomyomata during leuprolide acetate treatment, Fertil Steril 52:152, 1989.

85. **Schwartz LB, Diamond MP, Schwartz PE,** Leiomyosarcomas: clinical presentation, Am J Obstet Gynecol 168:180, 1993.

86. **Har-Toov J, Brenner SH, Jaffa A, Yavetz H, Peyser MR, Lessing JB,** Pregnancy during long-term gonadotropin-releasing hormone agonist therapy associated with clinical pseudomenopause, Fertil Steril 59:446, 1993.

5 Neuroendocrinology

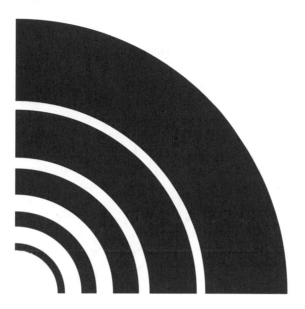

There are two major sites of action within the brain which are important in the regulation of reproductive function, the hypothalamus and the pituitary gland. In the past, the pituitary gland was viewed as the master gland. Then a new concept emerged in which the pituitary was relegated to a subordinate role as part of an orchestra, with the hypothalamus as the conductor, responding to both peripheral and central nervous system messages and exerting its influence by means of neurotransmitters transported to the pituitary by a portal vessel network. However, developments over the past 10–15 years indicate that the complex sequence of events known as the menstrual cycle is controlled by the sex steroids and peptides produced within the very follicle destined to ovulate. The hypothalamus and its direction are essential for the operation of the entire mechanism, but the endocrine function that leads to ovulation is brought about by endocrine feedback on the anterior pituitary.

A full understanding of this feature of reproductive biology will benefit the clinician who faces problems in gynecologic endocrinology. With this understanding, the clinician can comprehend the hitherto mysterious, but significant, effects of stress, diet, exercise, and other diverse influences on the pituitary-gonadal axis. Furthermore, we will be prepared to make advantageous use of the numerous neuropharmacologic agents that are the dividends of neuroendocrine research. To these ends, this chapter offers a clinically oriented review of the current status of reproductive neuroendocrinology.

Hypothalamic-Hypophyseal Portal Circulation

The hypothalamus is at the base of the brain just above the junction of the optic nerves. In order to influence the anterior pituitary gland, the brain requires a means of transmission or connection. A direct nervous connection does not exist. The blood supply of the anterior pituitary, however, originates in the capillaries that richly lace the median eminence area of the hypothalamus. The superior hypophyseal arteries form a dense network of capillaries within the median eminence, which then drain into the portal vessels that descend along the pituitary stalk to the anterior pituitary. The direction of the blood flow in this hypophyseal portal circulation is from the brain to the pituitary. Section of the neural stalk which interrupts this portal circulation leads to inactivity and atrophy of the gonads, along with a decrease in adrenal and thyroid activity to basal levels. With regeneration of the portal vessels, anterior pituitary function is restored. Thus, the anterior pituitary gland is under the influence of the hypothalamus by means of neurohormones released into this portal circulation. There also exists retrograde flow so that pituitary hormones can be delivered directly to the hypothalamus, creating the opportunity for pituitary feedback upon the hypothalamus. An additional blood supply is provided by short vessels which originate in the posterior pituitary that in turn receives its arterial supply from the inferior hypophyseal arteries.

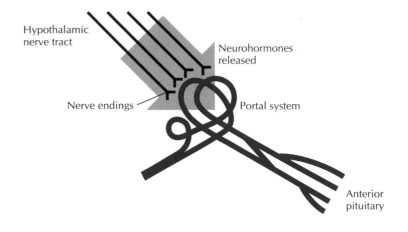

The Neurohormone Concept

A considerable body of evidence indicates that influence of the pituitary by the hypothalamus is achieved by materials secreted in the cells of the hypothalamus and transported to the pituitary by the portal vessel system. In addition to the stalk section experiments cited above, transplantation of the pituitary to ectopic sites (e.g., under the kidney capsule) results in failure of gonadal function. With retransplantation to an anatomic site under the median eminence, followed by regeneration of the portal system, normal pituitary function is regained. This retrieval of gonadotropic function is not accomplished if the pituitary is transplanted to other sites in the brain. Hence, there is something very special about the blood draining the basal hypothalamus. An exception to this overall pattern of positive influence is the control of prolactin secretion. Stalk secretion and transplantation cause release of prolactin from the anterior pituitary, implying a negative hypothalamic control. Furthermore, cultures of anterior pituitary tissue release prolactin in the absence of hypothalamic tissue or extracts.

Neuroendocrine agents originating in the hypothalamus have positive stimulatory effects on growth hormone, thyroid-stimulating hormone (TSH), adrenocorticotropin hormone (ACTH), as well as the gonadotropins, and represent the individual neurohormones of the hypothalamus. The neurohormone that controls gonadotropins is called gonadotropin releasing hormone (GnRH). The neurohormone that controls prolactin is called prolactin inhibiting hormone and is probably dopamine. Human corticotropin releasing hormone (CRH) is a 41 amino acid peptide which, besides being the principal regulator of ACTH secretion, also activates the sympathetic nervous system. CRH

Gonadotropin releasing hormone—
a decapeptide

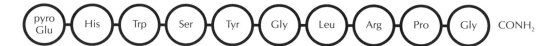

suppresses gonadotropin secretion, an action mediated by endorphin inhibition of GnRH. CRH is found in many tissues outside the central nervous system, including pancreas, gastrointestinal tract, liver, placenta, and adrenal gland.

In addition to their effects on the pituitary, behavioral effects within the brain have been demonstrated for several of the releasing hormones. Thyrotropin releasing hormone (TRH) antagonizes the sedative action of a number of drugs and also has a direct antidepressant effect in humans. GnRH evokes mating behavior in male and female animals.[1]

Initially, it was believed that there were two separate releasing hormones for follicle-stimulating hormone (FSH) and luteinizing hormone (LH). It is now apparent that there is a single neurohormone (GnRH) for both gonadotropins. GnRH is a small peptide with 10 amino acids with some variation in the amino acid sequence among various mammals. Purified or synthesized GnRH stimulates both FSH and LH secretion. The divergent patterns of FSH and LH in response to a single GnRH are due to the modulating influences of the endocrine environment, specifically the feedback effects of steroids on the anterior pituitary gland.

The classic neurotransmitters are secreted at the nerve terminal. Brain peptides require gene transcription, translation, and posttranslational processing, all within the neuronal cell body, the final product being transported down the axon to the terminal for secretion. Small neuroendocrine peptides share common large precursor polypeptides, called polyproteins or polyfunctional peptides. These proteins can serve as precursors for more than one biologically active peptide.

The gene that encodes for the 92 amino acid precursor protein for GnRH is located on the short arm of chromosome 8.[2] The precursor protein for GnRH contains (in the following order) a 23 amino acid signal sequence, the GnRH decapeptide, a 3 amino acid proteolytic processing site, and a 56 amino acid sequence called GAP (GnRH-associated peptide).[3] GAP is a potent inhibitor of prolactin secretion as well as a stimulator of gonadotropins; however, a physiologic role for GAP has not been established. Its primary role may be to provide appropriate conformational support for GnRH.

It is now apparent that GnRH has autocrine/paracrine functions throughout the body. It is present in both neural and nonneural tissues, and receptors are present in many extrapituitary tissues (such as the ovarian follicle and the placenta). Although GnRH is identical in all mammals, other nonmammalian forms exist, indicating that the GnRH molecule has existed for at least 500 million years.[4]

Prolactin Secretion

Prolactin gene expression occurs in the lactotrophs of the anterior pituitary gland, in decidualized endometrium, and the myometrium. The prolactin secreted in these various sites is identical, but there are differences in mRNA indicating differences in prolactin gene regulation.

Transcription of the prolactin gene is regulated by a transcription factor (named Pit-1) which binds to the 5' promoter region and which is specific for the pituitary and also necessary for growth hormone.[5] In addition, prolactin gene transcription is regulated by the interaction of estrogen and glucocorticoid receptors with 5' flanking sequences. Mutations in the sequences of these flanking regions or in the gene for the Pit-1 protein can result in the failure to secrete prolactin. The Pit-1 gene is also involved in differentiation and growth of anterior pituitary cells, and therefore mutations in this gene can lead not only to absent secretion of growth hormone and prolactin but to an absence of their trophic cells in the pituitary.

The main function of prolactin in mammals is lactogenesis, while in fish prolactin is important for osmoregulation. The prolactin gene from the Chinook salmon contains coding sequences that are similar to those in mammals, and it is regulated similarly in the pituitary.[6] Pit-1, the pituitary specific transcription factor, therefore, appears to be highly conserved among species.

Prolactin gene expression is further regulated by other species specific factors. Prolactin gene transcription is stimulated by estrogen and mediated by estrogen-receptor binding to estrogen responsive elements. This activation by estrogen requires interaction with Pit-1, in a manner not yet determined. Proximal promoter sequences are also activated by peptide hormones binding to cell surface receptors, e.g., TRH and growth factors. In addition, various agents that control cyclic AMP and calcium channels can stimulate or inhibit prolactin promoter activity.

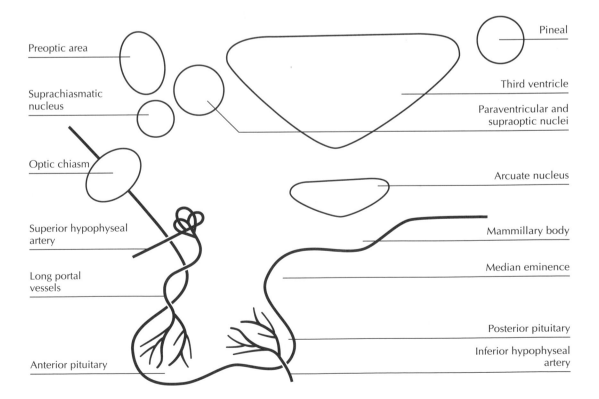

As noted, pituitary secretion of prolactin is chiefly under the inhibitory control of hypothalamic dopamine released into the portal circulation. The action of dopamine in the pituitary is mediated by receptors that are coupled to the inhibition of adenylate cyclase activity. Dopamine-regulated prolactin gene transcription, therefore, involves modulation of the promoter activity by cyclic AMP, intracellular calcium, and phosphatidyl inositol. Pit-1 binding sites are involved in this dopamine response. Molecular studies indicate that Pit-1 participates in mediating both stimulatory and inhibitory hormone signals for prolactin gene transcription.

The secretion of prolactin is inhibited and stimulated by the association and dissociation of dopamine from its receptors.[7] Other factors are also involved in the regulation of prolactin secretion, especially TRH, vasoactive intestinal peptide (VIP), and perhaps GnRH. These factors interact with each other, affecting the overall lactotroph responsiveness.

The Hypothalamus and GnRH Secretion

The hypothalamus is the part of the diencephalon at the base of the brain that forms the floor of the third ventricle and part of its lateral walls. Within the hypothalamus are peptidergic neural cells that secrete the releasing and inhibiting hormones. These cells share the characteristics of both neurons and endocrine gland cells. They respond to signals in the bloodstream, as well as to neurotransmitters within the brain, in a process known as neurosecretion. In neurosecretion, a neurohormone or neurotransmitter is synthesized on the ribosomes in the cytoplasm of the neuron, packaged into a granule in the Golgi apparatus, and then transported by active axonal flow to the neuronal terminal for secretion into a blood vessel or across a synapse.

The cells which produce GnRH originate from the olfactory area. By migration during embryogenesis, the cells move along cranial nerves connecting the nose and the forebrain to their primary location, the arcuate nucleus of the hypothalamus.[8] The GnRH neurons appear in the medial olfactory placode (a thickened plate of ectoderm from which a sense organ develops) and enter the brain with the nervus terminalis, a cranial nerve that projects from the nose to the septal-preoptic nuclei in the brain.[9] This amazing

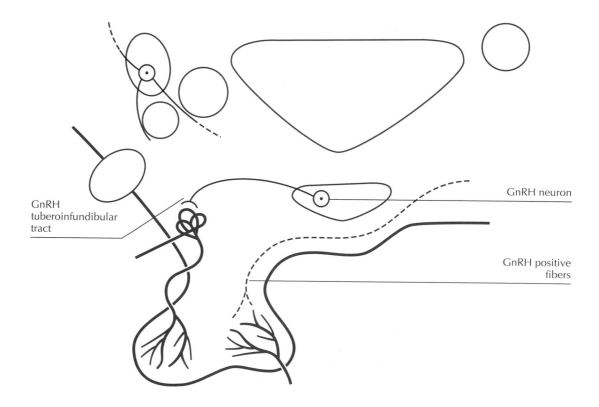

GnRH tuberoinfundibular tract

GnRH neuron

GnRH positive fibers

journey accounts for Kallmann's syndrome, an association between an absence of GnRH and a defect in smell (a failure of both olfactory axonal and GnRH neuronal migration from the olfactory placode). The mutations responsible for this syndrome involve a single gene on the short arm of the X chromosome in the Xp22.3 region, which encodes a protein (homologous to members of the fibronectin family) responsible for cell adhesion and protease inhibition, functions necessary for neuronal migration.[10,11] Location on the X chromosome explains why the syndrome occurs 5 to 7 times more frequently in males than in females.

In primates, the primary network of GnRH cell bodies is located within the medial basal hypothalamus.[12] Most of these cell bodies can be seen within the arcuate nucleus where GnRH is synthesized in GnRH neurons. The delivery of GnRH to the portal circulation is via an axonal pathway, the GnRH tuberoinfundibular tract.

Fibers, identified with immunocytochemical techniques using antibodies to GnRH, can also be visualized in the posterior hypothalamus, descending into the posterior pituitary, and in the anterior hypothalamic area projecting to sites within the limbic system.[12] However, lesions that interrupt GnRH neurons projecting to regions other than the median eminence do not affect gonadotropin release. Only lesions of the arcuate nucleus in the monkey lead to gonadal atrophy and amenorrhea.[13] Therefore, the arcuate nucleus can be viewed with the median eminence as a unit, the key locus within the hypothalamus for GnRH secretion into the portal circulation. The other GnRH neurons may be important for a variety of behavioral responses. Using hybridization techniques, messenger RNA for GnRH has been localized to the same sites previously identified by immunoreactivity.

GnRH Secretion

The half-life of GnRH is only 2–4 minutes. Because of this rapid degradation, combined with the enormous dilution upon entry into the peripheral circulation, biologically effective amounts of GnRH do not escape the portal system. Therefore, control of the reproductive cycle depends upon constant release of GnRH. This function, in turn, depends upon the complex and coordinated interrelationships among this releasing hormone, other neurohormones, the pituitary gonadotropins, and the gonadal steroids. The interplay among these substances is governed by feedback effects, both positive stimulatory and negative inhibitory. *The long feedback loop* refers to the feedback effects of circulating levels of target gland hormones, and this occurs both in the hypothalamus and the pituitary. *The short feedback loop* indicates a negative feedback of pituitary hormones on their own secretion, presumably via inhibitory effects on releasing hormones in the hypothalamus. *Ultrashort feedback* refers to inhibition by the releasing hormone on its own synthesis. These signals as well as signals from higher centers in the central nervous system may modify GnRH secretion through an array of neurotransmitters, primarily dopamine, norepinephrine, and endorphin but also serotonin and melatonin. GnRH neurons lack estradiol receptors; therefore, steroid hormone regulation is believed to be mediated through this collection of neurotransmitters.

Dopamine and norepinephrine are synthesized in the nerve terminals by decarboxylation of dihydroxyphenylalanine (DOPA), which in turn is synthesized by hydroxylation of tyrosine. Dopamine is the immediate precursor of norepinephrine, but dopamine itself functions as a key neurotransmitter in the hypothalamus and the pituitary.

A most useful concept is to view the arcuate nucleus as the central site of action, releasing GnRH into the portal circulation in pulsatile fashion. In a classic series of experiments, it was demonstrated that normal gonadotropin secretion requires pulsatile GnRH discharge within a critical range in frequency and amplitude.[14]

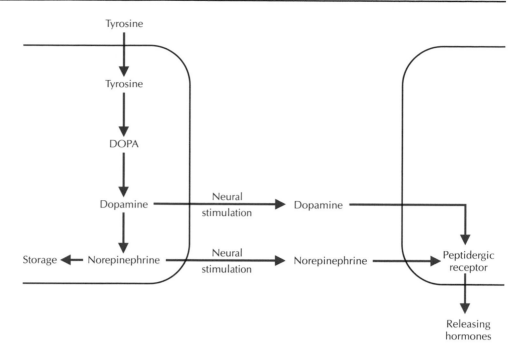

Experimental manipulations have indicated that the critical range of GnRH pulsatile secretion is rather narrow. The administration (to monkeys) of 1 μg GnRH per minute for 6 minutes every hour (1 pulse per hour) produces a portal blood concentration about equal to the peak concentration of GnRH in human portal blood, about 2 ng/mL. Increasing the frequency to 2 and 5 pulses per hour extinguishes gonadotropin secretion. A similar decline in gonadotropin secretion is obtained by increasing the dose of GnRH. Decreasing the pulse frequency decreases LH secretion but increases FSH secretion.

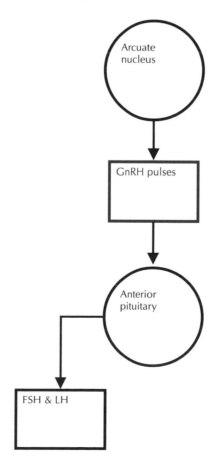

Like GnRH, gonadotropins are also secreted in pulsatile fashion, and indeed, the pulsatile pattern of gonadotropin release is believed to reflect the pulsatile GnRH pattern.[15,16] Initiation of the pulsatile pattern of gonadotropin secretion occurs just before puberty with nighttime increases in LH. After puberty, pulsatile secretion is maintained throughout the 24-hour period, but it varies in both amplitude and frequency. In puberty, arcuate activity begins with a low frequency of GnRH release and proceeds through a cycle of acceleration of frequency, characterized by passage from total inactivity, to nocturnal activation, to the full adult pattern. The progressive changes in FSH and LH reflect this activation of GnRH pulsatile secretion.

Timing of GnRH Pulses

The measurement of LH pulses is utilized as an indication of GnRH pulsatile secretion (the long half-life of FSH precludes its use for this purpose).[17] The characteristics of LH pulses (and presumably of GnRH pulses) during the menstrual cycle are as follows:[18]

LH pulse mean amplitude:

Early follicular phase:	6.5 IU/L.
Mid follicular phase:	5.1 IU/L.
Late follicular phase:	7.2 IU/L.
Early luteal phase:	14.9 IU/L.
Mid luteal phase:	12.2 IU/L.
Late luteal phase:	7.6 IU/L.

LH pulse mean frequency:

Early follicular phase:	94 minutes.
Late follicular phase:	71 minutes.
Early luteal phase:	103 minutes.
Late luteal phase:	216 minutes.

Pulsatile secretion is more frequent but smaller in amplitude during the follicular phase compared to the luteal phase. It should be emphasized that these numbers are not inviolate. There is considerable variability between and within individuals and a large normal range exists.[19] Despite the handicap of the long half-life, it has been ascertained that FSH secretion is correlated with LH secretion.

The anterior pituitary gland also appears to have a pulsatile pattern of its own. Although pulses of significant amplitude are linked to GnRH, small amplitude pulses of high frequency represent spontaneous secretion (at least as demonstrated in isolated pituitary glands in vitro).[20] It is not known whether this has any importance in vivo, and at the present time, the major secretory pattern is thought to reflect GnRH.

Control of GnRH Pulses

Normal menstrual cycles require the maintenance of the pulsatile release of GnRH within a critical range of frequency and amplitude. This pulsatile release is mediated by a catecholaminergic mechanism and can be modified by gonadal steroids and a variety of brain peptides.

The Dopamine Tract. Cell bodies for dopamine synthesis can be found in the arcuate and periventricular nuclei. The dopamine tuberoinfundibular tract arises within the medial basal hypothalamus and projects to the median eminence.

The administration of dopamine by intravenous infusion to men and women is associated with a suppression of circulating prolactin and gonadotropin levels.[21] Dopamine does not exert a direct effect on gonadotropin secretion by the anterior pituitary; thus, this effect is mediated through GnRH release in the hypothalamus. Athough the exact

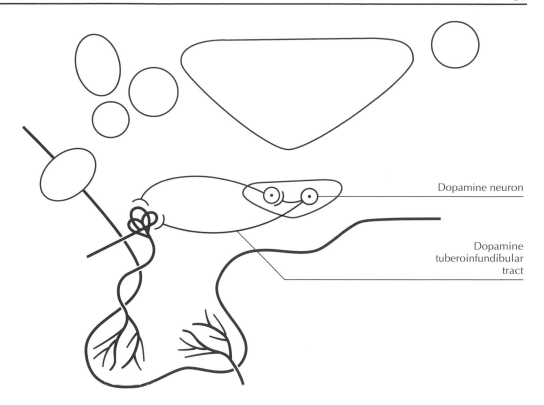

Dopamine neuron

Dopamine tuberoinfundibular tract

chemical nature of the endogenous prolactin inhibiting hormone is still not known, evidence is rather overwhelming that dopamine is the hypothalamic inhibitor of prolactin secretion. It is directly secreted into the portal blood, thus behaving like a neurohormone. Therefore, dopamine may directly suppress arcuate GnRH activity, and also be transported via the portal system to directly and specifically suppress pituitary prolactin secretion. The hypothalamic tuberoinfundibular dopamine pathway is not the only dopamine pathway in the CNS, and it is only one of two major dopamine pathways in the hypothalamus. But it is this pathway that directly participates in the regulation of prolactin secretion. Ergot derivatives, such as bromocriptine, used clinically to treat high prolactin levels, activate dopaminergic receptors and directly inhibit the secretion of prolactin in a fashion identical to dopamine. Whether the peptide associated with GnRH (GAP) plays a role in physiologic prolactin regulation is not known.

Many studies, including specific *in vitro* systems, have indicated that dopamine stimulates the release of GnRH from the hypothalamus.[22] This appears to be a paradox, but it simply indicates that the ultimate GnRH response reflects the complex interactions of steroids and neurotransmitters. For an understanding of clinical problems, it is best to view dopamine as an inhibitor of both GnRH and prolactin.

The story is further complicated by an apparent direct stimulation of prolactin secretion by GnRH.[23] This action is thought to represent a paracrine interaction between the pituitary gonadotropes and lactotropes, occurring independently of FSH and LH.

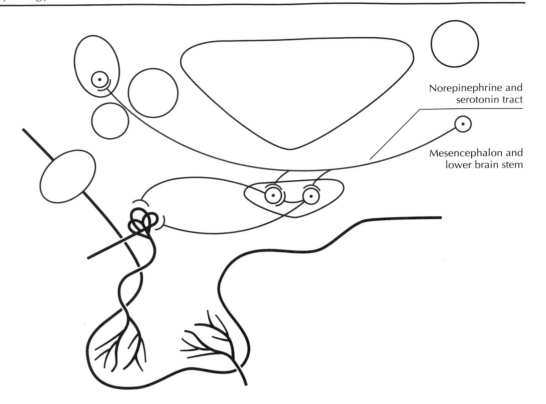

Norepinephrine and
serotonin tract

Mesencephalon and
lower brain stem

The Norepinephrine Tract. Most of the cell bodies that synthesize norepinephrine are located in the mesencephalon and lower brainstem. These cells also synthesize serotonin. Axons for amine transport ascend into the medial forebrain bundle to terminate in various brain structures including the hypothalamus.

The current concept is that the biogenic catecholamines modulate GnRH pulsatile release. Norepinephrine is thought to exert stimulatory effects on GnRH, while dopamine and serotonin exert inhibitory effects. Little is known, however, about the role of serotonin. The probable mode of action of catecholamines is to influence the frequency (and perhaps the amplitude) of GnRH discharge. Thus, pharmacologic or psychologic factors that affect pituitary function probably do so by altering catecholamine synthesis or metabolism, and thus the pulsatile release of GnRH.

Pituitary Gonadotropin Secretion

The gene for the α-subunit of the gonadotropins is expressed in both the pituitary and placenta. The β-subunit for human chorionic gonadotropin (HCG) is expressed in the placenta but not in the pituitary, while the βLH-subunit, as expected, is expressed in the pituitary but not in the placenta. The entire gene for the human βFSH-subunit has been sequenced.[24] Studies of gonadotropin gene expression confirm the relationships established by earlier studies. The sex steroids decrease and castration increases the rate of gonadotropin gene transcription as reflected by the levels of specific messenger RNAs. In addition, the sex steroids can act at the membrane level, affecting the interaction of GnRH with its receptor.[25]

Both LH and FSH are secreted by the same cell, the gonadotrope, localized primarily in the lateral portions of the pituitary gland and responsive to the pulsatile stimulation by GnRH. GnRH is calcium dependent in its mechanism of action and utilizes inositol 1,4,5-triphosphate (IP_3) and 1,2-diacylglycerol (1,2-DG) as second messengers to stimulate protein kinase activity[26] (Chapter 2). These responses require a G protein receptor, and are associated with cyclical release of calcium ions from intracellular stores and the opening of cell membrane channels to allow entry of extracellular calcium. Thus both protein kinase and calmodulin are mediators of GnRH action. GnRH receptors

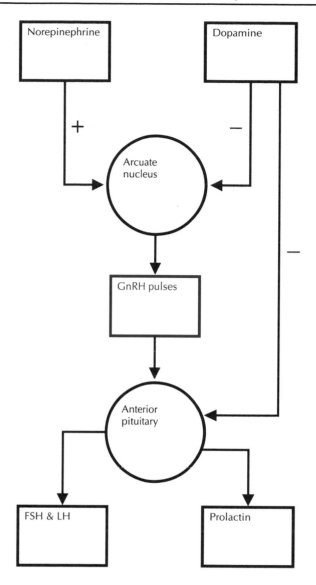

are regulated by many agents, including GnRH itself, inhibin, activin, and the sex steroids. A decreased gonadotropin response to continued excessive GnRH stimulation is not due to a loss of GnRH receptors alone but includes desensitization and uncoupling of the receptors (discussed in Chapter 2).

Synthesis of gonadotropins takes place on the rough endoplasmic reticulum. The hormones are packaged into secretory granules by the Golgi cisternae of the Golgi apparatus and then stored as secretory granules. Secretion requires migration (activation) of the mature secretory granules to the cell membrane where an alteration in membrane permeability results in extrusion of the secretory granules in response to GnRH. The rate limiting step in gonadotropin synthesis is the GnRH-dependent availability of the beta-subunits.

Binding of GnRH to its receptor in the pituitary activates multiple messengers and responses. The immediate event is a secretory release of gonadotropins, while delayed responses prepare for the next secretory release. One of these delayed responses is the self-priming action of GnRH that leads to even greater responses to subsequent GnRH pulses due to a complex series of biochemical and biophysical intracellular events. This self-priming action is important to achieve the large surge in secretion at midcyle; it requires estrogen exposure, and it can be augmented by progesterone. This important action of progesterone depends upon estrogen exposure (for an increase in progesterone receptors) and activation of the progesterone receptor by GnRH stimulated phosphory-lation. This latter action is an example of cross-talk between peptide and steroid hormone receptors.

Five different types of secretory cells coexist within the anterior pituitary gland: gonadotrophs, lactotrophs, thyrotrophs, somatotrophs, and corticotrophs. Autocrine and paracrine interactions combine to make anterior pituitary secretion subject to more complicated control than simply reaction to hypothalamic releasing factors and modu-lation by feedback signals. Substantial experimental evidence exists to indicate stimulatory and inhibitory influences of various substances on the pituitary secretory cells; however, the exact physiologic roles for these substances have been difficult to confirm.[27] Angiotensin II and activin are at least two brain peptides believed to have active regulatory functions within the anterior pituitary. Even GnRH can be of pituitary origin and influence local activity.

Brain Peptides

There are many peptides that can function as neurotransmitters, but most are active only in local regulatory autocrine and paracrine roles.[27] Although pituitary hormone synthesis and secretion are largely controlled by classic hormonal messenger systems, consider-able local intercellular communication exists as well. Examples of brain peptides include the following.

Neurotensin
A brain peptide that is vasodilatory, alters pituitary hormone release, and lowers body temperature.

Cholecystokinin
An intestinal hormone that is found in the brain and may be involved in the regulation of behavior, satiety, and fluid intake.

Vasoactive Intestinal Peptide (VIP)
High levels of this peptide are found in the cerebral cortex, and it is also found in the hypothalamus and pituitary. VIP causes vasodilation, stimulates conversion of glycogen to glucose, enhances lipolysis and insulin secretion, stimulates pancreatic and intestinal secretion, and inhibits the production of gastric acid. VIP is synthesized in the pituitary lactotrophs and increases prolactin secretion.

Angiotensin II
Several components of the renin-angiotensin system are present in the brain. Receptors for angiotensin II are found on various pituitary cell types, suggesting local effects on the secretion of pituitary hormones. In addition, angiotensin II in the hypothalamus appears to influence norepinephrine and dopamine effects on the releasing factors that control gonadotropin and prolactin secretion.

Endothelins
This family of peptides was originally isolated from vascular endothelial cells, but endothelins are widespread and are known to be secreted and active within the anterior pituitary gland. Endothelin can cause the release of vasopressin from the posterior pituitary and gonadotropins from the anterior pituitary, and inhibit prolactin response.

Somatostatin
This hypothalamic peptide inhibits the release of growth hormone, prolactin, and TSH from the pituitary. It is also a typical gut-brain peptide, being found in neurons throughout the brain, stomach, intestine, and pancreas. It inhibits secretion of glucagon, insulin, and gastrin. It is also located in sensory neurons and may be a transmitter of pain sensation.

Neuropeptide Y

The secretion and gene expression of neuropeptide Y in hypothalamic neurons is regulated by gonadal steroids.[28] Neuropeptide Y stimulates pulsatile release of GnRH and in the pituitary potentiates gonadotropin response to GnRH. It thus may facilitate pulsatile secretion of GnRH and gonadotropins. In the absence of estrogen, neuropeptide Y inhibits gonadotropin secretion. Because undernutrition is associated with an increase in neuropeptide Y and increased amounts have been measured in cerebrospinal fluid of women with anorexia and bulimia nervosa, it has been proposed that neuropeptide Y is at least one link between nutrition and reproductive function.[29,30]

Growth Factors

The ubiquitous growth factors appear to modulate pituitary hormone production and secretion. Messenger RNA coding for several growth factors is readily found in CNS tissue, including the pituitary gland.

Activin and Inhibin

Activin and inhibin are peptide members of the transforming growth factor-β family.[31] Inhibin consists of two dissimilar peptides (known as alpha- and beta-subunits) linked by disulfide bonds. Two forms of inhibin (inhibin A and inhibin B) have been purified, each containing an identical alpha-subunit and distinct but related beta-subunits. Thus, there are three subunits for inhibins: alpha, beta-A, and beta-B. Each subunit is a product of different messenger RNA; therefore, each is derived from its own large precursor molecule. Inhibin is secreted by granulosa cells, but messenger RNA for the alpha and beta chains has also been found in pituitary gonadotropes.[32] Inhibin selectively inhibits FSH, but not LH, secretion.

Activin, also derived from granulosa cells, but present as well in the pituitary gonadotropes, contains two subunits that are identical to the beta-subunits of inhibins A and B. Activin augments the secretion of FSH and inhibits prolactin and growth hormone responses.[33–35] The roles for inhibin and activin in regulating the events of the menstrual cycle are discussed in Chapter 6.

The Two Forms of Inhibin

Inhibin-A:	Alpha-Beta$_A$
Inhibin-B:	Alpha-Beta$_B$

The Three Forms of Activin

Activin-A:	Beta$_A$-Beta$_A$
Activin-AB:	Beta$_A$-Beta$_B$
Activin-B:	Beta$_B$-Beta$_B$

Follistatin

Follistatin is a peptide secreted by a variety of pituitary cells, including the gonadotrophs.[36] This peptide has also been called FSH-suppressing protein because of its main action: inhibition of FSH synthesis and secretion and the FSH response to GnRH. Follistatin also binds to activin and in that fashion decreases the activity of activin.[37]

Galanin

Galanin is released into the portal circulation in pulsatile fashion, and it is also produced by the lactotrophs in the pituitary. It positively influences LH secretion.[38] Galanin secretion is inhibited by dopamine and somatostatin and stimulated by TRH and estrogen.

The Endogenous Opiates

The most fascinating peptide group is the endogenous opioid peptide family.[39] β-Lipotropin is a 91 amino acid molecule which was first isolated from the pituitary in 1964. Its function remained a mystery for more than 10 years until receptors for opioid compounds were identified, and by virtue of their existence, it was postulated that endogenous opioid compounds must exist and serve important physiological roles. Endorphin was a word coined to denote morphine-like action and endogenous origin in the brain.

Opiate production is regulated by gene transcription and the synthesis of precursor peptides and at a posttranslational level where the precursors are processed into the various bioactive smaller peptides.[40] All opiates derive from one of 3 precursor peptides.

Proopiomelanocortin (POMC) — the source of endorphins.
Proenkephalin A and B — the source of several enkephalins.
Prodynorphin — yields dynorphins.

POMC was the first precursor peptide to be identified. It is made in the anterior and intermediate lobes of the pituitary, in the hypothalamus and other areas of the brain, in the sympathetic nervous system, and in other tissues including the gonads, the placenta, the gastrointestinal tract, and the lungs. The highest concentration is in the pituitary gland.

Proopiomelanocortin is split into 2 fragments, an ACTH intermediate fragment and β-lipotropin. β-Lipotropin has no opioid activity but is broken down in a series of steps to β-melanocyte-stimulating hormone (β-MSH), enkephalin, and α-, γ-, and β-endorphins. Melanocyte-stimulating hormone acts in lower animals to stimulate melanin granules within cells, causing darkening of the skin. In humans, there is no known function.

Enkephalin and the α- and γ-endorphins are as active as morphine on a molar basis, while β-endorphin is 5–10 times more potent. In the adult pituitary gland, the major products are ACTH and β-lipotropin, with only small amounts of endorphin. Thus, ACTH and β-lipotropin blood levels show similar courses, and they are major secretion products of the anterior pituitary in response to stress. In the intermediate lobe of the pituitary (which is prominent only during fetal life), ACTH is cleaved to CLIP (corticotropin-like intermediate lobe peptide) and β-MSH. In the placenta and adrenal medulla, POMC processing yields α-MSH-like and β-endorphin peptides. β-Endorphin has also been detected in the ovaries and in the testes.

In the brain, the major products are the opiates, with little ACTH. In the hypothalamus the major products are β-endorphin and α-MSH in the region of the arcuate nucleus and the ventromedial nucleus. The pituitary system is a system for secretion into the circulation while the hypothalamic system allows for distribution via axons to regulate other brain regions and the pituitary gland.

β-Endorphin is appropriately considered a neurotransmitter, a neurohormone, and a neuromodulator. β-Endorphin influences a variety of hypothalamic functions, including regulation of reproduction, temperature, cardiovascular and respiratory function, as well as extrahypothalamic functions such as pain perception and mood. POMC gene expression in the anterior pituitary is controlled mainly by adrenal hormones, stimulated by CRH (corticotropin releasing hormone) and influenced by the feedback effects of glucocorticoids. In the hypothalamus, regulation of POMC gene expression is via the sex steroids. In the absence of sex steroids, little, if any, secretion occurs.

Proenkephalin A is produced in the adrenal medulla, the brain, the posterior pituitary, the spinal cord, and the gastrointestinal tract. It yields several enkephalins: methionine-

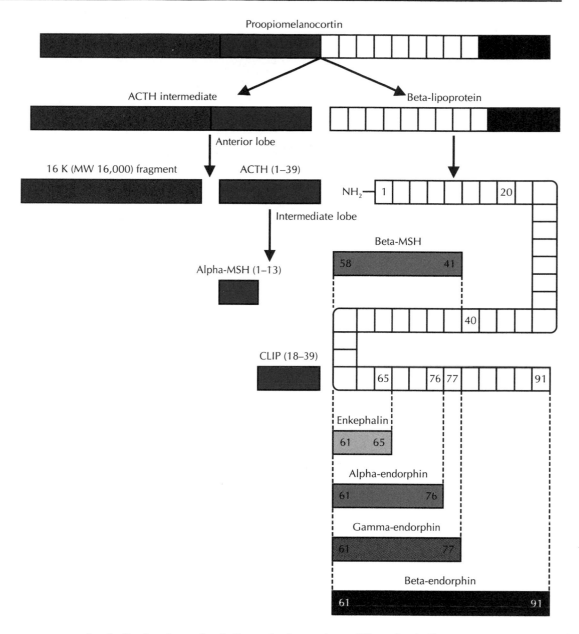

enkephalin, leucine-enkephalin, and other variants. The enkephalins are the most widely distributed endogenous opioid peptides in the brain and are probably mainly involved as inhibitory neurotransmitters in the modulation of the autonomic nervous system. Prodynorphin, found in the brain (concentrated in the hypothalamus) and the gastrointestinal tract, yields dynorphin, an opioid peptide with high analgesic potency and behavioral effects, as well as α-neoendorphin, β-neoendorphin, and leumorphin. The last 13 amino acids of leumorphin constitute another opioid peptide, rimorphin. The prodynorphin products probably function in a fashion similar to endorphin.

It is simpler to say that there are 3 classes of opiates: enkephalins, endorphin, and dynorphin.

Opioid peptides are able to act through different receptors, although specific opiates bind predominantly to one of the various receptor types. Naloxone, used in most human studies, does not bind exclusively to any one receptor type, and thus results with this antagonist are not totally specific. Localization of opioid receptors explains many of the pharmacological actions of the opiates. Opioid receptors are found in the nerve endings of sensory neurons, in the limbic system (site of euphoric emotions), in brainstem centers

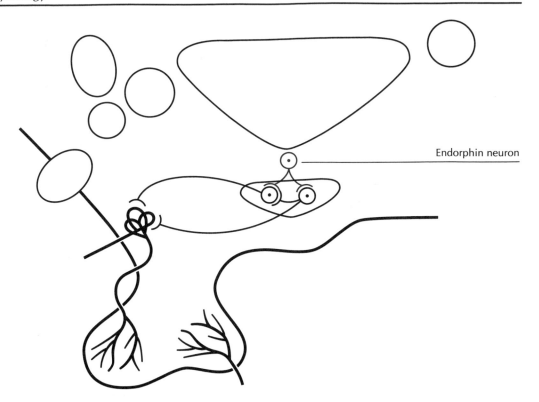

Endorphin neuron

for reflexes such as respiration, and widely distributed in the brain and the spinal cord.

Opioid Peptides and the Menstrual Cycle

The opioid tone is an important part of menstrual function and cyclicity.[41] Although estradiol alone increases endorphin secretion, the highest levels of endorphin occur with sequential therapy of both estradiol and progesterone (in ovariectomized monkeys). Endogenous endorphin levels, therefore, increase throughout the cycle from nadir levels during menses to highest levels during the luteal phase. Normal cyclicity thus requires sequential periods of high (luteal phase) and low (during menses) hypothalamic opioid activity.

A reduction in LH pulse frequency is linked to increased endorphin release.[42] Naloxone increases both the frequency and the amplitude of LH pulses. *Thus, the endogenous opiates inhibit gonadotropin secretion by suppressing the hypothalamic release of GnRH.* Opiates have no effect on the pituitary response to GnRH. The gonadal steroids modify endogenous opioid activity, and the negative feedback of steroids on gonadotropins appears to be mediated by endogenous opiates. Because the fluctuating levels of endogenous opiates in the menstrual cycle are related to the changing levels of estradiol and progesterone, it is attractive to speculate that the sex steroids directly stimulate endogenous opioid receptor activity. There is an absence of opioid effect on postmenopausal and oophorectomized levels of gonadotropins, and the response to opiates is restored with the administration of estrogen, progesterone, or both.[43] Both estrogen and progesterone alone increase endogenous opiates, but estrogen enhances the action of progesterone, which explains the maximal suppression of GnRH and gonadotropin pulse frequency during the luteal phase.[44,45] Experiments with naloxone administration suggest that the suppression of gonadotropins during pregnancy and the recovery during the postpartum period reflect steroid-induced opioid inhibition, followed by a release from central opioid suppression.

The principal endogenous opiates affecting GnRH release are β-endorphin and dynorphin, and it is probable that the major effect is modulation of the catecholamine pathway, principally norepinephrine. The action does not involve dopamine receptors, acetylcholine receptors, or alpha-adrenergic receptors. On the other hand, endorphin may affect GnRH release directly, without the involvement of any intermediary neuroamine.

Because α-MSH counteracts the effects of β-endorphin, posttranslational processing of POMC can affect hypothalamic-pituitary function by altering the amounts of α-MSH and β-endorphin.[46] This introduces another potential site for neuroendocrine regulation of reproductive function. Gonadal hormones likely have multiple sites for feedback signals.

A change in opioid inhibitory tone is not important in the changes of puberty because the responsiveness to naloxone does not develop until after puberty. A change in opioid tone does seem to mediate the hypogonadotropic state seen with elevated prolactin levels, exercise, and other conditions of hypothalamic amenorrhea, while endogenous opioid inhibition does not seem to play a causal role in delayed puberty or hereditary problems such as Kallmann's syndrome.[47,48] Treatment of patients with hypothalamic amenorrhea (suppressed GnRH pulsatile secretion) with a drug (naltrexone) which blocks opioid receptors restores normal function (ovulation and pregnancy).[49] Thus, the reduced GnRH secretion associated with hypothalamic amenorrhea is mediated by an increase in endogenous opioid inhibitory tone.

Experimental evidence indicates that corticotropin-releasing hormone (CRH) directly inhibits hypothalamic GnRH secretion, probably by augmenting endogenous opioid secretion. Women with hypothalamic amenorrhea demonstrate hypercortisolism, suggesting that this could be the pathway by which stress interrupts reproductive function.[50] Mathematical analysis of the associations among FSH, LH, β-endorphin and cortisol pulses support the existence of significant functional coupling between the neuro-regulatory systems that control the gonadal and adrenal axes.[51] Cumming concludes that most studies indicate an exercise-induced increase in endogenous opiates, but a significant impact on mood remains to be substantiated.[52] He notes that *runners' high* is more common in California than in Canada (euphoria is hard to come by when running in below freezing temperatures).

Administration of morphine, enkephalin analogs, and β-endorphin causes release of prolactin. The effect is mediated by inhibition of dopamine secretion in the tuberinfundibular neurons in the median eminence. Most studies have reported no effect of naloxone on basal, stress-induced, or pregnant levels of prolactin nor on secretion by prolactinomas. Thus a physiological role for endogenous opioid regulation of prolactin does not appear to exist in men and women. However, suppression of GnRH secretion associated with hyper-prolactinemia does appear to be mediated by endogenous opiates.[53]

Every pituitary hormone appears to be modulated by opiates. Physiologic effects are important with ACTH, gonadotropins, and possibly vasopressin. Opioid compounds have no direct action on the pituitary, nor do they alter the action of releasing hormones on the pituitary.

POMC-like mRNA is present in the ovary and the placenta.[54] Expression is regulated by gonadotropins in the ovary but not in the placenta. Reasons for endorphin presence in these tissues are not yet apparent. High concentrations of all of the members of the POMC family are found in human ovarian follicular fluid, but only β-endorphin shows significant changes during the menstrual cycle, reaching highest levels just before ovulation.[55]

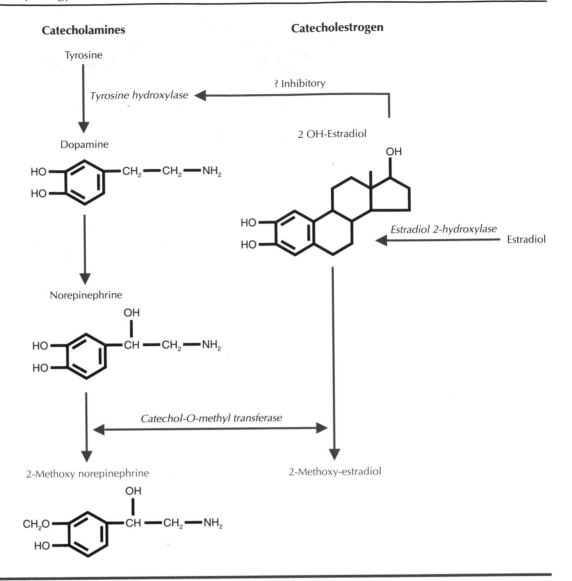

Catecholamines

Tyrosine

Tyrosine hydroxylase

Dopamine

Norepinephrine

Catechol-O-methyl transferase

2-Methoxy norepinephrine

Catecholestrogen

? Inhibitory

2 OH-Estradiol

Estradiol 2-hydroxylase ← Estradiol

2-Methoxy-estradiol

Catecholestrogens	The enzyme that converts estrogens to catecholestrogens (2-hydroxylase) is richly concentrated in the hypothalamus; hence there are higher concentrations of catecholestrogens than estrone and estradiol in the hypothalamus and pituitary gland. Catecholestrogens have two faces, a catechol side and an estrogen side. Because catecholestrogens have two faces, they have the potential for interacting with both catecholamine and estrogen-mediated systems.[56] To be specific, catecholestrogens can inhibit tyrosine hydroxylase (which would decrease catecholamines) and compete for catechol-*o*-methyltransferase (which would increase catecholamines). Since GnRH, estrogens, and catecholestrogens are located in similar sites, it is possible that catecholestrogens may serve to interact between catecholamines and GnRH secretion. However, these functions remain speculative because a definite role for catecholsteroids has not been established.

Summary: Control of GnRH Pulses	The key concept is that normal menstrual function requires GnRH pulsatile secretion in a critical range of frequency and amplitude.[16,17,57] The normal physiology and pathophysiology of the menstrual cycle, at least in terms of central control, can be explained by mechanisms which affect the pulsatile secretion of GnRH. The pulses of GnRH appear to be directly under the influence of a dual catecholaminergic system: norepinephrine facilatory and dopamine inhibitory. In turn, the catecholamine system can be influenced by endogenous opioid activity. The feedback effects of steroids may be

mediated through this system via catecholsteroid messengers or directly by influencing the various neurotransmitters.

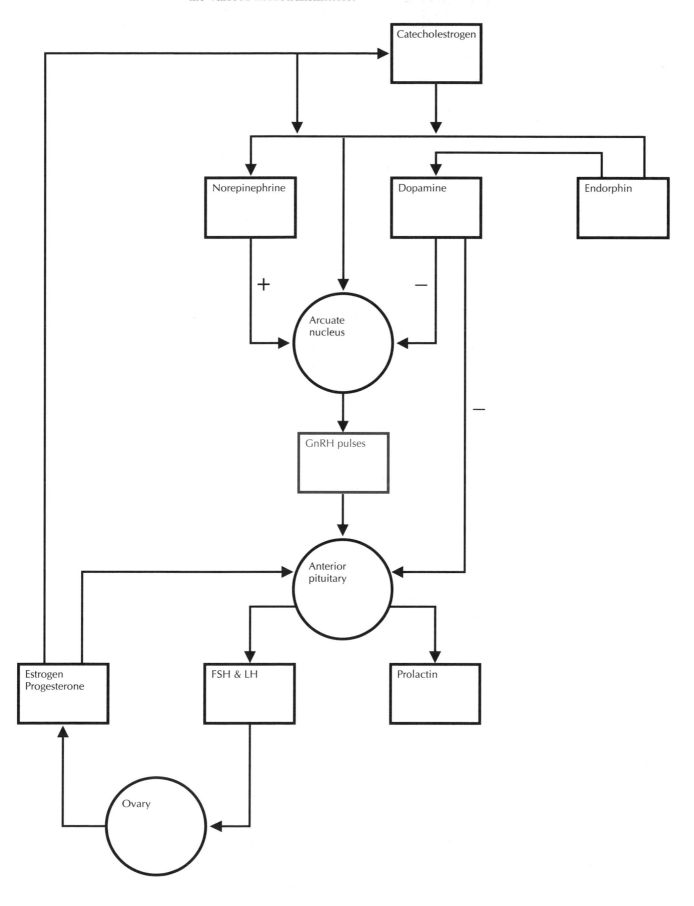

GnRH Agonists in Clinical Use

Position	1	2	3	4	5	6	7	8	9	10
Native GnRH	pGlu	His	Trp	Ser	Tyr	Gly	Leu	Arg	Pro	Gly-NH$_2$
Leuprolide						D-Leu				NH-Ethylamide
Buserelin						D-Ser (tertiary butanol)				NH-Ethylamide
Nafarelin						D-Naphthylalanine (2)				
Histrelin						D-His (tertiary benzyl)				NH-Ethylamide
Goserelin						D-Ser (tertiary butanol)				Aza-Gly
Deslorelin						D-Trp				NH-Ethylamide
Tryptorelin						D-Trp				

GnRH Agonists and Antagonists

The short half-life of GnRH is due to rapid cleavage of the bonds between amino acids 5–6, 6–7, and 9–10. By altering amino acids at these positions, analogues of GnRH can be synthesized with different properties. Thousands of GnRH analogues have been produced. Substitution of amino acids at the 6 position or replacement of the C-terminal glycine-amide (inhibiting degradation) produces agonists. The GnRH agonists are administered either intramuscularly or subcutaneously or by intranasal absorption. An initial agonistic action (the so-called flare effect) is associated with an increase in the circulating levels of FSH and LH. This response is greatest in the early follicular phase when GnRH and estradiol have combined to create a large reserve pool of gonadotropins. After 1–3 weeks, down-regulation and densensitization of the pituitary produce a hypogonadotropic, hypogonad state. The initial response is due to a loss of receptors, while the sustained response is due to desensitization and the uncoupling of the receptor from its effector system. Furthermore, postreceptor mechanisms lead to secretion of biologically inactive gonadotropins, which, however, can still be detected by immunoassay.

Gonadotropin releasing hormone

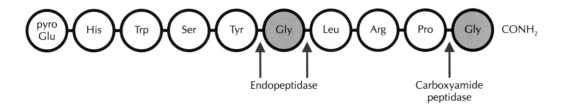

GnRH agonists

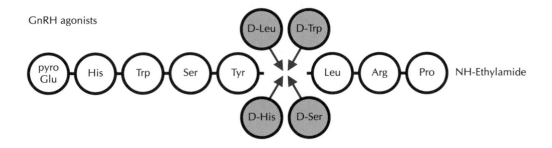

Suppression of pituitary secretion of gonadotropins by a GnRH agonist can be utilized for the treatment of endometriosis, uterine leiomyomas, precocious puberty, or the prevention of menstrual bleeding in special clinical situations (e.g., in thrombocytopenic patients). Various tumors contain receptors for GnRH, such as breast, pancreatic, and ovarian, and therefore, there exists a potential for treatment.

GnRH antagonists are synthesized by multiple amino acid substitutions. GnRH antagonists bind to the GnRH receptor and provide competitive inhibition of the naturally occurring GnRH. Thus GnRH antagonists produce an immediate decline in gonadotropin levels with an immediate therapeutic effect. The early products either lacked potency or were associated with undesirable side effects due to histamine release. New analogs continue to be developed and tested, aimed toward the control of fertility.[42] The combination of a GnRH antagonist and testosterone holds promise as a male contraceptive agent.

The GnRH analogues cannot escape destruction if administered orally. Higher doses administered subcutaneously can achieve nearly equal effects as observed with intravenous treatment; however, the smaller blood peaks are slower to develop and take longer to return to baseline. Other forms of administration include nasal spray, sustained release implants, and injections of biodegradable microspheres. With the nasal route, absorption enhancers have to be added to increase bioavailability; these agents produce considerable nasal irritation. Goserelin consists of a small biodegradable cylinder which is inserted subcutaneously and monthly using a prepackaged syringe. The depot formulation of leuprolide is administered intramuscularly and monthly.

Tanycytes

A significant pathway for hypothalamic influence may be via the cerebrospinal fluid (CSF). Tanycytes are specialized ependymal cells whose ciliated cell bodies line the third ventricle over the median eminence. The cells terminate on portal vessels, and they can transport materials from ventricular CSF to the portal system, e.g., substances from the pineal gland, or vasopressin, or oxytocin. Tanycytes change morphologically in response to steroids and exhibit morphological changes during the ovarian cycle.

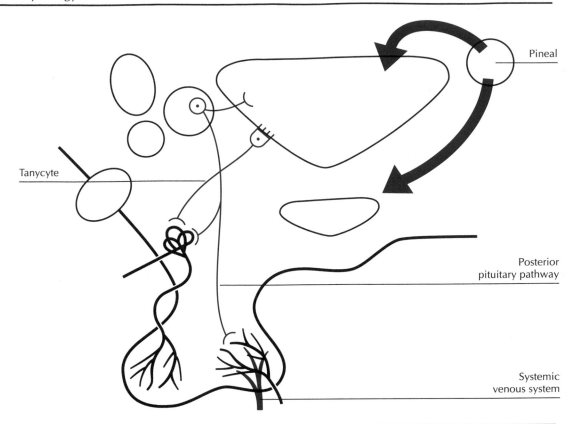

The Posterior Pituitary Pathway

The posterior pituitary is a direct prolongation of the hypothalamus via the pituitary stalk, whereas the anterior pituitary arises from pharyngeal epithelium that migrates into position with the posterior pituitary. Separate neurosecretory cells in both the supraoptic and paraventricular nuclei make vasopressin and oxytocin as parts of large precursor molecules that also contain the transport peptide, neurophysin.[58] Both oxytocin and vasopressin consist of 9 amino acid residues. In the human, vasopressin contains arginine, unlike animals that have lysine vasopressin. The neurophysins are polypeptides with a molecular weight of about 10,000. There are two distinct neurophysins, estrogen-stimulated neurophysin known as neurophysin I, and nicotine-stimulated neurophysin, known as neurophysin II.

The genes for oxytocin and vasopressin are closely linked on the same chromosome. The transcriptional activity of these genes is regulated by endocrine factors, such as the sex steroids and thyroid hormone, through hormone-response elements located upstream. The neurons secrete two large protein molecules, a precursor called pro-pressophysin, which contains vasopressin and its neurophysin, and a precursor called pro-oxyphysin, which contains oxytocin and its neurophysin.[59] Neurophysin I is specifically related to oxytocin, and neurophysin II accompanies vasopressin. Because of this unique packaging, the hormones and their neurophysins are stored together and released at the same time into the circulation. The neurophysins are cleaved from their associated neurohormones during axonal transport from the neuronal cell bodies in the supraoptic and paraventricular nuclei to the posterior pituitary. The only known function for the neurophysins is axonal transport for oxytocin and vasopressin.

The posterior pathway is complex and not limited to the transmission of vasopressin and oxytocin to the posterior pituitary. The transportation of vasopressin and oxytocin to the posterior pituitary occurs via nerve tracts which emanate from the supraoptic and paraventricular nuclei and descend through the median eminence to terminate in the posterior pituitary. However, these hormones are also secreted into the cerebrospinal fluid and directly into the portal system. Therefore, vasopressin and oxytocin can reach

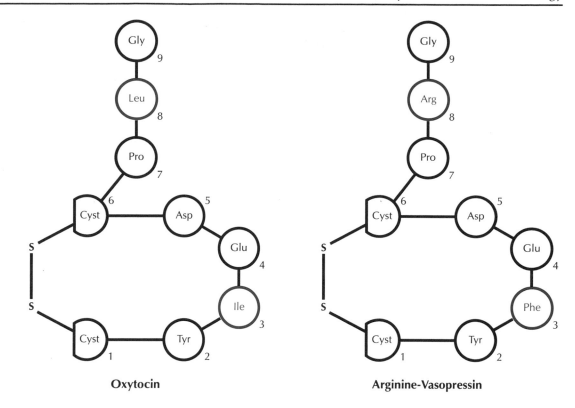

Oxytocin **Arginine-Vasopressin**

the anterior pituitary and influence, in the case of vasopressin, ACTH secretion, and in the case of oxytocin, gonadotropin secretion. Vasopressin cooperates with corticotropin releasing hormone to cause an increased yield of ACTH. Vasopressin and oxytocin-like materials are also found in the ovary, the oviduct, the testis, and the adrenal gland, suggesting that these neurohypophyseal peptides have roles as paracrine or autocrine hormones.[60] The concentrations of these substances in the cerebrospinal fluid exhibit a circadian rhythm (with peak levels occurring during the day), suggesting a different mechanism for CSF secretion compared to posterior pituitary release.[61]

Neurophysin II is called nicotine neurophysin because the administration of nicotine or hemorrhage increases the circulating levels. Neurophysin I is called estrogen neurophysin because estrogen administration increases the levels in the peripheral blood, and peak levels of both neurophysin I and oxytocin are found at the time of the LH surge.[62] The rise in estrogen neurophysin begins 10 hours after the rise in estrogen amd precedes that of the LH surge, and the elevation of neurophysin lasts longer than the LH surge. Because GnRH and oxytocin are competing substrates for hypothalamic degradation enzymes, it has been hypothesized that oxytocin in the portal blood at the midcycle may inhibit the metabolism of GnRH, thus increasing the amount of GnRH available. Furthermore, oxytocin may have direct actions on the pituitary, ovary, uterus, and fallopian tube during ovulation.

Neurophysin-containing pathways have been traced from the hypothalamic nuclei to various centers in the brainstem and the spinal cord. In addition, behavioral studies suggest a role for vasopressin in learning and memory. Administration of vasopressin has been associated with improvement in memory in brain-damaged human subjects, and enhanced cognitive responses (learning and memory) in both young, normal individuals and depressed patients.

Both oxytocin and vasopressin circulate as the free peptides with a rapid half-life (initial component less than 1 minute, second component of 2–3 minutes). Three major stimuli for vasopressin secretion are changes in osmolality of the blood, alterations in blood volume, and psychogenic stimuli such as pain and fear. The osmoreceptors are located in the hypothalamus; the volume receptors are in the left atrium, aortic arch, and carotid sinus. Angiotensin II also produces a release of vasopressin, suggesting another mechanism for the link between fluid balance and vasopressin. Cortisol may modify the osmotic threshold for the release of vasopressin.

The major functions of vasopressin involve the regulation of osmolality and blood volume. Vasopressin is a powerful vasoconstrictor and antidiuretic hormone. Vasopressin release increases when plasma osmolality rises and is inhibited by water loading (resulting in diuresis). Diabetes insipidus is a condition marked by loss of water because of a lack of vasopressin action in the tubules of the kidney, secondary to a defect in synthesis or secretion of vasopressin. The opposite condition is the continuous and autonomous secretion of vasopressin, the syndrome of inappropriate ADH (antidiuretic hormone) secretion. This syndrome, with its resultant retention of water, is associated with a variety of brain disorders as well as the production of vasopressin and its precursor by malignant tumors.

Oxytocin stimulates muscular contractions in the uterus and myoepithelial contractions in the breast. Thus it is involved in parturition and the letdown of milk. The release of oxytocin is so episodic that it is described as spurts. Ordinarily, there are about 3 spurts every 10 minutes. Oxytocin is released during coitus, probably by the Ferguson reflex (vaginal and cervical stimulation) but also by olfactory, visual, and auditory pathways. Perhaps oxytocin has some role in muscle contractions during orgasm.[63] In the male, release of oxytocin during coitus may contribute to sperm transport during ejaculation.

Maternal plasma oxytocin increases with gestational age, as do amniotic fluid levels. Fetal urine and meconium contain large amounts of oxytocin. Maternal levels increase from the first stage to the second stage of labor but decline during the third stage. The major mechanism is thought to be the Ferguson reflex.

Umbilical artery levels of oxytocin are always higher than umbilical vein levels, except when oxytocin is administered. Since oxytocin readily crosses the placenta, it is likely that during normal labor fetal oxytocin crosses into the maternal compartment, and during oxytocin administration there is a reverse movement into the fetal compartment. It is uncertain whether fetal oxytocin plays a role during labor.[64]

Oxytocin is released in response to suckling, mediated through impulses generated at the nipple and transmitted via the 3rd, 4th, and 5th thoracic nerves to the spinal cord to the hypothalamus. In addition to causing milk ejection, the reflex is responsible for the uterine contractions associated with breastfeeding. Opioid peptides inhibit oxytocin release, and this may be the means by which stress, fear, and anger inhibit milk output in lactating women.

The Brain and Ovulation

Classic studies in a variety of rodents indicated the presence of feedback centers in the hypothalamus that responded to steroids with the release of GnRH. The release of GnRH was the result of the complex, but coordinated, relationships among the neurohormones, the pituitary gonadotropins, and the gonadal steroids designated by the time-honored terms positive and negative feedback.

FSH levels were thought to be largely regulated by a negative inhibitory feedback relationship with estradiol. In the case of LH, there existed both a negative inhibitory feedback relationship with estradiol and a positive stimulatory feedback with high levels of estradiol. The feedback centers were located in the hypothalamus, and they were called the tonic and cyclic centers. The tonic center controlled the day-to-day basal level of gonadotropins and was responsive to the negative feedback effects of steroids. The cyclic center in the female brain was responsible for the midcycle surge of gonadotropins, a response mediated by the positive feedback of estrogen. Specifically, the midcycle surge of gonadotropins was thought to be due to an outpouring of GnRH in response to the positive feedback action of estradiol on the cyclic center of the hypothalamus.

This classic concept was not inaccurate. The problem was that the concept accurately described events in the rodent, but the mechanism is different in the primate.

In the primate, the "center" for the midcycle surge of gonadotropins has moved from the hypothalamus to the pituitary. Experiments in the monkey have demonstrated that GnRH, originating in the hypothalamus, plays a permissive role. Its pulsatile secretion is an important prerequisite for normal pituitary function,[57] but the feedback responses regulating gonadotropin levels are controlled by ovarian steroid feedback on the anterior pituitary cells.

The present concept is derived from experiments in which the medial basal hypothalamus (MBH) is either destroyed[14] or the hypothalamus is surgically separated from the pituitary.[65] In a typical (and now classic) experiment, lesion of the MBH by radiofrequency waves was followed by loss of LH levels as the source of GnRH was eliminated.[13] Administration of GnRH in a pulsatile fashion by an intravenous pump restored LH secretion. The administration of estradiol was then able to produce both negative and positive feedback responses, clearly actions that must be directly on the anterior pituitary because the hypothalamus was absent and GnRH was being administered in a steady and unchanging frequency and dose.

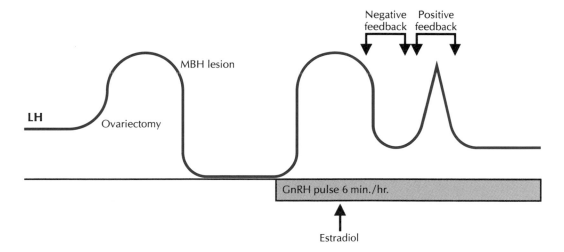

Administration of GnRH intravenously as a bolus produces an increase in blood levels of LH and FSH within 5 minutes, reaching a peak in about 20–25 minutes for LH and 45 minutes for FSH. Levels return to pretreatment values after several hours. When administered by constant infusion at submaximal doses, there is first a rapid rise with a peak at 30 minutes, followed by a plateau or fall between 45 and 90 minutes, then a second and sustained increase at 225–240 minutes. This biphasic response suggests the presence of two functional pools of pituitary gonadotropins.[66] The readily releasable pool (secretion) produces the initial response, and the later response is dependent upon a second, reserve pool of stored gonadotropins.

There are three principal positive actions of GnRH on gonadotropin elaboration.

1. Synthesis and storage (the reserve pool) of gonadotropins.

2. Activation, movement of gonadotropins from the reserve pool to a pool ready for direct secretion, a self-priming action.

3. Immediate release (direct secretion) of gonadotropins.

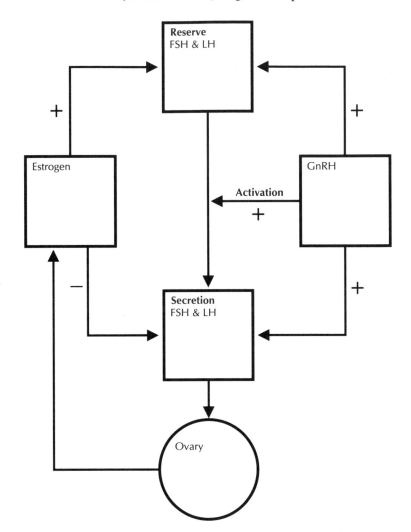

Secretion, synthesis, and storage change during the cycle. At the beginning of the cycle, when estrogen levels are low, both secretion and storage levels are low. With increasing levels of estradiol, a greater increase occurs in storage, with little change in secretion. Thus, in the early follicular phase, estrogen has a positive effect on the synthesis and storage response, building up a supply of gonadotropins in order to meet the requirements of the midcycle surge. Premature release of gonadotropins is prevented by a negative (inhibitory) action of estradiol on the pituitary secretory response to GnRH.

As the midcycle approaches, subsequent responses to GnRH are greater than initial responses, indicating that each response not only induces release of gonadotropins but also activates the storage pool for the next response. This sensitizing or priming action of GnRH also involves an increase in the number of its own receptors and requires the presence of estrogen.[67,68]

Because the midcycle surge of LH can be produced in the experimental monkey in the absence of a hypothalamus, and in the face of unchanging GnRH, the ovulatory surge of LH is now believed to be a response to positive feedback action of estradiol on the anterior pituitary. When the estradiol level in the circulation reaches a critical concentration and this concentration is maintained for a critical time period, the inhibitory action on LH secretion changes to a stimulatory action. The mechanism of this steroid action is not known with certainty, but experimental evidence suggests that the positive feedback action involves an increase in GnRH receptor concentration, while the negative feedback of estrogen operates through an uncertain, but different, system.[69,70]

What a logical mechanism! The midcycle surge must occur at the right time of the cycle to ovulate a ready and waiting mature follicle. What better way to achieve this extreme degree of coordination and timing than by the follicle itself, through the feedback effects of the sex steroids originating in the follicle destined to ovulate.

GnRH is increased in the peripheral blood of women and the portal blood of monkeys at midcycle. While this increase may not be absolutely necessary (as demonstrated in the monkey experiments), studies do indicate that activity is occurring in both the hypothalamus and the pituitary.[71,72] Therefore, although the system can operate with only an unwavering, permissive action of GnRH, fine tuning probably takes place by means of simultaneous effects on GnRH pulsatile secretion and pituitary response to GnRH. This is supported by gonadotropin gene expression studies, indicating steroid effects at both the hypothalamus and the pituitary. The upstream region of the LH-subunit gene (in the rat) binds the estrogen receptor, providing a means for direct steroid hormone modulation in the pituitary.[73] The human GnRH gene contains a hormone responsive element that binds estrogen and its receptor.[74] However, studies have failed to detect the presence of estrogen receptors in GnRH neurons and this hormone responsive element may be regulated by other substances.

Influencing the hypothalamic frequency of GnRH secretion can in turn influence pituitary response to GnRH. Faster or slower frequencies of GnRH pulses result in lower GnRH receptor numbers in the pituitary.[75] Thus a critical peak frequency is necessary for peak numbers of GnRH receptors and the peak midcycle response. Here is a method for the fine tuning at both the hypothalamus (pulse frequency) and the pituitary (receptor number). Indeed, turning off the surge may involve down-regulation because of excessive GnRH. Studies in sheep indicate that a surge of GnRH at the time of the LH surge is associated with a switch from episodic secretion to continuous secretion into the portal circulation, producing the high exposure known to result in down-regulation.[76]

Another aspect of gonadotropin secretion is clinically important. A disparity exists between the quantity of LH measured during the midcycle surge as determined by immunoassay and bioassay. More LH is secreted at midcycle in a molecular form with greater biological activity.[77] There is a well-established relationship between the activity and half-life of glycoprotein hormones and molecular composition (see Chapter 2, under "Heterogeneity" of tropic hormones). The estrogen influence on gonadotropin synthesis is an additional method for maximizing the biologic effects of the midcycle surge. The bioactivity is also very dependent upon pulsatile stimulation by GnRH.

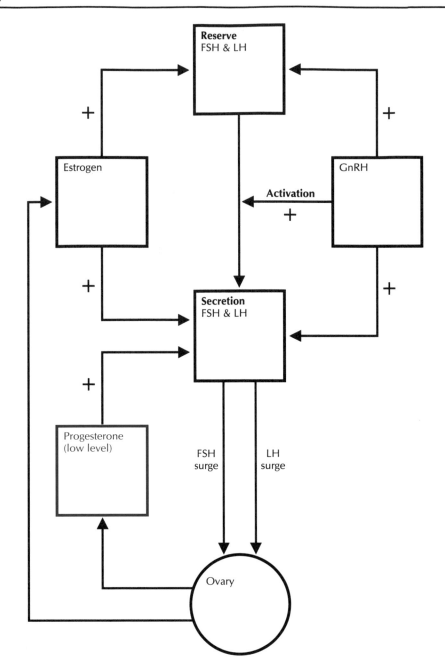

The midcycle surge of FSH has an important clinical purpose. A normal corpus luteum requires the induction of an adequate number of LH receptors on granulosa cells, a specific action of FSH. In addition, FSH accomplishes important intrafollicular changes necessary for the physical expulsion of the ovum. The midcycle surge of FSH, therefore, plays a critical role in ensuring ovulation and a normal corpus luteum. Emerging progesterone secretion, just prior to ovulation, is the key.

Progesterone, at low levels and in the presence of estrogen, augments the pituitary secretion of LH and is responsible for the FSH surge in response to GnRH.[78–81] As the rising levels of LH produce the morphologic change of luteinization in the ovulating follicle, the granulosa layer begins to secrete progesterone directly into the bloodstream. The process of luteinization is inhibited by the presence of the oocyte, and therefore progesterone secretion is relatively suppressed, ensuring that only low levels of progesterone reach the brain.

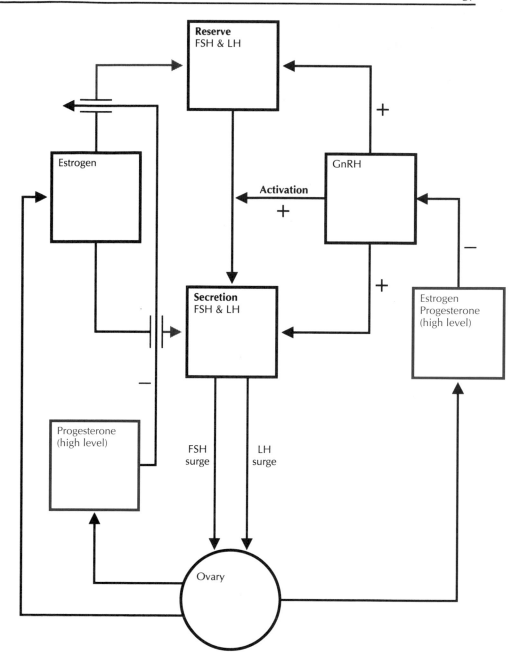

After ovulation, rapid and full luteinization is accompanied by a marked increase in progesterone levels, which, in the presence of estrogen, exercise a profound negative feedback action to suppress gonadotropin secretion. This action of progesterone takes place in two locations.[82–84] First, there definitely is a central action to decrease GnRH.[85] Progesterone fails to block estradiol-induced gonadotropin discharges in monkeys with hypothalamic lesions if pulsatile GnRH replacement is provided. Therefore, high levels of progesterone inhibit ovulation at the hypothalamic level. In addition, progesterone can also block estrogen-induced responses to GnRH at the pituitary level. In contrast, the facilatory action of low levels of progesterone is exerted only at the pituitary on the response to GnRH.

Summary: Key Points

1. Pulsatile GnRH secretion must be within a critical range for frequency and concentration (amplitude).

2. GnRH has only positive actions on the anterior pituitary: synthesis and storage, activation, and secretion of gonadotropins. The gonadotropins are secreted in a pulsatile fashion in response to the similar pulsatile release of GnRH.

3. Low levels of estrogen enhance FSH and LH synthesis and storage, have little effect on LH secretion, and inhibit FSH secretion.

4. High levels of estrogen induce the LH surge at midcycle, and high steady levels of estrogen lead to sustained elevated LH secretion.

5. Low levels of progesterone acting at the level of the pituitary gland enhance the LH response to GnRH and are responsible for the FSH surge at midcycle.

6. High levels of progesterone inhibit pituitary secretion of gonadotropins by inhibiting GnRH pulses at the level of the hypothalamus. In addition, high levels of progesterone antagonize pituitary response to GnRH by interfering with estrogen action.

The Pineal Gland

Although no physiologic role has been firmly established in the human, the reproductive functions of the hypothalamus may also be under inhibitory control of the brain via the pineal gland. The pineal arises as an outgrowth of the roof of the third ventricle, but soon after birth it loses all afferent and efferent neural connections with the brain. Instead the parenchymal cells receive a new and unusual sympathetic innervation which allows the pineal gland to be an active neuroendocrine organ that responds to photic and hormonal stimuli and exhibits circadian rhythms.[86,87]

The neural pathway begins in the retina and passes through the inferior accessory optic tracts and the medial forebrain bundle to the upper cord. Preganglionic fibers terminate at the superior cervical ganglion, and postganglionic symathetic nerves terminate directly on pineal cells. Interruption of this pathway gives the same effect as darkness, which is an increase in pineal biosynthetic activity.

Hydroxyindole-*o*-methyltransferase (HIOMT), an enzyme essential for melatonin synthesis, is found mainly in pineal parenchymal cells, and its products are essentially unique to the pineal. Norepinephrine stimulates tryptophan entry into the pineal cell and also adenylate cyclase activity in the membrane. The resulting increase in cyclic AMP leads to *N*-acetyltransferase activity, the rate-limiting step in melatonin synthesis. Thus, melatonin synthesis is controlled by norepinephrine stimulation of adenylate cyclase, and the norepinephrine is liberated by sympathetic stimulation due to the absence of light. HIOMT is also found in the retina where melatonin may serve to regulate the pigment in retinal cells, and in the intestine. However, pinealectomy completely eliminates detectable levels of melatonin in the circulation. Calcification of the pineal gland is common. It is frequently present in young children, and almost all elderly people have pineal calcification.

The association of hyperplastic pineal tumors with decreased gonadal function, and destructive tumors with precocious puberty, suggested that the pineal is the source of gonadal inhibiting substances. However, pineal mechanisms cannot be absolutely essential for gonadal function. Normal reproductive function returns to the pinealectomized rat several weeks after pinealectomy; blind women have normal fertility, and pinealectomy in a primate did not affect pubertal development.[88]

Darkness ⟶ Increased Melatonin ⟶ Decreased GnRH

A rat in constant light develops a small pineal with decreased HIOMT and melatonin, while the ovarian weight increases. A rat in constant dark has the opposite result, increased pineal size, HIOMT, and melatonin, with decreased ovarian weight and pituitary function. A rhythm is established in pineal HIOMT activity by the presence or absence of light. Short days and long nights result in gonadal atrophy, and this is the major mechanism governing seasonal breeding.[89] Possible roles in humans may be to give circadian rhythmicity to other functions such as temperature and sleep. In all vertebrates tested so far, there is a daily and seasonal rhythm in melatonin secretion: high values during the dark and low during light, greater secretion in the winter compared to the summer. Desynchronization with travel across time zones may contribute to the symptom complex known as jet lag.

The pineal, therefore, serves as an interface between the environment and hypothalamic-pituitary function. In order to correctly interpret day length, animals require a daily rhythm in melatonin secretion. This coordination of temporal, environmental information is especially important in seasonal breeders. This pineal rhythm appears to require the suprachiasmatic nucleus, perhaps the site at which pineal function and light changes are coordinated.

Melatonin is synthesized and secreted by the pineal gland and circulates in the blood like a classical hormone. It affects distant target organs, especially the neuroendocrine centers of the central nervous system. Whether melatonin is secreted primarily into the CSF or blood is still debated, but most evidence favors blood. Melatonin may reach the hypothalamus from the CSF by way of tanycyte transport.

The gonadal changes associated with melatonin are mediated via the hypothalamus and suggest a general suppressive effect on GnRH pulsatile secretion and reproductive function. In humans, melatonin blood levels are highest in the first year of life (with highest levels at night), then decrease with age, eventually releasing, some claim, the suppression of GnRH prior to puberty.[89] This hypothesis is challenged by the association of blindness in human females with an age of menarche that is earlier than normal.[90] On the other hand, there is a seasonal distribution in human conception in northern countries with a decrease in conception rates during the dark winter months.[91] Some report melatonin levels to be lowest at the time of the midcycle ovulatory surge; others do not.[92,93]

Pineal activity can be viewed as the net balance between hormone and neuron mediated influences. The pineal contains receptors for the active sex hormones, estradiol, testosterone, dihydrotestosterone, progesterone, and prolactin. Furthermore, the pineal converts testosterone and progesterone to the active 5α-reduced metabolites, and androgens are aromatized to estrogens. The pineal also appears to be unique in that a catecholamine neurotransmitter (norepinephrine), interacting with cell membrane receptors, stimulates cellular synthesis of estrogen and androgen receptors. In general, however, the sympathetic activity producing the circadian rhythm takes precedence over hormonal effects.

Despite a variety of suggestive leads, there is no definitive evidence for a role of the pineal in humans. Nevertheless the important relationship between light exposure and circadian rhythms continues to focus attention on the pineal gland as a coordinator.[94] In addition, the pineal can disrupt normal gonadal function. A male with delayed puberty due to hypogonadotropism has been described, who had an enlarged, hyperfunctional pineal gland.[95] Over time, his melatonin levels spontaneously decreased, and normal pituitary-gonadal function developed. Elevated nocturnal levels of melatonin have been reported in patients with hypothalmic amenorrhea and women with anorexia nervosa.[96]

A possible influence of the pineal gland may be the synchronization of menstrual cycles noted among women who spend time together. A significant increase in synchronization of cycles among roommates and among closest friends occurred in the first 4 months of residency in a dormitory of a women's college.[97] A similar increase in synchrony has been observed in women coworkers in occupations characterized by levels of interdependency that were equal to or greater than the levels of encountered job stress.[98] However, efforts to replicate these results have not always been successful.[99]

A number of other indoles (also derivatives of tryptophan) have been identified in the pineal gland. Biologic roles for these indoles remain elusive, but one in particular has been extensively investigated. Arginine vasotocin differs from oxytocin by a single amino acid in position 8 and from vasopressin by a single amino acid in position 3. In general, arginine vasotocin has an inhibitory action on the gonads and pituitary secretion of prolactin and LH. Nevertheless a precise role continues to be evasive.

Gonadotropin Secretion through Fetal Life, Childhood, and Puberty

We have often considered the endocrine events during puberty as an awakening, a beginning. However, endocrinologically, puberty is not a beginning, but just another stage in a development that began at conception. The development of the anterior pituitary in the human starts between the 4th and 5th weeks of fetal life, and by the 12th week of gestation the vascular connection between the hypothalamus and the pituitary is functional. Gonadotropin production has been documented throughout fetal life, during childhood, and into adult life.[100] Remarkable levels of FSH and LH, similar to postmenopausal levels, can be measured in the fetus. GnRH is detectable in the hypothalamus by 10 weeks of gestation, and by 10–13 weeks when the vascular connection is complete, FSH and LH are being produced in the pituitary. The peak pituitary concentrations of FSH and LH occur at about 20–23 weeks of intrauterine life, and peak circulating levels occur at 28 weeks.

The increasing production rate of gonadotropins until midgestation reflects the growing ability of the hypothalamic-pituitary axis to perform at full capacity. Beginning at midgestation, there is an increasing sensitivity to inhibition by steroids and a resultant decrease in gonadotropin secretion. Full sensitivity to steroids is not reached until late in infancy. The rise in gonadotropins after birth reflects loss of the high levels of placental steroids. Thus, in the first year of life there is considerable follicular activity in the ovaries in contrast to later in childhood when gonadotropin secretion is suppressed. Furthermore, the postnatal rise in gonadotropins is even greater in infants born prematurely.

Testicular function in the fetus can be correlated with the fetal hormone patterns. Initial testosterone production and sexual differentiation are in response to the fetal levels of HCG, whereas further testosterone production and masculine differentiation appear to be maintained by the fetal pituitary gonadotropins. Decreased testosterone levels in late gestation probably reflect the decrease in gonadotropin levels. The fetal generation of Leydig cells somehow avoids down-regulation and responds to high levels of HCG and LH by increased steroidogenesis and cell multiplication. This generation of cells is replaced by the adult generation which becomes functional at puberty and responds to high levels of HCG and LH with down-regulation and decreased steroidogenesis.

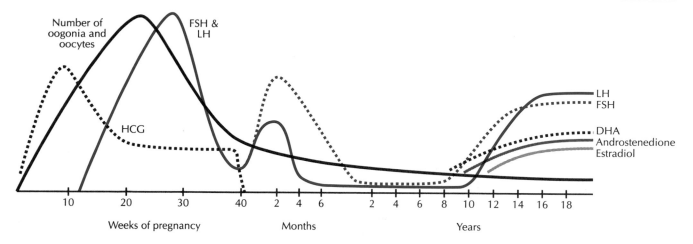

There is a sex difference in fetal gonadotropin levels. There are higher pituitary and circulating FSH and pituitary LH levels in female fetuses. The lower male levels are probably due to testicular testosterone and inhibin production. In infancy, the postnatal FSH rise is more marked and more sustained in females, while LH values are not as high. This early activity is accompanied by inhibin levels comparable to the low range observed during the follicular phase of the menstrual cycle.[101] After the postnatal rise, gonadotropin levels reach a nadir during early childhood (by about 6 months of age in males and 1–2 years in females) and then rise slightly between 4 and 10 years. This childhood period is characterized by low levels of gonadotropins in the pituitary and in the blood, little response of the pituitary to GnRH, and maximal hypothalamic suppression.

The precise signal that initiates the events of puberty is unknown.[102] In girls, the first steroids to rise in the blood are dehydroepiandrosterone (DHA) and its sulfate (DHAS) beginning at 6–8 years of age, at the same time that FSH begins to increase. Estrogen levels, as well as LH, do not begin to rise until 10–12 years of age. If the onset of puberty is triggered by the first hormone to increase in the circulation, then a role for adrenal steroids must be considered. However, there is no evidence to suggest that the adrenal steroids are necessary for the proper timing of puberty, and adrenarche appears to be independent, not controlled by the same mechanism which turns on the gonads.[103] Neither is there a definite relationship demonstrated between melatonin secretion and puberty. Because the studies have focused on the amount of melatonin secreted rather than the rhythm of secretion, this question remains open.

Prior to puberty, gonadotropin levels are low but still associated with pulses (although quite irregular).[104] The clinical onset of puberty is preceded by an increase in pulse frequency, amplitude, and regularity, especially during the night.[104,105] At the time of appearance of secondary sex characteristics, the mean LH levels are 2 to 4 times higher during sleep than during wakefulness. This pattern is not present before or after puberty and is an early sign of changes taking place in the hypothalamus, where there is increasing coordination of GnRH neurons with increasing GnRH pulsatile secretion. This pattern can be detected in individuals who develop increasing and decreasing degrees of hypothalamic suppression (such as in individuals with worsening and improving anorexia nervosa). FSH levels plateau by midpuberty, while LH and estradiol levels continue to rise until late puberty. Biologically active LH has been found to rise proportionately more than immunoactive LH with the onset of puberty.

The rise of gonadotropins at puberty appears to be independent of the gonads in that the same response can be observed in patients with gonadal dysgenesis (who lack functional steroid-producing gonadal tissue). Adolescent girls with Turner syndrome (45,X) also demonstrate augmented gonadotropin secretion during sleep.[106] Thus, maturation at puberty must involve changes in the hypothalamus that are independent of ovarian steroids.

The maturational change in the hypothalamus is followed by an orderly and predictable sequence of events. Increased GnRH secretion leads to increased pituitary responsiveness to GnRH (a combination of steroid influence on the pituitary and a frequency effect of GnRH pulses on GnRH receptor numbers), leading to increasing production and secretion of gonadotropins. Increased gonadotropins are responsible for follicular growth and development in the ovary and increased sex steroid levels. The rising estrogen contributes to achieving an adult pattern of pulsatile GnRH secretion, finally leading to cyclic menstrual patterns.

The trend toward lowering of the menarcheal age and the period of acceleration of growth has halted. In a 10-year prospective study of middle class contemporary American girls, the mean age of menarche was 12.83 with a range of 9.14–17.70 years.[107] The age of onset of puberty is variable and influenced by genetic factors, socioeconomic conditions, and general health. The earlier menarche today compared to the past is undoubtedly due to improved nutrition and better health. It has been suggested that initiation of growth and menarche occur at a particular body weight (48 kg) and percent of body fat (17%).[108] It is thought that this relationship reflects a required stage of metabolism. Although this hypothesis of a critical weight is a helpful concept, the extreme variability in onset of menarche indicates that there is no particular age or size at which an individual girl should be expected to experience menarche.

In the female, the typical sequence of events is growth initiation, thelarche, pubarche, and finally menarche. This generally begins sometime between 8 and 14 years of age. The length of time involved in this evolution is usually 2–4 years. During this time span, puberty is said to occur. Individual variation in the order of appearance of this sequence is great. For example, growth of pubic hair and breast development are not always correlated.

Puberty is due to the reactivation of the hypothalamic-pituitary axis, once fully active during fetal life but suppressed during childhood. If the systems are potentially responsive, what holds function in check until puberty? The hypothalamic-pituitary-gonadal system is operative prior to puberty but is extremely sensitive to steroids and therefore suppressed. The changes at puberty are due to a gradually increasing gonadotropin secretion that takes place because of a decrease in the sensitivity of the hypothalamic centers to the negative-inhibitory action of gonadal steroids. This can be pictured as a slowly rising set point of decreased sensitivity, resulting in increasing GnRH pulsatile secretion, leading to increasing gonadotropin production and ovarian stimulation, and finally to increasing estrogen levels. The reason that FSH is the first gonadotropin to rise at puberty is that arcuate activity begins with a low frequency of GnRH pulses. This is associated with a rise in FSH and little change in LH. With acceleration of frequency, FSH and LH reach adult levels. In addition, there is a qualitative change as a greater increase occurs in the bioactive forms of the gonadotropins.

Negative feedback of steroids, however, cannot be the sole explanation for the low gonadotropin levels in children. Agonadal children show the same decline in gonadotropins from age 2 to 6 as do normal children.[109] This indicates an intrinsic CNS inhibitory mechanism independent of gonadal steroids. Therefore, the restraint of puberty can be viewed as the result of two forces:

1. A CNS inhibitory force, a mechanism suppressing GnRH pulsatile secretion.

2. A very sensitive negative feedback of gonadal steroids (6–15 times more sensitive before puberty).

Because agonadal children show a rise in gonadotropins at pubertal age following suppression to a nadir during childhood, the dominant mechanism must be a CNS inhibitory force. The initial maturational change in the hypothalamus would then be a decrease in this inhibitory influence. A search for this mechanism continues. Some have argued that, rather than a chronic state of inhibition prior to puberty, the GnRH neurons exist in an unrestrained but uncoordinated pattern of activity that prevents adequate secretion.

The development of the positive feedback response to estrogen occurs later. This explains the well-known finding of anovulation in the first months (as long as 18 months) of menstruation. There are frequent exceptions, however, and ovulation can occur even at the time of menarche.

Don't think of puberty as being turned on by a controlling center in the brain but rather as a functional summary of all the influences. This is more a concept than an actual locus of action.

The overall result of this change in the hypothalamus is the development of secondary sex characteristics, attainment of adult set point levels, and the ability to reproduce. Neoplastic and vascular disorders that alter hypothalamic sensitivity can reverse the prepubertal threshold restraint and lead to precocious puberty.

References

1. **Kendrick KM, Dixson AF,** Luteinizing hormone releasing hormone enhances proceptivity in a primate, Neuroendocrinology 41:449, 1985.

2. **Hayflick JS, Adelman JP, Seeburg PH,** The complete nucleotide sequence of the human gonadotropin-releasing hormone gene, Nucleic Acids Res 17:6403, 1989.

3. **Nikolics K, Mason AJ, Szonyi E, Ramachandran J, Seeburg PH,** A prolactin-inhibiting factor within the precursor for human gonadotropin-releasing hormone, Nature 316:511, 1985.

4. **Sherwood NM, Lovejoy DA, Coe IR,** Origin of mammalian gonadotropin-releasing hormones, Endocr Rev 14:241, 1993.

5. **Elsholtz HP,** Molecular biology of prolactin: cell-specific and endocrine regulators of the prolactin gene, Seminars Reprod Endocrinol 10:183, 1992.

6. **Xiong F, Chin RA, Hew CL,** A gene encoding chinook salmon *(Oncorhynchus tschawytscha)* prolactin: gene structure and potential cis-acting regulatory elements, Mol Marine Biol Biotechnol 1:155, 1992.

7. **Martinez de la Escalera G, Weiner RI,** Dissociation of dopamine from its receptor as a signal in the pleiotropic hypothalamic regulation of prolactin secretion, Endocrin Rev 13:241, 1992.

8. **Schwanzel-Fukuda M, Pfaff DW,** Origin of luteinizing hormone-releasing hormone neurons, Nature 338:161, 1989.

9. **Ronnekleiv OK, Resko JA,** Ontogeny of gonadotropin-releasing hormone-containing neurons in early fetal development of rhesus macaques, Endocrinology 126:498, 1990.

10. **Bick D, Franco B, Sherin RJ, Heye B, Pike L, Crawford J, Maddalena A, Incerti B, Pragliola A, Meitinger T, Ballabio A,** Brief report: intragenic deletion of the *KALIG-1* gene in Kallmann's syndrome, New Engl J Med 326:1752, 1992.

11. **Hardelin J-P, Levilliers J, Young J, Pholsena M, Legovis R, Kirk J, Bouloux P, Petit C, Schaison G,** Xp22.3 deletions in isolated familial Kallmann's syndrome, J Clin Endocrinol Metab 76:827, 1993.

12. **Silverman AJ, Antunes JL, Abrams G, Nilaver G, Thau R, Robinson JA, Ferin M, Krey LC,** The luteinizing hormone-releasing pathways in the rhesus (maccaca mulatta) and pigtailed (maccaca nemestrina) monkeys: new observations using thick unembedded sections, J Comp Neurol 211:309, 1982.

13. **Nakai Y, Plant TM, Hess DL, Keogh EJ, Knobil E,** On the sites of the negative and positive feedback actions of estradiol in the control of gonadotropin secretion in the rhesus monkey, Endocrinology 102:1008, 1978.

14. **Knobil E,** The neuroendocrine control of the menstrual cycle, Recent Prog Horm Res 36:53, 1980.

15. **Van Vugt DA, Diefenbach WP, Ferin M,** Gonadotropin-releasing hormone pulses in third ventricular cerebrospinal fluid of ovariectomized rhesus monkeys: correlation with luteinizing hormone pulses, Endocrinology 117:1550, 1985.

16. **Gross KM, Matsumoto AM, Southworth MB, Bremner WJ,** Evidence for decreased luteinizing hormone-releasing hormone frequency in men with selective elevations of follicle-stimulating hormone, J Clin Endocrinol Metab 60:197, 1985.

17. **Reame N, Sauder SE, Kelch RP, Marshall JC,** Pulsatile gonadotropin secretion during the human menstrual cycle: evidence for altered frequency of gonadotropin-releasing hormone secretion, J Clin Endocrinol Metab 59:328, 1984.

18. **Filicori M, Santoro N, Merriam GR, Crowley WF Jr,** Characterization of the physiological pattern of episodic gonadotropin secretion throughout the human menstrual cycle, J Clin Endocrinol Metab 62:1136, 1986.

19. **Veldhuis JD, Evans WS, Johnson ML, Wills MR, Rogol AD,** Physiological properties of the luteinizing hormone pulse signal: impact of intensive and extended venous sampling paradigms on its characterization in healthy men and women, J Clin Endocrinol Metab 62:881, 1986.

20. **Gambacciani M, Liu JH, Swartz WH, Tueros VS, Yen SSC, Rasmussen DD,** Intrinsic pulsatility of luteinizing hormone release from the human pituitary in vitro, Neuroendocrinology 45:402, 1987.

21. **Andersen AN, Hagen C, Lange P, Boesgaard S, Djursing H, Eldrup E, Micic S,** Dopaminergic regulation of gonadotropin levels and pulsatility in normal women, Fertil Steril 47:391, 1987.

22. **Rasmussen DD, Liu JH, Wolf PL, Yen SSC,** Gonadotropin-releasing hormone neurosecretion in the human hypothalamus: *in vitro* regulation by dopamine, J Clin Endocrinol Metab 62:479, 1986.

23. **Christiansen E, Veldhuis JD, Rogol AD, Stumpf P, Evans WS,** Modulating actions of estradiol on gonadotropin-releasing hormone-stimulated prolactin secretion in postmenopausal individuals, Am J Obstet Gynecol 157:320, 1987.

24. **Jameson JL, Becker CB, Lindell CM, Habener JF,** Human follicle-stimulating hormone β-subunit encodes multiple messenger ribonucleic acids, Mol Endocrinol 2:806, 1988.

25. **Ravindra R, Aronstam RS,** Progesterone, testosterone, and estradiol-17β inhibit gonadotropin-releasing hormone stimulation of G protein GTPase activity in plasma membranes from rat anterior pituitary lobe, Acta Endocrinol 126:345, 1992.

26. **Tse A, Hille B,** GnRH-induced Ca^{2+} oscillations and rhythmic hyperpolarizations of pituitary gonadotropes, Science 255:462, 1992.

27. **Schwartz J, Cherny R,** Intercellular communication within the anterior pituitary influencing the secretion of hypophysial hormones, Endocrin Rev 13:453, 1992.

28. **Sahu A, Phelps CP, White JD, Crowley WR, Kalra SP, Kalra PS,** Steroidal regulation of hypothalamic neuropeptide Y release and gene expression, Endocrinology 130:3331, 1992.

29. **Kaye WH, Berrettini W, Gwirtsman H, George DT,** Altered cerebrospinal fluid neuropeptide Y and peptide YY immunoreactivity in anorexia and bulimia nervosa, Arch Gen Psychiatry 47:548, 1990.

30. **McShane TM, May T, Miner JL, Keisler DH,** Central actions of neuropeptide-Y may provide a neuromodulatory link between nutrition and reproduction, Biol Reprod 46:1151, 1992.

31. **Massague J,** The TGF-β family of growth and differentiation factors, Cell 49:437, 1987.

32. **Roberts V, Meunier H, Vaughan J, Rivier J, Rivier C, Vale W, Sawchenko P,** Production and regulation of inhibin subunits in pituitary gonadotropes, Endocrinology 124:552, 1989.

33. **Kitaoka M, Kojima I, Ogata E,** Activin-A: a modulator of multiple types of anterior pituitary cells. Biochem Biophys Res Commun 157:48, 1988.

34. **Billestrup N, Gonzalez-Manchon C, Potter E, Vale W,** Inhibition of somatotroph growth and growth hormone biosynthesis by activin in vitro, Mol Endocrinol 4:356, 1990.

35. **Corrigan AZ, Bilezikjian LM, Carroll RS, Bald LN, Schmelzer CH, Fendly BM, Mason AJ, Chin WW, Schwall RH, Vale W,** Evidence for an autocrine role of activin B within rat anterior piuitary cultures, Endocrinology 128:1682, 1991.

36. **Kaiser UB, Lee BL, Carroll RS, Unabia G, Chin WW, Childs GV,** Follistatin gene expression in the pituitary: localization in gonadotrophs and folliculostellate cells in diestrous rats, Endocrinology 130:3048, 1992.

37. **Kogawa K, Nakamura T, Sugiono K, Takio K, Titani K, Sugino H,** Activin-binding protein is present in pituitary, Endocrinology 128:1434, 1991.

38. **Lopez FJ, Merchenthaler I, Ching M, Wisniewski MG, Negro-Vilar A,** Galanin: a hypothalamic-hypophysiotropic hormone modulating reproductive functions, Proc Natl Acad Sci USA 88:4508, 1991.

39. **Howlett TA, Rees LH,** Endogenous opioid peptides and hypothalamo-pituitary function, Ann Rev Physiol 48:527, 1986.

40. **Bacchinetti F, Petraglia F, Genazzani AR,** Localization and expression of the three opioid systems, Seminars Reprod Endocrinol 5:103, 1987.

41. **Gindoff PR, Ferin M,** Brain opioid peptides and menstrual cyclicity, Seminars Reprod Endocrinol 5:125, 1987.

42. **Rabinovici J, Rothman P, Monroe SE, Nerenberg C, Jaffe RB,** Endocrine effects and pharmacokinetic characteristics of a potent new gonadotropin-releasing hormone antagonist (Ganirelix) with minimal histamine-releasing properties: studies in postmenopausal women, J Clin Endocrinol Metab 75:1220, 1992.

43. **Shoupe D, Montz FJ, Lobo RA,** The effects of estrogen and progestin on endogenous opioid activity in oophorectomized women, J Clin Endocrinol Metab 60:178, 1985.

44. **Casper RF, Alapin-Rubilovitz S,** Progestins increase endogenous opioid peptide activity in postmenopausal women, J Clin Endocrinol Metab 60:34, 1985.

45. **Marunicic M, Casper RF,** The effect of luteal phase estrogen antagonism on luteinizing hormone pulsatility and luteal function in women, J Clin Endocrinol Metab 64:148, 1987.

46. **Shalts E, Feng Y-J, Ferin M, Wardlaw SL,** α-Melanocyte-stimulating hormone antagonizes the neuroendocrine effects of corticotropin-releasing factor and interleukin-1α in the primate, Endocrinology 131:132, 1992.

47. **Petraglia F, D'Ambrogio G, Comitini G, Facchinetti F, Volpe A, Genazzani AR,** Impairment of opioid control of luteinizing hormone secretion in menstrual disorders, Fertil Steril 43:534, 1985.

48. **Khoury SA, Reame NE, Kelch RP, Marshall JC,** Diurnal patterns of pulsatile luteinizing hormone secretion in hypothalamic amenorrhea: reproducibility and responses to opiate blockade and α_2-adrenergic agonist, J Clin Endocrinol Metab 64:755, 1987.

49. **Wildt L, Leyendecker G, Sir-Petermann T, Waibel-Treber S,** Treatment with naltrexone in hypothalamic ovarian failure: induction of ovulation and pregnancy, Hum Reprod 8:350, 1993.

50. **Suh BY, Liu JH, Berga SL, Quigley ME, Laughlin GA, Yen SSC,** Hypercortisolism in patients with functional hypothalamic amenorrhea, J Clin Endocrinol Metab 66:733, 1988.

51. **Veldhuis JD, Johnson ML, Seneta E, Iranmanesh A,** Temporal coupling among luteinizing hormone, follicle stimulating hormone, β-endorphin and cortisol pulse episodes in vivo, Acta Endocrinol 126:193, 1992.

52. **Cumming DC, Wheeler GD,** Opioids in exercise physiology, Seminars Reprod Endocrinol 5:171, 1987.

53. **Sarkar DK, Yen SSC,** Hyperprolactinemia decreases the luteinizing hormone-releasing hormone concentration in pituitary portal plasma: a possible role for β-endorphin as a mediator, Endocrinology 116:2080, 1985.

54. **Chen CC, Chang C, Krieger DT, Bardin CW,** Expression and regulation of proopiomelanocortin-like gene in the ovary and placenta: comparison with the testis, Endocrinology 118:2382, 1986.

55. **Petraglia F, Di Meo G, Storchi R, Segre A, Facchinetti F, Szalay S, Volpe A, Genazzani AR,** Proopiomelanocortin-related peptides and methionine enkephalin in human follicular fluid: changes during the menstrual cycle, Am J Obstet Gynecol 157:142, 1987.

56. **Fishman J, Norton B,** Brain catecholestrogens: formation and possible functions, Adv Biosci 15:123, 1975.

57. **Mais V, Kazer RR, Cetel NS, Rivier J, Vale W, Yen SSC,** The dependency of folliculogenesis and corpus luteum function on pulsatile gonadotropin secretion in cycling women using a gonadotropin-releasing hormone antagonist as a probe, J Clin Endocrinol Metab 62:1250, 1986.

58. **Dierick K, Vandesdande F,** Immunocytochemical demonstration of separate vasopressin-neurophysin and oxytocin neurophysin neurons in the human hypothalamus, Cell Tissue Res 196:203, 1979.

59. **Brownstein MJ, Russel JT, Gainer H,** Synthesis, transport, and release of posterior pituitary hormones, Science 207:373, 1980.

60. **Kasson BG, Adashi EY, Hsueh AJW,** Arginine vasopressin in the testis: an intragonadal peptide control system, Endocr Rev 7:156, 1986.

61. **Perlow MJ, Reppert SM, Artman HA, Fisher DA, Seif SM, Robinson AG,** Oxytocin, vasopressin and estrogen-stimulated neurophsyin: daily patterns of concentration in cerebrospinal fluid, Science 216:1416, 1983.

62. **Amico JA, Seif SM, Robinson AG,** Elevation of oxytocin and the oxytocin-associated neurophysin in the plasma of normal women during midcycle, J Clin Endocrinol Metab 53:1229, 1981.

63. **Carmichael MS, Humbert R, Dixen J, Palmisano G, Greenleaf W, Davidson JM,** Plasma oxytocin increases in the human sexual response, J Clin Endocrinol Metab 64:27, 1987.

64. **Dawood MY, Raghavan KS, Pociask C, Fuchs F,** Oxytocin during human pregnancy and parturition, Obstet Gynecol 51:138, 1978.

65. **Ferin M, Rosenblatt H, Carmel PW, Antunes JL, Vande Wiele RL,** Estrogen-induced gonadotropin surges in female rhesus monkeys after pituitary stalk section, Endocrinology 104:50, 1979.

66. **Yen SSC, Lein A,** The apparent paradox of the negative and positive feedback control system on gonadotropin secretion, Am J Obstet Gynecol 126:942, 1976.

67. **Hoff JD, Lasley BL, Yen SSC,** The functional relationship between priming and releasing actions of luteinizing hormone-releasing hormone, J Clin Endocrinol Metab 49:8, 1979.

68. **Urban RJ, Veldhuis JD, Dufau ML,** Estrogen regulates the gonadotropin-releasing hormone-stimulated secretion of biologically active luteinizing hormone, J Clin Endocrinol Metab 72:660, 1991.

69. **Adams TE, Norman RL, Spies HG,** Gonadotropin-releasing hormone receptor binding and pituitary responsiveness in estradiol-primed monkeys, Science 213:1388, 1981.

70. **Menon M, Peegel H, Katta V,** Estradiol potentiation of gonadotropin-releasing hormone responsiveness in the anterior pituitary is mediated by an increase in gonadotropin-releasing hormone receptors, Am J Obstet Gynecol 151:534, 1985.

71. **Chappel SC, Resko JA, Norman RL, Spies HG,** Studies on rhesus monkeys on the site where estrogen inhibits gonadotropins: delivery of 17-estradiol to the hypothalamus and pituitary gland, J Clin Endocrinol Metab 52:1, 1981.

72. **Xia L, Van Vugt D, Alston EJ, Luckhaus J, Ferin M,** A surge of gonadotropin-releasing hormone accompanies the estradiol-induced gonadotropin surge in the Rhesus monkey, Endocrinology 131:2812, 1992.

73. **Shupnik MA, Weinmann CM, Notides AC, Chin WW,** An upstream region of the rat luteinizing hormone β gene binds estrogen receptor and confers estrogen responsiveness, J Biol Chem 264:80, 1989.

74. **Radovick S, Ticknor CM, Nakayama Y, Notides AC, Rahman A, Weintraub BD, Cutler GB Jr, Wondisford FE,** Evidence for direct estrogen regulation of the human gonadotropin-releasing hormone gene, J Clin Invest 88:1649, 1991.

75. **Katt JA, Duncan JA, Herbon L, Barkan A, Marshall JC,** The frequency of gonadotropin-releasing hormone stimulation determines the number of pituitary gonadotropin-releasing hormone receptors, Endocrinology 116:2113, 1985.

76. **Moenter SM, Brand RC, Karsch FJ,** Dynamics of gonadotropin-releasing hormone (GnRH) secretion during the GnRH surge: insights into the mechanism of GnRH surge induction, Endocrinology 130:2978, 1992.

77. **Marut EL, Williams RF, Cowan BD, Lynch A, Lerner SP, Hodgen GD,** Pulsatile pituitary gonadotropin secretion during maturation of the dominant follicle in monkeys: estrogen positive feedback enhances the biological activity of LH, Endocrinology 109:2270, 1981.

78. **Liu JH, Yen SSC,** Induction of midcycle gonadotropin surge by ovarian steroids in women: a critical evaluation, J Clin Endocrinol Metab 57:797, 1983.

79. **Collins RL, Hodgen GD,** Blockade of the spontaneous midcycle gonadotropin surge in monkeys by RU 486: a progesterone antagonist or agonist? J Clin Endocrinol Metab 63:1270, 1986.

80. **Turgeon JL, Waring DW,** The timing of progesterone-induced ribonucleic acid and protein synthesis for augmentation of luteinizing hormone secretion, Endocrinology 129:3234, 1991.

81. **Waring DW, Turgeon JL,** A pathway for luteinizing hormone releasing-hormone self-potentiation: cross-talk with the progesterone receptor, Endocrinology 130:3275, 1992.

82. **Wildt L, Hutchison JS, Marshall G, Pohl CR, Knobil E,** On the site of action of progesterone in the blockade of the estradiol-induced gonadotropin discharge in the rhesus monkey, Endocrinology 109:1293, 1981.

83. **Batra SK, Miller WL,** Progesterone decreases the responsiveness of ovine pituitary cultures to luteinizing hormone-releasing hormone, Endocrinology 117:1436, 1985.

84. **Araki S, Chikazawa K, Motoyama M, Ijima K, Abe N, Tamada T,** Reduction in pituitary desensitization and prolongation of gonadotropin release by estrogen during continuous administration of gonadotropin-releasing hormone in women: its antagonism by progesterone, J Clin Endocrinol Metab 60:590, 1985.

85. **Kasa-Vuvu JZ, Dahl GE, Evans NP, Thrun LA, Moenter SM, Padmanaghan V, Karsch FJ,** Progesterone blocks the estradiol-induced gonadotropin discharge in the ewe by inhibiting the surge of gonadotropin-releasing hormone, Endocrinology 131:208, 1992.

86. **Tamarkin L, Baird CJ, Almeida OFX,** Melatonin: a coordinating signal for mammalian reproduction? Science 227:714, 1985.

87. **Reiter RJ,** Pineal melatonin: cell biology of its synthesis and of its physiological interactions, Endocr Rev 12:151, 1991.

88. **Plant TM, Zorub DS,** Pinealectomy in agonadal infantile male rhesus monkeys (Macaca mulatta) does not interrupt initiation of the prepubertal hiatus in gonadotropin secretion, Endocrinology 118:227, 1986.

89. **Silman R,** Melatonin and the human gonadotrophin-releasing hormone pulse generator, J Endocrinol 128:7, 1991.

90. **Zacharias L, Wurtman RJ,** Blindness: its relation to age of menarche, Science 144:1154, 1964.

91. **Rojansky N, Brzezinski A, Schenker JG,** Seasonality in human reproduction: an update, Hum Reprod 7:735, 1992.

92. **Zimmermann RC, Schumacher M, Schroder S, Weise H-C, Baars S,** Melatonin and the ovulatory luteinizing hormone surge, Fertil Steril 54:612, 1990.

93. **Berga SL, Yen SSC,** Circadian pattern of plasma melatonin concentrations during four phases of the human menstrual cycle, Neuroendocrinol 51:606, 1990.

94. **Sack RL, Lewy AJ, Blood ML, Keith LD, Nakagawa H,** Circadian rhythm abnormalities in totally blind people: incidence and clinical significance, J Clin Endocrinol Metab 75:127, 1992.

95. **Puig-Domingo M, Webb SM, Serrano J, Peinado M-A, Corcoy R, Ruscalleda J, Reiter RJ, de Leiva A,** Brief report: melatonin-related hypogoandotropic hypogonadism, New Engl J Med 327:1356, 1992.

96. **Berga SL, Mortola JF, Yen SSC,** Amplification of nocturnal melatonin secretion in women with functional hypothalamic amenorrhea, J Clin Endocrinol Metab 66:242, 1988.

97. **McClintock MK,** Menstrual synchrony and suppression, Nature 229:244, 1971.

98. **Matteo S,** The effect of job stress and job interdependency on menstrual cycle length, regularity and synchrony, Psychoneuroendocrinology 12:467, 1987.

99. **Wilson HC, Kiefhaber SH, Gravel V,** Two studies of menstrual synchrony: negative results, Psychoneuroendocrinology 16:353, 1991.

100. **Huhtaniemi IT, Warren DW,** Ontogeny of pituitary-gonadal interactions: current advances and controversies, Trends Endocrinol Metab 1:356, 1990.

101. **Burger HG, Yamada Y, Bangah ML, McCloud PI, Warne GL,** Serum gonadotropin, sex steroid, and immunoreactive inhibin levels in the first two years of life, J Clin Endocrinol Metab 72:682, 1991.

102. **Reiter EO, Grumbach MM,** Neuroendocrine control mechanisms and the onset of puberty, Ann Rev Physiol 44:595, 1982.

103. **Sklar CA, Kaplan SL, Grumbach MM,** Evidence for dissociation between adrenarche and gonadarche: studies in patients with idiopathic precocious puberty, gonadal dysgenesis, isolated gonadotroph deficiency, and constitutionally delayed growth and adolescence, J Clin Endocrinol Metab 51:548, 1980.

104. **Dunkel L, Alfthan H, Stenman U-H, Selstam G, Rosberg S, Albertsson-Wikland K,** Developmental changes in 24-hour profiles of luteinizing hormone and follicle-stimulating hormone from prepuberty to midstages of puberty in boys, J Clin Endocrinol Metab 74:890, 1992.

105. **Oerter KE, Uriarte MM, Rose SR, Barnes KM, Cutler GB,** Gonadotropin secretory dynamics during puberty in normal girls and boys, J Clin Endocrinol Metab 71:1251, 1990.

106. **Boyar RM, Ramsey J, Chapman J, Fevere M, Madden J, Marks JF,** Luteinizing hormone and follicle-stimulating hormone secretory dynamics in Turner's syndrome, J Clin Endocrinol Metab 47:1078, 1978.

107. **Zacharias L, Rand WM, Wurtman RJ,** A prospective study of sexual development and growth in American girls: the statistics of menarche, Obstet Gynecol Survey 31:325, 1976.

108. **Frisch RE,** Body fat, menarche, and reproductive ability, Seminars Reprod Endocrinol 3:45, 1985.

109. **Ross JL, Loriaux DL, Cutler GB,** Developmental changes in neuroendocrine regulation of gonadotropin secretion in gonadal dysgenesis, J Clin Endocrinol Metab 57:288, 1983.

6　Regulation of the Menstrual Cycle

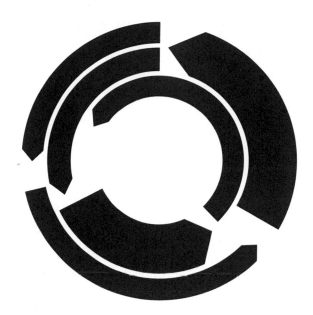

Many superstitious beliefs have surrounded menstruation throughout recorded history. Indeed, attitudes and ideas about this aspect of female physiology have changed slowly. Hopefully, the scientific progress of the last few decades, which has revealed the dynamic relationships between the pituitary and gonadal hormones and the cyclic nature of the normal reproductive process, will yield a new understanding. The hormone changes correlated with the morphologic and autocrine/paracrine events in the ovary make the coordination of this system one of the most remarkable events in biology.

The diagnosis and management of abnormal menstrual function must be based upon an understanding of the physiologic mechanisms involved in the regulation of the normal cycle. To understand the normal menstrual cycle, it is helpful to divide the cycle into 3 phases: the follicular phase, ovulation, and the luteal phase. We will examine each of these phases, concentrating on the changes in ovarian and pituitary hormones, what governs the pattern of hormone changes, and the effects of these hormones on the ovary, pituitary, and hypothalamus in regulating the menstrual cycle.

The Follicular Phase

During the follicular phase an orderly sequence of events takes place which ensures that the proper number of follicles is ready for ovulation. In the human ovary the end result of this follicular development is (usually) one surviving mature follicle. This process, which occurs over the space of 10–14 days, features a series of sequential actions of hormones and autocrine/paracrine peptides on the follicle, leading the follicle destined to ovulate through a period of initial growth from a primordial follicle through the stages of the preantral, antral, and preovulatory follicle.

The Primordial Follicle

The primordial germ cells originate in the endoderm of the yolk sac, allantois, and hindgut of the embryo, and by 5–6 weeks of gestation, they have migrated to the genital ridge. A rapid mitotic multiplication of germ cells occurs at 6–8 weeks of pregnancy, and by 16–20 weeks, the maximal number of oocytes is reached: a total of 6–7 million in both ovaries.[1] The primordial follicle consists of an oocyte, arrested in the diplotene stage of meiotic prophase, surrounded by a single layer of spindle-shaped granulosa cells.

Follicular growth is a process, best described by Peters as a continuum.[2] Until their numbers are exhausted, follicles begin to grow and undergo atresia under all physiologic circumstances. Growth and atresia are not interrupted by pregnancy, ovulation, or periods of anovulation. This dynamic process continues at all ages, including infancy and around the menopause. From the maximal number at 16–20 weeks of pregnancy, the number of oocytes will irretrievably decrease. The rate of decrease is proportional to the total number present; thus, the most rapid decrease occurs before birth, resulting in a decline from 6–7 million to 2 million at birth and to 300,000 at puberty. From this large reservoir, fewer than 500 follicles will ovulate during a woman's reproductive years.

The mechanism for determining which follicles and how many will start growing during any one cycle is unknown. The number of follicles that starts growing each cycle appears to be dependent upon the size of the residual pool of inactive primordial follicles.[2] Reducing the size of the pool (e.g., unilateral oophorectomy) causes the remaining follicles to redistribute their availability over time. It is possible that the follicle which is singled out to play the leading role in a particular cycle is the beneficiary of a timely match of follicle "readiness" and appropriate tropic hormone stimulation. The first follicle able to respond to stimulation may achieve an early lead that it never relinquishes.

The follicle destined to ovulate is recruited in the first few days of the cycle.[3] There is a school of thought which argues that the early growth of follicles occurs over the time span of several menstrual cycles and that the ovulatory follicle is one of a cohort recruited during the late luteal phase.[4] This hypothesis estimates that the total duration of time to achieve preovulatory status is 85 days. To fit this concept, the majority of growth (until a late stage) would have to be independent of gonadotropin stimulation. It is more useful (and in our view more consistent with human data) to assign a shorter duration of growth and development, with early response to the luteal-follicular change in follicle-stimulating hormone (FSH) as the critical feature.

The first visible signs of follicular recruitment are when the oocyte increases in size and when the granulosa cells become cuboidal rather than squamous in shape. At this same time, in response to FSH, small gap junctions develop between the granulosa cells and the oocyte. The gap junctions serve as the pathway for nutritional and metabolite interchange between the granulosa cells and the oocyte. With multiplication of the cuboidal granulosa cells, the primordial follicle becomes a primary follicle. The granulosa layer is separated from the stromal cells by a basement membrane called the basal lamina. The surrounding stromal cells differentiate into concentric layers designated the theca interna (closest to the basal lamina) and the theca externa (the outer portion).

The initiation of follicular growth is independent of gonadotropin stimulation. This conclusion is supported by the persistence of this initial growth in gonadotropin-deficient mutant mice.[5] In the vast majority of instances this growth is limited and rapidly followed by atresia. The general pattern of limited growth and quick atresia is interrupted at the beginning of the menstrual cycle when a group of follicles responds to a hormonal change and is propelled to further growth. The most important hormonal event at this time is a rise in FSH. The decline in luteal phase steroidogenesis and inhibin secretion allows the rise in FSH which rescues a group of follicles from atresia.[6]

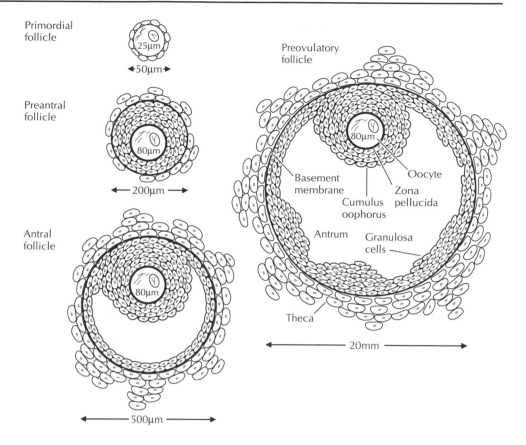

Primordial follicle

25μm

◄50μm►

Preantral follicle

80μm

◄ 200μm ►

Antral follicle

80μm

◄ 500μm ►

Preovulatory follicle

80μm

Basement membrane

Cumulus oophorus

Oocyte

Zona pellucida

Antrum

Granulosa cells

Theca

◄ 20mm ►

Follicular Growth and Development Based on Nonprimate and Primate Data

The following discussion of events which mark the growth and development of the ovarian follicle from the preantral stage to ovulation is based upon a formulation that assigns a key role to estradiol functioning as a classic hormone to transmit messages to the brain and as a local regulator within the follicle. This description has been challenged. The belief that the follicular estrogen concentration plays a paramount role within the follicle is based upon evidence (estrogens augment FSH action) derived from rat experiments. There is no similar evidence derived from primate studies. Let us first describe the traditional conventional wisdom regarding ovarian follicular growth and development derived from 10–15 years of scientific pursuit; then we will consider the differences in primates. **Local autocrine/paracrine peptides probably have replaced steroid hormones as the principal regulators within primate ovarian follicles.**

The Preantral Follicle

Once growth is initiated, the follicle progresses to the preantral stage as the oocyte enlarges and is surrounded by a membrane, the zona pellucida. The granulosa cells undergo a multilayer proliferation as the thecal layer continues to organize from the surrounding stroma. This growth is dependent upon gonadotropins and is correlated with increasing production of estrogen.

The granulosa cells of the preantral follicle have the ability to synthesize all 3 classes of steroids; however, significantly more estrogens than either androgens or progestins are produced. An aromatase enzyme system acts to convert androgens to estrogens and appears to be a factor limiting ovarian estrogen production. Aromatization is induced or activated through the action of FSH. The binding of FSH to its receptor and activation of the adenylate cyclase mediated signal is followed by expression of multiple mRNAs which encode proteins responsible for cell proliferation, differentiation, and function. Thus FSH both initiates steroidogenesis (estrogen production) in granulosa cells and stimulates granulosa cell growth.[7]

Specific receptors for FSH are present on preantral granulosa cells and, in the presence of FSH, the preantral follicle can aromatize limited amounts of androgens and generate its own estrogenic microenvironment.[8] Estrogen production is, therefore, also limited by FSH receptor content. The administration of FSH will raise and lower the concentration of its own receptor on granulosa cells (up- and down-regulation) both in vivo and in vitro.[9] This action of FSH is modulated by growth factors.[10] FSH receptors appear in the plasma membrane of granulosa cells immediately upon the initial growth of the follicle and quickly reach a concentration of approximately 1,500 receptors per granulosa cell.[11]

FSH operates through the G protein, adenylate cyclase system (described in Chapter 2), that is subject to down-regulation and modulation by many factors, including a calcium-calmodulin intermediary. Although steroidogenesis in the ovarian follicle is mainly regulated by the gonadotropins, multiple signaling pathways are involved which respond to many factors besides the gonadotropins. Besides the adenylate cyclase enzyme system, these pathways include ion gate channels, tyrosine kinase receptors, and the phospholipase system of second messengers. These pathways are utilized by a multitude of regulating factors, including the growth factors, prostaglandins, and peptides such as gonadotropin releasing hormone (GnRH), angiotensin II, tissue necrosis factor, and vasoactive intestinal peptide. The binding of luteinizing hormone (LH) to its receptor in the ovary is also followed by activation of the adenylate cyclase-cyclic AMP pathway in the G protein mechanism. Continuous exposure of receptors to gonadotropins results in down-regulation, involving loss of receptors by internalization, desensitization of the receptor by autophosphorylation of the cytoplasmic segment of the receptor, and uncoupling of the regulatory and catalytic subunits of the adenylate cyclase enzyme (described in Chapter 2).

FSH combines with estrogen to synergistically exert (at least in the nonprimate) a mitogenic action on granulosa cells to stimulate their proliferation. Together, FSH and estrogen promote a rapid accumulation of FSH receptors, reflecting in part the increase in the number of granulosa cells. The early appearance of estrogen within the follicle allows the follicle to respond to relatively low concentrations of FSH, an autocrine function for estrogen within the follicle. As growth proceeds, the granulosa cells differentiate into several subgroups of different cell populations. This appears to be determined by the position of the cells relative to the oocyte.

There is a system of communication that exists within follicles. Not every cell has to contain receptors for the gonadotropins. Cells with receptors can transfer a signal (presumably by gap junctions) which causes protein kinase activation in cells which lack receptors.[12] Thus, hormone-initiated action can be transmitted throughout the follicle despite the fact that only a subpopulation of cells binds the hormone.

The role of androgens in early follicular development is complex. Specific androgen receptors are present in the granulosa cells.[13] The androgens serve not only as substrate for FSH-induced aromatization but, in low concentrations, can further enhance aromatase activity. When exposed to an androgen-rich environment, preantral granulosa cells favor the conversion of androgens to more potent 5α-reduced androgens rather than to estrogens.[14] These androgens cannot be converted to estrogen and, in fact, inhibit aromatase activity.[15] They also inhibit FSH induction of LH receptor formation, another essential step in follicular development.[16]

The fate of the preantral follicle is in delicate balance. At low concentrations, androgens enhance their own aromatization and contribute to estrogen production. At higher levels, the limited capacity of aromatization is overwhelmed, and the follicle becomes androgenic and ultimately atretic.[17] Follicles will progress in development only if emerging when FSH is elevated and LH is low. Those follicles arising at the end of the luteal phase or early in the subsequent cycle would be favored by an environment in which aromatization in the granulosa cell can prevail. ***The success of a follicle depends upon its ability to convert an androgen microenvironment to an estrogen microenvironment.***[18]

Summary of Events in the Preantral Follicle

1. Initial follicular growth occurs independently of hormone influence.

2. FSH stimulation propels follicles to the preantral stage.

3. FSH-induced aromatization of androgen in the granulosa results in the production of estrogen.

4. Together, FSH and estrogen increase the FSH receptor content of the follicle.

The Antral Follicle

Under the synergistic influence of estrogen and FSH there is an increase in the production of follicular fluid that accumulates in the intercellular spaces of the granulosa, eventually coalescing to form a cavity, as the follicle makes its gradual transition to the antral stage. The accumulation of follicular fluid provides a means whereby the oocyte and surrounding granulosa cells can be nurtured in a specific endocrine environment for each follicle.

In the presence of FSH, estrogen becomes the dominant substance in the follicular fluid. Conversely, in the absence of FSH, androgens predominate.[19,20] LH is not normally present in follicular fluid until the midcycle. If LH is prematurely elevated in plasma and antral fluid, mitotic activity in the granulosa decreases, degenerative changes ensue, and intrafollicular androgen levels rise. Therefore, the dominance of estrogen and FSH is essential for sustained accumulation of granulosa cells and continued follicular growth. Antral follicles with the greatest rates of granulosa proliferation contain the highest estrogen concentrations and the lowest androgen:estrogen ratios, and are the most likely to house a healthy oocyte. An androgenic milieu antagonizes estrogen-induced granulosa proliferation and, if sustained, promotes degenerative changes in the oocyte.

The steroids present in follicular fluid can be found in concentrations several orders of magnitude higher than those in plasma and reflect the functional capacity of the surrounding granulosa and theca cells. The synthesis of steroid hormones is functionally compartmentalized within the follicle — the two cell system.[11,17,20,21]

The Two-Cell, Two-Gonadotropin System

Although each compartment (theca and granulosa) retains the ability to produce progestins, androgens, and estrogens, the aromatase activity of the granulosa far exceeds that observed in the theca. In human preantral and antral follicles, LH receptors are present only on the theca cells and FSH receptors only on the granulosa cells.[22,23] Thecal interstitial cells, located in the theca interna, have approximately 20,000 LH receptors in their cell membranes. In response to LH, thecal tissue is stimulated to produce androgens that can then be converted, through FSH-induced aromatization, to estrogens in the granulosa cells.

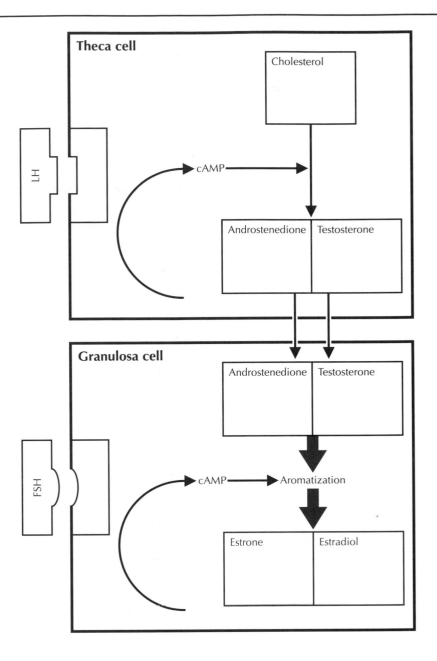

The interaction between the granulosa and theca compartments, with resulting accelerated estrogen production, is not fully functional until later in antral development. Like
preantral granulosa cells, the granulosa of small antral follicles exhibits an in vitro
tendency to convert significant amounts of androgen to the more potent 5α-reduced
form. In contrast, granulosa cells isolated from large antral follicles readily and
preferentially metabolize androgens to estrogens. The conversion from an androgen
microenvironment to an estrogen microenvironment (a conversion essential for further
growth and development) is dependent upon a growing sensitivity to FSH brought about
by the action of FSH and the enhancing influence of estrogen.

As the follicle develops, theca cells begin to express the genes for LH receptors,
P450scc, and 3β-hydroxysteroid dehydrogenase.[24] Insulin-like growth factor-I (IGF-I)
synergizes with LH to increase enzyme gene transcription; however IGF-I does not
stimulate steroidogenesis. The separately regulated (by LH) entry of cholesterol into
mitochondria, utilizing internalization of LDL-cholesterol, is essential for steroidogenesis. ***Therefore, ovarian steroidogenesis is always LH-dependent.***

As the follicle emerges, the theca cells are characterized by their expression of P450c17, the enzyme step which is rate-limiting for the conversion of 21-carbon substrate to androgens. Granulosa cells do not express this enzyme and thus are dependent upon androgens from the theca in order to make estrogen. Increasing expression of the aromatization system (P450arom) is a marker of increasing maturity of granulosa cells.

The importance of the two-cell, two-gonadotropin system in the primate is supported by the response of women with a deficiency in gonadotropins to treatment with recombinant (pure) FSH.[25,26] Follicles developed (confirming the essential role of FSH, and the lesser role for LH, in recruitment and initial growth), but estradiol production was severely limited. Some aromatization occurred, producing early follicular phase estradiol levels, but the usual robust steroidogenesis was impossible without the presence of LH to provide thecal production of androgen substrate. This same response has been observed in experiments that use a GnRH antagonist to produce LH-deficient monkeys and then administer recombinant, pure human FSH.[27] These results indicate that only FSH is required for folliculogenesis.

Selection of the Dominant Follicle

The successful conversion to an estrogen dominant follicle marks the "selection" of a follicle destined to ovulate, the process whereby, with rare exception, only a single follicle succeeds. This selection process is to a significant degree the result of two estrogen actions: 1) a local interaction between estrogen and FSH within the follicle (in the nonprimate model), and 2) the effect of estrogen on pituitary secretion of FSH. While estrogen exerts a positive influence on FSH action within the maturing follicle, its negative feedback relationship with FSH at the hypothalamic-pituitary level serves to withdraw gonadotropin support from the other less developed follicles. The fall in FSH leads to a decline in FSH-dependent aromatase activity, limiting estrogen production in the less mature follicles. Even if a lesser follicle succeeds in achieving an estrogen microenvironment, decreasing FSH support would interrupt granulosa proliferation and function, promote a conversion to an androgenic microenvironment, and thereby induce irreversible atretic change. Indeed, the first event in the process of atresia is a reduction in FSH receptors in the granulosa layer.

The loss of oocytes (and follicles) through atresia is a response to changes in many factors. Certainly gonadotropin stimulation and withdrawal are important, but ovarian steroids and autocrine/paracrine factors are also involved. The consequence of these unfavorable changes, atresia, is a process called ***apoptosis***, programmed cell death. This process is heralded by alterations in mRNAs required for cell proteins which maintain follicle integrity.[28] This type of "natural death" is a physiologic process, in contrast to the pathologic cell death of necrosis.

An asymmetry in ovarian estrogen production, an expression of the emerging dominant follicle, can be detected in ovarian venous effluent on day 5 of the cycle, corresponding with the gradual fall of FSH levels observed at the midfollicular phase and preceding the increase in diameter that marks the physical emergence of the dominant follicle.[29] This is a crucial time in the cycle. Exogenous estrogen, administered even after selection of the dominant follicle, disrupts preovulatory development and induces atresia by reducing FSH levels below the sustaining level. Because the lesser follicles have entered the process of atresia, loss of the dominant follicle during this period of time requires beginning over, with recruitment of another set of preantral follicles.[30]

The negative feedback of estrogen on FSH serves to inhibit the development of all but the dominant follicle. The selected follicle remains dependent upon FSH and must complete its preovulatory development in the face of declining plasma levels of FSH. The dominant follicle, therefore, must escape the consequences of FSH suppression induced by its own accelerating estrogen production. The dominant follicle has two significant advantages, a greater content of FSH receptors acquired because of a rate of granulosa proliferation that surpasses that of its cohorts and enhancement of FSH action because of its high intrafollicular estrogen concentration (the nonprimate model) or because of local autocrine/paracrine peptides (the primate model). As a result, the stimulus for aromatization, FSH, can be maintained, while at the same time it is being withdrawn from among the less developed follicles. A wave of atresia among the lesser follicles, therefore, is seen to parallel the rise in estrogen.

The accumulation of a greater mass of granulosa cells is accompanied by advanced development of the thecal vasculature. By day 9, thecal vascularity in the dominant follicle is twice that of other antral follicles.[31] This can allow a preferential delivery of gonadotropins to the follicle permitting the dominant follicle to retain FSH responsiveness and sustain continued development and function despite waning gonadotropin levels. The monkey ovary expresses a potent growth factor (vascular endothelial growth factor) that induces angiogenesis, and this expression is observed at the two development points when proliferation of capillaries is important: the emerging dominant follicle and the early corpus luteum.[32]

In order to respond to the ovulatory surge and to become a successful corpus luteum, the granulosa cells must acquire LH receptors. FSH induces LH receptor development on the granulosa cells of the large antral follicles. Here again either estrogen (the nonprimate) or local autocrine/paracrine peptides (primate) serve as the chief coordinator.

In the nonprimate model, with increasing concentrations of estrogen within the follicle, FSH changes its focus of action, from its own receptor to the LH receptor.[33] The combination of a capacity for continued response despite declining levels of FSH and a high local estrogen environment in the dominant follicle provides optimal conditions for LH receptor development. LH can induce the formation of its own receptor in FSH-primed granulosa cells, but the primary mechanism utilizes FSH stimulation and estrogen enhancement.[34,35] The role for estrogen goes beyond synergism and enhancement; it is obligatory. Inhibition of estrogen synthesis prevents FSH-stimulated increases in LH receptors.[36]

Although prolactin is always present in follicular fluid, there is no evidence to suggest that prolactin is important during normal ovulatory cycles in the primate.

The Feedback System
Through its own estrogen and peptide production, the dominant follicle assumes control of its own destiny. By altering gonadotropin secretion through feedback mechanisms it optimizes its own environment to the detriment of the lesser follicles.

As reviewed in Chapter 5, gonadotropin releasing hormone (GnRH) plays an obligatory role in the control of gonadotropin secretion, but the pattern of gonadotropin secretion observed in the menstrual cycle is the result of feedback modulation of steroids and peptides originating in the dominant follicle, acting directly on the hypothalamus and anterior pituitary.[3] Experimental evidence suggests that the estrogen positive feedback pituitary mechanism involves an increase in GnRH receptor concentration.[37] In addition, a surge in GnRH accompanies the LH surge, indicating that estrogen positive feedback operates at both pituitary and hypothalamic sites.[38] The negative feedback action on the pituitary operates through a different and uncertain system. Estrogen exerts its inhibitory effects in both the hypothalamus and the anterior pituitary, decreasing both GnRH pulsatile secretion and GnRH pituitary response.[39] Progesterone also operates in two sites. Its inhibitory action is at the hypothalamic level, and, like estrogen, its positive action is directly on the pituitary.[40]

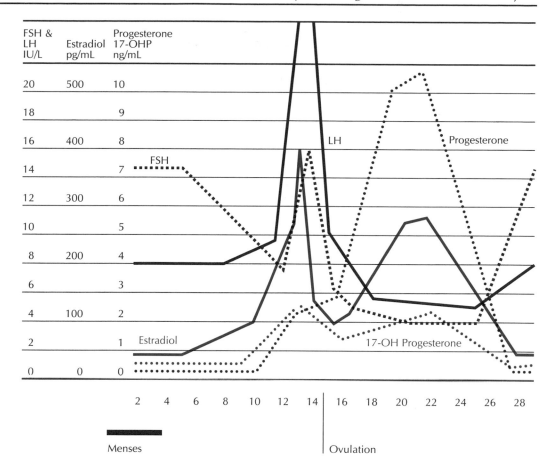

The secretion of FSH is very sensitive to the negative inhibitory effects of estrogen even at low levels. At higher levels, estrogen combines with inhibin for a suppression of FSH that is profound and sustained. In contrast, the influence of estrogen on LH release varies with concentration and duration of exposure. At low levels, estrogen commands a negative feedback relationship with LH. At higher levels, however, estrogen is capable of exerting a positive stimulatory feedback effect on LH release.

The transition from suppression to stimulation of LH release occurs as estradiol rises during the midfollicular phase. There are two critical features in this mechanism: 1) the concentration of estradiol and 2) the length of time during which the estradiol elevation is sustained. In women, the estradiol concentration necessary to achieve a positive feedback is more than 200 pg/mL (730 pmol/L), and this concentration must be sustained for approximately 50 hours.[41] The estrogen stimulus must be applied until after the surge actually begins. Otherwise, the LH surge is abbreviated or fails to occur at all.

Within the well-established monthly pattern, the gonadotropins are secreted in a pulsatile fashion with a frequency and magnitude that vary with the phase of the cycle. The pulsatile pattern is directly due to a similar pulsatile secretion of GnRH, but amplitude and frequency modulation (mean values below) is probably the consequence of steroid feedback on both hypothalamus and anterior pituitary.[42–44] ***Pulsatile secretion is more frequent but smaller in amplitude during the follicular phase compared to the luteal phase, with a slight increase in frequency observed as the follicular phase progresses to ovulation.***

LH Pulse Frequency:

Early follicular phase	—	94 minutes.
Late follicular phase	—	71 minutes.
Early luteal phase	—	103 minutes.
Late luteal phase	—	216 minutes.

LH Pulse Amplitude:

Early follicular phase	—	6.5 IU/L.
Midfollicular phase	—	5.1 IU/L.
Late follicular phase	—	7.2 IU/L.
Early luteal phase	—	14.9 IU/L.
Midluteal phase	—	12.2 IU/L.
Late luteal phase	—	7.6 IU/L.

The pulsatile pattern of FSH is not easily discerned because of its relatively longer half-life compared to LH, but the experimental data indicate that FSH and LH are secreted simultaneously and that GnRH stimulates the secretion of both gonadotropins. Only 36–48 hours before menses, gonadotropin secretion is characterized by infrequent LH pulses and low FSH levels typical of the late luteal phase.[43] During the transition from the previous luteal phase to the next follicular phase, GnRH and the gonadotropins are released from the inhibitory effects of estradiol, progesterone, and inhibin. A progressive and fairly rapid increase in GnRH pulse secretion is associated with a preferential secretion of FSH compared to LH. The frequency of GnRH and LH pulses increases 4.5-fold during this period of time, accompanied by a 3.5-fold increase in FSH secretion and a lesser 2-fold increase in LH.[45]

The GnRH pulse frequency changes in the luteal phase correlate with duration of exposure to progesterone, while pulse amplitude changes appear to be influenced by changes in progesterone levels.[42] Both estradiol and progesterone are required to achieve the low, suppressed secretory pattern of GnRH during the luteal phase.[46] The studies suggest that steroids influence the hypothalamic release of GnRH for frequency changes and the pituitary for action on amplitude of the gonadotropin pulses. The inhibitory action of luteal phase steroids appears to be mediated by an increase in hypothalamic endogenous opioid peptides. Both estrogen and progesterone can increase endogenous opiates, and administration of clomiphene (an estrogen antagonist) during the luteal phase increases the LH pulse frequency with no effect on amplitude.[47] Thus, estrogen appears to enhance the stimulatory action of progesterone in the luteal phase on endogenous opioid peptides, creating relatively high levels of endogenous opiates during the luteal phase.

Plasma endorphin begins to rise in the 2 days before the LH peak, coinciding with the midcycle gonadotropin surge.[48] The maximal level is reached just after the LH peak, coinciding with ovulation. Levels then gradually decline until the nadir is reached during menses and the early follicular phase. Monkeys have their highest beta-endorphin levels in the hypophyseal portal blood at midcycle.[49] Normal cyclicity requires sequential periods of high (midcycle and luteal phase) and low (during menses) hypothalamic opioid activity.

There is another important action of estrogen. A disparity exists between the patterns of FSH and LH secretion as determined by immunoassay and bioassay, indicating that more biologically active gonadotropins are secreted at midcycle than at other times in the cycle.[50] This quality, bioactivity vs immunoactivity, is determined by the molecular structure of the gonadotropin molecule, a concept referred to in Chapter 2 as heterogeneity of the tropic hormones. There is a well-established relationship between the activity and half-life of glycoprotein hormones and their sialic acid content. The feedback effects of estrogen include modulation of sialylation and the size and activity of the gonadotropins subsequently released, as well as an augmentation of GnRH-stimulated secretory release of biologically active gonadotropin. It certainly makes sense to intensify the gonadotropin effect at midcycle. The positive feedback action of estrogen, therefore, both increases the quantity and the quality (the bioactivity) of FSH and LH.

There is a diurnal rhythm in FSH and LH secretion.[51] In contrast to the nocturnal rise seen with ACTH, thyroid-stimulating hormone (TSH), growth hormone, and prolactin, FSH and LH exhibit nocturnal decline, probably mediated by endogenous opiates. This diurnal rhythm for LH is present only in the early follicular phase, while FSH maintains a circadian rhythm throughout the menstrual cycle (and thus it is not influenced by steroid hormone feedback) and even in the postmenopausal period of life.

Inhibin-Activin-Follistatin

A family of peptides is synthesized by granulosa cells in response to FSH and secreted into the follicular fluid and ovarian venous effluent.[52–55] The expression of these peptides is not limited to the ovary; they are present in many tissues throughout the body serving as autocrine/paracrine regulators. Inhibin is an important inhibitor of FSH secretion. Activin stimulates FSH release in the pituitary and augments FSH action in the ovary. Follistatin suppresses FSH activity, probably by binding activin.

Inhibin consists of two dissimilar peptides (known as alpha- and beta-subunits) linked by disulfide bonds. Two forms of inhibin (inhibin-A and inhibin-B) have been purified, each containing an identical alpha-subunit and distinct but related beta-subunits. Thus, there are three subunits for inhibins: alpha, beta-A, and beta-B. Each subunit is a product of different messenger RNA, each derived from its own precursor molecule.

The 2 Forms of Inhibin:

Inhibin-A:	**Alpha-Beta$_A$**
Inhibin-B:	**Alpha-Beta$_B$**

FSH stimulates the secretion of inhibin from granulosa cells and, in turn, is suppressed by inhibin — a reciprocal relationship.[56,57] The secretion of inhibin is further regulated by local autocrine/paracrine control. GnRH and epidermal growth factor diminish FSH stimulation of inhibin secretion, while insulin-like growth factor-I enhances inhibin production. The inhibitory effects of GnRH and epidermal growth factor are consistent with their known ability to decrease FSH-stimulated estrogen production and LH receptor formation. The action of GnRH lends some support for an endogenous ovarian GnRH-like substance (which is found in follicular fluid) and which is involved in inhibin production.

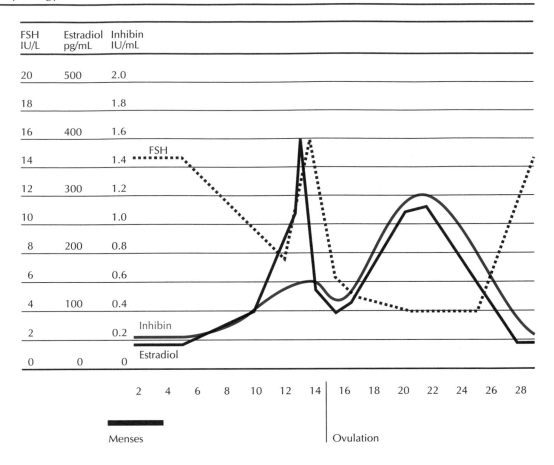

FSH IU/L	Estradiol pg/mL	Inhibin IU/mL
20	500	2.0
18		1.8
16	400	1.6
14		1.4
12	300	1.2
10		1.0
8	200	0.8
6		0.6
4	100	0.4
2		0.2
0	0	0

The secretion of inhibin into the circulation further amplifies the withdrawal of FSH from other follicles, another mechanism by which an emerging follicle secures dominance. Inhibin rises slowly but steadily throughout the follicular phase to reach a midcycle peak that coincides with the gonadotropin surge.[56,57] With development of the follicle into a corpus luteum, inhibin expression comes under the control of LH. The circulating levels of inhibin drop slightly from the midcycle peak, then rise to reach a level at the midluteal phase that is at least two times greater than the midcycle peak.[58] After conception, even higher circulating levels of inhibin are achieved. There is some question whether the luteal levels of immunoactive inhibin represent true inhibin bioactivity or whether inactive subunits of inhibin are being measured.

Inhibin has multiple, diverse inhibitory effects on gonadotropin secretion.[59] Inhibin can block the synthesis and secretion of FSH, prevent the up-regulation of GnRH receptors by GnRH, reduce the number of GnRH receptors present, and, at high concentrations, promote the intracellular degradation of gonadotropins.

Activin is a peptide that is related to inhibin but has an opposite action (the stimulation of FSH release and GnRH receptor number).[60,61] This peptide contains two subunits that are identical to the beta-subunits of inhibins A and B. Thus, when each of the beta-subunits of the inhibins is combined with an alpha-subunit, the resulting molecule, inhibin A or B, inhibits the release of FSH. If the beta-subunits are paired together, the molecule stimulates the release of FSH. Each inhibin and activin subunit is encoded by a distinct gene. The structure of the inhibin-activin genes is homologous to that of transforming growth factor-β, indicating that these products all come from the same gene family.[62] Another important member of this family is the antimüllerian hormone, as well as a protein active during insect embryogenesis, and a protein active in frog embryos.

The 3 Forms of Activin:

Activin-A:	**Beta$_A$-Beta$_A$**
Activin-AB:	**Beta$_A$-Beta$_B$**
Activin-B:	**Beta$_B$-Beta$_B$**

Activin is present in many cell types, regulating growth and differentiation. In the ovarian follicle, activin increases FSH binding in granulosa cells (by regulating receptor numbers) and augments FSH stimulation of aromatization and inhibin production.[54] Considerable evidence derived from human cells exists to indicate that inhibin and activin act directly on thecal cells to regulate androgen synthesis. Inhibin enhances the stimulatory action of LH and/or IGF-I, while activin suppresses this action. Inhibin in increasing doses can overcome the inhibitory action of activin. Prior to ovulation, activin suppresses granulosa progesterone production, perhaps preventing premature luteinization. There is a repertoire of cell transmembrane kinase receptors for activin, with differing binding affinities and domain structures.[63] This receptor heterogeneity allows the many different responses elicited by a single peptide.

In the male, activin inhibits and inhibin facilitates LH stimulation of androgen biosynthesis in Leydig cells. In addition, activin stimulates and inhibin decreases spermatogonial proliferation; inhibin is produced in the Sertoli cell, the locus that has the principal role in modulating spermatogenesis. Thus, activin and inhibin play similar autocrine/paracrine roles in both the male and female gonads.

The anterior pituitary expresses the inhibin/activin subunits, and locally produced activin-B augments FSH secretion. Activin-A has been demonstrated to directly stimulate the synthesis of GnRH receptors in pituitary cells.[64] The subunits are also expressed in the placenta where activin stimulates progesterone secretion, an action blocked by inhibin. The placenta contributes significant amounts to circulating inhibin during pregnancy. Levels rise to a peak at about 11 weeks of pregnancy, followed by a decline to a plateau that is maintained from 14 to 25 weeks, followed by a slow rise to the highest levels at term (4 times luteal levels).[65]

Follistatin is a single chain, glycosylated polypeptide produced in the pituitary but found primarily in preovulatory follicles. It is expressed by granulosa cells in response to FSH.[66] Its structure is distinct from that of inhibin and activin, and shows homology to epidermal growth factor. It modifies FSH activity by binding activin thus removing this enhancing agent from cellular activity.[54] It also possesses weak activity similar to inhibin. Thus, follistatin, like inhibin and activin, functions locally in the follicle and in the pituitary. Its circulating blood levels parallel estrogen and inhibin.

The pituitary secretion of FSH can be significantly regulated by the balance of activin and inhibin, with follistatin playing a role by inhibiting activin and enhancing inhibin activity. Within the ovarian follicle, activin and inhibin influence growth and development by modulating thecal and granulosal responses to the gonadotropins.

The inhibin-activin family of peptides (also including antimüllerian hormone and transforming growth factor-β) inhibits cell growth and can be considered as a class of tumor-suppressor proteins. Mice have been generated that are deficient in the inhibin alpha-subunit gene.[55] The mice that are homozygous and lack inhibin are susceptible to the development of gonadal stromal tumors which appear after normal sexual differentiation and development. Thus, the alpha-inhibin gene is a specific tumor-suppressor gene for the gonads. A contributing factor to this tumor development could be the high FSH levels associated with the deficiency in inhibin.

Growth Factors

Growth factors are polypeptides that modulate cell proliferation and differentiation, operating through binding to specific cell membrane receptors. They are not classic endocrine substances; they act locally and function in paracrine and autocrine modes. There are multiple growth factors, and most cells contain multiple receptors for the various growth factors.

Insulin-Like Growth Factors

The insulin-like growth factors (also called somatomedins) are peptides that have structural and functional similarity to insulin and mediate growth hormone action.[67] Insulin-like growth factor-I (IGF-I) and insulin-like growth factor-II (IGF-II) are single chain polypeptides containing 3 disulfide bonds. IGF-I is encoded on the long arm of chromosome 12 and IGF-II on the short arm of chromosome 11 (which also contains the insulin gene). The genes are subject to a variety of promoters, and thus differential regulation can govern ultimate actions.

IGF-I mediates the growth promoting actions of growth hormone. The majority of circulating IGF-I is derived from the growth hormone dependent synthesis in the liver. However, IGF-I is synthesized in many tissues where production can be regulated in conjunction with growth hormone or *independently* by other factors.

IGF-II has little growth hormone dependence. It is believed to be more important in fetal growth and development. Both IGFs induce the expression of cellular genes responsible for cellular proliferation and differentiation.

Insulin-like Growth Factor Binding Proteins. There are 6 known nonglycosylated peptides which function as IGF binding proteins: IGFBP-1 to IGFBP-6.[68] These binding proteins serve to carry the IGFs in serum, prolong half-lives, and regulate tissue effects of the IGFs. The regulating action appears to be due to binding and sequestering of the IGFs, preventing their access to the cell membrane surface receptors, and thus not permitting the synergistic actions that result when gonadotropins and growth factors are combined. The IGFBPs may also exert direct actions on cellular functions, independently of growth factor functions. IGFBP-1 is the principal BP in amniotic fluid; IGFBP-3 is the main BP in serum and its synthesis, primarily in the liver, is dependent on growth hormone. Circulating levels of IGFBP-3 reflect the total IGF concentration (IGF-I plus IGF-II) and carry at least 90% of the circulating IGFs. These BPs do not bind insulin. The BPs change with age (decreasing levels of BP-3) and during pregnancy (decreasing BP-3 due to a circulating protease unique to pregnancy).

The IGF Receptors. The Type I receptor preferentially binds IGF-1 and can be called the IGF-I receptor. The Type II receptor in a similar fashion can be called the IGF-II receptor. IGF-I also binds to the insulin receptor but with low affinity. Insulin binds to the IGF-I receptor with moderate affinity. The IGF-I receptor and the insulin receptor are similar in structure: tetramers composed of two α-subunits and two β-subunits linked by disulfide bonds. The intracellular component of the β-subunit is a tyrosine kinase that is activated by autophosphorylation. The IGF-II receptor does not bind insulin. It is a single chain glycoprotein, with 90% of its structure extending extracellularly. This receptor functions as a receptor coupled to a G protein. The physiologic effects of IGF-I are mediated by its own receptor, but IGF-II can exert its actions via both receptors. In human cells, the IGF-I receptor is present in theca and granulosa cells and in luteinized granulosa cells. IGF-II receptor expression is marked in luteinized granulosa cells, and only IGF-II is found in the corpus luteum. Ovarian stromal tissue contains IGF-I receptors.

Early Follicular Phase

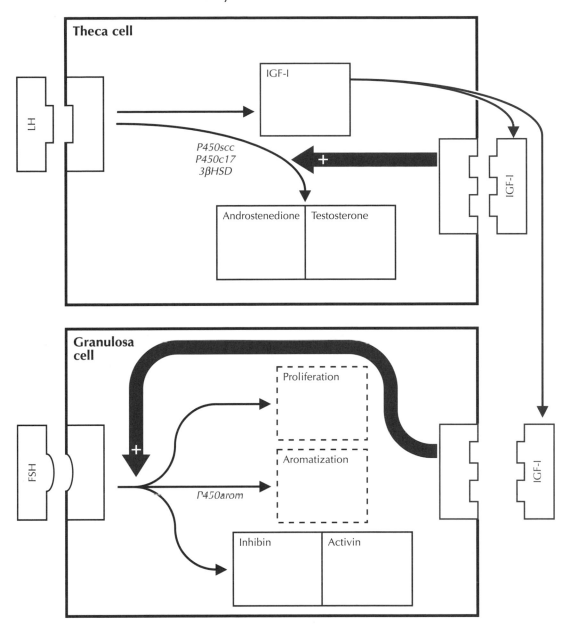

The Ovarian Actions of IGFs. IGF-I has been demonstrated to stimulate the following events in ovarian theca and granulosa cells: DNA synthesis, steroidogenesis, aromatase activity, LH receptor synthesis, and inhibin secretion. IGF-II stimulates granulosa mitosis. In human ovarian cells, IGF-I, in synergy with FSH, stimulates protein synthesis and steroidogenesis. After LH receptors appear, IGF-I enhances LH-induced progesterone synthesis and stimulates proliferation of granulosa-luteal cells. IGF-I, in synergy with FSH, is very active in stimulating aromatase activity in preovulatory follicles. Thus, IGF-I is involved in both estradiol and progesterone synthesis.

In animal experiments, the synthesis of IGF-I by granulosa cells is dependent upon FSH but enhanced by estradiol. Growth hormone also acts synergistically with FSH and estradiol to increase IGF synthesis. The story becomes confused when various growth factors and regulators are studied, because of their various stimulating and inhibiting effects. In the rat, the granulosa cell is the major site for IGF-I gene expression which is active only prior to ovulation. It is not detected in atretic follicles or in corpora lutea.

Preovulatory Follicle

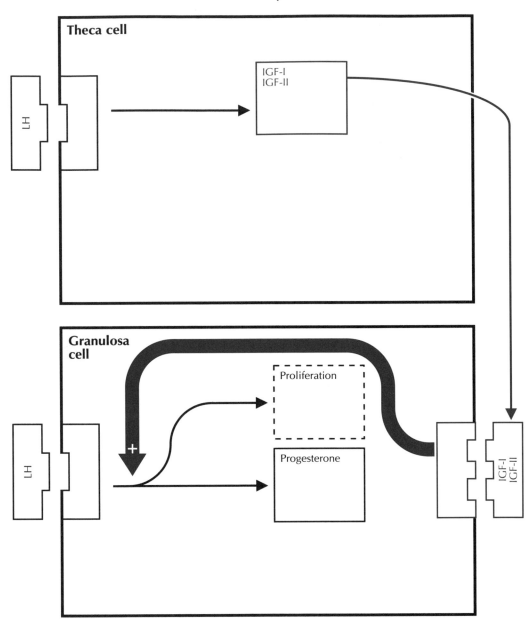

Again in the rat, IGF-II gene expression appears to be limited to the theca and interstitial cells. However, the site of IGF expression is different in primates.

In whole human ovary studies, IGF-I is of thecal origin in the preovulatory phase, which together with its known biochemical actions suggests that IGF-I moves from the theca to the granulosa to function in a paracrine fashion. IGF-II, on the other hand, is synthesized by luteinized granulosa and appears to function locally in an autocrine fashion.[69] Human thecal cells express mRNA transcripts which encode receptors for both IGF-I and insulin.[70] Thus IGF-I exerts a paracrine influence on granulosa cells and autocrine activity in the theca (augmenting LH stimulation of androgen production). These actions are augmented by growth hormone, which increases IGF production and thus indirectly enhances gonadotropin stimulation of ovarian follicles.[71]

This primate scenario is supported by finding high levels of IGF-I in the follicular fluid of developing follicles, with the highest levels present in dominant follicles. The IGF-

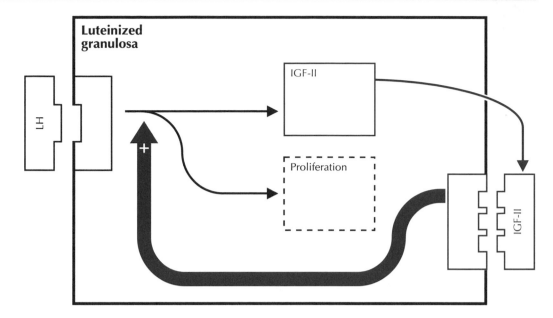

I levels in follicular fluid correlate with estradiol levels and undergo a further short increase after the LH surge. There are no menstrual cycle changes in the circulating levels of IGF-I and IGF-II; high levels in the dominant follicle are not associated with an increase in circulating levels.

Granulosa cells from women with anovulation (polycystic ovaries) produce estrogen equally in response to either IGF-I or FSH, and when applied together, a synergistic stimulation occurs.[72] This effect could not be produced with either insulin or IGF-II and supports a role for IGF-I in estrogen production during the follicular phase.

The 6 IGF binding proteins are synthesized in different amounts in various follicular tissues in response to gonadotropins, insulin, and IGF-I. In the rat, IGFBP-3 is made in the theca, stimulated by growth hormone, and inhibited by FSH and estradiol.[73] In the rat, low concentrations of FSH stimulate the expression of IGFBPs, while FSH at high concentrations inhibits IGFBP synthesis. It is proposed that this biphasic response allows an increase in IGF-I facilitation of mitosis during FSH-induced follicular growth, while IGF-I availability is limited during periods of low FSH when follicular steroidogenesis is the major effort.[74]

In studies with human tissue, IGFBP-1 inhibits IGF-1 mediated steroidogenesis and proliferation of luteinized granulosa cells. The synthesis of IGFBPs by human granulosa is inhibited by FSH, IGF-I, and IGF-II.[75,76] These findings fit with the overall idea that the BPs counteract the synergistic results of gonadotropins and growth factors. In general, IGFBP-1 expression is found in granulosa cells of growing follicles; IGFBP-3 in theca cells and the granulosa of the dominant follicle; IGFBP-2, -4, and -5 in granulosa of atretic follicles; and IGFBP-6 has not been found in the ovary.[77] The predominant binding protein in preovulatory follicles is IGFBP-3, that increases progressively in the follicle which emerges as the dominant follicle.[78] This suggests that -1 and -3 play a role in growing follicles, -2, -4, and -5 in atretic and failing follicles. IGFBP expression in polycystic ovaries is similar to that seen in atretic follicles. The decrease in IGFBP-3 that occurs in dominant follicles should allow an increase in IGF-I levels and activity. The increase in IGFBP-2 in failing follicles probably correlates with sequestering of IGF-I, depriving the follicle of an important force in gonadotropin augmentation.

Circulating levels of IGFBP-1 decrease in response to insulin, and thus circulating levels are decreased in women with anovulation and polycystic ovaries who have elevated levels of insulin.[79] These patients also have increased circulating levels of IGF-I, probably a consequence of LH-stimulated synthesis and secretion in theca cells. The level of IGFBP-1 in follicular fluid from polycystic ovaries is decreased; thus this BP is not playing a role inhibiting the action of IGF-I in polycystic ovaries. The levels of IGFBPs -2 and -4 in the follicular fluid from follicles in anovulatory patients are increased (as in atretic follicles).[77,80] Even though these changes may play a role in anovulatory pathophysiology, they are consistent with failure in development and thus may not be etiologic factors.

In addition to ovarian activities, IGF-I and its receptor and binding proteins operate in the pituitary gland. In the rat, the hyperplasia of various pituitary cell types appears to be mediated by estrogen regulation of the IGF-I system.[81] This mechanism is of special interest when considering the development of pituitary tumors, such as the prolactin secreting pituitary adenoma.

The insulin-like growth factor story is fascinating and compelling. However, its contribution may be facilitory and not essential. Laron-type dwarfism is characterized by a deficiency in IGF-I due to an abnormality in the growth hormone receptor. Despite low levels of IGF-I and high levels of IGFBP, a woman with Laron-type dwarfism responded to exogenous gonadotropin stimulation with the production of multiple, mature follicles with good estrogen production and fertilizable oocytes.[82] Another explanation for this observation is that IGF-II, rather than IGF-I, is the important factor in the human dominant follicle. This possibility is supported by evidence indicating that IGF-II is the most abundant IGF in human ovarian follicles.[83] Another possibility is that the Laron-type dwarf is deficient only in growth hormone-dependent IGF-I, and ovarian IGFs may not be totally dependent on growth hormone.

Summary of Insulin-Like Growth Factor Action in the Ovary

1. IGF-I stimulates granulosa cell proliferation, aromatase activity, and progesterone synthesis.

2. IGF-I is produced in theca cells; luteinized granulosa cells produce IGF-II. In the pig and rat, the sites are reversed; granulosa produces IGF-I and theca produces IGF-II.

3. Gonadotropins stimulate IGF production, and in animal experiments, this stimulation is enhanced by estradiol and growth hormone.

4. IGF-I receptors are present in theca and granulosa cells, and only IGF-II receptors are present in luteinized granulosa.

5. The most abundant IGF in human follicles is IGF-II.

6. FSH inhibits binding protein synthesis, and thus maximizes growth factor availability.

Epidermal Growth Factor

Epidermal growth factor is a mitogen for a variety of cells, and its action is potentiated by other growth factors. Granulosa cells, in particular, respond to this growth factor secretion by theca cells, in a variety of ways related to gonadotropin stimulation, including proliferation. Epidermal growth factor suppresses the up-regulation of FSH on its own receptor.[10]

Transforming Growth Factor

TGF-α is a structural analog of epidermal growth factor and can bind to the epidermal growth factor receptor. TGF-β utilizes a receptor distinct from the epidermal growth factor receptor. These factors are thought to be autocrine growth regulators. Inhibin and activin are derived from the same gene family. TGF-β, secreted by theca cells, enhances FSH induction of LH receptors on granulosa cells, an action which is opposite that of epidermal growth factor.[84] While this action can be viewed as a positive impact on granulosa cells, in the theca, TGF-β has a negative action, inhibiting androgen production.[85]

Fibroblast Growth Factor

This factor is a mitogen for a variety of cells and is present in all steroid producing tissues. Important roles in the ovarian follicle include stimulation of mitosis in granulosa cells, stimulation of angiogenesis, stimulation of plasminogen activator, inhibition of FSH up-regulation of its own receptor, and inhibition of FSH-induced LH receptor expression and estrogen production.[10,86] These actions are opposite of those of transforming growth factor-β.

Platelet-Derived Growth Factor

This growth factor modifies cyclic AMP pathways responding to FSH, especially those involved in granulosa cell differentiation. Both platelet-derived growth factor and epidermal growth factor may also modify prostaglandin production within the follicle.

Angiogenic Growth Factors

Vascularization of the follicle is influenced by peptides secreted into the follicular fluid.[87]

The Interleukin-1 System

Interleukin-1 is a member of the cytokine family of immunomediators. In the rat, it stimulates ovarian prostaglandin synthesis and perhaps plays a role in ovulation.[88]

Other Peptides

The follicular fluid is a veritable protein soup! It is composed of exudates from plasma and secretions from follicular cells. A variety of hormones can be found in the follicular fluid, as well as enzymes and peptides which play important roles in follicular growth and development, ovulation, and modulation of hormonal responses.

Follicular fluid contains *prorenin,* the inactive precursor of renin, in a concentration that is about 12 times higher than plasma levels.[89] It appears that LH stimulates its synthesis in the follicle, and there is a midcycle peak in prorenin plasma levels. The circulating levels of prorenin also increase (10-fold) during the early stages of pregnancy, the result of ovarian stimulation by the rise in human chorionic gonadotropin (HCG). These increases in prorenin from the ovary are not responsible for any significant changes in the plasma levels of the active form, renin. Possible roles for this ovarian prorenin-renin-angiotensin system include stimulation of steroidogenesis to provide androgen substrate for estrogen production, regulation of calcium and prostaglandin metabolism, and stimulation of angiogenesis. This system may affect vascular and tissue functions both within and outside the ovary.

Members of the proopiomelanocortin family are found in human follicular fluid.[90] Follicular levels of *ACTH* and β-*lipotropin* remain constant throughout the cycle, but β-*endorphin* levels peak just before ovulation. In addition, enkephalin is present in relatively unchanging concentrations.

Antimüllerian hormone is produced by granulosa cells and may play a role in oocyte maturation (it inhibits oocyte meiosis) and follicular development.[91,92] Antimüllerian hormone directly inhibits proliferation of granulosa and luteal cells, as well as epidermal growth factor-stimulated proliferation.

Follicular fluid prevents resumption of meiosis until the preovulatory LH surge either overcomes or removes this inhibition. This action is attributed to *oocyte maturation inhibitor (OMI)*. *Pregnancy-associated plasma protein A,* found in the placenta, is also present in follicular fluid. It may inhibit proteolytic activity within the follicle before ovulation. *Endothelin-1* is a peptide, originally isolated from vascular endothelial cells, which may be the substance previously known as luteinization inhibitor; endothelin gene expression is induced by the hypoxia associated with the avascular granulosa, and it inhibits LH-induced progesterone production.[93] It is uncertain whether *GnRH-like peptides* have a follicular role or represent sequestered GnRH. *Oxytocin* is found in preovulatory follicles and the corpus luteum, but its function is unknown. Growth hormone-binding protein is present in follicular fluid and similar in characteristics to the same binding protein in serum.

Summary of Events in the Antral Follicle

1. Follicular phase estrogen production is explained by the two cell, two gonadotropin mechanism.

2. Selection of the dominant follicle is established during days 5–7, and consequently, peripheral levels of estradiol begin to rise significantly by cycle day 7.

3. Estradiol levels, derived from the dominant follicle, increase steadily and, through negative feedback effects, exert a progressively greater suppressive influence on FSH release.

4. While directing a decline in FSH levels, the midfollicular rise in estradiol exerts a positive feedback influence on LH secretion.

5. The positive action of estrogen also includes modification of the gonadotropin molecule, increasing the quality (the bioactivity) as well as the quantity of LH at midcycle.

6. LH levels rise steadily during the late follicular phase, stimulating androgen production in the theca.

7. A unique responsiveness to FSH allows the dominant follicle to utilize the androgen as substrate and further accelerate estrogen production.

8. FSH induces the appearance of LH receptors on granulosa cells.

9. Follicular response to the gonadotropins is modulated by a variety of growth factors and autocrine/paracrine peptides.

10. Inhibin, and less importantly follistatin, secreted by the granulosa cells in response to FSH, directly suppresses pituitary FSH secretion.

11. Activin, originating in both granulosa and pituitary, augments FSH secretion and action.

Follicular Growth and Development in the Primate Ovary

Concern that the story for ovarian follicular growth and development might be different in the primate originated with the failure to find estrogen receptors in any of the significant ovarian compartments in the monkey: follicles, stromal tissue, interstitial tissue, or corpora lutea.[94] This finding in the monkey has been confirmed in human tissue by the failure to detect messenger RNA for the estrogen receptor in human granulosa cells (although estrogen receptor transcripts were present in mature oocytes).[95] It is possible that estradiol plays its important role without involving its receptor, but that is unlikely. In the animals in which studies constructed a regulating function for estradiol, estrogen receptors are present in the ovarian cells, and one would expect the usual receptor mechanism to be the means of estrogen action. In further monkey experiments, no reduction in total number or size of follicles resulted when estradiol production was effectively suppressed by treatment with an inhibitor of the aromatase enzyme system.[96] Oocyte development was not altered, although the subsequent fertilization rate was reduced by this treatment.

One possibility is that autocrine/paracrine peptides have replaced steroid hormones as the principal regulators in primate follicles. Consider the following actions that have been documented in primate ovaries:

1. *Inhibin and activin regulate androgen synthesis in human theca cells. Inhibin enhances and activin suppresses the stimulatory action of LH and/ or IGF-I, and inhibin can overcome the inhibitory action of activin on theca cells.[97,98]*

2. *In immature granulosa cells, activin augments FSH activities, especially aromatase activity (estrogen production).[99]*

3. *In luteinizing granulosa cells, activin has direct mitogenic activity and suppresses steroidogenesis in response to LH, while inhibin has no effect on LH-dependent aromatase in mature granulosa cells.[99,100]*

4. *In the follicular phase, granulosa production of inhibin is under the control of FSH, but during the late follicular phase a change occurs, culminating in LH control of luteal synthesis of inhibin.[101,102]*

Early Follicular Phase

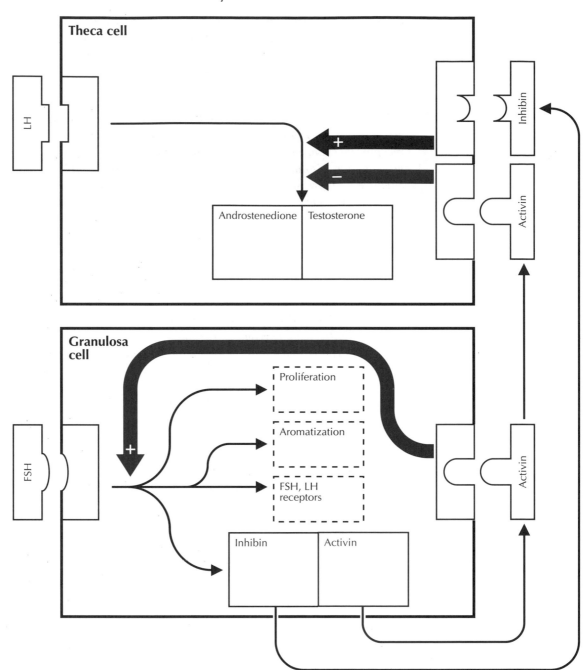

These actions may come together as follows. In the early follicular phase, activin produced by granulosa in immature follicles enhances the action of FSH on aromatase activity and FSH and LH receptor formation, while simultaneously suppressing thecal androgen synthesis. In the late follicular phase, increased production of inhibin by the granulosa (and decreased activin) promotes androgen synthesis in the theca in response to LH and IGF-I to provide substrate for even greater estrogen production in the granulosa. In the mature granulosa, activin serves to prevent premature luteinization and progesterone production.

The successful follicle is the one that acquires the highest level of aromatase activity and LH receptors in response to FSH. The successful follicle is characterized by the highest estrogen (for central feedback action) and the greatest inhibin production (for both local

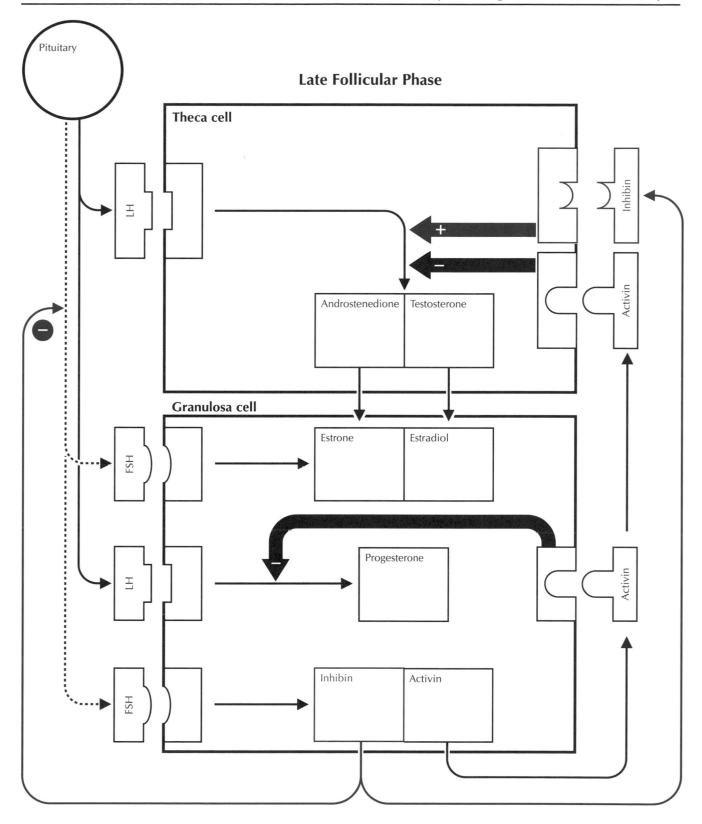

Late Follicular Phase

and central actions). This accomplishment occurs in synchrony with the appropriate activin expression. The highest level of gene activity encoding activin-B is found in immature antral follicles and the lowest level in preovulatory follicles. Thus the activin proteins (which enhance FSH activity) are produced in greatest amounts early in follicular development to enhance follicle receptivity to FSH.

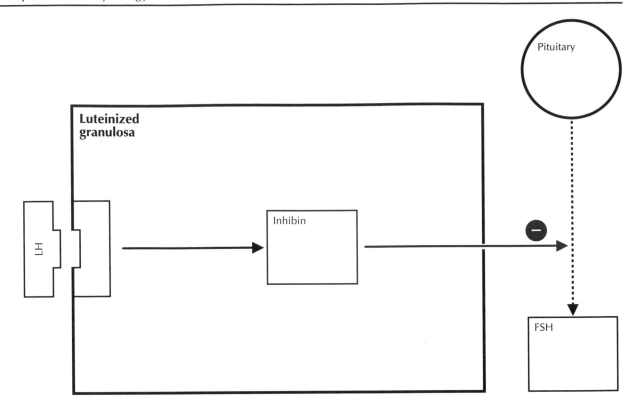

The right concentration of androgens in granulosa cells promotes aromatase activity and inhibin production and, in turn, inhibin promotes LH stimulation of thecal androgen synthesis. With development of the follicle, inhibin expression comes under control of LH. A key to successful ovulation and luteal function is conversion of the inhibin production to LH responsiveness to maintain FSH suppression centrally and enhancement of LH action locally.

A lesser role is assigned to the growth factors in view of the successful production of multiple, estrogen-producing follicles which yielded fertilizable oocytes in a woman with IGF-I deficiency treated with gonadotropins.[82] The growth factors assume an important, but perhaps not essential, role as facilitating agents. However, the successful pregnancy in a woman with IGF-I deficiency may indicate the greater importance of IGF-II. In addition, the IGFs in the ovary may not be growth hormone-dependent, and therefore IGF-I and/or IGF-II may also be important in primate ovarian follicles.

Summary of Events in the Primate Ovarian Follicle

1.   FSH stimulates inhibin and activin production by granulosa cells.

2.   Activin augments FSH activities: FSH receptor expression, aromatization, inhibin/activin production, and LH receptor expression.

3.   Inhibin enhances LH stimulation of androgen synthesis in the theca to provide substrate for aromatization to estrogen in the granulosa.

4.   With the appearance of LH receptors, inhibin production is maintained as it comes under control of LH.

5.   All functions are modulated by a host of growth factors, and IGF-II may be especially important.

The removal of estradiol from a local coordinating role in the primate ovarian follicle is a response directed by the monkey data, a failure to find evidence for the presence of estrogen receptors and successful follicular growth and development despite suppressed estrogen production.[94,96] Estrogen receptors in the granulosa cells of the baboon, however, have been identified by immunochemistry, and this was supported by the presence of estrogen receptor mRNA.[103] On the other hand, messenger RNA for the estrogen receptor was not detected in human granulosa cells (although expression of the estrogen receptor gene was detected in mature oocytes).[95] Are these species differences or a result of different laboratory techniques? A lesser role for estrogen in primates is supported by the demonstration of normal follicular growth and development with successful in vitro fertilization in women with 17α-hydroxylase deficiency (and therefore an inability to produce androgens and estrogens) given exogenous gonadotropins.[104,105] Ultimately time and further study especially of human tissue may well combine the primate and nonprimate stories, bringing appropriate understanding and recognition for the roles of both estradiol and the autocrine/paracrine peptides.

The Preovulatory Follicle

Granulosa cells in the preovulatory follicle enlarge and acquire lipid inclusions while the theca becomes vacuolated and richly vascular, giving the preovulatory follicle a hyperemic appearance. The oocyte resumes meiosis, approaching completion of its reduction division.

Approaching maturity, the preovulatory follicle produces increasing amounts of estrogen. During the late follicular phase, estrogens rise slowly at first, then rapidly, reaching a peak approximately 24–36 hours prior to ovulation.[106] The onset of the LH surge occurs when the peak levels of estradiol are achieved.[107] In providing the ovulatory stimulus to the selected follicle, the LH surge seals the fate of the remaining follicles, with their lower estrogen and FSH content, by further increasing androgen superiority.

Acting through its own receptors, LH promotes luteinization of the granulosa in the dominant follicle, resulting in the production of progesterone. The LH receptor, once expressed, inhibits further cell growth and focuses the cell's energy on steroidogenesis (actions enhanced by IGF-I).[108] An increase in progesterone can be detected in the venous effluent of the ovary bearing the preovulatory follicle as early as day 10 of the cycle.[29] This small but significant increase in the production of progesterone in the preovulatory period has immense physiologic importance. Prior to the emergence of this follicular progesterone, the circulating level of progesterone was derived from the adrenal gland.[109]

Although estrogen receptors cannot be detected in primate follicular cells, progesterone receptors begin to appear in the granulosa cells of the dominant follicle in the periovulatory period.[94] The traditional view has been that progesterone receptors are expressed in response to estrogen through an estrogen-receptor mediated mechanism. This is not the case with the primate ovarian follicle. Experimental data in the monkey provide excellent evidence that LH stimulates progesterone receptor expression in granulosa cells.[110] In vitro data with human cells suggest that the preovulatory progesterone and progesterone receptor expression directly inhibit granulosa cell mitosis, probably explaining the limitation of granulosa cell proliferation as these cells gain LH receptors.[111]

Progesterone affects the positive feedback response to estrogen in both a time and dose dependent manner. When introduced after adequate estrogen priming, progesterone facilitates the positive feedback response, in a direct action on the pituitary, and in the presence of subthreshold levels of estradiol can induce a characteristic LH surge.[112,113] Hence, the surprising onset of ovulation occasionally observed in an anovulatory, amenorrheic woman administered a progestin challenge. When administered before the estrogen stimulus, or in high doses (achieving a blood level greater than 2 ng/mL [6.4 nmol/L]), progesterone blocks the midcycle LH surge. Appropriately low levels of progesterone derived from the maturing follicle contribute to the precise synchronization of the midcycle surge.

In addition to its facilitory action on LH, progesterone at midcycle is significantly responsible for the FSH surge.[113] This action of progesterone can be viewed as a further step in ensuring completion of FSH action on the follicle, especially making sure that a full complement of LH receptors is in place in the granulosa layer. In certain experimental situations, incremental estradiol alone can elicit simultaneous surges of LH and FSH, suggesting that progesterone certainly enhances the effect of estradiol but may not be obligatory.[114] These actions of estrogen and progesterone require the presence and continuous action of GnRH.

The preovulatory period is associated with a rise in plasma levels of 17α-hydroxy-progesterone. This steroid does not appear to have a role in cycle regulation, and its appearance in the blood simply represents the secretion of an intermediate product. As such, however, it signals the LH stimulation of P450scc and P450c17, important enzyme activity for the production of theca androgens, the substrate for granulosa estrogen. After ovulation, some theca cells become luteinized as part of the corpus luteum and lose the ability to express P450c17. Other luteinized theca cells retain P450c17 activity and are believed to continue to produce androgens for aromatization to estrogens.

When the lesser follicles fail to achieve full maturity and undergo atresia, the theca cells return to their origin as a component of stromal tissue, retaining, however, an ability to respond to LH with P450 activity and steroid production. Because the products of thecal tissue are androgens, the increase in stromal tissue in the late follicular phase is associated with a rise in androgen levels in the peripheral plasma at midcycle. There is a 15% increase in androstenedione and a 20% increase in testosterone.[115] This response is enhanced by the rise in inhibin, known to augment LH stimulation of androgen production in thecal cells.

Androgen production at this stage in the cycle may serve two purposes: 1) a local role within the ovary to enhance the process of atresia, and 2) a systemic effect to stimulate libido.

Intraovarian androgens accelerate granulosa cell death and follicular atresia. The specific mechanism for this action is unclear, although it is attractive to suspect an interference with estrogen and the autocrine/paracrine factors in enhancing FSH activity. Therefore, androgens may play a regulatory role in ensuring that only a dominant follicle reaches the point of ovulation.

It is well known that libido can be stimulated by androgens. If the midcycle rise in androgens affects libido, then an increase in sexual activity should coincide with this rise. Early studies failed to demonstrate a consistent pattern in coital frequency in women because of the effect of male partner initiation. If only sexual behavior initiated by women is studied, a peak in female-initiated sexual activity is seen during the ovulatory phase of the cycle.[116] The coital frequency of married couples has also been noted to increase at the time of ovulation.[117] Therefore, the midcycle rise in androgens may serve to increase sexual activity at the time most likely to achieve pregnancy.

Summary of Events in the Preovulatory Follicle

1. Estrogen production becomes sufficient to achieve and maintain peripheral threshold concentrations of estradiol that are required in order to induce the LH surge.

2. Acting through its receptors, LH initiates luteinization and progesterone production in the granulosa layer.

3. The preovulatory rise in progesterone facilitates the positive feedback action of estrogen and may be required to induce the midcycle FSH peak.

4. A midcycle increase in local and peripheral androgens occurs, derived from the thecal tissue of lesser, unsuccessful follicles.

Ovulation

The preovulatory follicle, through the elaboration of estradiol, provides its own ovulatory stimulus. Considerable variation in timing exists from cycle to cycle, even in the same woman. A reasonable and accurate estimate places ovulation approximately 10–12 hours after the LH peak and 24–36 hours after peak estradiol levels are attained.[106,118] The onset of the LH surge appears to be the most reliable indicator of impending ovulation, occurring 34–36 hours prior to follicle rupture.[119] A threshold of LH concentration must be maintained for 14–27 hours in order for full maturation of the oocyte to occur.[120] Usually the LH surge lasts 48–50 hours.[119]

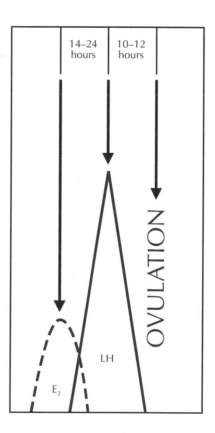

Because of the careful timing involved in in vitro fertilization programs, we have available some interesting data.[121] The LH surge tends to occur at approximately 3 A.M., beginning between midnight and 7:30 A.M. in two-thirds of women. Ovulation occurs primarily in the morning during Spring, and primarily in the evening during Autumn and Winter. From July to February in the northern hemisphere, about 90% of women ovulate between 4 and 7 P.M.; during Spring, half of the women ovulate between midnight and 11 A.M.

The gonadotropin surge stimulates a large collection of events that ultimately leads to ovulation, the physical release of the oocyte and its cumulus mass of granulosa cells.[122] This is not an explosive event; therefore, a complex series of changes must occur which cause the final maturation of the oocyte and the decomposition of the collagenous layer of the follicular wall.

The LH surge initiates the resumption of meiosis in the oocyte (meiosis is not completed until after the sperm has entered and the second polar body is released), luteinization of granulosa cells, expansion of the cumulus, and the synthesis of prostaglandins and other eicosanoids essential for follicle rupture. Premature oocyte maturation and luteinization are prevented by local factors. LH-induced cyclic AMP activity overcomes the local inhibitory action of oocyte maturation inhibitor (OMI) and luteinization inhibitor (LI). OMI originates from the granulosa cells, and its activity depends upon an intact cumulus oophorous. Activin also suppresses progesterone production by luteal cells, providing yet another means of preventing premature luteinization.[123,124]

With the LH surge, levels of progesterone in the follicle continue to rise up to the time of ovulation. The progressive rise in progesterone may act to terminate the LH surge as a negative feedback effect is exerted at higher concentrations. In addition to its central effects, progesterone increases the distensibility of the follicle wall. A change in the elastic properties of the follicular wall is necessary to explain the rapid increase in follicular fluid volume which occurs just prior to ovulation, unaccompanied by any significant change in intrafollicular pressure. The escape of the ovum is associated with degenerative changes of the collagen in the follicular wall so that just prior to ovulation the follicular wall becomes thin and stretched. FSH, LH, and progesterone stimulate the activity of proteolytic enzymes, resulting in digestion of collagen in the follicular wall and increasing its distensibility. The gonadotropin surge also releases histamine, and histamine alone can induce ovulation in some experimental models.

The proteolytic enzymes are activated in an orderly sequence.[125] The granulosa and theca cells produce plasminogen activator in response to the gonadotropin surge. Plasminogen is activated by either of two plasminogen activators: tissue-type plasminogen activator and urokinase-type plasminogen activator. These activators are encoded by separate genes and are also regulated by inhibitors.

Plasminogen activators produced by granulosa cells activate plasminogen in the follicular fluid to produce plasmin. Plasmin, in turn, generates active collagenase to disrupt the follicular wall. In rat models, plasminogen activator synthesis is triggered by LH stimulation (as well as growth factors and FSH), while plasminogen inhibitor synthesis is decreased.[126] Thus before and after ovulation, the inhibitor activity is high, while just at ovulation, activator activity is high and the inhibitors are at a nadir. The molecular regulation of these factors is necessary for the coordination that leads to ovulation. Plasminogen activator synthesis in granulosa cells is expressed only at the right preovulatory stage in response to LH. The inhibitor system, which is very active in the thecal and interstitial cells, prevents inappropriate activation of plasminogen and disruption of growing follicles. The inhibitor system has been demonstrated to be present in human granulosa cells and preovulatory follicular fluid and to be responsive to a paracrine

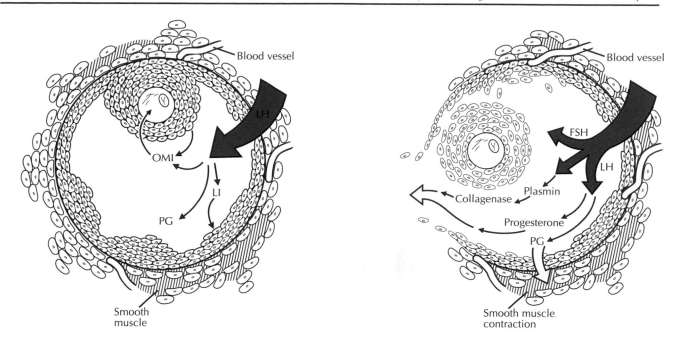

substance, epidermal growth factor.[127,128] Movement of the follicle destined to ovulate to the surface of the ovary is important in that the exposed surface of the follicle is now prone to rupture because it is separated from cells rich in the plasminogen inhibitor system. Ovulation is the result of proteolytic digestion of the follicular apex, a site called the stigma.

In the rat, the gene that encodes for plasminogen activator contains a promoter region which has several sequences for known transcription factors, such as the cyclic AMP-responsive element (CRE). The activation of this CRE (which involves the CRE binding protein) requires FSH stimulation. Thus, both gonadotropins appear to be involved in this process.

Prostaglandins of the E and F series and other eicosanoids (especially HETEs, hydroxy-eicosatetraenoic acid methyl esters) increase markedly in the preovulatory follicular fluid, reaching a peak concentration at ovulation.[129,130] Inhibition of the synthesis of these products from arachidonic acid blocks follicle rupture without affecting the other LH-induced processes of luteinization and oocyte maturation.[131] Prostaglandins may act to free proteolytic enzymes within the follicular wall, and the HETEs may promote angiogenesis and hyperemia (an inflammatory-like response).[130,132] Prostaglandins may also contract smooth muscle cells that have been identified in the ovary, thereby aiding the extrusion of the oocyte-cumulus cell mass. This role of prostaglandins is so well demonstrated that infertility patients should be advised to avoid the use of drugs that inhibit prostaglandin synthesis.[133]

Estradiol levels plunge as LH reaches its peak. This may be a consequence of LH down-regulation of its own receptors on the follicle. Thecal tissue derived from healthy antral follicles exhibits marked suppression of steroidogenesis when exposed to high levels of LH whereas exposure over a low range stimulates steroid production. The low midcycle levels of progesterone exert an inhibitory action on further granulosa cell multiplication, and the drop in estrogen may also reflect this local follicular role for progesterone. Finally, estrogen can exert an inhibitory effect on P450c17, a direct action on the gene that is not receptor-mediated.

The granulosa cells attached to the basement membrane enclose the follicle and become luteal cells. The cumulus granulosa cells attach to the oocyte. In the mouse, the cumulus cells are metabolically linked to the oocyte and respond to the FSH surge by secreting hyaluronic acid which disperses the cumulus cells prior to ovulation. This hyaluronic acid response depends upon maintenance of the link with the oocyte, indicating the secretion of a supporting factor. The oocyte further secretes factors that promote granulosa cell proliferation and maintain the structural organization of the follicle.[134] Proliferation of the cumulus cells is suppressed by FSH, while FSH stimulates mural granulosa cell proliferation, supported by the oocyte factor or factors.

The FSH peak, partially and perhaps totally dependent on the preovulatory rise of progesterone, has several functions. Plasminogen activator production is sensitive to FSH as well as LH. Expansion and dispersion of the cumulus cells allows the oocyte-cumulus cell mass to become free-floating in the antral fluid just before follicle rupture. The process involves the deposition of a hyaluronic acid matrix, the synthesis of which is stimulated by FSH. Finally, an adequate FSH peak ensures an adequate complement of LH receptors on the granulosa layer. It should be noted that a shortened or inadequate luteal phase is observed in cycles when FSH levels are low or selectively suppressed at any point during the follicular phase.

The mechanism that shuts off the LH surge is unknown. Within hours after the rise in LH, there is a precipitous drop in the plasma estrogens. The decrease in LH may be due to a loss of the positive stimulating action of estradiol or to an increasing negative feedback of progesterone. The abrupt fall in LH levels may also reflect a depletion in pituitary LH content due to down-regulation of GnRH receptors, either by alterations in GnRH pulse frequency or by changes in steroid levels.[135] Finally, LH may further be controlled by "short" negative feedback of LH upon the hypothalamus. Direct LH suppression of hypothalamic releasing hormone production has been demonstrated. It is likely that a combination of all of these influences contribute to the rapid decline in gonadotropin secretion. The abruptness of the LH surge has also suggested the presence of a surge inhibiting factor.

An adequate gonadotropin surge does not ensure ovulation. The follicle must be at the appropriate stage of maturity in order for it to respond to the ovulating stimulus. In the normal cycle, gonadotropin release and final maturation of the follicle coincide because the timing of the gonadotropin surge is controlled by the level of estradiol, which in turn is a function of follicular growth and maturation. Therefore, gonadotropin release and morphological maturity are usually coordinated and coupled in time. In the majority of human cycles, the requisite feedback relationships in this system allow only one follicle to reach the point of ovulation. Nonidentical multiple births may, in part, reflect the random statistical chance of more than one follicle fulfilling all the requirements for ovulation.

Summary of the Ovulatory Events

1. The LH surge stimulates resumption of reduction division in the oocyte, luteinization of the granulosa, and synthesis of progesterone and prostaglandins within the follicle.

2. Progesterone enhances the activity of proteolytic enzymes responsible, together with prostaglandins, for digestion and rupture of the follicular wall.

3. The progesterone-influenced midcycle rise in FSH serves to free the oocyte from follicular attachments, to convert plasminogen to the proteolytic enzyme, plasmin, and to ensure that sufficient LH receptors are present to allow an adequate normal luteal phase.

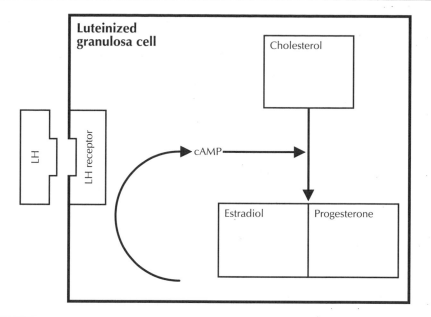

Luteal Phase

Before rupture of the follicle and release of the ovum, the granulosa cells begin to increase in size and assume a characteristic vacuolated appearance associated with the accumulation of a yellow pigment, lutein, which lends its name to the process of luteinization and the anatomical subunit, the corpus luteum. During the first 3 days after ovulation, the granulosa cells continue to enlarge. In addition, theca lutein cells may differentiate from the surrounding theca and stroma to become part of the corpus luteum. Dissolution of the basal lamina and rapid vascularization and luteinization make it difficult to distinguish the origin of specific cells.

Capillaries penetrate into the granulosa layer (under the influence of factors that induce angiogenesis), reach the central cavity, and often fill it with blood. By day 8 or 9 after ovulation, a peak of vascularization is reached, associated with peak levels of progesterone and estradiol in the blood. On occasion, this ingrowth of vessels and bleeding will result in unchecked hemorrhage and an acute surgical emergency which can present at any time during the luteal phase. Indeed, this is a significant clinical risk in women who are anticoagulated; such women should receive medication to prevent ovulation.

Normal luteal function requires optimal preovulatory follicular development. Suppression of FSH during the follicular phase is associated with lower preovulatory estradiol levels, depressed midluteal progesterone production, and a decrease in luteal cell mass.[136] Experimental evidence supports the contention that the accumulation of LH receptors during the follicular phase predetermines the extent of luteinization and the subsequent functional capacity of the corpus luteum. The successful conversion of the avascular granulosa of the follicular phase to the vascularized luteal tissue is also of importance. Because steroid production is dependent upon low-density lipoprotein (LDL) transport of cholesterol, the vascularization of the granulosa layer is essential to allow LDL-cholesterol to reach the luteal cells to provide sufficient substrate for progesterone production. One of the important jobs for LH is to regulate LDL receptor binding, internalization, and postreceptor processing; the induction of LDL receptor expression occurs in granulosa cells during the early stages of luteinization in response to the midcycle LH surge.[137,138] This mechanism supplies cholesterol to the mitochondria for utilization as the basic building block in steroidogenesis.

The lifespan and steroidogenic capacity of the corpus luteum are dependent on continued tonic LH secretion. Studies in hypophysectomized women have demonstrated that normal corpus luteum function requires the continuous presence of small amounts of

LH.[139] The dependence of the corpus luteum on LH is further supported by the prompt luteolysis that follows the administration of GnRH agonists or antagonists or withdrawal of GnRH when ovulation has been induced by the administration of pulsatile GnRH.[140] There is no evidence that other luteotropic hormones, such as prolactin, play a role in primates during the menstrual cycle.[141]

The corpus luteum is not homogeneous. Besides the luteal cells, also present are endothelial cells, macrophages, pericytes, and fibroblasts. But even the luteal cell population is not homogeneous, being composed of at least two distinct cell types, large and small cells. Large luteal cells produce peptides (relaxin and oxytocin) and are more active in steroidogenesis, with greater aromatase activity and more progesterone synthesis than small cells.[142] The small amount of oxytocin in the circulation throughout the menstrual cycle is derived from the pituitary, and the amount in the ovary is so small it is uncertain whether it plays an important role.[143]

Human granulosa cells (already luteinizing when recovered from in vitro fertilization patients) contain minimal amounts of P450c17 mRNA. This is consistent with the two cell explanation which assigns androgen production (and P450c17) to the cells derived from thecal cells. With luteinization, expression of P450scc and 3β-hydroxysteroid dehydrogenase markedly increases as expected, to account for the increasing production of progesterone, and the continued expression of mRNAs for these enzymes requires LH.[144] The aromatase system (P450arom), of course, continues to be active in luteinized granulosa cells.

In monkey studies, small and large luteal cells are stimulated by LH and HCG in the early luteal phase, but by the midluteal phase only the large cells respond.[145] Perhaps small cells become large cells during the lifespan of the corpus luteum, losing steroidogenic capacity as the corpus luteum ages. In the early luteal phase, small cells increase, then after the midluteal phase, the loss of large cells is predominant. This distinction based upon size may have little biologic meaning. Correlations between cellular origin, cellular appearance and size, and functions of steroid hormones and peptide factors remain to be unraveled.

Paraluteal cells are located in the periphery and along invaginations, while true luteal cells occupy the central tissue. Presumably the paraluteal cells are of theca origin and the luteal cells are of granulosa origin, continuing to work in a two cell mechanism, because the paraluteal cells produce androgen, and the luteal cells are more potent in the production of progesterone and estrogen.[146]

Progesterone levels normally rise sharply after ovulation, reaching a peak approximately 8 days after the LH surge. Progesterone acts both locally and centrally to suppress new follicular growth. If progesterone concentrations are monitored in ovarian venous effluents following luteectomy in the monkey, ovulation in the subsequent cycle uniformly occurs on the side opposite the higher progesterone level and contralateral to the previous corpus luteum.[147] If circulating progesterone levels are maintained after luteectomy, the subsequent ovulation again occurs in the ovary having a lower progesterone concentration in its venous effluent.[148] Under normal circumstances (i.e., regular, 28-day cycles), a woman may ovulate from alternate sides.[29,149] However, short-term ultrasonographic studies have failed to substantiate this pattern.

Initiation of new follicular growth during the luteal phase is further inhibited by the low levels of gonadotropins due to the negative feedback actions of estrogen, progesterone, and inhibin. Inhibin levels increase during the luteal phase, originating in the luteinized granulosa cells, and contribute to the achievement of a luteal nadir in FSH secretion.[56,58,150] While some have questioned the bioactivity of the luteal rise in immunoactive inhibin, the correlation of a rise in FSH with a decrease in inhibin after age 30 (while estradiol levels are unchanged) argues in favor of a connection between the cyclic changes in inhibin and FSH secretion. In contrast to inhibin, there is no change in circulating levels of activin during the menstrual cycle, indicating that activin has only autocrine/paracrine activity and no traditional endocrine function.[150]

The secretion of progesterone and estradiol during the luteal phase is episodic, and the changes correlate closely with LH pulses.[42,151] Because of this episodic secretion, relatively low midluteal progesterone levels, which some believe are indicative of an inadequate luteal phase, can be found in the course of totally normal luteal phases.

As noted, with the formation of the corpus luteum, inhibin production shifts from FSH to LH control.[152] Inhibin begins to rise with estradiol in the days before the midcycle LH peak. Despite the fall in estradiol, inhibin continues to rise. Thus inhibin and estradiol secretion by the granulosa are differentially regulated.[153] After the midcycle inhibin peak, inhibin falls to rise again to its highest levels in the miduteal phase. In the follicular phase, the inhibin response is due to FSH, while in the luteal phase, inhibin is regulated by LH.[102] The decrease in inhibin in the late luteal phase contributes to the important rise in FSH for the next cycle. The nadir circulating level of inhibin is reached the day after the onset of menses and is maintained for the first 5 days of the succeeding cycle.[154] The maximal suppression of gonadotropins and GnRH occurs at the midluteal phase when concentrations of estradiol, progesterone, and inhibin are at their highest levels.

In the normal cycle the time period from the LH midcycle surge to menses is consistently close to 14 days. For practical purposes, luteal phases lasting between 11 and 17 days can be considered normal.[155] The incidence of short luteal phases is about 5–6%. It is well known that significant variability in cycle length among women is due to the varying number of days required for follicular growth and maturation in the follicular phase. The luteal phase cannot be extended indefinitely even with progressively increasing LH exposure, indicating that the demise of the corpus luteum is due to an active luteolytic mechanism.

The corpus luteum rapidly declines 9–11 days after ovulation, and the mechanism of the degeneration remains unknown. In certain nonprimate mammalian species, a luteolytic factor originating in the uterus (prostaglandin $F_{2\alpha}$) regulates the lifespan of the corpus luteum. No definite luteolytic factor has been identified in the primate menstrual cycle, and removal of the uterus in the primate does not affect the ovarian cycle; however, the morphological regression of luteal cells may be induced by the estradiol produced by the corpus luteum. There is evidence to support a role for estrogen in the decline of the corpus luteum. The premature elevation of circulating estradiol levels in the early luteal phase results in a prompt fall in progesterone concentrations. Direct injections of estradiol into the ovary bearing the corpus luteum induce luteolysis while similar treatment of the contralateral ovary produces no effect.

An absence of estrogen receptors in luteal tissue[94] argues either against a luteolytic role for estrogen or a receptor-independent mechanism of action. Progesterone receptors are present in luteal tissue, but the formation of progesterone receptors in primate granulosa cells is a response to LH, and not the classic estrogen-receptor mediated mechanism as it operates in the endometrium.[94,110,156]

There is another possible role for the estrogen produced by the corpus luteum. In view of the known estrogen requirement for the synthesis of progesterone receptors in endometrium, luteal phase estrogen may be necessary to allow the progesterone-induced changes in the endometrium after ovulation. Inadequate progesterone receptor content

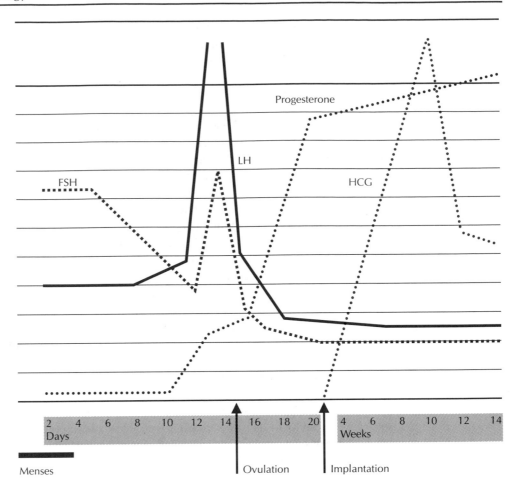

Progesterone

LH

FSH

HCG

| 2 | 4 | 6 | 8 | 10 | 12 | 14 | 16 | 18 | 20 | 4 | 6 | 8 | 10 | 12 | 14 |
Days

Weeks

Menses

Ovulation

Implantation

due to inadequate estrogen priming of the endometrium is an additional possible mechanism for infertility or early abortion, another form of luteal phase deficiency.

Auletta postulated that prostaglandin $F_{2\alpha}$ produced within the ovary bearing the corpus luteum or within the corpus luteum serves as the luteolytic agent, and the production of the prostaglandin is initiated by the luteal estrogen.[157] Experiments using inhibitors of prostaglandin synthesis have not been helpful because luteal tissue also produces members of the prostaglandin family that have stimulating effects (such as PGE and prostacyclin).[158] Also controversial is the contention that local oxytocin or a related peptide plays a role in luteolysis.

When ovulation is induced by the administration of GnRH, normal luteal phase demise occurs despite no change in treatment, arguing against a change in LH as the luteolytic mechanism. In addition, LH receptor binding affinity does not change throughout the luteal phase; thus the decline in steroidogenesis must reflect deactivation of the system (producing a refractoriness of the corpus luteum to LH), perhaps through the uncoupling of the G protein adenylate cyclase system. This is supported by studies in the monkey in which alteration in LH pulse frequency or amplitude did not provoke luteolysis.[159]

Unlike the biphasic pattern demonstrated by the circulating level of progesterone (a decrease after ovulation and then a new higher peak at the midluteal phase), the mRNA levels for the two major enzymes involved in progesterone synthesis (cholesterol side-chain cleavage and 3β-hydroxysteroid dehydrogenase) are maximal at ovulation and decline throughout the luteal phase.[160] This suggests that the lifespan of the corpus luteum is established at the time of ovulation, and luteal regression is inevitable unless the corpus luteum is rescued by the human chorionic gonadotropin (HCG) of pregnancy.

The survival of the corpus luteum is prolonged by the emergence of a new stimulus of rapidly increasing intensity, HCG. This new stimulus first appears at the peak of corpus luteum development (9–13 days after ovulation), just in time to prevent luteal regression.[161] HCG serves to maintain the vital steroidogenesis of the corpus luteum until approximately the 9th or 10th week of gestation, by which time placental steroidogenesis is well established. In some pregnancies placental steroidogenesis will be sufficiently established by the 7th week of gestation.

The decline in steroidogenesis in the late luteal phase of the cycle is accompanied by loss of the highly steroidogenic large cells and by a decline in the ability of the small cells to respond to LH. However, the remaining large cells are responsive to HCG, perhaps providing an important response for the rescue of the corpus luteum in early pregnancy.

Summary of Events in the Luteal Phase

1. Normal luteal function requires optimal preovulatory follicular development (especially adequate FSH stimulation) and continued tonic LH support.

2. Progesterone acts both centrally and within the ovary to suppress new follicular growth.

3. Regression of the corpus luteum may involve the luteolytic action of its own estrogen production, mediated by an alteration in local prostaglandin concentrations.

4. In early pregnancy HCG maintains luteal function until placental steroidogenesis is well established.

The Luteal-Follicular Transition

The interval extending from the late luteal decline of estradiol and progesterone production to the selection of the dominant follicle is a critical and decisive time, marked by the appearance of menses, but less apparent and very important are the hormone changes that initiate the next cycle. The critical factors include GnRH, FSH, LH, estradiol, progesterone, and inhibin.

Given the important role for FSH-mediated actions on the granulosa cells, it is appropriate that the changes are directed to a selective increase in FSH which begins approximately 2 days before the onset of menses.[154,162,163] There are at least two influential changes that result in this important increase in FSH: a decrease in luteal steroids and inhibin and a change in GnRH pulsatile secretion.

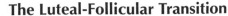

The Luteal-Follicular Transition

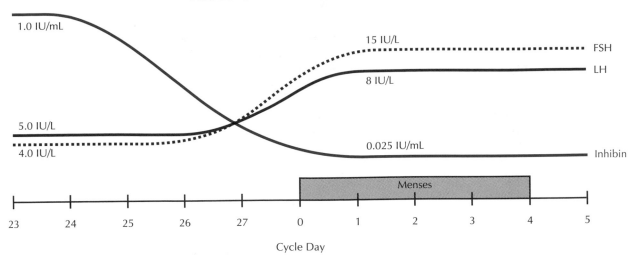

Inhibin, originating in the granulosa cells of the corpus luteum and now under the regulation of LH, peaks in the circulation at the midluteal period, and thus helps to suppress FSH secretion by the pituitary to the lowest levels reached during a menstrual cycle. The process of luteolysis, whatever the mechanism, with the resulting demise of the corpus luteum, affects inhibin secretion as well as steroidogenesis. Inhibin levels decline, reach their nadir on the first day of menses, and remain at this low level during the first 5 days of the cycle when FSH is essential for the growth of the emerging follicles.[154] Thus, an important suppressing influence on FSH secretion is removed from the anterior pituitary during the last days of the luteal phase. The selective action of inhibin on FSH (and not LH) is partly responsible for the greater rise in FSH seen during the luteal-follicular transition, compared to the change in LH. The administration of recombinant (pure) FSH to gonadotropin-deficient women has demonstrated that the early growth of follicles requires FSH, and that LH is not essential during this period of the cycle.[25,26]

The selective rise in FSH is also significantly influenced by a change in GnRH pulsatile secretion, previously strongly suppressed by the high estradiol and progesterone levels of the luteal phase.[46] A progressive and rapid increase in GnRH pulses (as assessed by the measurement of LH pulses) occurs during the luteal-follicular transition.[45] From the midluteal peak to menses, there is a 4.5-fold increase in LH pulse frequency (and presumably GnRH) from approximately 3 pulses/24 hours to 14 pulses/24 hours.[45] During this time period, the mean level of LH increases approximately 2-fold, from approximately a mean of 4.8 IU/L to 8 IU/L. The increase in FSH is, as noted, greater than that of LH. The pulse frequency increases 3.5-fold from the midluteal period to the time of menses, and FSH levels increase from a mean of approximately 4 IU/L to 15 IU/L.

An increase in GnRH pulse frequency from a low level of secretion has been associated with an initial selective increase in FSH in several experimental models, including the ovariectomized monkey with destruction of the hypothalamus. Treatment of hypogonadal women with pulsatile GnRH results first in predominance of FSH secretion (over LH). This experimental response and the changes during the luteal-follicular transition are similar to that observed during puberty, a predominance of FSH secretion as GnRH pulsatile secretion begins to increase.

The pituitary response to GnRH is also a factor. Estradiol suppresses FSH secretion by virtue of its classic negative feedback relationship at the pituitary level. The decrease in estradiol in the late luteal phase restores the capability of the pituitary to respond with an increase in FSH secretion.[164]

Summary of Events in the Luteal-Follicular Transition

1. The demise of the corpus luteum results in a nadir in the circulating levels of estradiol, progesterone, and inhibin.

2. The decrease in inhibin removes a suppressing influence on FSH secretion in the pituitary.

3. The decrease in estradiol and progesterone allows a progressive and rapid increase in the frequency of GnRH pulsatile secretion and a removal of the pituitary from negative feedback suppression.

4. The removal of inhibin and estradiol and increasing GnRH pulses combine to allow greater secretion of FSH compared to LH, with an increase in the frequency of the episodic secretion.

5. The increase in FSH is instrumental in rescuing a group of follicles from atresia, allowing a dominant follicle to begin its emergence.

The Normal Menstrual Cycle

Menstrual cycle length is determined by the rate and quality of follicular growth and development, and it is normal for the cycle to vary in individual women. Our best information comes from two longitudinal studies (with very similar results): the study of Vollman of more than 30,000 cycles recorded by 650 women and the study of Treloar of more that 25,000 woman-years in a little over 2,700 women.[165,166] The observations of Vollman and Treloar documented a normal evolution in length and variation in menstrual cycles.

Menarche is followed by approximately 5–7 years of increasing regularity as cycles shorten to reach the usual reproductive age pattern. In the 40s, cycles begin to lengthen again. The highest incidence of anovulatory cycles is under age 20 and over age 40.[165,167] At age 25, over 40% of cycles are between 25 and 28 days in length; from 25 to 35, over 60% are between 25 and 28 days. The perfect 28 day cycle is indeed the most common mode, but it totaled only 12.4% of Vollman's cycles. Overall, approximately 15% of reproductive age cycles are 28 days in length. Only 0.5% of women experience a cycle less than 21 days long, and only 0.9% a cycle greater than 35 days.[168] Most women have cycles that last from 24 to 35 days, but at least 20% of women experience irregular cycles.

The duration of the follicular phase is the major determinant of cycle length. Sherman and Korenman predicted in 1975 that a factor other than estrogen is the key — inhibin.[169] Cycle lengths are the shortest (with the least variability) in the late 30s, a time when subtle but real increases in FSH and decreases in inhibin are occurring.[170–172] This can be pictured as accelerated follicular growth (because of the changes in FSH and inhibin). At the same time, fewer follicles grow per cycle as a woman ages.[173] Approximately 2–4 years (6–8 years according to Trelolar) prior to menopause, the cycles lengthen again. Eventually menopause occurs because the supply of follicles is depleted.[174]

Women who present with "incipient" ovarian failure have elevated FSH levels and decreased levels of inhibin but normal levels of estradiol.[175] This indicates that inhibin levels are regulated independently of estradiol, and that inhibin is a more sensitive marker of ovarian follicular competence. The changes in the later reproductive years reflect lesser follicular competence as the better primordial follicles respond early in life,

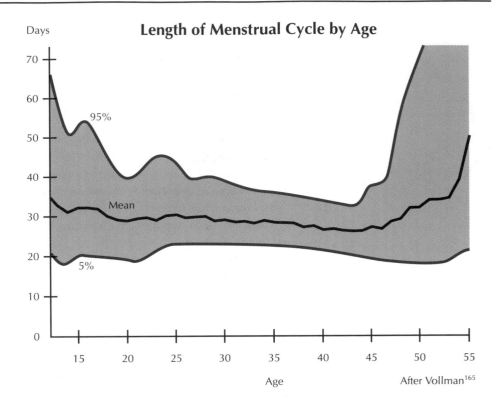

Days

Length of Menstrual Cycle by Age

Age

After Vollman[165]

leaving the lesser follicles for later. This is reflected in the decrease in fecundability that occurs with aging.

The rise in FSH during the later years is believed to represent declining inhibin production by the less competent ovarian follicles.[153] Inhibin levels are lower in the follicular phase in women 45–49 years old compared to younger women.[153] This decline begins early but accelerates after 40 years of age. The rise in FSH is not apparent until age 40, and there is no change in LH levels until menopause. The inability to suppress gonadotropins to a normal range during estrogen treatment of postmenopausal women reflects this loss of inhibin.

Despite these changes in the menstrual cycle that occur with aging, ovulation can still occur, and although luteal progesterone levels are lower, conception can still occur.[176]

References

1. **Baker TG,** A quantitative and cytological study of germ cells in the human ovaries, Proc R Soc London 158:417, 1963.

2. **Peters H, Byskov AG, Himelstein-Graw R, Faber M,** Follicular growth: the basic event in the mouse and human ovary, J Reprod Fertil 45:559, 1975.

3. **Mais V, Kazer RR, Cetel NS, Rivier J, Vale W, Yen SSC,** The dependency of folliculogenesis and corpus luteum function on pulsatile gonadotropin secretion in cycling women using a gonadotropin-releasing hormone antagonist as a probe, J Clin Endocrinol Metab 62:1250, 1986.

4. **Gougeon A,** Dynamics of follicular growth in the human: a model from preliminary results, Hum Reprod 1:81, 1986.

5. **Halpin DMG, Jones A, Fink G, Charlton HM,** Postnatal ovarian follicle development in hypogonadal (hpg) and normal mice and associated changes in the hypothalamic-pituitary axis, J Reprod Fertil 77:287, 1986.

6. **Vermesh M, Kletzky OA,** Longitudinal evaluation of the luteal phase and its transition into the follicular phase, J Clin Endocrinol Metab 65:653, 1987.

7. **Yong EL, Baird DT, Hillier SG,** Mediation of gonadotropin-stimulated growth and differentiation of human granulosa cells by adenosine-3',5'-monophosphate: one molecule, two messages, Clin Endocrinol 37:51, 1992.

8. **McNatty KP, Makris A, DeGrazia C, Osathanondh R, Ryan KJ,** The production of progesterone, androgens, and estrogens by granulosa cells, thecal tissue, and stromal tissue from human ovaries in vitro, J Clin Endocrinol Metab 49:687, 1979.

9. **LaPolt PS, Tilly JL, Aihara T, Nishimori K, Hsueh AJ,** Gonadotropin-induced up- and downregulation of ovarian follicle-stimulating hormone (FSH) receptor gene expression in immature rats: effects of pregnant mare's serum gonadotropin, human chorionic gonadotropin, and recombinant FSH, Endocrinology 130:1289, 1992.

10. **Tilly JL, LaPolt PS, Hsueh AJ,** Hormonal regulation of follicle-stimulating hormone receptor messenger ribonucleic acid levels in cultured rat granulosa cells, Endocrinology 130:1296, 1992.

11. **Erickson GF,** An analysis of follicle development and ovum maturation, Seminars Reprod Endocrinol 4:233, 1986.

12. **Fletcher WH, Greenan JRT,** Receptor mediated action without receptor occupancy, Endocrinology 116:1660, 1985.

13. **Hild-Petito S, West NB, Brenner RM, Stouffer RL,** Localization of androgen receptor in the follicle and corpus luteum of the primate ovary during the menstrual cycle, Biol Reprod 44:561, 1991.

14. **McNatty KP, Makris A, Reinhold VN, DeGrazia C, Osathanondh R, Ryan KJ,** Metabolism of androstenedione by human ovarian tissues in vitro with particular reference to reductase and aromatase activity, Steroids 34:429, 1979.

15. **Hillier SG, Van Den Boogard AMJ, Reichert LE, Van Hall EV,** Intraovarian sex steroid hormone interactions and the regulation of follicular maturation: aromatization of androgens by human granulosa cells in vitro, J Clin Endocrinol Metab 50:640, 1980.

16. **Jia XC, Kessel B, Welsh TH Jr, Hsueh AJW,** Androgen inhibition of follicle-stimulating hormone-stimulated luteinizing hormone receptor formation in cultured rat granulosa cells, Endocrinology 117:13, 1985.

17. **Erickson GF, Magoffin DA, Dyer CA, Hofeditz C,** The ovarian androgen producing cells: a review of structure/function relationships, Endocr Rev 6:371, 1985.

18. **Chabab A, Hedon B, Arnal F, Diafouka F, Bressot N, Flandre O, Cristol P,** Follicular steroids in relation to oocyte development and human ovarian stimulation protocols, Hum Reprod 1:449, 1986.

19. **McNatty KP, Smith DM, Makris A, Osathanondh R, Ryan KJ,** The microenvironment of the human antral follicle; inter-relationships among the steroid levels in antral fluid, the population of granulosa cells, and the status of the oocyte in vivo and in vitro, J Clin Endocrinol Metab 49:851, 1979.

20. **McNatty KP, Markris A, DeGrazia C, Osathanondh R, Ryan KJ,** Steroidogenesis by recombined follicular cells from the human ovary in vitro, J Clin Endocrinol Metab 51:1286, 1980.

21. **Hillier SG,** Paracrine control of follicular estrogen synthesis, Seminars Reprod Endocrinol 9:332, 1991.

22. **Kobayashi M, Nakano R, Ooshima A,** Immunohistochemical localization of pituitary gonadotropins and gonadal steroids confirms the two cells two gonadotropins hypothesis of steroidogenesis in the human ovary, J Endocrinol 126:483, 1990.

23. **Yamoto M, Shima K, Nakano R,** Gonadotropin receptors in human ovarian follicles and corpora lutea throughout the menstrual cycle, Horm Res 37(Suppl 1):5, 1992.

24. **Magoffin DA,** Regulation of differentiated functions in ovarian theca cells, Seminars Reprod Endocrinol 9:321, 1991.

25. **Schoot DC, Coelingh-Bennink HJT, Mannaerts BMJL, Lamberts SWJ, Bouchard P, Fauser BCJM,** Human recombinant follicle-stimulating homrone induces growth of preovulatory follicles without concomitant increase in androgen and estrogen biosynthesis in a woman with isolated gonadotropin deficiency, J Clin Endocrinol Metab 74:1471, 1992.

26. **Shoham Z, Mannaerts B, Insler V, Coelingh-Bennink H,** Induction of follicular growth using recombinant human follicle-stimulating hormone in two volunteer women with hypogonadotropic hypogonadism, Fertil Steril 59:738, 1993.

27. **Zeliniski-Wooten MB, Hutchison JS, Hess DL, Wolf DP, Stouffer RL,** Luteinizing hormone (LH) is not necessary for follicle growth and oocyte development in Rhesus monkeys, Abstract, Annual Meeting, American Fertility Society, 1993.

28. **Tilly JL, Kowalski KI, Schomberg DW, Hsueh AJ,** Apoptosis in atretic ovarian follicles is associated with selective decreases in messenger ribonucleic acid transcripts for gonadotropin receptors and cytochrome P450 aromatase, Endocrinology 131:1670, 1992.

29. **Chikasawa K, Araki S, Tameda T,** Morphological and endocrinological studies on follicular development during the human menstrual cycle, J Clin Endocrinol Metab 62:305, 1986.

30. **Clark JR, Dierschke DJ, Wolf RC,** Hormonal regulation of ovarian folliculogenesis in rhesus monkeys: III. Atresia of the preovulatory follicle induced by exogenous steroids and subsequent follicular development, Biol Reprod 25:332, 1981.

31. **Zeleznik AJ, Schuler HM, Reichert LE,** Gonadotropin-binding sites in the rhesus monkey ovary: role of the vasculature in the selective distribution of human chorionic gonadotropin to the preovulatory follicle, Endocrinology 109:356, 1981.

32. **Ravindranath N, Little-Ihrig L, Phillips HS, Ferrara N, Zeleznik AJ,** Vascular endothelial growth factor messenger ribonucleic acid expression in the primate ovary, Endocrinology 131:254, 1992.

33. **Richards JS, Jahnsen T, Hedin L, Lifka J, Ratoosh SL, Durica JM, Goldring NB,** Ovarian follicular development: from physiology to molecular biology, Recent Prog Horm Res 43:231, 1987.

34. **Jia XC, Hsueh AJW,** Homologous regulation of hormone receptors: luteinizing hormone increases its own receptors in cultured rat granulosa cells, Endocrinology 115:2433, 1984.

35. **Kessel B, Liu YX, Jia XC, Hsueh AJW,** Autocrine role of estrogens in the augmentation of luteinizing hormone receptor formation in cultured rat granulosa cells, Biol Reprod 32:1038, 1985.

36. **Knecht M, Brodie AMH, Catt KJ,** Aromatase inhibitors prevent granulosa cell differentiation: an obligatory role for estrogens in luteinizing hormone receptor expression, Endocrinology 117:1156, 1985.

37. **Adams TE, Norman RL, Spies HG,** Gonadotropin-releasing hormone receptor binding and pituitary responsiveness in estradiol-primed monkeys, Science 213:1388, 1981.

38. **Xia L, Van Vugt DL, Alston EJ, Luckhaus J, Ferin M,** A surge of gonadotropin-releasing hormone accompanies the estradiol-induced gonadotropin surge in the Rhesus monkey, Endocrinology 131:2812, 1992.

39. **Chappel SC, Resko JA, Norman RL, Spies HG,** Studies on Rhesus monkeys on the site where estrogen inhibits gonadotropins: delivery of 17-estradiol to the hypothalamus and pituitary gland, J Clin Endocrinol Metab 52:1, 1981.

40. **Wildt L, Hutchinson JS, Marshall G, Pohl CR, Knobil E,** On the site of action of progesterone in the blockade of the estradiol-induced gonadotropin discharge in the rhesus monkey, Endocrinology 109:1293, 1981.

41. **Young JR, Jaffe RB,** Strength-duration characteristics of estrogen effects on gonadotropin response to gonadotropin-releasing hormone in women: II. Effects of varying concentrations of estradiol, J Clin Endocrinol Metab 42:432, 1976.

42. **Filicori M, Santoro N, Merriam GR, Crowley WF Jr,** Characterization of the physiological pattern of episodic gonadotropin secretion throughout the human menstrual cycle, J Clin Endocrinol Metab 62:1136, 1986.

43. **Rossmanith WG, Laughlin GA, Mortola JF, Johnson ML, Veldhuis JD, Yen SSC,** Pulsatile cosecretion of estradiol and progesterone by the midluteal phase corpus luteum: temporal link to luteinizing hormone pulses, J Clin Endocrinol Metab 70:990, 1990.

44. **Evans WS, Sollenberger MJ, Booth RA Jr, Rogol AD, Urban RJ, Carlsen EC, Johnson ML, Veldhuis JD,** Contemporary aspects of discrete peak-detection algorithms. II. The paradigm of the luteinizing hormone pulse signal in women, Endocr Rev 13:81, 1992.

45. **Hall JE, Schoenfeld DA, Martin KA, Crowley WF Jr,** Hypothalamic gonadotropin-releasing hormone secretion and follicle-stimulating hormone dynamics during the luteal-follicular transition, J Clin Endocrinol Metab 74:600, 1992.

46. **Nippold TB, Reame NE, Kelch RP, Marshall JC,** The roles of estradiol and progesterone in decreasing luteinizing hormone pulse frequency in the luteal phase of the menstrual cycle, J Clin Endocrinol Metab 69:67, 1989.

47. **Maruncic M, Casper RF,** The effect of luteal phase estrogen antagonism on luteinizing hormone pulsatility and luteal function in women, J Clin Endocrinol Metab 64:148, 1987.

48. **Laatikainen T, Raisanen I, Tulenheimo A, Salminen K,** Plasma β-endorphin and the menstrual cycle, Fertil Steril 44:206, 1985.

49. **Wehrenberg WB, Wardlaw SL, Frantz AG, Ferin M,** β-Endorphin in hypophyseal portal blood: variations throughout the menstrual cycle, Endocrinology 111:879, 1982.

50. **Urban RJ, Veldhuis JD, Dufau ML,** Estrogen regulates the gonadotropin-releasing hormone-stimulated secretion of biologically active luteinizing hormone, J Clin Endocrinol Metab 72:660, 1991.

51. **Mortola JF, Laughlin GA, Yen SSC,** A circadian rhythm of serum follicle-stimulating hormone in women, J Clin Endocrinol Metab 75:861, 1992.

52. **Rivier C, Rivier J, Vale W,** Inhibin-mediated feedback control of follicle-stimulating hormone secretion in the female rat, Science 234:205, 1986.

53. **Bicsak TA, Tucker EM, Cappel S, Vaughan J, Rivier J, Vale W, Hsueh AJW,** Hormonal regulation of granulosa cell inhibin biosynthesis, Endocrinology 119:2711, 1986.

54. **Xiao S, Robertson DM, Findlay JK,** Effects of activin and follicle-stimulating hormone (FSH)-suppressing protein/follistatin on FSH receptors and differentiation of cultured rat granulosa cells, Endocrinology 131:1009, 1992.

55. **Matzuk MM, Finegold MJ, Su J-GJ, Hsueh AJW, Bradley A,** α-Inhibin is a tumour-suppressor gene with gonadal specificity in mice, Nature 360:313, 1992.

56. **McLachlan RI, Robertson DM, Healy DL, Burger HG, De Kretser DM,** Circulating immunoreactive inhibin levels during the normal human menstrual cycle, J Clin Endocrinol Metab 65:954, 1987.

57. **Buckler HM, Healy DL, Burger HG,** Purified FSH stimulates inhibin production from the human ovary, J Endocrinol 122:279, 1989.

58. **Lenton EA, de Kretser DM, Woodward AJ, Robertson DM,** Inhibin concentrations throughout the menstrual cycles of normal, infertile, and older women compared with those during spontaneous conception cycles, J Clin Endocrinol Metab 73:1180, 1991.

59. **Farnworth PG, Wang Q-F, Findlay JK, Robertson DM, De Kretser DM, Burger HG,** The mechanism of action of inhibin, in Melmed S, Robbins, RJ, editors, *Molecular and Clinical Advances in Pituitary Disosrders,* Blackwell Scientific Publications, Boston, 1991, pp 129-139.

60. **Ling N, Ying S, Ueno N, Shimasaki S, Esch F, Hotta M, Guillemin R,** Pituitary FSH is released by a heterodimer of the β-subunits from the two forms of inhibin, Nature 321:779, 1986.

61. **Braden TD, Conn PM,** Activin-A stimulates the synthesis of gonadotropin-releasing hormone receptors, Endocrinology 130:2101, 1992.

62. **Mason AJ, Hayflick JS, Ling N, Esch F, Ueno N, Ying SY, Guillemin R, Niall H, Seeburg PH,** Complementary DNA sequences of ovarian follicular fluid inhibin show precursor structure and homology with transforming growth factor-β, Nature 318:659, 1985.

63. **Attisano L, Wrana JL, Cheifetz S, Massague J,** Novel activin receptors: distinct genes and alternative mRNA splicing generate a repertoire of serine/threonine kinase receptors, Cell 68:97, 1992.

64. **Braden TD, Conn PM,** Activin-A stimulates the synthesis of gonadotropin-releasing hormone receptors, Endocrinology 130:2101, 1992.

65. **Bilezikjian LM, Vale WW,** Local extragonadal roles of activins, Trends Endocrinol Metab 3:218, 1992.

66. **Robertson DM,** Follistatin/activin-binding protein, Trends Endocrinol Metab 3:65, 1992.

67. **Giudice LC,** Insulin-like growth factors and ovarian follicular development, Endocr Rev 13:641, 1992.

68. **Shimasaki S, Ling N,** Identification and molecular characterization of insulin-like growth factor binding proteins (IGFBP-1, -2, -3, -4, -5, and -6), Prog Growth Factor Res 3:243, 1992.

69. **Hernandez ER, Hurwitz A, Vera A, Pellicer A, Adashi EY, LeRoith D, Roberts CT Jr,** Expression of the genes encoding the insulin-like growth factors and their receptors in the human ovary, J Clin Endocrinol Metab 74:419, 1992.

70. **Bergh C, Carlsson B, Olsson J-H, Selleskog U, Hillensjo T,** Regulation of androgen production in cultured human thecal cells by insulin-like growth factor I and insulin, Fertil Steril 59:323, 1993.

71. **Barreca A, Artini PG, Del Monte P, Ponzani P, Pasquini P, Cariola G, Volpe A, Genazzani AR, Giordano G, Minuto F,** In vivo and in vitro effect of growth hormone on estradiol secretion by human granulosa cells, J Clin Endocrinol Metab 77:61, 1993.

72. **Erickson GF, Magoffin DA, Cragun JR, Chang RJ,** The effects of insulin and insulin-like growth factors-I and -II on estradiol production by granulosa cells of polycystic ovaries, J Clin Endocrinol Metab 70:894, 1990.

73. **Ricciarelli E, Hernandez ER, Tedeschi C, Botero LF, Kokia E, Rohan RM, Rosenfeld RG, Albiston AL, Herington AC, Adashi EY,** Rat ovarian insulin-like growth factor binding protein-3: a growth hormone-dependent theca-interstitial cell-derived antigonadotropin, Endocrinology 130:3092, 1992.

74. **Adashi EY, Resnick CE, Hurwitz A, Riciarelli E, Hernandez ER, Rosenfeld RG,** Ovarian granulosa cell-derived insulin-like growth factor binding proteins: modulatory role of follicle-stimulating hormone, Endocrinology 128:754, 1991.

75. **Grimes RW, Samaras SE, Barber JA, Shimasaki S, Ling N, Hammond JM,** Gonadotropin and cyclic-AMP modulation of insulin-like growth factor-binding protein production in ovarian granulosa cells, Am J Physiol 262:E497, 1992.

76. **Dor J, Costritsci N, Pariente C, Rabinovici J, Mashiach S, Lunenfeld B, Kaneti H, Seppala M, Roistinen R, Karasik A,** Insulin-like growth factor-I and follicle-stimulating hormone suppress insulin-like growth factor binding protein-1 secretion by human granulosa-luteal cells, J Clin Endocrinol Metab 75:969, 1992.

77. **El-Roeiy A, Roberts VJ, Shimasaki S, Ling N, Yen SSC,** Localization and expression of insulin-like growth factor binding proteins (IGFBP's) 1-6 in normal and polycystic (PCO) human ovaries, Abstract, Annual Meeting, American Fertility Society, 1992.

78. **San Roman GA, Magoffin DA,** Insulin-like growth factor-binding proteins in healthy and atretic follicles during natural menstrual cycles, J Clin Endocrinol Metab 76:625, 1992.

79. **Cataldo NA, Giudice LC,** Follicular fluid insulin-like growth factor binding protein profiles in polycystic ovary syndrome, J Clin Endocrinol Metab 74:695, 1992.

80. **Cataldo NA, Giudice LC,** Insulin-like growth factor binding protein profiles in human ovarian follicular fluid correlate with follicular functional status, J Clin Endocrinol Metab 74:821, 1992.

81. **Michels KM, Lee W-H, Seltzer A, Saavedra JM, Bondy CA,** Up-regulation of pituitary [^{125}I]insulin-like growth factor-I (IGF-I) binding and IGF binding protein-2 and IGF-I gene expression by estrogen, Endocrinology 132:23, 1993.

82. **Dor J, Ben-Shlomo I, Lunenfeld B, Pariente C, Levran D, Karasik A, Seppala M, Mashiach S,** Insulin-like growth factor-I (IGF-I) may not be essential for ovarian follicular development: evidence from IGF-I deficiency, J Clin Endocrinol Metab 74:539, 1992.

83. **El-Roeiy A, Chen X, Roberts VJ, LeRoith D, Roberts CT Jr, Yen SSC,** Expression of insulin-like growth factor-I (IGF-I) and IGF-II and the IGF-I, IGF-II, and insulin receptor genes and localization of the gene products in the human ovary, J Clin Endocrinol Metab 77:1411, 1993.

84. **Dodson WC, Schomberg DW,** The effect of transforming growth factor-β on follicle-stimulating hormone-induced differentiation of cultured rat granulosa cells, Endocrinology 120:512, 1987.

85. **Hernandez ER, Hurwitz A, Payne DW, Dharmarajan AM, Purchio AF, Adashi EY,** Transforming growth factor-beta 1 inhibits ovarian androgen production: gene expression, cellular localization, mechanisms(s), and site(s) of action, Endocrinology 127:2804, 1990.

86. **Oury F, Faucher C, Rives I, Bensaid M, Bouche G, Darbon J-M,** Regulation of cyclic adenosine 3',5'-monophosphate-dependent protein kinase activity and regulatory subunit RIIB content by basic fibroblast growth factor (bFGF) during granulosa cell differentiation: possible implication of protein kinase C in bFGF action, Biol Reprod 47:202, 1992.

87. **Frederick JL, Shimanuki T, diZerega GS,** Initiation of angiogenesis by human follicular fluid, Science 224:389, 1984.

88. **Kokia E, Hurwitz A, Ricciarelli E, Tedeschi C, Resnick CE, Mitchell MD, Adashi EY,** Interleukin-1 stimulates ovarian prostaglandin biosynthesis: evidence for heterologous contact-independent cell-cell interaction, Endocrinology 130:3095, 1992.

89. **Itskovitz J, Sealey JE,** Ovarian renin-renin-angiotensin system, Obstet Gynecol Survey 42:545, 1987.

90. **Petraglia F, Di Meo G, Storchi R, Segre A, Facchinetti F, Szalay S, Volpe A, Genazzani AR,** Proopiomelanocortin-related peptides and methionine enkephalin in human follicular fluid: changes during the menstrual cycle, Am J Obstet Gynecol 157:142, 1987.

91. **Kim JH, Seibel MM, MacLaughlin DT, Donahoe PK, Ransil BJ, Hametz PA, Richards CJ,** The inhibitory effects of müllerian-inhibiting substance on epidermal growth factor induced proliferation and progesterone production of human granulosa-luteal cells, J Clin Endocrinol Metab 75:911, 1992.

92. **Seifer DB, MacLaughlin DT, Penzias AS, Behrman HR, Asmundson L, Donahoe PK, Haning RV Jr, Flynn SD,** Gonadotropin-releasing hormone agonist-induced differences in granulosa cell cycle kinetics are associated with alterations in follicular fluid Müllerian-inhibiting substance and androgen content, J Clin Endocrinol Metab 76:711, 1993.

93. **Tedeschi C, Hazum E, Kokia E, Ricciarelli E, Adashi EY, Payne DW,** Endothelin-1 as a luteinization inhibitor: inhibition of rat granulosa cell progesterone accumulation via selective modulation of key steroidogenic steps affecting both progesterone formation and degradation, Endocrinology 131:2476, 1992.

94. **Hild-Petito S, Stouffer RL, Brenner RM,** Immunocytochemical localization of estradiol and progesterone receptors in the monkey ovary throughout the menstrual cycle, Endocrinology 123:2896, 1988.

95. **Wu T-CJ, Wang L, Wan Y-JY,** Detection of estrogen receptor messenger ribonucleic acid in human oocytes and cumulus-oocyte complexes using reverse transcriptase-polymerase chain reaction, Fertil Steril 59:54, 1993.

96. **Zelinski-Wooten, MB, Hess DL, Baughman WL, Molskness TA, Wolf DP, Stouffer RL,** Adminstration of an aromatase inhibitor during the late follicular phase of gonadotropin-treated cycles in Rhesus monkeys: effects on follicle development, oocyte maturational, and subsequent luteal function, J Clin Endocrinol Metab 76:988, 1993.

97. **Hillier SG, Yong EL, Illingworth PJ, Baird DT, Schwall RH, Mason AJ,** Effect of recombinant activin on androgen synthesis in cultured human thecal cells, J Clin Endocrinol Metab 72:1206, 1991.

98. **Hillier SG, Yong EL, Illingworth PJ, Baird DT, Schwall RH, Mason AJ,** Effect of recombinant inhibin on androgen synthesis in cultured human thecal cells, Mol Cell Endocrinol 75:R1, 1991.

99. **Miro F, Hillier SG,** Relative effects of activin and inhibin on steroid hormone synthesis in primate granulosa cells, J Clin Endocrinol Metab 75:1556, 1992.

100. **Rabinovici J, Spencer SJ, Doldi N, Goldsmith PC, Schwall R, Jaffe RB,** Activin-A as an intraovarian modulator: actions, localization and regulation of the intact dimer in human ovarian cells, J Clin Invest 89:1528, 1992.

101. **Hillier SG, Wickings EJ, Illingworth PI, et al,** Control of immunoactive inhibin production by human granulosa cells, Clin Endocrinol 35:71, 1991.

102. **Brannian JD, Stouffer RL, Molskness TA, Chandrasekher YA, Sarkissian A, Dahl KD,** Inhibin production by Macaque granulosa cells from pre- and periovulatory follicles: regulation by gonadotropins and prostaglandin E$_2$, Biol Reprod 46:451, 1992.

103. **Billiar RB, Loukides JA, Miller MM,** Evidence for the presence of the estrogen receptor in the ovary of the baboon (Papio anubis), J Clin Endocrinol Metab 75:1159, 1992.

104. **Pellicer A, Miro F, Sampaio M, Gomez E, Bonilla-Maroles FM,** In vitro fertilization as a diagnostic and therapeutic tool in a patient with parital 17,20-desmolase deficiency, Fertil Steril 55:970, 1991.

105. **Rabinovici J, Blankstein J, Goldman B, Rudak E, Dor Y, Pariente C, Geier A, Lunenfeld B, Mashiach S,** In vitro fertilization and primary embryonic cleavage are possible in 17α-hydroxylase deficiency despite extremely low intrafollicular 17β-estradiol, J Clin Endocrinol Metab 68:693, 1989.

106. **Pauerstein CJ, Eddy CA, Croxatto HD, Hess R, Siler-Khodr TM, Croxatto HB,** Temporal relationships of estrogen, progesterone, and luteinizing hormone levels to ovulation in women and infrahuman primates, Am J Obstet Gynecol 130:876, 1978.

107. **Fritz MA, McLachlan RI, Cohen NL, Dahl KD, Bremner WJ, Soules MR,** Onset and characteristics of the midcycle surge in bioactive and immunoactive luteinizing hormone secretion in normal women: influence of physiological variations in periovulatory ovarian steroid hormone secretion, J Clin Endocrinol Metab 75:489, 1992.

108. **Yong EL, Baird DT, Yates R, Reichert LE Jr, Hillier SG,** Hormonal regulation of the growth and steroidogenic function of human granulosa cells, J Clin Endocrinol Metab 74:842, 1992.

109. **Judd S, Terry A, Petrucco M, White G,** The source of pulsatile secretion of progesterone during the human follicular phase, J Clin Endocrinol Metab 74:299, 1992.

110. **Aladin Chandrasekher Y, Brenner RM, Molskness TA, Yu Q, Stouffer RL,** Titrating luteinizing hormone surge requirements for ovulatory changes in primate follicles. II. Progesterone receptor expression in luteinizing granulosa cells, J Clin Endocrinol Metab 73:584, 1991.

111. **Chaffkin LM, Luciano AA, Peluso JJ,** Progesterone as an autocrine/paracrine regulator of human granulosa cell proliferation, J Clin Endocrinol Metab 75:1404, 1992.

112. **Collins RL, Hodgen GD,** Blockade of the spontaneous midcycle gonadotropin surge in monkeys by RU 486: a progesterone antagonist or agonist? J Clin Endocrinol Metab 63:1270, 1986.

113. **Couzinet B, Brailly S, Bouchard P, Schaison G,** Progesterone stimulates luteinizing hormone secretion by acting directly on the pituitary, J Clin Endocrinol Metab 74:374, 1992.

114. **Liu JH, Yen SSC,** Induction of midcycle gonadotropin surge by ovarian steroids in women: a critical evaluation, J Clin Endocrinol Metab 57:797, 1983.

115. **Judd LH, Yen SSC,** Serum androstenedione and testosterone levels during the menstrual cycle, J Clin Endocrinol Metab 38:475, 1973.

116. **Adams DB, Gold AR,** Rise in female-initiated sexual activity at ovulation and its suppression by oral contraceptives, New Engl J Med 229:1145, 1978.

117. **Hedricks C, Piccinino LJ, Udry JR, Chimbira THK,** Peak coital rate coincides with onset of luteinizing hormone surge, Fertil Steril 48:234, 1987.

118. **World Health Organization Task Force Investigators,** Temporal relationships between ovulation and defined changes in the concentration of plasma estradiol-17β, luteinizing hormone, follicle stimulating hormone, and progesterone, Am J Obstet Gynecol 138:383, 1980.

119. **Hoff JD, Quigley ME, Yen SSC,** Hormonal dynamics at midcycle: a reevaluation, J Clin Endocrinol Metab 57:792, 1983.

120. **Zelinski-Wooten MB, Hutchison JS, Chandrasekher YA, Wolf DP, Stouffer RL,** Administration of human luteinizing hormone (hLH) to Macaques after follicular development: further titration of LH surge requirements for ovulatory changes in primate follicles, J Clin Endocrinol Metab 75:502, 1992.

121. **Testart J, Frydman R, Roger M,** Seasonal influence of diurnal rhythms in the onset of the plasma luteinizing hormone surge in women, J Clin Endocrinol Metab 55:374, 1982.

122. **Yoshimura Y, Wallach EE,** Studies on the mechanism(s) of mammalian ovulation, Fertil Steril 47:22, 1987.

123. **Brannian JD, Woodruff TK, Mather JP, Stouffer RL,** Activin-A inhibits progesterone production by Macaque luteal cells in culture, J Clin Endocrinol Metab 75:756, 1992.

124. **Li W, Ho Yuen B, Leung PCK,** Inhibition of progestin accumulation by activin-A in human granulosa cells, J Clin Endocrinol Metab 75:285, 1992.

125. **Yoshimura Y, Santulli R, Atlas SJ, Fujii S, Wallach EE,** The effects of proteolytic enzymes on in vitro ovulation in the rabbit, Am J Obstet Gynecol 157:468, 1987.

126. **Peng X-R, Leonardsson G, Ohlsson M, Hsueh AJW, Ny T,** Gonadotropin induced transient and cell-specific expression of tissue-type plasminogen activator and plasminogen activator inhibitor type 1 leads to a controlled and directed proteolysis during ovulation, Fibrinolysis 6, Suppl4:151, 1992.

127. **Jones PBC, Vernon MW, Muse KN, Curry TE,** Plasminogen activator inhibitor in human preovulatory follicular fluid, J Clin Endocrinol Metab 68:1039, 1989.

128. **Piquette GN, Crabtree ME, El-Danasouri I, Milki A, Polan ML,** Regulation of plasminogen activator inhibitor-1 and -2 messenger ribonucleic acid levels in human cumulus and granulosa-luteal cells, J Clin Endocrinol Metab 76:518, 1993.

129. **Lumsden MA, Kelly RW, Templeton AA, Van Look PFA, Swanston IA, Baird DT,** Changes in the concentrations of prostaglandins in preovulatory human follicles after administration of hCG, J Reprod Fertil 77:119, 1986.

130. **Espey LL, Tanaka N, Adams RF, Okamura H,** Ovarian hydroxyeicodatetraenoic acids compared with prostanoids and steroids during ovulation in rats, Am J Physiol 260:E163, 1991.

131. **O'Grady JP, Caldwell BV, Auletta FJ, Speroff L,** The effects of an inhibitor of prostaglandin synthesis (indomethacin) on ovulation, pregnancy, and pseudopregnancy in the rabbit, Prostaglandins 1:97, 1972.

132. **Miyazaki T, Katz E, Dharmarajan AM, Wallach EE, Atlas SJ,** Do prostaglandins lead to ovulation in the rabbit by stimulating proteolytic enzyme activity? Fertil Steril 55:1182, 1991.

133. **Priddy AR, Killick SR, Elstein M, Morris J, Sullivan M, Patel L, Elder M,** The effect of prostaglandin synthetase inhibitors on human preovulatory follicular fluid prostaglandin, thromboxane, and leukotriene concentrations, J Clin Endocrinol Metab 71:235, 1990.

134. **Vanderhyden BC, Telfer EE, Eppig JJ,** Mouse oocytes promote proliferation of granulosa cells from preantral and antral follicles in vitro, Biol Reprod 46:1196, 1992.

135. **Katt JA, Duncan JA, Herbon L, Barkan A, Marshall JC,** The frequency of gonadotropin-releasing hormone stimulation determines the number of pituitary gonadotropin-releasing hormone receptors, Endocrinology 116:2113, 1985.

136. **Smith SK, Lenton EA, Cooke ID,** Plasma gonadotrophin and ovarian steroid concentrations in women with menstrual cycles with short luteal phase, J Reprod Fertil 75:363, 1985.

137. **Golos TG, Soto EA, Tureck RW, Strauss JF III,** Human chorionic gonadotropin and 8-bromo-adenosine 3',5'-monophosphate stimulate [^{125}I]low density lipoprotein uptake and metabolism by luteinized human granulosa cells in culture, J Clin Endocrinol Metab 61:633, 1985.

138. **Brannian JD, Shiigi SM, Stouffer RL,** Gonadotropin surge increases fluorescent-tagged low-density lipoprotein uptake by Macaque granulosa cells from preovulatory follicles, Biol Reprod 47:355, 1992.

139. **Vande Wiele RL, Bogumil J, Dyrenfurth I, Ferin M, Jewelewicz R, Warren M, Rizkallah R, Mikhail G,** Mechanisms regulating the menstrual cycle in women, Recent Prog Horm Res 26:63, 1970.

140. **Hutchison JS, Zeleznik AJ,** The rhesus monkey corpus luteum is dependent on pituitary gonadotropin secretion throughout the luteal phase of the menstrual cycle, Endocrinology 115:1780, 1984.

141. **Richardson DW, Goldsmith LT, Pohl CR, Schallenberger E, Knobil E,** The role of prolactin in the regulation of the primate corpus luteum, J Clin Endocrinol Metab 60:501, 1985.

142. **Maas S, Jarry H, Teichmann A, Rath W, Kuhn W, Wuttke W,** Paracrine actions of oxytocin, prostaglandin F$_{2\alpha}$, and estradiol within the human corpus luteum, J Clin Endocrinol Metab 74:306, 1992.

143. **Shukovski L,** Is there a function for ovarian oxytocin in primates? Reprod Fertil Dev 4:99, 1992.

144. **Ravindranath N, Little-Ihrig L, Benyo DF, Zeleznik AJ,** Role of luteinizing hormone in the expression of cholesterol side-chain cleavage cytochrome P450 and 3β-hydroxysteroid dehydrogenase Δ^{5-4} isomerase messenger ribonucleic acids in the primate corpus luteum, Endocrinology 131:2065, 1992.

145. **Brannian JD, Stouffer RL,** Progesterone production by monkey luteal cell subpopulations at different stages of the menstrual cycle: changes in agonist responsiveness, Biol Reprod 44:141, 1991.

146. **Brannian JD, Stouffer RL,** Cellular approaches to understanding the function and regulation of the primate corpus luteum, Seminars Reprod Endocrinol 9:341, 1991.

147. **diZerega GS, Lynch A, Hodgen GD,** Initiation of asymmetrical ovarian estradiol secretion in the primate ovarian cycle after luteectomy, Endocrinology 108:1233, 1981.

148. **diZerega GS, Hodgen GD,** The interovarian progesterone gradient: a spatial and temporal regulator of folliculogenesis in the primate ovarian cycle, J Clin Endocrinol Metab 54:495, 1982.

149. **Gougeon A, Lefevre B,** Histological evidence of alternating ovulation in women, J Reprod Fertil 70:7, 1984.

150. **Demura R, Suzuki T, Tajima S, Mitsuhashi S, Odagiri E, Demura H, Ling N,** Human plasma free activin and inhibin levels during the menstrual cycle, J Clin Endocrinol Metab 76:1080, 1993.

151. **Filicori M, Butler JP, Crowley WF,** Neuroendocrine regulation of the corpus luteum in the human: evidence for pulsatile progesterone secretion, J Clin Invest 73:1638, 1984.

152. **McLachlin RI, Cohen NL, Vale WE, Rivier JE, Burger HG, Bremmer WJ, Soules MR,** The importance of luteinizing hormone in the control of inhibin and progesterone secretion by the human corpus luteum, J Clin Endocrinol Metab 68:1078, 1989.

153. **MacNaughton J, Banah M, McCloud P, Hee J, Burger H,** Age related changes in follicle stimulating hormone, luteinizing hormone, oestradiol and immunoreactive inhibin in women of reproductive age, Clin Endocrinol 36:339, 1992.

154. **Roseff SJ, Bangah ML, Kettel LM, Vale W, Rivier J, Burger HG, Yen SSC,** Dynamic changes in circulating inhibin levels during the luteal-follicular transition of the human menstrual cycle, J Clin Endocrinol Metab 69:1033, 1989.

155. **Lenton EA, Landgren B, Sexton L,** Normal variation in the length of the luteal phase of the menstrual cycle: identification of the short luteal phase, Br J Obstet Gynaecol 91:685, 1984.

156. **Press MF, Greene GL,** Localization of progesterone receptor with monoclonal antibodies to the human progestin receptor, Endocrinology 122:1165, 1988.

157. **Auletta FJ, Flint APF,** Mechanisms controlling corpus luteum function in sheep, cows, nonhuman primates, and women especially in relation to the time of luteolysis, Endocr Rev 9:88, 1988.

158. **Zelinski-Wooten MB, Stouffer RL,** Intraluteal infusions of prostaglandins of the E, D, I, and A series prevent PGF2α-induced but not spontaneous luteal regression in rhesus monkeys, Biol Reprod 43:507, 1990.

159. **Zeleznik AJ, Little-Ihrig LL,** Effect of reduced luteinizing hormone concentrations on corpus luteum function during the menstrual cycle of rhesus monkeys, Endocrinology 125:2237, 1990.

160. **Bassett SG, Little-Ihrig LL, Mason JI, Zeleznik AJ,** Expression of messenger ribonucleic acids that encode for 3β-hydroxysteroid dehydrogenase and cholesterol side-chain cleavage enzyme throughout the luteal phase of the Macaque menstrual cycle, J Clin Endocrinol Mctab 72:362, 1991.

161. **Catt KJ, Dufau ML, Vaitukaitis JL,** Appearance of hCG in pregnancy plasma following the initiation of implantation of the blastocyst, J Clin Endocrinol Metab 40:537, 1975.

162. **Jia X-C, Kessel B, Yen SSC, Tucker EM, Hsueh AJW,** Serum bioactive follicle-stimulating hormone during the human menstrual cycle and in hyper- and hypogonadotropic states: application of a sensitive granulosa cell aromatase bioassay, J Clin Endocrinol Metab 62:1243, 1986.

163. **Schneyer AL, Sluss PM, Shitcomb RW, Hall JE, Crowley Jr WF, Freaman RG,** Development of a radioligand receptor assay for measuring follitropin in serum: application to premature ovarian failure, Clin Chem 37:508, 1991.

164. **Le Nestour E, Marraoui J, Lahlou N, Roger M, de Ziegler D, Bouchard PH,** Role of estradiol in the rise in follicle-stimulating hormone levels during the luteal-follicular transition, J Clin Endocrinol Metab 77:439, 1993.

165. **Vollman RF,** The menstrual cycle, in Friedman E, editor, *Major Problems in Obstetrics and Gynecology,* W.B. Saunders Co., Philadelphia, 1977.

166. **Treloar AE, Boynton RE, Borghild GB, Brown BW,** Variation of the human menstrual cycle through reproductive life, Int J Fertil 12:77, 1967.

167. **Collett ME, Wertenberger GE, Fiske VM,** The effect of age upon the pattern of the menstrual cycle, Fertil Steril 5:437, 1954.

168. **Munster K, Schmidt L, Helm P,** Length and variation in the menstrual cycle — a cross-sectional study from a Danish county, Br J Obstet Gynaecol 99:422, 1992.

169. **Sherman BM, Koreman SG,** Hormonal characteristics of the human menstrual cycle throughout reproductive life, J Clin Invest 55:699, 1975.

170. **Lenton EA, Landgren B, Sexton L, Harper R,** Normal variation in the length of the follicular phase of the menstrual cycle: effect of chronological age, Br J Obstet Gynecol 91:681, 1984.

171. **Lee SJ, Lenton EA, Sexton L, Cooke ID,** The effect of age on the cyclical patterns of plasma LH, FSH, oestradiol and progesterone in women with regular menstrual cycles, Hum Reprod 3:851, 1988.

172. **Hughes EG, Robertson DM, Handelsman DJ, Hayward S, Healy DL, de Kretser DM,** Inhibin and estradiol responses to ovarian hyperstimulation: effects of age and predictive value for in vitro fertilization outcome, J Clin Endocrinol Metab 70:358, 1990.

173. **Cha KY, Koo JJ, Ko JJ, Choi DH, Han SY, Yoon JK,** Pregnancy after IVF of human follicular ooctyes collected from nonstimulated cycles, their culture in vitro and their transfer in a donor occyte program, Fertil Steril 55:109, 1991.

174. **Richardson SJ, Senikas V, Nelson JF,** Follicular depletion during the menopausal transition — evidence for accelerated loss and ultimate exhaustion, J Clin Endocrinol Metab 65:1231, 1987.

175. **Buckler HM, Evans A, Mamlora H, Burger HG, Anderson DC,** Gonadotropin, steroid and inhibin levels in women with incipient ovarian failure during anovulatory and ovulatory 'rebound' cycles, J Clin Endocrinol Metab 72:116, 1991.

176. **Metcalf MG, Livesay JH,** Gonadotropin excretion in fertile women: effect of age and the onset of the menopausal transition, J Endocrinol 105:357, 1985.

7 Sperm and Egg Transport, Fertilization, and Implantation

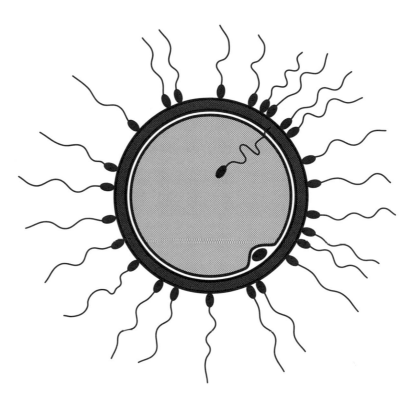

Among his many accomplishments, Galileo Galilei gave to science, in 1609, two important instruments, the telescope and the microscope.[1] Antonj van Leeuwenhoek was fascinated by Galileo's microscope. Leeuwenhoek was a draper and had no medical or scientific training, yet he became a Fellow of the Royal Society of London to which he submitted 375 scientific papers. In 1677, Leewenhoek described (fairly accurately) the "little animals of the sperm." It was another 198 years before Oscar Hertwig demonstrated fertilization, the union of sperm and egg.

The coming together of sperm and egg is one of the essentials of reproduction; however, the remote site of this event and the enclosed origins of the participants has made fertilization a difficult subject for study. This changed with the advent of in vitro fertilization. Greater understanding of sperm and egg development and union is one of the major benefits of the clinical application of the assisted reproductive technologies. This chapter will examine the mechanisms involved in sperm and egg transport, fertilization, and implantation.

Sperm Transport

The sperm reach the caudal epididymis approximately 72 days after the initiation of spermatogenesis. At this time, the head of the sperm contains a membrane bound nucleus capped by the acrosome, a large vesicle of proteolytic enzymes. The inner acrosomal membrane is closely opposed to the nuclear membrane, and the outer acrosomal membrane is next to the surface plasma membrane. The flagellum is a complex structure of microtubules and fibers, surrounded at the proximal end by mitochondria. Motility and the ability to fertilize are acquired gradually as the sperm pass into the epididymis.

The caudal epididymis stores sperm available for ejaculation. The ability to store functional sperm provides a capacity for repetitive fertile ejaculations. Preservation of optimal sperm function during this period of storage requires adequate testosterone levels in the circulation and maintenance of the normal scrotal temperature.[2] The importance of temperature is emphasized by the correlation of reduced numbers of sperm associated with episodes of body fever. The epididymis is limited to a storage role because sperm that have never passed through the epididymis and that have been obtained from the vasa efferentia in men with a congenital absence of the vas deferens can fertilize the human oocyte in vitro and result in pregnancy with live birth.[3]

Semen forms a gel almost immediately following ejaculation but then is liquefied in 20–30 minutes by enzymes derived from the prostate gland. The alkaline pH of semen provides protection for the sperm from the acid environment of the vagina. This protection is transient, and most sperm left in the vagina are immobilized within 2 hours. The more fortunate sperm, by their own motility, gain entrance into the tongues of cervical mucus that layer over the ectocervix. These are the sperm that enter the uterus; the seminal plasma is left behind in the vagina. This entry is rapid, and sperm have been found in mucus within 90 seconds of ejaculation.[4] The destruction of all sperm in the vagina 5 minutes after ejaculation does not interfere with fertilization in the rabbit, further attesting to the rapidity of transport.[5]

The exact mechanism for entry of sperm into the cervical mucus is unknown. Contractions of the female reproductive tract occur during coitus, and these contractions may be important for entry of sperm into the cervical mucus and further transport. Presumably successful entry is the result of combined female and male forces (the flagellar activity of the sperm). The success of therapeutic insemination, however, indicates that female coitus and orgasm are not essential for sperm transport.

The sperm swim and migrate through pores in the mucus microstructure that are smaller than the sperm head; therefore, the sperm must actively push their way through the mucus.[6] One cause of infertility, presumably, is impaired sperm movement that prevents this transport through the mucus. This movement is probably also influenced by the interaction between the mucus and the surface properties of the sperm head; for example, sperm antibodies on the sperm head inhibit sperm movement in the mucus.[7] Abnormal morphology of the sperm head is often associated with impaired flagellar function; however, abnormal head morphology alone can be a cause of poor mucus penetration.[8,9]

Uterine contractions propel the sperm upward, and in the human they can be found in the tube 5 minutes after insemination.[10] It is possible that the first sperm to enter the tube are at a disadvantage. In the rabbit these early sperm have only poor motility, and there is frequent disruption of the head membranes.[11] The sperm in this vanguard are unlikely to achieve fertilization. Other sperm that have colonized the cervical mucus, the cervical crypts, and the portion of the tubal isthmus nearest the uterus then make their way more slowly to the ampulla of the tube in order to meet the egg. Human sperm have been found in the fallopian tube as long as 80 hours after intercourse, and these sperm can still perform normally with zona-free hamster oocytes.[12] In animals, the fertilizable lifespan is usually one-half the motile lifespan. The number of sperm in the cervical mucus is relatively constant for 24 hours after coitus, and after 48 hours there are very few remaining in the mucus.[13]

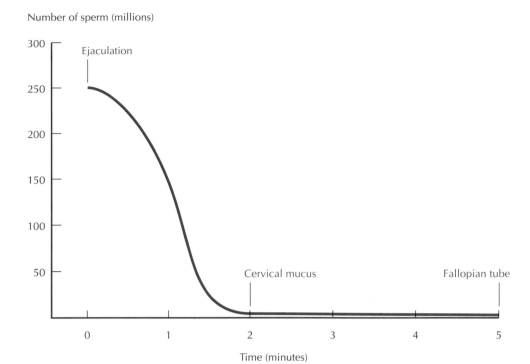

Number of sperm (millions)

The attrition in sperm numbers from vagina to tube is substantial. Of an average of 200 million to 300 million sperm deposited in the vagina, fewer than 200 achieve proximity to the egg. The major loss occurs in the vagina, with expulsion of semen from the introitus playing an important role. Other causes for loss are digestion of sperm by vaginal enzymes and phagocytosis of sperm along the reproductive tract. There are also reports of sperm burrowing into or being engulfed by endometrial cells. Sperm are not stored in the fallopian tube, and indeed many sperm continue past the oocyte to be lost into the peritoneal cavity. However, the cervix does serve as a reservoir providing a supply of sperm for up to 72 hours.

Within the fallopian tube, sperm display a new pattern of movement that has been called hyperactivated motility.[14] This motility may be influenced by an interaction with the tubal epithelium which results in greater speed and better direction.

Structure of the Cervical Mucus

The cervical mucus is a complex structure which is not homogeneous.[15] The mucus is secreted in granular form, and a networked structure of the mucus is formed in the cervical canal. Thus, not all areas of the cervical mucus are equally penetrable by the sperm. It is proposed, based upon animal studies, that the outward flow of the cervical mucus establishes a linear alignment of its structure that directs the sperm upward. Pressurization of the mucus by contractions of the uterus further aid this alignment and may contribute to the speed of sperm transport. The process of capacitation is initiated, and perhaps completed, during the sperm's passage through the cervix.

Capacitation

The discovery in 1951 that rabbit and rat spermatozoa must spend some hours in the female tract before acquiring the capacity to penetrate ova stimulated intensive research efforts to delineate the environmental conditions required for this change in the sperm to occur.[16,17] The process by which the sperm were transformed was called capacitation.[18] Attention was focused upon the hormonal and time requirements and the potential for in vitro capacitation.

Capacitation is characterized by 3 accomplishments:

1. The ability to undergo the acrosome reaction.

2. The ability to bind to the zona pellucida.

3. The acquisition of hypermotility.

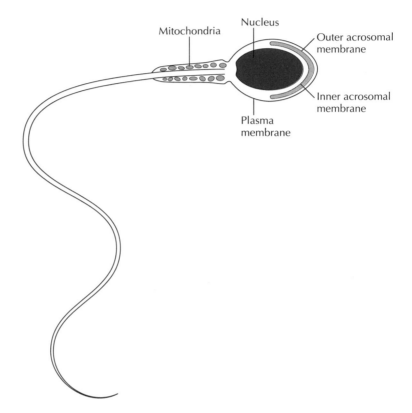

Capacitation changes the surface characteristics of sperm, as exemplified by removal of seminal plasma factors that coat the surface of the sperm, modification of their surface charge, and restriction of receptor mobility. This is associated with decreased stability of the plasma membrane and the membrane lying immediately under it, the outer acrosomal membrane. The membranes undergo further, more striking, modifications when capacitated sperm reach the vicinity of an ovum or when they are incubated in follicular fluid. There is a breakdown and merging of the plasma membrane and the outer acrosomal membrane, ***the acrosome reaction.***[19] This allows egress of the enzyme contents of the acrosome, the cap-like structure that covers the sperm nucleus. These enzymes, which include hyaluronidase, a neuraminidase-like factor, corona-dispersing enzyme, and a protease called acrosin, are all thought to play roles in sperm penetration of the egg investments. The changes in the sperm head membranes also prepare the sperm for fusion with the egg membrane. It is the inner acrosomal membrane that fuses with the oocyte plasma membrane. In addition, capacitation endows the sperm with hypermotility, and the increased velocity of the sperm may be the most critical factor in mediating zona penetration.[14] The acrosome reaction can be induced by zona pellucida proteins of the oocyte and by human follicular fluid in vitro.[20,21]

Although capacitation classically has been defined as a change sperm undergo in the female reproductive tract, it is apparent that sperm of some species, including the human, can acquire the ability to fertilize after a short incubation in defined media and without residence in the female reproductive tract. Therefore, success with assisted reproductive technologies is possible. In vitro capacitation requires a culture medium that is a balanced salt solution containing energy substrates such as lactate, pyruvate, and glucose and a protein such as albumin, or a biologic fluid such as serum or follicular fluid. Sperm washing procedures probably remove factors that coat the surface of the sperm, one of the initial steps in capacitation. The removal of cholesterol from the sperm membrane is believed to prepare the sperm membrane for the acrosome reaction.[22] The time required for in vitro capacitation is approximately 2 hours.[23] The hamster penetration test is a measure of the sperm's ability to undergo in vitro capacitation and the acrosome reaction.

The final dash to the oocyte is aided by the increased motility due to the state of hyperactivity. This change in motility can be measured by an increase in velocity and flagellar beat amplitude. Perhaps the increase in thrust gained by this hyperactivity is necessary for penetration of the oocyte.

Egg Transport

The oocyte, at the time of ovulation, is surrounded by granulosa cells (the cumulus oophorus) that attach the oocyte to the wall of the follicle. The zona pellucida, a noncellular porous layer of glycoproteins, separates the oocyte from the granulosa cells. The granulosa cells communicate metabolically with the oocyte by means of gap junctions between the oocyte plasma membrane and the cumulus cells. In response to the midcycle surge in luteinizing hormone (LH), maturation of the oocyte proceeds with the resumption of meiosis as the oocyte enters into the second meiotic division and arrests in the second metaphase. Just before ovulation, the cumulus cells retract their cellular contacts from the oocyte. The disruption of the gap junctions induces maturation and migration of the cortical granules to the outer cortex of the oocyte.[24] Prior to ovulation, the oocyte and its cumulus mass of cells prepare to leave their long residence in the ovary by becoming detached from the follicular wall.

Egg transport encompasses the period of time from ovulation to the entry of the egg into the uterus. The egg can be fertilized only during the early stages of its sojourn in the fallopian tube. Within 2–3 minutes of ovulation, the cumulus and oocyte are in the ampulla of the fallopian tube.

In rats and mice the ovary and distal portion of the tube are covered by a common fluid-filled sac. Ovulated eggs are carried by fluid currents to the fimbriated end of the tube. By contrast, in primates, including humans, the ovulated eggs adhere with their cumulus mass of follicular cells to the surface of the ovary. The fimbriated end of the tube sweeps over the ovary in order to pick up the egg. Entry into the tube is facilitated by muscular movements that bring the fimbriae into contact with the surface of the ovary. Variations in this pattern surely exist, as evidenced by women who achieve pregnancy despite having only one ovary and a single tube located on the contralateral side. Furthermore, eggs deposited in the cul-de-sac by transvaginal injection are picked up by the tubes.[25]

Although there can be a small negative pressure in the tube in association with muscle contractions, ovum pickup is not dependent upon a suction effect secondary to this negative pressure. Ligation of the tube just proximal to the fimbriae does not interfere with pickup.[26] The cilia on the surface of the fimbriae have adhesive sites, and these seem to have prime responsibility for the initial movement of the egg into the tube. This movement is dependent upon the presence of follicular cumulus cells surrounding the egg, because removal of these cells prior to egg pickup prevents effective egg transport.

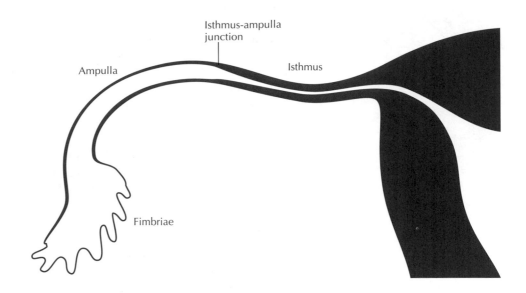

In the ampulla of the tube the cilia beat in the direction of the uterus. In women and monkeys this unidirectional beat is also found in the isthmus of the tube, whereas in the rabbit there are additional rows of cilia that beat in the direction of the ovary. The specific contribution of the cilia to egg transport in the ampulla and isthmus is an unresolved question. Most investigators have credited muscular contractions of the tubes as the primary force for moving the egg. However, interference with muscle contractility in the rabbit did not block egg transport.[27] Reversing a segment of the ampulla of the tube so that the cilia in this segment beat toward the ovary interferes with pregnancy in the rabbit without blocking fertilization. The fertilized ova are arrested when they come in contact with the transposed area.[28] This again suggests that ciliary beat is crucial for egg transport. Cilia play, in all likelihood, a less important role in the human. There are *fertile* women who have Kartagener's syndrome in which there is a congenital absence of dynein arms in cilia, and thus the cilia do not beat. This deficiency in the cilia is found in the fallopian tubes as well as in the respiratory tract.[29]

Muscular contractions of the tube are associated with a to-and-fro movement of the eggs rather than with a continuous forward progression. In most species transport of the ovum through the tube requires approximately 3 days.[30] The time spent within the various parts of the tube varies from one species to another. Transport through the ampulla is rapid in the rabbit, whereas in women it requires 30 hours for the egg to reach the ampullary-isthmic junction. The egg remains at this point another 30 hours, at which time it begins rapid transport through the isthmus of the tube.

Attempts to modify tubal function as a method for understanding its physiology have involved three major pharmacologic approaches: 1) altering levels of steroid hormones, 2) interference with or supplementation of adrenergic stimuli, and 3) treatment with prostaglandins. Although there is abundant literature on the effects of estrogen and progesterone on tubal function, it is clouded by the use of different hormones, different doses, and different timing of injections. Because of these variations it is difficult to obtain a coherent picture and to relate the experimental results to the in vivo situation. In general, pharmacologic doses of estrogen favor retention of eggs in the tube. This "tube locking" effect of estrogen can be partially reversed by treatment with progesterone.

The isthmus of the tube has an extensive adrenergic innervation. Surgical denervation of the tube, however, does not disrupt ovum transport. Prostaglandins (PG) of the E series relax tubal muscle, whereas those of the F series stimulate muscle activity of the

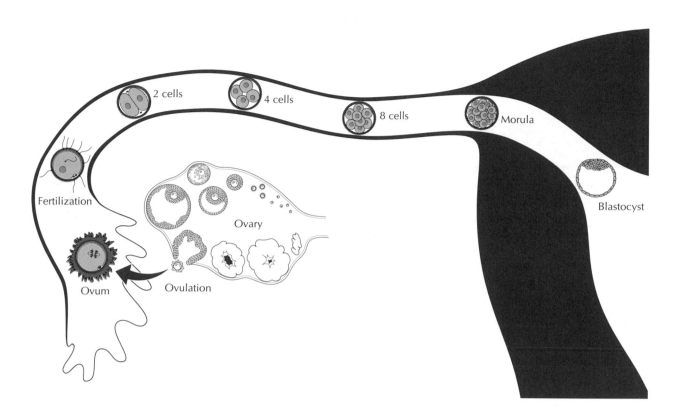

tube. Although $PGF_{2\alpha}$ stimulates human oviductal motility in vivo, it does not cause acceleration of ovum transport.

The effect on fertility of removal of different segments of the tube has been reviewed by Pauerstein and Eddy, who noted that excision of the ampullary-isthmic junction in rabbits did not block fertility.[31] This is equally true if small segments of the ampulla are removed, and pregnancy can occur even if the entire isthmus and uterotubal junction are excised. Although the fimbriae are thought to play a crucial role in fertility, spontaneous pregnancies have been reported following sterilization by fimbriectomy or following surgical repair of tubes whose fimbriated ends had been excised.[32,33]

In most species, a period of residence in the tube appears to be a prerequisite for full development. Rabbit eggs can be fertilized in the uterus, but they do not develop unless transferred to the tubes within 3 hours of fertilization.[34] This and other work implies that there may be a component in uterine fluid during the first 48 hours following ovulation that is toxic to the egg.[34] Indirect evidence of an inhospitable environment is also provided by studies indicating that there must be synchrony between development of the endometrium and the egg for successful pregnancy to occur.[35,36] If the endometrium is in a more advanced stage of development than the egg, fertility is compromised. Thus, it is conceptually useful to view the fallopian tube not as an active transport mechanism, but as a structure that provides an important holding action. This functional behavior is coordinated by the changing estrogen and progesterone levels after ovulation.

Successful pregnancies have occurred in the human following the Estes procedure, in which the ovary is transposed to the uterine cornua.[37] Eggs are ovulated directly into the uterus, completely bypassing the tube. Moreover, when fertilized donor eggs are transferred to women who are on hormone supplementation, there are a number of days during the treatment cycle when the blastocysts will implant. This crucial difference between animal and human physiology is of more than academic importance. There has been speculation concerning the use of drugs that could accelerate tubal transport as a means of providing contraception by ensuring that the egg would reach the uterus when it was in an unreceptive state. Although this may work in animals, it is of doubtful value in the human because perfect synchrony is not required.

Animal and human reproduction also differ in the occurrence of ectopic pregnancy. Ectopic pregnancies are rare in animals, and in rodents they are not induced even if the uterotubal junction is occluded immediately following fertilization. The embryos reach the blastocyst stage and then degenerate.

Fertilization

Following ovulation, the fertilizable lifespan of the rabbit egg is between 6 and 8 hours. The fertilizable life of the human ovum is unknown, but most estimates range between 12 and 24 hours. However, immature human eggs recovered for in vitro fertilization can be fertilized even after 36 hours of incubation. Equally uncertain is knowledge of the fertilizable lifespan of human sperm. The most common estimate is 48–72 hours, although motility can be maintained after the sperm have lost the ability to fertilize. Contact of sperm with the egg, which occurs in the ampulla of the tube, appears to be random; however, there is some evidence for sperm-egg communication which attracts sperm to the oocyte.[38,39]

Despite the evolution from external to internal fertilization over a period of about 100 million years, many of the mechanisms have remained the same.[40,41] The acellular zona pellucida that surrounds the egg at ovulation and remains in place until implantation has two major functions in the fertilization process:

1. The zona pellucida contains receptors for sperm which are, with some exceptions, relatively species-specific.

2. The zona pellucida undergoes the ***zona reaction*** in which the zona becomes impervious to other sperm once the fertilizing sperm penetrates, and thus it provides a bar to polyploidy.[42]

Penetration through the zona is rapid and possibly is mediated by acrosin, a trypsin-like proteinase that is bound to the inner acrosomal membrane of the sperm.[43] The pivotal role assigned to acrosin has been disputed. For example, manipulations that increase the resistance of the zona to acrosin do not interfere with sperm penetration, and thus sperm motility may be the critical factor.

The acrosome is a lysosome-like organelle in the anterior region of the sperm head, lying just beneath the plasma membrane. The acrosome contains many enzymes that are exposed by the acrosome reaction, the loss of the acrosome immediately before fertilization. This reaction requires an influx of calcium ions, the efflux of hydrogen ion, an increase in pH, and fusion of the plasma membrane with the outer acrosomal membrane, leading to the exposure and escape of the enzymes contained on the inner acrosomal membrane. Binding to the zona pellucida is required to permit a component of the zona to induce the acrosomal reaction. This component is believed to be a glycoprotein sperm receptor, which thus serves a dual function.

The initial contact between the sperm and the oocyte is a receptor-mediated process. The sperm receptors in the zona pellucida are glycoproteins, known as ZP1, ZP2, and ZP3, with ZP3 being the most abundant.[44] Structural alteration of these glycoproteins leads to a loss of receptor activity; inactivation of these receptors after fertilization is probably accomplished by one or more cortical granule enzymes. The zona pellucida is a porous structure, due to the many receptor glycoproteins assembled into long, interconnecting

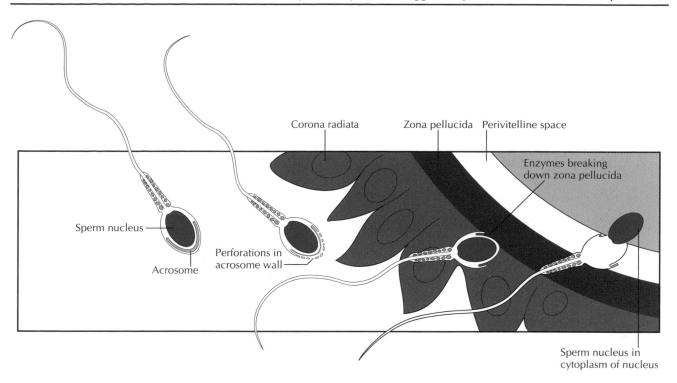

Corona radiata   Zona pellucida   Perivitelline space

Enzymes breaking down zona pellucida

Sperm nucleus

Perforations in acrosome wall

Acrosome

Sperm nucleus in cytoplasm of nucleus

filaments. The ZP3 gene is expressed only in growing oocytes. DNA sequence similarities of the ZP3 gene in various mammals indicates that this gene has been evolutionarily conserved and that the sperm-receptor interaction is a common mechanism among mammals.

The initial binding of the sperm to the zona requires recognition on the part of the sperm of the carbohydrate component of the species-specific glycoprotein receptor molecule. Once binding is accomplished, the acrosome reaction is triggered by the peptide chain component of the receptor glycoprotein. This interaction is analogous to the general principle of behavior for hormone-receptor binding and activity. In the case of sperm and oocyte, recognition of the oocyte zona receptor may involve an enzyme (galactosyl transferase and others) on the surface of the sperm which becomes exposed during capacitation. Formation of the enzyme-ZP3 complex, therefore, not only produces binding but also induces the acrosome reaction.

The initiation of the block to penetration of the zona (and the vitellus) by other sperm is mediated by the ***cortical reaction,*** a release of materials from the cortical granules, lysosome-like organelles which are found just below the egg surface.[45] As with other lysosome-like organelles, these materials include various hydrolytic enzymes. Changes brought about by these enzymes lead to the zona reaction, the hardening of the extracellular layer by cross-linking of proteins, and inactivation of sperm receptors. Thus the zona block to polyspermy is accomplished. The initial change in this zona block is a rapid depolarization of the oocyte membrane associated with a release of calcium ions from calmodulin. The increase in intracellular calcium acts as a signal or trigger to activate protein synthesis in the oocyte. The depolarization of the membrane initiates only a transient block to sperm entry. The permanent block is a consequence of the cortical reaction and release of enzymes, also apparently triggered by the increase in calcium.

Spermatozoa enter the perivitelline space at an angle. The postacrosomal region of the sperm head makes initial contact with the vitelline membrane (the egg plasma membrane). At first the egg membrane engulfs the sperm head, and subsequently there is fusion of egg and sperm membranes. This fusion is mediated by specific proteins. Two membrane proteins from the sperm head have been sequenced, one (PH-20) is involved in binding to the zona pellucida, and the other (PH-30) is involved in fusion with the oocyte.[46,47]

Fusion of the sperm and oocyte membrane triggers the cortical reaction, metabolic activation of the oocyte, and completion of meiosis. The second polar body is released at the time of fertilization and leaves the egg with a haploid complement of chromosomes. The addition of chromosomes from the sperm restores the diploid number to the now fertilized egg.

Fusion will occur only with sperm that have undergone the acrosome reaction. The chromatin material of the sperm head decondenses, and the male pronucleus is formed. The male and the female pronuclei migrate toward each other, and as they move into close proximity the limiting membranes break down, and a spindle is formed on which the chromosomes become arranged. Thus, the stage is set for the first cell division.

Embryonic genome activity in the human appears to begin after the first two rounds of cell division (the 4- and 8-cell stages). Early embryonic signals may be derived from a store of maternal mRNAs, termed the "maternal legacy."[48] An arrest of development in this pre-blastocyst cleavage stage is well-recognized. Perhaps not all of this loss is due to abnormalities in the embryo but to a failure to activate the embryonic genome. Perhaps better culture conditions in in vitro fertilization protocols might yield a higher rate of blastocyst formation.

The clinician is interested not only in how normal fertilization takes place but also in the occurrence of abnormal events that can interfere with pregnancy. It is worthwhile, therefore, to consider the failures that occur in association with in vivo fertilization. Studies in the nonhuman primate have involved monkeys and baboons. A surgical method was used to flush the uterus of regularly cycling rhesus monkeys, and 9 preimplantation embryos and 2 unfertilized eggs were recovered from 22 flushes. Two of the 9 embryos were morphologically abnormal and probably would not have implanted.[49] Hendrickx and Kraemer used a similar technique in the baboon and recovered 23 embryos, of which 10 were morphologically abnormal.[50] This suggests that in nonhuman primates some ovulated eggs are not fertilized and that many early embryos are abnormal and, in all likelihood, will be aborted. Similar findings have been reported in the human in the classic study of Hertig et al.[51] They examined 34 early embryos recovered by flushing and examination of reproductive organs removed at surgery. Ten of these embryos were morphologically abnormal, including 4 of the 8 preimplantation embryos. Because the 4 preimplantation losses would not have been recognized clinically, there would have been 6 losses recorded in the remaining 30 pregnancies.

By using sensitive pregnancy tests, it has been suggested that the total rate of pregnancy loss after implantation is approximately 30%.[52] When the loss of fertilized oocytes before implantation is included, approximately 46% of all pregnancies end before the pregnancy is clinically perceived.[53]

In the postimplantation period, if only clinically diagnosed pregnancies are considered, the generally accepted figure for spontaneous abortion in the first trimester is 15%. Approximately 50–60% of these abortions have chromosome abnormalities.[54] This suggests that a minimum of 7.5% of all human conceptions are chromosomally abnormal. The fact that only 1 in 200 newborns has a chromosome abnormality attests to the powerful selection mechanisms operating in early human gestation. In each ovulatory cycle, only 25% of normally fertile couples can achieve a live birth.

There is evidence for biologic selection against abnormal gametes and embryos throughout the reproductive process. Morphologically abnormal sperm are less successful than normal sperm in penetrating cervical mucus and in negotiating the uterotubal junction.[55] This selection does not seem to be operative against chromosomally abnormal sperm that are morphologically normal. Another protective mechanism is the attrition of sperm numbers that occurs between the vagina and the area of the tube that contains the egg. With only a small number of sperm making contact with the egg, there may be a decreased chance for penetration of the egg by more than one sperm.

In Vitro Fertilization and Embryo Loss

A number of the in vivo protective mechanisms are not present during in vitro fertilization. The filtering effects of the cervical mucus and the uterotubal junction are not available to remove grossly abnormal sperm. During in vitro fertilization, relatively large numbers of sperm are placed in the vicinity of the egg. This may increase the risk for penetration of the egg by more than one sperm. The zona blocking mechanisms are efficient enough, however, to prevent this from becoming a serious clinical problem.

The relatively low percentage of pregnancies achieved with in vitro fertilization to date is explainable to some extent by the high rate of embryo loss associated even with in vivo fertilization. This alone, however, does not completely account for the current results. Many of the losses result following transfer of embryos, and in some animals, this process is associated with a 50% embryo mortality. With increased experience the results should improve. It is clear, however, that there is a need for further understanding of the fertilization process and of implantation before we can feel confident that the in vitro environment is as physiologic as possible.

Implantation

Preparation for Implantation

The change from proliferative to secretory endometrium, described in detail in Chapter 4, is an essential part of achieving the receptive conditions required for implantation. This change is the histologic expression of many biochemical and molecular events. The endometrium is 10–14 mm thick at the time of implantation in the midluteal phase. By this time, secretory activity has reached a peak, and the endometrial cells are rich in glycogen and lipids. Understanding the dynamic endocrine behavior of the endometrium (Chapter 4) increases the appreciation for its active participation in the implantation process. The window of endometrial receptivity is restricted to days 16–19 (of a 28-day cycle).[36]

Early pregnancy factor (EPF) can be detected in the maternal circulation within 1–2 days after coitus results in a pregnancy.[56] EPF prior to implantation is apparently produced by the ovary in response to a signal from the embryo. After implantation, EPF is no longer secreted by the ovary but is derived from the embryo. EPF has immunosuppressive properties and is associated with cell proliferation and growth. Many other proteins, such as pregnancy-associated plasma protein-A and pregnancy associated endometrial protein, have been identified in trophoblast and the endometrium, but the biologic roles for these proteins remain to be determined.

Blastocysts grown in culture produce and secrete human chorionic gonadotropin (HCG).[57] Messenger RNA for HCG can be found in 6 to 8-cell human embryos.[58] Because the 8 to 12-cell stage is achieved about 3 days after fertilization, it is believed that the human embryo begins to produce HCG before implantation when it can be detected in the mother (about 6–7 days after ovulation). The embryo is capable, therefore, of preimplantation signaling, and higher levels of estradiol and progesterone can be measured in the maternal circulation even before maternal HCG is detectable,

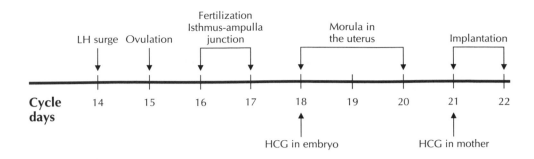

presumably due to stimulation of the corpus luteum by HCG delivered directly from the uterine cavity to the ovary.[59] Function of the corpus luteum is crucial during the first 7–9 weeks of pregnancy, and luteectomy early in pregnancy can precipitate abortion.[60] Similarly, early pregnancy loss in primates can be induced by injections of anti-HCG serum.[61]

In rodents and rabbits, implantation can be interrupted by injection of prostaglandin inhibitors.[62,63] Indomethacin prevents the increase in endometrial vascular permeability normally seen just prior to implantation. Additional evidence for a role by prostaglandins in the earliest stages of implantation is the finding of increased concentrations at implantation sites, similar to any inflammatory response.[64] The blastocysts of mice, rabbits, sheep, and cows produce prostaglandins, and prostaglandin release from human blastocysts and embryos has been demonstrated.[65] The endometrial cells are also a likely source of prostaglandin, and its synthesis may be stimulated by the tissue response that accompanies implantation. However, decidual synthesis of prostaglandins is significantly reduced compared to proliferative and secretory endometrium, apparently a direct effect of progesterone activity and perhaps a requirement in order to maintain the pregnancy.[64] Nevertheless, prostaglandin synthesis is increased at the implantation site, perhaps in response to blastocyst factors, e.g., platelet activating factor.[66] In the rabbit, platelet activating factor also induces the production of early pregnancy factor (discussed above).[67]

As discussed in Chapter 4, the many cytokines, peptides, and lipids secreted by the endometrium are inter-related through the stimulating and inhibiting actions of estrogen and progesterone, as well as the autocrine/paracrine activities of these substances on each other. The response to implantation certainly involves the many members of the growth factor family. Epidermal growth factor, for example, is highly concentrated in the implantation site in the mouse.[68]

Implantation

Implantation is defined as the process by which an embryo attaches to the uterine wall and penetrates first the epithelium and then the circulatory system of the mother to form the placenta. It is a process that is limited in both time and space. Implantation begins 2–3 days after the fertilized egg enters the uterus on day 18 or 19 of the cycle (3 or 4 days after ovulation).[69] Thus, implantation occurs 5–7 days after fertilization. The implantation site in the human uterus is usually in the upper, posterior wall in the midsagittal plane.

The human blastocyst remains in the uterine secretions for approximately 72 hours and then hatches from its zona pellucida in preparation for attachment. Implantation is marked initially by apposition of the blastocyst to the uterine epithelium. A prerequisite for this contact is a loss of the zona pellucida, which, in vitro, can be ruptured by contractions and expansions of the blastocyst. In vivo this activity is less critical, because the zona can be lysed by components of the uterine fluid. The exact nature and function of these components and related proteins that are thought to mediate the implantation process (implantation-initiating factor, fibronectin, uteroglobin and blasto-kinin) are uncertain.[70] Their production is, however, known to be dependent upon the secretion of ovarian steroid hormones. Even if the hormonal milieu and protein composition of the uterine fluid are hospitable to the implantation, it may not occur if the embryo is not at the proper stage of development. It has been inferred from this information that there must be developmental maturation of the surface of the embryo before it is able to achieve attachment and implantation.

Reports on changes in the surface charge of preimplantation embryos differ in their findings, and it is unlikely that changes in surface charge are solely responsible for adherence of the embryo to the surface of epithelial cells. Binding of the lectin concanavalin A to the embryo changes during the preimplantation period, an indication that the surface glycoproteins of the embryo are in transition.[71] It is reasonable to assume that these changes in configuration on the surface occur in order to enhance the ability of the embryo to adhere to the maternal surface.

As the embryo comes into close contact with the endometrium, the microvilli on the surface flatten and interdigitate with those on the luminal surface of the epithelial cells. A stage is reached where the cell membranes are in very close contact and junctional complexes are formed. The embryo can no longer be dislodged from the surface of the epithelial cells by flushing the uterus with physiologic solutions. Three types of subsequent interactions between the implanting trophoblast and the uterine epithelium have been described.[72] In the first, trophoblast cells intrude between uterine epithelial cells on their path to the basement membrane. In the second type of interaction, the epithelial cells lift off the basement membrane, an action which allows the trophoblast to insinuate itself underneath the epithelium. Last, fusion of trophoblast with individual uterine epithelial cells has been identified by electron microscopy in the rabbit.[73] This latter method of gaining entry into the epithelial layer raises interesting questions concerning the immunologic consequences of mixing embryonic and maternal cytoplasm.

Trophoblast has the ability to phagocytose a variety of cells but in vivo this activity seems largely confined to removal of dead endometrial cells, or cells that have been sloughed from the uterine wall. Similarly, despite the invasive nature of the trophoblast, destruction of maternal cells by enzymes secreted by the embryo does not seem to play a major role in implantation. The embryo does secrete a variety of enzymes (e.g., collagenase and plasminogen activators), and these may be important for digesting the intercellular matrix that holds the epithelial cells together. Studies in vitro have demonstrated the presence of plasminogen activator in mouse embryos and in human trophoblast, and its activity is important in the attachment and early outgrowth stages of implantation.[74,75] Urokinase and proteases, trophoblastic enzymes which convert plasminogen to plasmin, are inhibited by HCG, indicating regulation of this process by the embryo.[76]

The embryo at a somewhat later stage of implantation can digest, in vitro, a complex matrix composed of glycoproteins, elastin and collagen, all of which are components of the normal intercellular matrix.[77,78] Additional studies in vitro have shown that cells move away from trophoblast in a process called "contact inhibition."[79] Trophoblast then spreads to fill the spaces vacated by the cocultured cells. Once the intracellular matrix has been lysed, this movement of epithelial cells away from trophoblast would allow space for the implanting embryo to move through the epithelial layer. Trophoblast movement is aided by the fact that only parts of its surface are adhesive, and the major portion of the surface is nonadhesive to other cells.

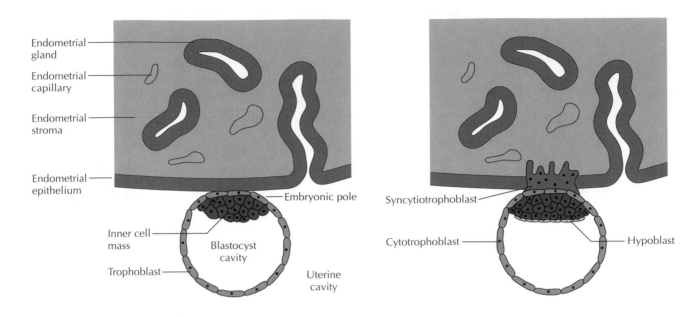

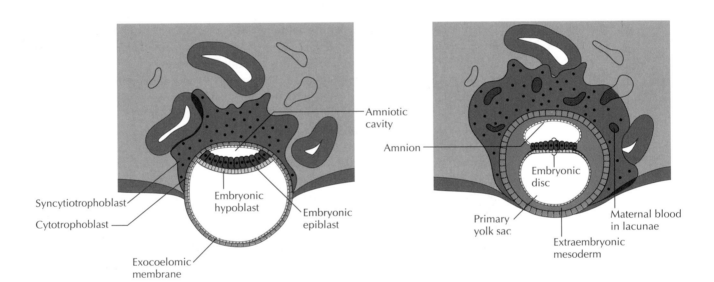

It is very likely that the highly proliferative phase of trophoblastic tissue during early embryogenesis is regulated by the many growth factors produced in both fetal and maternal tissues. Further penetration and survival depend upon factors that are capable of suppressing the maternal immune response to paternal antigens. The endometrial tissue makes a significant contribution to growth factor activity and immune suppression by synthesizing proteins in response to the blastocyst even before implantation.[80,81]

One of the great mysteries associated with implantation is the mechanism by which the mother rejects a genetically abnormal embryo or fetus. It is possible that the abnormal embryo cannot produce a signal in early pregnancy that can be recognized by the mother.

The embryonic signals will be effective only in a proper hormone milieu. Much of the knowledge concerning the hormone requirements for implantation in animals has been gained from studies of animals in delayed implantation. In a number of species, preimplantation embryos normally lie dormant in the uterus for periods of time which may extend for as long as 15 months before implantation is initiated. In other species, delayed implantation can be imposed by postpartum suckling or by performing ovariectomy on day 3 of pregnancy. This produces a marked decrease in synthesis of DNA and protein by the blastocyst. The embryo can be maintained at the blastocyst stage by injecting the mother with progesterone. Using this model, hormonal requirements for implantation have been determined. In mice there is a requirement for estrogen and progesterone followed by estrogen, which initiates implantation. In other species the nidatory stimulus of estrogen is not required, and progesterone alone is sufficient.

Although it is known that the hormone milieu of delayed implantation renders the embryo quiescent, it is not known whether this represents a direct effect on the embryo or whether there is a metabolic inhibitor present in uterine secretions that acts upon the embryo. Removal of the embryo from the uterus to culture dishes allows rapid resumption of normal metabolism, suggesting that there has, in fact, been a release from the inhibitory effects of a uterine product.

Limitation of Invasion

Many components of the inflammatory response appear to play roles in the process of implantation. Cytokine secretion from the lymphocyte infiltrate in the endometrium activates cellular lysis of trophoblast, perhaps an important process in limiting invasion.[82] Other suppressor cells are present to inhibit the maternal immune response to the implanting embryo. Autocrine/paracrine factors which have been identified in both trophoblast and endometrium include interleukin-2 and colony stimulating factor-1 (CSF-1).

Invasion by the trophoblast is limited by the formation of the decidual cell layer in the uterus. Fibroblast-like cells in the stroma are transformed into glycogen and lipid-rich cells. In the human, decidual cells surround blood vessels late in the nonpregnant cycle, but extensive decidualization does not occur until pregnancy is established. Ovarian steroids govern decidualization, and in the human a combination of estrogen and progesterone is critical. In animals, implantation is preceded by an increase in uterine stromal capillary permeability at the precise site where the blastocyst will attach. The localized nature of this reaction and of decidualization in rodents raises the possibility that a signal from the embryo might be an important triggering stimulus. Thus, maternal recognition of and preparation for pregnancy may depend upon receiving signals released by the embryo.

Boving suggested that the release of CO_2 by the embryo in the form of bicarbonate raises the pH of the embryo surface, which, in turn, increases its stickiness.[83] CO_2 may also act as a signal to induce a decidual response in the mother.

Histamine may initiate the decidual response.[84] Antihistamines given systemically or directly into the uterus prevent the decidual response in rats. This was disputed when other workers found that systemic antihistamines were not effective in preventing the decidual response. However, there are two different receptors for histamines, H1 and H2. These are not blocked by the same agents, and early experiments demonstrating a lack of effect of antihistamines may have utilized only a block to one receptor. Blockage of both receptors in rats is followed by a decrease in the number of implantation sites.[85] Mast cells in the uterus are a major source of histamine, but it is possible that the embryo can also synthesize histamine.[86] This would explain why the increase in capillary permeability and decidualization in the endometrium is localized to areas near the implanting embryo.

Unanswered Questions

Why is gamete production so wasteful? Billions of sperm are produced, but only a few are ever successful in fertilizing an egg. Does it relate to early forms of reproduction — e.g., those in fish, where the sperm are released into the sea and large numbers are needed to assure that a few reach the egg? Does the overpopulation of sperm allow selection processes to take place, ensuring that the more abnormal sperm are filtered out before the tube is reached? In the human female approximately 350 ova are ovulated during a woman's life, yet the ovaries contain millions of eggs at birth.

What is the purpose of capacitation? Is it needed to overcome the protective mechanisms that have been built into the sperm, specifically those that prevent premature release of acrosomal enzymes? Penetration by sperm of the egg is desirable, but invasion of other maternal cells might trigger immunologic reactions against sperm. Capacitation does free the sperm from some inhibitors, thus allowing the hypermotility that may be needed for zona penetration.

Why are there so many abnormal embryos? Current estimates are that 50% of embryos do not survive to term. Why is there a high rate of embryo loss, and, specifically, why is there a high selection against abnormal embryos? Is it because of intrinsic programming defects within the embryo or an inability of the embryo to produce a signal recognized by the mother, or does the maternal organism in some way recognize abnormality and react against it?

Why has embryo transfer in the human following in vitro fertilization resulted in a low number of takes? Can the uterine environment be manipulated in such a way as to increase successful implantation of in vitro fertilization eggs?

References

1. **Medvei VC,** *A History of Endocrinology,* MTP Press Limited, Lancaster, England, 1982.

2. **Foldesy RG, Bedford JM,** Biology of the scrotum. I. Temperature and androgens as determinants of the sperm storage capacity of the rat cauda epididymis, Biol Reprod 26:673, 1982.

3. **Silber SJ, Ord T, Balmaceda J, Patrizio P, Asch RH,** Congenital absence of the vas deferens. The fertilizing capacity of human epididymal sperm, New Engl J Med 323:1788, 1990.

4. **Sobrero AJ, MacLeod J,** The immediate postcoital test, Fertil Steril 13:184, 1962.

5. **Bedford JM,** The rate of sperm passage into the cervix after coitus in the rabbit, J Reprod Fertil 25:211, 1971.

6. **Yudin AI, Hanson FW, Katz DF,** Human cervical mucus and its interaction with sperm: fine structural view, Biol Reprod 40:661, 1989.

7. **Wang C, Baker HWG, Jennings MG, et al,** Interaction between human cervical mucus and sperm surface antibodies, Fertil Steril 44:484, 1985.

8. **Morales P, Katz DF, Overstreet JW, et al,** The relationship between the motility and morphology of spermatozoa in human semen, J Androl 9:241, 1988.

9. **Katz DF, Morales P, Samuels SJ, Overstreet JW,** Mechanisms of filtration of morphologically abnormal human sperm by cervical mucus, Fertil Steril 54:513, 1990.

10. **Settlage DSF, Motoshima M, Tredway DR,** Sperm transport from the external cervical os to the fallopian tubes in women: a time and quantitation study, Fertil Steril 24:655, 1973.

11. **Overstreet JW, Cooper GW,** Sperm transport in the reproductive tract of the female rabbit. I. Rapid transit phase and transport, Biol Reprod 19:101, 1978.

12. **Gould JE, Overstreet JW, Hanson FW,** Assessment of human sperm function after recovery from the female reproductive tract, Biol Reprod 31:888, 1984.

13. **Perloff WH, Steinberger E,** In vivo survival of spermatozoa in cervical mucus, Am J Obstet Gynecol 88:439, 1964.

14. **Katz DF, Drobnis EZ, Overstreet JW,** Factors regulating mammalian sperm migration through the female reproductive tract and oocyte vestments, Gamete Res 22:443, 1989.

15. **Overstreet JW, Katz DF, Yudin AI,** Cervical mucus and sperm transport in reproduction, Seminars Perinatol 15:149, 1991.

16. **Chang MC,** Fertilizing capacity of spermatozoa deposited into the fallopian tubes, Nature 168:697, 1951.

17. **Austin CR,** Observations on the penetration of the sperm into the mammalian egg, Aust J Sci Res (Ser B) 4:581, 1951.

18. **Zaneveld LJD, De Jonge CJ, Anderson RA, Mack SR,** Human sperm capacitation and the acrosome reaction, Hum Reprod 6:1265, 1991.

19. **Yanagimachi R,** Capacitation and the acrosome reaction, in Asch R, Balmaceda JP, Johnston I, editors, *Gamete Physiology,* Serono Symposia, USA, Norwell, Massachusetts, 1990, pp 31-42.

20. **Cross NL, Morales P, Overstreet JW, Hanson FW,** Induction of acrosome reactions by the human zona pellucida, Biol Reprod 38:235, 1988.

21. **Suarez SS, Wolf DP, Meizel S,** Induction of the acrosome reaction in human spermatozoa by a fraction of human follicular fluid, Gamete Res 14:107, 1986.

22. **Ravnik SE, Zarutskie PW, Muller CH,** Purification and characterization of a human follicular fluid lipid transfer protein that stimulates human sperm capacitation, Biol Reprod 47:1126, 1992.

23. **Overstreet JW, Gould JE, Katz DF,** In vitro capacitation of human spermatozoa after passage through a column of cervical mucus, Fertil Steril 34:604, 1980.

24. **Ducibella T,** Mammalian egg cortical granules and the cortical reaction, in Wassarman PM, editor, *Elements of Mammalian Fertilization,* CRC Press, Boca Raton, Florida, 1991, pp 206-231.

25. **Sharma V, Mason B, Riddle A, Campbell S,** Peritoneal oocyte and sperm transfer, Fifth World Congress on In Vitro Fertilization and Embryo Transfer, Norfolk, Virginia, April 5-10, 1987 (abstract).

26. **Clewe TH, Mastroianni L,** Mechanisms of ovum pickup: I. Functional capacity of rabbit oviducts ligated near the fimbriae, Fertil Steril 9:13, 1958.

27. **Halbert SA, Tam PY, Blandau RJ,** Egg transport in the rabbit oviduct: the roles of cilia and muscle, Science 191:1052, 1976.

28. **Eddy CA, Flores JJ, Archer DR, Pauerstein CJ,** The role of cilia in infertility: an evaluation by selective microsurgical modification of the rabbit oviduct, Am J Obstet Gynecol 132:814, 1978.

29. **Jean Y, Langlais J, Roberts KD, Chapdelaine A, Bleau G,** Fertility of a woman with nonfunctional ciliated cells in the fallopian tubes, Fertil Steril 31:349, 1979.

30. **Croxatto HB, Ortiz MS,** Egg transport in the fallopian tube, Gynecol Invest 6:215, 1975.

31. **Pauerstein CJ, Eddy CA,** The role of the oviduct in reproduction; our knowledge and our ignorance, J Reprod Fertil 55:223, 1979.

32. **Tompkins P,** Letter to the editor, Fertil Steril 31:696, 1979.

33. **Novy MJ,** Reversal of Kroener fimbriectomy sterilization, Am J Obstet Gynecol 137:198, 1980.

34. **Glass RH,** Fate of rabbit eggs fertilized in the uterus, J Reprod Fertil 31:139, 1972.

35. **Adams CE,** Consequences of accelerated ovum transport, including a re-evaluation of Estes' operation, J Reprod Fertil 55:239, 1979.

36. **Rosenwaks Z,** Donor eggs: their application in modern reproductive technologies, Fertil Steril 47:895, 1987.

37. **Ikle FA,** Pregnancy after implantation of the ovary into the uterus, Gynaecologia 151:95, 1961.

38. **Ralt D, Goldenberg M, Fetterolf P, Thompson D, Dor J, Mashiach S, Garbers DL, Eisenbach M,** Sperm attraction to a follicular factor(s) correlates with human egg fertilizability, Proc Natl Acad Sci USA 88:2840, 1991.

39. **Eisenbach M, Ralt D,** Precontact mammalian sperm-egg communication and role in fertilization, Am J Physiol 262:1095, 1992.

40. **Wassarman PM,** The biology and chemistry of fertilization, Science 235:553, 1987.

41. **Dietl JA, Rauth G,** Molecular aspects of mammalian fertilization, Hum Reprod 4:869, 1989.

42. **Hartmann JF, Gwatkin RBL,** Alteration of sites on the mammalian sperm surface following capacitation, Nature 234:479, 1971.

43. **Zaneveld LJD, Polakoski KL, Williams WL,** Properties of a proteolytic enzyme from rabbit sperm acrosomes, Biol Reprod 6:30, 1972.

44. **Shabanowitz RB, O'Rand MG,** Characterization of the human zona pellucida from fertilized and unfertilized eggs, J Reprod Fertil 82:151, 1988.

45. **Barros C, Yanagimachi R,** Induction of zona reaction in golden hamster eggs by cortical granule material, Nature 233:2368, 1971.

46. **Lathrop WF, Carmichael EP, Myles DG, Primakoff P,** cDNA cloning reveals the molecular structure of a sperm surface protein, PH-20, involved in sperm-egg adhesion and the wide distribution of its gene among mammals, J Cell Biol 111:1939, 1990.

47. **Blobel CP, Wolfsberg TG, Turck CW, Myles DG, Primakoff P, White JM,** A potential fusion peptide and an integrin ligand domain in a protein active in sperm-egg fusion, Nature 356:248, 1992.

48. **Artley JK, Braude PR,** Biochemistry of the preimplantation embryo, Assist Reprod Rev 3:13, 1993.

49. **Hurst PR, Jefferies K, Eckstein P, Wheeler AG,** Recovery of uterine embryos in rhesus monkeys, Biol Reprod 15:429, 1976.

50. **Hendrickx AG, Kraemer DC,** Preimplantation stages of baboon embryos, Anat Rec 162:111, 1968.

51. **Hertig AT, Rock J, Adams EC, Menkin MC,** Thirty-four fertilized ova, good, bad and indifferent from 210 women of known fertility, Pediatrics 23:202, 1959.

52. **Wilcox AJ, Weiberg CR, O'Connor JF, Baird DD, Schlatterer JP, Canfield RE, Armstrong EG, Nisula BC,** Incidence of early loss of pregnancy, New Engl J Med 319:189, 1988.

53. **Little AB,** There's many a slip 'twixt implantation and the crib; (editorial), New Engl J Med 319:241, 1988.

54. **Ohno M, Maeda T, Matsunobu A,** A cytogenetic study of spontaneous abortions with direct analysis of chorionic villi, Obstet Gynecol 77:394, 1991.

55. **Krzanowska H,** The passage of abnormal spermatozoa through the uterotubal junction of the mouse, J Reprod Fertil 38:81, 1974.

56. **Morton H, Rolfe BE, Cavanagh AC,** Early pregnancy factor, Seminars Reprod Endocrinol 10:72, 1992.

57. **Lopata A, Hay D,** The surplus human embryo: its potential for growth, blastulation, hatching, and human chorionic gonadotropin production in culture, Fertil Steril 51:984, 1989.

58. **Bonduelle M, Dodd R, Liebaers I, Steirteghem A, Williamson R, Akhurst R,** Chorionic gonadotropin-β mRNA, a trophoblast marker, is expressed in human 8-cell embryos derived from tripronucleate zygotes, Hum Reprod 3:909, 1988.

59. **Stewart DR, Overstreet JW, Nakajima ST, Lasley BL,** Enhanced ovarian steroid secretion before implantation in early human pregnancy, J Clin Endocrinol Metab 76:1470, 1993.

60. **Csapo AI, Pulkkinen MO, Wiest WO,** Effects of luteectomy and progesterone replacement therapy in early pregnant patients, Am J Obstet Gynecol 115:759, 1973.

61. **Stevens VC,** Potential control of fertility in women by immunization with HCG, Res Reprod 7:1, 1975.

62. **Hoffman LH, Davenport GR, Brash AR,** Endometrial prostaglandins and phospholipase activity related to implantation in rabbits: effects of dexamethasone, Biol Reprod 38:544, 1984.

63. **Kennedy TG,** Interactions of eicosanoids and other factors in blastocyst implantation, in Hiller K, editor, *Eicosanoids and Reproduction,* MTP Press, Lancaster, 1987, p.73.

64. **van der Weiden RMF, Helmerhorst FM, Keirse MJNC,** Influence of prostaglandins and platelet activating factor on implantation, Hum Reprod 6:436, 1991.

65. **Holmes PV, Sjogren A, Hamberger L,** Prostaglandin-E_2 released by pre-implantation human conceptuses, J Reprod Immunol 17:79, 1989.

66. **Harper MJK,** Platelet-activating factor: a paracrine factor in preimplantation stages of reproduction? Biol Reprod 40:907, 1989.

67. **Sueoka K, Dharmarajan AM, Miyazaki T, Atlas SJ, Wallach E,** Platelet activating factor-induced early pregnancy factor activity from the perfused rabbit ovary and oviduct, Am J Obstet Gynecol 159:1580, 1988.

68. **Brown MJ, Zogg JL, Schultz GS, Hilton FK,** Increased binding of epidermal growth factor at preimplantation sites in mouse uteri, Endocrinology 124:2882, 1989.

69. **Navot D, Scott RT, Droesch K, Veeck LL, Liu HS, Rosenwaks Z,** The window of embryo transfer and the efficiency of human conception in vitro, Fertil Steril 55:114, 1991.

70. **Kao L-C, Caltabiano S, Wu S, Strauss JF III, Kliman HJ,** The human villous cytotrophoblast: interactions with extracellular matrix proteins, endocrine function, and cytoplasmic differentiation in the absence of synctium formation, Dev Biol 130:693, 1988.

71. **Sobel JS, Nebel L,** Changes in concanavalin A agglutinability during development of the inner cell mass and trophoblast of mouse blastocyst in vitro, J Reprod Fertil 52:239, 1978.

72. **Schlafke S, Enders AC,** Cellular basis of interaction between trophoblast and uterus at implantation, Biol Reprod 12:41, 1975.

73. **Larsen JF,** Electron microscopy of the implantation site in the rabbit, Am J Anat 109:319, 1961.

74. **Strickland S, Reich E, Sherman MI,** Plasminogen activator in early embryogenesis: enzyme production by trophoblast and parietal endoderm, Cell 9:231, 1976.

75. **Queenan JT, Kao LC, Arboleda CE, Ulloa-Aguirre A, Golos TG, Cines DB, Strauss JF,** Regulation of urokinase-type plasminogen activator production by cultured human cytotrophoblasts, J Biol Chem 262:10903, 1987.

76. **Milwidsky A, Finci-Yeheskel Z, Yagel S, Mayer M,** Gonadotropin-mediated inhibition of proteolytic enzymes produced by human trophoblast in culture, J Clin Endocrinol Metab 76:1101, 1993.

77. **Glass RH, Aggeler J, Spindle A, Pedersen RA, Werb Z,** Degradation of extracellular matrix by mouse trophoblast outgrowths: a model for implantation, J Cell Biol 96:1108, 1983.

78. **Moll UM, Lane BL,** Proteolytic activity of first trimester human placenta: localization of interstitial collagenase in villous and extravillous trophoblast, Histochemistry 94:555, 1990.

79. **Glass RH, Spindle AI, Pedersen RA,** Mouse embryo attachment to substratum and the interaction of trophoblast with cultured cells, J Exp Zool 203:327, 1979.

80. **Clark DA, Slapsys RM, Croy BA, Kreck J, Rossant J,** Local active suppression by suppressor cells in the decidua: a review, Am J Reprod Immunol 6:78, 1984.

81. **Salmonsen LA, Doughton BW, Findlay JF,** The effect of the preimplantation blastocyst in vivo and in vitro on protein synthesis and secretion by cultured epithelial cells from sheep endometrium, Endocrinology 119:622, 1986.

82. **King A, Loke YW,** Trophoblast and JEG choriocarcinoma cells are sensitive to lysis by IL-2 stimulated decidual LGL, Cell Immunol 129:435, 1990.

83. **Boving BG,** Implantation, Ann NY Acad Sci 75:700, 1959.

84. **Shelesnyak MC,** Inhibition of decidual cell formation in the pseudopregnant rat by histamine antagonists, Am J Physiol 170:522, 1952.

85. **Brandon JM, Wallis RM,** Effect of mepyramine, a histamine H_1-, and burimamide, a histamine H_2- receptor antagonist, on ovum implantation in the rat, J Reprod Fertil 50:251, 1977.

86. **Dey SK, Johnson DC, Santos JG,** Is histamine production by the blastocyst required for implantation in the rabbit? Biol Reprod 21:1169, 1979.

8 The Endocrinology of Pregnancy

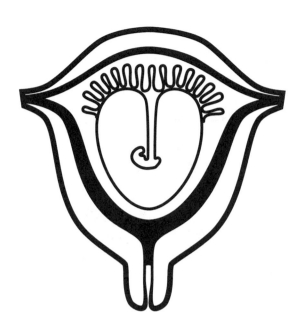

W ho is in charge of pregnancy, the mother or her fetus? For the fetus, one of the crucial aspects of intrauterine life is its dependency on the effective exchange of nutritional and metabolic products with the mother. It is not surprising that mechanisms exist by which a growing fetus can influence or control the exchange process and hence its environment. The methods by which a fetus can influence its own growth and development involve a variety of messages transmitted, in many cases, by hormones. Endocrine messengers from the conceptus can affect metabolic processes, uteroplacental blood flow, and cellular differentiation. Furthermore, a fetus may signal its desire and readiness to leave the uterus by hormonal initiation of parturition (discussed in Chapter 9). This chapter will review the mechanisms by which the fetus establishes influence over metabolic events during pregnancy. The important process of lactation is discussed in Chapter 17.

Steroid Hormones in Pregnancy

Steroidogenesis in the fetal-placental unit does not follow the conventional mechanisms of hormone production within a single organ. Rather, the final products result from critical interactions and interdependence of separate organ systems that individually do not possess the necessary enzymatic capabilities. It is helpful to view the process as consisting of a fetal compartment, a placental compartment, and a maternal compartment. Separately the fetal and placental compartments lack certain steroidogenic activities. Together, however, they are complementary and form a complete unit, which utilizes the maternal compartment as a source of basic building materials and as a resource for clearance of steroids.

Maternal Plasma Progesterone

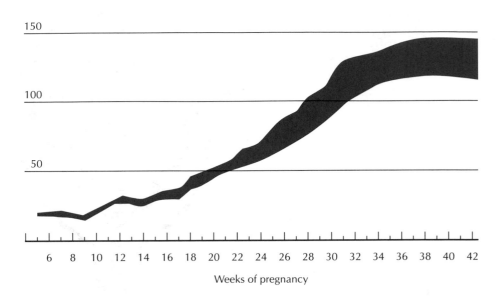

ng/mL

Weeks of pregnancy

Progesterone

In its key location as a way station between mother and fetus, the placenta can utilize precursors from either mother or fetus to circumvent its own deficiencies in enzyme activity. The placenta converts little, if any, acetate to cholesterol or its precursors. Cholesterol as well as pregnenolone are obtained from the maternal bloodstream for progesterone synthesis. The fetal contribution is negligible since progesterone levels remain high after fetal demise. Thus, the massive amount of progesterone produced in pregnancy depends upon placental-maternal cooperation.

Progesterone is largely produced by the corpus luteum until about 10 weeks of gestation. Indeed, until approximately the 7th week, the pregnancy is dependent upon the presence of the corpus luteum.[1] Exogenous support for an early pregnancy (until 10 weeks) requires 100 mg progesterone daily, associated with a maternal circulating level of approximately 10 ng/mL (32 nmol/L).[2] Despite this requirement, patients pregnant after ovarian stimulation with one of the techniques of assisted reproductive technology have concluded a successful pregnancy after experiencing extremely low progesterone levels.[3,4] Thus, individual variation is great, and very low circulating levels of progesterone can be encountered occasionally in women who experience normal pregnancies. The predictive value, therefore, of progesterone measurements is limited.

After a transition period of shared function between the 7th week and 10th week during which there is a slight decline in circulating maternal progesterone levels, the placenta emerges as the major source of progesterone and levels progressively increase.[2,5,6] At term, progesterone levels range from 100 to 200 ng/mL (320–640 nmol/L), and the placenta produces about 250 mg per day. Most of the progesterone produced in the placenta enters the maternal circulation.

In contrast to estrogen, progesterone production by the placenta is largely independent of the quantity of precursor available, the uteroplacental perfusion, fetal well-being, or even the presence of a live fetus. This is because the fetus contributes essentially no

252

precursor. The majority of placental progesterone is derived from maternal cholesterol that is readily available. At term a small portion (3%) is derived from maternal pregnenolone.

The cholesterol utilized for progesterone synthesis enters the trophoblast from the maternal bloodstream as low-density lipoprotein (LDL)-cholesterol, by means of the process of endocytosis (internalization) involving the LDL cell membrane receptors, a process enhanced in pregnancy by estrogen.[6-8] Hydrolysis of the protein component of LDL may yield amino acids for the fetus, and essential fatty acids may be derived from hydrolysis of the cholesterol esters. Unlike steroidogenesis elsewhere, it is not clear whether placental progesterone production requires the control of tropic hormones. While some evidence suggests tropic hormone support is not necessary, other evidence indicates that a small amount of human chorionic gonadotropin (HCG) must be present.[9,10]

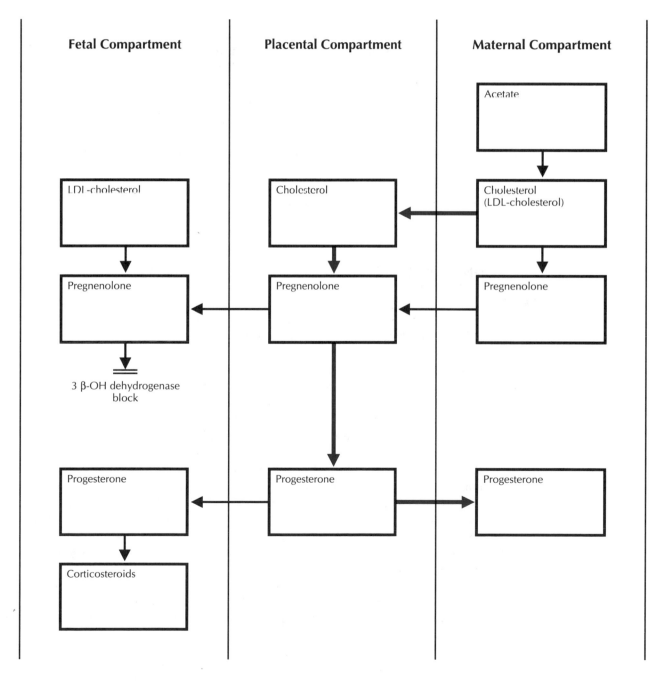

The human decidua and fetal membranes also synthesize and metabolize progesterone.[11] In this case, neither cholesterol nor LDL-cholesterol are significant substrates; pregnenolone sulfate may be the most important precursor. This local steroidogenesis may play a role in regulating parturition.

Amniotic fluid progesterone concentration is maximal between 10 and 20 weeks, then decreases gradually. Myometrial levels are about 3 times higher than maternal plasma levels in early pregnancy, remain high, and are about equal to the maternal plasma concentration at term.

In early pregnancy the levels of 17-hydroxyprogesterone rise, marking the activity of the corpus luteum. By the 10th week of gestation this compound has returned to baseline levels, indicating that the placenta has little 17-hydroxylase activity. However, beginning about the 32nd week there is a second, more gradual rise in 17-hydroxyprogesterone, due to placental utilization of fetal precursors.

There are two active metabolites of progesterone which increase significantly during pregnancy. There is about a 10-fold increase of the 5α-reduced metabolite, 5α-pregnane-3,20-dione.[12] This compound contributes to the refractory state in pregnancy against the pressor action of angiotensin II. The circulating level, however, is the same in normal and hypertensive pregnancies. The concentration of deoxycorticosterone (DOC) at term is 1,200 times the nonpregnant levels. Some of this is due to the 3–4-fold increase in cortisol binding globulin during pregnancy, but a significant amount is due to 21-hydroxylation of circulating progesterone in the kidney.[13] This activity is significant during pregnancy because the rate is proportional to the plasma concentration of progesterone. The fetal kidney is also active in 21-hydroxylation of the progesterone secreted by the placenta into the fetal circulation. At the present time there is no physiologic role known for DOC during pregnancy.

Progesterone has a role in parturition as will be discussed in Chapter 9. It has been suggested that progesterone is important in suppressing the maternal immunological response to fetal antigens, preventing maternal rejection of the trophoblast. Progesterone helps prepare and maintain the endometrium to allow implantation. The human corpus luteum makes significant amounts of estradiol, but it is progesterone and not estrogen that is required for successful implantation.[14] Since implantation normally occurs about 6–7 days after ovulation, and human chorionic gonadotropin (HCG) must appear by the 10th day after ovulation to rescue the corpus luteum, the blastocyst must successfully implant and secrete HCG within a narrow window of time. In the first 5–6 weeks of pregnancy, HCG stimulation of the corpus luteum results in the daily secretion of about 25 mg progesterone and 0.5 mg estradiol. Whereas estrogen levels begin to increase at 4–5 weeks due to placental secretion, progesterone production by the placenta does not significantly increase until about 10–11 weeks after ovulation.

Progesterone serves as the substrate for fetal adrenal gland production of gluco- and mineralocorticoids; however, most of the cortisol synthesis is derived from low-density lipoprotein cholesterol (LDL-cholesterol) obtained from the fetal circulation and synthesized in the fetal liver.[15,16] The fetal zone in the adrenal gland is extremely active, but produces steroids with a 3β-hydroxy-Δ^5 configuration like pregnenolone and dehydroepiandrosterone, rather than 3-keto-Δ^4 products such as progesterone. The fetus therefore lacks significant activity of the 3β-hydroxysteroid-dehydrogenase, Δ^{4-5} isomerase system. Thus, the fetus must borrow progesterone from the placenta to circumvent this lack in order to synthesize the biologically important corticosteroids. In return the fetus supplies what the placenta lacks: 19-carbon compounds to serve as precursors for estrogens.

Steroid levels have been compared in maternal blood, fetal blood, and amniotic fluid obtained at fetsocopy in women undergoing termination of pregnancy at 16–20 weeks gestation.[17] Cortisol, corticosterone, and aldosterone are definitely secreted by the fetal adrenal gland independently of the mother. The fetal arterial-venous differences confirm that placental progesterone is a source for fetal adrenal cortisol and aldosterone.

Estrogens

The basic precursors of estrogens are 19-carbon androgens. However, there is a virtual absence of 17-hydroxylation and 17–20 desmolase activity (P450c17) in the human placenta. As a result, 21-carbon products (progesterone and pregnenolone) cannot be converted to 19-carbon steroids (androstenedione and dehydroepiandrosterone). Like progesterone, estrogen produced by the placenta P450arom enzyme system must derive precursors from outside the placenta.

The androgen compounds utilized for estrogen synthesis in human pregnancy are, in the early months of gestation, derived from the maternal bloodstream. By the 20th week of pregnancy, the vast majority of estrogen excreted in the maternal urine is derived from fetal androgens. In particular, approximately 90% of estriol excretion can be accounted for by dehydroepiandrosterone sulfate (DHAS) production by the fetal adrenal gland.[18] The high output of DHAS by the fetal zone is due to low 3β-hydroxysteroid dehydrogenase gene expression.[19] Removed into cell culture conditions, this gene becomes active in response to ACTH.

The fetal endocrine compartment is characterized by rapid and extensive conjugation of steroids with sulfate. Perhaps this is a protective mechanism, blocking the biologic effects of potent steroids present in such great quantities. In order to utilize fetal precursors, the placenta must be extremely efficient in cleaving the sulfate conjugates brought to it via the fetal bloodstream. Indeed, the sulfatase activity in the placenta is rapid and quantitatively very significant. It is recognized that a deficiency in placental sulfatase is associated with low estrogen excretion, giving clinical importance to this metabolic step. This syndrome will be discussed in greater detail later in this chapter.

The fetal adrenal provides DHAS as precursor for placental production of estrone and estradiol. However, the placenta lacks a 16α-hydroxylation ability, and estriol with its 16α-hydroxyl group must be derived from an immediate fetal precursor. The fetal adrenal, with the aid of 16α-hydroxylation in the fetal liver, provides the 16α-hydroxy-dehydroepiandrosterone sulfate for placental estriol formation. After birth, neonatal 16-hydroxylation activity rapidly disappears. The maternal contribution of DHAS to total estrogen synthesis must be negligible because in the absence of normal fetal adrenal glands (as in an anencephalic infant) maternal estrogen levels and excretion are extremely low. The fetal adrenals secrete more than 200 mg of DHAS daily, about 10 times more than the mother.[20]

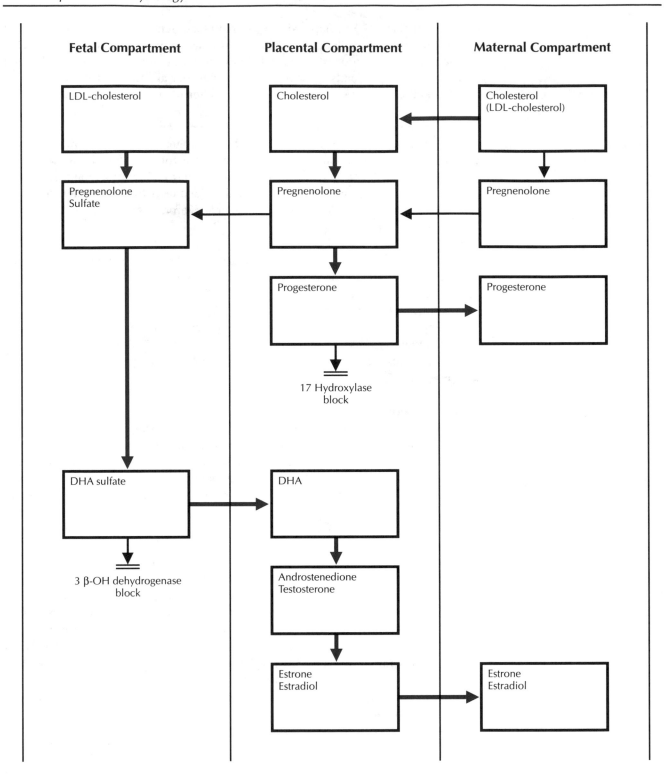

Fetal Compartment

Placental Compartment

Maternal Compartment

LDL-cholesterol

Cholesterol

Cholesterol
(LDL-cholesterol)

Pregnenolone
Sulfate

Pregnenolone

Pregnenolone

Progesterone

Progesterone

17 Hydroxylase
block

DHA sulfate

DHA

3 β-OH dehydrogenase
block

Androstenedione
Testosterone

Estrone
Estradiol

Estrone
Estradiol

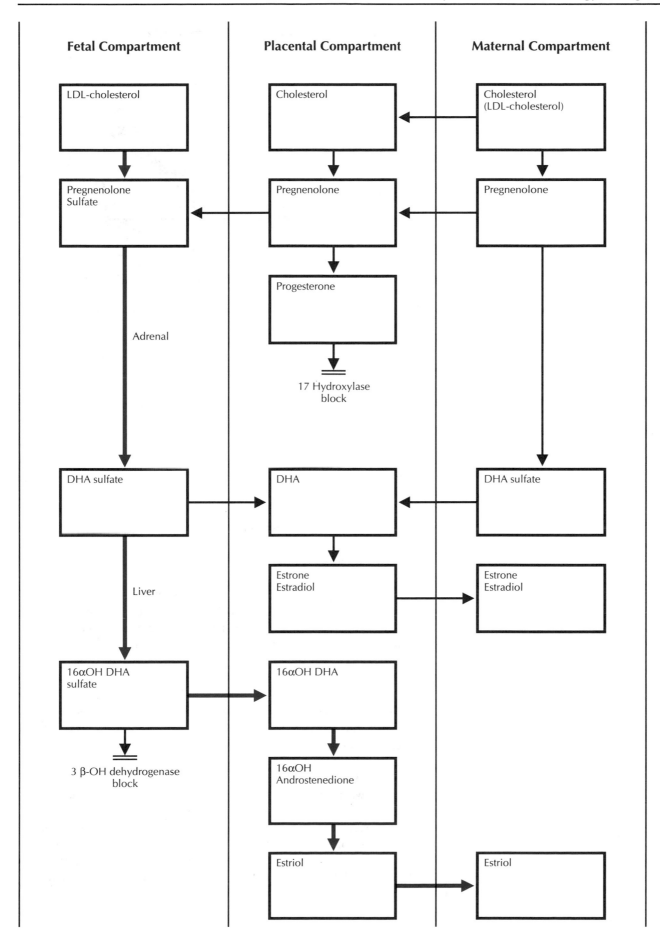

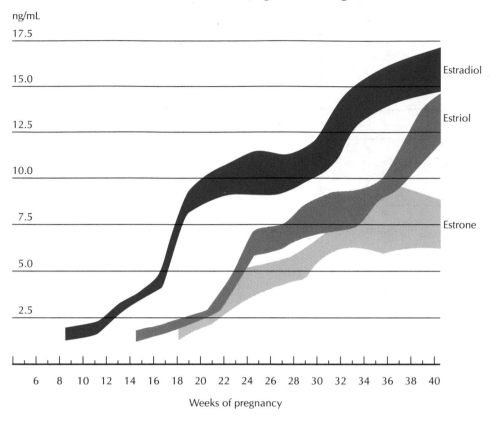

Maternal Plasma Unconjugated Estrogens

The profiles of the unconjugated compounds in the maternal compartment for the three major estrogens in pregnancy are:

1. A rise in estrone begins at 6–10 weeks, and individual values range from 2 to 30 ng/mL at term.[21] This wide range in normal values precludes the use of estrone measurements in clinical applications.

2. A rise in estradiol begins in weeks 6–8 when placental function becomes apparent.[2,22,23] Individual estradiol values vary between 6 and 40 ng/mL (20–150 nmol/L) at 36 weeks of gestation and then undergo an accelerated rate of increase.[21] At term, an equal amount of estradiol arises from maternal DHAS and fetal DHAS, and its importance in fetal monitoring is negligible.

3. Estriol is first detectable at 9 weeks when the fetal adrenal gland secretion of precursor begins. Estriol concentrations plateau at 31–35 weeks, and then increase again at 35–36 weeks.[24]

During pregnancy, estrone and estradiol excretion is increased about 100 times over nonpregnant levels. However, the increase in maternal estriol excretion is about a thousand-fold. The traditional view that estriol is a weak estrogen metabolite is not accurate. A weak estrogen provided in high concentrations can produce a biologic response equivalent to that of estradiol.[25] Because of its high production and concentration, estriol is an important hormone in pregnancy. The maternal level of estradiol is higher than the level in the fetus; in contrast, the estriol level in the fetus is greater than in the mother.

The estrogens presented to the maternal bloodstream are rapidly metabolized by the maternal liver prior to excretion into the maternal urine as a variety of more than 20 products. The bulk of these maternal urinary estrogens is composed of glucosiduronates conjugated at the 16-position. Significant amounts of the 3-glucosiduronate and the 3-sulfate-16-glucosiduronate are also excreted. Only approximately 8–10% of the maternal blood estriol is unconjugated.

The Fetal Adrenal Cortex

The fetal adrenal cortex is differentiated by 7 weeks into a thick inner fetal zone and a thin outer definitive zone, the source of cortisol and the forerunner of the adult cortex. Early in pregnancy, adrenal growth and development are remarkable, and the gland achieves a size equal to or larger than that of the kidney by the end of the first trimester. After the first trimester the adrenal glands slowly decrease in size until a second spurt in growth begins at about 34–35 weeks. The gland remains proportionately larger than the adult adrenal glands. After delivery, the fetal zone (about 80% of the bulk of the gland) rapidly involutes to be replaced by the adult definitive zone of the adrenal cortex. Thus, the specific steroidogenic characteristics of the fetus are associated with a specific morphologic change of the adrenal gland.

Fetal dehydroepiandrosterone (DHA) and DHAS production rises steadily concomitant with the increase in the fetal zone and adrenal weight.[26] The well-known increase in maternal estrogen levels is significantly influenced by the increased availability of fetal DHAS as a precursor. Indeed, the accelerated rise in maternal estrogen levels near term can be explained in part by an increase in fetal DHAS. The stimulus for the substantial adrenal growth and steroid production has been a puzzle.

Early in pregnancy, the adrenal gland can function without ACTH, perhaps in response to HCG. After 20 weeks, fetal ACTH is required. However, during the last 12–14 weeks of pregnancy when fetal ACTH levels are declining, the adrenal quadruples in size.[27] Because pituitary prolactin is the only fetal pituitary hormone to increase throughout pregnancy, paralleling fetal adrenal gland size changes, it has been proposed that fetal prolactin is the critical tropic substance. In experimental preparations, however, only ACTH exerts a steroidogenic effect. There is no fetal adrenal response to prolactin, HCG, growth hormone, melanocyte-stimulating hormone (MSH), or thyrotropin releasing hormone (TRH).[28,29] Furthermore, in patients treated with bromocriptine, fetal blood prolactin levels are suppressed, but DHAS levels are unchanged.[30] Nevertheless, interest in prolactin persists because both ACTH and prolactin can stimulate steroidogenesis in vivo in the fetal baboon.[31]

There is no question that ACTH is essential for the morphologic development and the steroidogenic mechanism of the fetal adrenal gland.[32,33] ACTH activates adenylate cyclase, leading to steroidogenesis. Soon the supply of cholesterol becomes rate limiting. Further ACTH action results in an increase in LDL receptors leading to an increased uptake of circulating LDL-cholesterol.[15] With internalization of LDL-cholesterol, hydrolysis by lysosomal enzymes of the cholesterol ester makes cholesterol available for steroidogenesis. For this reason, fetal plasma levels of LDL are low, and after birth newborn levels of LDL rise as the fetal adrenal involutes. In the presence of low levels of LDL-cholesterol, the fetal adrenal is capable of synthesizing cholesterol de novo.[34] Thus near term, both de novo synthesis and utilization of LDL-cholesterol are necessary to sustain the high rates of DHAS and estrogen formation. The tropic support of the fetal adrenal gland by ACTH from the fetal pituitary is protected by placental estrogen. The placenta prevents maternal cortisol from reaching the fetus by converting cortisol to cortisone. This 11β-hydroxysteroid dehydrogenase activity is stimulated by placental estrogen.[35]

Adrenal gland steroidogenesis involves autocrine and paracrine regulation. Fetal adrenal cells produce inhibin, and the alpha-subunit is preferentially increased by ACTH.[36,37] Inhibin consists of two dissimilar peptides, alpha- and beta-subunits, linked by disulfide bonds. Inhibin A and inhibin B each contain an identical alpha-subunit, but distinct beta-subunits. Activin contains two subunits which are identical to the beta-subunits of the inhibins.

The Two Forms of Inhibin

Inhibin-A:	Alpha-Beta$_A$
Inhibin-B:	Alpha-Beta$_B$

The Three Forms of Activin

Activin-A:	Beta$_A$-Beta$_A$
Activin-AB:	Beta$_A$-Beta$_B$
Activin-B:	Beta$_B$-Beta$_B$

Activin enhances ACTH-stimulated steroidogenesis while inhibiting mitogenesis in human fetal adrenal cells.[37] This effect on steroidogenic activity is not present in adult adrenal cells. In vitro, activin enhances a shift in fetal adrenal cells from ACTH stimulation of DHAS production to cortisol production. This shift is analogous to the shift that occurs after birth. Perhaps activin plays this role in the remodeling of the fetal zone in the newborn. A specific action for inhibin in fetal adrenal cells has not been described.

The insulin-like growth factors (IGF-I and IGF-II) are important in mediating the tropic effects of ACTH. IGF-II production in the fetal adrenal is very significant and is stimulated by ACTH. IGF-II is believed to be important in prenatal growth.[38] The abundance of IGF-II in the fetal adrenal gland implicates this growth factor as a mediator of ACTH-induced growth.[39] Both IGF-I and IGF-II are equally mitogenic in a cell culture system of fetal adrenal cells and enhance the proliferation stimulated by basic fibroblast growth factor and epidermal growth factor.[39] However, only transcription of IGF-II is stimulated by ACTH. Thus, the growth promoting effects of ACTH are mediated by various growth factors, with a principal role played by IGF-II. In this regard, the fetal adrenal differs from the adult adrenal where IGF-I is predominant.

The unique features of the fetal adrenal gland can be ascribed to its high estrogen environment. A series of tissue culture studies has demonstrated that hormonal peptides of pituitary or placental origin are not the factors which are responsible for the behavior of the fetal adrenal gland.[40–42] Estrogens at high concentration inhibit 3β-hydroxysteroid dehydrogenase-isomerase activity in the fetal adrenal gland and, in the presence of ACTH, enhance the secretion of dehydroepiandrosterone (DHA). Estradiol concentrations of 10–100 ng/mL (37–370 nmol/L) are required to inhibit cortisol secretion.[43] The total estrogen concentrations in the fetus are easily in this range. A study of the kinetics of 3β-hydroxysteroid dehydrogenase activity in human adrenal microsomes reveals that all steroids are inhibitory, and most notably, estrone and estradiol at levels found in fetal life cause almost total inhibition.[44] The hyperplasia of the fetal adrenal may be the result of the high ACTH levels due to the relatively low cortisol levels, a consequence of the enzyme inhibition.

The development of the adrenal gland during human fetal life and during the neonatal period is paralleled in the baboon.[45] The adrenal cortex of the fetal baboon is characterized by the same deficiency in 3β-hydroxysteroid dehydrogenase as is seen in the human, with the same diversion of steroidogenesis into production of DHAS. Treatment of the neonatal baboon with estrogens and progesterone did not halt the regression of the fetal zone and DHAS production, arguing against the hypothesis that the fetal zone is

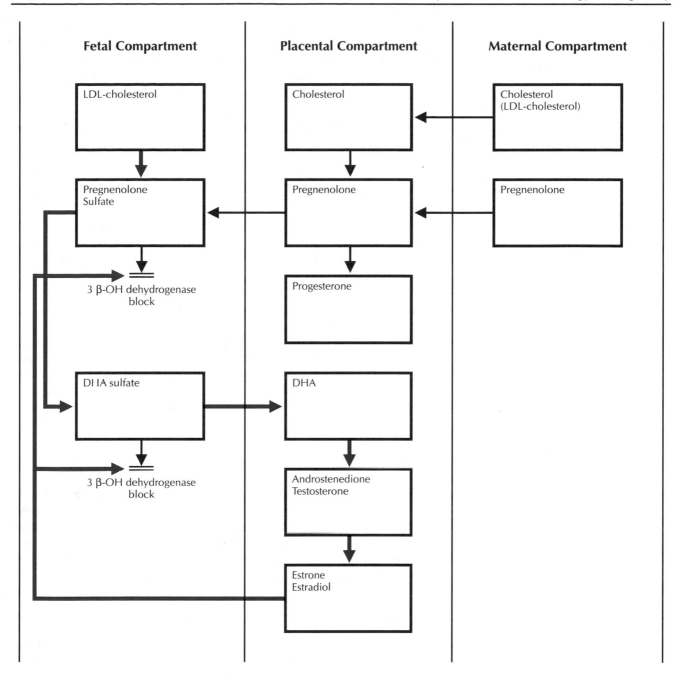

| **Fetal Compartment** | **Placental Compartment** | **Maternal Compartment** |

dependent upon an estrogen-induced deficiency in 3β-hydroxysteroid dehydrogenase. It continues to be uncertain, however, whether the internal microenvironment of the adrenal gland can be affected by the exogenous administration of steroids. In vitro studies of human fetal zone cells indicate that estradiol and IGF-II combine to direct steroidogenesis to DHAS in a mechanism not due to inhibition of 3β-hydroxysteroid dehydrogenase.[46] In addition, there is a virtual absence of estrogen receptors in the fetal zone of monkey adrenal glands.[47]

The principal mission of the fetal adrenal may be to provide DHAS as the basic precursor for placental estrogen production. Estrogen, in turn, feeds back to the adrenal to direct steroidogenesis along the Δ^5 pathway to provide even more of its precursor, DHAS. Thus far this is the only known function for DHAS. With birth and loss of exposure to estrogen, the fetal adrenal gland quickly changes to the adult type of gland.

Measurement of Estrogen in Pregnancy

Because pregnancy is characterized by a great increase in maternal estrogen levels, and estrogen production is dependent upon fetal and placental steroidogenic cooperation, the amount of estrogen present in the maternal blood or urine reflects both fetal and placental enzymatic capability and, hence, well-being. Attention focuses on estriol because 90% of maternal estriol is derived from fetal precursors. The end product to be assayed in the maternal blood or urine is influenced by a multitude of factors. Availability of precursor from the fetal adrenal gland is a prime requisite as well as the ability of the placenta to carry out its conversion steps. Maternal metabolism of the product as well as the efficiency of maternal renal excretion of the product can modify the daily amount of estrogen in the urine. Blood flow to any of the key organs in the fetus, placenta, and mother becomes important.[48,49] Fetal hypoxemia due to reduced uteroplacental blood flow is associated with a marked increase in adrenal androgen production in response to an increase in fetal ACTH and, in response to the availability of androgen precursors, an increase in maternal estrogen levels.[50] The response to acute stress is in contrast to the effect of chronic uteroplacental insufficiency which is associated with a reduction in fetal androgens and maternal estrogens. In addition, drugs or diseases can affect any level in the cascade of events leading up to assay of estrogen.

For years, measurement of estrogen in a 24-hour urine collection was the standard hormonal method of assessing fetal well-being. This was replaced by immunoassay of unconjugated estriol in the plasma.[51] Because of its short half-life (5–10 minutes) in the maternal circulation, unconjugated estriol has less variation than urinary or total blood estriol.

Normal Values and Interpretation

There are two essential aspects to the clinical use of estriol assays. First, a single specimen is meaningless. Daily assays must be performed to provide a serial assessment of sequential changes. Second, to be significant, there must be a decrease of approximately 40% from the mean of the three highest consecutive values.[51,52] While estrogen levels in the mother are related to the size of the fetal adrenal gland and its production of precursor, there is a poor correlation between birth weight and plasma estriol levels. Macrosomia is not always associated with high estriol levels. However, excessive adrenal activity as in congenital adrenal hyperplasia can be associated with unusually high levels.

Problems

Drugs that affect the maternal estrogen level include corticosteroids and antibiotics. Corticosteroids administered to the mother cross the placenta poorly, and large amounts (the equivalent of 75 mg cortisol daily) are required to suppress fetal adrenal production of estriol precursor. The synthetic steroids, dexamethasone and betamethasone, however, cross the placenta more easily, and maternal estriol assessment is not reliable for at least 1 week, and sometimes 2 weeks, after the last dose. Antibiotics which affect the flora of the maternal gastrointestinal tract depress maternal total estriol levels by interfering with the enterohepatic circulation. Such antibiotics inhibit hydrolysis of the biliary estriol conjugates in the gut, preventing their reabsorption and reconjugation, leading to loss of estriol in the feces. Total blood and urinary estriol decline, but unconjugated estriol is unaffected. Falsely elevated blood total estriols will be encountered in the presence of renal disease or when a patient is receiving oxytocin for the induction of labor because of the antidiuretic action of oxytocin, but the levels of unconjugated estriol will not be affected.

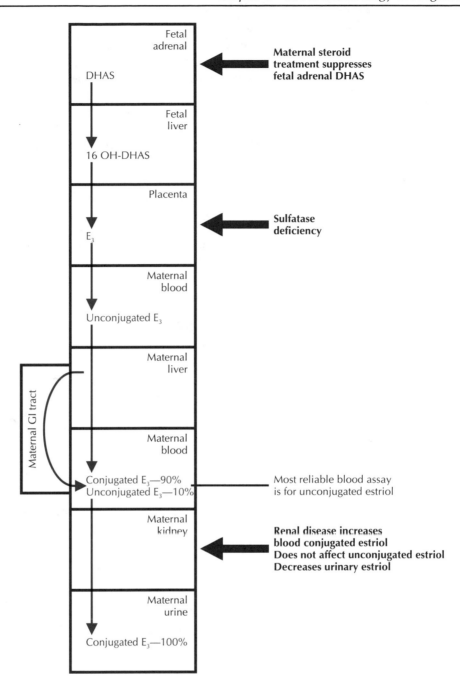

Maternal steroid treatment suppresses fetal adrenal DHAS

Sulfatase deficiency

Most reliable blood assay is for unconjugated estriol

Renal disease increases blood conjugated estriol
Does not affect unconjugated estriol
Decreases urinary estriol

Clinical Uses of Estriol Assays

Assessment of maternal estriol levels has been superseded by various biophysical fetal monitoring techniques such as nonstress testing, stress testing, and measurement of fetal breathing and activity. Nevertheless, in certain clinical situations the addition of estriol assays is useful. The combination of a low estriol and a positive stress test is ominous. Certainly patients should not be managed by estriols alone. While a low estriol and a positive stress test indicate a fetus in jeopardy, a low estriol with a negative stress test allows postponement of intervention. Modern screening for fetal aneuploidy (discussed later in the chapter) utilizes 3 markers in the maternal circulation: alpha fetoprotein, human chorionic gonadotropin, and unconjugated estriol.

Amniotic Fluid Estrogen Measurements

Amniotic fluid estriol is correlated with the fetal estrogen pattern rather than the maternal. Most of the estriol in the amniotic fluid is present as 16-glucosiduronate or as

3-sulfate-16-glucosiduronate. A small amount exists as 3-sulfate. Very little unconjugated estriol is present in the amniotic fluid because free estriol is rapidly transferred across the placenta and membranes. Estriol sulfate is low in concentration because the placenta and fetal membranes hydrolyze the sulfated conjugates, and the free estriol is then passed out of the fluid. Because the membranes and the placenta have no glucuronidase activity, the glucosiduronate conjugates are removed slowly from the fetus. The glucosiduronates therefore predominate in the fetal urine and the amniotic fluid. Because of the slow changes in glucosiduronates, measurements of amniotic fluid estriol have wide variations in both normal and abnormal pregnancies. An important clinical use for amniotic fluid estrogen measurements has not emerged.

Estetrol

Estetrol (15α-hydroxyestriol) is formed from fetal precursor, and is very dependent upon 15-hydroxylation activity in the fetal liver. The capacity for 15-hydroxylation of estrogens increases during fetal life, reaching a maximum at term. This activity then declines during infancy and is low, absent, or undetectable in adults. The clinical use of maternal blood and urine estetrol measurements is of no advantage over the usual estriol assessment.

Placental Sulfatase

There is an X-linked metabolic disease expressed by a placental sulfatase deficiency, and postnatally, ichthyosis, occurring in about 1 in 2,000–6,000 newborns.[53] Patients with the placental sulfatase disorder are unable to hydrolyze DHAS or 16α-hydroxy-DHAS, and, therefore, the placenta cannot form normal amounts of estrogen. A deficiency in placental sulfatase is usually discovered when patients go beyond term and are found to have extremely low estriol levels and no evidence of fetal distress. The patients usually fail to go into labor and require delivery by cesarean section. Most striking is the failure of cervical softening and dilatation; thus a cervical dystocia occurs that is resistant to oxytocin stimulation. There are many case reports of this deficiency, almost all detected by finding low estriol levels. All newborn children, with a few exceptions, have been male. The steroid sulfatase X-linked recessive ichthyosis locus has been mapped on the distal short arm portion of the X chromosome. There are no known geographic or racial factors which affect the gene frequency.

The characteristic steroid findings are as follows: extremely low estriol and estetrol in the mother with extremely high amniotic fluid DHAS and normal amniotic fluid DHA and androstenedione. The normal DHA and androstenedione with a high DHAS rule out congenital adrenal hyperplasia. The small amount of estriol which is present in these patients probably arises from 16-hydroxylation of DHAS in the maternal liver, thus providing 16-hydroxylated DHA to the placenta for aromatization to estriol. Measurement in maternal urine of steroids derived from fetal sulfated compounds is a simple and reliable means of prenatal diagnosis. Demonstration of a high level of DHAS in the amniotic fluid is reliable. To establish the diagnosis with certainty, a decrease in sulfatase activity should be demonstrated in an in vitro incubation of placental tissue. The clinician should keep in mind that fresh tissue is needed for this procedure as freezing lowers enzyme activity. Alternatively, steroid sulfatase activity can be assayed in leukocytes.

It is now recognized that steroid sulfatase deficiency is present in other tissues and can persist after birth. These children develop ichthyosis, characterized by hyperkeratosis (producing scales on the neck, trunk, and palms) and associated with corneal opacities, pyloric stenosis, and cryptorchidism. The skin fibroblasts have a low activity of steroid sulfatase, and scale formation that occurs early in the first year of life is thought to be due to an alteration in the cholesterol:cholesterol ester ratio (due to the accumulation of cholesterol sulfate). This inherited disorder thus represents a single entity: placental sulfatase deficiency and X-linked ichthyosis, both reflecting a deficiency of microsomal sulfatase. A family history of scaling in males (as well as repeated postdate pregnancies and cesarean sections) should prompt an effort to establish a diagnosis prenatally. Because the clinical use of estriol measurements has declined, there is no effective method to identify the presence of this problem in women with normal obstetrical histories.

Protein Hormones of Pregnancy

The two main trophoblastic layers consist of the cytotrophoblast, separate mononuclear cells prominent early in pregnancy and sparse late in pregnancy, and the syncytiotrophoblast, a continuous multinuclear layer on the surface of the villi. The cytotrophoblast is the basic placental stem cell from which the syncytiotrophoblasts arise by differentiation. The syncytiotrophoblast is, therefore, the functional cell of the placenta, the major site of hormone and protein production. Control of this important cellular differentiation is still not understood; however, the process is influenced by HCG and, undoubtedly, a variety of growth factors.[54] The releasing hormones, neurohormones, inhibin, and activin are produced in the cytotrophoblast. The surface of the syncytiotrophoblast is in direct contact with the maternal blood in the intervillous space. This may be a reason why placental proteins are secreted preferentially into the mother.

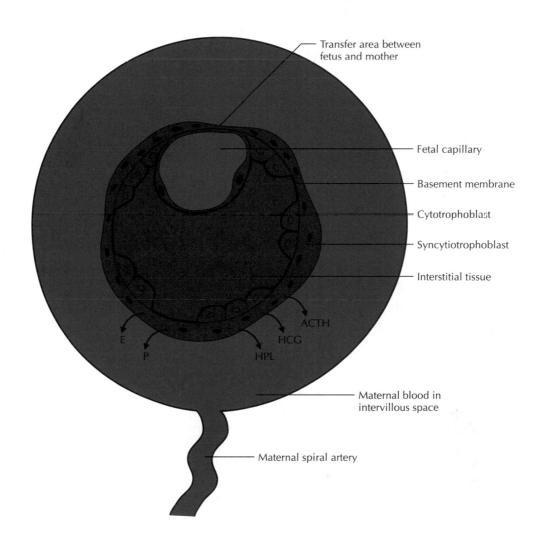

Transfer area between fetus and mother

Fetal capillary

Basement membrane

Cytotrophoblast

Syncytiotrophoblast

Interstitial tissue

ACTH
HCG
HPL
E
P

Maternal blood in intervillous space

Maternal spiral artery

Proteins Associated with Pregnancy

Fetal Compartment	Placental Compartment	Maternal Compartment

Alpha-fetoprotein	Hypothalamic-like hormones
	  GnRH
	  CRH
	  TRH
	  Somatostatin
	
	Pituitary-like hormones
	  HCG
	  HPL
	  HGH
	  HCT
	  ACTH
	
	Growth factors
	  IGF-I
	  Epidermal growth factor
	  Platelet-derived growth factor
	  Fibroblast growth factor
	  Transforming growth factor-β
	  Inhibin
	  Activin
	
	Cytokines
	  Interleukin-1
	  Interleukin-6
	  Colony stimulating factor-1
	
	Other
	  Opiates
	  Prorenin
	  Pregnancy-specific β₁-glycoprotein
	  Pregnancy-associated plasma protein A
		Decidual proteins
		  Prolactin
		  Relaxin
		  IGFBP-1
		  Interleukin-1
		  Colony stimulating factor-1
		  Progesterone-associated endometrial protein
		
		Corpus luteum proteins
		  Relaxin
		  Prorenin

Hypothalamic-like Releasing Hormones

The human placenta contains many releasing and inhibiting hormones, including gonadotropin releasing hormone (GnRH), corticotropin releasing hormone (CRH), thyrotropin releasing hormone (TRH) and somatostatin.[55] Because of the presence of hypothalamic-like releasing hormones in an organ that produces tropic hormones, we are motivated to construct a system of regulation analogous to the hypothalamic-pituitary axis. However, as we shall see, this proves to be very difficult.

Immunoreactive GnRH can be localized in the cytotrophoblast. Evidence indicates that placental GnRH regulates placental steroidogenesis and release of prostaglandins as well as HCG.[55–59] The highest amount of GnRH is produced early in pregnancy when the number of cytotrophoblasts is greatest and HCG secretion reaches its peak. The placental binding site for GnRH has a lower affinity than that of GnRH receptors in the pituitary, ovary, and testis.[60] This reflects the situation in which the binding site is in close proximity to the site of secretion for the regulatory hormone. A higher affinity is not necessary because of the large amount of GnRH available in the placenta, and the low affinity receptors avoid response to the low levels of circulating GnRH. GnRH release is increased by estrogen and activin, and inhibited by progesterone, endogenous opiates, and inhibin.

In addition to cytotrophoblasts, CRH is produced in the fetal membranes and the decidua. Its production is regulated by steroids, decreased by progesterone and, in contrast to the usual negative feedback action in the hypothalamus, increased by glucocorticoids.[61] These interactions are consistent with the increase in fetal and maternal ACTH and cortisol associated with the last weeks of pregnancy and labor. Placental CRH is further regulated (as in the hypothalamus) by an array of neuropeptides such as vasopressin, norepinephrine, angiotensin II, and oxytocin. CRH release is stimulated by activin and inhibited by inhibin.

Other releasing hormones that have been identified in the placenta are thyrotropin releasing hormone (TRH) and growth hormone releasing hormone. There is little known regarding the physiologic roles for these hormones.

Human Chorionic Gonadotropin (HCG)	Human chorionic gonadotropin is a glycoprotein, a peptide framework to which carbohydrate side chains are attached.[62] Alterations in the carbohydrate components (about one-third of the molecular weight) change the biologic properties. For example, the long half-life of HCG is approximately 24 hours as compared to 2 hours for luteinizing hormone (LH), a 10-fold difference which is due mainly to the greater sialic acid content of HCG. As with the other glycoproteins, follicle-stimulating hormone (FSH), LH, and thyroid-stimulating hormone (TSH), HCG consists of two noncovalently linked subunits, called alpha (α) and beta (β). The α-subunits in these glycoprotein hormones are identical, consisting of 92 amino acids. Unique biological activity as well as specificity in immunoassays is attributed to the molecular and carbohydrate differences in the β-subunits (see "Heterogeneity" in Chapter 2).

A single gene on chromosome 6 encodes the α-subunit for the four glycoprotein tropic hormones. The genes that encode for the beta-subunits of HCG, LH, and TSH are located in a cluster on chromosome 19.[63] There is one gene for β-LH, but there are 6 genes for the β-subunit of HCG, each with different promotor activity. Only two of the genes are actively transcribed, and it is not certain why there are two active genes for β-HCG. It may be necessary for the high output of HCG during pregnancy, and it may reflect the relatively recent and rapid evolution of the β-HCG cluster. Only primates and horses have genes for β-CG. In contrast to the primate, the equine β-CG gene is identical to the equine β-LH gene, i.e., a single gene produces the β-subunits for both LH and CG. The primate β-CG gene is thus believed to have evolved from an ancestral β-LH gene. The most logical reason for this evolvement is development of new control mechanisms for gene expression in the placenta producing a glycosylated gonadotropin with a longer half-life. In this process, a single base deletion caused a read-through mutation of a stop signal in the β-LH gene, leading to the extended carboxy terminal sequence of β-HCG.

The similarity of HCG to LH suggests that a similar regulatory system for HCG secretion is operative, specifically involving gonadotropin releasing hormone (GnRH). Placental tissue synthesizes GnRH that is identical to pituitary GnRH.[64] GnRH stimulates pulsatile HCG secretion in in vitro systems with placental tissue, although response requires a higher concentration of GnRH compared to the pituitary gland.[65] Similar responses can be demonstrated with other peptides, such as interleukin-1β.[66] HCG production and secretion are the product of complex interaction among the sex steroids, cytokines, GnRH, and growth factors.

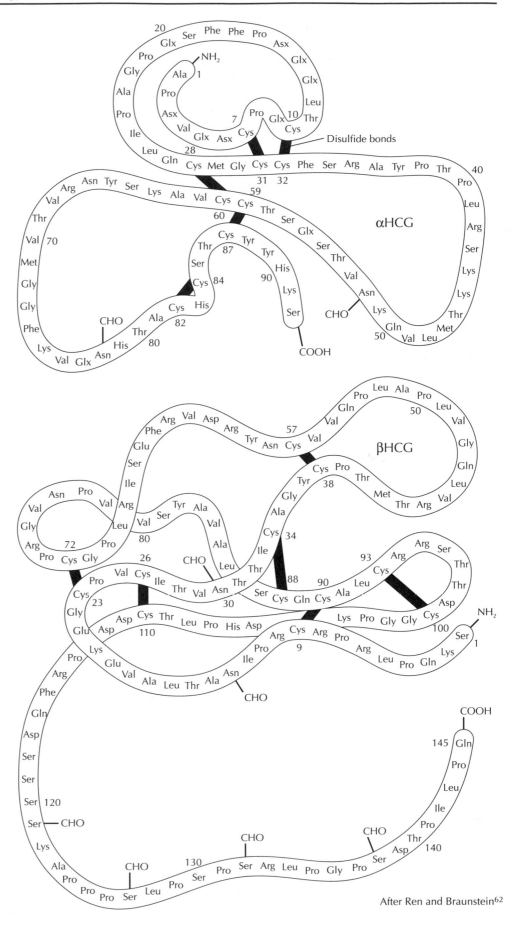

After Ren and Braunstein[62]

GnRH is synthesized by placental cells; GnRH receptors are present on placental cells, and GnRH stimulates the secretion of HCG and the steroid hormones in in vitro studies of placental cells.[67] The secretion and action of GnRH are modulated by many factors, but especially noteworthy is the stimulatory action of activin and the inhibitory influence of inhibin.[68] In addition, estrogen stimulates and progesterone reduces GnRH release.[69] As in the hypothalamus, endogenous opioid peptides inhibit GnRH release in the placenta. While a relatively clear story can be constructed into a working concept regarding the autocrine/paracrine interactions in the regulation of the menstrual cycle (Chapter 6), placental function is more complex, and a simple presentation of the many interactions cannot be produced. For example, epidermal growth factor stimulates HCG secretion, but also stimulates inhibin secretion in placental cells, and inhibin suppresses GnRH stimulation of HCG.[70] Inhibin secretion in the placenta is further stimulated by prostaglandins.[71]

Can the cytotrophoblast-syncytiotrophoblast relationship be compared to the hypothalamic-pituitary axis? It does appear that hypothalamic-like peptides (CRH, GnRH) originate in the cytotrophoblast and influence the syncytiotrophoblast to secrete pituitary-like hormones (HCG, HPL, ACTH). Unraveling the interaction is made more difficult by the incredible complexity of the syncytiotrophoblast, a tissue that produces and responds to steroid and peptide hormones, growth factors, and neuropeptides. The best we can say is that locally produced hormones, growth factors, and peptides work together to regulate placental function.

The carboxy-terminal 24 amino acids of the β-HCG subunit are unique and critical for the biologic activity of HCG. This uniqueness allows specific antisera to discriminate between HCG and LH. Despite this difference, HCG is biologically similar to LH. To this day, the only definitely known function for HCG is support of the corpus luteum, taking over for LH on about the 8th day after ovulation, one day after implantation, when β-HCG first can be detected in maternal blood. HCG has been detected at the 8-cell stage in the embryo using molecular biology techniques.[72]

Continued survival of the corpus luteum is totally dependent upon HCG, and, in turn, survival of the pregnancy is dependent upon steroids from the corpus luteum until the 7th week of pregnancy.[1] From the 7th week to the 10th week, the corpus luteum is gradually replaced by the placenta, and by the 10th week, removal of the corpus luteum will not be followed by steroid withdrawal abortion.

It is very probable, but not conclusively proven, that HCG stimulates steroidogenesis in the early fetal testes, so that androgen production will ensue and masculine differentiation can be accomplished.[73] It is also possible that the function of the inner fetal zone of the adrenal cortex depends upon HCG for steroidogenesis early in pregnancy. The β-HCG gene is expressed in fetal kidney and fetal adrenal, suggesting that HCG may affect the development and function of these organs.[74]

HCG is secreted by the syncytiotrophoblast. The maternal circulating HCG concentration is approximately 100 IU/L at the time of the expected but missed menses. A maximal level of about 100,000 IU/L in the maternal circulation is reached at 8–10 weeks of gestation. Why does the corpus luteum involute at the time that HCG is reaching its highest levels? One possibility is that a specific inhibitory agent becomes active at this time. Another is down-regulation of receptors by the high levels of HCG. In early pregnancy, down-regulation may be avoided because HCG is secreted in an episodic fashion.[75] For unknown reasons, the fetal testes escape desensitization; no receptor down-regulation takes place.[73]

HCG levels decrease to about 10,000–20,000 IU/L by 18–20 weeks and remain at that level to term. It is not certain why HCG levels are decreased in the second half of pregnancy. Advancing gestation is associated with increasing amounts of "nicked" HCG molecules in the maternal circulation.[76] These molecules are missing a peptide linkage on the beta-subunit, and therefore, they dissociate into free α- and β-subunits. At any one point in time the maternal circulation contains HCG, nicked HCG, free subunits, and fragments of HCG. The production of normal molecules is maximal in early gestation when the biologic actions of HCG are so important.

In the complex process of HCG regulation, several inhibiting factors have been identified, including inhibin and progesterone. The decline in HCG occurs at the time of increasing placental progesterone production, and a direct inhibition by this steroid could explain the lower levels of HCG after the 10th week of gestation.[77]

HCG levels close to term are higher in women bearing female fetuses. This is true of serum levels, placental content, urinary levels, and amniotic fluid concentrations. The mechanism and purpose of this difference are not known.

There are two clinical conditions in which blood HCG titers are very helpful: trophoblastic disease and ectopic pregnancies. Early pregnancy is characterized by the sequential appearance of HCG, followed by β-HCG and then α-HCG. The ratio of β-HCG to whole HCG remains constant after early pregnancy. Trophoblastic disease is distinguished by very high β-HCG levels (3–100 times higher than normal pregnancy). Ectopic production of alpha- and beta-HCG by nontrophoblastic tumors is rare. Previous studies with polyclonal antisera suggesting ectopic production were not accurate. The production of whole HCG in such tumors may not occur.

Following molar pregnancies the HCG titer should fall to a nondetectable level by 16 weeks in patients without persistent disease. Patients with trophoblastic disease show an abnormal curve (a titer greater than 500 IU/L) frequently by 3 weeks and usually by 6 weeks.[78,79] A diagnosis of gestational trophoblastic disease is made when the β-HCG plateaus or rises over a 2 week period, or a continued elevation is present 16 weeks after evacuation. In the United States, the rare occurrence of this disease mandates consultation with a certified subspecialist in gynecologic oncology. Following treatment, HCG should be measured monthly for at least a year, then twice yearly for 5 years.

In order to avoid unnecessary treatment (prophylactic chemotherapy) of the 80–85% of patients who undergo spontaneous remission, there is a need to identify those at high risk for persistent disease. An immunoassay for the free beta-subunit of HCG may serve this need in that persistent trophoblastic disease is associated with excessive production of the free beta-subunit.[80,81]

Virtually all ectopic pregnancies are associated with detectable HCG. The HCG level increases at different rates in normal and ectopic pregnancies, and the quantitative measurement of HCG combined with pelvic ultrasonography has had an enormous impact on the diagnosis and management of ectopic pregnancy. This important clinical problem is discussed fully in Chapter 32. The contributions of HCG measurement can be summarized as follows:

1. The quantitative measurement of HCG can assess pregnancy viability. A normal rate of rise usually indicates a normal pregnancy.

2. When the HCG titer exceeds 1,000–1,500 IU/L, vaginal ultrasonography should identify the presence of an intrauterine gestation.

3. Declining HCG levels are consistent with effective treatment, and persistent or rising levels indicate the presence of viable trophoblastic tissue.

With the use of modern sensitive assays, it is now appreciated that virtually all normal human tissues produce the intact HCG molecule. HCG can be detected in the blood of normal men and women, where it is secreted in a pulsatile fashion in parallel with LH, and apparently the source of this circulating HCG is the pituitary gland.[82,83] The concentration of this pituitary HCG normally reaches the sensitivity of the usual modern assay only in a rare postmenopausal woman with high LH levels. HCG produced in sites other than the placenta has little or no carbohydrate, and therefore it has a very short half-life and is rapidly cleared from the circulation.

Human Placental Lactogen (HPL)

Human placental lactogen (sometimes called human chorionic somatomammotropin), also secreted by the syncytiotrophoblast, is a single chain polypeptide of 191 amino acids held together by two disulfide bonds. It is very similar in structure to human growth hormone (HGH), but has only 3% of HGH somatotropin activity. The growth hormone-HPL gene family consists of 5 genes on chromosome 17. Two genes encode for HGH and 3 for HPL; however, only 2 of the HPL genes are active in the placenta, each producing the same HPL hormone.[84]

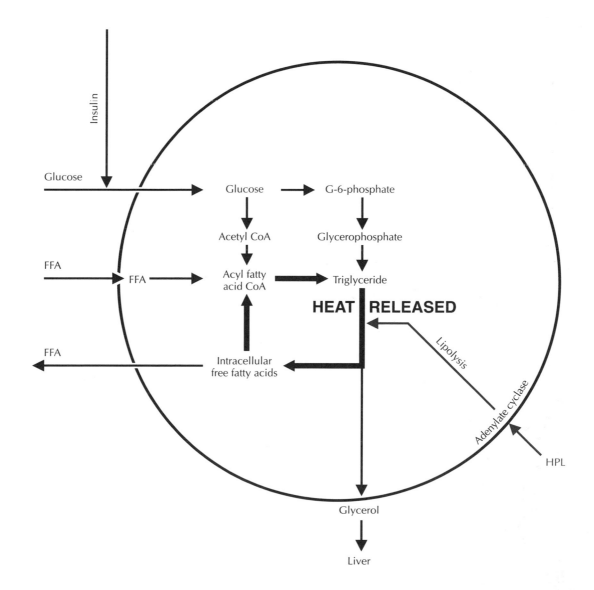

HPL Changes in the Fed State

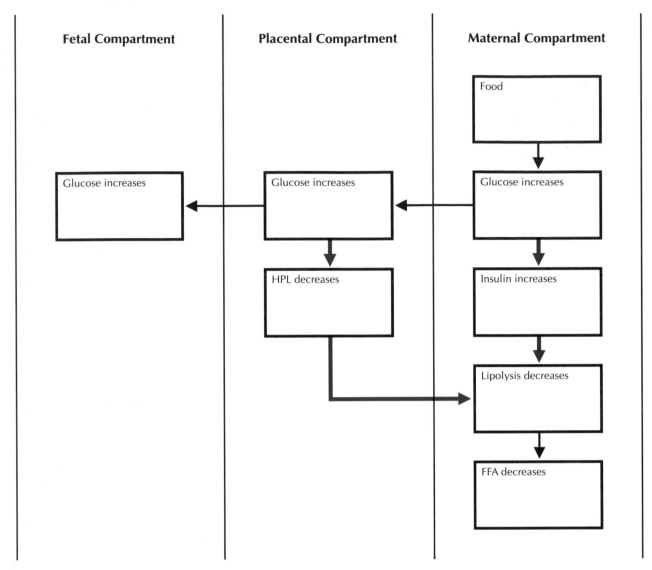

Although HPL has about 50% of the lactogenic activity of sheep prolactin in certain bioassays, its lactogenic contribution in human pregnancy is uncertain. Its half-life is short, about 15 minutes; hence its appeal as an index of placental problems. The level of HPL in the maternal circulation is correlated with fetal and placental weight, steadily increasing until plateauing in the last 4 weeks of pregnancy (5–7 μg/mL). There is no circadian variation, and only minute amounts of HPL enter the fetal circulation. Very high maternal levels are found in association with multiple gestations; levels up to 40 μg/mL have been found with quadruplets and quintuplets. An abnormally low level is anything less than 4 μg/mL in the last trimester.

Physiologic Function

In the mother, HPL stimulates IGF-I production and induces insulin resistance and carbohydrate intolerance. Experimentally, the maternal level of HPL can be altered by changing the circulating level (chronically, not acutely) of glucose. HPL is elevated with hypoglycemia and depressed with hyperglycemia. This information and studies in fasted pregnant women have led to the following formulation for the physiologic function of HPL.[85–91]

HPL Changes in the Fasting State

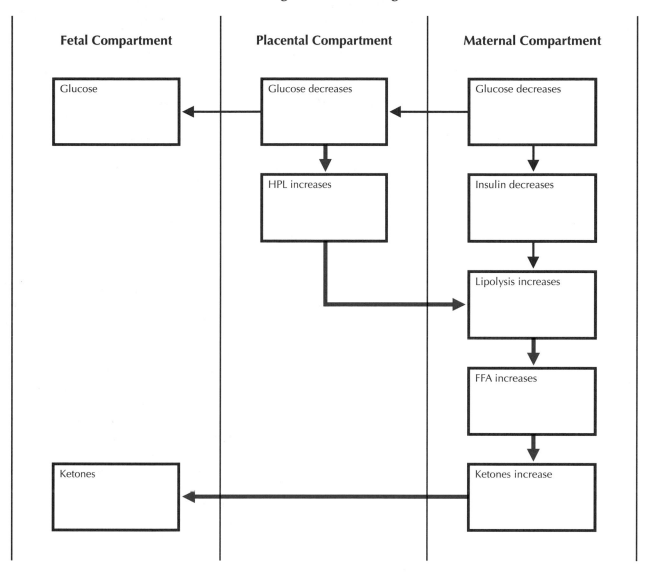

The metabolic role of HPL is to mobilize lipids as free fatty acids. In the fed state, there is abundant glucose available, leading to increased insulin levels, lipogenesis, and glucose utilization. This is associated with decreased gluconeogenesis, and a decrease in the circulating free fatty acid levels, as the free fatty acids are utilized in the process of lipogenesis to deposit storage packets of triglycerides (see Chapter 19, Obesity).

Pregnancy has been likened to a state of "accelerated starvation," characterized by a relative hypoglycemia in the fasting state.[87] This state is due to two major influences:

1. Glucose provides the major, although not the entire, fuel requirement for the fetus. A difference in gradient causes a constant transfer of glucose from the mother to the fetus.

2. Placental hormones, specifically estrogen and progesterone, and especially HPL, interfere with the action of maternal insulin. In the second half of pregnancy when HPL levels rise approximately 10-fold, HPL is a major force in the diabetogenic effects of pregnancy. The latter is characterized by increased levels of insulin associated with decreased cellular response (peripheral insulin resistance and hyperinsulinemia).

As glucose decreases in the fasting state, HPL levels rise. This stimulates lipolysis leading to an increase in circulating free fatty acids. Thus, a different fuel is provided for the mother so that glucose and amino acids can be conserved for the fetus. With sustained fasting, maternal fat is utilized for fuel to such an extent that maternal ketone levels rise. There is limited transport of free fatty acids across the placenta. Therefore, when glucose becomes scarce for the fetus, fetal tissues utilize the ketones which do cross the placenta. Thus, decreased glucose levels lead to decreased insulin and increased HPL, increasing lipolysis and ketone levels. HPL also may enhance the fetal uptake of ketones and amino acids. The mechanism for the insulin antagonism by HPL may be the HPL-stimulated increase in free fatty acid levels, which in turn directly interfere with insulin-directed entry of glucose into cells. These interactions significantly involve growth factors, particularly insulin-like growth factor, at the cellular level.

This mechanism can be viewed as an important means to provide fuel for the fetus between maternal meals. However, with a sustained state of inadequate glucose intake the subsequent ketosis may impair fetal brain development and function. Pregnancy is not the time to severely restrict caloric intake.

The lipid, lipoprotein, and apolipoprotein changes during pregnancy are positively correlated with changes in estradiol, progesterone, and HPL.[92] The lipolytic activity of HPL is an important factor because HPL is also linked to the maternal blood levels of cholesterol, triglycerides, phospholipids, and insulin-like growth factor-I.

When glucose is abundant as in pregnant women with diabetes mellitus, the flow of nutritional substrates (in this case, glucose and amino acids) is in the direction of the fetus. The subsequent hyperinsulinemia in the fetus becomes a strong stimulus to growth, perhaps compounded by maternal hyperinsulinemia caused by obesity as well as the hyperinsulinemia due to the peripheral resistance produced by the hormones of pregnancy.[93] Fetal undernutrition lowers fetal IGF-I levels, and this is associated with a high prevalence of insulin resistance later as adults.[94] In vitro studies indicate that HPL, despite its lower levels in the fetus, directly affects fetal tissue metabolism, including synergistic actions with insulin, especially on glycogen synthesis in the liver. The failure of fetal growth hormone to affect fetal growth (e.g., normal growth in anencephalics) further indicates that HPL may be the fetal growth hormone.

HPL Clinical Uses

Blood levels of HPL are related to placental function. While some studies indicated that HPL was valuable in screening patients for potential fetal complications, others did not support the use of HPL measurements. Even though utilization of the HPL assay can have an impact on perinatal care, fetal heart rate monitoring techniques are more reliably predictive and sensitive for assessing fetal well-being. Furthermore, totally uneventful pregnancies have been reported despite undetectable HPL.[95,96]

Previous suggestions that a low or declining level of HPL and a high level of HCG are characteristic of trophoblastic disease were not accurate. Because of the rapid clearance of HPL, aborting molar pregnancies are likely to have low levels of HPL, while the level of HCG is still high. However, intact molar pregnancies can have elevated levels of both HPL and HCG.[97]

Human Chorionic Growth Hormone

Little is known about the placental growth hormone. It is secreted by the syncytiotrophoblast into the maternal circulation, but it is not detected in the fetal circulation.[98] It is likely that placental growth hormone contributes to the regulation of IGF-I levels in the maternal circulation.

Human Chorionic Thyrotropin (HCT)

The human placenta contains two thyrotropic substances. One is called human chorionic thyrotropin (HCT), similar in size and action to pituitary TSH. The content in the normal placenta is very small. HCT differs from the other glycoproteins in that it does not appear to share the common α-subunit. Antiserum generated to α-HCG does not neutralize the biologic activities of HCT, but it does neutralize that of HCG and pituitary TSH.

Rarely, patients with trophoblastic disease have hyperthyroidism. Studies have indicated that HCG has intrinsic thyrotropic activity, suggesting that HCG is the second placental thyrotropic substance.[99-101] It has been calculated that HCG contains approximately 1/4000th of the thyrotropic activity of human TSH. In conditions with very elevated HCG levels, the thyrotropic activity can be sufficient to produce hyperthyroidism, but this may not be a simple HCG mechanism. The thyroid hormone changes in pregnancy and the role of HCG as a thyroid stimulator are discussed in Chapter 20.

Human Chorionic Adrenocorticotropin

The rise in maternal free cortisol that takes place throughout pregnancy is due to ACTH and corticotropin releasing hormone (CRH) production and secretion into the maternal circulation by the placenta.[102,103] The placental content of ACTH is higher than can be accounted for by the contribution of sequestered blood. In addition, cortisol levels in pregnant women are resistant to dexamethasone suppression, suggesting that there is a component of maternal ACTH and CRH that does not originate in the maternal pituitary gland. The placental production of ACTH in the syncytiotrophoblast (and the increase in maternal ACTH levels) is probably due to stimulation by the locally produced CRH in the cytotrophoblast.[104] One can speculate that placental ACTH and CRH raise maternal adrenal activity in order to provide the basic building blocks (cholesterol and pregnenolone) for placental steroidogenesis. There is no passage of ACTH between the fetal and maternal compartments.

The maternal ACTH response to the administration of CRH during pregnancy is blunted, indicating a high level of endogenous CRH and ACTH activity. Vasopressin stimulates ACTH secretion in the pituitary, both directly and indirectly by potentiating the action of CRH. In contrast to the blunted response to CRH during pregnancy, the ACTH response to vasopressin is increased.[105] This is further evidence that placental CRH produces a state of chronic stimulation for the maternal pituitary-adrenal axis. Thus, in contrast to nonpregnant women, CRH levels in maternal plasma are relatively high, rising in the second trimester to peak values at term.[106] Both maternal and fetal levels are further elevated in pathologic states such as premature labor, hypertension, fetal asphyxia, and intrauterine growth retardation.[107] Because CRH also stimulates prostaglandin synthesis in the placenta and fetal membranes, it is implicated in the premature labor that accompanies pathologic conditions.[108]

Alpha-Fetoprotein

Alpha-fetoprotein (AFP) is a relatively unique glycoprotein (590 amino acids and 4% carbohydrate) derived largely from fetal liver and partially from the yolk sac until it degenerates at about 12 weeks. In early pregnancy (5–12 weeks), amniotic fluid AFP is mainly from yolk sac origin, whereas maternal circulating AFP is mainly from the fetal liver.[109] Its function is unknown, but it is comparable in size to albumin and contains 39% sequence homology; it may serve as a protein carrier of steroid hormones in fetal blood. AFP may also be a modulator of cell proliferation, synergizing with various growth factors.[110]

Peak levels of AFP in the fetal blood are reached at the end of the first trimester; then levels decrease gradually until a rapid decrease begins at 32 weeks. Maternal blood levels are much lower than fetal levels, rising until week 32 (probably because of the great increase in trophoblast villous surface area during this time period) and then declining. Because AFP is highly concentrated in the fetal CNS, abnormal direct contact of CNS with the amniotic fluid (as with neural tube defects) results in elevated amniotic fluid and maternal blood levels. Other fetal abnormalities, such as intestinal obstruction, omphalocele, and congenital nephrosis are also associated with high levels of AFP in the amniotic fluid. Besides indicating a variety of fetal anomalies, elevated maternal AFP levels are also present with multiple pregnancies and associated with an increased risk of spontaneous abortion, stillbirth, neonatal death, and low birth weight (probably reflecting an increase in villous surface area in response to an adverse intrauterine environment).[111]

Multiple Marker Screening

Down syndrome is a very common genetic cause of abnormal development. The majority of cases are due to trisomy 21, an extra chromosome usually due to nondisjunction in maternal meiosis. A low maternal level of AFP is associated with trisomy 21. However, there is extensive overlap between normal and affected pregnancies responsible for a significant false positive rate. Several placental products are secreted in increased amounts in pregnancies with trisomy 21, including HCG and HPL, whereas the maternal circulating level of unconjugated estriol is lower in affected pregnancies. With trisomy 18, all markers are decreased. Modern screening for fetal aneuploidy combines three markers: AFP, HCG, and unconjugated estriol.[112,113] This protocol will also detect 85% of open neural tube defects.

The multiple marker screening protocol measures AFP, HCG, and unconjugated estriol in maternal serum at 16–18 weeks gestation, the optimal time for neural tube defect detection. Using the patient's age and the laboratory results, patients are provided a statistical estimation of risks for both neural tube defects and Down syndrome. Corrections are applied for race and weight. A pattern similar to that of Down syndrome has also been reported to be associated with hydropic fetal Turner syndrome.[114] The most critical factor for correct risk assessment is accurate gestational dating. A two-week error in dating can change the calculated risk for Down syndrome ten-fold. Therefore, ultrasound confirmation of gestational dating is essential. In addition, ultrasonography will indicate fetal number and assess the fetus for anomalies.

The multiple marker protocol is for screening a low risk population regardless of age. Amniocentesis is necessary for final diagnosis, and it should be kept in mind that multiple marker screening does not provide information regarding risk for chromosome disorders other than Down syndrome. Genetic amniocentesis is still recommended for all women 35 and older.

Relaxin

Relaxin is a peptide hormone produced by the corpus luteum of pregnancy, and not detected in men or nonpregnant women. It is composed of two short peptide chains (24 and 29 amino acids, respectively) linked by disulfide bridges. While it has been argued that the human corpus luteum is the sole source of relaxin in pregnancy, it has also been identified in human placenta, decidua, and chorion.[115–117] The maternal serum concentration rises during the first trimester when the corpus luteum is dominant and declines in the second trimester.[118] This suggests a role in maintaining early pregnancy, but its function is not really known. In animals, relaxin softens the cervix, inhibits uterine contractions, and relaxes the pubic symphysis. The cervical changes are comparable to those seen with human labor.[119] To examine the contribution of the corpus luteum, normally pregnant women were compared to women pregnant with donated oocytes (and therefore without corpora lutea).[120] Relaxin was undetectable in the women without functioning ovaries, confirming that its major source is the corpus luteum. No effect on prolactin secretion was observed, but it did appear that relaxin enhanced growth hormone secretion by the pituitary. Obviously relaxin is not necessary for the maintenance of pregnancy and labor because the rest of pregnancy and the outcomes did not differ between those women with circulating levels of relaxin and those with undetectable levels. However, recombinant relaxin is being tested for ripening of the cervix.

Prolactin

Following ovulation, the endometrium becomes a secretory organ and remains so throughout pregnancy. Decidualized endometrium secretes renin which may be involved in the regulation of water and electroytes in the amniotic fluid, and relaxin, which may influence prostaglandin production in the membranes. One of the best studied special endocrine functions of the decidual endometrium is the secretion of prolactin. Prolactin is synthesized by endometrium during a normal menstrual cycle, but this synthesis is not initiated until histologic decidualization begins about day 23.[121,122] The control of prolactin secretion by decidual tissue has not been definitively established. Some argue that once decidualization is established, prolactin secretion continues in the absence of either progesterone or estradiol, although there is evidence for an inhibitory feedback by decidual proteins (perhaps prolactin itself).[122,123] Others indicate that endometrial prolactin production requires the combined effects of progestin and estrogen hormones plus the presence of other placental and decidual factors including relaxin, IGF-I, and specific stimulatory and inhibitory proteins.[124]

During pregnancy, prolactin secretion is limited to the fetal pituitary, the maternal pituitary, and the uterus. Neither trophoblast nor fetal membranes synthesize prolactin, but both the myometrium and endometrium can produce prolactin. The endometrium requires the presence of progesterone to initiate prolactin, while progesterone suppresses prolactin synthesis in the myometrium. Prolactin derived from the decidua is the source of prolactin found in the amniotic fluid.[125] The prolactin in the fetal circulation is derived from the fetal pituitary.

Amniotic fluid concentrations of prolactin parallel maternal serum concentration until the 10th week of pregnancy, rise markedly until the 20th week, and then decrease. The maternal and fetal blood levels of prolactin are derived from the respective pituitary glands. Bromocriptine suppression of pituitary secretion of prolactin throughout pregnancy produces minimal maternal and fetal blood levels, yet there is normal fetal growth and development, and amniotic fluid levels are unchanged.[126] Fortunately decidual secretion of prolactin is unaffected by dopamine agonist treatment because decidual prolactin may be important for fluid and electrolyte regulation of the amniotic fluid. This decidual prolactin is transported across the membranes in a process which requires the intact state of amnion and chorion with adherent decidua.

No clinical significance can be attached to maternal and fetal blood levels of prolactin in abnormal pregnancies. Decidual and amniotic fluid prolactin levels are lower, however, in hypertensive pregnancies and in patients with polyhydramnios.[127,128] Prolactin receptors are present in the chorion laeve, and their concentration is lower in patients with polyhydramnios.[129] Prolactin reduces the permeability of the human amnion in the fetal to maternal direction. This receptor-mediated action takes place on the epithelium lining the fetal surface.[130] There is also evidence that prolactin derived from the fetal pituitary contributes to the regulation of fetal water and electrolyte balance by acting as an antidiuretic hormone.[131]

The increase in maternal levels of prolactin represents maternal pituitary secretion in response to estrogen. The mechanisms for pituitary secretion of prolactin are discussed in Chapters 2 and 17.

Growth Factors and Cytokines

The placenta synthesizes many proteins that are part of the normal composition of cells throughout the body. Local placental cytokine production is believed to be important for embryonic growth and in the maternal immune response essential for survival of the pregnancy.[132] Interleukin-1β is produced in the decidualized endometrium during pregnancy, and colony-stimulating factor-1 (CSF-1) is produced by both decidua and placenta. CSF-1 gene expression in response to interleukin-1β has been localized to mesenchymal fibroblasts from the core of placental villi.[133] Thus, a system of communication is present between maternal decidual and fetal tissue to provide growth factor support for the placenta which would include fetal hematopoiesis, a known response to CSF-1. The placenta also produces interleukin-6, and both interleukins stimulate HCG release by activation of the interleukin-6 receptor.[134] Thus, the interleukin-1 influence on HCG secretion is mediated by the interleukin-6 system. Both trophoblast derived interleukin-1 and tumor necrosis factor-α (TNF-α) synergistically release interleukin-6 and activate the interleukin-6 system to secrete HCG.[135]

The insulin-like growth factors, IGF-I and IGF-II, are involved in prenatal and postnatal growth and development. These growth factors do not cross the placenta into the fetal circulation; however, they may be involved in placental growth.[136] The maternal levels of IGF-I are significantly regulated by growth hormone dependent liver synthesis. The fetus can influence maternal IGF-I levels by means of the placental secretion of HPL.

The IGF binding proteins transport IGFs in the circulation, protect IGFs against metabolism and clearance, and importantly, affect the biologic activity of IGFs by modulating IGF availability at the cellular level. Pregnancy is marked by a rise in maternal levels of insulin-like growth factor binding protein-1 (IGFBP-1), beginning at the end of the first trimester and reaching a peak at term.[137] IGFBP-1 is now recognized to be the same as placental protein-12, a decidual protein. Thus IGFBP-1 originates in the decidua, regulated by progesterone, as well as in the liver. The prominence of IGFBP-1 in the pregnant state is in contrast to the nonpregnant state when IGFBP-3 is the main circulating IGFBP. During pregnancy, the levels of IGFBP-3 and IGFBP-2 decrease, apparently due to the activity of a pregnancy-associated serum protease.[137]

How these changes interact to regulate growth and development of different organs and tissues is a new area of research activity. For example, in the pregnant ewe and fetal lamb, glucose and other nutritional factors regulate the gene expression and therefore the circulating levels of IGF binding proteins.[138] Fasting and feeding increased and decreased, respectively, the IGFBP concentrations, perhaps partly a response to insulin levels and the effect of insulin on liver synthesis of IGFBPs. These changes are consistent with IGF and IGFBP involvement in the responses to nutrition and stress. Because IGFBP-1 appears to be the principal binding protein in pregnancy, attention is focused on the changes in IGF-I and IGFBP-1. IGF-I, produced in the placenta, regulates transfer of nutrients across the placenta to the fetus and thus enhances fetal growth; IGFBP-1, produced in the decidua, interferes with IGF-I action and inhibits fetal growth.[139] Thus newborn birth weight correlates directly with maternal levels of IGF-I and inversely with levels of IGFBP-1.

Epidermal growth factor (EGF) is synthesized by syncytiotrophoblast and probably is involved in the differentiation of cytotrophoblast into syncytiotrophoblast. EGF is well known as a mitogen. Other growth factors isolated from human placenta include platelet-derived growth factor, nerve growth factor, fibroblast growth factor, and transforming growth factor. These factors are probably all involved in the proliferation and growth associated with pregnancy.

Inhibin and Activin

The placenta produces inhibin which is responsible for the marked increase in maternal inhibin levels throughout pregnancy.[140,141] Inhibin originates in the syncytiotrophoblast, and its synthesis is stimulated by PGE_2 and $PGF_{2\alpha}$, the predominant placental prostaglandins.[141] Similar to their action in the ovarian follicle, inhibin and activin are regulators within the placenta for the production of GnRH, HCG, and steroids; as expected, activin is stimulatory, and inhibin is inhibitory.[68] GnRH and the subunits for inhibin and activin can be found in the same placental cells, in both cytotrophoblast and syncytiotrophoblast, but not in all cells.[142] Trophoblast synthesis and release of inhibin and activity are part of the complex placental story, involving many hormones and locally produced factors. The placental and decidual appearance of inhibin and activin occurs early in pregnancy in time for possible roles in embryogenesis and local immune responses.

Endogenous Opiates

Fetal and maternal endogenous opiates originate from the pituitary glands, and are secreted in parallel with ACTH, in response to corticotropin releasing hormone, which is in part derived from the placenta.[143] There is reason to believe that in pregnancy the intermediate lobe of the maternal pituitary gland is a major source of elevated circulating endorphin levels. However, the syncytiotrophoblast in response to CRH produces all of the products of proopiomelanocortin (POMC) metabolism, including β-endorphin and enkephalins. The placenta is richly endowed with G protein opioid receptors.[144] The presence of CRH in the placenta and placental opiate production in reponse to CRH indicate a CRH-endogenous opiate interaction similar to that in the hypothalamic-pituitary axis.[145]

The maternal blood levels of endogenous opiates increase progressively with advancing gestation. Maximal maternal values are reached during labor, coinciding with full cervical dilatation. The maternal levels also correlate with the degree of pain perception and use of analgesia. On the fetal side, hypoxia is a potent stimulus for endorphin release.

There are many hypotheses surrounding the function of endogenous opiates in pregnancy. These include roles related to stress, inhibition of oxytocin, vasopressin and gonadotropins, the promotion of prolactin secretion, and, of course, a natural analgesic agent during labor and delivery.

Prorenin

The circulating levels of prorenin, the inactive precursor of renin, increase (10-fold) during early pregnancy, the result of ovarian stimulation by HCG.[146,147] This increase in prorenin from the ovary is not associated with any significant change in the blood levels of the active form, renin. Possible roles for this ovarian prorenin-renin-angiotensin system include the following: stimulation of steroidogenesis to provide androgen substrate for estrogen production, regulation of calcium and prostaglandin metabolism, and stimulation of angiogenesis. This system may affect vascular and tissue functions both in and outside the ovary. Prorenin also originates in chorionic tissues and is highly concentrated in the amniotic fluid. The highest biologic levels of prorenin are found in gestational sacs in early pregnancy; its possible roles in embryonic growth and development remain speculative.[148]

Atrial Natriuretic Peptide

Atrial natriuretic peptide (ANP) is derived from human atrial tissue. It is a potent natriuretic, diuretic, and smooth muscle relaxant peptide that circulates as a hormone. Maternal ANP increases during labor, and cord levels on the arterial side suggest that ANP is a circulating hormone in the fetus.[149]

Other Proteins

The mother responds to a pregnancy even before implantation. Remarkably, early pregnancy factor (EPF) can be detected in the maternal circulation within 1–2 days after coitus results in a pregnancy.[150] It remains throughout pregnancy, but interestingly, disappears before parturition. EPF prior to implantation is apparently produced by the ovary in response to a signal from the embryo. After implantation, EPF is no longer secreted by the ovary but now is derived from the embryo. EPF is a protein associated with cell proliferation and growth and therefore is present in many nonpregnant tissues such as neoplasms. EPF has immunosuppressive properties and is abundant in platelets. We are just beginning to learn about this fetal and maternal protein.

Pregnancy-specific γ_1-glycoprotein (PSG) was previously known as Schwangerschafts-protein 1. The physiologic function of PSG produced by the placenta is unknown, but it has been used as a test for pregnancy and a marker for malignancies, including choriocarcinoma. Molecular studies have revealed that PSG consists of a family of closely related glycoproteins encoded by genes on chromsome 19.[151] The PSG family is closely related to the carcinoembryonic antigen (CEA) proteins. Pregnancy-associated plasma protein-A (PAPP-A) is a placental protein that is similar to a macroglobulin in the serum and still in search of specific functions. Progesterone associated endometrial protein, previously called placental protein 14, is now recognized to originate in secretory endometrium and decidua. No role for this protein has been described thus far.

Fetal Lung Maturation

The pulmonary alveoli are lined with a surface-active phospholipid-protein complex called pulmonary surfactant that is synthesized in the type II pneumocyte of mature lungs. It is this surfactant that decreases surface tension, thereby facilitating lung expansion and preventing atelectasis. In full-term fetuses, surfactant is present at birth in sufficient amounts to permit adequate lung expansion and normal breathing. In premature fetuses, however, surfactant is present in lesser amounts, and when insufficient, postnatal lung expansion and ventilation are frequently impaired, resulting in progressive atelectasis, the clinical syndrome of respiratory distress.

Phosphatidylcholine (lecithin) has been identified as the most active and most abundant lipid of the surfactant complex. The second most active and abundant material is phosphatidylglycerol (PG), which significantly enhances surfactant function. Both are present in only small concentrations until the last 5 weeks of pregnancy. Beginning at 20–22 weeks of pregnancy, a less stable and less active lecithin, palmitoylmyristoyl lecithin, is formed. Hence, a premature infant does not always develop respiratory distress syndrome; however, in addition to being less active, synthesis of this lecithin is decreased by stress and acidosis, making the premature infant more susceptible to respiratory distress. At about the 35th week of gestation, there is a sudden surge of dipalmitoyl lecithin, the major surfactant lecithin, which is stable and very active. Since secretion by the fetal lungs contributes to the formation of amniotic fluid and the sphingomyelin concentration of amniotic fluid changes relatively little throughout pregnancy, assessment of the lecithin/sphingomyelin (L/S) ratio in amniotic fluid at approximately 34–36 weeks of pregnancy can determine the amount of dipalmitoyl lecithin available and thus the degree to which the lungs will adapt to newborn life.

Gluck and colleagues were the first to demonstrate that the L/S ratio correlates with pulmonary maturity of the fetal lung.[152] In normal development, sphingomyelin concentrations are greater than those of lecithin until about gestational week 26. Prior to 34 weeks, the L/S ratio is approximately 1:1. At 34–36 weeks, with the sudden increase in lecithin, the ratio rises acutely. In general, a ratio of 2.0 or greater indicates pulmonary maturity and that respiratory distress syndrome will not develop in the newborn. Respiratory distress syndrome associated with a ratio greater than 2.0 usually follows a difficult delivery with a low 5-minute Apgar score, suggesting that severe acidosis can inhibit surfactant production. A ratio in the transitional range (1.0–1.9) indicates that respiratory distress syndrome may develop but that the fetal lung has entered the period of lecithin production, and a repeat amniocentesis in 1 or 2 weeks usually reveals a mature L/S ratio. The rise from low to high ratios may actually occur within 3–4 days.

An increase in the surfactant content of phosphatidylglycerol at 34–36 weeks marks the final maturation of the fetal lung. When the L/S ratio is greater than 2.0 and PG is present, the incidence of respiratory distress syndrome is virtually zero. The assessment of PG is especially helpful when the amniotic fluid is contaminated in that the analysis is not affected by meconium, blood, or vaginal secretions.

Abnormalities of pregnancy may affect the rate of maturation of the fetal lung, resulting either in an early mature L/S ratio or a delayed rise in the ratio. Accelerated maturation of the ratio is associated with hypertension, advanced diabetes, hemoglobinopathies, heroin addiction, and poor maternal nutrition. Delayed maturation is seen with diabetes without hypertension, and Rh sensitization. In general, accelerated maturation is associated with reductions in uteroplacental blood flow (and presumably increased fetal stress). With vigorous and effective control of maternal diabetes, the risk of respiratory distress syndrome in the newborns is not significantly different from infants born to nondiabetics.

Since Liggins observed survival of premature lambs following the administration of cortisol to the fetus, it has become recognized that fetal cortisol is the principal requisite for surfactant biosynthesis. This is true despite the fact that no increase in fetal cortisol can be demonstrated to correlate with the increases in fetal lung maturation. For that reason, fetal lung maturation can be best viewed as the result of not only cortisol, but the synergistic action of cortisol, prolactin, thyroxine, estrogens, prostaglandins, growth factors, and perhaps other yet unidentified agents. Insulin directly inhibits surfactant protein expression in fetal lung tissue, which explains the increase in respiratory distress syndrome associated with hyperglycemia in pregnancy (although this effect can be overcome by the stress associated with advanced diabetes).[153]

In general, maximal benefit in terms of enhanced fetal pulmonic maturity has been demonstrated with glucocorticoid administration under 32 weeks of gestational age, with some benefit between 32–34 weeks, and no benefit beyond 34 weeks. The optimal effect requires that 48 hours elapse after initiation of therapy, and this benefit is lost after 7 days. Most clinicians restrict antenatal steroid treatment for premature labor to pregnancies between 28–32 weeks. Although every case of respiratory distress syndrome and subsequent chronic lung disease cannot be prevented, a significant impact can be achieved on infant mortality, and the incidence and severity of respiratory distress syndrome. Additional treatment with thyrotropin releasing hormone (TRH) further reduces the incidence of chronic lung disease in glucocorticoid-treated very low birth weight infants.[154]

References

1. **Csapo AL, Pulkkinen MO, Wiest WG,** Effects of luteectomy and progesterone replacement in early pregnant patients, Am J Obstet Gynecol 115:759, 1973.

2. **Schneider MA, Davies MC, Honour JW,** The timing of placental competence in pregnancy after oocyte donation, Fertil Steril 59:1059, 1993.

3. **Azuma K, Calderon I, Besanko M, Maclachlan V, Healy DL,** Is the luteo-placental shift a myth? Analysis of low progesterone levels in sucessful Art pregnancies, J Clin Endocrinol Metab 77:195, 1993.

4. **Sultan KM, Davis OK, Liu H-C, Rosenwaks Z,** Viable term pregnancy despite "subluteal" serum progesterone levels in the first trimester, Fertil Steril 60:363, 1993.

5. **Mishell DR, Thorneycroft IH, Nagata Y, Murata T, Nakamura RM,** Serum gonadotropin and steroid patterns in early human gestation, Am J Obstet Gynecol 117:631, 1973.

6. **Tulchinsky D, Hobel CJ,** Plasma human and chorionic gonadotropin, estrogen, estradiol, estriol, progesterone and 17α-hydroxyprogesterone in human pregnancy, Am J Obstet Gynecol 117:884, 1973.

7. **Parker CR, Illingworth DR, Bissonnette J, Carr BR,** Endocrine changes during pregnancy in a patient with homozygous familial hypobetalipoproteinemia, New Engl J Med 314:557, 1986.

8. **Albrecht ED, Pepe GJ,** Placental steroid hormone biosynthesis in primate pregnancy, Endocrin Rev 11:124, 1990.

9. **Begum-Hasan J, Murphy BEP,** *In vitro* stimulation of placental progesterone production by 19-nortestosterone and C$_{19}$ steroids in early human pregnancy, J Clin Endocrinol Metab 75:838, 1992.

10. **Bhattacharyya S, Chaudhary J, Das C,** Antibodies to hCG inhibit progesterone production from human syncytiotrophoblast cells, Placenta 13:135, 1992.

11. **Mitchell BF, Challis JRG, Lukash L,** Progesterone synthesis by human amnion, chorion, and decidua at term, Am J Obstet Gynecol 157:349, 1987.

12. **Parker CR, Everett RB, Quirk JG, Whalley PJ, Gant NF,** Hormone production during pregnancy in the primigravid patient: I. Plasma levels of progesterone and 5α-pregnane-3,20-dione throughout pregnancy of normal women and women who developed pregnancy-induced hypertension. Am J Obstet Gynecol 135:778, 1979.

13. **Parker CR, Everett RB, Whalley PJ, Quirk JG, Gant NF, MacDonald PC,** Hormone production during pregnancy in the primigravid patient: II. Plasma levels of deoxycorticosterone throughout pregnancy of normal women and women who developed pregnancy-induced hypertension. Am J Obstet Gynecol 138:626, 1980.

14. **Rothchild I,** Role of progesterone in initiating and maintaining pregnancy, in Bardin CW, Milgrom E, Mauvais-Jarvis P, editors, *Progesterone and Progestins*, Raven Press, New York, 1983, pp 219-229.

15. **Carr BR, Simpson ER,** Lipoprotein utilization and cholesterol synthesis by the human fetal adrenal gland, Endocrin Rev 2:306, 1981.

16. **Carr BR, Simpson ER,** Cholesterol synthesis by human fetal hepatocytes: effect of lipoproteins, Am J Obstet Gynecol 150:551, 1984.

17. **Partsch C-J, Sippell WG, Mackenzie IZ, Aynsley-Green A,** The steroid hormonal milieu of the undisturbed human fetus and mother at 16-20 weeks gestation, J Clin Endocrinol Metab 73:969, 1991.

18. **Siiteri PK, MacDonald PC,** Placental estrogen biosynthesis during human pregnancy, J Clin Endocrinol Metab 26:751, 1966.

19. **Voutilainen R, Ilvesmaki V, Miettinen PJ,** Low expression of 3β-hydroxy-5-ene steroid dehydrogenase gene in human fetal adrenals *in vivo;* adrenocorticotropin and protein dinase C-dependent regulation in adrenocortical cultures, J Clin Endocrinol Metab 72:761, 1991.

20. **Madden JD, Gant NF, MacDonald PC,** Study of the kinetics of conversion of maternal plasma dehydroisoandrosterone sulfate to 16α-hydroxydehydroisoandrosterone sulfate, estradiol, and estriol, Am J Obstet Gynecol 132:392, 1978.

21. **Buster JE, Abraham GE,** The applications of steroid hormone radioimmunoassays to clinical obstetrics, Obstet Gynecol 46:489, 1975.

22. **Devroey P, Camus M, Palermo G, Smitz J, Van Waesberghe L, Wsanto A, et al,** Placental production of estradiol and progesterone after oocyte donation in patients with primary ovarian failure, Am J Obstet Gynecol 162:66, 1990.

23. **Salat-Baroux J, Cornet D, Alvarez S, Antoine JM, Mandelbaum J, Plachot M,** Hormonal secretions in singleton pregnancies arising from the implantation of fresh or frozen embryos after oocyte donation in women with ovarian failure, Fertil Steril 57:150, 1992.

24. **Buster JE, Sakakini J Jr, Killam AP, Scragg WH,** Serum unconjugated estriol levels in the third trimester and their relationship to gestational age, Am J Obstet Gynecol 125:672, 1975.

25. **Katzenellenbogen BS,** Biology and receptor interactions of estriol and estriol derivatives in vitro and in vivo, J Steroid Biochem 20:1033, 1984.

26. **Parker CR Jr, Leveno K, Carr BR, Hauth J, MacDonald PC,** Umbilical cord plasma levels of dehydroepiandrosterone sulfate during human gestation, J Clin Endocrinol Metab 54:1216, 1982.

27. **Winters AJ, Oliver C, Colston C, MacDonald PC, Porter JC,** Plasma ACTH levels in the human fetus and neonate as related to age and parturition, J Clin Endocrinol Metab 39:269, 1974.

28. **Walsh SW, Norman RL, Novy MJ,** In utero regulation of rhesus monkey fetal adrenals: effects of dexamethasone, adrenocorticotropin, thyrotropin-releasing hormone, prolactin, human chorionic gonadotropin, and α-melanocyte-stimulating hormone on fetal and maternal plasma steroids, Endocrinology 104:1805, 1979.

29. **Abu-Hakima M, Branchaud CL, Goodyer CG, Murphy BEP,** The effects of human chorionic gonadotropin on growth and steroidogenesis of the human fetal adrenal gland in vitro, Am J Obstet Gynecol 156:681, 1987.

30. **del Pozo E, Bigazzi M, Calaf J,** Induced human gestational hypoprolactinemia: lack of action on fetal adrenal androgen synthesis, J Clin Endocrinol Metab 51:936, 1980.

31. **Walker ML, Pepe GJ, Albrecht ED,** Regulation of baboon fetal adrenal androgen formation by pituitary peptides at mid- and late gestation, Endocrinology 122:546, 1988.

32. **McNulty WP, Novy MJ, Walsh SW,** Fetal and postnatal development of the adrenal glands in *Macaca mulatta,* Biol Reprod 25:1079, 1981.

33. **Pepe GJ, Albrecht ED,** Regulation of the primate fetal adrenal cortex, Endocrin Rev 11:151, 1990.

34. **Mason JI, Rainey WE,** Steroidogenesis in the human fetal adrenal: a role for cholesterol synthesized *de novo,* J Clin Endocrinol Metab 64:140, 1987.

35. **Baggia S, Albrecht ED, Pepe GJ,** Regulation of 11 beta-hydroxysteroid dehydrogenase activity in the baboon placenta by estrogen, Endocrinology 126:2742, 1990.

36. **Voutilainen R, Eramaa M, Ritvos O,** Hormonally regulated inhibin gene expression in human fetal and adult adrenals, J Clin Endocrinol Metab 73:1026, 1991.

37. **Spencer SJ, Rabinovici J, Mesiano S, Goldsmith PC, Jaffe RB,** Activin and inhibin in the human adrenal gland. Regulation and differential effects in fetal and adult cells, J Clin Invest 90:142, 1992.

38. **D'Ercole AJ,** Somatomedins/insulin-like growth factors and fetal growth, J Dev Physiol 9:481, 1987.

39. **Mesiano S, Mellon SH, Jaffe RB,** Mitogenic action, regulation, and localization of insulin-like growth factors in the human fetal adrenal gland, J Clin Endocrinol Metab 76:968, 1993.

40. **Fujieda K, Faiman C, Reyes FI, Winter JSD,** The control of steroidogenesis by human fetal adrenal cells in tissue culture: I. Responses to adrenocorticotropin, J Clin Endocrinol Metab 53:34, 1981.

41. **Fujieda K, Faiman C, Reyes FI, Thliveris J, Winter JSD,** The control of steroidogenesis by human fetal adrenal cells in tissue culture: II. Comparison of morphology and steroid production in cells of the fetal and definitive zones. J Clin Endocrinol Metab 53:401, 1981.

42. **Fujieda K, Faiman C, Reyes FI, Winter JSD,** The control of steroidogenesis by human fetal adrenal cells in tissue culture: III. The effects of various hormonal peptides. J Clin Endocrinol Metab, 53:690, 1981.

43. **Fujieda K, Faiman C, Reyes FI, Winter JSD,** The control of steroidogenesis by human fetal adrenal cells in tissue culture: IV. The effects of exposure to placental steroids, J Clin Endocrinol Metab 54:89, 1982.

44. **Byrne GC, Perry YS, Winter JSD,** Steroid inhibitory effects upon human adrenal 3β-hydroxysteroid dehydrogenase activity, J Clin Endocrinol Metab 62:413, 1986.

45. **Ducsay CA, Hess DL, McClellan MC, Novy MJ,** Endocrine and morphological maturation of the fetal and neonatal adrenal cortex in baboons, J Clin Endocrinol Metab 73:385, 1991.

46. **Mesiano S, Jaffe RB,** Interaction of insulin-like growth factor-II and estradiol directs steroidogenesis in the human fetal adrenal toward dehydroepiandrosterone sulfate production, J Clin Endocrinol Metab 77:754, 1993.

47. **Hirst J, West NB, Brenner RM, Novy MJ,** Steroid hormone receptors in the adrenal glands of fetal and adult Rhesus monkeys, J Clin Endocrinol Metab 75:308, 1992.

48. **Fritz MA, Stanczyk FZ, Novy MJ,** Relationship of uteroplacental blood flow to the placental clearance of maternal dehydroepiandrosterone through estradiol formation in the pregnant baboon, J Clin Endocrinol Metab 61:1023, 1985.

49. **Fritz MA, Stanczyk FZ, Novy MJ,** Maternal estradiol response to alterations in uteroplacental blood flow, Am J Obstet Gynecol 155:1317, 1986.

50. **Shepherd RW, Stanczyk FZ, Bethea CL, Novy MJ,** Fetal and maternal endocrine responses to reduced uteroplacental blood flow, J Clin Endocrinol Metab 75:301, 1992.

51. **Distler W, Gabbe SG, Freeman RK, Mestman JH, Goebelsmann U,** Estriol in pregnancy: V. Unconjugated and total plasma estriol in the management of pregnant diabetic patients, Am J Obstet Gynecol 130:424, 1978.

52. **Whittle MJ, Anderson D, Lowensohn RI, Mestman JH, Paul RH, Goebelsmann U,** Estriol in pregnancy: VI. Experience with unconjugated plasma estriol assays, Am J Obstet Gynecol 135:764, 1979.

53. **Bradshaw KD, Carr BR,** Placental sulfatase deficiency: maternal and fetal expression of steroid sulfatase deficiency and X-linked ichthyosis, Obstet Gynecol Survey 41:401, 1986.

54. **Shi QJ, Lei ZM, Rao CV, Lin J,** Novel role of human chorionic gonadotropin in differentiation of human cytotrophoblasts, Endocrinology 132:1387, 1993.

55. **Siler-Khodr TM, Khodr GS,** Production and activity of placental releasing hormones, in Novy MJ, Resko JA, editors, *Fetal Endocrinology,* Academic Press, New York, 1981, pp 183–210.

56. **Siler-Khodr TM, Kuehl TJ, Vickery BH,** Effects of a gonadotropin-releasing antagonist on hormone levels in the pregnant baboon and on fetal outcome, Fertil Steril 41:448, 1984.

57. **Siler-Khodr TM, Khodr GS, Harper MJK, Rhode J, Vickery BH, Nestor JJ Jr,** Differential inhibition of human placental prostaglandin release in vitro by a GnRH antagonist, Prostaglandins 31:1003, 1986.

58. **Siler-Khodr TM, Khodr GS,** Content of luteinizing hormone releasing factor in human placenta, Am J Obstet Gynecol 130:216, 1988.

59. **Belisle S, Guevin J-F, Bellabarba D, Lehoux J-G,** Luteinizing hormone-releasing hormone binds to enriched placental membranes and stimulates in vitro the synthesis of bioactive human chorionic gonadotropin, J Clin Endocrinol Metab 59:119, 1984.

60. **Iwashita M, Evans MI, Catt KJ,** Characterization of a gonadotropin-releasing hormone receptor site in term placenta and chorionic villi, J Clin Endocrinol Metab 62:127, 1986.

61. **Jones SA, Brooks AN, Challis JRG,** Steroids modulate corticotropin-releasing hormone production in human fetal membranes and placenta, J Clin Endocrinol Metab 68:825, 1989.

62. **Ren S-G, Braunstein GD,** Human chorionic gonadotropin, Seminars Reprod Endocrinol 10:95, 1992.

63. **Jameson JL, Hollenberg AN,** Regulation of chorionic gonadotropin gene expression, Endocrin Rev 14:203, 1993.

64. **Tan L, Rousseau P,** The chemical identity of the immunoreactive LHRH-like peptide biosynthesized in the placenta, Biochem Biophys Res Commun 109:1061, 1982.

65. **Merz WE, Erlewein C, Licht P, Harbarth P,** The secretion of human chorionic gonadotropin as well as the α- and β messenger ribonucleic acid levels are stimulated by exogenous gonadoliberin pulses applied to first trimester placenta in a superfusion culture system, J Clin Endocrinol Metab 73:84, 1991.

66. **Steele GL, Currie WD, Leung E, Ho Yuen B, Leung PCK,** Rapid stimulation of human chorionic goandotropin secretion by interleukin-1β from perifused first trimester trophoblast, J Clin Endocrinol Metab 75:783, 1992.

67. **Siler-Khodr TM, Khodr GS, Valenzuelea G, Rhode J,** Gonadotropin-releasing hormone effects on placental hormones during gestation. II. Progesterone, estrogen, estradiol and estriol, Biol Reprod 34:255, 1986.

68. **Petraglia F, Vaughn J, Vale W,** Inhibin and activin modulate the release of gonadotropin-releasing hormone, human chorionic gonadotropin, and progesterone from cultured placental cells, Proc Natl Acad Sci USA 86:5114, 1989.

69. **Petraglia F, Vaughan J, Vale W,** Steroid hormones modulate the release of immunoreactive gonadotropin-releasing hormone from cultured human placental cells, J Clin Endocrinol Metab 70:1173, 1990.

70. **Qu J, Brulet C, Thomas K,** Effect of epidermal growth factor in inhibin secretion in human placental cell culture, Endocrinology 131:2173, 1992.

71. **Qu J, Thomas K,** Prostaglandins stimulate the secretion of inhibin from human placental cells, J Clin Endocrinol Metab 77:556, 1993.

72. **Bonduelle ML, Dodd R, Liebaers I, Van SA, Williamson R, Akhurst R,** Chorionic gonadotrophin-beta mRNA, a trophoblast marker, is expressed in human 8-cell embryos derived from tripronucleate zygotes, Hum Reprod 3:909, 1988.

73. **Rabinovici J, Jaffe RB,** Development and regulation of growth and differentiated function in human and subhuman primate fetal gonads, Endocrin Rev 11:532, 1990.

74. **Rothman PA, Chao VA, Taylor MR, Kuhn RW, Jaffe RB, Taylor RN,** Extraplacental human fetal tissues express mRNA transcripts encoding the human chorionic gonadotropin-β subunit protein, Molec Reprod Dev 33:1, 1992.

75. **Nakajima ST, McAuliffe T, Gibson M,** The 24-hour pattern of the levels of serum progesterone and immunoreactive human chorionic gonadotropin in normal early pregnancy, J Clin Endocrinol Metab 71:345, 1990.

76. **Cole LA, Kardana A, Andrade-Gordon P, et al,** The heterogeneity of hCG: III. The occurrence, biological and immunological activities of nicked hCG, Endocrinology 129:1559, 1991.

77. **Maruo T, Matsuo H, Ohtani T, Hoshina M, Mochizuchi M,** Differential modulation of chorionic gonadotropin (CG) subunit messenger ribonucleic acid level and CG secretion by progesterone in normal placenta and choriocarcinoma cultured *in vitro*, Endocrinology 119:858, 1986.

78. **Schlaerth JB, Morrow CP, Kletzky OA, Nalick RH, D'Ablaing GA,** Prognostic characteristics of serum human chorionic gonadotropin titer regression following molar pregnancy. Obstet Gynecol 58:478, 1981.

79. **Yedema KA, Verheijen RH, Kenemans P, Schijf CP, Borm GF, Segers MJ, Thomas CM,** Identification of patients with persistent trophoblastic disease by means of a normal human chorionic gonadotropin regression curve, Am J Obstet Gynecol 168:787, 1993.

80. **Khazaeli MB, Hedayat MM, Hatach KD, To ACW, Soong S-J, Shingleton HM, Boots LR, LoBuglio AF,** Radioimmunoassay of free β-subunit of human chorionic gonadotropin as a prognostic test for persistent trophoblastic disease in molar pregnancy, Am J Obstet Gynecol 155:320, 1986.

81. **Khazaeli MB, Buchina ES, Pattillo RA, Soong S-J, Hatch KD,** Radioimmunoassay of free β-subunit of human chorionic gonadotropin in diagnosis of high-risk and low-risk gestational trophoblastic disease, Am J Obstet Gynecol 160:444, 1989.

82. **Odell WD, Griffin J,** Pulsatile secretion of human chorionic gonadotropin in normal adults, New Engl J Med 317:1688, 1987.

83. **Odell WD, Griffin J,** Pulsatile secretion of chorionic gonadotropin during the normal menstrual cycle, J Clin Endocrinol Metab 69:528, 1989.

84. **Walker WH, Fitzpatrick SL, Barrera-Saldana HA, Resendes-Perez D, Saunders GF,** The human placental lactogen genes: structure, function, evolution and transcriptional regulation, Endocrin Rev 12:316, 1991.

85. **Grumbach MM, Kaplan SL, Vinik A,** HCS, in Berson SA, Yalow RS, editors, *Peptide Hormones*, Vol 2B, North-Holland, Amsterdam, 1973, pp 797-819.

86. **Spellacy WN, Buhi WC, Schram JC, Birk SA, McCreary SA,** Control of human chorionic somatomammotropin levels during pregnancy, Obstet Gynecol 37:567, 1971.

87. **Felig P,** Maternal and fetal fluid homeostasis in human pregnancy, Am J Clin Nutr 26:998, 1973.

88. **Felig P, Lynch V,** Starvation in human pregnancy: hypoglycemia, hypoinsulinemia, and hyperketonemia, Science 170:990, 1970.

89. **Kim YJ, Felig P,** Plasma chorionic somatomammotropin levels during starvation in mid-pregnancy, J Clin Endocrinol Metab 32:864, 1971.

90. **Felig P, Kim YJ, Lynch V, Hendler R,** Amino acid metabolism during starvation in human pregnancy, J Clin Invest 51:1195, 1972.

91. **Handwerger S,** Clinical counterpoint: the physiology of placental lactogen in human pregnancy, Endocrin Rev 12:329, 1991.

92. **Desoye G, Schweditsch MO, Pfeiffer KP, Zechner R, Kostner GM,** Correlation of hormones with lipid and lipoprotein levels during normal pregnancy and postpartum, J Clin Endocrinol Metab 64:704, 1987.

93. **Kalkhoff RK,** Impact of maternal fuels and nutritional state on fetal growth, Diabetes 40 (Suppl 2):61, 1991.

94. **Barker DJP, Hales CN, Fall CHD, Osmond C, Phipps K, Clark PMS,** Type 2 non-insulin-dependent-diabetes mellitus, hypertension and hyperlipidaemia (syndrome X): relation to reduced fetal growth, Diabetologia 36:62, 1993.

95. **Nielsen PV, Pedersen H, Kampmann E,** Absence of human placental lactogen in an otherwise uneventful pregnancy, Am J Obstet Gynecol 135:322, 1979.

96. **Sideri M, de Virgiliis G, Guidobono F, et al,** Immunologically undetectable human placental lactogen in a normal pregnancy. Case report, Br J Obstet Gynaecol 90:771, 1983.

97. **Dawood MY, Teoh ES,** Serum human chorionic somatomammotropin in unaborted hydatidiform mole, Obstet Gynecol 47:183, 1976.

98. **Frankenne F, Closset J, Gomez F, Scippo ML, Smal J, Hennen G,** The physiology of growth hormones (GHs) in pregnant women and partial characterization of the placental GH variant, J Clin Endocrinol Metab 66:1171, 1988.

99. **Pekonen F, Althan H, Stenman U, Ylikorkala O,** Human chorionic gonadotropin (hCG) and thyroid function in early human pregnancy: circadian variation and evidence for intrinsic thyrotropic activity of hCG, J Clin Endocrinol Metab 66:853, 1988.

100. **Kimura M, Amino N, Tamaki H, Mitsuda N, Miyai K, Tanizawa O,** Physiologic thyroid activation in normal early pregnancy is induced by circulating hCG, Obstet Gynecol 75:775, 1990.

101. **Ballabio M, Poshyachinda M, Ekins RP,** Pregnancy-induced changes in thyroid function: role of human chorionic gonadotropin as putative regulator of maternal thyroid, J Clin Endocrinol Metab 73:824, 1991.

102. **Rees LH, Buarke CW, Chard T, Evans SW, Letchorth AT,** Possible placental origin of ACTH in normal human pregnancy, Nature 254:620, 1975.

103. **Goland RS, Wardlaw SL, Blum M, Tropper PJ, Stark RI,** Biologically active corticotropin-releasing hormone in maternal and fetal plasma during pregnancy, Am J Obstet Gynecol 159:884, 1988.

104. **Petraglia F, Sawchenko PE, Rivier J, Vale W,** Evidence for local stimulation of ACTH secretion by corticotropin-releasing factor in human placenta, Nature 328:717, 1987.

105. **Goland RS, Wardlaw SL, MacCarter G, Warren WB, Stark RI,** Adrenocorticotropin and cortisol responses to vasopressin during pregnancy, J Clin Endocrinol Metab 73:257, 1991.

106. **Laatikainen T, Virtanen T, Raiosanen I, Salminen K,** Immunoreactive corticotropin releasing factor and corticotropin in plasma during pregnancy, labor and puerperium, Neuropeptides 10:343, 1987.

107. **Wolfe CDA, Patel SP, Linton EA, et al,** Plasma corticotrophin-releasing factor (CRH) in abnormal pregnancy, Br J Obstet Gynaecol 95:1003, 1988.

108. **Jones SA, Challis JRG,** Local stimulation of prostaglandin production by corticotropin-releasing hormone in human fetal membranes and placenta, Biochem Biophys Res Commun 159:192, 1989.

109. **Jauniaux E, Gulbis B, Jurkovic D, Schaaps JP, Campbell S, Meuris S,** Protein and steroid levels in embryonic cavities in early human pregnancy, Hum Reprod 8:782, 1993.

110. **Keel BA, Eddy KB, Cho S, Gangrade BK, May JV,** Purified human alpha fetoprotein inhibits growth factor-stimulated estradiol production by porcine granulosa cells in monolayer culture, Endocrinology 130:3715, 1992.

111. **Williams MA, Hickok DE, Zingheim RW, Luthy DA, Kimelman J, Nyberg DA, Mahony BS,** Elevated maternal serum α-fetoprotein levels and midtrimester placental abnormalities in relation to subsequent adverse pregnancy outcomes, Am J Obstet Gynecol 167:1032, 1992.

112. **Phillips OP, Elias S, Shulman LP, Andersen RN, Morgan CD, Simpson JL,** Maternal serum screening for fetal Down syndrome in women less than 35 years of age using alpha-fetoprotein, hCG, and unconjugated estriol: a prospective 2-year study, Obstet Gynecol 80:353, 1992.

113. **Haddow JE, Palomaki GE, Knoght GJ, Williams J, Pulkkinen A, Canick JA, Saller DN Jr, Bowers GB,** Prenatal screening for Down's syndrome with use of maternal serum markers, New Engl J Med 327:588, 1992.

114. **Saller DN, Canick JA, Schwartz S, Blitzer MG,** Multiple-marker screening in pregnancies with hydropic and nonhydropic Turner syndrome, Am J Obstet Gynecol 167:1021, 1992.

115. **Weiss G, O'Byrne EM, Hochman J, Steinetz BG, Goldsmith L, Flitcraft JG,** Distribution of relaxin in women during pregnancy, Obstet Gynecol 52:569, 1978.

116. **Fields PA, Larkin LH,** Purification and immunohistochemical localization of relaxin in the human term placenta, J Clin Endocrinol Metab 52:79, 1981.

117. **Lopez Bernal A, Bryant-Greenwood GD, Hansell DJ, Hicks BR, Greenwood FC, Turnbull AC,** Effect of relaxin on prostaglandin E production by human amnion: changes in relation to the onset of labour, Br J Obstet Gynaecol 94:1045, 1987.

118. **Quagliarello J, Steinetz BG, Weiss G,** Relaxin secretion in early pregnancy, Obstet Gynecol 53:62, 1979.

119. **MacLennan AH, Katz M, Creasy R,** The morphologic characteristics of cervical ripening induced by the hormones relaxin and prostaglandin $F_{2\alpha}$ in a rabbit model, Am J Obstet Gynecol 152:691, 1985.

120. **Emmi AM, Skurnick J, Goldsmith LT, Gagliardi CL, Schmidt CL, Kleinberg D, Weiss G,** Ovarian control of pituitary hormone secretion in early human pregnancy, J Clin Endocrinol Metab 72:1359, 1991.

121. **Maslar IA, Ansbacher R,** Effects of progesterone on decidual prolactin production by organ cultures of human endometrium, Endocrinology 118:2102, 1986.

122. **Daly DC, Kuslis S, Riddick DH,** Evidence of short-loop inhibition of decidual prolactin synthesis by decidual proteins, Part I, Am J Obstet Gynecol 155:358, 1986.

123. **Daly DC, Kuslis S, Riddick DH,** Evidence of short-loop inhibition of decidual prolactin synthesis by decidual proteins, Part II, Am J Obstet Gynecol 155:363, 1986.

124. **Handwerger S, Brar A,** Placental lactogen, placental growth hormone, and decidual prolactin, Seminars Reprod Endocrinol 10:106, 1992.

125. **McCoshen JA, Barc J,** Prolactin bioactivity following decidual synthesis and transport by amniochorion, Am J Obstet Gynecol 153:217, 1985.

126. **Ho Yuen B, Cannon W, Lewis J, Sy L, Woolley S,** A possible role for prolactin in the control of human chorionic gonadotropin and estrogen secretion by the fetoplacental unit, Am J Obstet Gynecol 136:286, 1980.

127. **Luciano AA, Varner MW,** Decidual, amniotic fluid, maternal, and fetal prolactin in normal and abnormal pregnancies, Obstet Gynecol 63:384, 1984.

128. **Golander A, Kopel R, Lasebik N, Frenkel Y, Spirer Z,** Decreased prolactin secretion by decidual tissue of pre-eclampsia in vitro, Acta Endocrinol 108:111, 1985.

129. **Healy DL, Herington AC, O'Herlihy C,** Chronic polyhydramnios is a syndrome with a lactogen receptor defect in the chorion laeva, Br J Obstet Gynaecol 92:461, 1985.

130. **Raabe MA, McCoshen JA,** Epithelial regulation of prolactin effect on amnionic permeability, Am J Obstet Gynecol 154:130, 1986.

131. **Pullano JG, Cohen-Addad N, Apuzzio JJ, Ganesh VL, Josimovich JB,** Water and salt conservation in the human fetus and newborn. I. Evidence for a role of fetal prolactin, J Clin Endocrinol Metab 69:1180, 1989.

132. **Ben-Rafael Z, Orvieto R,** Cytokines—involvement in reproduction, Fertil Steril 58:1093, 1992.

133. **Harty JR, Kauma SW,** Interleukin-1β stimulates colony-stimulating factor-1 production in placental villous core mesenchymal cells, J Clin Endocrinol Metab 75:947, 1992.

134. **Masuhiro K, Matsuzaki N, Nishino E, Taniguchi T, Kameda T, Li Y, Saji F, Tanizawa O,** Trophoblast-derived interleukin-1 (IL-1) stimulates the release of human chorionic gonadotropin by activating IL-6 and IL-6-receptor system in first trimester human trophoblasts, J Clin Endocrinol Metab 72:594, 1991.

135. **Li Y, Matsuzaki N, Masuhiro K, et al,** Trophoblast-derived tumor necrosis factor induces release of human chorionic gonadotropin using interleukin-6 (IL-6) and Il-6-receptor-dependent system in the normal human trophoblasts, J Clin Endocrinol Metab 74:184, 1992.

136. **Pekonen F, Suikkari A-M, Makinen T, Rutanen E-M,** Different insulin-like growth factor binding species in human placenta and decidua, J Clin Endocrinol Metab 67:1250, 1988.

137. **Giudice LC, Farrell EM, Pham H, Lamson G, Rosenfeld RG,** Insulin-like growth factor binding proteins in maternal serum throughout gestation and in the puerperium: effects of a pregnancy-associated serum protease activity, J Clin Endocrinol Metab 71:806, 1990.

138. **Osborn BH, Fowlkes J, Han VKM, Fremark M,** Nutritional regulation of insulin-like growth factor-binding protein gene expression in the ovine fetus and pregnant ewe, Endocrinology 131:1743, 1992.

139. **Iwashita M, Kobayashi M, Matsuo A, Nakayama S, Mimuro T, Takeda Y, Sakamoto S,** Feto-maternal interactions of IGF-I and its binding proteins in fetal growth, Early Hum Dev 29:187, 1992.

140. **Abe Y, Hasegawa Y, Miyamoto K, Yamaguchi M, Andoh A, Ibuki Y,** High concentrations of plasma immunoreactive inhibin during normal pregnancy in women, J Clin Endocrinol Metab 71:133, 1990.

141. **Qu J, Ying S-Y, Thomas K,** Inhibin production and secretion in human placental cells cultured in vitro, Obstet Gynecol 79:705, 1992.

142. **Petraglia F, Woodruff TK, Botticelli G, Botticelli A, Genazzani AR, Mayo KE, Vale W,** Gonadotropin-releasing hormone, inhibin, and activin in human placenta: evidence for a common cellular localization, J Clin Endocrinol Metab 74:1184, 1992.

143. **Hung TT,** The role of endogenous opioids in pregnancy and anesthesia, Seminars Reprod Endocrinol 5:161, 1987.

144. **Xie G-X, Miyajima A, Goldstein A,** Expression cloning of cDNA encoding a seven-helix receptor from human placenta with affinity for opioid ligands, Proc Natl Acad Sci USA 89:4124, 1992.

145. **Margioris AN, Grino M, Protos P, Gold PW, Chrousos GP,** Corticotropin-releasing hormone and oxytocin stimulate the release of placental proopiomelanocortin peptides, J Clin Endocrinol Metab 66:922, 1988.

146. **Derkx FHM, Stuenkel C, Schalekamp MPA, Visser W, Huisveld IH, Schalekamp MADH,** Immunoreactive renin, prorenin, and enzymatically active renin in plasma during pregnancy and in women taking contraceptives, J Clin Endocrinol Metab 63:1008, 1986.

147. **Derkx FHM, Alberda AT, De Jong FH, Zeilmaker FH, Makovitz JW, Schalekamp MADH,** Source of plasma prorenin in early and late pregnancy: observations in a patient with primary ovarian failure, J Clin Endocrinol Metab 65:349, 1987.

148. **Itskovitz J, Rubattu S, Levron J, Sealey JE,** Highest concentrations of prorenin and human chorionic gonadotropin in gestational sacs during early human pregnancy, J Clin Endocrinol Metab 75:906, 1992.

149. **Yamaji T, Hirai N, Ishibashi M, Takaku F, Yanaihara T, Nakayama T,** Atrial natriuretic peptide in umbilical cord blood: evidence for a circulating hormone in human fetus, J Clin Endocrinol Metab 63:1414, 1986.

150. **Morton H, Rolfe BE, Cavanagh AC,** Early pregnancy factor, Seminars Reprod Endocrinol 10:72, 1992.

151. **Chou JY, Plouzek CA,** Pregnancy-specific β_1-glycoprotein, Seminars Reprod Endocrinol 10:116, 1992.

152. **Gluck L, Kulovich MV, Borer RC, Brenner PH, Anderson GG, Spellacy WN,** Diagnosis of respiratory distress syndrome by amniocentesis, Am J Obstet Gynecol 109:440, 1971.

153. **Dekowski SA, Snyder JM,** Insulin regulation of messenger ribonucleic acid for the surfactant-associated proteins in human fetal lung in vitro, Endocrinology 131:669, 1992.

154. **Ballard RA, Ballard PL, Creasy RK, Padbury J, Polk DH, Bracken M, Moya FR, Gross I, and the TRH Study Group,** Respiratory disease in very-low-birthweight infants after prenatal thyrotropin-releasing hormone and glucocorticoids, Lancet 339:510, 1992.

9 Prostaglandins

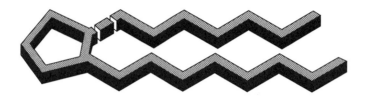

Prostaglandins play fundamental roles in the regulation of reproductive events. Given the name prostaglandins because of the erroneous belief they were the secretory products of only the prostate gland, these substances have widespread actions in keeping with their ubiquitous presence.

This chapter will review the fundamental biochemistry of prostaglandins and focus on the roles of prostaglandins in pregnancy, specifically physiologic control mechanisms in luteal regression, the fetal circulation, parturition, uteroplacental blood flow, and maternal blood pressure.

| Prostaglandin History | The historical evolution of the prostaglandin story is by now familiar. America can claim the first clue to the existence of prostaglandins because two New York gynecologists at Columbia University, Kurzrok and Lieb, reported, in 1930, the contractile effects of fresh human seminal fluid on strips of human uterus. This clue was overlooked, however, and the field was left for the pioneer work to come from Sweden and England, especially from the Karolinska Institute in Stockholm. |

Goldblatt in England, in 1933, and von Euler in Sweden, in 1934, independently discovered that extracts of seminal vesicles stimulated smooth muscle preparations and also had vasodepressor activity. A year later, in 1935, von Euler reported that this biologic activity was due to an acidic lipid which he named prostaglandin. Nothing further was done until the late 1950s. World War II was certainly one reason for this hiatus, but also techniques were not sufficiently sensitive to measure and study prostaglandins, which were available only in small amounts.

The supply problem was initially overcome by collecting large batches of sheep seminal vesicles and utilizing biosynthesis. This was an expensive and major logistic effort. The reward was the characterization and synthesis of prostaglandins in the early 1960s in the laboratory of Professor Sune Bergstrom, a student of von Euler. The discovery in 1970 that a coral (*Plexaura homomala*) off the coast of Florida contained large amounts of prostaglandin materials that could be used for the production of pure prostaglandins was a big boost for laboratory and clinical research. Shortly thereafter, total synthesis of prostaglandins was achieved, and supply was no longer a problem.

During the 1970s the reproductive world was startled by the work of Sultan Karim in Uganda. He was the first to use prostaglandins for the successful induction of labor and abortions, and this clinical application was responsible for a great surge of interest both clinically and in the laboratory. Subsequent history centered on the new members of the prostaglandin family: thromboxane, prostacyclin, and the leukotrienes. The 1982 Nobel Prize in medicine was awarded jointly to Sune Bergstrom for his work with prostaglandins, Bengt Samuelsson for the leukotrienes, and John R. Vane for prostacyclin.

An appreciation for the make-up of this remarkable biochemical family is essential in order to understand the current prostaglandin world.

Prostaglandin Biochemistry

Biosynthesis

The family of prostaglandins with the greatest biologic activity is that having two double bonds, derived from arachidonic acid.[1] Arachidonic acid can be obtained from two sources, directly from the diet (from meats) or by formation from its precursor linoleic acid, which is found in vegetables. In the plasma, 1–2% of the total free fatty acid content is free arachidonic acid. The majority of arachidonic acid is covalently bound in esterified form as a significant proportion of the fatty acids in phospholipids and in esterified cholesterol. Arachidonic acid is only a minor fatty acid in the triglycerides packaged in adipose tissue.

The rate-limiting step in the formation of the prostaglandin family is the release of free arachidonic acid. A variety of hydrolases may be involved in arachidonic acid release, but phospholipase A_2 activation is an important initiator of prostaglandin synthesis because of the abundance of arachidonate in the 2 position of phospholipids. Types of stimuli that activate such lipases include burns, infusions of hypertonic and hypotonic solutions, thrombi and small particles, endotoxin, snake venom, mechanical stretching, catecholamines, bradykinin, angiotensin, and the sex steroids.

"Eicosanoids" refer to all the 20-carbon derivatives, while "prostanoids" indicate only those containing a structural ring. After the release of arachidonic acid the synthetic path can go in two different directions: the lipoxygenase pathway or the cyclooxygenase (prostaglandin endoperoxide H synthetase) pathway. The leukotrienes are formed by 5-lipoxygenase oxygenation of arachidonic acid at C-5, forming an unstable intermediate, LTA_4.[2] LTB_4 is formed by hydration and LTC_4 by the addition of gluathione. The remaining leukotrienes are metabolites of LTC_4. The previously known slow reacting substance of anaphylaxis consists of a mixture of LTC_4, LTD_4, and LTE_4. The leukotrienes are involved in the defense reactions of white cells and participate in hypersensitivity and inflammatory responses. LTB_4 acts primarily on leukocytes (stimulation of leukocyte emigration from the bloodstream), while LTC_4, LTD_4, and LTE_4 affect smooth muscle cells (bronchoconstriction in the lungs and reduced contractility in the heart). All leukotrienes increase microvascular permeability. Thus, the leukotrienes are major agonists, synthesized in response to antigens and provoking asthma and airway obstruction. Leukotrienes are 100–1000 times more potent than histamine in the pulmonary airway.

The 12-lipoxygenase pathway leads to 12-hydroxyeicosatetraenoic acid (12-HETE). Little is known about 12-HETE other than its function as a leukostatic agent. An additional group of arachidonic acid products has been discovered, the lipoxins.[2] The lipoxins (LXA and LXB) inhibit natural killer cell cytotoxicity.

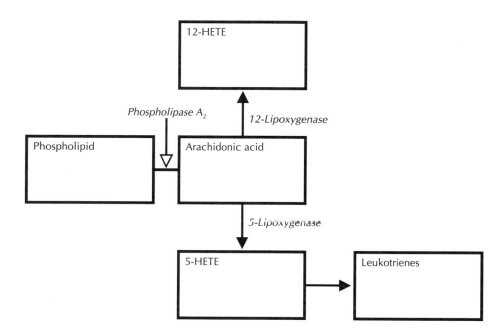

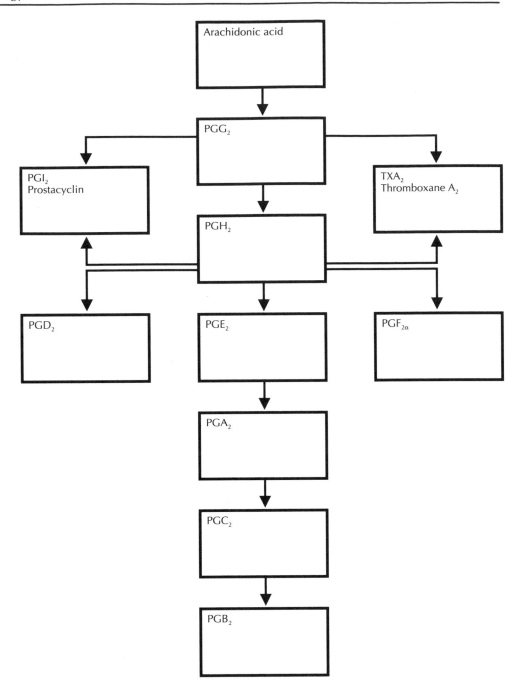

The cyclooxygenase pathway leads to the prostaglandins. The first true prostaglandin (PG) compounds formed are PGG_2 and PGH_2 (half-life of about 5 minutes), the mothers of all other prostaglandins. The numerical subscript refers to the number of double bonds. This number depends on which of the three precursor fatty acids has been utilized. Besides arachidonic acid, the other two precursor fatty acids are linoleic acid, which gives rise to the PG_1 series, and pentanoic acid, the PG_3 series. The latter two series are of less importance in physiology, hence the significance of the arachidonic acid family. The prostaglandins of original and continuing relevance to reproduction are PGE_2 and $PGF_{2\alpha}$ and possibly PGD_2. The α in $PGF_{2\alpha}$ indicates the α steric configuration of the hydroxyl group at the C-9 position. The A, B, and C prostaglandins either have little biologic activity or do not exist in significant concentrations in biologic tissues. In the original work, the prostaglandin more soluble in ether was named PGE, and the one more soluble in phosphate (spelled with an F in Swedish) buffer was named PGF. Later, naming became alphabetical.

**Thromboxane and
Prostacyclin**

Thromboxanes are not true prostaglandins due to the absence of the pentane ring, but prostacyclin (PGI_2) is a legitimate prostaglandin. Thromboxane (TX) (half-life about 30 seconds) and PGI_2 (half-life about 2–3 minutes) can be viewed as opponents, each having powerful biologic activity that counters or balances the other. TXA_2 is the most powerful vasoconstrictor known, while PGI_2 is a potent vasodilator. These two agents also have opposing effects on platelet function. Platelets, lungs, and the spleen predominately synthesize TXA_2, while the heart, stomach, and blood vessels throughout the body synthesize PGI_2. The lungs are a major source of prostacyclin. Normal pulmonary endothelium makes prostacyclin while TXA_2 appears in response to pathologic stimuli.[3] The pulmonary release of prostacyclin may contribute to the body's defense against platelet aggregation.

Let's take a closer look at platelets. The primary function of platelets is the preservation of the vascular system. Blood platelets stick to foreign surfaces or other tissues, a process called adhesion. They also stick to each other and form clumps; this process is called aggregation. Because platelets synthesize TXA_2, a potent stimulator of platelet aggregation, the natural tendency of platelets is to clump and plug defects and damaged spots. The endothelium, on the other hand, produces PGI_2 and its constant presence inhibits platelet aggregation and adherence, keeping blood vessels free of platelets and ultimately clots. Thus, prostacyclin has a defensive role in the body. It is 4 to 8 times more potent a vasodilator than the E prostaglandins, and it prevents the adherence of platelets to healthy vascular endothelium. However, when the endothelium is damaged, platelets gather, beginning the process of thrombus formation. Even in this abnormal situation, prostacyclin strives to fulfill its protective role because increased PGI_2 can be measured in injured endothelium, thrombosed vessels, and in the vascular tissues of hypertensive animals.

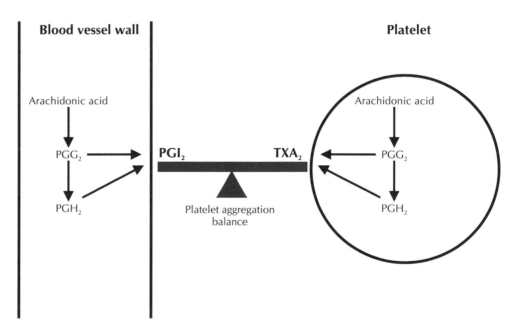

Conditions associated with vascular disease can be understood through the prostacyclin-thromboxane mechanism.[4] For example, atheromatous plaques and nicotine inhibit prostacyclin synthesis. Increasing the cholesterol content of human platelets increases the sensitivity to stimuli which cause platelet aggregation due to increased thromboxane production. The well-known association between low-density and high-density lipoproteins (LDL-cholesterol and HDL-cholesterol) and cardiovascular disease may also be partly explained in terms of PGI_2. LDL from men and postmenopausal women inhibits and HDL stimulates prostacyclin production.[5] Platelets from diabetics and from Class

A diabetic pregnant women make more TXA_2 than platelets from normal pregnant women. Smokers who use oral contraceptives have increased platelet aggregation and an inhibition of prostacyclin formation.[6] Incidentally, onion and garlic inhibit platelet aggregation and TXA_2 synthesis.[7] Perhaps the perfect contraceptive pill is a combination of progestin, estrogen, and some onion or garlic.

In some areas of the world there is a low incidence of cardiovascular disease. This can be directly attributed to diet and the protective action of prostacyclin.[8] The diet of Eskimos and Japanese has a high content of pentanoic acid and low levels of linoleic and arachidonic acids. Pentanoic acid is the precursor of prostaglandin products with 3 double bonds, and, as it happens, PGI_3 is an active agent while TXA_3 is either not formed, or it is inactive. The fat content of most common fish is 8–12% pentanoic acid, and more than 20% in the more exotic (and expensive) seafoods such as scallops, oysters, and caviar.

Metabolism

The metabolism of prostaglandins occurs primarily in the lungs, kidney, and liver. The lungs are important in the metabolism of E and F prostaglandins. Indeed, there is an active transport mechanism which specifically carries E and F prostaglandins from the circulation into the lungs. Any active prostaglandins in the circulation are metabolized during one passage through the lungs. Therefore, members of the prostaglandin family have a short half-life, and in most instances, exert autocrine/paracrine actions at the site of their synthesis. Because of the rapid half-lives, studies are often performed by measuring the inactive end products, for example 6-keto-$PGF_{1\alpha}$, the metabolite of prostacyclin, and TXB_2, the metabolite of thromboxane A_2.

Prostaglandin Inhibition

A review of prostaglandin biochemistry is not complete without a look at the inhibition of the biosynthetic cascade of products. Corticosteroids were previously thought to inhibit the prostaglandin family by stabilizing membranes and preventing the release of phospholipase. It is now recognized that corticosteroids induce the synthesis of proteins called lipocortins (or annexins) which block the action of phospholipase.[9] Thus far, steroids and some local anesthetic agents are the only substances known to work at this step.

Aspirin is an irreversible inhibitor, selectively acetylating the cyclooxygenase involved in prostaglandin synthesis. The other inhibiting agents, nonsteroidal anti-inflammatory agents such as indomethacin and naproxen, are reversible agents, forming a reversible bond with the active site of the enzyme. Acetaminophen inhibits cyclooxygenase in the central nervous system, accounting for its analgesic and antipyretic properties, but has no anti-inflammatory properties nor does it affect platelets. However, acetaminophen does reduce prostacyclin synthesis; the reason for this preferential effect is unkown.[10]

The analgesic, antipyretic, and anti-inflammatory actions of these agents are mediated by inhibition of the cyclooxygenase enzyme. Because of the irreversible nature of the inhibition by aspirin, aspirin exerts a long lasting effect on platelets, maintaining inhibition in the platelet for its lifespan (8–10 days). Prostacyclin synthesis in the endothelium recovers more quickly because the endothelial cells can resynthesize new cyclooxygenase. Platelets, lacking nuclei, cannot produce new enzyme. The sensitivity of the platelets to aspirin may explain the puzzling results in the early studies in which aspirin was given to prevent subsequent morbidity and mortality following thrombotic events. It takes only a little aspirin to effectively inhibit thromboxane synthesis in platelets. Going beyond this dose will not only inhibit thromboxane synthesis in platelets, but also the protective prostacyclin production in blood vessel walls. Controversy continues about what dose of aspirin and what frequency of administration are best. Some suggest that a dose of 3.5 mg/kg (about half an aspirin tablet) given at 3-day

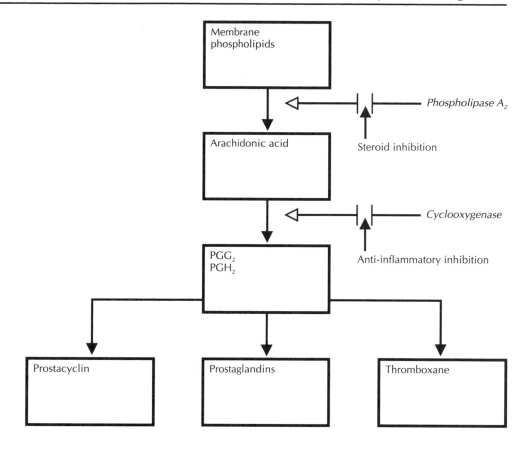

intervals effectively induces maximal inhibition of platelet aggregation without affecting prostacyclin production by the vessel walls.[11] Others indicate that the dose which effectively and selectively inhibits platelet cyclooxygenase is 20–40 mg daily.[12,13] The major handicap with the use of inhibitors of PG synthesis is that they strike blindly and with variable effect from tissue to tissue. Obviously drugs that selectively inhibit TXA_2 synthesis will be superior to aspirin in terms of antithrombotic effects.

Prostaglandins and Luteal Regression

Prostaglandin $F_{2\alpha}$ causes luteal regression in many species. It is the agent responsible for terminating the lifespan of the corpus luteum if fertilization fails to take place, so that a subsequent repeat ovulation can follow rapidly. The $PGF_{2\alpha}$ originates in the endometrium, and its synthesis is stimulated by the estrogen produced in growing follicles. It is transported directly to the corpus luteum through the vasculature connecting the ovary and the uterus, thus achieving an effective concentration at the corpus luteum and avoiding rapid clearance in the systemic circulation.

The mechanism of $PGF_{2\alpha}$-induced luteolysis is two-fold. First, there is a rapid anti-LH action followed by a loss of luteinizing hormone (LH) receptors in the corpus luteum.[14] The rapid action is expressed only in intact cells and appears to be the result of some mediator that blocks LH receptor activation of adenylate cyclase. The slower response is an indirect action, interfering with prolactin maintenance of LH receptors.

Luteolysis has not been demonstrated in the primate, and it is well-known that removal of the uterus does not interfere with normal ovulatory cycles. However, high doses of estrogen can induce luteolysis in the monkey and perhaps in the human. In the monkey, estrogen induces a drop in progesterone during the luteal phase, mirrored by a rise in F prostaglandin. Furthermore, indomethacin can block this effect of estrogen.[15] There is considerable evidence to support a role for estrogen in the decline of the human corpus luteum. The premature elevation of circulating estradiol levels in the early luteal phase results in a prompt fall in progesterone concentrations. Direct injections of estradiol into the ovary bearing the corpus luteum induces luteolysis, while similar treatment of the contralateral ovary produces no effect. Auletta postulates that prostaglandin $F_{2\alpha}$ produced within the ovary bearing the corpus luteum or within the corpus luteum serves as the luteolytic agent, and the production of the prostaglandin is initiated by the luteal estrogen.[16–18] However, the absence of estrogen receptors in luteal tissue argues against a luteolytic role in the primate for physiologic concentrations of estrogen (discussed in Chapter 6).

The human application of these findings can be found in the use of postcoital estrogen for contraception. High doses of estrogen can decrease progesterone levels in human cycles.[19] It is important to remember that the mechanism of estrogen is through $PGF_{2\alpha}$, and since the mechanism of $PGF_{2\alpha}$ is antagonism of LH action, human chorionic gonadotropin (HCG) can overcome this effect of estrogen. Hence, the effective action of estrogen when used for postcoital contraception is limited to the 7 days prior to implantation, before the corpus luteum is subject to rescue by HCG.

Prostaglandins and the Fetal Circulation

The predominant effect of prostaglandins on the fetal and maternal cardiovascular system is to maintain the ductus arteriosus, renal, mesenteric, uterine, placental, and probably the cerebral and coronary arteries in a relaxed or dilated state. The importance of the ductus arteriosus can be appreciated by considering that 59% of the cardiac output flows through this connection between the pulmonary artery and the descending aorta.

Control of ductal patency and closure is mediated through prostaglandins. The arterial concentration of oxygen is the key to the caliber of the ductus. With increasing gestational age, the ductus becomes increasingly responsive to increased oxygen. In this area, too, attention has turned to PGI_2 and TXA_2.

Fetal lamb ductus homogenates produce mainly PGI_2 when incubated with arachidonic acid. PGE_2 and $PGF_{2\alpha}$ are formed in small amounts and TXA_2 not at all. Although PGE_2 is less abundant than PGI_2 in the ductus, it is a more potent vasodilator of the ductus and is more responsive to oxygen (decreasing vasodilatation with increasing oxygen).[20] Thus, PGE_2 appears to be the most important prostaglandin in the ductus from a functional point of view, while PGI_2, the major product in the main pulmonary artery, appears to be the major factor in maintaining vasodilatation in the pulmonary bed. The ductus is dilated maximally in utero by production of prostaglandins, and a positive vasoconstrictor process is required to close it. The source of the vasoconstrictor is probably the lung. With increasing maturation, the lung shifts to TXA_2 formation. This fits with the association of ductal patency with prematurity. With the onset of pulmonary ventilation at birth leading to vascular changes that deliver blood to the duct directly from the lungs, TXA_2 can now serve as the vasoconstrictor stimulus. The major drawback to this hypothesis is the failure of inhibitors to affect the constriction response to oxygen.

Administration of vasodilating prostaglandins can maintain patency after birth, while preparing an infant for surgery to correct a congenital lesion causing pulmonary hypertension. Infants with persistent ductus patency may be spared thoracotomy by treatment with an inhibitor of prostaglandin synthesis. The use of indomethacin to close a persistent ductus in the premature infant is successful about 40% of the time.[20] An important factor is early diagnosis and treatment because with increasing postnatal age the ductus becomes less sensitive to prostaglandin inhibitors, probably because of more efficient clearance of the drug.[21] The highest incidence of successful indomethacin ductus closure has been with infants less than 30 weeks gestation and less than 10 days old.

This aspect of the use of prostaglandin inhibitors is of concern in considering the use of agents to inhibit premature labor. The drug half-life in the fetus and newborn is prolonged because the metabolic pathways are limited, and there is reduced drug clearance because of immature renal function. In utero constriction of the ductus can cause congestive heart failure and fetal pulmonary hypertension.[22] Prolonged ductus constriction leads to subendocardial ischemia and fibrotic lesions in the tricuspid valve muscles. Infants with persistent pulmonary hypertension have hypoxemia, cardio-megaly, and right to left shunting through the foramen ovale or the ductus. Infants of mothers given either indomethacin or salicylates chronically have been reported to have this syndrome. Duration of exposure and dosage are critical. It takes occlusion of the ductus for more than 2 weeks to produce fetal pulmonary hypertension and cardiac hypertrophy. This side effect is absent in pregnancies less than 27 weeks gestation; the ductus arteriosus begins to respond at 27–30 weeks, and after 30 weeks, this is an important side effect which can be minimized if long-term use is avoided.

Prostaglandins and Fetal Breathing

Prior to parturition, fetal breathing is very shallow. It is proposed that placental PGE_2 suppresses breathing by acting in the fetal brain.[23] Occlusion of the umbilical cord is rapidly followed by a loss of this PGE_2 influence and the onset of air breathing. The administration of indomethacin to fetal sheep increases, while infusion of PGE suppresses, fetal breathing movements. This may be the explanation for the decrease in fetal breathing movements observed during human labor (associated with an increase in prostaglandin levels).

Prostaglandins and Parturition

Perhaps the best example of the interplay among fetus, placenta, and mother is the initiation and maintenance of parturition. Endocrine changes in the uteroplacental environment are the principal governing factors accounting for the eventual development of uterine contractions. The sequence of events has been repeatedly reviewed in detail, where references to the original work are available.[24–26]

Extensive work in the sheep has implicated the fetal pituitary-adrenal axis in normal parturition. The sequence of events in the sheep begins about 10 days prior to labor with elevation of fetal cortisol in response to fetal pituitary ACTH. Fetal adrenalectomy or hypophysectomy prolongs pregnancy, while infusion of ACTH or glucocorticoids into the sheep fetus stimulates premature labor. Maternal stimulation of the fetal adrenal is not a factor because in sheep (and in women) there is little or no placental transfer of maternal ACTH into the fetal circulation. Thus, parturition in the ewe is initiated by a signal in the fetal brain activating ACTH secretion.

Increased cortisol secretion by the fetal adrenal gland starts a chain of events associated with labor. The sequence of events continues in the sheep with a decline in progesterone. This change is brought about by the induction of 17α-hydroxylase, 17,20-lyase enzyme activity (P450c17) in the sheep placenta.

Glucocorticoid treatment of sheep placental tissue specifically increases the rate of production of 17α,20α-dihydroxypregn-4-en-3-one. This dihydroxyprogesterone compound also has been identified in sheep placental tissue obtained after spontaneous labor. Thus, direct synthesis of progesterone does not decline, but increased metabolism to a 17-hydroxylated product results in less available progesterone. Progesterone withdrawal is associated with a decrease in the resting potential of myometrium, i.e., an increased response to electric and oxytocic stimuli. Conduction of action potential through the muscle is increased, and the myometrial excitability is increased.

Changes in Sheep Pregnancy

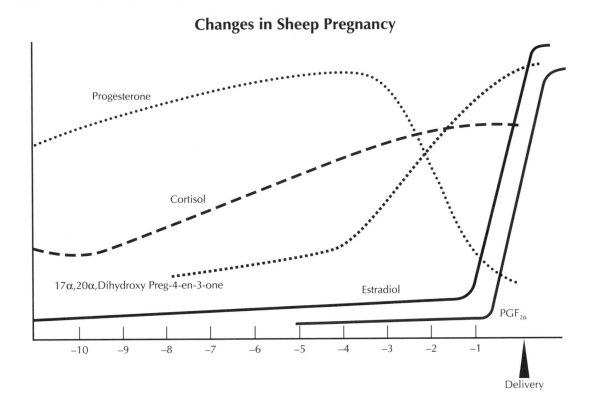

Progesterone

Cortisol

17α,20α,Dihydroxy Preg-4-en-3-one

Estradiol

$PGF_{2\alpha}$

-10   -9   -8   -7   -6   -5   -4   -3   -2   -1

Delivery

Dihydroxyprogesterone also serves as a precursor for the rise in estrogen levels which occurs a few days prior to parturition. Estrogens enhance rhythmic contractions as well as increasing vascularity and permeability, and the oxytocin response. Thus, progesterone withdrawal and estrogen increase lead to an enhancement of conduction and excitation.

The final event in the ewe is a rise in $PGF_{2\alpha}$ production hours before the onset of uterine activity. A cause-and-effect relationship between the rise in estrogen and the appearance of $PGF_{2\alpha}$ has been demonstrated in sheep. These events indicate that the decline in progesterone, the rise in estrogen, and the increase in $PGF_{2\alpha}$ are all secondary to direct induction of a placental enzyme by fetal cortisol.

The steroid events in human pregnancy are not identical to events in the ewe. In addition, there is a more extended time scale. Steroid changes in the sheep occur over the course of several days, while in human pregnancy the changes begin at approximately 34–36 weeks and occur over the last 5 weeks of pregnancy.

Cortisol rises dramatically in amniotic fluid, beginning at 34–36 weeks, and correlates with pulmonary maturation. Cord blood cortisol concentrations are high in infants born vaginally or by cesarean section following spontaneous onset of labor. In contrast, cord blood cortisol levels are lower in infants born without spontaneous labor, whether delivery is vaginal (induced labor) or by cesarean section (elective repeat section). In keeping with the extended time scale of events, administration of glucocorticoids is not followed acutely by the onset of labor in pregnant women (unless the pregnancy is past due).

It is unlikely that the cortisol increments in the fetus represent changes due to increased adrenal activity in the mother in response to stress. Although maternal cortisol crosses the placenta readily, it is largely (85%) metabolized to cortisone in the process. This, in fact, may be the mechanism by which suppression of the fetal adrenal gland by maternal steroids is avoided. In contrast to the maternal liver, the fetal liver has a limited capacity for transforming the biologically inactive cortisone to the active cortisol. On the other hand, the fetal lung does possess the capability of changing cortisone to cortisol, and this may be an important source of cortisol for the lung. Cortisol itself induces this conversion in lung tissue. Increased fetal adrenal activity is followed by changes in steroid levels as well as important developmental accomplishments (e.g., increased pulmonary surfactant production and the accumulation of liver glycogen).

But the increased levels of fetal cortisol associated with labor appear to be secondary to the stress of the process, and at the present time there is no evidence that fetal cortisol production triggers human parturition. In human parturition the important contribution of the fetal adrenal, rather than cortisol, is probably its effect on placental estrogen production. The common theme in human pregnancies associated with failure to begin labor on time is decreased estrogen production, e.g., anencephaly and placental sulfatase deficiency. In contrast, mothers bearing fetuses who cannot form normal amounts of cortisol, such as those with congenital adrenal hyperplasia, deliver on time.[27]

An increase in estrogen levels in maternal blood begins at 34–35 weeks of gestation, but a late increase just before parturition (as in the sheep) has not been observed in human pregnancy. Perhaps a critical concentration is the signal in human pregnancy rather than a triggering increase. Or the changes are taking place at a local level and are not reflected in the maternal circulation.[28] Although it has not been definitely demonstrated, increased or elevated estrogen levels are thought to play a key role in increasing prostaglandin production.

Progesterone maintenance of uterine quiescence and increased myometrial excitability associated with progesterone withdrawal are firmly established as mechanisms of parturition in lower species. In primates, the role of progesterone is less clear, largely because of the inability to demonstrate a definite decline in peripheral blood levels of progesterone prior to parturition. Nevertheless, pharmacologic treatment with progesterone or synthetic progestational agents has some effect in preventing premature labor.[29,30] There is also reason to believe that progesterone concentration is regulated locally, and progesterone withdrawal can be accomplished by a combination of binding and metabolism.[31] However, no strong evidence exists to support progesterone withdrawal (by any method, including binding or sequestration) as a mechanism in human parturition. Nevertheless, interruption of exposure to progesterone (e.g., with the antiprogesterone, RU486) leads to uterine contractions. Perhaps multiple mechanisms exist which affect in a subtle fashion the local concentration and actions of progesterone.

Evidence for a role of prostaglandin in parturition includes the following:

1.   Prostaglandin levels in maternal blood and amniotic fluid increase in association with labor.

2.   Arachidonic acid levels in the amniotic fluid also rise in labor, and arachidonate injected into the amniotic sac initiates parturition.

3.   Patients taking high doses of aspirin have a highly significant increase in the average length of gestation, incidence of postmaturity, and duration of labor.

4.   Indomethacin prevents the normal onset of labor in monkeys and stops premature labor in human pregnancies.

5. Stimuli known to cause the release of prostaglandins (cervical manipulation, stripping of membranes, and rupture of membranes) augment or induce uterine contractions.

6. Prostaglandins induce labor.

The precursor fatty acid for prostaglandin production in part may be derived from storage pools in the fetal membranes, the decidua, or both.[9] Phospholipase A_2 has been demonstrated in both human chorioamnion and uterine decidua. Although the precise mechanism for initiating prostaglandin synthesis, presumably by activation of the enzyme phospholipase A_2, remains unknown, the availability of arachidonic acid for prostaglandin production during parturition can be due to stimulation of hydrolysis of phosphatidylethanolamine and phosphatidylinositol in decidual, amnion, and chorion laeve tissues.[32–34] Microsomes from amnion, chorion laeve, and decidua vera tissues contain lipases that hydrolyze fatty acids esterified in the 2 position. Specific phospholipase activity combined with a diacylglycerol lipase which also has a specificity for arachidonic acid provides a mechanism for the release of arachidonic acid. The activity of these enzymes in fetal membranes and decidua vera tissue increases with increasing length of gestation.

The key may be the increasing formation of estrogen (both estradiol and estriol) in the maternal circulation as well as in the amniotic fluid or, more importantly, locally within the uterus. The marked rise in estrogen near term may affect the activity of the lipase enzymes, leading to the liberation of arachidonic acid. The activity of these phospholipases is increased by increasing concentrations of calcium, and therefore the regulation of intracellular calcium is an important mechanism.

The human fetal membranes and decidua are incredibly active. Human chorion and decidua produce estrogen utilizing a variety of substrates, especially estrone sulfate and dehydroepiandrosterone sulfate (DHAS), and this activity is increased around the time of parturition.[35,36] In addition, the human fetal membranes synthesize and metabolize progesterone.[37] The membranes contain a 17,20-hydroxysteroid dehydrogenase system. One active site converts 20α-dihydroxyprogesterone to progesterone, while another active site on this enzyme converts estrone to estradiol. Thus, this enzyme can play an important role in altering the estrogen/progesterone ratio. The membranes and the decidua contain distinct cell populations with different biochemical activities (which change with labor).[38] Steroidogenic and prostaglandin interactions among these cells could produce the changes necessary for parturition without affecting the concentrations of circulating hormones. In addition, relaxin derived from decidua and/or chorion may exert a paracrine action on amnion prostaglandin production.[39] Finally, the fetus may take a very direct role in this scenario by secreting substances into the amniotic fluid, which interact with the fetal membranes to signal the initiation of parturition.

With labor, the arachidonic acid pathway in the fetal membranes shifts in the cyclooxygenase direction with a large increase in the production of PGE_2. Specific protein inhibitors of prostaglandin synthetase have been demonstrated in placenta, amnion, and chorion, and these proteins cannot be found in tissue from patients who have established labor.[9,40] The link between infection and the onset of labor (especially preterm labor) may be due to the conversion by bacterial medium (with factors such as the interleukins) of arachidonic metabolism in the membranes and decidua to a condition associated with labor marked by the production of PGE_2.[9,41,42]

Undoubtedly, prostaglandin production during pregnancy reflects the usual complex interaction of a host of autocrine/paracrine factors. Platelet-activating factor stimulates prostaglandin production by the fetal membranes (apparently by regulating intracellular calcium concentrations); it can be released in the decidua by inflammation, and it can also be derived from the fetal lung.[43] Secretory products of the fetal membranes themselves are active stimulators of membrane prostaglandin production, including renin derived from chorion prorenin.[44] Decidual $PGF_{2\alpha}$ production is enhanced by bradykinin, epidermal growth factor and transforming growth factor-α, and these responses are further increased by interleukin-1β.[45,46] Prostaglandin production by amnion, chorion, and decidual cells is stimulated by cortiocotropin releasing hormone and modulated by progesterone.[47] The ubiquitous substances, activin and inhibin, are involved here as well. Amnion and chorion produce the activin and inhibin subunits, and activin stimulates prostaglandin PGE_2 release from amnion cells.[48]

During labor the maternal circulating levels of PGE_2, $PGF_{2\alpha}$, and the $PGF_{2\alpha}$-metabolite are increased, a change which can be directly attributed to uterine production in that the gradient across the uterus for these substances is also increased. This increase in production of prostaglandins within the uterus must be the key factor, because the concentration and affinity of prostaglandin receptors do not change at parturition.[49] Meanwhile, prostacyclin and its metabolite are not increased. Prostacyclin is produced (at least in vitro) by a variety of tissues involved in pregnancy: endometrium, myometrium, placenta, amnion, chorion, decidua. As will be discussed later, this prostacyclin is probably more important in the vascular responses of mother and fetus, and in all likelihood does not play a role in initiating or maintaining uterine contractions.

It is uncertain how much prostaglandin is derived from the amnion. Decidua produces both PGE_2 and $PGF_{2\alpha}$, but the amnion and chorion produce primarily PGE_2.[50] There is evidence for the transfer of prostaglandin E_2 across the membranes to the decidua and possibly the myometrium.[51] The paradox of PGE_2 production in the amnion being matched not by a PGE-metabolite in the maternal circulation, but by a $PGF_{2\alpha}$-metabolite, is explained by transfer across the membranes and conversion of PGE_2 to $PGF_{2\alpha}$ in the decidua.[52] However, continued study of this issue strongly indicates that prostaglandins produced on one side of the membranes do not contribute to the prostaglandins on the other side, arguing that uterine contractions must be primarily influenced by decidual or myometrial prostaglandins.[53]

Paul MacDonald emphasizes that the prostaglandins are involved in a series of events, and that the timing of their increased production argues against a primary role in the initiation of parturition.[54] The increase in prostaglandins may be a consquence of the inflammatory changes associated with labor and not a factor in the initiation of labor. MacDonald argues that parturition follows the interruption of the mechanisms that actively maintain uterine quiescence, perhaps by the endogenous production of a substance or substances acting as an antiprogesterone.

Using sensitive assays, an increase in maternal levels of oxytocin can be detected prior to parturition. Once labor has begun, oxytocin levels rise significantly, especially during the second stage. Thus, oxytocin may be important for developing the more intense uterine contractions. Extremely high concentrations of oxytocin can be measured in the cord blood at delivery, and release of oxytocin from the fetal pituitary may also be involved in labor. However, this is controversial, and studies in monkeys fail to indicate a role for fetal oxytocin in parturition.[55] Part of the contribution of oxytocin to parturition is the stimulation of prostaglandin synthesis in decidua and myometrium.[56] Cervical dilatation appears to be dependent upon oxytocin stimulation of prostaglandin production, probably in the decidua. The greater frequency of labor and delivery at night may be due to greater nocturnal oxytocin secretion.[57]

It is likely that oxytocin action during the inital stages of labor may depend on myometrial sensitivity to oxytocin in addition to the levels of oxytocin in the blood. The concentration of oxytocin receptors in the myometrium is low in the nonpregnant state and increases steadily throughout gestation (an 80-fold increase), and during labor the concentration doubles. This receptor concentration correlates with the uterine sensitivity to oxytocin. The mechanism for the increase is unknown, but it likely is due to a change in the prostaglandin and hormonal milieu of the uterus. In addition, oxytocin is synthesized in the amnion, chorion, and significantly, in the decidua.[57] The local production and effects of oxytocin, estrogen, and progesterone combine in a complicated process of autocrine, paracrine, and endocrine actions to result in parturition.

Animal studies have implicated the formation of low resistance pathways in the myometrium, called *gap junctions,* as an important action of steroids and prostaglandins during labor.[58] In the gap junction, a pore forms which allows communication from cytoplasm to cytoplasm between two cells. The pore is a cylinder-shaped channel formed of 6 special proteins called *connexins.* Either substances or electrical current (ions) can follow this pathway without leakage into extracellular space. Thus, gap junctions provide a means of communication between myometrial cells, allowing enhancement of electrical conductivity and synchronization of activity. Gap junction formation is related to the estrogen/progesterone ratio (estrogen is stimulatory and progesterone is inhibitory) and to the presence of the stimulating prostaglandins, PGE_2 and $PGF_{2\alpha}$. Therefore it is not surprising that the number of gap junctions increases in the final weeks of pregnancy, especially just before labor. The modulation of the number and the permeability of gap junctions is another contributing factor in the control of uterine contractility.

The final contraction of uterine muscle results from increased free calcium concentrations in the myofibril, the result of prostaglandin action, an action opposed to that of progesterone which promotes calcium binding in the sarcoplasmic reticulum.[59] Thus, prostaglandins and oxytocin increase while progesterone decreases intracellular calcium levels. The intracellular calcium concentration is affected by cellular entry and exit of calcium as well as binding in the sarcoplasmic reticulum. It is the intracellular concentration of calcium which determines the rate of myosin phosphorylation and the contractile state of the myometrium. Tocolytic therapy (the use of beta-adrenergic agents) stimulates adenylate cyclase activity which increases the levels of cellular cyclic AMP, which in turn decreases intracellular calcium concentration as well as inhibiting actin-myosin interaction by modulating kinase phosphorylation.

Ducsay and colleagues propose that the coordination of this complex relationship of physiologic, endocrine, and molecular mechanisms is expressed in rhythms.[60] Both mother and fetus experience 24-hour rhythms in hormone secretions, and uterine activity is correlated with day and night (photoperiod regulation). The coordination and enhancement of this rhythmicity play a role in parturition. Improved detection and measurement of this activity could contribute to better prevention and treatment of preterm labor.

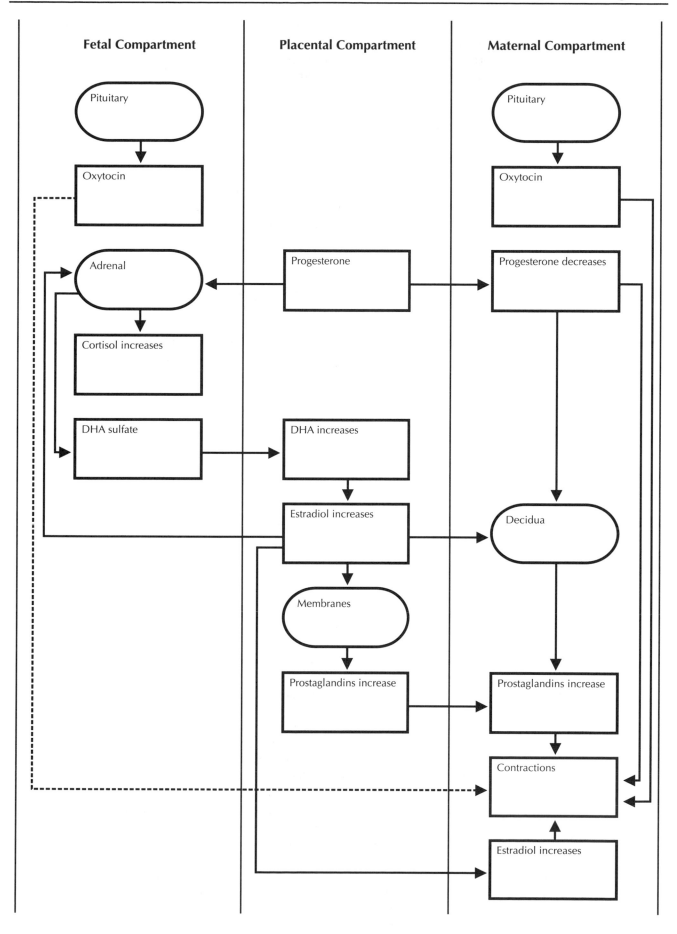

Treatment of Labor with Prostaglandin Inhibition

The key role for prostaglandins in parturition raises the potential for treatment of premature labor with inhibitors of prostaglandin synthesis. The concern has been that such treatment would result in intrauterine closure of the ductus arteriosus and pulmonary hypertension. Clinical studies, however, indicate that use of the nonsteroidal anti-inflammatory agents for short periods of time (3 days) yields good results and does not result in this complication.[61] Beyond 34 weeks, the fetus is more sensitive to this action, and treatment should be limited to pregnancies less than 32 weeks and with caution from 32–34 weeks. Perhaps it is the treatment of choice for the inhibition of labor during a maternal transport. If the drug is failing, it should not be maintained because increased blood loss can occur at delivery. Because indomethacin inhibits the synthesis of all members of the prostaglandin family, including the vasodilating prostacyclin, it should be used with caution in hypertensive patients.[62]

Treatment of pregnant women with indomethacin reduces the amniotic fluid volume due to a decrease in fetal urine output. This is reversible with a decrease in dose. This treatment has been used for polyhydramnios with good response and no effect on the newborn despite treatment for 2 to 11 weeks.[63]

Sulindac is just as effective as a tocolytic but does not affect urine output and amniotic fluid.[64] It may have less of an impact on the fetal ductus arteriosus.

Induction of Labor and Cervical Ripening

Pharmacologically and physiologically, prostaglandins have two direct actions associated with labor: ripening of the cervix and a direct oxytocic action. Successful parturition requires organized changes in both the upper uterus and in the cervix. The cervical changes are in response to the estrogen/progesterone ratio and the local release of prostaglandins. Whether relaxin plays a role in human parturition is not established; however, recombinant relaxin is being tested for cervical ripening.

Ripening of the cervix is the result of a change which includes an increase in hyaluronic acid and water and a decrease in dermatan sulfate and chondroitin sulfate (these compounds hold the collagen fibers in a rigid structure). How prostaglandins operate in this change is unknown, but enzyme activation must be involved. For ripening of the cervix, PGE_2 is very effective, while $PGF_{2\alpha}$ has little effect. The purpose of achieving ripening of the cervix is to increase the success rate with induction of labor and lower the proportion of cesarean sections. Intravaginal prostaglandin E_2 administered as tablets, suppositories, and mixed in gels has been very effective for cervical ripening. The commercial formulation currently available in the U.S. consists of 0.5 mg PGE_2 dissolved in a triacetin viscous gel base, also containing a colloid silicone dioxide, provided in a prefilled syringe for application (Prepidil Gel, The Upjohn Company).[65]

A major clinical application for the induction of labor in the United States is the use of intravaginal PGE_2 in cases of fetal demise and anencephalic fetuses. Based on our own experience, certain precautions have been developed. The patient should be well hydrated with an electrolyte solution to counteract the induced vasodilatation and decreased peripheral resistance. If satisfactory uterine activity is established, the next application should be withheld. And, finally, because there is a synergistic effect when oxytocin is used shortly after prostaglandin administration, there should be a minimum of 6 hours between the last prostaglandin dose and beginning oxytocin augmentation.

Prostaglandins are used to induce term labor. Intravenous prostaglandins are not an acceptable method due to the side effects achieved by the high dosage necessary to reach the uterus. The intravaginal and oral administration of PGE_2 is as effective as intravenous oxytocin, even including patients with previous cesarean sections.[66,67] These methods, plus intracervical administration, are in routine use in many parts of the world.

Therapeutic Abortion

Prostaglandins are effective for postcoital contraception and first trimester abortion but impractical due to the high incidence of side effects, including an unacceptable rate of incomplete abortions. For midtrimester abortions, intraamniotic prostaglandin, intramuscular methyl esters, and vaginal PGE suppositories are available. The major clinical problems have been the efficacy in accomplishing complete expulsion and the high level of systemic side effects. Overall, there is a higher risk of hemorrhage, fever, infection, antibiotic administration, readmission to the hospital, and more operative procedures when compared to saline abortions. These complications can be minimized if care is paid to two aspects of the clinician's technique. First, laminaria should be used to reduce the incidence of cervical injury and the need for retreatment. Second, aggressive management of the third stage is necessary. Removing the placenta with ring forceps, inspecting the cervix, and exploring the uterine cavity are necessary immediately after expulsion of the fetus. This aggressive management will minimize the most troublesome side effects, which are due to retained tissue.

The combination of prostaglandin's oxytocic action with the antiprogesterone effect of RU486 has proved to be a safe and effective medical treatment for the induction of therapeutic abortion prior to 9 weeks gestation.[68,69]

An orally active methyl ester of prostaglandin E_1 is only 20% effective as an abortifacient when administered by itself. Combining the prostaglandin with RU486 achieves greater than 95% efficacy, safely and inexpensively.

Prostaglandins and Postpartum Hemorrhage

When routine methods of management for postpartum hemorrhage caused by uterine atony have failed, an analogue of prostaglandin $F_{2\alpha}$ has been used with excellent results (80–90% successful).[70] Prostin 15 M is (15-S)-15-methyl prostaglandin $F_{2\alpha}$-tromethamine. The dose is 0.25–0.5 mg, repeated up to 4 times and given with equal efficacy either intramuscularly or directly into the myometrium. It can also be used after the replacement of an inverted uterus. Failures are usually associated with infections or magnesium sulfate therapy. It should not be used in patients with severe hypertension or symptomatic asthma. Diarrhea is a frequent side effect.

Prostaglandins, Uteroplacental Blood Flow, and Maternal Blood Pressure

A change must take place in the maternal vascular system to accommodate the volume and flow changes during pregnancy. The maternal plasma volume begins to increase about the 6th week of pregnancy. It rapidly expands during the second trimester but increases only slightly in the last trimester until term. There is a greater increment in plasma volume compared to the red cell volume in normal pregnancy (mean plasma volume increase of 1074 mL vs. 350 mL increase in red cell volume).[71] In order to accommodate the increase in volume (and cardiac output) without a significant increase in the maternal blood pressure, there must be a decrease in the peripheral vascular resistance. There are two mechanisms for the decrease in resistance. One is the increasing fraction of the cardiac output which passes through the uteroplacental circulation; the other is vasodilatation in the maternal vascular tree. Maintenance of normal maternal blood pressure and also maintenance of uteroplacental blood flow (and therefore effective exchange functions across the placenta) depend upon vasodilatation, both in the systemic maternal circulation and locally with the uteroplacental unit. Prostacyclin may mediate this important function.

Preeclampsia as a Chronic Disease

For an economy of words, it continues to be useful to use "preeclampsia" interchangeably with pregnancy-induced hypertension. A more important change in our thinking has been the acceptance of the concept of preeclampsia as a chronic problem throughout pregnancy, not an acute disease arising at the time of hypertension. Besides the vasospasm and hypertension, preeclampsia is associated with increased activation of platelets and the coagulation system in the microvasculature. The endothelium is a target of the alterations in preeclampsia and is important role in the pathogenesis of preeclampsia.[72] Altered endothelial cell function and endothelial cell injury are responsible for the characteristic pathologic lesions of preeclampsia.

Measuring the metabolic clearance rate of dehydroepiandrosterone sulfate (DHAS), Gant et al demonstrated a decline in DHAS clearance prior to the development of clinically evident preeclampsia.[73] Subsequently, the same group showed that the pressor response to angiotensin II was different as early as 22 weeks in a group of primigravid women who went on to develop near term the typical clinical manifestations of preeclampsia.[74] Even the routine measurement of blood pressure, by a standardized technique that included a 5-minute rest period, was able to delineate a group of women who later became hypertensive, in that they had higher blood pressures throughout pregnancy.[75] Doppler blood flow studies confirm that in women destined to develop preeclampsia, changes occur early in pregnancy.[76]

The above studies indicate that preeclampsia is caused by or associated with a disturbance in a homeostatic mechanism responsible for maintenance of blood pressure and uteroplacental blood flow. A syndrome resembling preeclampsia can be produced in the pregnant monkey by chronic reduction of lower aortic pressure.[77] The metabolic requirements of the fetus are best served by maintaining an adequate blood flow. In pregnancy, there is a need beyond the ordinary organ's concern with cellular function; there is the obligation of meeting the demands of the growing fetus. Preeclampsia is associated with a 40–60% reduction in blood flow through the uteroplacental unit in women, but it has been impossible to determine whether this is a primary or secondary event. If preeclampsia is due to the development of impaired blood flow over a period of time, it would seem that the clinical symptoms of the disease would be a late occurrence, and subclinical abnormalities should be detectable earlier in pregnancy (as in the above studies). Indeed, it has been demonstrated that clearance of DHAS reflects a decrease in uteroplacental blood flow and, therefore, reduced uteroplacental blood flow precedes the appearance of hypertension.[78] Because the unique requirement for preeclampsia is the presence of placental tissue, attention focuses on the placental origin of blood borne factors that initiate the pathophysiologic changes associated with preeclampsia.

Prostaglandins and Preeclampsia

Two properties of certain classes of prostaglandins are noteworthy in searching for the mechanism of vasodilatation and regulation of blood flow in pregnancy. First, E prostaglandins and prostacyclin are potent vasodilators, decreasing the peripheral resistance and systemic blood pressure by directly relaxing the smooth muscle of the arterial walls. Second, the majority of the activity of these prostaglandins appears to be limited to the immediate vicinity of the synthesizing tissue itself.

Initially, attention was focused on E and F prostaglandins. The important observations in the monkey,[79–81] the sheep,[82] the dog,[83] and the rabbit,[84] were as follows:

1. Angiotensin II increased uterine blood flow.

2. Angiotensin II increased PGE production by the pregnant uterus.

3. Inhibition of prostaglandin synthesis lowered basal blood flow, blocked the blood flow and PGE response to angiotensin II, and raised the systemic blood pressure.

These findings are consistent with a role for E prostaglandins in maintaining the resting uteroplacental and maternal vasomotor tone and in moderating resistance to flow in response to vasoconstrictors. In the experiments in monkeys in the third trimester, angiotensin II-induced hypertension following treatment with indomethacin failed to increase uterine artery blood flow as had been noted after the initial infusion of angiotensin.

The entire renin-angiotensin-aldosterone system is increased in pregnancy, presumably due to a direct stimulation of substrate (angiotensinogen) synthesis by estrogen. It appears that this increase is the basic mechanism for producing the increased blood volume of pregnancy. The demonstration that blood vessels produce prostaglandins led to the speculation that vascular prostaglandins were responsible for the concomitant vasodilatation associated with the increased renin-angiotensin-aldosterone activity.[85] A pregnant woman's blood pressure at any point in time then reflected the balance of these various forces. A role for prostaglandins was supported by the demonstration that the administration of indomethacin or aspirin decreased the amount of angiotensin necessary to produce a pressor response in pregnant women.[85] This is consistent with the conclusion that pressor responsiveness to angiotensin II during pregnancy is determined by the degree of vascular resistance to the pressor agent. A hypothesis was then suggested linking estrogen, the renin-angiotensin system, and prostaglandins.[86]

Estrogen can be viewed as a principal messenger for ensuring normal growth and development. Estrogen increases uterine blood flow, apparently via the mediation of a vasodilating prostaglandin. The major precursor for placental estrogen production is DHAS, secreted by the fetal adrenal gland. What regulates estrogen production has been an important question in placental physiology. This question appears to be answered, with the concept that the fetal adrenal-placental unit governs its own rate of estrogen production (see chapter 8). The amount of precursor available for estrogen production may be the major rate-limiting factor. Estrogen itself circulates back to the fetus to increase the production of its precursor by suppressing the activity of the enzyme, 3β-hydroxysteroid dehydrogenase, thus diverting the steroidogenic pathway to DHAS. This mechanism (still an unproven hypothesis) allows ever increasing levels of estrogen production. The rising levels of estrogen increase the activity of the aldosterone system to expand blood volume, and at the same time may stimulate prostacyclin production within fetal and maternal blood vessels to maintain vasodilatation and blood flow.

Prostacyclin and Preeclampsia

The emergence of prostacyclin as a vasodilator even more potent than E prostaglandins directed attention to this member of the prostaglandin family. In addition, it was appreciated that the prostacyclin metabolite migrates with E prostaglandins in separation systems. Therefore, previous studies implicating E prostaglandins may have been dealing with prostacyclin.

It is proposed that a fundamental disturbance in preeclampsia is an imbalance between the vasodilator and vasoconstrictor members of the prostaglandin family, prostacyclin (PGI$_2$) and thromboxane A$_2$ (TXA$_2$). Many investigators have reported a general decrease in prostacyclin associated with preeclampsia.[87-89] Lower levels of this potent vasodilator and inhibitor of platelet activity could explain three of the most significant clinical consequences of preeclampsia: hypertension, platelet consumption, and reduced uteroplacental blood flow.

For years, investigators have implicated disseminated intravascular coagulation (DIC) as an important component of the symptom complex associated with preeclampsia. Pritchard has argued strongly that thrombocytopenia in preeclampsia is not an etiologic factor, but a consequence of a disease that is most consistent with platelet adherence at sites of vascular endothelial damage.[90] A closer analysis reveals that the thrombocytopenia associated with preeclampsia is most similar to that seen with various microangiopathies, a consequence of abnormal platelet-endothelial interaction.[91] Indeed modern assessments indicate that preeclampsia is associated with high fibronectin, low antithrombin III, and low alpha$_2$-antiplasmin, suggesting endothelial injury, clotting, and fibrinolysis, respectively.[92] The most marked resolution associated with delivery occurs with fibronectin, a marker for endothelial injury.

As with blood pressure measurement, DHAS clearance, and angiotensin II pressor response, decreased platelet counts, when studied in a carefully controlled manner, also precede the development of hypertension. Early platelet consumption may be seen with preeclampsia before deterioration of urate clearance or elevation of blood pressure. The failure of heparin therapy to affect the clinical course of preeclampsia supports the fact that DIC is not the mechanism of the thrombocytopenia. Indeed, the reason that hypertension does not accompany coagulation disorders associated with intrauterine fetal demise and abruption placentae may be that these classic problems are due to infusion of thromboplastin and DIC, and not to an endothelial disorder. The pathologic appearance of blood vessels in the placental bed in preeclampsia bears significant resemblance to the blood vessels associated with microangiopathic syndromes.[93] Patients with the hemolytic uremic syndrome and thrombotic thrombocytopenic purpura share a common problem: defective prostacyclin activity.[94–96]

The precise problem may be more a reflection of the thromboxane/prostacyclin balance. Both thromboxane and prostacyclin production are increased during pregnancy, but the increase in prostacyclin far exceeds the increase in thromboxane.[13] At the same time that a reduction in prostacyclin precedes the clinical development of preeclampsia, an increase in thromboxane biosynthesis can be detected.[97,98] This imbalance can be a consequence of endothelial cell injury altering the prostacyclin-thromboxane relationship with a subsequent activation of platelets and microangiopathy. The underlying mechanism for the initial changes that lead to this imbalance continue to be unknown. It is likely that these changes also involve the endothelial relaxing factor (nitric oxide) and the endothelial vasoconstrictor (endothelin) as well.[99,100] The imbalance between thromboxane and prostacyclin is further associated with increased levels of lipid peroxides, compounds which can damage endothelial cells and inhibit prostacyclin production.[101] The lipid peroxides could arise from increased oxygen radical formation secondary to the placental increase in thromboxane cyclooxygenase activity. Low dose aspirin treatment effectively and selectively inhibits both thromboxane and lipid peroxide in the maternal circulation.[102]

A low dose of aspirin (40–80 mg daily) that selectively inhibits platelet cyclooxygenase results in a marked reduction in thromboxane levels in maternal blood (but not in fetal blood), with minimal but transient impact on prostacyclin metabolites and no impairment of prostacyclin synthesis in the umbilical artery.[103] Low doses of aspirin that inhibit thromboxane production (in platelets and perhaps in trophoblastic tissue), unbalancing the ratio in favor of prostacyclin, offer prophylaxis against preeclampsia.[104–106] The measurement of the pressor response to angiotensin II indicates that pregnant women with preeclampsia can have an underlying imbalance of thromboxane and prostacyclin corrected by low dose aspirin.[107,108] This dose of aspirin appears to be safe for the fetus because it takes 100 mg daily to decrease levels of thromboxane in cord bloods (leaving prostacyclin unaffected) and 500 mg to inhibit both thromboxane and prostacyclin in the fetus.[109] Low dose aspirin (60 mg per day) has been demonstrated to be effective in some clinical trials, but not all, in preventing preeclampsia and intrauterine growth retardation.[106,110] This treatment is especially indicated for women with a previous history of significant preeclampsia. Large scale clinical trials are underway to determine efficacy and adverse effects.

In a sheep model of preeclampsia, a specific inhibitor of thromboxane synthetase increased uterine blood flow and glomerular filtration rate, decreased proteinuria, and restored platelet counts to normal.[111] During the hypertension, both prostacyclin and thromboxane decreased (as measured by their metabolites), and after treatment with the inhibitor, prostacyclin increased even higher than baseline while thromboxane did not change. Finally, part of the beneficial impact of magnesium therapy for preeclampsia can be attributed to an effect on prostacyclin. Magnesium increases prostacyclin production in cultured human umbilical endothelial cells, and so does the plasma from preeclamptic patients undergoing magnesium sulfate treatment.[112]

Evidence is accumulating to link prostacyclin and thromboxane to the clinical and pathological manifestations of preeclampsia. Having recognized and accepted the concept that preeclampsia is a chronic disease, the current challenge is to discover a practical method for early diagnosis, long before the irreversible end stage represented by the classical triad of hypertension, proteinuria, and edema develops. Accurate early diagnosis would open the door for pharmacologic intervention.

References

1. **Ramwell PW, Foegh M, Loeb R, Leovey EMK,** Synthesis and metabolism of prostaglandins, prostacyclin, and thromboxanes: the arachidonic acid cascade, Seminars Perinatol 4:3, 1980.

2. **Samuelsson B, Dahlen S-E, Lindgren JA, Rouzer CA, Serhan CN,** Leukotrienes and lipoxins: structures, biosynthesis, and biological effects, Science 237:1171, 1987.

3. **Gryglewski RJ, Korbut R, Oetkiewicz A, Splawinski J, Wojtaszek B, Swies J,** Lungs as a generator of prostacyclin — hypothesis on physiological significance, Arch Pharmacol 304:45, 1979.

4. **Moncada S, Vane JR,** Arachidonic acid metabolites and the interactions between platelets and blood vessel walls, New Engl J Med 300:1142, 1979.

5. **Beitz J, Muller G, Forster W,** Effect of HDL and LDL from pre and post menopausal women on prostacyclin synthesis, Prostaglandins 30:179, 1985.

6. **Mileikowsky GN, Nadler JL, Huey F, Francis R, Roy S,** Evidence that smoking alters prostacyclin formation and platelet aggregation in women who use oral contraceptives, Am J Obstet Gynecol 159:1547, 1988.

7. **Makheja A, Vanderhoek JY, Bailey JM,** Inhibition of platelet aggregation and thromboxane synthesis by onion and garlic, Lancet 1:781, 1979.

8. **Fischer S, Weber PC,** The prostacyclin/thromboxane balance is favourably shifted in Greenland Eskimos, Prostaglandins 32:235, 1986.

9. **Olson DM, Zakart T,** Intrauterine tissue prostaglandin synthesis: regulatory mechanisms, Seminars Reprod Endocrin 11:234, 1993.

10. **Green K, Drvota V, Vesterqvist O,** Pronounced reduction of *in vivo* prostacyclin synthesis in humans by acetaminophen (paracetamol), Prostaglandins 37:311, 1989.

11. **Masotti G, Poggesi L, Galanti G, Abbate R, Neri Serneri GG,** Differential inhibition of prostacyclin production and platelet aggregation by aspirin, Lancet 2:1213, 1979.

12. **Bochner F, Lloyd J,** Is there an optimal dose and formulation of aspirin to prevent arterial thrombo-embolism in man? Clin Sci 71:625, 1986.

13. **Fitzgerald DJ, Mayo G, Catella F, Entman SS, FitzGerald GA,** Increased thromboxane biosynthesis in normal pregnancy is mainly derived from platelets, Am J Obstet Gynecol 157:325, 1987.

14. **Auletta FJ, Flint APF,** Mechanisms controlling corpus luteum function in sheep, cows, primates and women especially in relation to the time of luteolysis, Endocrin Rev 9:88, 1988.

15. **Auletta FJ, Agins H, Scommegna A,** Prostaglandin $F_{2\alpha}$ mediation of the inhibitory effect of estrogen on the corpus luteum of the rhesus monkey, Endocrinology 103:1183, 1978.

16. **Auletta FJ, Caldwell BV, Speroff L,** Estrogen-induced luteolysis in the rhesus monkey: reversal with indomethacin, Prostaglandins 11:745, 1976.

17. **Auletta FJ, Kamps DL, Pories S, Bisset J, Gibson M,** An intra-ovarian site for the luteolytic action of prostaglandin $F_{2\alpha}$ in the rhesus monkey, Prostaglandins 27:285, 1984.

18. **Auletta FJ, Kamps DL, Wesley M, Gibson M,** Luteolysis in the rhesus monkey: ovarian venous estrogen, progesterone, and prostaglandin $F_{2\alpha}$-metabolite, Prostaglandins 27:299, 1984.

19. **Gore BC, Caldwell BV, Speroff L,** Estrogen-induced human luteolysis, J Clinol Endocrin Metab 36:615, 1973.

20. **Coceani F, Olley PM, Lock JE,** Prostaglandins, ductus arteriosus, pulmonary circulation: current concepts and clinical potential, Eur J Clin Pharmacol 18:75, 1980.

21. **Brash AR, Hickey DE, Graham TP, Stahlman MT, Oates JA, Cotton RB,** Pharmacokinetics of indomethacin in the neonate: relation of plasma indomethacin levels to response of the ductus arteriosus, New Engl J Med 305:67, 1981.

22. **Rudolph AM,** The effects of nonsteroidal antiinflammatory compounds on fetal circulation and pulmonary function, Obstet Gynecol 58:635, 1981.

23. **Thorburn GD,** The placenta, PGE_2 and parturition, Early Hum Dev 29:63, 1992.

24. **Mitchell MD,** Mechanisms of human parturition: role of prostaglandins and related compounds, Adv Prostaglandin Thromboxane Leukotriene Res 15:613, 1985.

25. **Casey ML, MacDonald PC,** The initiation of labor in women: regulation of phospholipid and arachidonic acid metabolism and of prostaglandin production, Seminars Perinatol 10:270, 1986.

26. **Mitchell MD,** Current topic: the regulation of placental eicosanoid biosynthesis, Placenta 12:557, 1991.

27. **Price HV, Cone BA, Keogh M,** Length of gestation in congenital adrenal hyperplasia, J Obstet Gynaecol Br Common 78:430, 1971.

28. **Davidson BJ, Murray RD, Challis JRG, Valenzuela GJ,** Estrogen, progesterone, prolactin, prostaglandin E_2, prostaglandin $F_{2\alpha}$, 13,14-dihydro-15-keto-prostaglandin $F_{2\alpha}$, and 6-keto-prostaglandin $F_{1\alpha}$ gradients across the uterus in women in labor and not in labor, Am J Obstet Gynecol 157:54, 1987.

29. **Femini M, Borenstein R, Dreazen E, Apelman Z, Mogilner BM, Kessler I, Lancet M,** Pevention of premature labor by 17α-hydroxyprogesterone caproate, Am J Obstet Gynecol 151:574, 1985.

30. **Erny R, Pigne A, Prouvost C, Gamerre M, Malet C, Serment H, Barrat J,** The effects of oral administration of progesterone for premature labor, Am J Obstet Gynecol 154:525, 1986.

31. **Khan-Dawood FS,** In vitro conversion of pregnenolone to progesterone in human term placenta and fetal membranes before and after onset of labor, Am J Obstet Gynecol 157:1333, 1987.

32. **Okazaki T, Sagawa N, Okita JR, Bleasdale JE, MacDonald PC, Johnston JM,** Diacylglycerol metabolism and arachidonic acid release in human fetal membranes and decidua vera, J Biol Chem 256:7316, 1981.

33. **Okazaki T, Sagawa N, Bleasdale JE, Okita JR, MacDonald PC, Johnston JM,** Initiation of human parturition: XIII. Phospholipase C, phospholipase A_2, and diacylglycerol lipase activities in fetal membranes and decidua vera tissues from early and late gestation, Biol Reprod 25:103, 1981.

34. **DiRenzo GC, Johnston JM, Okazaki T, Okita JR, MacDonald PC, Bleasdale JE,** Phosphatidylinositol specific phospholipase C in fetal membranes and uterine decidua, J Clin Invest 67:847, 1981.

35. **Romano WM, Lukash LA, Challis JRG, Mitchell BF,** Substrate utilization for estrogen synthesis by human fetal membranes and decidua, Am J Obstet Gynecol 155:1170, 1986.

36. **Chibbar R, Hobkirk R, Mitchell BF,** Sulfohydrolase activity for estrone sulfate and dehydroepiandrosterone sulfate in human fetal membranes and decidua around the time of parturition, J Clin Endocrinol Metab 62:90, 1986.

37. **Mitchell BF, Challis JRG, Lukash L,** Progesterone synthesis by human amnion, chorion, and decidua at term, Am J Obstet Gynecol 157:349, 1987.

38. **Challis JRG, Vaughan M,** Steroid synthetic and prostaglandin metabolizing activity is present in different cell populations from human fetal membranes and decidua, Am J Obstet Gynecol 157:1474, 1987.

39. **Lopez Bernal A, Bryant-Greenwood GD, Hansell DJ, Hicks BR, Greenwood FC, Turnbull AC,** Effect of relaxin on prostaglandin E production by human amnion: changes in relation to the onset of labour, Br J Obstet Gynaecol 94:1045, 1987.

40. **Mortimer G, Hunter IC, Stimson WH, Govan ADT,** A role for amniotic epithelium in control of human parturition, Lancet 1:1074, 1985.

41. **Bennett PR, Rose MP, Myatt L, Elder MG,** Preterm labor: stimulation of arachidonic acid metabolism in human amnion cells by bacterial productions, Am J Obstet Gynecol 156:649, 1987.

42. **Romero R, Avila C, Brekus CA, Morotti R,** The role of systemic and intrauterine infection in preterm parturition, Ann NY Acad Sci 622:355, 1991.

43. **Morris C, Khan H, Sullivan MHF, Elder MG,** Effects of platelet-activating factor on prostaglandin E_2 production by intact fetal membranes, Am J Obstet Gynecol 166:1228, 1992.

44. **Lundin-Schiller S, Mitchell MD,** Renin increases human amnion cell prostaglandin E_2 biosynthesis, J Clin Endocrinol Metab 73:436, 1991.

45. **Mitchell MD,** The regulation of decidual prostaglandin biosynthesis by growth factors, phorbol esters, and calcium, Biol Reprod 44:871, 1991.

46. **Schrey MP, Monaghan H, Holt JR,** Interaction of paracrine factors during labour: interleukin-1β causes amplification of decidua cell prostaglandin $F_{2\alpha}$ production in response to bradykinin and epidermal growth factor, Prostaglandins Leukotrienes Essential Fatty Acids 45:137, 1992.

47. **Jones SA, Brooks AN, Challis JRG,** Steroids modulate corticotropin-releasing hormone production in human fetal membranes and placenta, J Clin Endocrinol Metab 68:825, 1989.

48. **Petraglia F, Anceschi MM, Calza L, Garuti GC, Fusaro P, Giardino L, Genazzani AR, Vale W,** Inhibin and activin in human fetal membranes: evidence for a local effect on prostaglandin release, J Clin Endocrinol Metab 77:542, 1993.

49. **Giannopoulis G, Jackson K, Kredentser J, Tulchinsky D,** Prostaglandin E_2 and F_2 receptors in human myometrium during the menstrual cycle and in pregnancy and labor, Am J Obstet Gynecol 153:904, 1985.

50. **Okazaki T, Casey ML, Okita JR, MacDonald PC, Johnston JM,** Initiation of human parturition: XII. Biosynthesis and metabolism of prostaglandins in human fetal membranes and uterine decidua vera, Am J Obstet Gynecol 139:373, 1981.

51. **Nakla S, Skinner K, Mitchell BF, Challis JRG,** Changes in prostaglandin transfer across human fetal membranes obtained after spontaneous labor, Am J Obstet Gynecol 155:1337, 1986.

52. **Niesert S, Christopherson W, Korte K, Mitchell MD, MacDonald PC, Casey ML,** Prostaglandin E_2 9-ketoreductase activity in human decidua vera tissue, Am J Obstet Gynecol 155:1348, 1986.

53. **Mitchell BF, Rogers K, Wong S,** The dynamics of prostaglandin metabolism in human fetal membranes and decidua around the time of parturition, J Clin Endocrinol Metab 77:759, 1993.

54. **MacDonald PC, Casey ML,** The accumulation of prostaglandins (PG) in amniotic fluid is an aftereffect of labor and not indicative of a role for PGE_2 or $PGF_{2\alpha}$ in the initiation of human parturition, J Clin Endocrinol Metab 76:1332, 1993.

55. **Hirst JJ, Haluska GJ, Cook MJ, Novy MJ,** Plasma oxytocin and nocturnal uterine activity: maternal but not fetal concentrations increase progressively during late pregnancy and delivery in Rhesus monkeys, Am J Obstet Gynecol 169:415, 1993.

56. **Wilson T, Liggins GC, Whittaker DJ,** Oxytocin stimualtes the release of arachidonic acid and prostaglandin $F_{2\alpha}$ from human decidual cells, Prostaglandins 35:771, 1988.

57. **Hirst JJ, Chibbart R, Mitchell BF,** Role of oxytocin in the regulation of uterine activity during pregnancy and in the initiation of labor, Seminars Reprod Endocrin 11:219, 1993.

58. **Burghardt RC, Barhoumi R, Dookwah H,** Endocrine regulation of myometrial gap junctions and their role in parturition, Seminars Reprod Endocrin 11:250, 1993.

59. **Carsten ME, Miller JD,** A new look at uterine muscle contraction, Am J Obstet Gynecol 157:1303, 1987.

60. **Ducsay CA, Seron-Fere M, Germain AM, Valenzuela GJ,** Endocrine and uterine activity rhythms in the perinatal period, Seminars Reprod Endocrin 11:285, 1993.

61. **Van den Veyyer IB, Moise KJ Jr,** Prostaglandin synthetase inhibitors in pregnancy, Obstet Gynecol Survey 48:493, 1993.

62. **Sorensen TK, Easterling TR, Carlson KL, Brateng DA, Benedetti TJ,** The maternal hemodynamic effect of indomethacin in normal pregnancy, Obstet Gynecol 79:661, 1992.

63. **Cabrol D, Landesman R, Muller J, Uzan M, Sureau C, Saxena BB,** Treatment of polyhydramnios with prostaglandin synthetase inhibitor (indomethacin), Am J Obstet Gynecol 157:422, 1987.

64. **Carlan SJ, O'Brien WF, O'Leary TD, Mastrogiannis D,** Randomized comparative trial of indomethacin and sulindac for the treatment of refractory preterm labor, Obstet Gynecol 79:223, 1992.

65. **Bernstein P,** Prostaglandin E_2 gel for cervical ripening and labor induction: a multicentre placebo-controlled trial, Can Med Assoc J 145:1249, 1991.

66. **Ray DA, Garite TJ,** Prostaglandin E_2 for induction of labor in pateints with premature rupture of membranes at term, Am J Obstet Gynecol 166:836, 1992.

67. **Sanchez-Ramos L, Kaunitz AM, Del Valle GO, Delke I, Schroeder PA, Briones DK,** Labor induction with the prostaglandin E_1 methyl analogue misoprostol versus oxytocin: a randomized trial, Obstet Gynecol 81:332, 1993.

68. **Norman JE, Thong KJ, Baird DT,** Uterine contractility and induction of abortion in early pregnancy by misoprostol and mifepristone, Lancet 338:1233, 1991.

69. **Peyron R, Aubeny E, Targosz V, Silvestre L, Renault M, Elkik F, Leclerc P, Ulmann A, Baulieu EE,** Early termination of pregnancy with mifepristone (RU 486) and the orally active prostaglandin misoprostol, New Engl J Med 328:1509, 1993.

70. **O'Leary JA,** Prostaglandins and postpartum hemorrhage, Seminars Reprod Endocrinol 3:247, 1985.

71. **Brinkman CR,** Physiology and pathophysiology of maternal adjustments to pregnancy, in Aladjem S, Brown AK, editors, *Clinical Perinatology*, C. V. Mosby, St. Louis, 1975.

72. **Roberts JM, Redman CWG,** Pre-eclampsia: more than pregnancy-induced hypertension, Lancet 341:1447, 1993.

73. **Gant NP, Hutchinson HT, Siiteri PK, MacDonald PC,** Study of the metabolic clearance of dehydroisoandrosterone sulfate in pregnancy, Am J Obstet Gynecol 111:555, 1971.

74. **Gant NF, Daley GL, Chand S, Whalley PJ, MacDonald PC,** A study of angiotensin II pressor response throughout primigravid pregnancy, J Clin Invest 52.2682, 1973.

75. **Gallery EDM, Ross M, Hunyor SN, Gyory AX,** Predicting the development of pregnancy-associated hypertension, the place of standardized blood pressure measurement, Lancet 1:1273, 1977.

76. **Cohen-Overbeck T, Pearce JM, Campbell S,** The antenatal assessment of utero-placental and feto-placental blood flow using Doppler ultrasound, Ultrasound Med Biol 11:329, 1985.

77. **Combs CA, Katz MA, Kitzmiller JL, Brescia RJ,** Experimental preeclampsia produced by chronic constriction of the lower aorta: validation with longitudinal blood pressure measurements in conscious rhesus monkeys, Am J Obstet Gynecol 169:215, 1993.

78. **Fritz MA, Stanczyk FZ, Novy MJ,** Relationship of uteroplacental blood flow to the placental clearance of maternal dehydroepiandrosterone through estradiol formation in the pregnant baboon, J Clin Endocrinol Metab 61:1023, 1985.

79. **Franklin GO, Dowd AJ, Caldwell BV, Speroff L,** The effect of angiotensin II intravenous infusion on plasma renin activity and prostaglandins A, E, and F levels in the uterine vein of the pregnant monkey, Prostaglandins 6:271, 1974.

80. **Speroff L, Haning RV Jr, Ewaschuk EJ, Alberino SL, Kieliszek FX,** Uterine artery blood flow studies in the pregnant monkey, in Lindheimer MD, Katz AL, Zuspan FP, editors, *Hypertension in Pregnancy*, John Wiley, New York, 1976, pp 315-327.

81. **Speroff L, Haning RV Jr, Levin RM,** The effect of angiotensin II and indomethacin on uterine artery blood flow in pregnant monkeys, Obstet Gynecol 50:611, 1977.

82. **McLaughlin MK, Brennan SC, Chez RA,** Effects of indomethacin on sheep uteroplacental circulations and sensitivity to angiotensin II, Am J Obstet Gynecol 132:430, 1978.

83. **Terragno NA, Terragno DA, Pacholxzyk D, McGiff JC,** Prostaglandins and the regulation of uterine blood flow in pregnancy, Nature 249:57, 1974.

84. **Venuto RC, O'Dorisio T, Stein JH, Ferris TF,** Uterine prostaglandin E secretion and uterine blood flow in the pregnant rabbit, J Clin Invest 55:193, 1975.

85. **Everett RB, Worley RJ, MacDonald PC, Gant NF,** Effect of prostaglandin synthetase inhibitors on pressor response to angiotensin II in human pregnancy, J Clin Endocrinol Metab 46:1007, 1978.

86. **Speroff L, Dorfman GS,** Prostaglandins and pregnancy hypertension, Clin Obstet Gynecol 4:635, 1977.

87. **Goodman RP, Killam AP, Brash AR, Branch RA,** Prostacyclin production during pregnancy: comparison of production during normal pregnancy and pregnancy complicated by hypertension, Am J Obstet Gynecol 142:817, 1982.

88. **Ylikorkala O, Pekonen F, Viinikka L,** Renal prostacyclin and thromboxane in normotensive and preeclamptic pregnant women and their infants, J Clin Endocrinol Metab 63:1307, 1986.

89. **Fitzgerald DJ, Entman SS, Mulloy K, FitzGerald GA,** Decreased prostacyclin biosynthesis preceding the clinical manifestations of pregnancy-induced hypertension, Circulation 75:956, 1987.

90. **Pritchard JA, Cunningham FG, Mason RA,** Coagulation changes in eclampsia: their frequency and pathogenesis, Am J Obstet Gynecol 124:855, 1976.

91. **Bern MM, Driscoll SG, Leavitt T Jr,** Thrombocytopenia complicating pre-eclampsia, Obstet Gynecol 57:28S, 1981.

92. **Saleh AA, Bottoms SF, Welch RA, Ali AM, Mariona FG, Mammen EF,** Preeclampsia, delivery, and the hemostatic system, Am J Obstet Gynecol 157:331, 1987.

93. **De Wolf F, Robertson WB, Brosens I,** The ultrastructure of acute atherosis in hypertensive pregnancy, Am J Obstet Gynecol 123:154, 1975.

94. **Jorgensen KA, Pedersen RS,** Familial deficiency of prostacyclin production stimulating factor in the hemolytic uremic syndrome of childhood, Thromb Res 21:311, 1981.

95. **Machin SJ, Defreyn G, Chamone DAF, Vermylen J,** Plasma 6-keto-$PGF_{1\alpha}$ levels after plasma exchange in thrombotic thrombocytopenic purpura, Lancet 1:661, 1980.

96. **Remuzzi G, Imperti L, DeGaetano G,** Prostacyclin deficiency in thrombotic microangiopathy, Lancet 2:1422, 1981.

97. **Fitzgerald DJ, Rocki W, Murray R, Mayo G, Fitzgerald GA,** Thromboxane A_2 synthesis in pregnancy-induced hypertension, Lancet 335:751, 1990.

98. **Van Assche FA, Spitz B, Hanssens M, Van Geet C, Arnout J, Vermylen J,** Increased thromboxane formation in diabetic pregnancy as a possible contributor to preeclampsia, Am J Obstet Gynecol 168:84, 1993.

99. **Myatt L, Brewer A, Brockman DE,** The action of nitric oxide in the perfused human fetal-placental circulation, Am J Obstet Gynecol 164:687, 1991.

100. **Taylor RN, Varma M, Teng NNH, Roberts JM,** Women with preeclampsia have higher plasma endothelin levels than women with normal pregnancies, J Clin Endocrinol Metab 71:1675, 1990.

101. **Wang Y, Walsh SW, Kay HH,** Placental lipid peroxides and thromboxane are increased and prostacyclin is decreased in women with preeclampsia, Am J Obstet Gynecol 167:946, 1992.

102. **Walsh SW, Wang Y, Kay HH, McCoy MC,** Low-dose aspirin inhibits lipid peroxides and thromboxane but not prostacyclin in pregnant women, Am J Obstet Gynecol 167:926, 1992.

103. **Ritter JM, Farquhar C, Rodin A, Thom MH,** Low dose aspirin treatment in late pregnancy differentially inhibits cyclo-oxygenase in maternal platelets, Prostaglandins 34:717, 1987.

104. **Beaufils M, Donsimoni R, Uzan S, Colau JC,** Prevention of preeclampsia by early antiplatelet therapy, Lancet 2:240, 1985.

105. **Wallenburg HCS, Dekker GA, Makovitz JW, Rotmans P,** Low-dose aspirin prevents pregnancy-induced hypertension and preeclampsia in angiotensin-sensitive primigravidae, Lancet 1:1, 1986.

106. **Dekker GA, Sibai BM,** Low-dose aspirin in the prevention of preeclampsia and fetal growth retardation: rationale, mechanisms, and clinical trials, Am J Obstet Gynecol 168:214, 1993.

107. **Brown CEL, Gant NF, Cox K, Spitz B, Rosenfeld CR, Magness RR,** Low-dose aspirin. II. Relationship of angiotensin II pressor responses, circulating eicosanoids, and pregnancy outcome, Am J Obstet Gynecol 163:1853, 1990.

108. **Wallenburg HCS, Dekker GA, Makovitz JW, Rotmans N,** Effect of low-dose aspirin on vascular refractoriness in angiotensin-sensitive primigravid women, Am J Obstet Gynecol 164:1169, 1991.

109. **Ylidordala O, Makila U, Kaapa P, Viinikka L,** Maternal ingestion of acetylsalicylic acid inhibits fetal and neonatal prostacyclin and thromboxane in humans, Am J Obstet Gynecol 155:345, 1986.

110. **Italian Study of Aspirin in Pregnancy,** Low-dose aspirin in prevention and treatment of intrauterine growth retardation and pregnancy-induced hypertension, Lancet 341:396, 1993.

111. **Keith JC, Miller K, Eggleston MK, Kutruff J, Howerton T, Konczal C, McDaniels C,** Effects of thromboxane synthetase inhibition on maternal-fetal homeostasis in gravid ewes with ovine pregnancy-induced hypertension, Am J Obstet Gynecol 161:1305, 1989.

112. **Watson K, Moldow CG, Ogburn PL, Jacob HS,** Magnesium sulfate: rationale for its use in preeclampsia, Proc Natl Acad Sci USA 83:1075, 1986.

Part II

Clinical Endocrinology

10 Normal and Abnormal Sexual Development

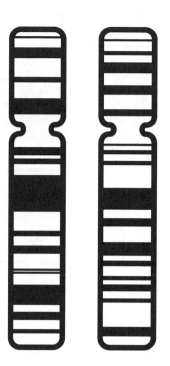

Abnormalities of sexual differentiation are seen infrequently in an individual physician's practice. There are, however, few practitioners who have not been challenged at least once by a newborn with ambiguous genitalia or by a young woman with primary amenorrhea on a genetic basis. The categorization of the various syndromes in this area has been confusing, requiring constant reference to multiple textbooks, and dependence upon memory of eponym-laden, seemingly endless lists of syndromes. Happily, this "catalogue" state of affairs has changed; major advances in reproductive science have yielded clarification and consolidation. As a result, an informed basis for clinical practice has emerged and is readily applicable.

This chapter will present classification of the major problems and our clinical approach to diagnosis. Normal sexual differentiation will be considered in order to provide a basis of understanding for the various types of abnormal development. This is followed by a section on the diagnosis and management of ambiguous genitalia. Some subjects are discussed in other chapters, but brief descriptions will be repeated here in order to present a complete picture. It will be seen that analysis of phenotypic ambiguity follows a fundamental, pervasive theme: too little androgen effect in males, too much androgen effect in females. Whereas androgen biologic "availability" may be excessive in females because of abnormally high levels of intake or production, reduced androgen effects in males can be the result of defects in synthesis, peripheral and target organ conversion, abnormalities in androgen receptor or receptor-DNA interactions, as well as defective gonadal development and function.

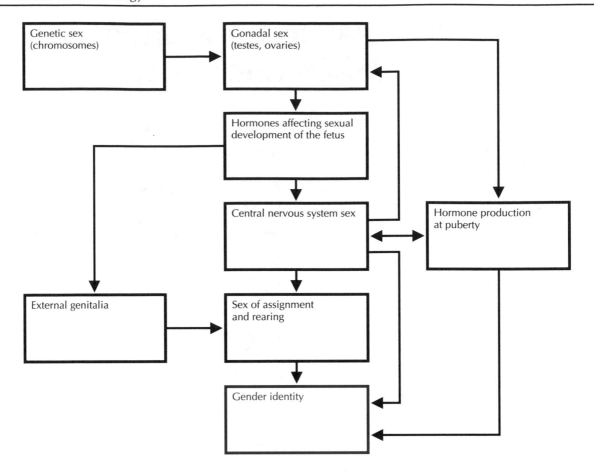

Normal Sexual Differentiation

The gender identity of a person (whether an individual identifies as a male or a female) is the end result of genetic, hormonal, and morphologic sex as influenced by the environment of the individual. It includes all behavior with any sexual connotation, such as body gestures and mannerisms, habits of speech, recreational preferences, and content of dreams. Sexual expression, both homosexual and heterosexual, can be regarded as the result of all influences on the individual, both prenatal and postnatal. Specifically, gender identity is the result of the following determinants: genetic sex, gonadal sex, the internal genitalia, the external genitalia, the secondary sexual characteristics that appear at puberty, and the role assigned by society in response to all of these developmental manifestations of sex.

Prenatally, sexual differentiation follows a specific sequence of events. First is the establishment of the genetic sex. Second, under the control of the genetic sex the gonads differentiate, determining the hormonal environment of the embryo, the differentiation of internal duct systems, and the formation of the external genitalia. It has become apparent that the embryonic brain is also sexually differentiated, perhaps via a control mechanism very similar to that which determines the sexual development of the external genitalia. The inductive influences of hormones on the central nervous system may have an effect on the patterns of hormone secretion and sexual behavior in the adult.[1]

Gonadal Differentiation

In human embryos, the gonads begin development during the 5th week of gestation as protuberances overlying the mesonephric ducts. The migration of primordial germ cells into these gonadal ridges occurs between weeks 4 and 6 of gestation. Although germ cells do not induce gonadal development, if the germ cells fail to arrive, gonads do not develop and only the fibrous streak of gonadal agenesis will exist (Chapter 3). At 6 weeks of fetal life the gonads are indifferent but bipotential, possessing both cortical and

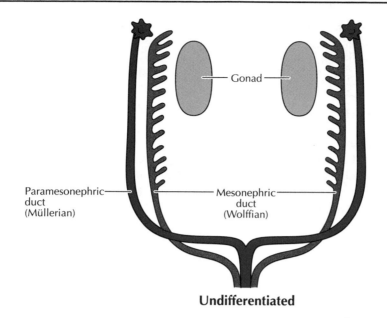

Undifferentiated

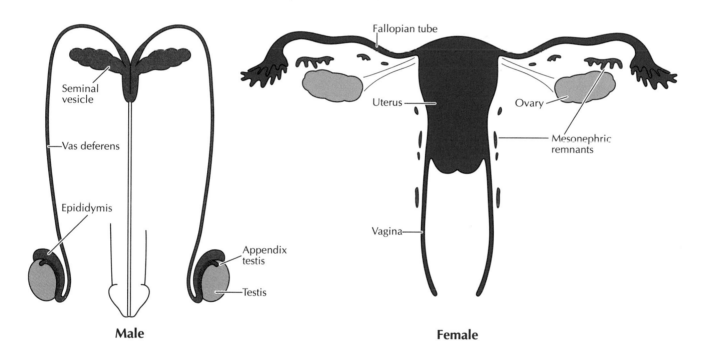

Male

Female

medullary areas, and are capable of differentiation into either testes or ovaries. They are composed of germ cells, special epithelia (potential granulosa/Sertoli cells), mesenchyme (potential theca/Leydig cells), and the mesonephric duct system. Wolffian and müllerian ducts exist side by side; external genitalia are undifferentiated.[2] Subsequent sexual differentiation requires direction by various genes, with a single gene determinant on the Y chromosome (testes determining factor — TDF) necessary for testicular differentiation.[3]

The distal end of the short arm of the Y chromosome is called the pseudoautosomal region because during meiosis the homologous distal short arms of the X and Y chromosomes pair, and interchange of genetic material occurs. The genes in the pseudoautosomal regions are doubly present in both sexes, and therefore escape X inactivation. Gene deletions in this area of the X chromosome (Xp22.3) are associated with various conditions, known as contiguous gene syndromes: short stature, mental retardation, X-linked ichthyosis, Kallmann's syndrome. The testis-determing gene is located on the distal short arm of the Y, immediately adjacent to the pseudoautosomal region. Loss of the TDF gene causes gonadal dysgenesis. Transfer of the TDF gene to the X results in an XX male.

Since the identification of the Y chromosome's importance to male differentiation over 3 decades ago, three proteins have been suggested as the Y-encoded, gene expressed, testis determining factor. The first was the H-Y histocompatibility antigen and the second ZFY (a zinc finger protein). Both were abandoned because of inconsistencies of expression in various cell types (in XX males and XY females), as well as absent expression in indisputable males with testes. More recently, SRY has been isolated, the sex-determining region on the short arm of the Y chromosome.[4] It is a single copy gene located in the smallest Y chromosome region capable of sex reversal. It is expressed in the genital ridge only during the appropriate time of embryonic development when testicular cords form; it is deleted or mutated in cases of human XY females, and present in 46,XX males, and it can sex-reverse XX mice into males.[5–7] The protein product contains an 80 amino acid domain with a motif shared by a newly recognized family of transcription factors (the high mobility group) that bind to DNA and regulate gene transcription. Investigations of the DNA binding properties of the SRY high mobility group (HMG) box in the promoter regions of P450 aromatase (conversion of testosterone to estradiol which is down-regulated in the male embryo) and antimüllerian hormone (responsible for regression of the müllerian ducts) support the hypothesis that SRY directly controls male development through sequence-specific regulation of target genes.[8]

SRY participation in morphogenesis and pattern formation leading to a testis from the bipotential genital ridge is a model "genetic switch" between alternative inherent programs. Whereas testes formation is an active event, female sex determination is the default pathway occurring if SRY is absent or deficient. Proteins other than SRY are required for proper gonadogenesis.[9] In the human, autosomal genes are essential for gonadal development. These autosomal genes regulate migration of the germ cells and coding of the steroidogenic enzymes. The formation of the testicle precedes any other sexual development in time, and a functionally active testis controls subsequent sexual development. Testicular hormones activate or repress genes to direct development away from an otherwise predetermined course of female differentiation.

Testicular differentiation begins at 6–7 weeks; first with Sertoli cells which aggregate to form spermatogenic cords, then seminiferous tubules, followed by Leydig cell formation a week later. Human chorionic gonadotropin (HCG) stimulation produces Leydig cell hypertrophy, and peak fetal testosterone levels are seen at 15–18 weeks.[9]

In an XX individual, without the active influence of a Y chromosome, the bipotential gonad develops into an ovary about 2 weeks later than testicular development. The cortical zone develops and contains the germ cells, while the medullary portion regresses with its remnant being the rete ovarii, a compressed nest of tubules and Leydig cells in the hilus of the ovary. The germ cells proliferate by mitosis, reaching a peak of 5–7 million by 20 weeks. By 20 weeks, the fetal ovary achieves mature compartmentalization with primordial follicles containing oocytes, initial evidence of follicle maturation and atresia, and an incipient stroma. Degeneration (atresia) begins even earlier, and by birth, approximately 1–2 million germ cells remain. These have become surrounded by a layer of follicular cells, forming primordial follicles with oocytes which have entered the first meiotic division. Meiosis is arrested in the prophase of the first meiotic division until reactivation of follicular growth that may not occur until years later. Excessively rapid atresia (germ cell attrition) in gonadal dysgenesis (45,X) accounts for the streak gonad seen in these cases.[10] A complete 46,XX chromosomal complement is necessary for normal ovarian development.[11] The second X chromosome, therefore, contains elements essential for ovarian maintenance.

Duct System Differentiation

Caspar Wolff described the mesonephros in 1759 in his doctoral dissertation when he was 26 years old.[12] The paired structures of the mesonephros of the early vertebrate embryo were named wolffian bodies by the 19th century embryologist, Rathke, in recognition of Wolff's initial discovery and description. Johannes Müller, a German physiologist with a prodigious academic output, described the embryology of the genitalia in 1830. The paramesonephric ducts received his name, not because of his original contributions, but because of his ability to synthesize current knowledge in his effective writings. His physiology text was a standard in many European countries.

Renal development goes through 3 stages: pronephric, mesonephric, and metanephric. The mesonephric ducts remain for development as internal genitalia. At this stage the mesonephric ducts are called the wolffian ducts. The paired paramesonephric ducts are the müllerian ducts. The wolffian and müllerian ducts are discrete primordia which temporarily coexist in all embryos during the ambisexual period of development (up to 8 weeks). Thereafter, one type of duct system persists normally and gives rise to special ducts and glands, whereas the other disappears during the 3rd fetal month, except for nonfunctional vestiges.

Hormonal control of mammalian somatic sex differentiation was established by the classic experiments of Alfred Jost.[13] In Jost's landmark studies, the active role of male determining factors was defined as the directing feature of sex differentiation. This principle applies not only to the internal ducts but to the gonad, external genitalia, and perhaps even the brain. The critical factors in determining which of the duct structures stabilize or regress are the secretions from the testes: antimüllerian hormone (AMH), also known as müllerian inhibiting substance or müllerian inhibiting factor, and testosterone.

AMH is a member of the transforming growth factor-β family of glycoprotein differentiation factors that include inhibin and activin.[14,15] The gene for AMH has been mapped to the short arm of chromosome 19. AMH is synthesized by Sertoli cells soon after testicular differentiation and is responsible for the ipsilateral regression of the müllerian ducts by 8 weeks, before the emergence of testosterone and stimulation of the wolffian ducts.[16] Despite its presence in serum up to puberty, lack of regression of the uterus and tubes is the only consistent expression of AMH gene mutations. In the absence of AMH, the fetus will develop fallopian tubes, uterus, and upper vagina from the paramesonephric ducts (the müllerian ducts). *This development requires the prior appearance of the mesonephric ducts, and for this reason, abnormalities in the renal system are associated with abnormalities in development of the tubes, uterus, and upper vagina.*

AMH may have extra müllerian functions. AMH exerts an inhibitory effect on oocyte meiosis, plays a role in the descent of the testes, and inhibits surfactant accumulation in the lungs.[17] Proteolytic cleavage of AMH produces fragments which have the ability to inhbit growth of various tumors (a potential therapeutic application). Testicular descent occurs in stages. Transabdominal movement of the testes is the result of rapid gubernacular growth, apparently under AMH control. Movement through the inguinal canal is mediated by androgens.

AMH is detectable in the serum of males during infancy, childhood, adolescence, and adulthood. In contrast, AMH is not measureable until the second decade of life in females. This difference allows serum measurement to be a sensitive marker for the presence of testicular tissue in intersex anomalies.[18]

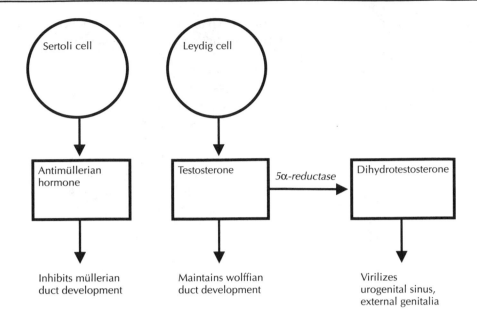

Testosterone is secreted by the fetal testes soon after Leydig cell formation (at 8 weeks) and rapidly rises to peak concentrations at 15–18 weeks. This testosterone secretion stimulates development of the wolffian duct system into epididymis, vas deferens, and seminal vesicles. Testosterone levels in the male fetus correlate with Leydig cell development, overall gonadal weight, 3β-hydroxysteroid dehydrogenase activity, and chorionic gonadotropin (HCG) concentrations. As HCG declines (approximately 20 weeks) the fetal pituitary luteinizing hormone (LH) assumes control of Leydig cell testosterone secretion; anencephalics and other forms of congenital hypopituitarism display diminished androgen effects on internal and external genitalia.

The wolffian ducts receive testosterone signals directly from nearby Leydig cells as well as the general fetal circulation. This local paracrine effect is essential to the stimulation of ipsilateral differentiation into the epididymis, vas deferens, and seminal vesicles. Duct system differentiation will proceed, therefore, according to the nature of the adjacent gonad. The wolffian ducts do not form dihydrotestosterone, so the direct high concentration is crucial for normal development.[19] Because of this local paracrine action, wolffian development cannot be stimulated in females exposed to adrenal or exogenous androgens.

The internal genitalia possess the intrinsic tendency to feminize. In the absence of a Y chromosome and a functional testis, the lack of AMH allows retention of the müllerian system and development of fallopian tubes, uterus, and upper vagina. In the absence of testosterone, the wolffian system regresses. In the presence of a normal ovary or the absence of any gonad, müllerian duct development takes place.

External Genitalia Differentiation

In the bipotential state (6th gestational week), the external genitalia consist of a genital tubercle, a urogenital sinus, and two lateral labioscrotal swellings. Unlike the internal genitalia where both duct systems initially coexist, the external genitalia are neutral primordia able to develop into either male or female structures depending on gonadal steroid hormone signals. Normally, this differentiation is under the active influence of androgen from the Leydig cells of the testis. The genital tubercle forms the penis, labioscrotal folds fuse to form a scrotum, and folds of the urogenital sinus form the penile urethra. The testis begins androgen secretion by 8–9 weeks; masculinization of the external genitalia is manifest 1 week later and is completed by 14 weeks. To achieve this morphologic change, external genitalia target tissue cells must convert testosterone to dihydrotestosterone (DHT) by the intracellular enzyme 5α-reductase. In the male, DHT mediates the following androgen events: temporal hairline recession, growth of facial and body hairs, development of acne, and development of the external genitalia and prostate.

In the absence of this androgen effect (the absence of a Y chromosome, the presence of an ovary, the absence of a gonad, abnormalities in androgen receptor or postreceptor events, or defects of the 5α-reductase enzyme), the folds of the urogenital sinus remain open, forming the labia minora, the labioscrotal folds form the labia majora, the genital tubercle forms the clitoris, and the urogenital sinus differentiates into the vagina and the urethra. Thus, the lower vagina is formed as part of the external genitalia.

Bipotential Stage

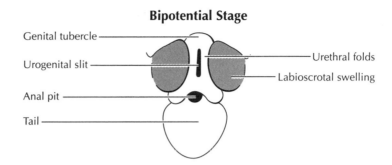

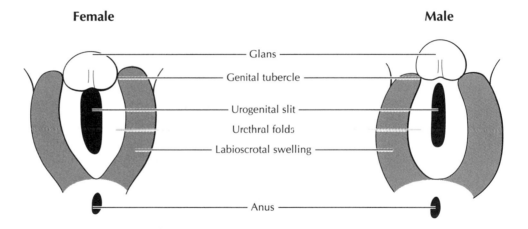

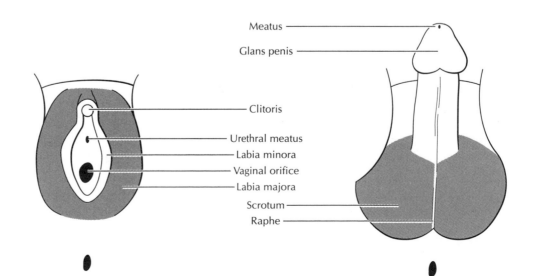

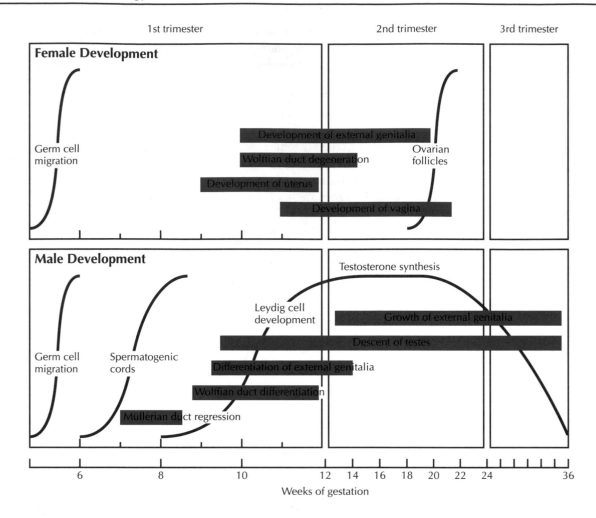

1st trimester **2nd trimester** **3rd trimester**

Female Development

Germ cell migration

Development of external genitalia

Wolffian duct degeneration

Development of uterus

Development of vagina

Ovarian follicles

Male Development

Testosterone synthesis

Leydig cell development

Germ cell migration

Spermatogenic cords

Growth of external genitalia

Descent of testes

Differentiation of external genitalia

Wolffian duct differentiation

Müllerian duct regression

6   8   10   12 14 16 18 20 22 24   36

Weeks of gestation

Exposure to androgens at critical time periods leads to variable masculinization. Androgen exposure at 9–14 weeks superimposes variable external ambiguity on the basic female phenotype (clitoral hypertrophy, hypospadias, scrotalization of nonfused labia). By the same token, incompletely masculinized genitalia will result if sufficient local androgen concentration or activity is not achieved by the 12th week in the male. Because of shared common tissue origin, male-female external genital structural ambiguities reflect abnormal androgen impact: males too little, females too much.

Central Nervous Differentiation

At the same time the presence or absence of androgens is playing a critical role in genitalia development, the neuroendocrine mechanism of the central nervous system is also being influenced. Androgens present in sufficient amounts during the appropriate critical stage of development may program the central nervous system (CNS) to induce the potential for male sexual behavior.[20–22] Experimental and analytical evidence suggests that a behavioral effect can be traced to this early androgen influence. Inappropriate fetal hormonal programming may contribute, therefore, to the spectrum of psychosexual behavior seen in humans. In addition, gender role is heavily influenced by assignment of sex of rearing followed by social interaction based upon genital appearance and the development of secondary sexual characteristics.

Abnormal Sexual Differentiation	The standard classification of individuals with intersexuality (hermaphroditism) proceeds according to gonadal morphology. In this terminology, a *true hermaphrodite* possesses both ovarian and testicular tissue. A *male pseudohermaphrodite* has testes, but external and sometimes internal genitalia take on female phenotypic aspects. A *female pseudohermaphrodite* has ovaries, but genital development displays masculine characteristics. These classifications are modified to reflect gonadal abnormalities due to abnormal sex chromosome constitution or abnormalities of phenotype attributable to an inappropriate fetal hormone environment. Hypospadias in the absence of any other deformity is not included in this classification:

Disorders of Fetal Endocrinology

Female pseudohermaphroditism (partial virilization)
    Congenital adrenal hyperplasia
        21-Hydroxylase deficiency (P450c21)
        11β-Hydroxylase deficiency (P450c11β)
        3β-Hydroxysteroid dehydrogenase deficiency
    Drug intake
    Maternal disease
    Placental aromatase deficiency

Male pseudohermaphroditism (inadequate virilization)
    Antimüllerian hormone defect
    Impaired androgenization
    Androgen insensitivity syndromes
    5α-Reductase deficiency
    Testosterone biosynthesis defects
    P450scc deficiency
    3β-Hydroxysteroid dehydrogenase deficiency
    17α-Hydroxylase deficiency (P450c17)
    17β-Hydroxysteroid dehydrogenase deficiency

Disorders of Gonadal Development

Male pseudohermaphroditism
    Primary gonadal defect
    Y Chromosome defect

True hermaphroditism

Gonadal dysgenesis
    Turner syndrome
    Mosaicism
    Structural abnormality — X chromosome
    Normal karyotype

Masculinized Females (Female Pseudohermaphrodites)	Masculinized females possess ovaries and are female by genetic sex (XX), but the external genitalia are not those of a normal female. Of all infants with ambiguous genitalia, 40–45% have adrenal hyperplasia. Rarer causes of female pseudohermaphroditism are excess maternal androgen caused by drug ingestion, tumor secretion, or possibly placental aromatase deficiency.

Congenital Adrenal Hyperplasia (the Adrenogenital Syndrome)

Congenital adrenal hyperplasia in females is characterized by masculinized external genitalia, and is diagnosed by demonstrating excessive androgen production by the adrenal cortex, caused by either tumor or hyperplasia.[23,24] The syndrome may appear in utero or develop postnatally.

Depending on the time of onset, quantity available, and duration of exposure, the presence of excessive androgens is manifested by varying degrees of fusion of the labioscrotal folds, clitoral enlargement, and anatomical changes of the urethra and vagina. Generally, the urethra and vagina share a urogenital sinus formed by the fusion of labial folds. This sinus opens at the base of the clitoris, which is usually enlarged. The degree of urogenital sinus deformity is related to the timing in prenatal development of the onset of masculinizing androgen effect. Because there is no anomalous secretion of antimüllerian hormone in females with congenital adrenal hyperplasia, the fallopian tubes, uterus, and upper vagina develop normally. Since wolffian duct development and maintenance depend on high local androgen levels provided by the male gonad, the excessive androgens of adrenal hyperplasia origin cannot stimulate this process, and no wolffian development is retained. The external genitalia on the other hand can be substantially altered by adrenal hyperplasia. After the 10th week, when the vagina and urethra have separated, the emerging excess androgen effect may be limited to clitoral hypertrophy. High androgen levels earlier than the 12th week of fetal age, however, can cause progressive fusion of the labia (anteriorly-posteriorly), formation of an urogenital sinus, and even variable closure of the urethra along the phallus (hypospadias). The absence of palpable testes may be the only clinical marker suggesting female pseudohermaphroditism.

Only the external genitalia are affected because internal genitalia differentiation is completed by the 10th week of gestation, while the adrenal cortex begins function by the 12th week. Since the female external genitalia phenotype is not completed until 140 days of fetal age, early androgen excess (7–12 weeks) may fully masculinize, whereas late (18–20 weeks) androgen may create limited ambiguity of the basically female appearance of the urogenital sinus and genital folds. The size of the clitoris depends on the quantity rather than timing of androgen excess. Cases of incorrect sex assignment in the female are due to the similarity between these external genitalia and hypospadias and bilateral cryptorchidism in a male infant.

If untreated, the female with adrenal hyperplasia will develop signs of progressive virilization postnatally. Pubic hair will appear by age 2–4, followed by axillary hair, then body hair and beard. Bone age is advanced by age 2, and because of early epiphyseal closure, height in childhood is achieved at the expense of shortened stature in adulthood. Progressive masculinization continues with the development of the male habitus, acne, deepened voice, and primary amenorrhea and infertility.

In addition to sexual changes, patients can present with metabolic disorders such as salt wasting, hypertension, or rarely, hypoglycemia. An electrolyte imbalance of the salt-losing type is usually apparent within a few days of birth and occurs in approximately two-thirds of patients with virilizing adrenal hyperplasia. Beginning with a refusal to feed, failure to thrive, apathy, and vomiting, the infant goes on to an Addisonian-like crisis with hyponatremia, hyperkalemia, and acidosis. Rapid diagnosis and treatment are necessary to save these infants. Less frequent is hypertension, which occurs in approximately 5% of patients with virilizing adrenal hyperplasia.

Virilizing adrenal hyperplasia is the result of an inherited abnormality of steroid biosynthesis which results in an inability to synthesize glucocorticoids. The hypothalamic-pituitary axis reacts to the low level of cortisol by elevated ACTH secretion in a homeostatic response to achieve normal levels of cortisol production. This stimulation induces a hyperplastic adrenal cortex which produces androgens as well as corticoid precursors in abnormal quantities. Therefore, one can see a well-compensated infant who has achieved normal cortisol levels but at the expense of extensive masculinization. In summary, the clinical picture resulting from a specific enzyme deficiency is due to the effects of both the inadequate production of cortisol/aldosterone and excess accumulation of precursors, with diversion into biosynthetic pathways yielding androgens.

The most common enzymatic defects are the 21-hydroxylase (P450c21), the 11β-hydroxylase (P450c11), and the 3β-hydroxysteroid dehydrogenase types. Very rarely, blocked synthesis of cortisol can be due to a defect in either of the two other enzymes involved in the cortisol/androgen biosynthetic pathways: P450scc and P450c17. These steps are common to the adrenal cortex, ovary, and testes. With respect to their gonadal impact, however, the resulting diminished production of androgens leads to incomplete genital development in genetic males but no change in the basic female pattern of females.

Enzyme Defect in Adrenal Only: Deficient 21-Hydroxylase (P450c21). The 21-hydroxylase block is the most common form of congenital adrenal hyperplasia (90% of cases), the most frequent cause of sexual ambiguity, and the most frequent endocrine cause of neonatal death. With severe uncompensated blocks of this type, salt wasting and shock accompany significant virilization. In less severe variations, when sufficient cortisol can be produced, virilization due to excess androgen is still present in utero, at birth, or later in life. Three different clinical forms are recognized: the salt-wasting, the simple virilizing, and the late-onset (also known as nonclassic, attenuated, or acquired adrenal hyperplasia). The first and second are associated with female pseudohermaphroditism at birth, while the third usually becomes apparent at adolescence or beyond and causes hirsutism, menstrual irregularities, and infertility.

Developments in molecular biology and genetics have greatly expanded our understanding of this condition.[25] As a result of the close genetic linkage between 21-hydroxylase deficiency and the human leukocyte antigen (HLA) complex located on the short arm of chromosome 6, we have learned the following:

1. The disorder is inherited as a monogenic autosomal recessive trait.

2. HLA typing can be used to determine the carrier status of family members and for early prenatal diagnosis prior to virilization.

3. Two 21-hydroxylase genes exist, designated CYP21A and CYP21B, located on chromosome 6 between HLA-B and DR, and are in tandem duplication with the genes encoding the fourth component of complement. Only CYP21B is active in adrenal steroidogenesis; CYP21A is not involved (a pseudogene because its product is enzymatically inactive).

4. A variety of mutations affecting CYP21B (deletions, gene conversion [material from CYP21A to CYP21B], point mutations) lead to 21-hydroxylase deficiency.

By combined HLA genotyping and ACTH stimulation testing (see 17-OHP nomogram in Chapter 14) of families that contained patients with late-onset and classic disease, a concept of allelic variants at the 21-hydroxylase locus evolved.[26,27] Salt-wasting, simple virilizing, and late-onset alleles, respectively, caused the most, less, and the least deficiency of 21-hydroxylase. Some family members exhibited abnormal responses to ACTH, and, although some of these had clinical evidence of androgen excess, others were entirely normal and represented a "cryptic" form of 21-hydroxylase deficiency.

Finally, heterozygotes for either the mild or severe deficiency allele exhibited the mildest enzyme deficiency and were clinically asymptomatic.

In summary, a useful classification has been proposed.[26] There are 3 alleles for 21-hydroxylase deficiency:

1. 21-hydroxylase deficiency[normal].

2. 21-hydroxylase deficiency[mild].

3. 21-hydroxylase deficiency[severe].

The correspondence between the extent of DNA mutations categorized as severe, moderate, or mild, and the clinical expression of 21-hydroxylase deficiency is imperfect. Furthermore, the clinical dicta that severity recurs within families and is related to the degree of 17-hydroxyprogesterone elevations are not absolute. In general, however, classical disease results when an individual is homozygous for the severe allele. All of the recent terms (late-onset, attenuated, acquired, nonclassical, including the cryptic form) refer to individuals who are either homozygous for the mild allele or carry one mild and one severe allele. Simple virilizing denotes a reduction of cortisol production alone, while in salt wasting, production of both cortisol and aldosterone is impaired. Despite the absence of symptoms, individuals with cryptic 21-hydroxylase deficiency are biochemically indistinguishable from those with the late onset form and carry the same genotypes. Heterozygotes for either the mild or severe deficiency allele also possess a normal allele and are unaffected carriers.

Enzyme Defect in Adrenal Only: Deficient 11β-Hydroxylase (P450c11). The final step in cortisol synthesis is blocked in this condition. In classic 11β-hydroxylase deficiency, 11-deoxycortisol is not converted to cortisol. Accumulated precursors are shunted into androgen biosynthesis with virilization similar to that seen with 21-hydroxylase deficiency. However, a parallel defect also exists so that deoxycorticosterone (DOC) is not converted to corticosterone. This pathway is used in the zona glomerulosa to synthesize aldosterone, and the degree to which aldosterone levels are affected lends clinical heterogeneity to the classic presentation of 11β-hydroxylase deficiency (virilization, hypertension, volume overload).

Usually as a result of 11β-hydroxylase deficiency, metabolically active precursors of corticosterone and cortisol add to excess androgen synthesis as further liabilities of ACTH-induced hyperplasia. Hypertension and hypokalemic alkalosis are induced by elevated DOC with reduced renin and aldosterone. Virilization is caused by androgens of the "deoxy" type (dehydroepiandrosterone [DHA], dehydroepiandrosterone sulfate [DHAS], and androstenedione). The diagnosis is confirmed by high plasma DOC and compound S (11-deoxycortisol) levels.

About two-thirds of untreated patients with 11β-hydroxylase deficiency become hypertensive, usually of mild to moderate degree (150/90 mm Hg) and only after several years of life. A mild nonclassic form of 11β-hydroxylase deficiency, as in 21-hydroxylase defects, has also been documented; it is characterized by mild biochemical abnormalities, and the patients are only mildly virilized and rarely hypertensive.

Contrary to 21-hydroxylase deficiency, the 11β-hydroxylase deficiency locus is remote from the HLA complex. The gene for the enzyme is on the long arm of chromosome 8, and the deficiency is inherited in autosomal recessive fashion.[28]

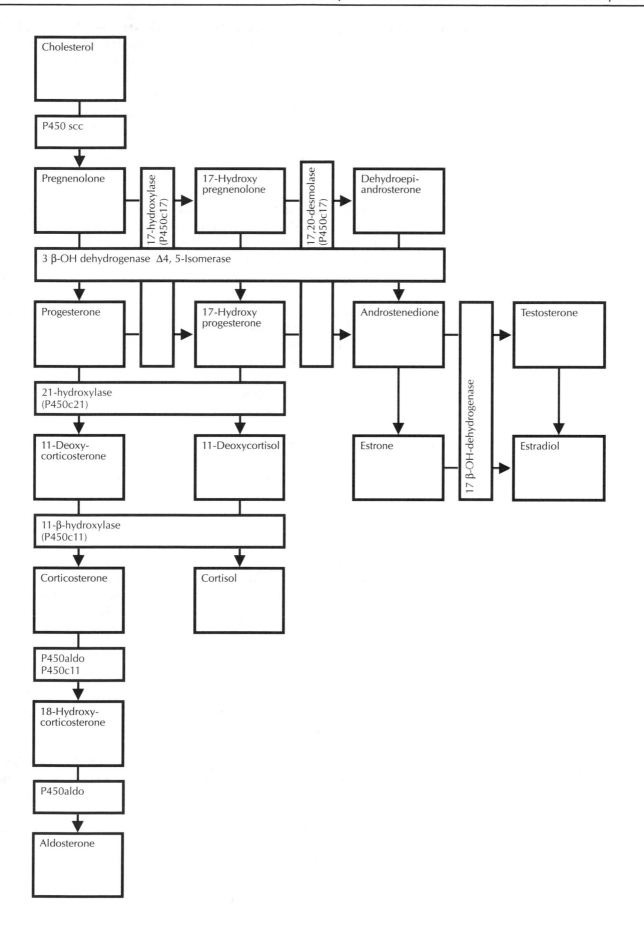

Enzyme Defect in Adrenal and Ovary: Deficient 17α-Hydroxylase (P450c17).
With block of the 17α-hydroxylase enzyme (P450c17), synthesis of cortisol, androgens, and estrogens is curtailed. Only the non-17-hydroxylated corticoids, DOC and corticosterone, are formed.[29] The molecular basis for this enzyme deficiency is due to a variety of mutations which result in multiple base deletions and duplications in the gene on chromosome 10.[30] The resulting syndrome is composed of hypertension (due to hypernatremia and hypervolemia), hypokalemia, infantile female external genitalia, which do not mature at puberty, and primary amenorrhea with elevated follicle-stimulating hormone (FSH) and luteinizing hormone (LH). Genital ambiguity is a problem only in male infants.

Enzyme Defects in Adrenal and Ovary: Deficient 3β-Hydroxysteroid Dehydrogenase. Lack of this essential step in the formation of all biologically active steroids affects both the adrenal cortex and the ovary and is also inherited in autosomal recessive fashion. Thus, there is decreased synthesis of glucocorticoids, mineralocorticoids, androgens, and estrogens. These infants are severely ill at birth and rarely survive. The external genitalia ambiguity results from the massive increase in DHA that is androgenic when available in excess, and also can be utilized to form more potent androgens in peripheral tissues. Thus, females may be slightly virilized and males incompletely masculinized with a variable degree of hypospadias. As in 21-hydroxylase deficiency, milder nonclassic cases may be common with mild hirsutism and elevated DHA (and DHAS) being the only distinguishing features. The spectrum of clinical phenotypes also includes both salt wasting and non-salt wasting forms. The degree of the enzyme defect cannot be extrapolated from the degree of external genitalia ambiguity.

Enzyme Defects in Adrenal and Ovary: Deficient 20-22-Desmolase (P450scc). A block in this step prevents conversion of cholesterol to pregnenolone, the necessary precursor to all biologically active steroids. The adrenals are enlarged and filled with cholesterol esters. Predictably, the internal and external genitalia are female, and death occurs.

Epidemiology

Only the 21-hydroxylase deficiency has been studied sufficiently, in part because it is not only the most frequent cause of genital ambiguity and congenital adrenal hyperplasia but also because of the high prevalence of the nonclassical, late onset forms of the disease. The genetic defect in virilizing adrenal hyperplasia is an autosomal recessive gene. Within families, the clinical picture is uniform, the type of syndrome (simple, salt-wasting, hypertensive) is usually but not always the same in affected siblings. The ratio in offspring of unaffected parents is one affected to three nonaffected individuals. Treated patients have a 1:100 to 1:200 chance of producing an affected infant. Males and females are at equal risk. On the basis of worldwide screening, the overall incidence of 21-hydroxylase deficiency is 1 per 14,000 births. The highest frequency for congenital adrenal hyperplasia is in Alaskan Yupik Eskimos.

The classic form is a relatively common inborn error of metabolism. One out of every 100 Caucasians is likely to be a genetic carrier of the classic type, and neonatal screening tests indicate an incidence of 1 in 14,000, which is equivalent to phenylketonuria.

For the nonclassic types, frequency rates established by the usual methodology (neonatal screening, case surveys) are likely to markedly underestimate what may be one of the most common autosomal recessive disorders in humans. Extrapolations from ACTH testing suggest the following frequency:[31]

	Nonclassical Disease	Heterozygous Carrier
Eastern European Jews	1 in 30	1 in 3
Hispanics	1 in 40	1 in 4
Slavs	1 in 50	1 in 5
Italians	1 in 333	1 in 9
Others	1 in 1000	1 in 14

Prenatal Diagnosis

The diagnosis of congenital adrenal hyperplasia due to 21-hydroxylase deficiency can be obtained prenatally by demonstrating elevated levels of 17-OHP, 21-deoxycortisol, and androstenedione in the amniotic fluid. 17-OHP may be elevated only in the salt losing form of adrenal hyperplasia, but androstenedione is increased with all forms. HLA genotyping of amniotic cells can yield confirmation by showing that the fetus is HLA identical to an affected sibling. The 11β-hydroxylase deficiency is associated with elevated levels of 11-deoxycortisol in amniotic fluid and tetrahydro-11-deoxycortisol in maternal urine, but this defect is not linked to HLA because the gene coding for this enzyme is found on the long arm of chromosome 8.[32]

Prenatal diagnosis of the 21-hydroxylase deficiency by chorion villus biopsy utilizing DNA probes offers the timely options of termination or in utero therapy.[33] With chorion villus biopsy, diagnosis can be made and therapy instituted before the critical period of fetal genital differentiation with avoidance of genital ambiguity in affected female fetuses. In addition, masculinization of the fetal brain can be avoided which might have an impact on gender identity and adult sexual behavior. Despite the very real limitations

Prenatal Treatment and Diagnosis of 21-Hydroxylase Deficiency

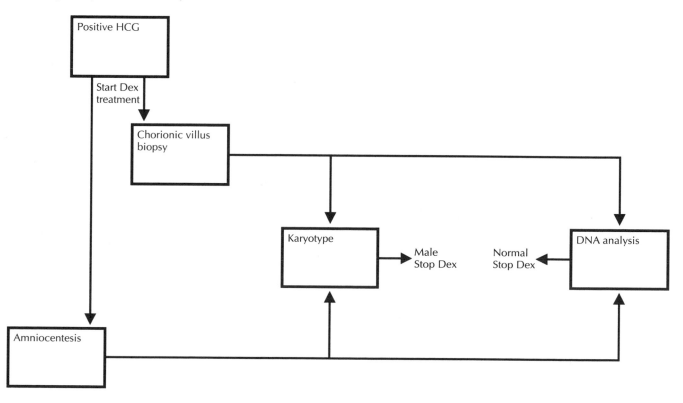

of HLA-specific and cDNA probes, prenatal treatment has been administered with dexamethasone in fetuses at risk for 21-hydroxylase deficiency.[34–37] Using multiple daily doses of dexamethasone (total no greater than 1.5 mg/day), complete prevention has been achieved in some newborns and diminished virilization in others. No congenital malformations, fetal death, or low birth weight or height have resulted from pregnancy-long cortisol derivative therapy. However, this treatment is associated with significant maternal side effects, such as severe striae with permanent scarring, hyperglycemia, hypertension, gastrointestinal symptoms, and emotional lability.[38] A reduction in dosage during the second half of pregnancy is recommended; dosage can be titered by maintaining the maternal serum estriol levels in the normal range. Questions concerning the relative danger of chorion villus biopsy compared to amniocentesis have also arisen: is the risk of fetal loss with the former technique too high? In patients who prefer amniocentesis and who have been started on dexamethasone treatment at 5–6 weeks gestation, dexamethasone can be discontinued for 5 days prior to amniocentesis, allowing 17-OHP and androstenedione in the amniotic fluid to reach diagnostic levels.[39] Given that only one in four siblings are at risk and one-half will be males (who do not suffer genital ambiguity from the excess androgen associated with 21-hydroxylase deficiency) then only 1 of 8 fetuses require treatment.

Diagnosis

For years the demonstration of a metabolic defect and its location depended upon the study of urinary steroid excretion. Today, the immunoassay of blood 17-hydroxy-progesterone (17-OHP) has become the primary assessment for the diagnosis and management of congenital adrenal hyperplasia. With the 21-hydroxylase and 11β-hydroxylase deficiencies, the 17-OHP level will be 50–400-fold above normal.

During delivery of affected infants, the concentration of 17-OHP is elevated in cord blood (1,000–3,000 ng/dL [30–90 nmol/L]), but it rapidly decreases to 100–200 ng/dL (3–6 nmol/L) after 24 hours. A delay in measurement gains accuracy. In contrast to 17-ketosteroids in the urine where the delay must be several days, with 17-OHP the delay need be only a day or two. In affected infants, 17-OHP ranges from 3,000 to 40,000 ng/dL (90–1,200 nmol/L). Measurement of 17-OHP is the basis for the newborn screening programs currently in place in many countries and some states in the U.S.

In adults, 17-OHP must be measured first thing in the morning to avoid later elevations due to the diurnal pattern of ACTH secretion. The baseline 17-OHP level should be less than 200 ng/dL (6 nmol/L). Levels greater than 200 ng/dL, but less than 800 ng/dL (24 nmol/L), require ACTH testing (discussed in Chapter 14). Levels over 800 ng/dL (24 nmol/L) are virtually diagnostic of the 21-hydroxylase deficiency. The DHAS level is usually normal. The hallmarks of late-onset adrenal hyperplasia are elevated levels of 17-OHP and a dramatic increase after ACTH stimulation. The elevated levels of 17-OHP are often not impressive (e.g., overlapping with those found in women with polycystic ovaries due to anovulation), and a simple ACTH stimulation test must be utilized.

Of course, in patients with 3β-hydroxysteroid dehydrogenase or 17-hydroxylase blocks, the 17-OHP level will not be elevated. With the 3β-hydroxysteroid dehydrogenase block, the blood levels of DHA and DHA sulfate (DHAS) will be markedly increased. In the 11β-hydroxylase deficiency, in addition to elevated 17-OHP, elevation of 11-deoxycortisol is diagnostic. In this deficiency, plasma renin activity will be low, whereas in 21-hydroxylase and 3β-hydroxysteroid dehydrogenase deficiencies plasma renin activity is elevated in the salt losing forms.

Treatment

Treatment of adrenal hyperplasia is to supply the deficient hormone, cortisol. This decreases ACTH secretion and lowers production of androgenic precursors. The addition of salt-retaining hormone to glucocorticoid therapy has improved the control of the disease. When the plasma renin activity is normalized, ACTH and androgen levels are further decreased, and a decrease in the glucocorticoid dose is also possible. Therefore, the modern management of hormonal control requires the measurement of the blood levels of 17-OHP, androstenedione, testosterone, and plasma renin activity.[23] The drugs of choice are hydrocortisone (approximately 10 mg per day) and 9-fluorohydrocortisone (approximately 100 µg/day). This method of treatment and monitoring applies to all forms of adrenal hyperplasia. The standard dose of cortisol is 12–18 mg/m^2 or 3.5–5 mg/m^2 of prednisone, but larger doses given on alternate days (14 mg/m^2 of prednisone, about 20 mg) can maintain adrenal androgen suppression and perhaps achieve better growth and pubertal development, despite higher levels of 17-hydroxyprogesterone.[40] The 17-OHP level should be maintained in the range of 500 to 4,000 ng/dL, thereby avoiding both overtreatment and undertreatment. Minor stresses will cause brief elevations of adrenal androgens but usually do not require readjustment of dosage. With major stress, such as surgery, additional hormonal support is necessary.

The surgical treatment of the anatomical abnormalities should be carried out in the first few years of life, when the patient is still too young to remember the procedure and too young to have developed psychological problems centered about the abnormal external genitalia. If clitoridectomy is necessary, the clitoral recession procedure, conserving the glans and its innervation, should be employed. It is important to know that women who undergo total clitoral amputations have no subsequent impairment of erotic responsiveness or capacity for orgasm. Significant vaginal reconstruction, if necessary, is best accomplished after puberty when mature compliance is possible.

Normal reproduction is possible with replacement therapy of the cortisol deficiency. Unfortunately poor compliance with therapy and less than satisfactory surgical reconstruction of the vagina result in decreased fertility and sexuality.[41] Greater attention to these factors is needed to improve the sexual experience and fertility of these women. Many cases come to cesarean section because normal anatomy of the perineum may be obscured by scar tissue from earlier plastic surgery; therefore, greater blood loss and the risk of a hematoma with a vaginal delivery are significant factors. A masculine pelvis is not expected since the adult form and size of the inlet of the pelvis are assumed largely during the growth spurt in puberty. However, a small pelvis might be anticipated if the bone age is up to age 13–14 when treatment is initiated. Fertility in women with late onset adrenal hyperplasia is only slightly reduced, dependent upon the degree of hormonal dysfunction (which is promptly corrected with glucocorticoid therapy).[42]

The maintenance steroid dose usually does not need to be changed during pregnancy. The dosage of steroids used in the treatment of this syndrome replaces the approximate amount normally produced and, therefore, is a physiologic dose. At these low doses, teratogenic effects would be unlikely, and none have been noted. The need for additional steroids during the stress of labor and delivery is obvious and is usually met by the administration of cortisone acetate intramuscularly and cortisol intravenously. Infection and impaired wound healing have not been problems. Aside from the liability associated with genetic transmission of this syndrome, the children born to patients with adrenal hyperplasia have been normal. The newborn should be closely observed for adrenal insufficiency due to steroid crossover and suppression of the fetal adrenal in utero.

Treatment Problems

Overtreatment causes Cushing's syndrome and poor growth; undertreatment is associated with short stature, hirsutism, and infertility. In some cases, undertreatment and increased androgen secretion lead to premature pubertal maturation that may require treatment with a gonadotropin-releasing hormone (GnRH) agonist. The adult height achieved by most patients is less than normal, testimony to overtreatment and undertreatment (which both compromise growth). Mineralocorticoid therapy should be maximized (maintaining the plasma renin activity at its lower limit of normal) to eliminate hypovolemia as a stimulus for ACTH secretion. A treatment approach is being investigated that adds an antiandrogen and an aromatase inhibitor in an effort to avoid hypercortisolism and block excess sex steroid action on growth.

Masculinization Due to Elevated Androgens in Maternal Circulation

Masculinization of the female fetus, although in most cases due to fetal virilizing adrenal hyperplasia, may be produced by an androgen-secreting maternal tumor or may be due to the intake of exogenous androgenic substances, such as progestins and danazol. When not caused by an error in the metabolism of the fetal adrenal gland, virilization is not progressive, blood steroids are not elevated, and no hormonal therapy is needed. Subsequent development will be normal. Therefore, surgical correction of abnormalities in the external genitalia is the only indicated treatment.

The occurrence of an androgen-secreting tumor in a mother during pregnancy is rarely seen. On the other hand, the iatrogenic cause of masculinization is a well-known story. The majority of these cases resulted from antenatal maternal treatment of threatened or recurrent abortion with various progestin compounds. In view of the lack of evidence for positive results with such therapy, the use of progestin compounds in pregnancy is contraindicated.

Placental Aromatase Deficiency

A placental deficiency in aromatase activity would allow an accumulation of the fetal androgen precursors utilized in placental estrogen synthesis. This condition is associated with virilization of the mother during pregnancy, low estrogen levels in the mother, and a female newborn with masculinization.[43] Accurate prenatal diagnosis requires a loading test with DHA and DHAS. A patient with a placental sulfatase deficiency will increase her estrogen levels in response to DHA and not to DHAS. A patient with an aromatase deficiency will respond to neither steroid.

Incompletely Masculinized Males

Incompletely masculinized males are male by genetic sex (XY) and possess testicles, but the external genitalia are not normally male. Male pseudohermaphrodites may arise in one of three ways:

1. Defective responses in androgen dependent tissues — Androgen Insensitivity Syndromes.

2. Abnormal androgen synthesis.

3. Absent or defective antimüllerian hormone.

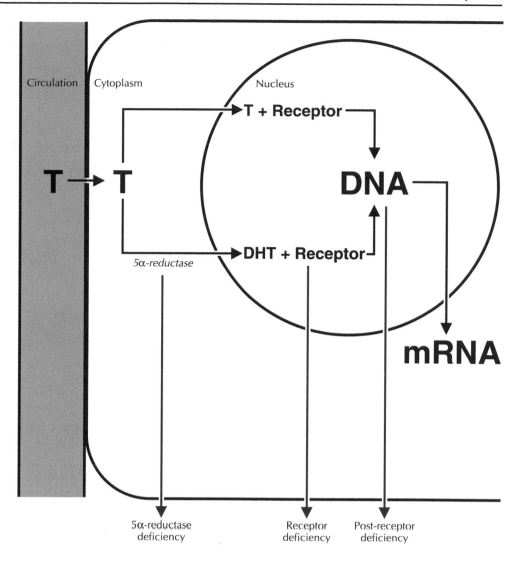

Syndromes of Androgen Insensitivity

Factors that influence the response to androgens in specific target cells include the following:

1. The intracellular concentration of androgen.
2. The relative binding affinity of these steroids to their nuclear androgen receptors.
3. The binding capacity of the receptor.
4. The nuclear content of androgen receptors.
5. The cellular concentrations of catabolic and/or synthetic enzymes (e.g., 5α-reductase, aromatase, 17β-hydroxysteroid dehydrogenase).
6. The adequacy of the nuclear (chromatin) acceptor site.
7. The adequacy of regulatory molecules controlling chromatin "read" of the androgen message.
8. RNA processing and translation.
9. The quality of the protein gene product.

Defects in androgenization of targets doubtless occur as a result of failure in any of these steps. Three major clinical conditions are worthy of detailed review.

Androgen Insensitivity Syndromes

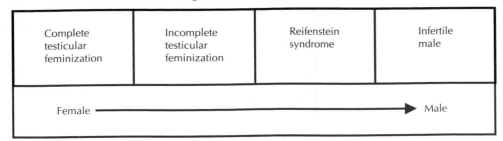

Phenotypic Spectrum

Complete Androgen Insensitivity — Testicular Feminization

Complete androgen insensitivity was first described in detail by Morris at Yale, who provided the descriptive term, testicular feminization.[44] The phenotype of this condition (also discussed in Chapter 12) is female, despite the normal male karyotype 46,XY. There is a congenital insensitivity to androgens, transmitted by means of a maternal X-linked recessive gene responsible for the androgen intracellular receptor. Therefore, androgen induction of wolffian duct development does not occur. However, anti-müllerian hormone activity is present, and the individual does not have müllerian development (a natural experiment that indicates the presence of an antimüllerian hormone). Frequently the testes have descended to the inguinal ring because AMH mediates the transabdominal descent of the testes. The vagina is short (derived from the urogenital sinus only) and ends blindly. The uterus and tubes are absent. The testes are normally developed but abnormally positioned. Testosterone production is normal or slightly increased. There is no problem of sex assignment because there is no trace of androgen activity. The diagnosis is likely when an individual presents following breast development at puberty, with primary amenorrhea, scanty or absent pubic and axillary hair, a short vagina, and an absent cervix and uterus. Males with enzyme defects that prevent testosterone synthesis will have a female phenotype, but breast development does not occur. Androgen insensitivity accounts for about 10% of all cases of primary amenorrhea, third most common after gonadal dysgenesis and congenital absence of the vagina. The hormone profile in these individuals is typical: high LH, normal to slightly elevated male testosterone levels, high estradiol (for men), and normal to elevated FSH.

An absent uterus in a normal appearing female is encountered in only two conditions: androgen insensitivity and müllerian agenesis (the Mayer-Rokitansky-Kuster-Hauser syndrome). The latter is easily diagnosed because of the presence of pubic and axillary hair and a normal 46,XX karyotype.

The "complete" form indicates that there is no androgen response; therefore, normal external female development occurs, and these infants should be reared as females. The testes (azoospermic with hyperplastic Leydig cells) may be present in the inguinal canals. Children with inguinal hernias and/or inguinal masses should be suspected of testicular feminization. There is no virilization at puberty because of the lack of androgen response. In contrast to dysgenetic gonads with a Y chromosome, the occurrence of gonadal tumors is relatively late, rarely before age 25, and the overall incidence is less, about 5%.[45,46] Therefore, gonadectomy should be performed at approximately age 16–18, to allow endogenous hormonal changes and a smooth transition through puberty. Individuals with complete androgen insensitivity perform less well in tests of visual-spatial ability, suggesting that androgens exert an organizing effect in the brain during development.[47]

Because of the importance of prophylactic gonadectomy, detection of this syndrome demands careful investigation for other affected family members. This syndrome

The Androgen Insensitivity Syndromes[48]

	5α-reductase	Complete	Incomplete	Reifenstein	Infertile
Inheritance	Autosomal recessive	X-linked recessive	X-linked recessive	X-linked recessive	X-linked recessive
Spermatogenesis	Decreased	Absent	Absent	Absent	Decreased
Müllerian	Absent	Absent	Absent	Absent	Absent
Wolffian	Male	Absent	Male	Male	Male
External	Female	Female	Female clitoromegaly	Male hypospadias	Male
Breasts	Male	Female	Female	Gynecomastia	Gynecomastia

follows an X-limited recessive pattern of inheritance. Apparent sisters of affected individuals have a 1 in 3 chance of being XY. Female offspring of a normal sister of an affected individual have a 1 in 6 chance of being XY. About a third of the patients have negative family histories and presumably represent new mutations.

Incomplete Androgen Insensitivity

A spectrum of disorders, all due to an X-linked recessive trait, are known as incomplete forms of testicular feminization. It is one-tenth as common as the complete syndrome.[48] The clinical presentation ranges from almost complete failure of virilization to essentially complete phenotypic masculinization. Between these poles exist examples of mild clitoromegaly and slight labial fusion to significant genital ambiguity. Reifenstein's syndrome is now applied to all the intermediate forms that were initially given individual names (such as Lubs syndrome). Recently, males have been described whose only indication of androgen insensitivity was azoospermic or severe oligospermic infertility. Indeed the incidence may approach 40% or more of men with infertility due to azoospermia or severe oligospermia. However, the defect in androgen receptor function may be so subtle that some affected men are fertile.[49] The undervirilized fertile male syndrome is another manifestation of this androgen receptor disorder. The diversity of presentation represents variable manifestations of the same mutant gene. The biochemical abnormality lies in the degree of function of the androgen receptor or postreceptor events.

Molecular analysis of the androgen receptor gene in individuals with androgen insensitivity has demonstrated a spectrum of disorders in which both the complete and partial forms result from androgen receptor gene mutations.[50] The gene encoding the androgen receptor is localized to the q11–12 region (the long arm) of the X chromosome and encodes a receptor protein comprised of discrete functional domains which mediate steroid binding, DNA binding, and transcriptional activation of target genes.[51]

Two types of defective androgen receptor function are recognized: abnormalities of androgen binding and abnormalities of DNA binding. The molecular defects responsible for these deficiencies have been identified and characterized. These include major structural abnormalities of the androgen receptor gene in which complete deletion of the gene or deletions of the exons encoding the androgen binding domain or the DNA binding domain each result in the clinical picture of complete androgen insensitivity.[52–54] In addition, point mutations that result in a defective receptor or alter receptor mRNA and cause reduced receptor protein production also result in complete androgen insensitivity.[55] On the other hand, single base mutations that change a single amino acid yield subjects displaying either complete or partial androgen insensitivity.[56] Alterations in receptor function, therefore, range from complete loss to subtle qualitative changes in the stimulation and transcription of androgen dependent target genes. Less understandable, however, is the poor correlation between receptor levels (and androgen binding affinity) with the degree of masculinization seen in partial androgen insensitivity. Nevertheless, the same mode of inheritance, despite differences in androgen receptor functioning, indicates that all forms originate in changes in the structural gene responsible for the androgen receptor.

Sex assignment may be a problem when ambiguous genitalia exist because of a partial response of the receptor. If sex assignment is female, early gonadectomy is performed to avoid neoplasia. In Reifenstein syndrome, the phallus may be large enough to allow a male sex assignment at birth, despite the perineal hypospadias. After puberty, however, the inadequate androgen receptor resource becomes evident and feminization with gynecomastia occurs. The receptor function is inadequate to respond to the surge of androgen at puberty; without androgen effect, estrogen activity prevails. These individuals are infertile and cannot react to exogenous androgen. The karyotype is male XY, distinguishing it from other feminizing syndromes of puberty in phenotypic males (e.g., Klinefelter's syndrome).

The endocrine profiles of both the complete and incomplete forms are similar: high blood levels of testosterone, normal to elevated FSH levels, mildly elevated LH (due to absence of negative androgen feedback), and high levels of estradiol (increased testicular response to LH and increased peripheral conversion).

5α-Reductase Deficiency

This form of familial incomplete male (46,XY) pseudohermaphroditism is due to an autosomal recessive trait that leads to a deficiency of the 5α-reductase enzyme (and, in some individuals, enzyme that is present but unstable) and is characterized by severe perineal hypospadias and underdevelopment of the vagina.[57] In the past it was known as pseudovaginal perineoscrotal hypospadias (PPH). It differs from the incomplete forms of testicular feminization because, at puberty, masculinization occurs (the breasts remain male). Normal testicular function occurs, and there is no lack of response to endogenous or exogenous androgen. At birth, however, the external genitalia are similar to that of incomplete testicular feminization; i.e., hypospadias, varying failure of fusion of labioscrotal folds and a urogenital opening, or separate urethral and vaginal openings. The cleft in the scrotum appears to be a vagina (there are no müllerian ducts), and these patients have been reared as girls with an enlarged clitoris. At birth, steroid levels are normal, ruling out adrenal disorders.

Diagnosis can be established by demonstrating an elevated T:DHT ratio based upon the blood levels of testosterone and dihydrotestosterone, especially after HCG stimulation. The karyotype is XY, and, as with other incompletely masculinized males, the sex assignment is female if the phallus is inadequate. Gonadectomy is necessary to avoid not only neoplasia but the virilization that is certain to appear at puberty. The deficiency is believed to be due to the homozygous state, manifest clinically only in males. Homozygous 46,XX females have normal fertility.

At least 3 "types" of enzyme deficiency have been described in affected families:

1. Abnormally low concentration of enzyme.

2. Reduced enzyme activity due to enzyme instability.

3. Normal enzyme concentration but defective affinity for testosterone and/or essential cofactors leading to reduced enzyme activity.

Two 5α-reductase genes have been cloned.[58] One isoenzyme is encoded on chromosome 5; mutations in the other isoenzyme encoded on chromosome 2 are responsible for male pseudohermaphroditism due to 5α-reductase deficiency. This deficiency in females does not affect fertility and contributes to the high incidence of the disorder. The relatively easy switch of individuals reared as girls to boys at puberty suggests that the other 5α-reductase gene is operative in the brain.

Study of this syndrome points out important lessons in intersexuality. In this condition, the wolffian duct virilizes in a normal male fashion, but the urogenital sinus and genital tubercle persist as female structures. The failure is due to inadequate DHT formation intracellularly in these external genitalia tissues at the time the normal male fetus virilizes. In the 5α-reductase deficiencies, the seminal vesicles, ejaculatory ducts, epididymis, and vas deferens which are all testosterone-dependent are present, whereas the DHT-dependent structures, external genitalia, urethra, and prostate do not develop along male lines. Affected men have less facial and body hair, less temporal hairline recession and no problems with acne. However, spermatogenesis, muscle mass, male libido, deepening of the voice do occur in these men. DHT presence is a requirement only in the fetus, as indicated by the significant genital virilization these patients undergo at puberty and thereafter.[59] These individuals require surgical correction of hypospadias and cryptorchidism. Whereas the conversion from male to female role is exceedingly traumatic psychologically, the reversal of sex identity (female to male) some of these patients in the past have undergone at puberty was apparently uncomplicated.[20] In one such case, a "double-life" was conducted. Although functioning in all public respects as a female, one 5α-reductase individual conducted numerous and prolonged heterosexual affairs, which were quite satisfactory, albeit clandestine. He had known of his male sexual identity since puberty but delayed medical assistance for fear that exposure would bring shame and guilt to his religiously devoted elderly "old world" mother. He decided to keep his secret until his mother died. He finally sought diagnostic help at age 65, however, because his mother at age 93 continued to enjoy good health.

Abnormal Androgen Synthesis

Defective male development may stem from a secretory failure of the testes during the critical period of sex differentiation. In addition to the obvious specific and often familial defects in enzymatic steps leading to testosterone biosynthesis, a variety of other intrinsically testicular problems can lead to male pseudohermaphroditism. In all, the following conditions account for 4% of male pseudohermaphroditism:

1. Aberrations in testicular organogenesis (dysgenetic testes).

2. Defective synthesis, secretion, or response to antimüllerian hormone.

3. Testicular unresponsiveness to LH with Leydig cell hypoplasia.

Defects in testosterone synthesis can be at any one of the four required enzymatic reactions that lead from cholesterol to testosterone: P450scc, 3β-hydroxysteroid dehydrogenase, P450c17, and 17β-hydroxysteroid dehydrogenase. These defects are inherited as autosomal recessive traits, and the phenotypes range from partial to complete male pseudohermaphroditism.

Patients with male pseudohermaphroditism who are considered variants of testicular feminization upon partial virilization at puberty may actually have a defect in androgen synthesis. The diagnosis is made by demonstrating elevated blood levels of androstenedione and estrogens, while the blood level of testosterone is low or low-normal. When the enzyme involves a reaction that is active in the adrenal gland (all but the 17βhydroxysteroid dehydrogenase), the adrenal blocks are usually severe with adrenal failure and death in the newborn period.

The male pseudohermaphrodite due to deficient testicular 17β-hydroxysteroid dehydrogenase activity has male internal genitalia and no müllerian structures. The characteristic clinical findings in these patients are external female genitalia at birth with testes usually located in the inguinal canal. Paradoxically, at puberty they may virilize (enlarged phallus, male body hair and muscle mass, voice changes) and/or feminize with gynecomastia depending on the extent of peripheral conversion of elevated androstenedione to either testosterone and/or estrogen.[60] These patients have elevated circulating levels of androstenedione and estrone and low levels of testosterone. In individuals being raised as girls, early gonadectomy is required to avoid virilization at puberty and testicular neoplasia.

Gonadotropin Resistant Testes

Male pseudohermaphrodites, due to agenesis or abnormal differentiation of Leydig cells, are characterized by reduced responsiveness to LH/HCG, deficiency in the availability or function of receptors or post-receptor elements, such as regulatory guanyl nucleotides, cyclic AMP, crucial phosphokinases, cholesterol uptake, and esterase enzymes. All these cases could be termed "gonadotropin resistant testes." In general, the characteristics of the syndrome include basically female but ambiguous genitalia, male cryptorchid testes with degenerated Leydig cells, no müllerian ducts but present vas deferens and epididymis, elevated gonadotropins (FSH rises further after gonadectomy, indicating the presence of inhibin).[61] Although an absence or deficiency of LH receptors is postulated, an environmentally or autoimmune produced disappearance of the receptors or the Leydig cells is possible.

Abnormal Antimüllerian Hormone

Hernia Uterine Inguinale (Uterine Hernia Syndrome). Individuals with this syndrome appear to be normal males, but relatively well-differentiated müllerian duct structures are found, usually a uterus and tubes in an inguinal hernia sac. This is due to a failure of AMH function either as a result of failure of Sertoli cell secretion of this polypeptide or an inability of the müllerian ducts to respond to AMH. It is inherited as a recessive trait, either X-linked or autosomal. Fertility is usually preserved. Other instances in which some müllerian duct retention is found include dysgenetic testes, ovotestes, mixed gonadal dysgenesis, müllerian duct and utricular cysts, and prenatal diethylstilbestrol (DES) exposure.

Abnormal Gonadogenesis

The proper development and eventual function of the gonad depends on the presence of germ cells, the appropriate sex chromosome constitution, and appropriate gonadal ridge somatic cells. Errors in meiotic division can cause aneuploidy and abnormal sex chromosomes. These occur by nondisjunction, anaphase lag, translocation, breakage, rearrangements, or deletions. Mitosis can also be marred by nondisjunction and anaphase lag leading to mosaicism. Two or more different cell lines can persist and appear in different tissues. Finally, abnormal gonadogenesis may occur as a result of structural or disease related catastrophes leading to loss of fetal gonadal function.

Bilateral Dysgenesis of the Testes (Swyer Syndrome)
Affected individuals have an XY karyotype but normal (infantile) female external and internal genitalia.[62] There are fibrous bands in place of the gonads yielding primary amenorrhea and lack of secondary sexual development at puberty. It is a matter of prudent practice to avoid the possibility of virilization or neoplasm; therefore, removal of these band areas is advocated as soon as the diagnosis is made. Presumably, testes failed to develop or were eliminated (testicular regression) before internal or external

A Clarification of Terminology

Event	Time of Event (Days After Fertilization)	Nomenclature	Müllerian Duct	Wolffian Duct	External Genitalia
Early embryonic testicular regression	Before 43	Pure gonadal dysgenesis	Present	Absent	Female
Late embryonic testicular regression	43–59	Swyer syndrome	Present	Absent	Female
Early fetal testicular regression	60–69	Agonadism	Present	Absent	Ambiguous
	70–75	Testicular dysgenesis	Present	Present	Ambiguous
	75–84	Testicular regression	Absent	Present	Ambiguous
Midfetal testicular regression	90–120	Rudimentary testis	Absent	Present	Male infantile
Late fetal testicular regression	After 140	Vanishing testis, anorchia	Absent	Present	Male infantile

genital differentiation.[63] Estrogen and progestin sequential therapy supports female secondary sex development.

True Agonadism

The pathogenesis of this condition, in view of a normal XY sex chromosome complement, must be complete testicular degeneration sometime between 6 and 12 weeks of pregnancy. If testicular loss is early, there is inadequate androgen stimulation (minimal wolffian development and female external genitalia), and müllerian ducts are preserved. The presence of a normal vagina, uterus, and tubes distinguishes this syndrome from testicular feminization variants. However, if testes loss occurs late, no gonads will be present, external genitalia will be ambiguous (but primarily female), and rudimentary components of both müllerian and wolffian internal ducts will be present.[63] Surgical removal of the streaks is required as a precaution against neoplasia.

Anorchia

Affected XY individuals have infantile unambiguous male external genitalia, and male wolffian ducts and lack müllerian ducts. There are, however, no detectable testes. Early testis function did occur (wolffian presence, AMH function) but was not sustained in sufficient amounts or duration to develop a normal size phallus. It is frequently called "the disappearing testis syndrome." Sex of assignment depends on the extent of external genitalia development.

True Hermaphrodites

Hermaphroditus, the Greek god with bisexual attributes, was the son-daughter of Hermes, the god of athletics, secrets, and occult philosophy, and Aphrodite, the goddess of love. The bisexual theme was immortalized in countless statues by the Greeks and Romans, depicting a normal woman with normal male external genitalia (not a combination commonly encountered in real life). Pliny (23–79 A.D.) was the first to apply the term hermaphrodite to humans, presenting a description in his massive work, *Historia Naturalis.*

Abnormal sexual differentiation can occur as a result of a mixture of gonadal sex (true hermaphroditism) or complete uncertainty of gonadal sex (gonadal dysgenesis with some virilization).[64] A true hermaphrodite possesses both ovarian and testicular tissue.

Both types may be contained in one gonad (ovotestis) or less often, one side may be an ovary, the other a testis. The internal structures correspond to the adjacent gonad. In the majority, external genitalia are ambiguous with sufficient male character to allow male sex assignment. However, three-fourths develop gynecomastia and half menstruate after puberty. Sixty percent are genetic females (XX), few are XY, the rest are mosaics with at least one cell line XX. 46,XX individuals without SRY may have a mutation of an autosomal gene that permits testicular determination in the absence of the testis determining factor.[65]

Gonadal Dysgenesis

Gonadal dysgenesis with bilateral rudimentary streak gonads due to an abnormality in or absence of one of the X chromosomes in all cell lines is called Turner syndrome. Approximately 60% of Turner patients have the total loss of one X chromosome; the remainder have either a structural abnormality in one of the X chromosomes or mosaicism with an abnormal X. Henry Turner, born in 1892, became chief of endocrinology and associate dean of the University of Oklahoma school of medicine. Turner's clinical description of this syndrome was presented to the annual meeting of the Association for the Study of Internal Secretions in 1938.

In the absence of gonadal development, these individuals are phenotypic females. The well-known characteristics are short stature (142–147 cm, 56–58 inches), sexual infantilism, and streak gonads. The streak gonad is composed of white fibrous stromal tissue, 2–3 cm long and about 0.5 cm wide, containing no ova or follicular derivatives. Other congenital problems in this syndrome are a webbed neck, a high arched palate, cubitus valgus, a broad shield-like chest with widely spaced nipples, a low hairline on the neck, short fourth metacarpal bones, disproportionately short legs, and renal abnormalities (horseshoe kidney, unilateral pelvic kidney, rotational abnormalities, and partial or complete duplication of the collecting system). Autoimmune disorders are common, such as Hashimoto's thyroiditis, Addison's disease, alopecia, and vitiligo. Hypothyroidism is present in about 10% of patients. Mild insulin resistance and hearing loss are also common. One-third of patients with Turner syndrome have cardiovascular abnormalities, including bicuspid aortic valves, coarctation of the aorta, mitral valve prolapse, and aortic aneurysms. Usually the diagnosis is not made until puberty when amenorrhea and lack of sexual development become apparent. At birth, however, lymphedema (due to hypoplasia of superficial vessels) of the extremities may indicate the condition. It is important to assess the aorta, aortic root, and aortic valve with ultrasonography at least in infancy and again during the teens. Patients with Turner syndrome have normal intelligence; however, there may be difficulty with mathematical ability, visual-motor coordination, and spatial-temporal processing.

About 98% of conceptuses with only one X chromosome abort. The remaining 2% account for an incidence of Turner syndrome in about 1 in 2,000–5,000 liveborn girls.

Because of the high incidence of assorted abnormalites in patients with Turner syndrome, the following evaluations should be performed, some only once at the time of diagnosis, and others annually as part of on-going surveillance: thyroid function testing (annually) and antibodies (at least once), intravenous pyelogram or renal ultrasonography (once if normal), echocardiography, audiometry, and annual evaluation of the lipid profile and glucose metabolism.

The presence of menstrual function and reproduction in a patient with Turner phenotype must be due to a mosaic complement, such as a 46,XX line in addition to 45,X. When pregnancy does occur in an X deficient subject, the incidence of aneuploidy in the conceptus is almost 50%.

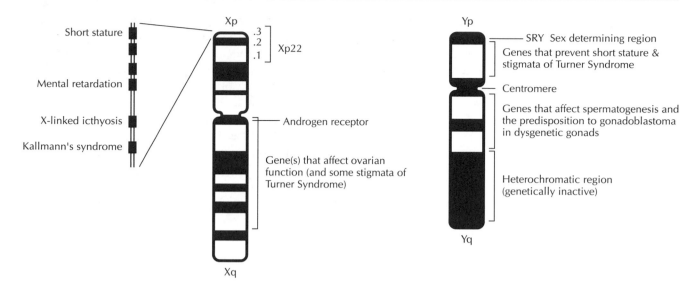

A large variety of mosaic patterns is seen with gonadal dysgenesis. From analysis of the various combinations, it is apparent that short stature is related to loss of regions on the short arm of one X chromosome. Distal long arm deletions of one of the X chromosomes are associated with amenorrhea (usually secondary after some ovarian function) and streak gonads, but the patients are not always growth compromised nor do they display other Turner somatic malformations. Long arm deletions near the centromere are associated with primary amenorrhea. Thus, loss of material from the short arms of the X chromosome leads to short stature and the other stigmata of Turner syndrome. This suggests that normal ovarian development requires two loci, one on the long arm and one on the short arm; loss of either results in gonadal failure. Thyroid autoimmunity is common in Turner syndrome, but Hashimoto's thyroiditis may be specific to 46,XXqi cases.

Just as X chromosome monosomy, with deletion of the second X chromosome, results in Turner's phenotype, the same will apply to loss of the Y chromosome. The 45,X karyotype derived from leukocyte culture does not guarantee that a mosaic does not exist with a gonadal line containing XY. For this reason, annual pelvic examinations and appropriate screening are required to detect incipient signs of gonadal neoplasia as an adnexal mass. If a presumed 45,X patient develops breasts or sexual hair without exogenous therapy, a gonadoblastoma or dysgerminoma should be considered and ruled out. Heterosexual signs require scrutiny in all 45,X individuals. ***Expert consultation should be obtained to pursue further analysis with X- and Y-specific DNA probes.***

The term "gonadal dysgenesis" is frequently used to describe all subjects with female genitalia, normal müllerian structures and streak gonads. Not all possess the spectrum of Turner phenotype anomalies, and some show none of these characteristics. The latter groups are referred to as "pure gonadal dysgenesis." Ovarian determination and subsequent internal and external genitalia development proceed normally. However, at variable times thereafter, the gonads undergo accelerated germ cell loss, and premature degeneration of the ovaries ensues. A similar morphologic consequence of premature ovarian degeneration exists in 46,XX gonadal dysgenesis. In these instances, a mutation in an autosomal gene is considered the likely etiologic factor, inherited in autosomal recessive fashion.[46] Perrault syndrome is the combination of XX gonadal dysgenesis and neurosensory deafness.

Subjects with 46,XY karyotype also have gonadal dysgenesis, most, but not all, with the pure gonadal dysgenesis form without Turner stigmata.[66] The 46,XY gonadal dysgenesis patients are diagnosed in early adolescence with delayed pubertal development. As expected they show elevated gonadotropins, normal female levels of androgen, and low levels of estrogens, female external genitalia, a uterus, and fallopian tubes. On occasion, slight clitoral enlargement can be seen, due probably to hilar cell stimulation of HCG production. Similarly, minimal breast enlargement reflects peripheral aromatization of androgen. Menstrual function suggests tumor development in the streak gonad. These streaks often display ovarian stroma but no follicles. Their propensity to tumor development is significant, a 20–30% incidence. Patients with mosaic patterns in the karyotype have a reduced risk of tumor, but it still amounts to 15–20%. The most common tumor is the often bilateral gonadoblastoma, but dysgerminomas and even the more threatening embryonal carcinoma are also seen. Intraabdominal testes should be removed as early in life as possible because of the known risk of tumor development. If well visualized, streak gonads can be removed by laparoscopy.[67–69] The uterus and tubes should be retained for the possibility of pregnancy with donor oocytes.

The etiology of this defect is thought to be a short arm Y chromosome deletion involving SRY, a mutation in other genes that inhibit SRY function, or a XXqi mutation of SRY.[7] There is evidence to suggest that some cases of 46,XY gonadal dysgenesis are due to impaired function of a gene on the X chromosome that is necessary for normal SRY function.[70] The absence of Turner stigmata in these patients suggests the preservation of a nearby gene that protects XY individuals from developing Turner stigmata.[71] In 46,XY partial gonadal dysgenesis individuals there is some testicular development, and therefore, they present as newborns with ambiguous genitalia.[72] The degree of external masculinization and the relative proportions of müllerian and wolffian duct structures present correlate with the extent of testes differentiation.

Curiously, to date analysis of a large number of 46,XY partial gonadal patients has not demonstrated mutation of the coding region of the SRY gene. The association of this form of gonadal dysgenesis with duplications of the short arm of the X chromosome, and various inherited syndromes of multiple congenital anomalies (Wilms tumor-chromosome 11 and abnormalities of chromosome 9), indicate the role of several genes other than SRY in testes development. Males who have a 46,XX karyotype usually have SRY present, probably by translocation from the Y to an X chromosome.[71] Some subjects, however, lack SRY, indicating that more than one genetic defect yields 46,XX maleness.

Multiple X females (47,XXX) have normal development and reproductive function, although mental retardation may be more frequent. Secondary amenorrhea and/or eunuchoidism can be seen.

Mixed Gonadal Dysgenesis   Mosaicism involving the Y chromosome can be associated with abnormalities of sex differentiation. Of the variety of karyotypes possible from loss of the Y by nondisjunction, 45,X/46,XY is the most common. A wide variety of phenotypes is displayed by these individuals from newborns with ambiguous genitalia to normal fertile males or normal female phenotype with bilateral streak gonads. Most have short stature, and one-third have other Turner stigmata.

In the "typical" mixed gonadal dysgenesis case presenting with abnormal sex differentiation the usual gonadal pattern is a streak gonad on one side and a dysgenetic or normal appearing testis on the other side of the abdomen. Müllerian and wolffian duct development correlates with the character of the ipsilateral gonad. All possible permutations combining streaks, and dysgenetic and apparently normal testes have been encountered. The diversity of presentation is presumed to reflect the relative proportion of 45,X and 46,XY cells in the gonadal ridge. The incidence of gonadal tumors is 25%.

The application of molecular biology methods allows markers for DNA sequences on the Y chromosome to seek out similar sequences on patients' sex chromosomes. In one series of 40 Turner syndrome patients, one patient had identifiable Y chromosome material using polymerase chain reaction of the gene from SRY region of the Y chromosome.[73] In 3 of 18 patients (none of whom had evidence of Y chromosomal material by cytogenetic analysis), Y chromosomal segments from the SRY region were detected by polymerase chain amplification and Southern blot analysis.[74] The short coming of this method is that polymerase chain reaction and in situ hybridization identify only those DNA sequences that correspond to the probes used in the analysis. There may be a sequence from a Y chromosome that does not correspond to the selected probes. A totally reliable method awaits identification of the gene responsible for tumor formation or the complete mapping of the Y chromosome sequences. Until then, patients with gonadal dysgenesis having any Y chromosome fragments must be considered to be at risk for gonadal tumors and virilization at puberty.

Surgical Removal of Gonadal Tissue

There is no debate that gonadal tissue having any Y chromosome component in phenotypic females requires removal as soon as the diagnosis is made to avoid the risk of malignant gonadal tumors. There is one exception to this rule. Because gonadal tumors occur relatively late in patients with complete androgen insensitivity, surgery is delayed until after puberty. An accomplished laparoscopist can attempt this procedure, with the option of laparotomy if the gonads prove to be inaccessible. Streak gonads have been removed in this fashion, as well as the testes in androgen insensitivity.[67-69] With androgen insensitivity, the gonads can be close to the external iliac artery and herniated into the inguinal canals. The procedure is more difficult, and care must be taken to extract the gonad from the inguinal canal to secure complete excision. It may also be necessary to make a small abdominal incision or a culdotomy to extract the gonad in order to avoid morcellation.

The uterus and tubes should be preserved for the possibility of pregnancy with donor oocytes.

Hormone Treatment of Patients without Ovaries

When ovaries are absent in individuals being reared as females, either because of surgery or streak gonads, hormonal treatment will be necessary at puberty and thereafter. Estrogen will initiate and sustain maturation and function of secondary sexual characteristics, and promote the achievement of the full height potential. The adolescent increase in bone density is a very important determinant of an indivdual's later risk for osteoporosis. This alone is sufficient reason for treatment.[75] Very small amounts of estrogen will promote growth and development. Start at about age 10 with unopposed estrogen (0.3 mg conjugated estrogens or 0.5 mg estradiol daily). After 6 months to 1 year, move to a sequential program with 0.625 mg conjugated estrogens or 1.0 mg estradiol daily and 10 mg medroxyprogesterone acetate for the first 12 days each month (if a uterus is present). Adequacy of treatment can be assessed by following bone age changes, although this is unnecessary in most cases. In patients with genetic shortness in stature (e.g., Turner syndrome), estrogen treatment is not started until bone age is 11–12 to avoid epiphysial closure and to allow a longer period of time for long bone growth.

Stimulation of Growth

Short stature occurs in virtually all patients with a 45,X karyotype and nearly all patients with Turner syndrome who have other karyotypes.[76] This growth impairment begins in utero, is apparent throughout childhood, and results in a short adult height (a mean of 143 cm).[77] This attenuation of growth is partly due to insufficient growth hormone secretion due to the deficiency in sex steroids and also to an end organ resistance to insulin-like growth factor-I.[78] Anabolic steroids have been used to stimulate growth, especially in patients with Turner syndrome. Short-term growth can be stimulated by anabolic steroids; however, the effect on final adult height is equivocal because epiphyseal maturation is also enhanced. Furthermore, virilizing side effects are a drawback. The combination of low doses of estrogen and recombinant growth hormone offer the best prospect. Treatment with growth hormone (50 μg/kg/day) yields significant growth acceleration that can be sustained for at least 6 years, achieving an adult height of over 150 cm (59 inches), which is a low normal range for women.[79] The future may see effective use of growth hormone-releasing hormone for this purpose. It is worth noting that adolescents with Turner syndrome being treated with growth hormone do not lose bone mineral density prior to estrogen treatment; hence, it is unnecessary to begin estrogen treatment at an early age (when it might counteract the goal of growth hormone therapy, achieving maximal height).[76]

The Possibility of Pregnancy

In women who have variants of gonadal dysgenesis and who menstruate, pregnancy can occur. However, there is a 30% incidence of congenital anomalies in the offspring, including spina bifida and Down syndrome. Sex chromsome abnormalities are frequent in the children born to mosaic mothers.[80] Prenatal diagnosis by amniocentesis or chorionic villus biopsy is highly advised. Assisted reproductive technology with donated oocytes yields excellent results in women with streak gonads (see Chapter 31).

Noonan's Syndrome

Both affected males and females have apparently normal chromosome complements and normal gonadal function. The phenotypic appearance of the female is that of a patient with Turner syndrome: short stature, webbed neck, shield chest, and cardiac malformations. The cardiac lesions, however, are different. Pulmonic stenosis is most frequent in Noonan syndrome as opposed to aortic coarctation in Turner syndrome. Apparently this syndrome results from a second mutant gene or genes.[81] In the past these patients have been referred to as male Turner's or Turner's with normal chromosomes. Noonan's are fertile and transmit the trait as an autosomal dominant with variable expression.

Diagnosis of Ambiguous Genitalia

Ambiguous external genitalia in a newborn infant represents not only a major diagnostic challenge, but a social and medical emergency. The physician is involved in a pressure-filled situation because of the necessity for making such an influential decision as the sex of sexual rearing. Rapid and organized evaluation must be initiated to assign the appropriate gender, identify a possible life-threatening medical condition, and begin necessary medical, surgical, and psychological interventions.[82] Input from a team of experts in endocrinology, genetics, neonatology, psychology, surgery, and urology is essential. Nevertheless, the primary physician should be the sole contact with the family. Diagnostic procedures may delay the decision, but it is well-recognized that a period of delay is far better than later reversal of the sex assignment. Naming of the child should be delayed until a gender is firmly assigned. Parental education and guidance are essential in this anxiety-ridden situation.

The most important point to remember when confronted with a newborn infant with ambiguous genitalia, or an apparently male infant with bilateral cryptorchidism, is that the prime diagnosis until ruled out is congenital adrenal hyperplasia. The reason is clear: adrenal hyperplasia is the only condition which is life-threatening. Signs of adrenal failure such as vomiting, diarrhea, dehydration, and shock may develop rapidly. Furthermore, most infants with ambiguous genitalia are virilized females, and most of these have congenital adrenal hyperplasia.

The history of a previously affected relative may aid in the diagnosis of testicular feminization or any of its variants. Similarly, the history of a sibling with genital ambiguity or the history of a previous neonatal death in a sibling strongly suggest the possibility of adrenal hyperplasia. A history of maternal exposure to androgenic compounds may be difficult to elicit. The mother may be unaware of the nature of her medications, and the obstetrician should be consulted to determine if medication was used for threatened or recurrent abortion or endometriosis.

Although the appearance of the external genitalia in intersex infants may be similar regardless of etiology, and a definitive diagnosis unachievable by physical examination alone, certain useful clues can be discerned.

Are gonads palpable? Palpation of the genital and inguinal regions is the most important part of the physical examination. Gonads in the inguinal regions or in scrotal folds are almost certainly testes. Ovaries are not found in scrotal folds or in the inguinal regions. The testicles, however, may be intraabdominal. If testicles are not palpable, the infant should be considered to have congenital adrenal hyperplasia until demonstrated otherwise.

What is the phallus length and diameter? Measured from the pubic ramus to the tip of the glans, a stretched penile length of less than 2.5 cm is 2.5 standard deviations below the mean for infants at 40 weeks of gestational age (2.0 cm for 36 weeks and 1.5 cm for 32 weeks).[82] The normal newborn clitoris measures less than 1 cm long; a normal newborn penis measures 2.8–4.2 cm in length.

What is the position of the urethral meatus? The urethral meatus can range from a mild hypospadias to an opening in the perineal area into a urogenital sinus. Hypospadias is almost always accompanied by chordee, which is a ventral curvature of the phallus resulting from a shortened urethra.

To what degree are the labioscrotal folds fused? The findings can range from unfused labia majora of a normal female through labia with variable degrees of posterior fusion, a bifid scrotum, to a fully fused normal appearing male scrotum. The distance from the anus to the edge of the vagina divided by the distance from the anus to the base of the clitoris is a ratio which is less than 0.5 in normal females. A ratio greater than 0.5 indicates some degree of labioscrotal fusion.

Is there a vagina, vaginal pouch, or urogenital sinus? Does the rectal exam suggest a midline structure that might be a uterus? A uterus can be palpable, especially shortly after birth when the uterus is a little enlarged in response to maternal estrogen.

Further important physical signs include evidence of hyperpigmentation due to the melanocyte stimulation associated with high levels of ACTH in adrenal hyperplasia, dehydration, hypotension, hypertension, and the manifestations of Turner syndrome such as webbed neck, low hairline, edema of hands and feet, and cardiac and renal anomalies. Careful examination of the phallus may differentiate between a clitoris and a penis. The penis has a midline ventral frenulum, while the clitoris has two folds which extend from the lateral aspects of the clitoris to the labia minora.

All patients with ambiguous genitalia require pelvic ultrasonography (to detect a uterus and ovaries or undescended testes) and a retrograde injection of contrast media into the urogenital orifice to outline the urethra and/or vaginal anatomy, the existence of a urogenital sinus, and the presence of a cervix.[83] Magnetic imaging of the newborn pelvis can supplant both of these procedures.[84]

Rapid testing of blood leukocytes for karyotype analysis, serum electrolytes, serum androgens (androstenedione, testosterone, dehydroepiandrosterone, dehydroepiandrosterone sulfate), 17-hydroxyprogesterone, 11-deoxycorticosterone, and 11-deoxycortisol is an essential laboratory component in the evaluation of intersex. In selected circumstances, ACTH testing and genital skin biopsy provide specific amplifying information.

Differential Diagnosis

The presence or absence of palpable gonads, the presence or absence of a uterus, and the karyotype places the patient in one of four categories: female pseudohermaphroditism, male pseudohermaphroditism, true hermaphroditism, or gonadal dysgenesis.

Clinical signs of adrenal failure indicate that the newborn has some form of adrenal enzyme defect regardless of the steroid pattern. The diagnosis is certain if such an infant is hyperkalemic and hyponatremic (due to aldosterone deficiency) or hypertensive and hypokalemic (secondary to elevated deoxycorticosterone).

In the absence of maternal androgen excess, the diagnosis of genetic females with excess androgen (female pseudohermaphroditism) must distinguish 3 forms of congenital virilizing adrenal hyperplasia.The diagnosis of 21-hydroxylase deficiency is confirmed by finding an elevated level of 17-hydroxyprogesterone in the serum. Elevated levels of 11-deoxycorticosterone and 11-deoxycortisol are found in 11β-hydroxylase deficiency, while the precursors to cortisol and androgen, 17-hydroxypregnenolone and dehydroepiandrosterone, are high in the 3β-hydroxysteroid dehydrogenase deficiency. Marginal basal aberrations can be accentuated by an ACTH stimulation test.

Male pseudohermaphroditism (genetic males with too little androgen) can be the result of one of the relatively rare enzyme disorders. Five derive from enzymatic errors in the biosynthesis of testosterone. Patients with P450scc deficiency have no measurable cortisol or androgen precursors. P450c17 deficient patients display elevated progesterone, whereas individuals with 3β-hydroxysteroid dehydrogenase deficiency have elevated DHA and 17-hydroxypregnenolone levels. Again, ACTH testing can be useful in amplifying compensated defects. A testosterone biosynthetic error which leads to deficient masculinization involves an enzyme not required for glucocorticoid or mineralocorticoid synthesis. Thus no evidence of adrenal insufficiency with electrolyte disturbance is seen in 17β-hydroxysteroid dehydrogenase deficiency. Using HCG stimulation testing, elevated androstenedione and DHA are abnormally high. In Leydig cell hypoplasia, HCG stimulation reveals very low circulating testosterone and its precursors, but no adrenal defects, confirming a specific cellular defect in the testes.

HCG stimulation tests and cultures of genital skin fibroblasts are useful in the laboratory differentiation of 5α-reductase deficiency and partial androgen insensitivity in the newborn. An elevated ratio of testosterone to dihydrotestosterone after HCG stimulation suggests 5α-reductase deficiency that can be confirmed in culture. On the other hand, patients with androgen insensitivity will have normal ACTH and HCG stimulation tests and abnormal androgen binding or androgen receptor gene mutations in cultured cells.

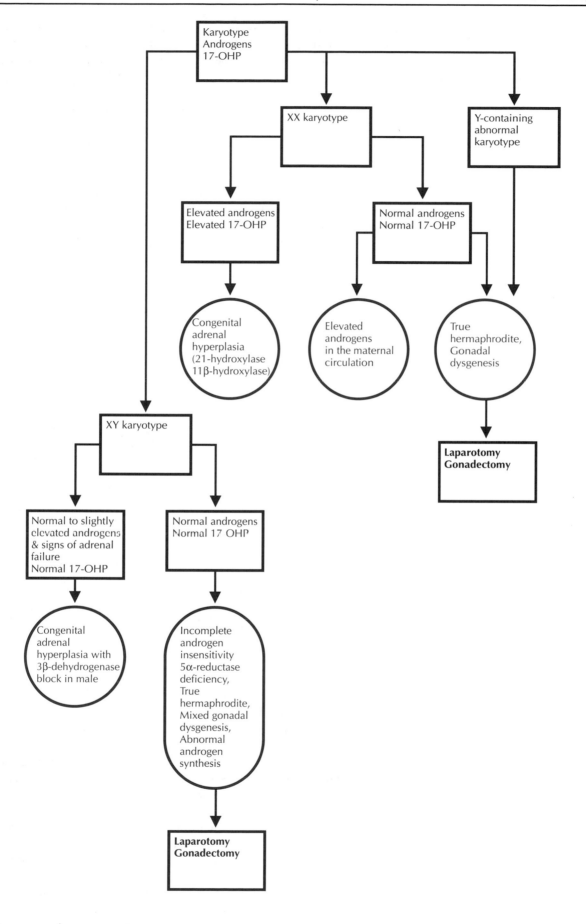

Although laparotomy is not necessary for assignment of sex, it may be the only way to arrive at a definitive diagnosis. Laparotomy is indicated in the following situations (laparoscopic evaluation is inadequate because gonads may be small and hidden in the inguinal canal).

1. The XX infant with ambiguous genitalia, normal androgens, in apparent good health, and no history of maternal androgen exposure. This is either a true hermaphrodite or a variant of mixed gonadal dysgenesis, and gonadectomy is indicated.

2. The XY patient with ambiguous genitalia, without palpable gonads, and normal androgens. The possibilities are incompletely masculinized males (variants of testicular feminization), a true hermaphrodite, mixed gonadal dysgenesis, and 5α-reductase deficiency. Sex of rearing will be female, and gonadectomy is necessary to avoid virilization at puberty and the propensity to develop gonadal neoplasia.

Only laparotomy, gonadal biopsy, and/or gonadectomy confirm the diagnosis of true hermaphroditism and individuals with ambiguous genitalia and 46,XY or 45X/46,XY karyotypes. It should be emphasized that evaluations for mutations in the SRY gene are powerful research tools, but these tests are not currently available for clinical determinations.[85]

Assignment of Sex of Rearing

In a newborn who presents a problem of correct sex assignment, it is better to delay than to reverse the sex assignment at a later date. Generally, the decision can be made within a few days, at most a few weeks. In dealing with the parents, terms with unfortunate connotations, such as hermaphrodite, should be avoided. An easy way to explain ambiguous genital development to parents is to indicate that the genitals are unfinished, rather than abnormal from a sexual point of view. Chromosome discrepancies are probably best left unmentioned.

When all the information is in place, gender assignment will rest on:

1. Future fertility,

2. The projected appearance of genitalia after puberty,

3. Penile adequacy for coital function.

The future fertility in all masculinized females is unaffected. With proper treatment, reproduction is possible, since the internal genitalia and gonads are those of a normal female. Therefore, all masculinized females should be reared as females.

The only other category of patients with ambiguous genitalia with reproductive capability consists of males with 1) isolated hypospadias, 2) the male with repaired isolated cryptorchidism, and 3) the male with the uterine hernia syndrome.

All other patients with ambiguous genitalia will be sterile. Except for salt-wasting adrenal hyperplasia, the physician's prime concern is not with physical survival, but to enable the patient to grow into a psychologically normal, healthy, and well-adjusted adult. The sex of assignment depends upon only one judgment: can the phallus ultimately develop into a penis adequate for intercourse. The success of a penis is dependent upon erectile tissue, and the genitalia should not only be serviceable but also erotically sensitive. Technically, the construction of female genitalia is easier, and therefore the physician must be convinced that a functional penis is possible.[86,87]

All decisions regarding sex of rearing and the overall treatment program should be made early in life. If a case has been neglected, sex reassignments must be made according to the gender identity in which a child has developed. Reassignment of sex can probably be made safely up to age 18 months.

Socialization and hormone therapy are important for gender identity and sexual function. Future gender role and identity can be in accord with assigned sex if 4 conditions are met:

1. The parents are comfortable in their ability to raise their child and their resolution of any doubts or uncertainty about the sex of the child. In this acceptance and adaptation, the parents must have participated in and agreed to the sex reassignment decision. Ambiguous names should be discouraged to assure normal gender identity.

2. Genital reconstruction should take place as early as possible, certainly well before 18 months. Thereafter, sex reassignment is difficult and adjustment impaired.

3. Properly timed hormonal and/or additional surgical interventions must be provided at puberty.

4. The patient should be informed about his or her condition as deemed age-appropriate.

Sex Testing in Athletics

Gender verification tests were introduced into competitive sports in the 1960s because of the concern that individuals might masquerade as the opposite sex to gain a competitive advantage. Sex testing can be based on chromosomal or other histological assays, hormone measurements, or anatomical criteria. Such testing could identify 3 potential groups of problem athletes: transsexuals who have undergone sex change operations, impersonators, and individuals with intersex conditions. Neither sex changed individuals nor masqueraders have been a problem in athletic events. However, sex testing creates the possibility of public exposure and embarrassment for intersex individuals. In addition, sex testing has the potential for revealing to an unaffected individual an underlying diagnosis in a shocking, difficult manner. For all of these reasons, it is argued that physical examination alone should suffice, and any individual with a female phenotype should be allowed to compete as a woman.[88] Even individuals with mild disorders would be able to pass the physical examination requirement. Sex testing of athletes is unnecessary and fraught with potential harm.

References

1. **Money J, Schwartz M, Lewis VG,** Adult erotosexual status and fetal hormonal masculinization and demasculinization: 46,XX congenital virilizing adrenal hyperplasia and 46,XY androgen-insensitivity syndrome compared, Psychoneuroendocrinology 9:405, 1984.

2. **Van Wagenen G, Simpson ME,** *Embryology of the Ovary and Testis, Homo Sapiens and Mucaca Mulatta,* Yale University Press, New Haven, Connecticut, 1965.

3. **Sinclair AH, Berta P, Palma MS, Hawkins JR, Griffiths BL, Smith MJ, Foster JW, Frischauf A-M, Lovell-Badge R, Goodfellow PN,** A gene from the human sex determining region encodes a protein with homology to a conserved DNA binding motif, Nature 346:240, 1990.

4. **Berta P, Hawkins JR, Sinclair AH, Taylor A, Griffiths BL, Goodfellow PN, Fellows M,** Genetic evidence equating SRY and the testes-determining factor, Nature 348:448, 1990.

5. **Jager RJ, Anvret M, Hall K, Scherer G,** A human XY female with a frame shift mutation in the candidate testis-determining gene SRY, Nature 348:452, 1990.

6. **Moore CCD, Grumbach MM,** Sex determination and gonadogenesis: a transcription cascade of sex chromosome and autosome genes, Seminars Perinatol 16:266, 1992.

7. **Muller J, Schwartz M, Skakkebaek NE,** Analysis of the sex-determining region of the Y chromosome (SRY) in sex reversed patients: point-mutation in SRY causing sex-reversion in a 46,XY female, J Clin Endocrinol Metab 75:331, 1992.

8. **Haqq CM, King C-Y, Donahoe PK, Weiss MA,** SRY recognizes conserved DNA sites in sex-specific promoters, Proc Natl Acad Sci USA 90:1097, 1993.

9. **Wilson JD, Griffin JE, George FW, Leshin M,** The role of gonadal steroids in sexual differentiation, Recent Prog Horm Res 37:1, 1981.

10. **Singh RP, Carr DH,** The anatomy and histology of XO human embryos and fetuses, Anat Rec 155:369, 1966.

11. **Krauss CM, Turksoy RN, Atkins L, McGlaughlin C, Brown LG, Page DC,** Familial premature ovarian failure due to an interstitial deletion of the long arm of the X chromosome, New Engl J Med 317:125, 1987.

12. **Speert H,** *Obstetric and Gynecologic Milestones,* The Macmillin Company, New York, 1958.

13. **Jost A, Vigier B, Prepin J, Perchellet JP,** Studies on sex differentiation in mammals, Recent Prog Horm Res 29:1, 1973.

14. **Picard JY, Josso N,** Purification of testicular anti müllerian hormone allowing direct visualization of the pure glycoprotein and determination of yield and purification factor, Mol Cell Endocrinol 34:23, 1984.

15. **Pepinsky RB, Sinclair LK, Chow EP, Mattaliano RJ, Manganaro TF, Donahoe PK, Cate RL,** Proteolytic processing of müllerian inhibiting substance produces a transforming growth factor-beta-like fragment, J Biol Chem 263:18961, 1988.

16. **Taguchi O, Cunha GR, Lawrence WD, Robboy SJ,** Timing and irreversibility of müllerian duct inhibition in the embryonic reproductive tract of the human male, Dev Biol 106:394, 1984.

17. **Lee MM, Donahoe PK,** Müllerian inhibiting substance: a gonadal hormone with multiple functions, Endocrin Rev 14:152, 1993.

18. **Gustafson ML, Lee MM, Asmundson L, MacLaughlin DT, Donahoe PK,** Müllerian inhibiting substance in the diagnosis and management of intersex and gonadal abnormalities, J Pediatr Surg 28:439, 1993.

19. **Siiteri PK, Wilson JD,** Testosterone formation and metabolism during male sexual differentiation in the human embryo, J Clin Endocrinol Metab 38:113, 1974.

20. **Imperato-McGinley J, Peterson RE, Gaultier T, Sturla E,** Androgens and the evolution of male gender identity among male pseudohermaphrodites with 5α-reductase deficiency. New Engl J Med 300:1233, 1979.

21. **LeVay S,** A difference in hypothalamic structure between heterosexual and homosexual men, Science 253:1034, 1991.

22. **Hofman MA, Swaab DF,** Sexual dimorphism of the human brain: myth and reality, Exp Clin Endocrinol 98:161, 1991.

23. **White PC, New MI, DuPont B,** Congenital adrenal hyperplasia, New Engl J Med 316:1519,1580, 1987.

24. **New MI,** Female pseudohermaphroditism, Seminars Perinatol 16:289, 1992.

25. **Speiser PW, Dupont J, Zhu D, Serrat J, Buegeleisen M, Tusie-Luna MT, Lesser M, New MI, White PC,** Disease expression and molecular genotype in congenital adrenal hyperplasia due to 21-hydroxylase deficiency, J Clin Invest 90:584, 1992.

26. **Kohn B, Levine LS, Pollack MS, Pang S, Lorezen F, Levy DJ, Lerner AJ, Gian FR, DuPont B, New MI,** Late onset steroid 21-OH deficiency: a variant of classical congenital adrenal hyperplasia. J Clin Endocrinol Metab 55:817, 1982.

27. **Spenser PW, New MI,** Genotype and hormonal phenotype in nonclassical 21-OH deficiency, J Clin Endocrinol Metab 64:86, 1987.

28. **Chua CH, Szabo P, Vitek A, Grzeschik K-H, John M, White PC,** Cloning of cDNA encoding steroid 11 beta-hydroxylase (P450c11), Proc Natl Acad Sci USA 84:7193, 1987.

29. **Biglieri EG, Herron MA, Brust N,** 17-Hydroxylation deficiency in man. J Clin Invest 45:1946, 1966.

30. **Yanase T, Sanders D, Shibata A, Matsui N, Simpson ER, Waterman MR,** Combined 17α-hydroxylase/17,20-lyase deficiency due to a 7-basepair duplication in the N-terminal region of the cytochromoe $P450_{17\alpha}$ (CYP17) gene, J Clin Endocrinol Metab 70:1325, 1990.

31. **Sherman SL, Aston CE, Morton NE, Speiser PW, New MI,** A segregation and linkage study of classical and nonclassical 21 hydroxylase deficiency, Am J Hum Genet 42:830, 1988.

32. **Rosler A, Weshler N, Leiberman E, Hochberg Z, Weidenfeld J, Sack J, Chemke J,** 11β-hydroxylase deficiency congenital adrenal hyperplasia: update of prenatal diagnosis, J Clin Endocrinol Metab 66:830, 1988.

33. **Reindollar RH, Lewis JB, White PC, Fernhoff PM, McDonough PG, Whitney JB III,** Prenatal diagnosis of 21-hydroxylase deficiency by the complementary deoxyribonucleic acid probe for cytochrome $P-450_{C-21OH}$, Am J Obstet Gynecol 158:545, 1988.

34. **Petersen KE, Damkjaer-Nielsen M, Buus O, Couillin P,** Congenital adrenal hyperplasia. Prenatal treatment, Pediatr Res 20:1201, 1986.

35. **Forest MG, Betull H, David M,** Antenatal treatment of congenital adrenal hyperplasia due to 21 hydroxylase deficiency: a multicenter study, Ann Endocrinol (Paris) 48:31, 1987.

36. **Speiser PW, Laforgia N, Kato K, Pareira J, Khan R, Yang SY, Whorwood C, White PC, Elias S, Schriock E, Schriock E, Simpson JL, Taslimi M, Najjar J, May S, Mills G, Crawford C, New MI,** First trimester prenatal treatment and molecular genetic diagnosis of congenital adrenal hyperplasia (21-hydroxylase deficiency), J Clin Endocrinol Metab 70:838, 1990.

37. **Karaviti L, Mercado AB, Mercado MB, Speiser PW, Buegeleisen M, Crawford C, Antonian L, White PC, New MI,** Prenatal diagnosis/treatment in families at risk for infants with steroid 21-hydroxylase deficiency (congenital adrenal hyperplasia), J Steroid Biochem Mol Biol 41:445, 1992.

38. **Pang S, Clark AT, Freeman LC, Dolan LM, Immken L, Mueller OT, Stiff D, Shulman DI,** Maternal side effects of prenatal dexamethasone therapy for fetal congenital adrenal hyperplasia, J Clin Endocrinol Metab 75:249, 1992.

39. **Dorr HG, Sippell WG,** Prenatal dexamethasone treatment in pregnancies at risk for congenital adrenal hyperplasia due to 21-hydroxylase deficiency: effect on midgestational amniotic fluid steroid levels, J Clin Endocrinol Metab 76:117, 1993.

40. **Linder B, Feuillan P, Chrousos GP,** Alternate day prednisone therapy in congenital adrenal hyperplasia: adrenal androgen suppression and normal growth, J Clin Endocrinol Metab 69:191, 1989.

41. **Mulaikal RM, Migeon CJ, Rock JA,** Fertility rates in female patients with congenital adrenal hyperplasia due to 21-hydroxylase deficiency, New Engl J Med 316:178, 1987.

42. **Feldman S, Billaud L, Thalabard J-C, Raux-Demay M-C, Mowszowicz I, Kuttenn F, Mauvais-Jarvis P,** Fertility in women with late-onset adrenal hyperplasia due to 21-hydroxylase deficiency, J Clin Endocrinol Metab 74:635, 1992.

43. **Shozu M, Akasofu K, Harada T, Kubota Y,** A new cause of female pseudohermaphroditism: placental aromatase deficiency, J Clin Endocrinol Metab 72:560, 1991.

44. **Morris JM, Mahesh BV,** The syndrome of testicular feminization in male pseudohermaphrodites, Am J Obstet Gynecol 65:1192, 1953.

45. **Manuel M, Katayama KP, Jones Jr HW,** The age of occurrence of gonadal tumors in intersex patients with a Y chromosome. Am J Obstet Gynecol 124:293, 1976.

46. **Simpson JL,** Genetics of sexual differentiation, in Rock JA, Carpenter SE, editors, *Pediatric and Adolescent Gynecology,* Raven Press, New York, 1992, pp 1-37.

47. **Imperato-McGinley J, Pichardo M, Gautier T, Voyer D, Bryden MP,** Cognitive abilities in androgen-insensitive subjects: comparison with control males and females from the same kindred, Clin Endocrinol 34:341, 1991.

48. **Griffin JE,** Androgen resistance — the clinical and molecular spectrum, New Engl J Med 326:611, 1992.

49. **Grino PB, Griffin JE, Cushard WG Jr, Wilson JD,** A mutation of the androgen receptor associated with partial androgen resistance, familial gynecomastia, and fertility, J Clin Endocrinol Metab 66:754, 1988.

50. **McPhaul MJ, Marcelli M, Zoppi S, Griffin JE, Wilson JD,** Genetic basis of endocrine disease 4: the spectrum of mutations in the androgen receptor gene that causes androgen resistance, J Clin Endocrinol Metab 76:17, 1993.

51. **Lubahn DB, Brown TR, Simental JA, Higgs HN, Migeon CJ, Wilson EM, French FS,** Sequence of intron/exon junctions of the coding region of the human androgen receptor gene and identification of a point mutation in a family with complete androgen insensitivity, Proc Natl Acad Sci USA 86:9534, 1989.

52. **Brown TR, Lubahn DB, Wilson EM, Joseph DR, French FS, Migeon CJ,** Deletion of the steroid binding domain of the human androgen receptor gene in one family with complete androgen insensitivity syndrome: evidence for further heterogeneity in this syndrome, Proc Natl Acad Sci USA 85:8151, 1988.

53. **Trifero M, Gottlieb B, Pinsky L,** The 56/58 K Da androgen binding protein in male genital skin fibroblasts with a deleted androgen receptor gene, Mol Cell Endocrinol 75:37, 1991.

54. **Quigley CA, Evans BA, Simental JA, Marschke KB, Sar M, Lubahn DB, Davies P, Hughes IA, Wilson EM, French FS,** Complete androgen insensitivity due to deletion of exon C of the androgen receptor gene highlights the functional importance of the second zinc finger of the androgen receptor in vivo, Mol Endocrinol 6:1103, 1992.

55. **Marcelli M, Tilley WD, Wilson CM, Wilson JD, Griffin JE, McPhaul MJ,** A single nucleotide substitution introduces a premature termination codon into the androgen receptor gene of a patient with receptor negative androgen resistance, J Clin Invest 85:1522, 1990.

56. **Zoppi S, Marcelli M, Deslypere J-P, Griffin JE, Wilson JD, McPhaul MJ,** Amino acid substitutions in the DNA-binding domain of the human androgen receptor are a frequent cause of receptor binding positive androgen resistance, Mol Endocrinol 6:409, 1992.

57. **Peterson RE, Imperato-McGinley J, Gautier T, Sturia E,** Male pseudohermaphroditism due to steroid 5α-reductase deficiency, Am J Med 62:170, 1977.

58. **Thigpen AE, Davis DL, Gautier T, Imperato-McGinley J, Russell DW,** Brief report: The molecular basis of steroid 5α-reductase deficiency in a large Dominican kindred, New Engl J Med 327:1216, 1992.

59. **Wilson JD, George FW, Griffin JE,** The hormonal control of sexual development, Science 211:1278, 1981.

60. **Castro-Magana M, Angulo M, Uy J,** Male hypogonadism with gynecomastia caused by late-onset deficiency of testicular 17-ketosteroid reductase, New Engl J Med 328:1297, 1993.

61. **Perez-Palacios G, Scaglia HE, Kofman-Alfaro S,** Inherited male pseudohermaphroditism due to gonadotropin unresponsiveness, Acta Endocrinol 98:148, 1981.

62. **Swyer GIM,** Male pseudohermaphroditism: a hitherto undescribed form, Br Med J II:709, 1955.

63. **Coulam CB,** Testicular regression syndrome. Obstet Gynecol 53:44, 1979.

64. **Simpson JL,** True hermaphroditism: etiology and phenotypic considerations. Birth Defects 14:9, 1978.

65. **Berkovitz GD, Fechner PY, Marcantonio SM, Bland G, Stetten G, Goodfellow PN, Smith KD, Migeon CJ,** The role of the sex-determining region of the Y chromosome (SRY) in the etiology of 46,XX true hermaphroditism, Hum Genet 88:411, 1992.

66. **Berkovitz GD, Fechner PY, Zacur HW, Rock JA, Snyder HM, Migeon CJ, Perlman EJ,** Clinical and pathologic spectrum of 46,XY gonadal dysgenesis: its relevance to the understanding of sex differentiation, Medicine 70:375, 1991.

67. **Droesch K, Droesch J, Chumas J, Bronson R,** Laparoscopic gonadectomy for gonadal dysgenesis, Fertil Steril 53:360, 1990.

68. **Shalev E, Zabari A, Romano S, Luboshitzky R,** Laparoscopic gonadectomy in 46XY female patient, Fertil Steril 57:459, 1992.

69. **Gililland J, Cummings D, Hibbert ML, Crain T, Rozanski T,** Laparoscopic orchiectomy in a patient with complete androgen insensitivity, J Laparoendoscopic Surg 3:51, 1993.

70. **Fechner PY, Marcantonio SM, Ogata T, Rosales TO, Smith KD, Goodfellow PN, Migeon CJ, Berkovitz GD,** Report of a kindred with X-linked (or autosomal dominant sex-linked) 46,XY partial gonadal dysgenesis, J Clin Endocrinol Metab 76:1248, 1993.

71. **Fisher EMC, Beer-Romero P, Brown LG, Ridley A, McNeil JA, Lawrence JB, Willard HF, Bieber FR, Page DC,** Homologous ribosomal protein genes on the human X and Y chromosome: escape from X inactivation and possible implications for Turner syndrome, Cell 63:1205, 1990.

72. **Fechner PY, Marcantonio SM, Jaswaney V, Stetten G, Goodfellow PN, Migeon CJ, Smith KD, Berkovitz GD,** The role of the sex-determining region Y gene in the etiology of 46,XX maleness, J Clin Endocrinol Metab 76:690, 1993.

73. **Medlej R, Lobaccaro JM, Berta P, Belon C, Leheup B, Toublanc JE, Weill J, Chevalier C, Dumas R, Sultan C,** Screening for Y-derived sex determining gene SRY in 40 patients with Turner syndrome, J Clin Endocrinol Metab 75:1289, 1992.

74. **Kocova M, Siegel SF, Wenger SL, Lee PA, Trucco M,** Detection of Y chromosome sequences in Turner's syndrome by Southern blot analysis of amplified DNA, Lancet 342:140, 1993.

75. **Neely EK, Marcus R, Rosenfeld RG, Bachrach LK,** Turner syndrome adolescents receiving growth hormone are not osteopenic, J Clin Endocrinol Metab 75:861, 1993.

76. **Park E, Bailey JD, Cowell CA,** Growth and maturation of patients with Turner's syndrome, Pediatr Res 17:1, 1983.

77. **Lyon AL, Preece MA, Grant DB,** Growth curve for girls with Turner syndrome, Arch Dis Child 60:932, 1985.

78. **Zadik Z, Landau H, Chen M, Altman Y, Lieberman E,** Assessment of growth hormone (GH) axis in Turner's syndrome using 24-hour integrated concentrations of GH, insulin-like growth factor-I, plasma GH-binding activity, GH binding to IM9 cells, and GH response to pharmacological stimulation, J Clin Endocrinol Metab 75:412, 1992.

79. **Rosenfeld RG, Frane J, Attie KM, et al,** Six-year results of a randomized, prospective trial of human growth hormone and oxandrolone in Turner's syndrome, J Pediatr 121:49, 1992.

80. **Kaaneko N, Kawagoe S, Hizoi M,** Turner's syndrome — review of the literature with reference to a successful pregnancy outcome, Gynecol Obstet Invest 29:81, 1990.

81. **Allanson JE, Hall JG, Hughes HE, Preus M, Witt RD,** Noonan syndrome: the changing phenotype, Am J Med Genet 21:507, 1985.

82. **Myers-Seifer CH, Charest NJ,** Diagnosis and management of patients with ambiguous genitalia, Seminars Perinatol 16:332, 1992.

83. **Siegel MJ,** Pediatric gynecologic sonography, Radiology 179:593, 1991.

84. **Hricak H, Chang YCF, Thurnher S,** Vagina: evaluation with MR imaging. Part I: Normal anatomy and congenital anomalies, Radiology 169:169, 1988.

85. **Hawkins JR, Taylor A, Goodfellow PN, Migeon CJ, Smith KD, Berkovitz GD,** Evidence for increased prevalence of SRY mutations in XY females with complete rather than partial gonadal dysgenesis, Am J Hum Genet 51:979, 1992.

86. **Coran AG, Porley TZ,** Surgical management of ambiguous genitalia in the infant and child, J Pediatr Surg 26:812, 1991.

87. **Donahue PK, Powell DM, Lee MK,** Clinical management of intersex abnormalities, Curr Probl Surg 28:515, 1992.

88. **Ljungqvist A, Simpson JL,** Medical examination for health of all athletes replacing the need for gender verification in international sports: the International Amateur Athletic Federation plan, JAMA 267:850, 1992.

11   Abnormal Puberty and Growth Problems

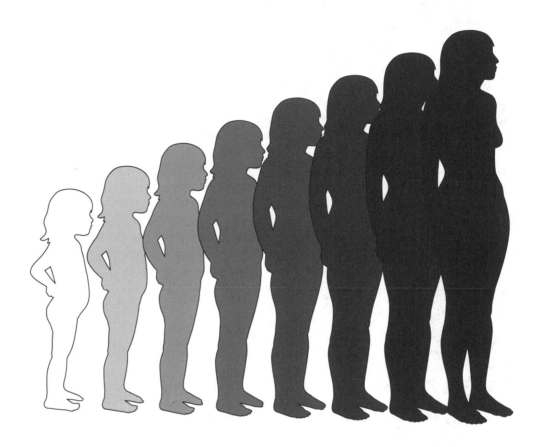

I n many societies throughout history, puberty has been a time of celebration. The changes of puberty announce the acquisition of fertility. However, it is precisely these psychological, social, and cultural forces that make this a stressful, difficult transition for many individuals. Unfortunately, the earlier age of puberty in modern times has made it difficult to cope with an earlier sexuality. Early teenage pregnancies are a relatively new problem (previously they were a biological impossibility). This change in modern life, probably due to improved nutrition and living conditions, makes it all the more important to understand puberty.

The ability to diagnose and manage disorders of female pubescence requires a thorough understanding of the physical and hormonal events which mark the evolution of the child into a sexually mature adult capable of reproduction. Abnormalities in this process of developmental endocrinology either lead to premature, attenuated, or retarded (delayed) puberty. This chapter reviews the important landmarks and mechanisms of normal female maturation as well as the abnormalities which lead to precocious or delayed puberty.

The Physiology of Puberty

The Period of Infancy and Childhood

The hypothalamus, anterior pituitary gland, and gonads of the fetus, neonate, the prepubertal infant and child are all capable of secreting hormones in adult concentrations. Even during fetal life, serum concentrations of follicle-stimulating hormone (FSH) and luteinizing hormone (LH) reach adult levels at midgestation but fall thereafter as the high level of pregnancy steroid hormones exerts inhibitory feedback.[1] Separation of the newborn from its sources of maternal and placental estrogen and progesterone releases newborn FSH and LH from this negative feedback. A prompt rise in gonadotropin secretion follows that, in female neonates, may reach levels greater than those in the normal adult menstrual cycle.[2] As a result, transient estradiol secretion equivalent to the level of the midfollicular phase of the menstrual cycle is induced and is associated with waves of ovarian follicle maturation and atresia. Full negative feedback is rapidly attained; ovarian steroids and gonadotropins decline and remain at very low levels until at least 8 years of age. During this period, the hypothalamic-pituitary system controlling gonadotropins (the "gonadostat") is highly sensitive to negative feedback of estrogen (estradiol concentration in these years remains low at 10 pg/mL [40 pmol/L]). Studies on gonadal dysgenesis and other hypogonadal infants indicate that the "gonadostat" is 6–15 times more sensitive to negative feedback at this period than in the adult.[3] Therefore, gonadotropin secretion is in part restrained by even extraordinarily low levels of estrogen.

This reduction in the infant's gonadotropins is not entirely due to exquisite sensitivity to negative feedback. Low levels of FSH and LH even exist in hypogonadal children (with gonadal dysgenesis) between the ages of 5 and 11 years and are similar to the low levels in normal infants of this age.[4] Because gonadotropin releasing hormone (GnRH) infusion stimulates moderate LH and FSH secretion in these agonadal subjects, a central nonsteroidal suppressor of endogenous GnRH and gonadotropin synthesis appears to be operative.[5]

Although peptide hormone concentrations are low throughout infancy and the prepubertal child, FSH and LH display evidence of pulsatile control of secretion.[6–8] As noted, pituitary gonadotropins react with small but significant responses to exogenously administered GnRH, which although quantitatively less than those achieved in puberty are nevertheless capable of inducing the immature gonad to respond with modest steroid secretion. Immaturity of the various endocrine components is not the rate-limiting factor in the onset of puberty.

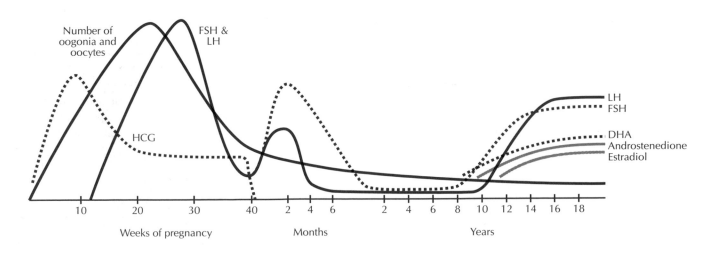

The Prepubertal Period

As puberty approaches, three critical changes in the low endocrine homeostatic function of childhood emerge:

1. Adrenarche.

2. Decreasing repression of the "gonadostat."

3. Gradual amplification of the peptide-peptide and peptide-steroid interactions leading to "gonadarche."

Adrenarche

The growth of pubic and axillary hair is due to an increased production of adrenal androgens at puberty. Thus, this phase of puberty is often referred to as adrenarche (or pubarche). *Premature adrenarche* by itself is occasionally seen; i.e., pubic and axillary hair without any other sign of sexual development. *Premature thelarche* (breast development) without other signs of puberty is very rare, but does occur. Increased adrenal cortical function, expressed by a rise in circulating dehydroepiandrosterone (DHA), dehydroepiandrosterone sulfate (DHAS), and androstenedione, occurs progressively in late childhood from about age 6–7 to adolescence (13–15 years of age).[9] This steroid secretion is associated with an increase in size and differentiation of the inner zone (zona reticularis) of the cortex. Generally, the beginning of adrenarche precedes by 2 years the linear growth spurt, the rise in estrogens and gonadotropins of early puberty, and menarche at midpuberty. Because of this temporal relationship, activation of adrenal androgen secretion has been suggested as a possible initiating event in the ontogeny of the pubertal transition.

Considerable evidence, however, supports a *dissociation* of the control mechanisms that initiate adrenarche and those governing GnRH-pituitary-ovarian maturation ("gonadarche").[10] Premature adrenarche (precocious appearance of pubic and axillary hair before age 8 years) is not associated with a parallel abnormal advancement of gonadarche.[11] In hypergonadotropic hypogonadism (gonadal dysgenesis) or in hypogonadotropic states such as Kallmann's syndrome, adrenarche occurs despite the absence of gonadarche. When adrenarche is absent, as in children with cortisol-treated Addison's disease (hypoadrenalism), gonadarche still occurs. Finally, in true precocious puberty occurring before 6 years of age, gonadarche precedes adrenarche.

Plasma levels of adrenal androgens change without corresponding changes in cortisol and ACTH during fetal life, puberty, and aging. Furthermore, in other circumstances such as chronic disease, surgical stress, recovery from secondary adrenal insufficiency, and anorexia nervosa, changes in ACTH-induced cortisol secretion are not accompanied by corresponding changes in plasma adrenal androgen levels.[12] Thus, adrenarche does not appear to be under direct control of gonadotropins or ACTH.

A pituitary adrenal androgen stimulating factor formed by cleavage of a high molecular weight precursor, proopiomelanocortin (POMC), which also contains ACTH and β-lipotropin, acting on an ACTH prepared and maintained adrenal, has been suggested as the agent stimulating adrenarche. A large glycoprotein has been identified that also displayed adrenal androgen stimulating activity.[13] However, in a study confirming the dissociation between plasma adrenal androgens and cortisol in children and adolescents with Cushing's disease and ectopic ACTH producing tumors, all known proopiomelanocortin-related peptides, including ACTH, β-endorphin, and β-lipotropin did not have a determinative role in the initiation of adrenarche.[14] Studies fail to demonstrate a relationship between melatonin secretion and adrenarche.[15] A study of the kinetics of the 3β-hydroxysteroid dehydrogenase enzyme in human adrenal microsomes suggests that the changes in adrenal secretion from fetal life to adulthood can be explained by local steroid inhibition of key enzymes within the adrenal, acting to a variable degree in different layers of the cortex and at different stages of development.[16] It is fair to say that the factors controlling adrenarche remain obscure.

Decreasing Repression of the "Gonadostat"

Regardless of its relation to adrenarche, factors which induce gonadarche in late prepuberty involve derepression of the central nervous system (CNS)-pituitary gonadostat, progressive responsiveness of the anterior pituitary to exogenous (and presumably endogenous) GnRH, and follicle reactivity to FSH and LH.

For approximately 8 years, from early infancy to the prepubertal period, LH and FSH are suppressed to very low levels. The mechanisms for this restraint on gonadotropin secretion are a highly sensitive negative feedback of low level gonadal estrogen on hypothalamic and pituitary sites, and an intrinsic central inhibitory influence on GnRH that reduces basal gonadotropin concentrations even in agonadal children. Gonadal dysgenesis patients display marked elevations of gonadotropins for the first 2–3 years of life. Thereafter, a striking decline in concentrations of FSH and LH occurs, reaching a nadir at 6–8 years. By age 10–11 (at the time puberty would have occurred), however, gonadotropins are elevated once again to the postmenopausal range. The overall pattern of basal gonadotropin secretion in agonadal children is qualitatively similar to that observed in normal females.

Whereas negative feedback inhibition may play the more important role in early childhood, the central intrinsic inhibitor becomes functionally dominant in midchildhood and persists up to prepuberty. Suppression of, or damage to, the neural source of this inhibition has been postulated in the pathogenesis of the precocious puberty secondary to hypothalamic lesions that compress or destroy posterior hypothalamic areas.[17] Thus, normal pubertal timing of gonadarche, with the reactivation of gonadotropin synthesis and secretion, results from the combined reduction in intrinsic suppression of GnRH and decreased sensitivity to the negative feedback of estrogen.[18]

It has been suggested that the reversal of central intrinsic suppression is due to a reduction in melatonin secretion by the pineal gland. In lower animals affected by photoperiodicity, pineal melatonin appears to inhibit hypothalamic-pituitary gland secretion. While melatonin may play a role in the altered timing of puberty associated with pineal tumors and in the pathophysiology of central precocious puberty, there is no evidence that it is important in the physiologic onset of normal puberty in humans.[19] In two large studies of circadian rhythms of serum melatonin from infancy to adulthood (1–18 years) the decline in the nocturnal surge of melatonin, thought to have been exclusively related to the pubertal conversion, was observed to begin in infancy and progressively decline through pubescence.[20,21] Pinealectomy in agonadal primates does not prevent the inhibition of FSH and LH seen during transition from infancy to childhood nor the return of gonadotropins with the advent of puberty.[22]

The fascinating search for the factor(s) involved in the derepression of the "gonadostat" so crucial to the timing of puberty continues. POMC-related peptides do not appear to change during the transitional period.[23] The ontogeny of the GnRH gene and its expression, so elegantly demonstrated in rodents, is yet to be extended to the primate.

Human growth hormone and other growth promoting peptides have been investigated in primate pubescence. It appears that both the nongonadal (central) control and estradiol feedback inhibition of basal gonadotropins begin and follow sustained elevation of serum growth hormone unrelated to a specific increment or threshold level of body growth or body weight.[24]

Alteration and Amplification of GnRH-Gonadotropin and Gonadotropin-Ovarian Steroid Interactions

FSH and LH levels increase during the progress through the stages of puberty. Rhythmic pulses of GnRH given to immature rhesus monkeys will initiate activity of the pituitary-gonadal apparatus, supporting the primacy of endogenous GnRH in the establishment and maintenance of puberty. Similar effects have been demonstrated in prepubertal girls.[25] Normal pubertal maturation in girls is also accompanied by changes in the pattern of gonadotropin responses to the hypothalamic releasing hormone GnRH. FSH responses to GnRH are initially pronounced but decrease steadily throughout the onset of puberty. In contrast, LH responses are low in prepubertal girls and increase strikingly during puberty.[26] This is the basis of the observation that in general FSH rises initially and plateaus in midpuberty while LH tends to rise more slowly and reaches adult levels in late puberty. The increased amplitude and frequency of pulsatile GnRH are believed to provoke progressively enhanced responses of FSH and LH secretion. GnRH acts as a self-primer on the gonadotrope cells of the anterior pituitary by inducing cell surface receptors specific for GnRH and necessary for its action (up-regulation). Thus, gonadotrope cells increase their capacity to respond to GnRH first by synthesis and later by secretion of gonadotropins. As gonadotropin secretion appears, ovarian follicle steroid synthesis is stimulated and estrogen secretion rises.

Elsewhere (Chapters 5 and 6), the evidence for the dichotomous effects of estrogen feedback on the anterior pituitary has been reviewed. Suffice to say, by midpuberty estrogen enhances LH secretory responses to GnRH (positive feedback) while combining with inhibin to maintain relative inhibition (negative feedback) of FSH response.

The amplification of peptide-steroid interactions during pubescence is not restricted to the GnRH impact on gonadotropin or steroid feedback on the pituitary and hypothalamus. As pubertal transition advances there is a disproportionate rise of biologically potent LH beyond the increase seen in immunologic LH. This marked increase in the bioactive to immunoactive ratio is due to molecular alterations in the glycosylation pattern of LH, as reviewed in Chapter 2 under "Heterogeneity."[27]

The onset of significant GnRH pulses first occurs during sleep. There is sleep-associated release of LH in both sexes that correlates with the timing (early puberty) of LH responses to exogenous GnRH. The early stages of puberty are associated with a marked nocturnal augmentation of FSH and LH pulses (both amplitude and frequency); this difference between nighttime and daytime switches by late puberty with an increase in daytime and a decrease in sleep pulsatility.[7,28] It should be noted that day-night differences exist before puberty, but the differences become more marked with the onset of puberty. This change is not abrupt with the onset of puberty. Very sensitive assays can detect an increase in FSH and LH (both day and night) in the months preceeding the beginning of breast development.[28]

Sleep-related LH pulses also are seen in children with idiopathic precocious puberty, in anorexia nervosa patients during intermediate stages of exacerbation and recovery, and also in agonadal patients during the pubertal age period when their gonadotropins are returning from midchildhood reductions.[29] GnRH pulses appear and are maintained independent of steroid feedback.

Puberty

The cascade of events initiated by the release of pulsatile GnRH from prepubertal feedback and central negative inhibition results in increased levels of gonadotropins and steroids with appearance of secondary sexual characteristics and eventual adult function (menarche and, later, ovulation). Between the ages of 10 and 16 the endocrine sequence observed includes, first, increased pulsatile patterns of LH during sleep, followed by similar pulses of less amplitude occurring throughout the 24-hour day. Episodic peaks of estradiol result and menarche appears. By mid to late puberty, maturation of the positive feedback relationship between estradiol and LH is established, leading to ovulatory cycles.

Timing of Puberty

Although the major determinant of the timing of puberty is genetic, other factors appear to influence the time of initiation and the rate of progression of puberty: geographic location, exposure to light, general health and nutrition, and psychologic factors. For example, children with a family history of early puberty start early.[30] Children closer to the equator, at lower altitudes, those in urban areas, and mildly obese children start earlier than those in Northern latitudes, at higher elevations above sea level, in rural areas, and normal weight children, respectively. There is a fairly good correlation between the times of menarche of mothers and daughters and between sisters.[30]

The decline in the age of menarche displayed by children in developed countries undoubtedly reflects improved nutritional status and healthier living conditions. Frisch believes that a critical body weight (47.8 kg) must be reached by a girl to achieve menarche.[31] Possibly more important than total weight is the shift in body composition to a greater percent fat (from 16.0 to 23.5%), which in turn is influenced by the nutritional state.[32] Indeed, moderately obese girls (20–30% over normal weight) have earlier menarche than normal weight girls. Conversely, anorectics and intense exercisers (low weight or low percent fat component of weight) have delayed menarche or secondary amenorrhea. That other factors are involved is indicated by the delayed menarche experienced by morbidly obese girls (greater than 30% overweight), diabetics, and intense exercisers of normal weight. Intriguingly, blind girls experience earlier menarche.[33] Furthermore, girls with idiopathic central precocious puberty may undergo menarche at a total body fat of 19%: children with hypothyroidism display sexual precocity despite a total body fat of 29%, while girls with no signs of puberty may have measured total body fat of 27%.[34] It is reasonable to hypothesize that central mechanisms bring about maturation of the hypothalamic-pituitary-ovarian axis which in turn stimulates growth to the critical weight as well as the increases in body fat composition. However, not all auxologic studies have found a relationship between the onset of puberty and either body fat mass or body fat distribution.[35] Evidence suggests that growth acceleration is due to estrogen and concomitant increases in growth hormone production and secondary stimulation of insulin-like growth factor-I levels.[36]

Stages of Pubertal Development

On the average, the pubertal sequence of accelerated growth, breast development, adrenarche, and menarche requires a period of 4.5 years (range 1.5 to 6 years). The largest body of data was accumulated in healthy European girls; current North American standards are approximately 6 months earlier for each stage.[37–43] Secondary sex characteristics develop slightly earlier in black girls compared to white girls.

In general, the first sign of puberty is an acceleration of growth followed by breast budding (thelarche) (median age 9.8 years). Breast development follows a well-recognized sequence of events. Breast budding is a change distinguished by enlargement and elevation of the nipples and areolae. This is followed by elevation of the breast by the building of the breast mound. Just prior to the formation of the final adult contours, the areolae form a secondary mound.

Although the sequence may be reversed, adrenarche usually appears after the breast bud (median 10.5 years) with axillary hair growth 2 years later. In approximately 20% of children, pubic hair growth is the first sign of puberty. Menarche is a late event (median 12.8 years), occurring after the peak of growth has passed.

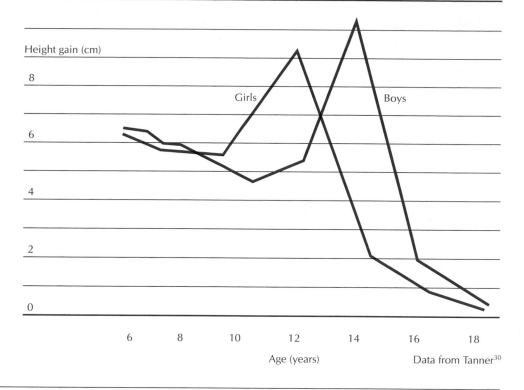

Height gain (cm)

Girls   Boys

Age (years)

Data from Tanner[30]

Growth

An adolescent girl's growth spurt occurs 2 years earlier (at 11–12 years) than that of a boy, and in 1 year, her rate of growth doubles, yielding a height increment of between 6 and 11 cm (2.4–4.3 inches).[44] The average girl reaches this growth peak about 2 years after breast budding and 1 year prior to menarche. Hormonal requirements for this increased growth velocity include growth hormone and gonadal estrogen. The pubertal growth spurt is associated with an increase in the circulating levels of growth hormone and insulin-like growth factor-I. Adrenal androgens are not involved because cortisol-repleted Addisonian patients display normal pubertal growth patterns.

In a remarkable study of African pygmies, it was discovered that the short stature of adult pygmies is due primarily to a failure of growth to accelerate during puberty, and that the principal factor responsible for normal pubertal growth is insulin-like growth factor-I (IGF-I).[45] Growth hormone exerts its action through a locally produced mediator, insulin-like growth factor-I. In addition, growth hormone can directly stimulate epiphyseal cartilage growth. Normal growth at puberty requires the concerted action of growth hormone, insulin-like growth factor-I, and sex steroids. The increase in circulating insulin-like growth factor-I at puberty correlates with sexual development and results from the interaction between sex steroids and growth hormone. Specifically, the increase in sex steroids in turn increases the secretion of growth hormone, which stimulates the production of insulin-like growth factor-I.[46] However, studies also indicate that the sex steroids can have a direct effect on bone growth independent of growth hormone.[47] Thus, Laron-type dwarfs (who have a genetic defect in the growth hormone receptor and cannot stimulate IGF-I secretion) can undergo a growth spurt at puberty in response to the sex steroids. However, normal pubertal growth velocities require the combined action of the sex steroids and growth hormone. The sex steroid hormones also limit the ultimate height attained by stimulating epiphyseal fusion.

The most abundant hormone produced by the pituitary gland is growth hormone, which is secreted not as a single substance but as one predominant form and one smaller variant.[48] Growth hormone is encoded by 5 genes located on chromosome 17q22-q24. One gene is for the predominant form in the pituitary; 3 of the genes are expressed in the placenta. The pituitary gene is regulated by growth hormone-releasing hormone, thyroid hormone, and glucocorticoids. Besides the stimulation of IGF-I in cartilage, growth hormone also stimulates IGF-I production in a variety of tissues throughout the body, especially in the liver (the main source of circulating IGF-I).

Like the gonadotropins, growth hormone is secreted in pulsatile fashion, and during puberty, the amplitude of the pulses increases, especially during sleep. Your grandmother was right when she said: "sleep and you'll grow." The age at which an increase in pulse amplitude first occurs corresponds to the the age of most rapid growth. Slower growing children secrete fewer and smaller pulses of growth hormone. The pulsatile pattern of growth hormone secretion is regulated by stimulation from growth hormone releasing hormone and inhibition from somatropin release-inhibiting hormone, both released into the hypothalmic-pituitary portal circulation from hypothalamic nuclei. This mechanism is influenced at multiple levels by estrogens and androgens. Prior to puberty, the sex steroid hormones are not involved with growth hormone secretion, beyond a low maintenance effect on secretion. At puberty, however, the dynamics of growth hormone secretion are critically dependent on the gonadal sex steroid hormones. Growth hormone secretion must be very sensitive to the stimulatory effect of estrogens because growth hormone levels increase before any signs of sexual development appear.

The amounts of estrogen required to stimulate long-bone cortical growth are incredibly small. Doses of 100 nanograms of estradiol per kilogram body weight per day increase the amplitude of growth hormone pulsatile secretion and produce maximal growth in agonadal recipients. These doses are insufficient to cause breast budding, vaginal cornification, or an increase in sex hormone binding globulin.[49,50] These low dose effects are consistent with the observation that girls attain peak height velocity early in puberty at a serum estradiol concentration of 20 pg/mL (80 pmol/L) which is one-sixth the mean level of adult women. Furthermore, at low doses, estrogen stimulates growth hormone-induced IGF-I secretion, while high doses suppress IGF-I levels.

Osteoporosis and vertebral fractures are less common in black compared to white women. Vertebral bone density increases rapidly and significantly during adolescence, and the increase is greater in black girls, providing one explanation for the racial difference in osteoporosis.[51] The pubertal increase in bone density ranges from 10% to 20%, an accumulation which provides 10–20 years of protection against the normal age-related loss of skeletal mass. Calcium supplementation during adolescence results in a significant increase in bone density and skeletal mass, providing even greater protection against future osteoporosis.[52] Optimal growth has both immediate and long-term consequences. Adolescents with abnormal menstrual function (suppressed estrogen levels) should not be ignored, but properly evaluated and treated. The influence of the sex steroid levels on bone mass is underscored by the fact that the maximal gain occurs in the two years after menarche.

Menarche

As mentioned previously, environmental factors are important in the onset of puberty. Improved living standards and nutrition in the mother antenatally, and in children postnatally, have played a significant role in producing taller, heavier children with earlier maturation. Studies of identical twins and nonidentical twins indicate that the age at menarche is chiefly controlled by genetic factors when the environment is optimal. In affluent cultures, the trend toward lowering of the menarcheal age and puberty halted around 1960.[38] In the 1700s, the mean age of voice change in the Boys' Bach Choir in Leipzig was 18, now it is 13.5 years. Recent studies have indicated an upward trend in the age of menarche, perhaps a response to some environmental deterioration.[53]

Age at menarche (years)

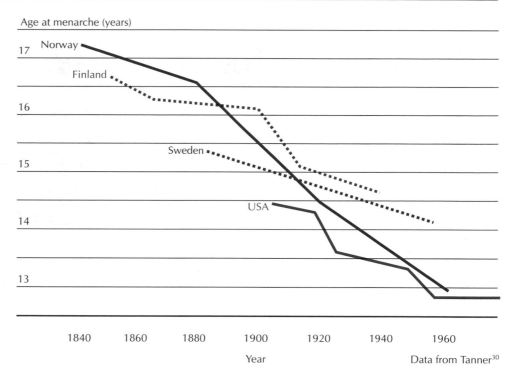

Data from Tanner[30]

The relationship between menarche and the growth spurt is relatively fixed: menarche occurs after the peak in growth velocity has passed. Hence slower growth, totaling no more than 6 cm (2.4 inches) is noted after initiation of menses.

The normal age range of menarche in U.S. girls is 9.1–17.7 years with a median of 12.8.[38,39] The final endocrine hallmark of puberty is the development of positive estrogen feedback on the pituitary and hypothalamus. This feedback stimulates the midcycle surge of LH required for ovulation. Thus, the menses following menarche are usually anovulatory, irregular, and occasionally heavy. Anovulation lasts as long as 12–18 months after menarche, but there are reports of pregnancy before menarche. Ovulation increases in frequency as puberty progresses, but it is common for 25–50% of adolescents to still be anovulatory 4 years after menarche.[40,41]

Summary of Pubertal Events

The onset of puberty is an evolving sequence of maturational steps. The hypothalamic-pituitary-gonadal system differentiates and functions during fetal life and early infancy. Thereafter, it is suppressed to low activity levels during childhood by a combination of hypersensitivity of the "gonadostat" to estrogen negative feedback and an intrinsic CNS inhibitor. All the components located below GnRH (below the CNS) are competent to respond at all ages (as will be seen in the pathogenesis of precocious puberty). After a decade of functional GnRH insufficiency (between late infancy and the onset of puberty), GnRH secretion is resumed and gonadarche (the reactivation of the CNS-pituitary-ovarian apparatus) appears. Prolongation of intrinsic CNS suppression or disability in any of the components of the gonadarche cascade leads to delayed or absent pubescence.

1. FSH and then LH levels rise moderately before the age of 10 and are followed by a rise in estradiol. An increase in LH pulses is first seen only in sleep but gradually extends throughout the day. In the adult, they occur at roughly 1.5–2 hourly intervals.

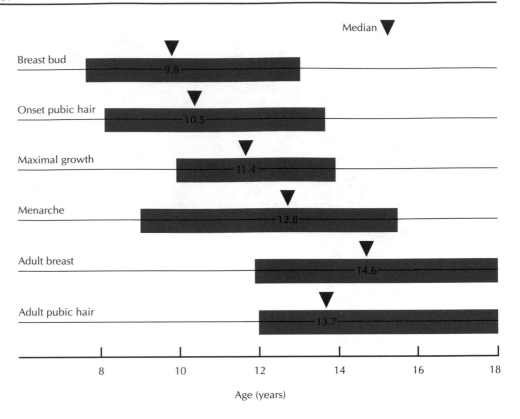

2. As gonadal estrogen increases (gonadarche), breast development, female fat distribution, and vaginal and uterine growth occur. Skeletal growth rapidly increases as a result of initial gonadal secretion of low levels of estrogen, which increases the secretion of growth hormone, which in turn stimulates the production of IGF-I.

3. Adrenal androgen (adrenarche) and, to a lesser degree, gonadal androgen secretion cause pubic and axillary hair growth. Adrenarche plays little if any part in skeletal growth. While temporarily related to gonadarche, adrenarche is an independent, functionally unrelated biological event.

4. At midpuberty, sufficient gonadal estrogen secretion proliferates the endometrium, and the first menses (menarche) occurs.

5. Postmenarchal cycles are initially anovulatory. Sustained, predictable positive LH surge responses to estradiol are late pubertal events.

Blood Hormone Concentrations During Female Puberty[54-60]

Tanner Stage	FSH IU/L	LH IU/L	Estradiol pg/mL	DHA ng/dL
Stage 1	0.9–5.1	1.8–9.2	<10	19–302
Stage 2	1.4–7.0	2.0–16.6	7–37	45–1904
Stage 3	2.4–7.7	5.6–13.6	9–59	125–1730
Stage 4	1.5–11.2	7–14.4	10–156	153–1321
Adult: follicular	3–20	5–25	30–100	162–1620

Precocious Puberty

Puberty is the biologic transition between immature and adult reproductive function. Its timing, endocrine milieu, and physical expressions have been characterized sufficiently to set clinically reasonable time limits for the normal appearance of female maturity and to allow recognition of the pathogenesis and pathophysiology of most of the causes of premature or delayed pubescence.

If one accepts the mean ±2.5 standard deviations as encompassing the normal range, then pubertal changes before the age of 8 are regarded as precocious. Increased growth is often the first change in precocious puberty. This is usually followed by breast development and growth of pubic hair. On occasion, adrenarche, thelarche, and linear growth occur simultaneously. Menarche, however, can be the first sign.

Traditionally, precocious puberty has been divided into two classifications:

1. **GnRH-Dependent Precocious Puberty.** Complete, isosexual, central (or specifically GnRH- and gonadotropin-dependent) precocity — also known as *true precocious puberty*. These terms all refer to early activation of the hypothalamic-pituitary-gonadal axis.

2. **GnRH-Independent Precocious Puberty.** Incomplete, isosexual or heterosexual, peripheral or *precocious pseudopuberty*. Sexual maturation in these instances may be due to extra pituitary secretion of human chorionic gonadotropin (HCG) or sex steroid secretion independent of hypothalamic-pituitary gonadotropin stimulation. Thus, this mechanism is GnRH-independent.

In clinical practice, these classifications are of little practical use. Precocity occurs in girls 5 times more frequently than boys, and almost three-quarters of precocity in girls is idiopathic. Nevertheless, in the face of any precocious development, the clinician is obligated to rule out a serious disease process in central or peripheral sites. In girls over 4 years old a specific etiology is rarely found. In younger girls, a CNS lesion is usually present.

Sexual development does not require ovulatory capability. Evaluation of a patient's possible fertility, for example, with basal body temperatures or progesterone assays, is an unnecessary procedure. More importantly, complete sexual precocity with potential fertility and adult levels of gonadotropins does not rule out the possibility of a serious disease process (e.g., a CNS tumor). While it is true that the most common form of sexual precocity in females is idiopathic or constitutional precocity (true sexual precocity), this must be a diagnosis by exclusion with prolonged follow-up in an effort to detect slowly developing lesions of the brain, ovary, or adrenal gland.

Classification and Relative Occurrence of Precocious Puberty[61–63]

	Female	Male
GnRH-Dependent (True Precocity)		
Idiopathic	74.0%	41.0%
CNS problem	7.0%	26.0%
GnRH-Independent (Precocious Pseudopuberty)		
Ovarian (cyst or tumor)	11.0%	—
Testicular	—	10.0%
McCune-Albright syndrome	5.0%	1.0%
Adrenal feminizing	1.0%	0.0%
Adrenal masculinizing	1.0%	22.0%
Ectopic gonadotropin production	0.5%	0.5%

A classification of sexual precocity is presented to provide a guide to the possible conditions and the relative incidences encountered. It should be noted that a GnRH-dependent cause is found in up to 80% of girls, with a lesser occurrence in boys. Ovarian tumors, adrenal disease, and the McCune-Albright syndrome make up the majority of noncentral precocity in girls.

Particular attention should be given to the following possibilities: drug ingestion, cerebral problems such as cranial trauma or encephalitis, retarded growth with symptoms of hypothyroidism, and a pelvic or abdominal mass. A left hand-wrist film (for use with atlases) should be obtained for bone age. Determination of thyroid function is indicated, and blood levels of gonadotropins and steroids should be measured. Imaging of the brain is indicated in patients with precocious puberty, even in the face of a normal overall evaluation, including normal routine skull x-rays. Other procedures should be dictated by the clinical findings. Virilization, of course, demands a full adrenal evaluation.

GnRH-Dependent Precocious Puberty (Precocious Development Due to Stimulation of Gonadotropin Secretion, True Precocious Puberty)

The signs of *constitutional* sexual precocity are due to premature maturation of the hypothalamic-pituitary-ovarian axis, resulting in production of gonadotropins and sex steroids. These patients experience an increase in growth that is associated with pubertal levels of insulin-like growth factor-I. Constitutional precocity runs in families and usually occurs very close to the "borderline" age of 8 years. On the other hand, *idiopathic* precocious puberty does not run in families and occurs much earlier in childhood. It must be reemphasized that these benign diagnoses should be made only by exclusion and deserve long-term follow-up, because cerebral abnormalities may not become apparent until adulthood.

Clinical presentation of true precocity may not follow the usual progression of breast and pubic hair growth, acceleration of growth rate and then menses. It is not unusual for adrenarche or menarche to be the first sign (or an adult body odor) with others following. This progression is variable, usually slower in idiopathic cases, but telescoped in precocity due to central disease.

Sexual precocity is consistent with normal reproductive life and it is not associated with premature menopause. The most serious effect of precocity is the resultant adult short stature. Because the skeleton is very sensitive to even the lowest levels of estrogen, these children are transiently tall for their age, but as a result of early epiphyseal fusion, eventually short stature results. Fifty percent are less than 5 feet tall (152 cm).

Intellectual and psychosocial development are also commensurate with chronologic age rather than stage of puberty. Expectations of emotional, social, sexual, and intellectual competence corresponding to their pubertal state leave these youngsters and their families with potentially serious difficulties on all levels of social and emotional function.

A number of CNS problems, including abnormal skull development due to rickets, can cause true precocious development. Various tumors can induce precocity, including hamartomas in the hypothalamus (the most common lesion in very young girls), craniopharyngioma, astrocytoma, glioma, neurofibroma, ependymoma, and suprasellar teratoma — all usually near the hypothalamus. Pineal tumors, for unknown reasons, have been seen only in male precocious puberty. Nontumorous causes include encephalitis, meningitis, hydrocephalus, and von Recklinghausen's disease. An injury to the skull may stimulate sexual development.[64] The mechanism is unknown, and a latent period of 1–2 months is usually seen. A hamartoma is a hyperplastic congenital malformation in the floor of the third ventricle that usually produces precocity in the first few years of life; magnetic resonance imaging is the most sensitive method for the detection of small tumors like a hamartoma. Patients with true precocious puberty and known CNS lesions or a history of cranial irradiation should be evaluated for growth hormone deficiency because of the recognized association of these defects.[47]

There is no unifying pathophysiologic mechanism linking this diverse spectrum of etiologies for central precocity. Increased intracerebral pressure and a predilection for posterior hypothalamic lesions have suggested numerous theories. The finding that transforming growth factor-α (TGF-α) accumulates in areas of brain injury as a result of trauma-induced activation of gene expression in glial cells presents an intriguing model in that TGF-α stimulates GnRH release.[65] Hamartomas can produce gonadotropin releasing hormone pulses, just as the normal hypothalamic tissue from which they are derived.

Ectopic gonadotropin production is a rare cause of sexual precocity accounting for less than 0.5% of cases. The most common tumors producing human chorionic gonadotropin (HCG) are chorioepithelioma and dysgerminoma of the ovary, and liver hepatoblastoma.[66,67] Tumor spread may be present at the time of pubertal development; pelvic and abdominal masses accompanied by ascites are usually detectable.

True sexual precocity occurs in a small number of children with long-standing hypothyroidism. In addition to short stature (but not bone age acceleration), galactorrhea may be present. The sella turcica is frequently enlarged, but with thyroid replacement pubertal development will stop and even regress. The sella films will return to normal. Although reported cases have been severe and therefore clinically obvious, laboratory evaluation of thyroid function is indicated in all cases of sexual precocity.

GnRH-Independent Precocious Puberty (Development Due to Availability of Sex Steroids, Precocious Pseudopuberty)

Eleven percent of girls with precocious puberty have an ovarian tumor. The tumor is usually an estrogen-producing neoplasm or cyst. Five percent of granulosa cell tumors and 1% of theca cell tumors occur before puberty. However, gonadoblastomas, teratomas, lipoid cell tumors, cystadenomas and even ovarian cancers have been reported as causes of precocity. Bleeding is irregular and menorrhagic — clearly anovulatory. A pelvic mass is readily palpable in 80% of cases. The palpation of a pelvic or abdominal mass demands surgical exploration. Increasing use has been made of pelvic ultrasonography and whole body (abdominal) imaging for the work-up of precocious puberty. In addition to estrogen and androgens, these tumors can secrete HCG.

A feminizing adrenal tumor is very rare (1% of cases) and is associated with increased blood levels of DHAS.

Drug ingestion should be suspected in all cases of precocity, especially when there is dark pigmentation of the nipples and breast areolae, an effect of certain synthetic estrogens such as stilbestrol. Common sources are oral contraceptives, anabolic steroids, and hair or facial creams.

McCune-Albright syndrome (polyostotic fibrous dysplasia) accounts for 5% of female precocity and consists of multiple disseminated cystic bone lesions that easily fracture, cafe au lait skin spots of various sizes and shapes, and sexual precocity. In addition, this syndrome can be associated with ovarian cysts, growth hormone and prolactin secreting adenomas, hyperthyroidism, adrenal hypercortisolism, and osteomalacia. Premature menarche may be the first sign of the syndrome. Skeletal abnormalities may become evident following the onset of puberty. The combination of multiple bone fractures, cafe au lait patches, and premature development should lead to the diagnosis. But remember that the manifestations of this syndrome can be varied and sometimes subtle. A technetium-99 bone scan may be necessary to demonstrate the areas of bony fibrous dysplasia.

Sexual precocity in McCune Albright syndrome is now demonstrated to be the result of autonomous early production of estrogen by the ovaries.[68] FSH and LH levels are low, respond poorly to GnRH stimulation, and there is an absence of nocturnal gonadotropin pulsations (all unlike central precocity). In addition, Cushing's disease, acromegaly, hyperparathyroidism, and hyperthyroidism have been reported in this syndrome. The protean manifestations of this disorder suggested that the pathophysiology results from a basic defect in cellular regulation at the level of the G protein-cAMP-kinase function in affected tissues.[69] A mutation in the alpha-subunit of the G protein (as described in Chapter 2) has been identified in all affected tissues in patients with McCune-Albright syndrome. This mutation attenuates GTPase activity which is necessary to terminate adenylate cyclase activation; thus, affected tissues have autonomous activity. Somatic mosaicism of the alpha-subunit accounts for the fact that this mutation is not lethal and for the variation in site and activity throughout the body. This mutation can also occur in nonendocrine tissues in patients with McCune-Albright syndrome, thus explaining the occurrence of hepatitis, intestinal polyps, and cardiac arrhythmias. It is possible that this mechanism is responsible for childhood diseases other than McCune-Albright syndrome. For this reason, it has been suggested that this genetic disorder should be called inherited $G_s\alpha$ deficiency.[70]

Eventual fertility is unimpaired, and adult height is usually normal. These positive factors must be considered in the choice of management of the syndrome. In keeping with the autonomous nature of the gonadal activity, treatment with a GnRH analogue fails to suppress gonadal hormone secretion or reverse the sexual precocity.[71]

Yet another example of precocity due to GnRH-independent gonadal secretion of estrogen is by autonomous benign ovarian follicular or luteal cysts.[72] These children demonstrate an absence of gonadotropin pulsations, variable responses to GnRH, and a lack of suppression of puberty by a long-acting GnRH agonist. The cysts may enlarge and involute and then recur so that signs of sexual precocity and vaginal bleeding remit and exacerbate.[73] The cysts are unusually large and therefore palpable. GnRH testing is useful in differentiating the autonomous (nonreactive) cyst from those secondary to the FSH and LH stimulation of central true precocity (reactive).

It is now understood that nearly every cause of peripheral precocious puberty may *secondarily activate* the hypothalamic-pituitary-gonadal axis with development and superimposition of a central GnRH-dependent true precocity process. Presumably the central mechanism controlling the onset of puberty can be activated once a critical threshold of somatic development has been achieved by the premature production of estrogen *regardless* of source of secretion. This explains the previously paradoxical observations of continuing progressive puberty despite effective treatment of specific causative disease as well as the variable effectiveness of GnRH agonist therapy in McCune-Albright and the syndrome of recurrent ovarian cyst formation. GnRH testing to determine the level of activation will dictate the need for additional GnRH agonist suppression, inhibition of steroidogenesis, or peripheral aromatase inhibition therapy in these cases.

Laboratory Findings in Disorders Producing Precocious Puberty

	Gonadal Size	Basal FSH/LH	Estradiol or Testosterone	DHAS	GnRH Response
Idiopathic	Increased	Increased	Increased	Increased	Pubertal
Cerebral	Increased	Increased	Increased	Increased	Pubertal
Gonadal	Unilat. incr.	Decreased	Increased	Increased	Flat
Albright	Increased	Decreased	Increased	Increased	Flat
Adrenal	Small	Decreased	Increased	Increased	Flat

Special Cases of Precocious Development

Special cases of precocious development include the isolated appearance of one sexual characteristic: premature adrenarche or pubarche (pubic hair), premature thelarche (breast development), or premature isolated menarche. These cases present a special dilemma for the concerned clinician. Are they benign, self-limited variants of normal sexual development that do not require treatment or the first sign of a potentially accelerating process in which early exhaustive diagnosis and long-term therapy may be necessary?

Typically linear growth and skeletal maturation are not advanced, and baseline hormone levels are normal for age and sexual development. However, there is a spectrum of conditions of premature sexual maturation defined by idiopathic central precocious puberty at one end and isolated premature thelarche or premature adrenarche at the other. Between these poles are examples of mixed atypical problems with variable tendencies for stability or progression. Guidelines are emerging that address the issues of when sophisticated diagnostic testing (ACTH stimulation, GnRH testing, ultrasonography, bone assessments) is indicated.

Premature Thelarche

Premature thelarche usually occurs in the first few years of life and is usually self-limited, requiring no therapy. Follow-up has revealed that these children experience normal puberty and growth and, eventually, normal reproduction.[74] The breast growth may regress after a few months, wax and wane for years, or last until puberty. Premature thelarche can be unilateral.

Premature Menarche

Isolated premature menarche without other evidence of maturation is an exceedingly rare presentation of precocity; infection, the presence of a foreign body, abuse and trauma, and local neoplasms should be considered. Normal growth, development, and fertility are not affected.[75]

Premature Adrenarche

Premature adrenarche is the consequence of an early modest increase in the adrenal androgens, androstenedione, dehydroepiandrosterone and dehydroepiandrosterone sulfate. An adrenal enzyme deficit should be excluded by appropriate laboratory testing, but it is rarely discovered in a prepubertal child who presents only with early growth of pubic hair.[76,77] Thus, an ACTH stimulation test is not necessary; a measurement of the circulating level of 17-hydroxyprogesterone will suffice. Treatment is not necessary because the transient acceleration in growth and bone maturation has no major influence on puberty or final height.[78] Surveillance of these patients should be continued because, although not certain, it has been suggested that they have an increased incidence of anovulation and hirsutism.[79] Sparse hair growth on the vulva does not represent precocious pubarche.

An ACTH stimulation test should be performed in patients who have an advanced bone age and circulating androgen levels that are greater than those seen in the early stages of puberty. ACTH testing of all children with premature adrenarche will yield results in some that are consistent with mild errors of steroidogenesis. However, even if present, these mild enzyme changes do not require treatment, and hence, exact diagnosis is not necessary. Treatment is indicated only for unequivocal cases of 21-hydroxylase deficiency, in whom baseline 17-hydroxyprogesterone levels will be diagnostic.

Diagnosis of Precocious Puberty	The cause of precocious development may be obvious by findings in the history or physical examination. Familial occurrence helps to exclude certain disease processes (tumors). Clinically, the nature of precocity dictates certain diagnostic priorities.

1. **Rule out life-threatening disease.** This includes neoplasms of the CNS, ovary, and adrenal.

2. **Define the velocity of the process.** Is it progressing or stabilized? Management decisions hinge on this determination. Isolated, nonendocrine causes of vaginal bleeding (trauma, foreign body, vaginitis, genital neoplasm) must be excluded.

Differential Diagnostic Steps

Physical Diagnosis:
Record of growth, Tanner stages, height and weight percentiles.
External genitalia changes.
Abdominal, pelvic, neurologic examination.
Signs of androgenization.
Special findings: McCune-Albright, hypothyroidism.

Laboratory Diagnosis:
Bone age.
Head CT scan or MRI, ultrasonography of abdomen and pelvis.
FSH, LH, HCG assay.
Thyroid function tests (TSH and free T_4).
Steroids (serum DHAS, testosterone, estradiol, progesterone, 17-hydroxy-progesterone).
GnRH testing.

If the full signs of sexual precocity are present, and basal or GnRH-stimulated gonadotropins are in the pubertal range, a pituitary source of gonadotropins is suspected. Any abnormality on neurologic exam or imaging points toward cerebral precocious puberty.

If these are all normal, idiopathic sexual precocity is the most likely diagnosis. It should be emphasized that basal serum gonadotropins may be in the prepubertal range in the early stages of idiopathic or cerebral precocious puberty; with time and progression of sexual development these will rise to the pubertal range. However, an ectopic source of HCG should be considered if serum gonadotropins are suppressed while estradiol is markedly elevated; a situation easily confirmed by an immunoassay specific for the β-subunit of HCG. The rare feminizing adrenal tumor may be present if the laboratory picture is more one of elevated adrenal androgens with only slightly elevated serum estradiol and suppressed serum gonadotropins. Abdominal and pelvic ultrasonography or magnetic resonance imaging (MRI) is indicated.

When signs of sexual precocity are associated with accelerated growth and skeletal maturation, in the absence of virilization, the etiology may be an ovarian tumor or cyst. A pelvic mass is usually palpable. In this situation, serum FSH and LH are suppressed, while serum estradiol is usually elevated. An elevated serum progesterone suggests an ovarian luteoma. Pelvic ultrasound or imaging can help to confirm the presence of an ovarian mass. Laparotomy is indicated to confirm the diagnosis and carry out surgical resection.

Adrenal hyperplasia or a virilizing adrenal or ovarian tumor must be considered if signs of sexual precocity are accompanied by virilization. With elevation of serum 17-hydroxyprogesterone (17-OHP) and adrenal androgens, the diagnosis of 21-hydroxylase deficient adrenal hyperplasia is established, whereas an elevation of serum 11-deoxy-cortisol leads to the diagnosis of 11-hydroxylase deficient adrenal hyperplasia. If these two serum hormones are normal, while serum DHAS or androstenedione is elevated, an adrenal tumor or a virilizing ovarian tumor is suspect. Ultrasound examination and abdominal imaging can be utilized to further localize the tumor.

Breast development usually correlates with a bone age of 11 and menarche with a bone age of 13. If breast and genital development, pubic hair growth, and vaginal bleeding are seen in a short child with a *delayed* bone age, primary hypothyroidism is the most likely diagnosis. This can be confirmed by finding a low serum T_4 and elevated TSH concentration. Serum FSH and LH levels may be in the pubertal range, but these will decrease following thyroid treatment. Galactorrhea may be present along with elevated serum prolactin concentrations. These return to normal with thyroid treatment.

Tanner Staging

	Breast	Pubic Hair
Stage 1 (prepubertal)	Elevation of papilla only	No pubic hair
Stage 2	Elevation of breast and papilla as small mound, areola diameter enlarged. Median age: 9.8 years	Sparse, long, pigmented hair chiefly along labia majora. Median age: 10.5 years
Stage 3	Further enlargement without separation of breast and areola. Median age: 11.2 years	Dark, coarse, curled hair sparsely spread over mons. Median age: 11.4 years
Stage 4	Secondary mound of areola and papilla above the breast. Median age: 12.1 years	Adult-type hair, abundant but limited to the mons. Median age: 12.0 years
Stage 5	Recession of areola to contour of breast. Median age: 14.6 years	Adult-type spread in quantity and distribution. Median age: 13.7 years

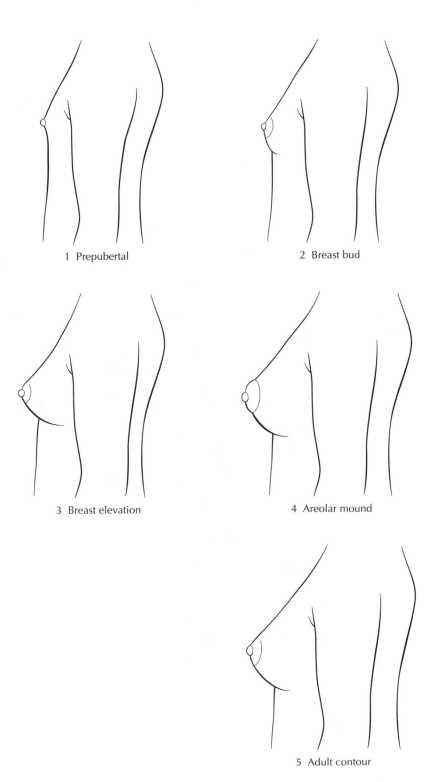

1 Prepubertal

2 Breast bud

3 Breast elevation

4 Areolar mound

5 Adult contour

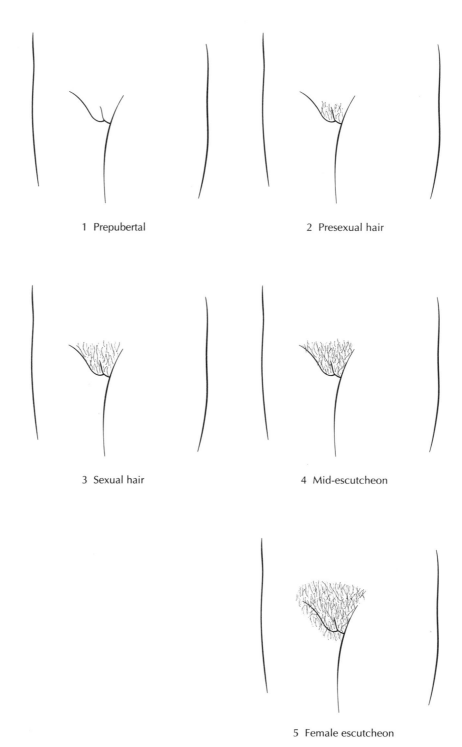

1 Prepubertal

2 Presexual hair

3 Sexual hair

4 Mid-escutcheon

5 Female escutcheon

Treatment of Precocious Development

The objectives of management and treatment of precocious puberty include:

1. Diagnose and treat intracranial disease.

2. Arrest maturation until normal pubertal age.

3. Attenuate and diminish established precocious characteristics.

4. Maximize eventual adult height.

5. Avoidance of abuse, reduction of emotional problems, and contraception if necessary.

A number of therapies have been used to achieve these goals. These have included medroxyprogesterone acetate, cyproterone acetate, and danazol. In addition to undesirable side effects, bone maturation and growth were not regularly or sufficiently controlled. Major progress has been made with the use of GnRH analogues for the treatment of true precocious puberty.

The short half-life of GnRH is due to rapid cleavage of bonds between amino acids 5–6, 6–7, and 9–10. Substitution of amino acids at position 6 and replacement of the c-terminal glycine amide has produced effective GnRH agonists. Agents can be chosen that are administered subcutaneously, intranasally daily, or in long-acting depot forms.

GnRH Agonists in Clinical Use

Position	1	2	3	4	5	6	7	8	9	10
Native GnRH	pGlu	His	Trp	Ser	Tyr	Gly	Leu	Arg	Pro	Gly-NH$_2$
Leuprolide						D-Leu				NH-Ethylamide
Buserelin						D-Ser (tertiary butanol)				NH-Ethylamide
Nafarelin						D-Naphthylalanine (2)				
Histrelin						D-His (tertiary benzyl)				NH-Ethylamide
Goserelin						D-Ser (tertiary butanol)				Aza-Gly
Deslorelin						D-Trp				NH-Ethylamide
Tryptorelin						D-Trp				

After an initial short-term "flare" stimulation of gonadotropin release, down-regulation and desensitization follow, yielding profound reduction in gonadotropins, steroid production, and biologic effects. Substantial regression of pubertal characteristics, amenorrhea, and reduction in growth velocity are rapidly achieved and maintained within the first year of treatment.[80] Final bone height is increased but is dependent upon the stage at which medication is begun, the bone age at which the drug is stopped, and the adequacy of the dose regimen.[81,82] Even individuals with advanced bone ages will achieve greater growth because suppression of gonadal steroids will delay epiphyseal fusion and prolong the duration of growth. The dose can be monitored by measuring estradiol levels; the objective is to maintain an estradiol less than 10 pg/mL (40 pmol/L). Because many commercial estradiol assays lack sensitivity in this range, it may be necessary to confirm adequate suppression by demonstrating a lack of gonadotropin response to the administration of GnRH. In general, children require higher doses of GnRH agonists to achieve suppression compared to adults. Even with treatment, adrenarche will probably continue, true to its independent control system.

Sustained release pellets (goserelin) or sustained release injections (leuprolide) allow once a month dosing.[83] Treatment is maintained until the epiphyses are fused or until appropriate pubertal and chronological ages are matched. Discontinuation of therapy is followed by prompt reactivation of the pubertal process and the development of regular ovulatory function in a pattern similar to that of normal adolescents.[84] GnRH agonist treatment is also recommended for GnRH-secreting hamartomas of the hypothalamus.[85] The progress of the tumor can be monitored by imaging, and risky surgery can be avoided.

GnRH agonist treatment is not effective for noncentral forms of precocious puberty such as McCune-Albright syndrome, GnRH-independent sexual precocity, or congenital adrenal hyperplasia. However, should patients with McCune-Albright syndrome or congenital adrenal hyperplasia mature their hypothalamic-pituitary-gonadal axis and develop true sexual precocity, then supplementary GnRH agonist therapy is helpful.[86,87] Primary treatment in these cases is directed toward suppression of gonadal steroidogenesis. Medroxyprogesterone acetate can be utilized in depot form to suppress LH secretion, or testolactone, an aromatase inhibitor, can be administered.

If a specific etiology for precocious puberty is identified, treatment is aimed at curing the underlying disorder. Neurosurgical excision of hypothalamic, pituitary, cerebral, or pineal tumors must be individualized in each patient. If these tumors are small and do not extend around or into vital brain structures, their removal may be successful. If complete surgical excision is not possible, radiation therapy should be considered. Although many tumors are said not to be radiosensitive, this may be the only treatment available, although new chemotherapy protocols are of benefit with some tumors. The tumors that secrete ectopic HCG, such as choriocpithcliomas, tcratomas, hcpatomas, should be managed in a manner consistent with current specific treatment protocols for HCG-secreting neoplasms.

If an ovarian or adrenal tumor is identified, surgical excision is the treatment of choice. In the case of an ovarian cyst, it may be difficult to know whether the cyst is an autonomous source of estrogens or whether its growth is secondary to gonadotropin stimulation. GnRH testing is useful in resolving this question. If multiple bilateral cysts are discovered, these are usually secondary to central gonadotropin secretion. If the cyst is solitary and the contralateral ovary appears immature, then cyst resection is justified. With primary hypothyroidism, thyroid replacement will prevent further progression of sexual precocity. If adrenal hyperplasia is identified, treatment with appropriate doses of glucocorticoids (and mineralocorticoids if salt-wasting is present) will also prevent further progression of pubertal development. If these patients have a bone age of 11–12 years, glucocorticoid therapy may result in onset of true sexual precocity.

Careful consideration must be given to the management of psychosocial problems in all children with precocious puberty. As mentioned previously, these children have intellectual, behavioral and psychosexual maturation in keeping with their chronological age, not their physical or pubertal age. They do not have early heterosexual activity or abnormal sexual libido. Unfortunately, parents, teachers, and peers may have unrealistic expectations of their intellectual and athletic abilities, and these children may even inappropriately be labeled as retarded. Careful explanation of these considerations must be given to parents. The children should be counseled that their secondary sexual characteristics are normal albeit early. If the child is bright, advancement in school may be possible with special tutoring and this may prove beneficial. Children with precocious puberty may place a stress on the marital or family relationship, and in these situations formal psychological counseling can be useful.

Prognosis

The prognosis for precocious puberty depends on the underlying cause. With primary hypothyroidism, the prognosis is excellent. Children with adrenal hyperplasia tend to be short as adults. Removal of benign ovarian tumors and adrenal tumors carries a good prognosis, while malignant carcinomas often have metastatic disease at the time of presentation, with consequent poor prognosis. Approximately 20% of granulosa cell tumors are malignant, and the prognosis is guarded for recurrences as late as 25 years after removal. Approximately 25% of ovarian Sertoli-Leydig cell tumors are malignant.

With CNS causes of sexual precocity, the prognosis again depends on the exact etiology. If tumors of the CNS are completely resectable, the prognosis is good; however, this tends to be the exception rather than the rule. Some tumors, though, such as hamartomas, are slow growing and may only be discovered during a routine autopsy following death due to other causes. Other tumors, such as craniopharyngiomas, are developmental remnants rather than true neoplasms, and with partial resection and radiation therapy patients may go into remission for many years. With other conditions, such as congenital cysts, hydrocephalus, encephalitis, McCune-Albright syndrome, and neurofibromatosis, the prognosis is related to associated neurologic deficits.

Psychometric testing indicates that girls with precocious puberty have higher verbal IQ scores. Behavioral testing demonstrates that a majority of girls do not have problems; a minority may show a tendency toward social difficulties related to apparent age and physical maturation, such as depression, social withdrawal, moodiness, aggression and hyperactivity. However, with the exception of short stature as an adult, the prognosis for idiopathic sexual precocity remains good if the children enter adult life without psychosexual scars. The mean height in adult women is approximately 152 cm (5 feet). Even with prompt GnRH agonist treatment final adult height is likely to be compromised because some stimulation to epiphyseal closure will already have occurred before treatment is initiated. One can consider adding growth hormone to patients who appear to be falling short of their predicted height, however the expense of growth hormone is a factor and the impact is not yet well established. Most women have normal menstrual cycles and fertility, and they do not have premature menopause.[88]

Delayed Puberty

Since there is such a wide variation in normal development it is difficult to define the patient with abnormally delayed sexual maturation. Nearly all U.S. white girls and all U.S. black girls have entered puberty by age 13.[39] However, some evaluation is needed whenever a patient and parents are concerned enough to seek a clinician's advice. Patients who have not developed signs of puberty by age 17 are very likely to have a specific problem and not physiological delay of puberty.

Delayed puberty is a rare condition in girls, and a genetic problem or hypothalamic-pituitary disorder must be suspected. In addition, anatomic abnormalities of the target organ (uterus and endometrium) or outflow tract are unique but important elements to consider in amenorrheic but otherwise normal pubertal adolescents.

The history and physical examination are very useful in the diagnostic work-up of delayed puberty. Special note should be taken of past general health, height and weight records, and the height and pubertal milestone experience of older siblings and parents, and relevant behavior such as extreme exercise or abnormal eating habits. Physiological delayed puberty tends to be familial. On physical examination, in addition to body measurements and Tanner staging of any secondary sexual characteristics present, a search for signs of hypothyroidism, gonadal dysgenesis, hypopituitarism, or chronic illness should be made. Persistent deciduous teeth are typical of hypothyroidism. The absence of pubic hair in a patient with a uterus and vagina indicates hypopituitarism. The absence of pubic hair in a patient with a vaginal pouch indicates that the patient has androgen insensitivity syndrome.

The failure of growth in stature suggests several possibilities. Isolated growth hormone deficiency is associated with somewhat delayed sexual maturity. Menarche may eventually occur, albeit delayed, but with bone age still several years below chronologic age. More global pituitary hormone deficiency will result in total pubertal delay. Finally, gonadal dysgenesis (45,X) will be associated with decreased height and sexual infantilism with normal to slightly reduced bone age and hypergonadotropism.

Neurologic examination is important; evidence of intracranial disease, restricted visual fields, or absent sense of smell are key findings. Anatomic defects of the müllerian ducts must be sought, especially when a disparity between normal puberty and absent menses is encountered.

As will be seen in the discussion of the work-up, the diverse etiologic possibilities for delayed puberty are best classified by the level of gonadotropin encountered. The distribution of diagnostic frequencies in the three categories — hypergonadotropic hypogonadism, hypogonadotropic hypogonadism and eugonadism — is listed on the following page, representing the findings in 326 patients.[89]

Laboratory Assessments of Delayed Puberty

Laboratory work-up of delayed puberty usually includes x-rays for bone age, skull imaging (if hypogonadotropic), gonadotropin and prolactin levels, appropriate adrenal and gonadal steroid measurements, and assessment of thyroid function. In addition, general laboratory screening for systemic disorders is worthwhile. Evaluation according to the program outlined in Chapter 12 will lead to the proper diagnosis. Patients with elevated gonadotropins require a karyotype.

Hypergonadotropic Hypogonadism

If gonadotropins are increased into the postmenopausal range (hypergonadotropic hypogonadism), then some type of gonadal deficiency usually is the basis of delayed maturation. In sickle cell disease, approximately 20% of patients have delayed puberty and hypergonadotropism. A 17α-hydroxylase deficiency in steroid synthesis (affecting both adrenals and ovaries) will cause hypergonadotropic delayed puberty *and hypertension.*

The most common disorder of this type is gonadal dysgenesis. In the 45,X patient, the typical phenotypic stigmata of Turner syndrome will be displayed. However, these may be minimal or absent in sex chromosome mosaicism or structural deletions of the X chromosome. A Y-bearing cell line requires gonadal excision as prophylaxis against the risk of gonadal malignancy. Intersex patients (Chapter 10) can present with delayed puberty.

A hypergonadotropic 46,XX individual presents interesting possibilities. If hypertension, sexual infantilism, and an elevated serum progesterone are found, 17α-hydroxylase deficiency in steroid synthesis is likely. Acquired ovarian damage from torsion or inflammation should be ruled out. Finally, the 46,XX patient may have pure gonadal dysgenesis (gonadal streaks) or the resistant ovary syndrome. See the discussion in Chapter 12 under "Premature Ovarian Failure."

383

Relative Frequency of Delayed Pubertal Abnormalities[89]

Hypergonadotropic Hypogonadism		**43.0%**
Ovarian failure, abnormal karyotype		26.0%
Ovarian failure, normal karyotype		17.0%
46, XX	15.0%	
46, XY	2.0%	
Hypogonadotropic Hypogonadism		**31.0%**
Reversible		18.0%
Physiologic delay	10.0%	
Weight loss/anorexia	3.0%	
Primary hypothyroidism	1.0%	
Congenital adrenal hyperplasia	1.0%	
Cushing's syndrome	0.5%	
Prolactinomas	1.5%	
Irreversible		13.0%
GnRH deficiency	7.0%	
Hypopituitarism	2.0%	
Congenital CNS defects	0.5%	
Other pituitary adenomas	0.5%	
Craniopharyngioma	1.0%	
Malignant pituitary tumor	0.5%	
Eugonadism		**26.0%**
Müllerian agenesis		14.0%
Vaginal septum		3.0%
Imperforate hymen		0.5%
Androgen insensitivity syndrome		1.0%
Inappropriate positive feedback		7.0%

Hypogonadotropic Hypogonadism

Decreased secretion of LH (less than 6 IU/L), associated with depressed FSH, is seen in hypothalamic amenorrhea, amenorrhea and anosmia — Kallmann's syndrome, pituitary (tumor) disorders, hyperprolactinemia, or nonpathologic constitutional (physiologic) delay in development. Physiological delayed puberty can be regarded as a physiologic variant in development. The typical patient with physiological delay is short with appropriate bone maturation delay. Physiological delay accounts for only 10% of cases with delayed puberty, emphasizing the need to seek another diagnosis. As previously noted, physiological delay is frequently seen in a familial pattern with the expectation of a late but otherwise normal growth pattern and adult reproductive function.

Poor nutrition (anorexia nervosa, malabsorption, chronic illness, regional ileitis, renal disease) can lead to hypogonadotropic delayed growth and development. Exercise and/or stress-induced amenorrhea can also delay puberty. Unfortunately, illegal drug use (especially marijuana) must be considered.

In the presence of normal olfaction and normal prolactin levels, exclusion of pituitary, parapituitary, or hypothalamic tumor by specialized neuroradiologic procedures is necessary. If tumor or vascular malformation is not found, the diagnosis is (by exclusion) physiological delayed puberty.

Craniopharyngioma. This tumor is the most common neoplasm associated with delayed puberty. Craniopharyngioma is a tumor of Rathke's pouch, originating from the pituitary stalk with suprasellar extension. The peak incidence is between ages 6 and 14.[90] Imaging reveals an abnormal sella and calcifications in 70% of cases. Treatment consists of a combination of surgery and irradiation.

Eugonadism

Müllerian tube segmental discontinuities, müllerian agenesis, or androgen insensitivity syndrome will present as delayed menarche despite normal development of an adult female phenotype (Chapter 12). Müllerian agenesis accounts for one-seventh of cases of prolonged primary amenorrhea. Other obstructive anomalies of the müllerian ducts are less frequently seen. Anovulation and polycystic ovaries, and androgen-producing adrenal disease, can present as primary amenorrhea. Virilization raises the possibility of adrenal hyperplasia or an intersex problem.

Treatment of Sexual Infantilism (Delayed Puberty)

The first priority in therapy is removal or correction of primary etiology when possible. In this regard, thyroid therapy for hypothyroidism, growth hormone for isolated growth hormone deficiency, and treatment of ileitis are examples of specific therapy. In XY individuals, properly timed gonadectomy followed by sex hormone treatment is required. In physiological delay, reassurance that the anticipated development will occur is the only management step needed, especially when there is a family history of delayed puberty. Early hormone treatment is worthwhile in order to minimize psychological stress.

In hypogonadism, hormonal therapy will initiate and sustain maturation and function of secondary sexual characteristics and promote the achievement of full height potential. The importance of the adolescent increase in bone density should not be underrated. This is sufficient reason to recommend hormone treatment.

Hormone treatment should conform to what we have learned about the early stages of puberty. Very small amounts of estrogen will promote growth and development. Start with unopposed estrogen, 0.3 mg conjugated estrogens or 0.5 mg estradiol daily. After 6 months to 1 year, move to a sequential program with 0.625 mg conjugated estrogens or 1.0 mg estradiol daily and 10 mg medroxyprogesterone acetate for the first 12 days each month. Patients with physiological delay of puberty will continue development on their own when bone age has advanced to 13 years.

Monthly menstruation is an important experience for adolescents. Regular and visible bleeding serves to reinforce the young patient's identification with the feminine gender role. However, remember that the doses used for this therapy will not protect against pregnancy in the event the hypothalamic-pituitary-ovarian axis is activated. In a sexually active patient, it would be wiser to use oral contraception to provide the missing estrogen.

Treatment with pulsatile GnRH is both a logical and effective means of inducing a physiologic puberty.[91] However, this treatment regimen is not practical. Although its expense is an important consideration, the technical aspects associated with the parenteral administration of GnRH pulses make this method too cumbersome and difficult.

Growth Problems in Normal Adolescents

Perhaps the worst thing about an adolescent growth problem is that it makes the individual "different." It is probably true that more than anyone else the adolescent does not like to be different. Therefore, excessive or insufficient growth is not a problem to be dismissed lightly, and psychologic support and reassurance are key features in the management of such problems. A willingness to listen to problems, together with an adult-to-adult attitude, will place the adolescent-physician relationship at the proper level of mutual respect.

The basic and essential laboratory procedure is a left hand-wrist x-ray for bone age. The Bayley-Pinneau tables predict future adult height, utilizing the bone age and present height.[92] To use the tables, one needs a measurement of height, the patient's age, and an x-ray of the left hand and wrist for bone age. All of the hand epiphyses and those of the distal end of the arm are used to determine the skeletal age. The Bayley-Pinneau tables begin at the end of this chapter.

To estimate a patient's adult height, use the tables as follows. Go down the left column to the patient's present height, follow this horizontal row to the column under the bone age which is given by 6-month intervals across the top. The number at the intersection represents the predicted adult height. The predicted height can be easily extrapolated if figures do not fall at the 1-inch or 6-month intervals used on the tables.

It is important to use the table suitable for the rate of maturing. If the bone age is within 1 year of the chronologic age, use the table for average girls; if the bone age is accelerated 1 year or more, use the table for accelerated girls; if the bone age is retarded 1 year or more, use the table for retarded girls.

The tables are for use with bone age films of the hand and wrist only in conjunction with the Greulich-Pyle Atlas. Use with bone age determined by any other method is less accurate.

Short Stature
Thorough medical history and physical examination will eliminate the usual disorders associated with short stature: malnutrition, chronic urinary tract disease, chronic infectious disease, hypothyroidism, mental illness, panhypopituitarism, and gonadal dysgenesis. In the history, the heights and weights of parents, siblings, and relatives should be obtained along with timing of growth in the family, dietary history, daily activities, and sleep habits. Normal history and examination in an individual with a bone age only 1 year behind the chronologic age suggest a constitutional pattern that does not require treatment.

Endocrine disease is an uncommon basis for impairment of growth. Congenital hypothyroidism is the most frequent problem of this type, followed by hypopituitarism, hypothyroidism with onset during childhood, and excess cortisol.

It is unlikely that a patient with congenital hypothyroidism will present undiagnosed and untreated as an adolescent. However, juvenile hypothyroidism must be suspected in an adolescent with obesity and short stature and normal early childhood development. Similarly, an adolescent with hypopituitarism due to a slow growing pituitary tumor may present with a failure to develop secondary sexual characteristics and a failure to grow. Cortisol excess may be due to Cushing's disease (rare in childhood) or to therapy with corticosteroids. Excess endogenous or exogenous corticosteroids suppress skeletal maturation and growth. Moderate overdosage of cortisol; e.g., when treating children with adrenal hyperplasia, may suppress growth.

Treatment of Short Stature. Support and observation are indicated if the physician concludes that an adolescent suffers from a delay of normal growth and no disease process is present. Reassurance is essential if the bone age is more than 1 year below the chronologic age, but the family history reveals a consistent pattern of retarded but eventual normal growth. It is helpful to point out the x-ray, indicating that the individual has 1 year or more of unused potential in which to catch up with her friends.

Hormone treatment can be considered when continued failure to grow is evident in the absence of disease. Presently the use of growth hormone is limited to use in growth hormone deficiency. Illicit sources of growth hormone have been administered by parents and young people eager to "grow" to achieve greater athletic prowess. This dangerous practice all too often leads to growth but of fragile bones unsupported by the sought-after muscular capacities.

Anabolic-androgenic steroids are illegally utilized by both adolescent males and females to increase athletic performance and even in an effort to look better.[93] Response to these agents ranges from increased strength and libido (virilization and menstrual dysfunction in women) to liver diseases, impotence, and oligospermia. Excessive androgen use by adolescents can prevent individuals from reaching their genetic height potential. Although not well-studied, most experts believe that there are significant psychological and behavioral effects (such as enhanced aggression), as well as psychological dependence. In addition, adolescents who use anabolic steroids are more likely to use other drugs and to share needles (a major risk factor for human immunodeficiency virus infection).[94]

Fortunately, it is rare to see a female adolescent complaining of short stature. More commonly it is an adolescent boy who is sensitive to reduced growth, and in whom the use of testosterone may be indicated. In cases of gonadal failure, estrogen can be used in a female to stimulate epiphyseal growth, bringing the bone age to match the chronologic age. Conjugated estrogens (0.3 mg) or estradiol (0.5 mg) administered daily are effective in hypogonadal individuals (this is a much smaller dose than previously used). Patients should be observed at monthly intervals to document the pattern of growth and development. Hormone treatment may be discontinued when the bone age matches the chronologic age.

Tall Stature
This is rarely a problem in boys. Basketball has provided a ready outlet, and fortunately participation in sports is now appealing to girls as well. But girls who are the daughters of very tall parents may come for help. The Bayley-Pinneau tables are accurate in predicting the height of tall girls. A predicted height greater than 6 feet probably deserves treatment.

A hand-wrist x-ray for bone age is necessary. The degree of development of secondary sexual characteristics is important, because the more mature a girl is, the less effective treatment is in influencing her eventual height.

Treatment of Tall Stature. It is difficult to make a decision for treatment, and parental participation in the decision is essential. In a case where some success can be achieved, the patient is relatively young and may find it hard to know what to think about the future problem.

Because the adolescent growth spurt precedes menarche, treatment must begin before menarche in order to be optimally successful. This would be as early as 8 or 9 years, and certainly before the age of 12. However, treatment begun after menarche may still achieve up to an inch of growth reduction.[95,96] Once begun, treatment must continue until epiphyses are fused. If treatment is stopped earlier, further growth will occur. The parents and patient must be informed of possible problems with menorrhagia, breast symptoms, water retention, etc.

Conjugated estrogens can be given in a dose of 2.5–5 mg daily, and medroxy-progesterone acetate, 10 mg, is added on the 1st through the 12th each month to ensure consistent and predictable menstrual bleeding. Hand-wrist films should be taken every 6 months until epiphyseal closure is demonstrated. In view of the sensitivity of growth physiology to low levels of estrogen, it is not certain that these high doses are necessary. It would be reasonable to consider the usual replacement dose (0.625–1.25 mg conjugated estrogens), especially if the high doses elicit unpleasant symptoms.

References

1. **Kaplan SL, Grumbach MM, Aubert ML,** The ontogenesis of pituitary hormones and hypothalamic factors in the human fetus: maturation of central nervous system regulation of anterior pituitary function, Recent Prog Horm Res 32:161, 1976.

2. **Burger HG, Yfamada Y, Bangah ML, McCloud PI, Warne GL,** Serum gonadotropin, sex steroid, and immunoreactive inhibin levels in the first two years of life, J Clin Endocrinol Metab 72:682, 1991.

3. **Winter JSD, Faiman C,** The development of cyclic pituitary-gonadal function in adolescent females, J Clin Endocrinol Metab 37:714, 1973.

4. **Conte FA, Grumbach MM, Kaplan SL, Reiter EO,** Correlation of LHRF induced LH and FSH release from infancy to 19 years with the changing pattern of gonadotropin secretion in agonadal patients: relation to restraint of puberty, J Clin Endocrinol Metab 50:165, 1980.

5. **Roth JC, Kelch RP, Kaplan SL, Grumbach MM,** FSH and LH response to luteinizing hormone-releasing factor in prepubertal and pubertal children, adult males and patients with hypogonadotropic and hypergonadotropic hypogonadism, J Clin Endocrinol Metab 37:680, 1973.

6. **Jakacki RI, Kelch RP, Sander SE, Lloyd JS, Hopwood NJ, Marshall JC,** Pulsatile secretion of luteinizing hormone in children, J Clin Endocrinol Metab 53:453, 1982.

7. **Oerter KE, Uriarte MM, Rose SR, Barnes KM, Cutler GB Jr,** Gonadotropin secretory dynamics during puberty in normal girls and boys, J Clin Endocrinol Metab 71:1251, 1990.

8. **Dunkel L, Alfthan H, Stenman U-H, Selstam G, Rosberg S, Albertsson-Wikland K,** Developmental changes in 24-hour profiles of luteinizing hormone and follicle-stimulating hormone from prepuberty to midstages of puberty in boys, J Clin Endocrinol Metab 74:890, 1992.

9. **Sizonenko PC, Paunier L, Carmignac D,** Hormonal changes during puberty: IV. Longitudinal study of adrenal androgen secretion, Horm Res 7:288, 1976.

10. **Counts DR, Pescovitz OH, Barnes, KM, Hench KD, Chrousos GP, Sherins RJ, Comite F, Loriaux DL, Cutler GB Jr,** Dissociation of adrenarche and gonadarche in precocious puberty and in isolated hypogonadotropic hypogonadism, J Clin Endocrinol Metab 64:1174, 1987.

11. **Sklar CA, Kaplan SL, Grumbach MM,** Evidence for dissociation between adrenarche and gonadarche: studies in patients with idiopathic precocious puberty, gonadal dysgenesis, isolated gonadotropin deficiency, and constitutionally delayed growth and adolescence, J Clin Endocrinol Metab 51:548, 1980.

12. **Zumoff B, Walsh BT, Katz JL,** Subnormal plasma dehydroiso-androsterone to cortisol ratio in anorexia nervosa: a second hormonal parameter of ontogenetic regression, J Clin Endocrinol Metab 56:668, 1983.

13. **Parker LN, Lifrak AT, Odell WD,** A 60,000 molecular weight glycoprotein stimulates adrenal androgen secretion, Endocrinology 113:2092, 1983.

14. **Hauffa BP, Kaplan SL, Grumbach MM,** Dissociation between plasma adrenal androgens and cortisol in Cushing's disease and ectopic ACTH producing tumor: relation to adrenarche, Lancet 1:1373, 1984.

15. **Cavallo A,** Melatonin secretion during adrenarche in normal human puberty and in pubertal disorders, J Pineal Res 12:71, 1992.

16. **Byrne GC, Perry YS, Winter JSD,** Steroid inhibitory effects upon human adrenal 3β-hydroxysteroid dehydrogenase activity, J Clin Endocrinol Metab 62:413, 1986.

17. **Terasawa E, Noonan JJ, Nass TE, Loose MD,** Posterior hypothalamic lesions advance the onset of puberty in the female rhesus monkey, Endocrinology 115:224, 1984.

18. **Foster DL, Ryan KD,** Endocrine mechanisms governing transition into adulthood: a marked decrease in inhibitory feedback action of estradiol on tonic secretion of LH in the lamb during puberty, Endocrinology 105:896, 1979.

19. **Waldhauser F, Boepple PA,** The pubertal growth spurt in eight patients with true precocious puberty and growth hormone deficiency: evidence for a direct role of sex steroids, J Clin Endocrinol Metab 71:975, 1990.

20. **Attanasio A, Borrelli P, Gupta D,** Circadian rhythms in serum melatonin from infancy to adolescence, J Clin Endocrinol Metab 61:388, 1985.

21. **Cavallo A, Richards GE, Smith ER,** Relation between nocturnal melatonin profile and hormonal markers of puberty in humans, Horm Res 37:185, 1992.

22. **Plant TM, Zorub DS,** Pinealectomy in agonadal infantile male rhesus monkeys does not interrupt initiation of the prepubertal hiatus in gonadotropin secretion, Endocrinology 118:227, 1986.

23. **Genazzani AR, Fachinetti F, Petraglia F, Pintor C, Corda R,** Hyperendorphinemia in obese children and adolescents, J Clin Endocrinol Metab 62:36, 1986.

24. **Wilson ME, Gordon TP, Collins DC,** Ontogeny of LH secretion and first ovulation in seasonal breeding rhesus monkeys, Endocrinology 118:293, 1986.

25. **Marshall JC, Kelch RP,** Low dose pulsatile GnRH in anorexia nervosa: a model of human pubertal development, J Clin Endocrinol Metab 49:712, 1979.

26. **Job JC, Garnier PE, Chaussain JL, Milhaud G,** Elevation of serum gonadotropins (LH and FSH) after releasing hormone (LH-RH) injection in normal children and in patients with disorders of puberty, J Clin Endocrinol Metab 35:473, 1972.

27. **Burstein S, Schaff-Blass E, Blass J, Rosenfield R,** Changing ratio of bioactive to immunoactive LH through puberty, J Clin Endocrinol Metab 61:508, 1985.

28. **Apter D, Butzow TL, Laughlin GA, Yen SSC,** Gonadotropin-releasing hormone pulse generator activity during pubertal transition in girls: pulsatile and diurnal patterns of circulating gonadotropins, J Clin Endocrinol Metab 76:940, 1993.

29. **Kapen S, Boyar RM, Hellman L, Weltzman ED,** 24-Hour patterns of LH secretion in humans: ontogenic and sexual consideration, Prog Brain Res 42:103, 1975.

30. **Tanner JM,** *Growth at Adolescence,* 2nd edition, Blackwell Scientific Publications, Oxford, 1962.

31. **Frisch RE,** Body fat, menarche, and reproductive ability, Seminars Reprod Endocrinol 3:45, 1985.

32. **Maclure M, Travis LB, Willett W, MacMahon B,** A prospective cohort study of nutrient intake and age at menarche, Am J Clin Nutr 54:649, 1991.

33. **Zacharias L, Wurtman RJ,** Blindness: its relation to age of menarche, Science 144:1154, 1964.

34. **Crawford JD, Osler DC,** Body composition at menarche: the Frisch Revelle hypothesis revisited, Pediatrics 56:449, 1975.

35. **de Ridder CM, Thijssen JHH, Bruning PF, Van den Brande JL, Zonderland ML, Erich WBM,** Body fat mass, body fat distribution, and pubertal development: a longitudinal study of physical and hormonal sexual maturation of girls, J Clin Endocrinol Metab 75:442, 1992.

36. **Harris DA, Van Vliet G, Egli LA, Grumbach MM, Kaplan SL, Styne DM, Vainsel M,** Somatomedin-C in normal puberty and in true precocious puberty before and after treatment with a potent luteinizing hormone-releasing hormone agonist, J Clin Endocrinol Metab 61:152, 1985.

37. **Marshall WA, Tanner JM,** Variations in the pattern of pubertal changes in girls, Arch Dis Child 44:291, 1969.

38. **Zacharias L, Rand WM, Wurtman RJ,** A prospective study of sexual development and growth in American girls: the statistics of menarche, Obstet Gynecol Survey 31:325, 1976.

39. **Harlan WR, Harlan EA, Grillo GP,** Secondary sex characteristics of girls 12 to 17 years of age: the U.S. Health Examination Survey, J Pediatr 96:1074, 1980.

40. **Read G, Wilson D, Hughes I, Griffiths K,** The use of salivary progesterone assays in the assessment of ovarian function in postmenarcheal girls, J Endocrinol 102:265, 1984.

41. **Vuorento T, Huhtaniemi I,** Daily levels of salivary progesterone during menstrual cycle in adolescent girls, Fertil Steril 58:685, 1992.

42. **Lee PA,** Normal ages of pubertal events among American males and females, J Adolesc Health Care 1:26, 1980.

43. **Beller FK, Borsos A, Kieback D, Csoknyay J, Lampe L,** Geschlechtsentwicklung: die entwicklung der sekundaren geschlechtsmerkmale — die Tannerstadien 25 jahre spater, Zentlrabl Gynakol 113:499, 1991.

44. **Fried RI, Smith EE,** Postmenarcheal growth patterns, J Pediatr 61:562, 1962.

45. **Merimee TJ, Zapf J, Hewlett B, Cavalli-Sforza LL,** Insulin-like growth factors in pygmies, New Engl J Med 316:906, 1987.

46. **Mansfield MJ, Rudlin CR, Crigler JF Jr, Karol KA, Crawford JD, Boepple PA, Crowley WF Jr,** Changes in growth and serum growth hormone and plasma somatomedin-C levels during suppression of gonadal sex steroid secretion in girls with central precocious puberty, J Clin Endocrinol Metab 66:3, 1988.

47. **Attie KM, Ramierez NR, Conte FA, Kaplan SL, Grumbach MM,** The pubertal growth spurt in eight patients with true precocious puberty and growth hormone deficiency: evidence for a direct role of sex steroids, J Clin Endocrinol Metab 71:975, 1990.

48. **Kerrigan JR, Rogol AD,** The impact of gonadal steroid hormone action on growth hormone secretion during childhood and adolescence, Endocr Rev 13:281, 1992.

49. **Ross JL, Long LM, Skerda M, Cassorla F, Kurtz D, Loriaux DL, Cutler GB Jr,** Effect of low doses of estradiol on 6-month growth rates and predicted height in patients with Turner syndrome, J Pediatr 109:950, 1986.

50. **Bohnet HG,** New aspects of oestrogen/gestagen-induced growth and endocrine changes in individuals with Turner syndrome, Eur J Pediatr 145:275, 1986.

51. **Gilsanz V, Roe TF, Mora S, Costin G, Goodman WG,** Changes in vertebral bone density in black girls and white girls during childhood and puberty, New Engl J Med 325:1597, 1991.

52. **Lloyd T, Andon MB, Rollings N, Martel JK, Landis JR, Demers LM, Eggli DF, Kiesselhorst K, Kulen HE,** Calcium supplementation and bone mineral density in adolescent girls, JAMA 270:841, 1993.

53. **Dann TC, Roberts DF,** Menarcheal age in University of Warwick young women, J Biosoc Sci 25:531, 1993.

54. **Sizonenko PC, Paunier L,** Hormonal changes in puberty III: correlation of plasma dehydro-epiandrosterone, testosterone, FSH and LH with stage of puberty and bone age in normal boys and girls and in patients with Addison's disease or hypogonadism or premature or late adrenarche, J Clin Endocrinol Metab 41:894, 1975.

55. **Hung W, August GP, Glasgow AM,** *Pediatric Endocrinology,* Medical Examination Publishing Co., Garden City, 1978.

56. **Jenner MR, Kelch RP, Kaplan SL, Grumbach MM,** Hormonal changes in puberty. IV. Plasma estradiol, LH and FSH in prepubertal children, pubertal females, and in precocious puberty, premature thelarche, hypogonadism and in a child with a feminizing ovarian tumor, J Clin Endocrinol Metab 34:521, 1972.

57. **Raiti S, Johanson A, Light C, Migeon CJ, Blizzard RM,** Measurement of immunologically reactive follicle stimulating hormone in serum of normal male children and adults, Metabolism 18:234, 1969.

58. **Johanson J, Guyda H, Light C, Migeon CJ, Blizzard RM,** Serum luteinizing hormone by radioimmunoassay in normal children, J Pediatr 74:416, 1969.

59. **Frasier SD, Gafford F, Horton R,** Plasma androgens and adolescence, J Clin Endocrinol Metab 29:1404, 1969.

60. **Lee PA, Migeon CJ,** Puberty in boys: correlation of plasma levels of gonadotropins (LH, FSH), androgens (testosterone, androstenedione, dehydroepiandrosterone and its sulfate), estrogens (estrone and estradiol) and progestins (progesterone and 17-hydroxyprogesterone), J Clin Endocrinol Metab 41:556, 1975.

61. **Jolly H,** *Sexual precocity,* Charles C Thomas, Springfield, Illinois, 1955.

62. **Wilkins L,** *The Diagnosis and Treatment of Endocrine Disorders in Childhood and Adolescence,* 3rd edition, Charles C Thomas, Springfield, Illinois,1965.

63. **Stein DT,** New developments in the diagnosis and treatment of sexual precocity, Am J Med Sci 303:53, 1992.

64. **Maxwell M, Karacostas D, Ellenbogen RG, Brzezinski A, Zervas NT, Black PM,** Precocious puberty following head injury, J Neurosurg 73:123, 1990.

65. **Junier MP, Ma YJ, Costa ME, Hoffman G, Hill DF, Ojeda SR,** Transforming growth factor-α contributes to the mechanism by which hypothalamic injury induces precocious puberty, Proc Natl Acad Sci USA 88:9743, 1991.

66. **Pomariede R, Finidori J, Cernichow P, Pfister A, Hirsch JF, Rappaport R,** Germinoma in a boy with precocious puberty: evidence of HCG secretion by the tumoral cells, Child Brain 11:298, 1984.

67. **Navarro C, Corretser JM, Sancho A, Rovira J, Morales L,** Paraneoplastic precocious puberty. Report of a new case with hepatoblastoma and review of the literature, Cancer 56:1725, 1985.

68. **Lee PA, Van Dop C, Migeon CJ,** McCune-Albright syndrome: long-term follow-up, JAMA 256:290, 1986.

69. **Schwindenger WF, Francomano CA, Levine MA,** Identification of a mutation in the gene encoding the alpha subunit of the stimulatory G protein adenylcyclase in McCune-Albright syndrome, Proc Natl Acad Sci USA 89:5152, 1992.

70. **Miric A, Vechio JD, Levine MA,** Heterogeneous mutations in the gene encoding the α-subunit of the stimulatory G protein of adenyl cyclase in Albright hereditary osteodystrophy, J Clin Endocrinol Metab 76:1560, 1993.

71. **Comite F, Shawker TH, Pescovitz OH, Loriaux DL, Cutler GB Jr,** Cyclical ovarian function resistant to treatment with an analogue of luteinizing hormone releasing hormone in McCune-Albright syndrome, New Engl J Med 311:1032, 1984.

72. **Lightner ES, Kelch RP,** Treatment of precocious pseudopuberty associated with ovarian cysts, Am J Dis Child 138:126, 1984.

73. **Millar DM, Blake JM, Stringer DA, Hara H, Babiak C,** Prepubertal ovarian cyst formation: 5 years' experience, Obstet Gynecol 81:434, 1993.

74. **Van Winter JT, Noller KL, Zimmerman D, Melton LJ,** Natural history of premature thelarche in Olmsted County, Minnesota 1940 to 1984, J Pediatr 116:278, 1990.

75. **Murram D, Dewhurst J, Grant DB,** Premature menarche: a follow-up study, Arch Dis Child 58:142, 1983.

76. **Saenger P, Rester EO,** Premature adrenarche: a normal variant of puberty, J Clin Endocrinol Metab 74:236, 1992.

77. **Morris AH, Reiter EO, Geffner ME, Lippe BM, Itami RM, Mayes DM,** Absence of nonclassical congenital adrenal hyperplasia in patients with precocious adrenarche, J Clin Endocrinol Metab 69:709, 1989.

78. **Ibanez L, Virdis R, Potau N, Zampolli M, Ghizzoni L, Albisu MA, Carrascosa A, Bernasconi S, Vicens-Calvet E,** Natural history of premature pubarche: an auxological study, J Clin Endocrinol Metab 74:254, 1992.

79. **Ibanez L, Potau N, Virdis R, Zampolli M, Terzi C, Gussinye M, Carrascosa A, Vicens-Calvet E,** Postpubertal outcome in girls diagnosed of premature pubarche during childhood: increased frequency of functional ovarian hyperandrogenism, J Clin Endocrinol Metab 76:1599, 1993.

80. **Wheeler MD, Styne DM,** The treatment of precocious puberty, Endocrinol Metab Clin North Am 20:183, 1991.

81. **Manasco PK, Pescovitz OH, Hill SC, Jones JM, Barnes KM, Hench KD, Loriaux DL, Cutler CG,** Six-year results of luteinizing hormone releasing hormone (LHRH) agonist treatment in children with LHRH-dependent precocious puberty, J Pediatr 115:105, 1989.

82. **Cook JS, Doty KL, Conn PM, Hansen JR,** Assessment of depot leuprolide acetate dose adequacy for central precocious puberty, J Clin Endocrinol Metab 74:1206, 1992.

83. **Parker KL, Baine-Bailon RG, Lee PA,** Depot leuprolide acetate dosage for sexual precocity, J Clin Endocrinol Metab 73:50, 1991.

84. **Jay N, Mansfield MJ, Blizzard RM, Crowley WF Jr, Schoenfeld D, Rhubin L, Boepple PA,** Ovulation and menstrual function of adolescent girls with central precocious puberty after therapy with gonadotropin-releasing hormone agonists, J Clin Endocrinol Metab 75:890, 1992.

85. **Mahachoklertwattana P, Kaplan S, Grumbach MM,** The luteinizing hormone-releasing hormone-secreting hypothalamic hamartoma is a congenital malformation: natural history, J Clin Endocrinol Metab 77:118, 1993.

86. **Mansfield MJ, Beardsworth DE, Loughlin JS, Crawford JD, Bode HH, Rivier J, Vale W, Kushner DC, Crigler JF Jr, Crowley WF Jr,** Long-term treatment of central precocious puberty with a long-acting analogue of luteinizing hormone-releasing hormone. effects on somatic growth and skeletal maturation, New Engl J Med 309:1286, 1983.

87. **Pescovitz OH, Comite F, Cassorla F, Dwyer AJ, Poth MA, Sperling MA, Hench K, McNemar A, Skerda M, Loriaux DL, Cutler GB Jr,** True precocious puberty complicating congenital adrenal hyperplasia: treatment with a luteinizing hormone-releasing hormone analog, J Clin Endocrinol Mctab 58:857, 1984.

88. **Murran D, Dewhurst J, Grant DB,** Precocious Puberty: a follow-up study, Arch Dis Child 59:77, 1984.

89. **Reindollar RH, Tho SPT, McDonough PG,** Delayed puberty: an updated study of 326 patients, Trans Am Gynecol Obstet Soc 8:146, 1989.

90. **Thomsett JJ, Conte FA, Kaplan SL, Grumbach MM,** Endocrine and neurologic outcome in childhood craniopharyngioma: review of effect of treatment in 42 patients, J Pediatr 97:728, 1980.

91. **Stanhope R, Pringle PJ, Brook CGD, Adams J, Jacobs HS,** Induction of puberty by pulsatile gonadotropin releasing hormone, Lancet 2:552, 1987.

92. **Bayley N, Pinneau SR,** Tables for predicting adult height from skeletal age: revised for use with the Greulich-Pyle hand standards, J Pediatr 40:423, 1952.

93. **Rogol AD, Yesalis CE III,** Clinical review 31: anabolic-androgenic steroids and athletes: what are the issues? J Clin Endocrinol Metab 74:465, 1992.

94. **DuRant RH, Rickert VI, Ashworth CS, Newman C, Slavens G,** Use of multiple drugs among adolescents who use anabolic steroids, New Engl J Med 328:922, 1993.

95. **Schoen EJ, Solomon IL, Warner D, Wingerd J,** Estrogen treatment of tall girls, Am J Dis Child 125:71, 1973.

96. **Norman H, Wettenhall B, Cahill C, Roche AF,** Tall girls: a survey of 15 years of management and treatment, Adolesc Med 86:602, 1975.

Bayley-Pinneau Table for Average Girls
(J Pediatr 40:423, 1952)

To predict height, find vertical column corresponding to skeletal age and horizontal row for the present height. The number at the intersection is the predicted height in inches. If figures do not fall at the whole inch or 6-month intervals, the predicted height must be extrapolated.

Skeletal Age		6/0	6/6	7/0	7/6	8/0	8/6	9/0	9/6	10/0	10/6	11/0	11/6	12/0
Height in inches	37	51.4												
	38	52.8	51.5											
	39	54.2	52.8	51.5										
	40	55.6	54.2	52.8	51.8									
	41	56.9	55.6	54.2	53.1	51.9								
	42	58.3	56.9	55.5	54.4	53.2	51.9							
	43	59.7	58.3	56.8	55.7	54.4	53.1	52.0						
	44	61.1	59.6	58.1	57.0	55.7	54.3	53.2	52.1	51.0				
	45	62.5	61.0	59.4	58.3	57.0	55.6	54.4	53.3	52.2				
	46	63.9	62.3	60.8	59.6	58.2	56.8	55.6	54.5	53.4	52.0			
	47	65.8	63.7	62.1	60.9	59.5	58.0	56.8	55.7	54.5	53.2	51.9	51.4	51.0
	48	66.7	65.0	63.4	62.2	60.8	59.3	58.0	56.9	55.7	54.3	53.0	52.5	52.1
	49	68.1	66.4	64.7	63.5	62.0	60.5	59.3	58.1	56.8	55.4	54.1	53.6	53.1
	50	69.4	67.8	66.1	64.8	63.3	61.7	60.5	59.2	58.0	56.6	55.2	54.7	54.2
	51	70.8	69.1	67.4	66.1	64.6	63.0	61.7	60.4	59.2	57.7	56.3	55.8	55.3
	52	72.2	70.5	68.7	67.4	65.8	64.2	62.9	61.6	60.3	58.8	57.4	56.9	56.4
	53	73.6	71.8	70.0	68.7	67.1	65.4	64.1	62.8	61.5	60.0	58.5	58.0	57.5
	54		73.2	71.3	69.9	68.4	66.7	65.3	64.0	62.6	61.1	59.6	59.1	58.6
	55		74.5	72.7	71.2	69.6	67.9	66.5	65.2	63.8	62.2	60.7	60.2	59.7
	56			74.0	72.5	70.9	69.1	67.7	66.4	65.0	63.3	61.8	61.3	60.7
	57				73.8	72.2	70.4	68.9	67.5	66.1	64.5	62.9	62.4	61.8
	58					73.4	71.6	70.1	68.7	67.3	65.6	64.0	63.5	62.9
	59					74.7	72.8	71.3	69.9	68.4	66.7	65.1	64.6	64.0
	60						74.1	72.6	71.1	69.6	67.9	66.2	65.6	65.1
	61							73.8	72.3	70.8	69.0	67.3	66.7	66.2
	62								73.5	71.9	70.1	68.4	67.8	67.2
	63								74.6	73.1	71.3	69.5	68.9	68.3
	64									74.2	72.4	70.6	70.0	69.4
	65										73.5	71.7	71.1	70.5
	66										74.7	72.9	72.2	71.6
	67											74.0	73.3	72.7
	68												74.4	73.8
	69													74.8
	70													
	71													
	72													
	73													
	74													

12/6	13/0	13/6	14/0	14/6	15/0	15/6	16/0	16/6	17/0	17/6	18/0	
												37
												38
												39
												40
												41
												42
												43
												44
												45
												46
												47
51.0												48
52.1	51.1											49
53.1	52.2	51.3	51.0									50
54.2	53.2	52.4	52.0	51.7	51.5	51.4	51.2	51.2	51.1	51.0	51.0	51
55.3	54.3	53.4	53.1	52.7	52.5	52.4	52.2	52.2	52.1	52.0	52.0	52
56.3	55.3	54.4	54.1	53.8	53.5	53.4	53.2	53.2	53.1	53.0	53.0	53
57.4	56.4	55.4	55.1	54.8	54.5	54.4	54.2	54.2	54.1	54.0	54.0	54
58.4	57.4	56.5	56.1	55.8	55.6	55.4	55.2	55.2	55.1	55.0	55.0	55
59.5	58.5	57.5	57.1	56.8	56.6	56.4	56.2	56.2	56.1	56.0	56.0	56
60.6	59.5	50.5	50.2	57.0	57.6	57.4	57.2	57.2	57.1	57.0	57.0	57
61.6	60.5	59.5	59.2	58.8	58.6	58.4	58.2	58.2	58.1	58.0	58.0	58
62.7	61.6	60.6	60.2	59.8	59.6	59.4	59.2	59.2	59.1	59.0	59.0	59
63.8	62.6	61.6	61.2	60.9	60.6	60.4	60.2	60.2	60.1	60.0	60.0	60
64.8	63.7	62.6	62.2	61.9	61.6	61.4	61.2	61.2	61.1	61.0	61.0	61
65.9	64.7	63.7	63.3	62.9	62.6	62.4	62.2	62.2	62.1	62.0	62.0	62
67.0	65.8	64.7	64.3	63.9	63.6	63.4	63.3	63.2	63.1	63.0	63.0	63
68.0	66.8	65.7	65.3	64.9	64.6	64.4	64.3	64.2	64.1	64.0	64.0	64
69.1	67.8	66.7	66.3	65.9	65.7	65.5	65.3	65.2	65.1	65.0	65.0	65
70.1	68.9	67.8	67.3	66.9	66.7	66.5	66.3	66.2	66.1	66.0	66.0	66
71.2	69.9	68.8	68.4	68.0	67.7	67.5	67.3	67.2	67.1	67.0	67.0	67
72.3	71.0	69.8	69.4	69.0	68.7	68.5	68.3	68.2	68.1	68.0	68.0	68
73.3	72.0	70.8	70.4	70.0	69.7	69.5	69.3	69.2	69.1	69.0	69.0	69
74.4	73.1	71.9	71.4	71.0	70.7	70.5	70.3	70.2	70.1	70.0	70.0	70
	74.1	72.9	72.4	72.0	71.7	71.5	71.3	71.2	71.1	71.0	71.0	71
		73.9	73.5	73.0	72.7	72.5	72.3	72.2	72.1	72.0	72.0	72
		74.9	74.5	74.0	73.7	73.5	73.3	73.2	73.1	73.0	73.0	73
					74.7	74.5	74.3	74.2	74.1	74.0	74.0	74

Bayley-Pinneau Table for Accelerated Girls

To predict height, find vertical column corresponding to skeletal age and horizontal row for the present height. The number at the intersection is the predicted height in inches. If figures do not fall at the whole inch or 6-month intervals, the predicted height must be extrapolated.

Skeletal Age		7/0	7/6	8/0	8/6	9/0	9/6	10/0	10/6	11/0	11/6	12/0
Height in inches	37	52.0										
	38	53.4	51.9									
	39	54.8	53.3	52.0								
	40	56.2	54.6	53.3	51.9							
	41	57.6	56.0	54.7	53.2	51.9						
	42	59.0	57.4	56.0	54.5	53.2	51.9					
	43	60.4	58.7	57.3	55.8	54.4	53.2	51.9				
	44	61.8	60.1	58.7	57.1	55.7	54.4	53.1	51.4			
	45	63.2	61.5	60.0	58.4	57.0	55.6	54.3	52.6	54.0		
	46	64.6	62.8	61.3	59.7	58.2	56.9	55.6	53.7	52.1	51.6	51.1
	47	66.0	64.2	62.7	61.0	59.5	58.1	56.8	54.9	53.2	52.7	52.2
	48	67.4	65.6	64.0	62.3	60.8	59.3	58.0	56.1	54.4	53.9	53.3
	49	68.8	66.9	65.3	63.6	62.0	60.6	59.2	57.2	55.5	55.0	54.4
	50	70.2	68.3	66.7	64.9	63.3	61.8	60.4	58.4	56.6	56.1	55.5
	51	71.6	69.7	68.0	66.1	64.6	63.0	61.6	59.6	57.8	57.2	56.6
	52	73.0	71.0	69.3	67.4	65.8	64.3	62.8	60.7	58.9	58.4	57.7
	53	74.4	72.4	70.7	68.7	67.1	65.5	64.0	61.9	60.0	59.5	58.8
	54		73.8	72.0	70.0	68.4	66.7	65.2	63.1	61.2	60.6	59.9
	55			73.3	71.3	69.6	68.0	66.4	64.3	62.3	61.7	61.0
	56			74.7	72.6	70.9	69.2	67.6	65.4	63.4	62.8	62.2
	57				73.9	72.2	70.5	68.8	66.6	64.6	64.0	63.3
	58					73.4	71.7	70.0	67.8	65.7	65.1	64.4
	59					74.7	72.9	71.3	68.9	66.8	66.2	65.5
	60						74.2	72.5	70.1	68.0	67.3	66.6
	61							73.7	71.3	69.1	68.5	67.7
	62							74.9	72.4	70.2	69.6	68.8
	63								73.6	71.3	70.7	69.9
	64								74.8	72.5	71.8	71.0
	65									73.6	72.9	72.1
	66									74.7	74.1	73.3
	67											74.4
	68											
	69											
	70											
	71											
	72											
	73											
	74											

12/6	13/0	13/6	14/0	14/6	15/0	15/6	16/0	16/6	17/0	17/6	
											37
											38
											39
											40
											41
											42
											43
											44
											45
											46
											47
51.9											48
53.0	51.9	50.9									49
54.1	52.9	51.9	51.4	51.0							50
55.2	54.0	53.0	52.5	52.0	51.7	51.5	51.4	51.3	51.1	51.0	51
56.3	55.0	54.0	53.5	53.1	52.7	52.5	52.4	52.3	52.1	52.0	52
57.4	56.1	55.0	54.5	54.1	53.8	53.5	53.4	53.3	53.1	53.0	53
58.4	57.1	56.1	55.6	55.1	54.8	54.5	54.4	54.3	54.1	54.0	54
59.5	58.2	57.1	56.6	56.1	55.8	55.5	55.4	55.3	55.1	55.0	55
60.6	59.3	58.2	57.6	57.1	56.8	56.5	56.4	56.3	56.1	56.0	56
61.7	60.3	59.2	58.6	58.2	57.8	57.6	57.4	57.3	57.1	57.0	57
62.8	61.4	60.2	59.7	59.2	58.8	58.6	58.4	58.3	58.1	58.0	58
63.9	62.4	61.3	60.7	60.2	59.8	59.6	59.4	59.3	59.1	59.0	59
64.9	63.5	62.3	61.7	61.2	60.9	60.6	60.4	60.3	60.1	60.0	60
66.0	64.6	63.3	62.8	62.2	61.9	61.6	61.4	61.3	61.1	61.0	61
67.1	65.6	64.4	63.8	63.3	62.9	62.6	62.4	62.3	62.1	62.0	62
68.2	66.7	65.4	64.8	64.3	63.9	63.6	63.4	63.3	63.1	63.0	63
69.3	67.7	66.5	65.8	65.3	64.9	64.6	64.4	64.3	64.1	64.0	64
70.3	68.8	67.5	66.9	66.3	65.9	65.7	65.5	65.3	65.1	65.0	65
71.4	69.8	68.5	67.9	67.3	66.9	66.7	66.5	66.3	66.1	66.0	66
72.5	70.9	69.6	68.9	68.4	68.0	67.7	67.5	67.3	67.1	67.0	67
73.6	72.0	70.6	70.0	69.4	69.0	68.7	68.5	68.3	68.1	68.0	68
74.7	73.0	71.7	71.0	70.4	70.0	69.7	69.5	69.3	69.1	69.0	69
	74.1	72.7	72.0	71.4	71.0	70.7	70.5	70.3	70.1	70.0	70
		73.7	73.0	72.4	72.0	71.7	71.5	71.4	71.1	71.0	71
		74.8	74.1	73.5	73.0	72.7	72.5	72.4	72.1	72.0	72
				74.5	74.0	73.7	73.5	73.4	73.1	73.0	73
						74.4	74.5	74.4	74.1	74.0	74

Bayley-Pinneau Table for Retarded Girls

To predict height, find vertical column corresponding to skeletal age and horizontal row for the present height. The number at the intersection is the predicted height in inches. If figures do not fall at the whole inch or 6-month intervals, the predicted height must be extrapolated.

Skeletal Age		6/0	6/6	7/0	7/6	8/0	8/6	9/0	9/6	10/0	10/6	11/0	11/6
Height in inches	38	51.8											
	39	53.2	51.9										
	40	54.6	53.3	51.9									
	41	55.9	54.6	53.2	52.0								
	42	57.3	55.9	54.5	53.3	52.2	51.0						
	43	58.7	57.3	55.8	54.6	53.5	52.2	51.1					
	44	60.0	58.6	57.1	55.8	54.7	53.5	52.3	51.3				
	45	61.4	59.9	58.4	57.1	56.0	54.7	53.5	52.4	51.5			
	46	62.8	61.3	59.7	58.4	57.2	55.9	54.7	53.6	52.6	51.3		
	47	64.1	62.6	61.0	59.6	58.5	57.1	55.9	54.8	53.8	52.5	51.2	
	48	65.5	63.9	62.3	60.9	59.7	58.3	57.1	55.9	54.9	63.6	52.3	51.8
	49	66.9	65.2	63.6	62.2	60.9	59.5	58.3	57.1	56.1	54.7	53.4	52.9
	50	68.2	66.6	64.9	63.5	62.2	60.8	59.5	58.3	57.2	55.8	54.5	54.0
	51	69.6	67.9	66.2	64.7	63.4	62.0	60.6	59.4	58.4	56.9	55.6	55.1
	52	70.9	69.2	67.5	66.0	64.7	63.2	61.8	60.6	59.5	58.0	56.6	56.2
	53	72.3	70.6	68.8	67.3	65.9	64.4	63.0	61.8	60.6	59.2	57.7	57.2
	54	73.7	71.9	70.1	68.5	67.2	65.6	64.2	62.9	61.8	60.3	58.8	58.3
	55		73.2	71.4	69.8	68.4	66.8	65.4	64.1	62.9	61.4	59.9	59.4
	56		74.6	72.7	71.1	69.7	68.0	66.6	65.3	64.1	62.5	61.0	60.5
	57			74.0	72.3	70.9	69.3	67.8	66.4	65.2	63.6	62.1	61.6
	58				73.6	72.1	70.5	69.0	67.6	66.4	64.7	63.2	62.6
	59				74.9	73.4	71.7	70.2	68.8	67.5	65.8	64.3	63.7
	60					74.6	72.9	71.3	69.9	68.7	67.0	65.4	64.8
	61						74.1	72.5	71.1	69.8	68.1	66.4	65.9
	62							73.7	72.3	70.9	69.2	67.5	67.0
	63							74.7	73.4	72.1	70.3	68.6	68.0
	64								74.6	73.2	71.4	69.7	69.1
	65									74.4	72.5	70.8	70.2
	66										73.7	71.9	71.3
	67										74.8	73.0	72.4
	68											74.1	73.4
	69												74.5
	70												
	71												
	72												
	73												
	74												

12/0	12/6	13/0	13/6	14/0	14/6	15/0	15/6	16/0	16/6	17/0	
											38
											39
											40
											41
											42
											43
											44
											45
											46
											47
51.5											48
52.6	51.6										49
53.6	52.7	51.9	51.2								50
54.7	53.7	52.9	52.2	51.9	51.6	51.3	51.2	51.1	51.1	51.0	51
55.8	54.8	53.9	53.2	52.9	52.6	52.3	52.2	52.1	52.1	52.0	52
56.9	55.8	55.0	54.2	53.9	53.6	53.3	53.2	53.1	53.1	53.0	53
57.9	56.9	56.0	55.3	54.9	54.6	54.3	54.2	54.1	54.1	54.0	54
59.0	58.0	57.1	56.3	56.0	55.6	55.3	55.2	55.1	55.1	55.0	55
60.1	59.0	58.1	57.3	57.0	56.6	56.3	56.2	56.1	56.1	56.0	56
61.2	60.1	59.1	58.3	58.0	57.6	57.3	57.2	57.1	57.1	57.0	57
62.2	61.1	60.2	59.4	59.0	58.6	58.3	58.2	58.1	58.1	58.0	58
63.3	62.2	61.2	60.4	60.0	59.7	59.4	59.2	59.1	59.1	59.0	59
64.4	63.2	62.2	61.4	61.0	60.7	60.4	60.2	60.1	60.1	60.0	60
65.5	64.3	63.3	62.4	62.1	61.7	61.4	61.2	61.1	61.1	61.0	61
66.5	65.3	64.3	63.5	63.1	62.7	62.4	62.2	62.1	62.1	62.0	62
67.6	66.4	65.3	64.5	64.1	63.7	63.4	63.3	63.1	63.1	63.0	63
68.7	67.4	66.4	65.5	65.1	64.7	64.4	64.3	64.1	64.1	64.0	64
69.7	68.5	67.4	66.5	66.1	65.7	65.4	65.3	65.1	65.1	65.0	65
70.8	69.5	68.5	67.6	67.1	66.7	66.4	66.3	66.1	66.1	66.0	66
71.9	70.6	69.5	68.6	68.2	67.7	67.4	67.3	67.1	67.1	67.0	67
73.0	71.7	70.5	69.6	69.2	68.8	68.4	68.3	68.1	68.1	68.0	68
74.0	72.7	71.6	70.6	70.2	69.8	69.4	69.3	69.1	69.1	69.0	69
	73.8	72.6	71.6	71.2	70.8	70.4	70.3	70.1	70.1	70.0	70
	74.8	73.6	72.7	72.2	71.8	71.4	71.3	71.1	71.1	71.0	71
		74.7	73.7	73.3	72.8	72.4	72.3	72.1	72.1	72.0	72
			74.7	74.3	73.8	73.4	73.3	73.1	73.1	73.0	73
					74.8	74.4	74.3	74.1	74.1	74.0	74

12   Amenorrhea

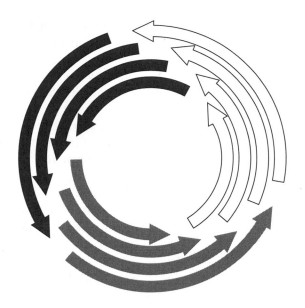

Few problems in gynecologic endocrinology are as challenging or taxing to the clinician as amenorrhea. The physician must be concerned with an array of potential diseases and disorders involving, in many instances, unfamiliar organ systems, some carrying morbid and even lethal consequences for the patient. Not infrequently, the otherwise confident and experienced physician dismisses the problem as too complex for a busy practice and refers the patient to a "specialist" in the field. In doing so, the nonavailability of sophisticated laboratory techniques is often cited as necessitating the costly and frequently inconvenient transfer of the patient.

The intent of this chapter is to provide a simple mechanism for differential diagnosis of amenorrhea of all types and chronology, utilizing procedures available to all physicians. Strict adherence to this design will unerringly pinpoint the organ system locus of disorder leading to the presenting symptom of amenorrhea. Once this is accomplished, the detailed evidence confirming the diagnosis can be sought and the assistance of appropriate specialists (neurosurgeon, internist, endocrinologist, psychiatrist) confidently chosen. In the end, the patient receives the most reliable diagnosis and therapy at minimum cost and optimum convenience. The majority of patients with amenorrhea have relatively simple problems that can be managed easily by the patients' primary care physicians.

The "workup" to be described is not new. With minor modifications, it has been continuously and successfully applied for several decades. Before presenting the diagnostic workup in detail, it is necessary to provide a definition of amenorrhea, designating the appropriate selection of patients. In addition, a brief review of the physiologic mechanisms by which a menstrual flow is produced is presented to clarify the logic of the various steps in the diagnostic procedures.

Definition of Amenorrhea

Any patient fulfilling the following criteria should be evaluated as having the clinical problem of amenorrhea:

1. No period by age 14 in the absence of growth or development of secondary sexual characteristics.

2. No period by age 16 regardless of the presence of normal growth and development with the appearance of secondary sexual characteristics.

3. In a woman who has been menstruating, the absence of periods for a length of time equivalent to a total of at least 3 of the previous cycle intervals or 6 months of amenorrhea.

Having affirmed the traditional criteria, let us now point out that strict adherence to these criteria can result in improper management of individual cases. There is no reason to defer the evaluation of a young girl who presents with the obvious stigmata of Turner syndrome. Similarly, the 14 year old girl with an absent vagina who is otherwise completely normal should not be told to return in 2 years. A patient deserves a considerate evaluation whenever her anxieties, or those of her parents, bring her to a physician. Finally, the possibility of pregnancy should always be considered.

Another tradition has been to categorize amenorrhea as primary or secondary in nature. While these stipulations are inherent in the classic definitions noted above, experience has shown that premature categorization of this sort leads to diagnostic omission in certain instances, and frequently, unnecessary and expensive diagnostic procedures. Because the prescribed workup to be detailed here applies comprehensively to all amenorrheas, the classic definitions are not retained.

Basic Principles in Menstrual Function

The clinical demonstration of menstrual function depends on visible external evidence of the menstrual discharge. This requires an intact outflow tract that connects the internal genital source of flow with the outside. As such, the outflow tract requires patency and continuity of the vaginal orifice, the vaginal canal, and the endocervix with the uterine cavity. The presence of a menstrual flow depends on the existence and development of the endometrium lining the uterine cavity. This tissue is stimulated and regulated by the proper quantity and sequence of the steroid hormones, estrogen and progesterone. The secretion of these hormones originates in the ovary, but more specifically in the evolving spectrum of follicle development, ovulation, and corpus luteum function. This essential maturation of the follicular apparatus is guided by the stimuli provided by the sequence and magnitude of the gonadotropins, follicle-stimulating hormone (FSH) and luteinizing hormone (LH), originating in the anterior pituitary. The secretion of these hormones is in turn dependent upon gonadotropin releasing hormone (GnRH), the specific peptide releasing hormone produced in the basal hypothalamus and blood borne via the portal vessels of the stalk to receptive cells within the anterior pituitary. The entire system is regulated by a complex mechanism which integrates biophysical and biochemical information comprised of interactive levels of hormonal signals, autocrine/paracrine factors, and target cell receptor function in the uterus, ovary, pituitary, hypothalamus, and other central nervous system (CNS) sources.

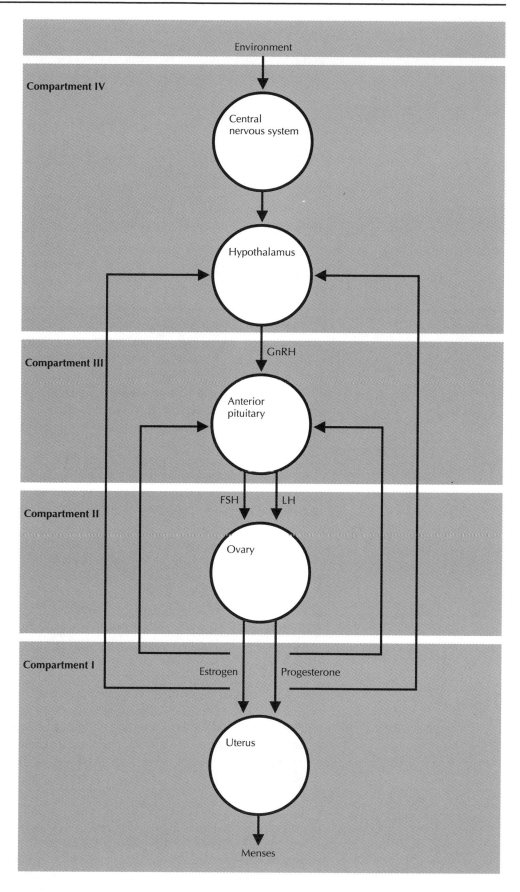

The basic principles underlying the physiology of menstrual function permit formulation of several discrete compartmental systems on which proper menstruation depends. It is useful to employ a diagnostic evaluation that segregates causes of amenorrhea into the following compartments:

Compartment I:
Disorders of the outflow tract or uterine target organ.

Compartment II:
Disorders of the ovary.

Compartment III:
Disorders of the anterior pituitary.

Compartment IV:
Disorders of CNS (hypothalamic) factors.

Evaluation of Amenorrhea

A careful history and physical examination should seek the following: evidence for psychological dysfunction or emotional stress, family history of apparent genetic anomalies, signs of a physical problem with a focus on nutritional status, abnormal growth and development, the presence of a normal reproductive tract, and evidence for CNS disease. A patient with amenorrhea is then exposed to a combined therapeutic and laboratory dissection according to the depicted flow diagrams. Because a significant number of patients with amenorrhea also have galactorrhea (nonpuerperal breast secretion), and there are similarities in the evaluation of these two conditions, the workup as described is appropriate for patients who have amenorrhea, galactorrhea, or both. Galactorrhea is an important clinical physical sign, whether it is spontaneous or present only with careful expression by the examiner, unilateral or bilateral, persistent or intermittent. Galactorrhea is also considered in Chapter 17.

Amenorrhea and galactorrhea need be the sole pertinent initial items of information. Although additional data are undoubtedly available at this time, derived from history and physical examination and evaluation of other endocrine glands such as the thyroid and adrenal, these items should not be utilized for diagnostic purposes until the entire workup is completed. Experience has shown that premature diagnostic bias at this point, while frequently accurate, not uncommonly leads to erroneous judgments as well as inappropriate, costly, and useless testing.

Step 1

The initial step in the workup of the amenorrheic patient after excluding pregnancy begins with a measurement of thyroid-stimulating hormone (TSH), a prolactin level, and a progestational challenge. The initial step in the patient presenting with galactorrhea, regardless of menstrual history, also includes TSH and prolactin measurement but adds a coned-down, lateral x-ray view of the sella turcica. The x-ray can be safely omitted in those patients who have galactorrhea, but also have regular, ovulatory menstrual cycles.

Only a few patients presenting with amenorrhea and/or galactorrhea will have hypothyroidism which is not clinically apparent. Although it seems rather extravagant to measure TSH in such a large number of patients for such a small return, because treatment for hypothyroidism is so simple and is rewarded by such a prompt return of ovulatory cycles, and, if galactorrhea is present, by a disappearance of the breast secretions (a slower process that can take several months), TSH measurement is warranted.

The duration of the hypothyroidism is important with regard to the mechanism of the galactorrhea; the longer the duration the higher the incidence of galactorrhea and the higher the prolactin levels.[1] This is thought to be associated with declining hypothalamic content of dopamine with on-going hypothyroidism. This would lead to an unopposed thyrotropin-releasing hormone (TRH) stimulatory effect on the pituitary cells which secrete prolactin. In our experience, prolactin levels associated with primary hypothyroidism have always been less than 100 ng/mL (4,440 pmol/L).

Constant stimulation by hypothalamic releasing hormones can result in hypertrophy or hyperplasia of the pituitary. The x-ray picture of a tumor (distortion, expansion, or erosion of the sella turcica) can be seen, therefore, with primary hypothyroidism and in patients with elevated GnRH and gonadotropin secretion due to premature ovarian failure.[2] Patients with primary hypothyroidism and hyperprolactinemia can present with either primary or secondary amenorrhea.[3]

The purpose of the progestational challenge is to assess the level of endogenous estrogen and the competence of the outflow tract. A course of a progestational agent totally devoid of estrogenic activity is administered. There are two choices: parenteral progesterone in oil (200 mg) or orally active medroxyprogesterone acetate, 10 mg daily for 5 days. The usc of an orally active agent avoids an unpleasant intramuscular injection (although this might be necessary when compliance is a concern). Other hormonal preparations, such as oral contraceptives, are not appropriate since they do not exert a purely progestational effect.

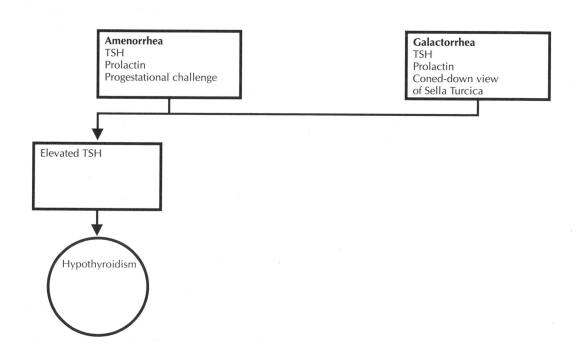

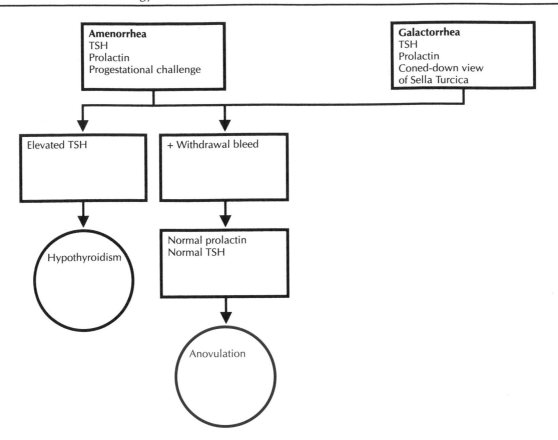

Within 2–7 days after the conclusion of progestational medication, the patient will either bleed or not bleed. If the patient bleeds, a diagnosis of anovulation has been reliably and securely established. The presence of a functional outflow tract and a uterus lined by reactive endometrium sufficiently prepared by endogenous estrogen is confirmed. With this demonstration of the presence of estrogen, minimal function of the ovary, pituitary, and CNS is established. In the absence of galactorrhea, with a normal prolactin level, and a normal TSH, further evaluation is unnecessary.

How much bleeding constitutes a positive withdrawal response? The appearance of only a few blood spots following progestational medication implies marginal levels of endogenous estrogen. Such patients should be followed closely and periodically re-evaluated, since the marginally positive response may progress to a clearly negative response, placing the patient in a new diagnostic category. Bleeding in any amount beyond a few spots is considered a positive withdrawal response.

There are two rare situations associated with a negative withdrawal response despite the presence of adequate levels of endogenous estrogen. In both situations, the endometrium is decidualized, and therefore it will not be shed following the withdrawal of exogenous progestin. The first condition finds the endometrium decidualized in response to high androgen levels, e.g., due to the anovulatory state (with polycystic ovaries). In the second unusual clinical situation, the endometrium is decidualized by high progesterone levels associated with a specific adrenal enzyme deficiency.

All anovulatory patients require therapeutic management, and with this minimal evaluation, therapy can be planned immediately. Because of the short latent period in the progression from normal endometrial tissue to atypia to cancer, clinicians are sensitive to the issue of endometrial cancer. But all too often, the clinician believes that this is a problem limited to older age. The critical feature is the duration of exposure to constant, unopposed estrogen. Therefore even young women, anovulatory for relatively long periods of time, can develop endometrial cancer. If there is any concern, evaluation of the endometrium (with aspiration curettage) is in order. On the other hand, the latent phase for breast cancer is long, perhaps as long as 20 years. It is only recently that data have emerged indicating that women who are anovulatory when they are young may have an increased risk of breast cancer when they are postmenopausal.[4] This could reflect exposure to unopposed estrogen or it could be the consequence of infertility and the absence of the protection against breast cancer that pregnancy early in the reproductive years confers. However, some studies have not observed a link between anovulation and the risk of breast cancer (discussed with full references in Chapter 17).

Minimal therapy of anovulatory women requires the monthly administration of a progestational agent. An easily remembered program is to prescribe 10 mg medroxyprogesterone acetate daily for the first 10 days of each month. Experience with the endometrium in estrogen therapy programs has established the importance of a time period of at least 10 days to provide adequate protection against the growth promoting effects of constant estrogen. When reliable contraception is essential, the use of low dose oral contraceptive pills in the usual cyclic fashion is appropriate. Attempts to demonstrate a relationship between pill use and subsequent postpill amenorrhea have not been successful. Anovulation with amenorrhea or oligomenorrhea should not be viewed as a contraindication to the use of oral contraception.

If, at any time, an anovulatory patient fails to have withdrawal bleeding on a monthly progestin program, this is a sign (providing the patient is not pregnant) that she has moved to the negative withdrawal bleed category, and the remainder of the workup must be pursued. The progestational challenge will occasionally trigger an ovulation in an anovulatory patient. The tip-off will be a later withdrawal bleed, 14 days after the progestational challenge!

In the absence of galactorrhea and if the serum prolactin level is normal (less than 20 ng/mL [888 pmol/L] in most laboratories), further evaluation for a pituitary tumor is unnecessary provided the patient has undergone a withdrawal bleed. Random single samples for prolactin are sufficient, because variations in the amplitude of the spikes of secretion and the sleep-related and food-related increases appear to be attenuated in both functional and tumor hyperprolactinemic states. If the prolactin is elevated, imaging evaluation of the sella turcica is essential (as discussed below). At this point in the workup, the following statement is a useful clinical rule of thumb: *A positive withdrawal bleeding response to progestational medication, the absence of galactorrhea, and a normal prolactin level together effectively rule out the presence of a significant pituitary tumor.*

Ectopic production of prolactin is rarely encountered. Increased prolactin secretion should draw attention to the pituitary gland. However, to be complete, we should mention case reports with ectopic secretion associated with pituitary tissue in the pharynx, bronchogenic carcinoma, renal cell carcinoma, a gonadoblastoma, and a woman with amenorrhea and hyperprolactinemia due to a prolactinoma in the wall of an ovarian dermoid cyst.[5,6]

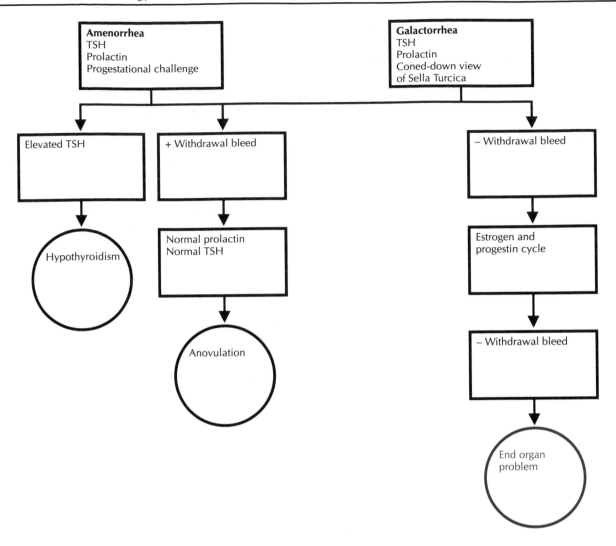

Step 2

If the course of progestational medication does not produce withdrawal flow, either the target organ outflow tract is inoperative or preliminary estrogen proliferation of the endometrium has not occurred. Step 2 is designed to clarify this situation. Orally active estrogen is administered in quantity and duration certain to stimulate endometrial proliferation and withdrawal bleeding provided that a completely reactive uterus and patent outflow tract exist. An appropriate dose is 1.25 mg conjugated estrogens daily for 21 days. The terminal addition of an orally active progestational agent (medroxyprogesterone acetate 10 mg daily for the last 5 days) is necessary to achieve withdrawal. In this way the capacity of Compartment I is challenged by exogenous estrogen. In the absence of withdrawal flow, a validating second course of estrogen is a wise precaution.

As a result of the pharmacologic test of Step 2, the patient with amenorrhea will either bleed or not bleed. If there is no withdrawal flow, the diagnosis of a defect in the Compartment I systems (endometrium, outflow tract) can be made with confidence. If withdrawal bleeding does occur, one can assume that Compartment I systems have normal functional abilities if properly stimulated by estrogen.

From a practical point of view, in a patient with normal external and internal genitalia by pelvic examination, and in the absence of a history of infection or trauma (such as curettage), an abnormality of the outflow tract is unlikely. Outflow tract problems include either destruction of the endometrium, generally the result of an overzealous curettage or the result of an infection, or primary amenorrhea resulting from the discontinuity or disruption of the müllerian tube. ***Abnormalities in the systems of Compartment I are not commonly encountered, and in the absence of a reason to suspect a problem, Step 2 can be omitted.***

Step 3

With the elucidation of the amenorrheic patient's inability to provide adequate stimulatory amounts of estrogen, the physiologic mechanisms responsible for the elaboration of this steroid must be tested. In order to produce estrogen, ovaries containing a normal follicular apparatus and sufficient pituitary gonadotropins to stimulate that apparatus are required. Step 3 is designed to determine which of these two crucial components (gonadotropins or follicular activity) is functioning improperly.

This step involves an assay of the level of gonadotropins in the patient. Because Step 2 involved administration of exogenous estrogen, endogenous gonadotropin levels may be artificially and temporarily altered from their true baseline concentrations. Hence, a delay of 2 weeks following Step 2 must ensue before doing Step 3, the gonadotropin assay. One should keep in mind that the midcycle surge of LH is approximately 3 times the baseline level. Therefore, if the patient does not bleed 2 weeks after the blood sample was obtained, a high level can be safely interpreted as abnormal.

Step 3 is designed to determine whether the lack of estrogen is due to a fault in the follicle (Compartment II) or in the CNS-pituitary axis (Compartments III and IV). The result of the gonadotropin assay in the amenorrheic woman who does not bleed following a progestational agent will be abnormally high, abnormally low, or in the normal range.

Clinical State	Serum FSH	Serum LH
Normal adult female	5–30 IU/L, with the ovulatory midcycle peak about 2 times the base level	5–20 IU/L, with the ovulatory midcycle peak about 3 times the base level
Hypogonadotropic state: Prepubertal, hypothalamic and pituitary dysfunction	Less than 5 IU/L	Less than 5 IU/L
Hypergonadotropic state: Postmenopausal, castrate and ovarian failure	Greater than 30 IU/L	Greater than 40 IU/L

High Gonadotropins

The association between castrate or postmenopausal levels of gonadotropins and ovarian failure is very reliable. However, there are rare situations in which high gonadotropins can be accompanied by ovaries that contain follicles.

1. On rare occasions, tumors can produce gonadotropins. This situation is usually associated with lung cancer and is so infrequent that, with a normal history and physical examination, routine chest x-ray is not warranted in amenorrheic patients.

2. There have been a handful of reports of a single gonadotropin deficiency. The importance of measuring both FSH and LH can be appreciated since a high level of one and a baseline level of the other would reveal this rare condition.

3. Elevated gonadotropins can be due to a gonadotropin-secreting pituitary adenoma. However, gonadotropin-secreting adenomas are not associated with hypogonadism (amenorrhea) and, therefore, are hard to diagnose.[7–9] There is no specific symptom or symptom complex associated with hypersecretion of gonadotropins. Thus, these tumors are usually diagnosed because of tumor growth that results in headaches and visual disturbances. Previously it was believed that these tumors were very rare and more common in men. This belief was due to the difficulty in recognizing these adenomas, especially in women. However, tumors of the pituitary are relatively common, and most are not nonsecreting, but in fact they arise from gonadotroph cells and they are active.[10] In addition to secreting FSH and, rarely, LH, these tumors secrete high levels of the α-subunit of the glycopeptide hormones, and sometimes only the α-subunit. Patients suspected of having pituitary tumors should have their gonadotropin and α-subunit levels measured. Gonadotropin-secreting tumors usually require surgery, but they may respond to bromocriptine.[7]

4. During the perimenopausal period it is normal for FSH levels to begin to rise even before bleeding has ceased.[11] This is true whether the perimenopausal period is premature at age 25–35 or at the usual time. This increase in FSH is associated with a decrease in inhibin. During the perimenopausal period the remaining follicles may be viewed as the least sensitive of all follicles because they have remained in place and failed to respond to gonadotropins for many years. The rise in FSH prior to menopause is due to the declining inhibin production by the less competent ovarian follicles. Attention must be paid to this situation because a period of elevated levels of FSH can be followed by a pregnancy. The value of measuring both FSH and LH is again emphasized because this special perimenopausal condition is associated with a high FSH but a normal LH.

5. In the resistant or insensitive ovary syndrome the patient with amenorrhea has elevated gonadotropins despite the presence of ovarian follicles. It is believed that this condition represents an absence of gonadotropin receptors on the follicles or a postreceptor signaling defect.[12] In these cases laparotomy is the only definitive way to evaluate the ovaries, because follicles are contained deep within the ovary, yielding only to a full thickness biopsy.[13] Because this condition is very rare, and the chance of achieving pregnancy is probably impossible even with large doses of exogenous gonadotropins, laparotomy is *not* recommended for every patient with amenorrhea and high gonadotropins. One might consider the use

of transvaginal ultrasonography, and if follicles can be definitely outlined by the ultrasonographer, stimulation can be attempted with exogenous gonadotropins.

6. Secondary amenorrhea caused by premature ovarian failure can be due to autoimmune disease.[14] The ovaries contain normal-appearing primordial follicles, but developing follicles contain lymphocytes and plasma cells in the theca cell and granulosa cell layers. Most commonly, evidence of abnormal thyroid function is detected, and therefore, complete thyroid testing (with antibodies) is necessary in all patients with premature ovarian failure. The extensive polyglandular syndrome that includes hypoparathyroidism, adrenal insufficiency, thyroiditis, and moniliasis is rare. Other rare conditions associated with premature ovarian failure include myasthenia gravis, idiopathic thrombocytopenic purpura, rheumatoid arthritis, vitiligo, and autoimmune hemolytic anemia. Classically premature ovarian failure precedes adrenal failure, and thus a case can be made for continuing adrenal surveillance. Frequently, various endocrine disorders will be present among family members. Very rare pregnancies have been reported in women with ovarian failure and autoimmune disease, Ovulation has been restored temporarily with corticosteroid treatment, and at least one patient had a temporary spontaneous return of menstrual ovarian activity.[15] Because pregnancy is extremely unlikely, consideration should be given to donor oocytes. However, an impressive pregnancy rate has been reported by one group combining suppression with a GnRH agonist, corticosteroid treatment, and induction of ovulation with high doses of exogenous gonadotropins.[16]

7. In patients with galactosemia, an abnormal carbohydrate component of the gonadotropin molecules may render FSH and LH inactive.[17] On the other hand, the problem in patients with galactosemia may be primarily gonadal; fewer oogonia may be the result of a direct effect of galactose on germ cell migration to the genital ridge.[18]

8. The final rare clinical situation associated with high gonadotropins is the patient with an enzymatic deficiency in both ovaries and the adrenal gland, the 17-hydroxylase deficiency (P450c17). A patient with a deficiency of 17-hydroxylase is readily detectable because she would present with absent secondary sexual development (sex steroids cannot be produced due to the enzyme block in the adrenal glands and the ovaries), and hypertension, hypokalemia, and high blood levels of progesterone.

The Need for Chromosome Evaluation

All patients under the age of 30 who have been assigned the diagnosis of ovarian failure on the basis of elevated gonadotropins must have a karyotype determination. The presence of mosaicism with a Y chromosome requires excision of the gonadal areas because the presence of any testicular component within the gonad carries with it a significant chance of malignant tumor formation. These are highly malignant secondary tumors from germ cells: gonadoblastomas, dysgerminomas, yolk sac tumors, and choriocarcinoma. Approximately 30% of patients with a Y chromosome will not develop signs of virilization. Therefore, even the normal appearing adult woman with elevated gonadotropin levels must be karyotyped. Even if the karyotype is normal, as an added precaution all patients with ovarian failure should have an annual pelvic examination. Such preventive care is also indicated because these patients will be on hormone therapy. Over the age of 30, amenorrhea with high gonadotropins is best labeled premature menopause. Genetic evaluation is unnecessary because it is essentially unheard of to have a gonadal tumor appear in these patients after the age of 30. These tumors usually appear before age 20.[19]

The clinician and patient should give consideration to whether it is worth obtaining an expensive karyotype to seek identification of chromosomal abnormalities that have clinical implications for other family members. Deletions of the X chromosome can be responsible for premature ovarian failure. Accurate diagnosis of these deletions is not essential for decision-making regarding the patient; however, the presence of such abnormalities within a family is associated with infertility due to premature ovarian failure. Having this information can influence the family planning decisions of family members. We recommend that women with premature ovarian failure who are less than 63 inches tall (160 cm) be karyotyped because of the close conjunction of the genes responsible for stature and normal ovarian function.

Premature Ovarian Failure: A Clinical Dilemma

Patients with elevated gonadotropin levels can be reliably diagnosed as having ovarian failure and can be considered sterile. In the past this was a diagnosis made with great confidence, and careful explanation was given to the patient indicating that future pregnancy was impossible. However, rare cases have been reported of patients presenting with secondary amenorrhea and elevated gonadotropins who several months later demonstrated resumption of normal function.[20,21] This has been associated with the use of estrogen therapy, suggesting that the estrogen may activate receptor formation on follicles, and the high gonadotropins may thus stimulate follicular growth and development. On the other hand, temporary recovery of ovarian function may be the reason for apparent success with treatment. In some patients, return of normal ovarian function with pregnancy has occurred spontaneously. While resumption of normal function is extremely rare, it is now necessary to tell patients who fit into this category that there is a very remote possibility of future pregnancy (but it should be emphasized this is very unlikely). In addition the feasibility of pregnancy with the transfer of a fertilized donated ovum should be presented as a possible option (Chapter 31).

Because a number of cases of ovarian failure have been reported with autoimmune disorders, a reasonable approach is to perform a few selected blood tests for autoimmune disease:

Calcium
Phosphorus
A.M. cortisol
Free T_4
TSH
Thyroid antibodies
Complete blood count and sedimentation rate
Total protein, albumin:globulin ratio
Rheumatoid factor
Antinuclear antibody

Testing for ACTH reserve (with metyrapone, see Chapter 33) seems debatable if clinical appearance and other laboratory tests are normal. Periodic surveillance for adrenal failure is in order because ovarian failure usually precedes adrenal failure.

It has been suggested that blood gonadotropins and estradiol should be measured weekly on 4 occasions.[21] If FSH is not higher than LH (an FSH:LH ratio less than 1.0), and if estradiol is greater than 50 pg/mL (180 pmol/L), induction of ovulation can be considered. Prior to treatment with exogenous gonadotropins, there may be some advantage to first bring the elevated gonadotropins down to normal range with administration of

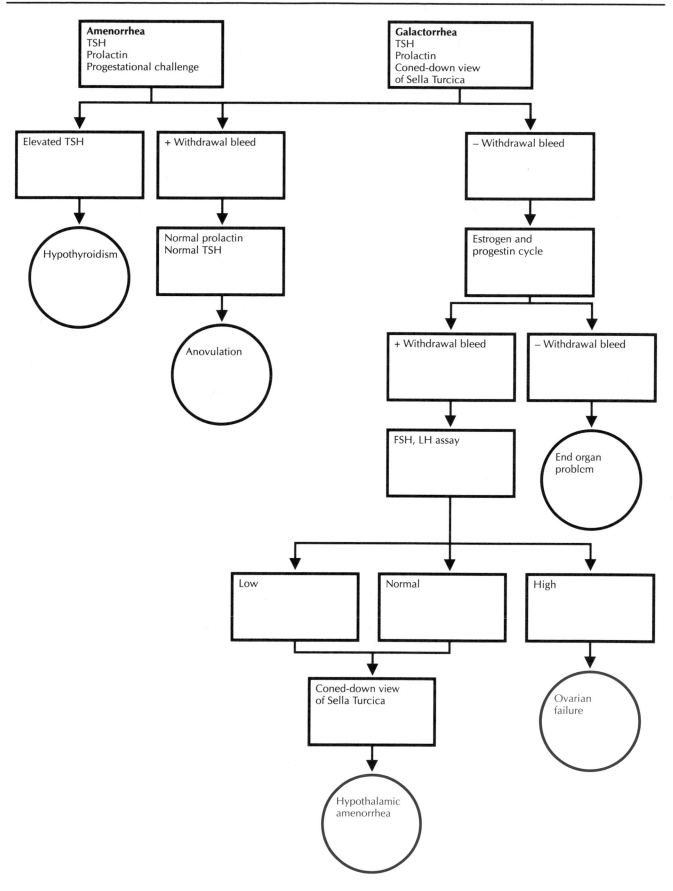

estrogen or a GnRH agonist. However, the experience with this approach has been unrewarding.

It seems appropriate to offer the patient a choice between a full thickness ovarian biopsy and empirical treatment. In our view, empirical treatment appears to outweigh the cost and risk of laparotomy, since only a very rare woman with hypergonadotropic amenorrhea can be expected to conceive. In other words, even if there is some gonadotropic and estradiol evidence of follicular activity, the response to exogenous gonadotropin stimulation has been very disappointing.

Transvaginal ultrasonography can identify ovarian follicular activity in some of these patients. However, the meaning of this finding is uncertain. Are patients with ovarian follicles present on ultrasonography more likely to respond to treatment and achieve pregnancy? In time, clinical studies should provide us with an answer.

This clinical problem requires scientific study. Ovarian failure may be the consequence of more than one abnormal condition. One recognized example is ovarian failure due to an accelerated rate of follicular atresia leading to the premature depletion of the follicular supply. Other cases may be due to a failure in the gonadotropin receptor mechanism. Unsuccessful binding can be due to defective receptors, blockage of receptors (e.g., by autoantibodies), or to genetic mutations that direct the production of gonadotropins of altered structure which are incapable of binding. Molecular studies of these patients should bring important clinical clarification in the coming years.

Normal Gonadotropins

Why is it that hypoestrogenic (negative progestational withdrawal) patients will frequently have normal circulating levels of FSH and LH as measured by immunoassay? If normal gonadotropins were truly present in the circulation, follicular growth should be maintained and estrogen levels would be adequate to provide a positive withdrawal bleed. The answer to this paradox lies in the heterogeneity of the glycoprotein hormones (as discussed in Chapter 2).

The molecules of gonadotropins produced by these amenorrheic patients have increased amounts of sialic acid in the carbohydrate portion. Therefore, the molecules are qualitatively altered and biologically inactive. The antibodies in the immunoassay, however, are able to recognize a sufficient portion of the molecule to return a normal answer. Another very rare possibility is an inherited disorder of gonadotropin synthesis leading to the production of immunologically active but biologically inactive hormones.[22]

The significant clinical point is the following: FSH and LH levels in the normal range in a patient with a negative progestational withdrawal test are consistent with pituitary-CNS failure. Indeed, this is the most commonly encountered clinical situation. Extremely low or nondetectable gonadotropins are seldom found, usually only with large pituitary tumors or in patients with anorexia nervosa. Further evaluation, therefore, is in order and follows the recommendations for low gonadotropins.

Low Gonadotropins

If the gonadotropin assay is abnormally low, or in the normal range, one final localization is required to distinguish between a pituitary (Compartment III) or CNS-hypothalamic (Compartment IV) cause for the amenorrhea. This is achieved by imaging evaluation of the sella turcica for signs of abnormal change.

Imaging of the Sella Turcica

The diagnostic modality of choice is either thin section coronal computerized tomography (CT scan) with intravenous contrast enhancement or magnetic resonance imaging (MRI). CT scanning (capable of high resolution 1 mm cuts) is able to evaluate the contents of the sella turcica as well as the suprasellar area; however, total accuracy is not achieved.[23] Magnetic resonance imaging is even more sensitive than the CT scan, but it is also more expensive, and it requires a lengthy period of time to obtain the images. MRI provides highly accurate assessments without biologic hazard, and it is better for evaluation of extrasellar extensions and the empty sella turcica.[24] Most neuroradiologists and neurosurgeons prefer MRI, as do we. The intention of this workup is to be conscious of cost and to isolate those few patients who require sophisticated but expensive imaging.

There has been growing conservatism in the management of small prolactin-secreting pituitary tumors because of an appreciation that the majority of these tumors never change.[25,26] We have adopted the conservative approach of close surveillance, recommending dopamine agonist treatment for those tumors that display rapid growth, or those tumors which are already large, and reserving surgery only for those tumors that are unresponsive to medical therapy. This means that small tumors (microadenomas are less than 10 mm in diameter) need not be treated at all. Hence, the initial x-ray evaluation for amenorrheic patients with or without galactorrhea is the coned-down lateral view of the sella turcica. This will detect the presence of a large tumor, although an incredibly rare suprasellar extension might escape this method. The coned-down lateral view of the sella is also a good screen for other lesions, such as a craniopharyngioma. Combining this screening technique with the prolactin assay, we are able to select those few patients who require more sensitive sellar imaging. If the prolactin level is greater than 100 ng/mL (4,440 pmol/L), or if the coned-down view of the sella turcica is abnormal, we recommend CT scan evaluation or MRI. *A double floor of the sella is often seen on the coned-down view and, in the absence of enlargement and/or demineralization, is interpreted as a normal variation rather than asymmetrical depression of the sellar floor by a tumor.*

The presence of visual problems and/or headaches should also encourage CT scan or MRI evaluation. Headaches are definitely correlated with the presence of a pituitary adenoma.[27] Although they are usually bifrontal, retroorbital, or bitemporal, no locations or features are specific for pituitary tumors.

The prolactin level of 100 ng/mL (4,440 pmol/L) for determining a more aggressive approach has been empirically chosen. Both in our own experience, and that of others, large tumors are most frequently associated with prolactin levels greater than 100. *Large masses associated with prolactin levels less than 100 ng/mL are more likely to be tumors other than prolactin-secreting adenomas, causing stalk compression and interruption of the normal dopamine regulation of prolactin secretion. These tumors will be associated with abnormal changes present in the coned-down view of the sella turcica.*

If imaging rules out an empty sella syndrome, or a suprasellar problem, treatment is dictated by the patient's desires, the size of the tumor, and the rapidity of growth of the tumor.

The above approach to the problem of pituitary tumors implies that patients with prolactin levels less than 100 ng/mL and with normal coned-down views of the sella turcica can be offered a choice between treatment and surveillance. An annual prolactin level and a periodic coned-down view (at first annually, then at increasing intervals) are indicated for continued observation to detect an emerging and slow-growing tumor.

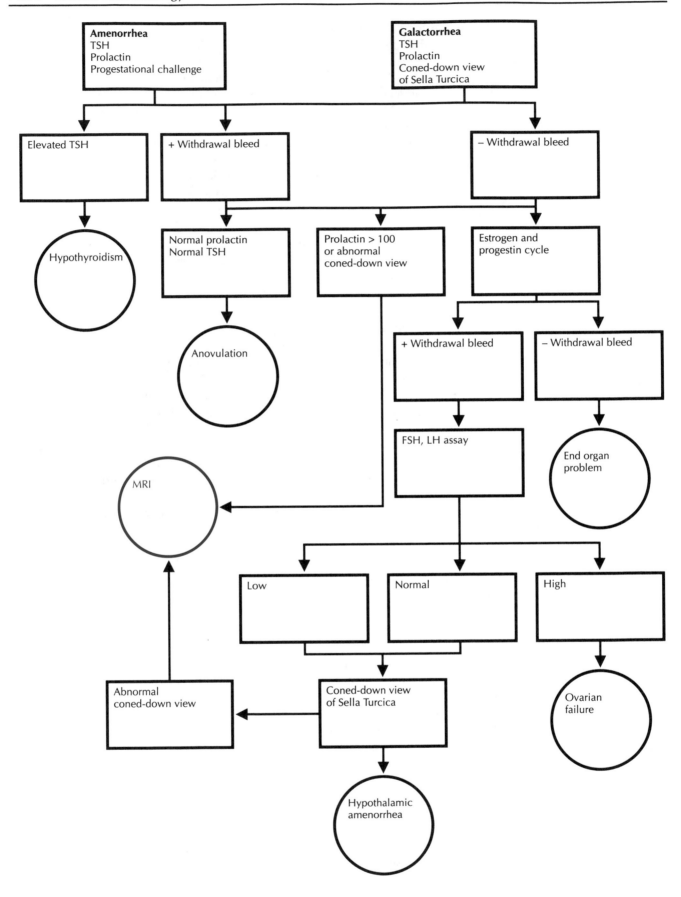

Dopamine agonist therapy is recommended for patients wishing to achieve pregnancy and for those patients who have galactorrhea to the point of discomfort. Thus far, long-term therapy with a dopamine agonist has not been proven to be successful in producing a complete reversal of the problem (with either permanent suppression of elevated prolactin levels or elimination of small tumors). Thus, a very strong argument can be made for a "need not to know" the presence of a pituitary microadenoma. If treatment and management are not changed, it is not necessary to document the presence of a microadenoma.

Reasons Why the Diagnosis of Microadenoma Is Not Necessary
1. Very common occurrence.
2. Very rarely grow during pregnancy.
3. Significant recurrence rate after surgery.
4. Natural course unaffected by dopamine agonist treatment.
5. No contraindication to hormone therapy or oral contraception.

Evaluation of the Abnormal Sella Turcica and/or High Prolactin
The high incidence of pituitary tumors in patients with amenorrhea has prompted a search for a reliable method of diagnosing the condition. Expectations for the utilization of endocrine testing to discriminate between disorders of the hypothalamus and the anterior pituitary have not been realized. These endocrine maneuvers include GnRH stimulation, TRH stimulation, and other steps to alter prolactin, growth hormone, and ACTH secretion. TRH stimulation of the prolactin response is the most consistently abnormal response (a blunter response of prolactin), but some patients with tumors respond normally. Variability in response to all maneuvers is the rule.

Frankly, the endocrine maneuvers yield no more useful information than the two major screening procedures, the blood prolactin and the coned-down view of the sella turcica. Visual field examination is not useful in screening for pituitary tumors because abnormalities are seen only with large tumors which are evident by prolactin, x-ray evaluation, and/or visual symptoms and headaches.

If the coned-down view is abnormal and/or the prolactin level is over 100, further evaluation and treatment require consultation with expert endocrine resources. These patients are rare, and accumulated experience which can provide the necessary clinical judgment can be found only with the referral resource. On the other hand, our workup easily deals with the vast majority of patients, and the few who require a multi-disciplinary team approach are readily identified.

Hypogonadotropic Hypogonadism

Patients with amenorrhea and without galactorrhea who have reached this point in the workup and have normal x-rays are classified as *hypothalamic amenorrhea.* The mechanism of the amenorrhea is suppression of pulsatile GnRH secretion below its critical range. This is a diagnosis by exclusion because we can identify probable causes (e.g., anorexia and weight loss) but we cannot test, manipulate, or measure the hypothalamus to prove our diagnosis.

Specific Disorders within Compartments

With only modest effort, expense, and time the problem of amenorrhea has been dissected into compartments of dysfunction which positively correlate with specific organ systems. At this point, with the specific anatomic locus of the defect defined, the clinician can now undertake steps to elucidate the specific disorder leading to amenorrhea. Congenital abnormalities are limited to amenorrhea that presents in the pubertal period of life. In a collection of 262 patients with secondary amenorrhea of adult onset, the following diagnostic frequencies were most often observed:[28]

Compartment I	
Asherman's syndrome	7.0%
Compartment II	
Abnormal chromosomes	0.5%
Normal chromosomes	10.0%
Compartment III	
Prolactin tumors	7.5%
Compartment IV	
Anovulation	28.0%
Weight loss/anorexia	10.0%
Hypothalamic suppression	10.0%
Hypothyroidism	1.0%

Compartment I: Disorders of the Outflow Tract or Uterus

Asherman's Syndrome

Secondary amenorrhea follows destruction of the endometrium (Asherman's syndrome).[29] This condition generally is the result of an overzealous postpartum curettage resulting in intrauterine scarification. A typical pattern of multiple synechiae is seen on a hysterogram. Diagnosis by hysteroscopy is more accurate and will detect minimal adhesions that are not apparent on a hysterogram. In the presence of normal ovarian function, the basal body temperature will be biphasic. The adhesions may partially or completely obliterate the endometrial cavity, the internal cervical os, the cervical canal, or combinations of these areas. Surprisingly, despite stenosis or atresia of the internal os, hematometra does not inevitably occur. The endometrium, perhaps in response to a buildup of pressure, becomes refractory, and simple cervical dilatation cures the problem. Asherman's syndrome also can occur following uterine surgery, including cesarean section, myomectomy, or metroplasty. Very severe adhesions have been noted following postpartum curettage and postpartum hypogonadism, e.g., in Sheehan's syndrome.

Patients with Asherman's syndrome can present with other problems besides amenorrhea, including abortions, dysmenorrhea, or hypomenorrhea. They can even have normal menses. Infertility can be present with mild adhesions, an association not readily explainable. Patients with repeated abortions, infertility, or pregnancy wastage should have investigation of the endometrial cavity by hysterogram or hysteroscopy.

Impairment of the endometrium resulting in amenorrhea can be caused by tuberculosis, a condition that is rare in the United States. Diagnosis is made by culture of the menstrual discharge or tissue obtained by endometrial biopsy. Uterine schistosomiasis is another rare cause of end organ failure, and eggs may be found in urine, feces, rectal scrapings, menstrual discharge, or endometrium. We have seen the syndrome following intrauterine device (IUD)-related infections and severe, generalized pelvic infections.

Asherman's syndrome in the past was treated with a dilatation and curettage to break up the synechiae and, if necessary, an on-the-table hysterogram to ensure a free uterine cavity. Hysteroscopy with direct lysis of adhesions by cutting, cautery, or laser yields better results than the "blind" dilatation and curettage. Following operation, a method should be utilized to prevent the sides of the uterine cavity from adhering. Previously an IUD was used for this purpose; however, a pediatric Foley catheter appears to be a better option. The bag is filled with 3 ml fluid, and the catheter is removed after 7 days. A broad-spectrum antibiotic is started preoperatively and maintained for 10 days. An inhibitor of prostaglandin synthesis can be used if uterine cramping is a problem. The patient is treated for 2 months with high stimulatory doses of estrogen (e.g., conjugated estrogens 2.5 mg daily 3 weeks out of 4 with medroxyprogesterone acetate 10 mg daily added during the 3rd week). When the initial attempt fails to re-establish menstrual flow, repeated attempts are worthwhile. Persistent treatment with repeated procedures may be necessary to regain reproductive potential. Approximately 70–80% of patients with this condition have achieved a successful pregnancy. Pregnancy is frequently complicated, however, by premature labor, placenta accreta, placenta previa, and/or postpartum hemorrhage.

Müllerian Anomalies

In primary amenorrheas, discontinuity by segmental disruptions of the müllerian tube should be ruled out. Thus, imperforate hymen, obliteration of the vaginal orifice, and lapses in continuity of the vaginal canal must be ruled out by direct observation. The cervix or the entire uterus may be absent. Far less common, the uterus may be present, but the cavity absent, or, in the presence of a cavity, the endometrium may be congenitally lacking. With the exception of the latter abnormalities, the clinical problem of amenorrhea due to obstruction is compounded by the painful distention of hematocolpos, hematometra, or hematoperitoneum. In all instances an effort must be made to incise and drain from below at the points of closure of the müllerian tube. Even in complicated circumstances re-establishment of müllerian duct continuity usually can be achieved surgically. The unfortunate consequences of operative extirpation of painful masses from above with damage to bladder, ureter, and rectum, as well as irretrievable loss of distended but otherwise healthy reproductive organs, are rare but well-remembered.

Knowing what to expect prior to attempting surgical correction is a great advantage. Magnetic resonance imaging (MRI) can be utilized to accurately delineate the anatomical abnormality.[30] A correct preoperative diagnosis will certainly facilitate the planning and execution of surgery.

Müllerian Agenesis

Lack of müllerian development *(Mayer-Rokitansky-Kuster-Hauser syndrome)* is the diagnosis for the individual with primary amenorrhea and no apparent vagina.[31] This is a relatively common cause of primary amenorrhea, more frequent than congenital androgen insensitivity and second only to gonadal dysgenesis. These patients have an absence or hypoplasia of the vagina. The uterus may be normal, but lacking a conduit to the introitus, or there may only be rudimentary, bicornuate cords present. If a partial endometrial cavity is present, cyclic abdominal pain may be a complaint. Because of the similarity to some types of male pseudohermaphroditism, it is worthwhile to demonstrate the normal female karyotype. Ovarian function is normal and can be documented with basal body temperatures or peripheral levels of progesterone. Growth and development are normal. Although usually sporadic, occasional occurrence may be noted within a family.

Further evaluation should include radiologic studies. Approximately one-third of patients have urinary tract abnormalities, and 12% or more have skeletal anomalies, most involving the spine. Renal tract abnormalities include ectopic kidney, renal agenesis, horseshoe kidney, and abnormal collecting ducts. When the presence of a uterine structure is suspected on examination, ultrasound can be utilized to depict the size and symmetry of the structure. When the anatomic picture on ultrasonography is not certain, MRI is indicated.[32,33] Laparoscopic visualization of the pelvis is not necessary. MRI is more accurate than ultrasonography and less expensive and invasive than laparoscopy. Extirpation of the müllerian remnants is certainly not necessary unless they are causing a problem such as uterine fibroid growth, hematometra, endometriosis, or symptomatic herniation into the inguinal canal.

Because of the difficulties and complications experienced in surgical series, we favor, when possible, an alternative to the surgical construction of an artificial vagina. Instead, we encourage the use of progressive dilatation as initially described by Frank[34] and later by Wabrek et al.[35] Beginning first in a posterior direction, and then after 2 weeks changing upward to the usual line of the vaginal axis, pressure with commercially available vaginal dilators is carried out for 20 min daily to the point of modest discomfort. Utilizing increasingly larger dilators, a functional vagina can be created in approximately 6–12 weeks. Plastic syringe covers can be used instead of the expensive commercial glass dilators. Operative treatment should be reserved for those women in whom the Frank method is unacceptable, or fails, or when a well-formed uterus is present and fertility might be preserved. The symptoms of retained menstruation should identify these patients. One recommendation is to perform an initial laparotomy to evaluate the cervical canal; if the cervix is atretic, the uterus should be removed.[36] If it is the relatively simple problem of an imperforate hymen or a transverse vaginal septum, surgery is indicated. Most have recommended against trying to preserve fertility in the presence of complete vaginal agenesis. The morbidity subsequent to this surgery argues for removal of the müllerian structures at the time of construction of a neovagina.

Patients with a transverse vaginal septum, which is a failure of canalization of the distal third of the vagina, usually present with symptoms of obstruction and urinary frequency. A transverse septum can be differentiated from an imperforate hymen by a lack of distention at the introitus with Valsalva's maneuver.

Distal obstruction of the genital tract is the only condition in this category which can be considered an emergency. Delay in surgical treatment can lead to infertility due to inflammatory changes and endometriosis. Definitive surgery should be accomplished as soon as possible. Diagnostic needling should be avoided because a hematocolpos can be converted into a pyocolpos.

Reassurance and support are necessary to carry a patient through these procedures. Problems with body image and sexual enjoyment can be avoided, and, although infertile, a full and normal life as a woman can be achieved. Furthermore, genetic offspring can be achieved by collection of oocytes from the genetic mother, fertilization by the genetic father, and placement into a surrogate carrier.[37]

Androgen Insensitivity (Testicular Feminization)

Complete androgen insensitivity (testicular feminization) is the likely diagnosis when a blind vaginal canal is encountered and the uterus is absent (discussed in detail in Chapter 10). This is the third most common cause of primary amenorrhea after gonadal dysgenesis and müllerian agenesis. The patient with testicular feminization is a male pseudohermaphrodite. The adjective male refers to the gonadal sex; thus, the individual has testes and an XY karyotype. Pseudohermaphrodite means that the genitalia are

Differences between Müllerian Agenesis and Testicular Feminization

	Müllerian Agenesis	Testicular Feminization
Karyotype	46,XX	46,XY
Heredity	Not known	Maternal X-linked recessive; 25% risk of affected child, 25% risk of carrier
Sexual hair	Normal female	Absent to sparse
Testosterone level	Normal female	Normal to slightly elevated male
Other anomalies	Frequent	Rare
Gonadal neoplasia	Normal incidence	5% incidence of malignant tumors

opposite of the gonads; thus, the individual is phenotypically female but with absent or meager pubic and axillary hair.

The male pseudohermaphrodite is a genetic and gonadal male with failure of virilization. Failures in male development can be considered a spectrum with incomplete forms of androgen insensitivity being represented by some androgen response. Transmission of this disorder is by means of an X-linked recessive gene that is responsible for the androgen intracellular receptor (see chapter 10 for a discussion of the androgen receptor defect). Clinically the diagnosis should be considered in:

1. A female child with inguinal hernias because the testes are frequently partially descended;

2. A patient with primary amenorrhea and an absent uterus;

3. A patient with absent body hair.

These patients appear normal at birth except for the possible presence of an inguinal hernia, and most patients are not seen by a physician until puberty. Growth and development are normal, although overall height is usually greater than average, and there may be an eunuchoidal tendency (long arms, big hands and feet). The breasts, although large, are abnormal; actual glandular tissue is not abundant, nipples are small, and the areolae are pale. More than 50% have an inguinal hernia, the labia minora are usually underdeveloped, and the blind vagina is less deep than normal. Rudimentary fallopian tubes are composed of fibromuscular tissue with only occasional epithelial lining. Horseshoe kidneys have been reported.

The testes may be intra-abdominal, but often are in a hernia. They are similar to any cryptorchid testis except that they may be nodular. After puberty, the testis displays immature tubular development, and tubules are lined by immature germ cells and Sertoli cells. There is no spermatogenesis. The incidence of neoplasia in these gonads is high. In 50 reported cases, there were 11 malignancies, 15 adenomas, and 10 benign cysts: a 22% incidence of malignancy and a 52% incidence of neoplasia.[38] More recent series indicate a lower overall incidence of gonadal tumors, about 5%.[39,40] Therefore, once full development is attained after puberty, the gonads should be removed at about age 16–18, and the patient placed on hormone therapy. ***This is the only exception to the rule that gonads with a Y chromosome should be removed as soon as a diagnosis is made.*** There are two reasons: first, the development achieved with hormone treatment does not seem to match the smooth pubertal changes due to endogenous hormones, and second, gonadal tumors in these patients have not been encountered prior to puberty. Removal of gonadal tissue can be accomplished by a skilled operator through the laparoscope, reserving the option of laparotomy if the gonads are inaccessible.[41]

When testicular feminization was first studied, it was found that the urinary 17-ketosteroids were normal, and it was suggested that there might be a resistance to androgen action rather than an absence of androgens — a congenital androgen insensitivity. Indeed, the plasma levels of testosterone are in the normal to high male range, and the plasma clearance and metabolism of testosterone are normal. Thus, these patients produce testosterone, but they do not respond to androgens, either their own or those given locally or systemically. Therefore, the critical steps in sexual differentiation which require androgens fail to take place, and development is totally female. Because antimüllerian hormone is present, development of the müllerian duct is inhibited, hence the absence of uterus, tubes, and upper vagina.

This syndrome is marked by a unique combination:

1.   Normal female phenotype.

2.   Normal male karyotype, 46,XY.

3.   Normal or slightly elevated male blood testosterone levels and a high LH.

Cases of *incomplete androgen insensitivity* (one-tenth as common as the complete syndrome) represent individuals with some androgen effect. These individuals may have clitoral enlargement, or a phallus may even be present. Axillary hair and pubic hair develop along with breast growth. Gonadectomy should not be deferred in such cases because it will obviate unwanted further virilization. Patients with a deficit in testicular 17β-hydroxysteroid dehydrogenase activity will have impaired testosterone production and present clinically as incomplete androgen insensitivity. Since treatment (gonadectomy) is the same, precise diagnosis is not essential.

Conventional wisdom warns against unthinking and needless disclosure of the gonadal and chromosomal sex to a patient with complete androgen insensitivity. Although infertile, these patients are certainly completely female in their gender identity, and this should be reinforced rather than challenged. There are exceptions to every rule, however, and certain situations may call for a more straightforward, accurate discussion. One example in our own practice was a student nurse who pointed out that she would much rather have learned the facts from her parents and physician than from the textbooks she was reading in school.

Compartment II: Disorders of the Ovary

Problems in gonadal development can present with either primary or secondary amenorrhea. 30–40% of primary amenorrhea cases have gonadal streaks due to abnormal development: gonadal dysgenesis. These patients can be grouped according to the following karyotypes:

50% — 45,X
25% — Mosaics
25% — 46,XX

Women with gonadal dysgenesis can also present with secondary amenorrhea. The karyotypes associated with this presentation are, in order of decreasing frequency:

46,XX (most common).
Mosaics (e.g., 45,X/46,XX).
Deletions of X short and long arms.
47,XXX
45,X

The finding of a normal karyotype, the most common situation, is most perplexing. Simpson suggests that maldevelopment is the result of an autosomal recessive defect in meiosis, a failure of synapses, an event which is very common in plants and animals.[42] Gonadal dysgenesis associated with a normal karyotype is also linked to neurosensory deafness (Perrault syndrome). Auditory evaluation should be considered in all 46,XX gonadal dysgenesis cases.

Turner Syndrome

Turner syndrome (an abnormality in or an absence of one of the X chromosomes) is a well-known and thoroughly studied entity. The characteristics of short stature, webbed neck, shield chest, and increased carrying angle at the elbow, combined with hyper-gonadotropic hypoestrogenic amenorrhea, make a diagnosis possible on the most superficial evaluation. However, special attention must be given to the less common variations of this syndrome. Autoimmune disorders, cardiovascular abnormalities, and various renal anomalies must be ruled out. A karyotype should be performed on all patients with elevated gonadotropins despite the appearance of a typical case of Turner syndrome. The presence of a pure syndrome, 45,X chromosome single cell line, should be confirmed. This expensive test cannot be viewed just as a step toward academic perfection. Forty percent of individuals who appear to have Turner syndrome are mosaics or have structural aberrations in the X or Y chromosome.

Mosaicism

The presence of mosaicism (multiple cell lines of varying sex chromosome composition) must be ruled out for a very important reason. The presence of a Y chromosome in the karyotype requires excision of the gonadal areas because the presence of any medullary (testicular) component within the gonad is a predisposing factor to tumor formation and to heterosexual development (virilization). Only in the patient with the complete form of androgen insensitivity can laparotomy be deferred until after puberty, because the individual is resistant to androgens and gonadal tumors occur late. In all other patients with a Y chromosome, gonadectomy should be performed as soon as the diagnosis is made to avoid virilization and early tumor formation. One should be aware that approximately 30% of patients with a Y chromosome will not develop signs of virilization. Therefore, even the normal appearing adult patient with elevated serum levels of gonadotropins must be karyotyped to detect a silent Y chromosome so that prophylactic gonadectomy can be performed before neoplastic changes occur. The fully stained and banded karyotype continues to be the best method to detect the presence of testicular tissue or other mosaic combinations. When standard cytogenetic analysis is uncertain, expert consultation should be obtained to pursue further analysis with X- and Y-specific DNA probes.[43]

The impact of mosaicism, even in the absence of a Y-containing line, is significant. With an XX component (e.g., XX/XO), functional cortical (ovarian) tissue can be found within the gonad, leading to a variety of responses, including some degree of female development, and, on occasion, even menses and reproduction. These individuals may appear normal, attaining normal stature before premature menopause is experienced. More commonly, these patients are short. Most patients with missing sex chromosome material are less than 63 inches (160 cm) in height. The menopause is early, because the functioning follicles undergo an accelerated rate of atresia.

This complex array of gonadal dysgenesis variations, from the typical pure form to an otherwise normal appearing and functioning woman with premature menopause, is the result of a variety of mosaicism which produces a complex mixture of cortical and medullary gonadal tissue. The clinical importance of this information justifies obtaining karyotypes in all cases of elevated gonadotropins in women under age 30. All patients with absent ovarian function and quantitative alterations in the sex chromosomes are categorized as having *gonadal dysgenesis* (Chapter 10).

XY Gonadal Dysgenesis

A female patient with an XY karyotype who has a palpable müllerian system, normal female testosterone levels, and lack of sexual development has *Swyer's syndrome.* Tumor transformation in the gonadal ridge can occur at any age, and extirpation of the gonadal streaks should be performed as soon as the diagnosis is made.

Gonadal Agenesis

No complicated clinical problems accompany the gonadal failure due to agenesis. Without precise information, only conjecture about the causes of absent development can be made. Thus, viral and metabolic influences in early gestation are suspected. Nevertheless, the final result is irretrievable — hypergonadotropic hypogonadism. In the absence of gonadal function, development is female. Surgical removal of the gonadal streaks is necessary to avoid the possibility of neoplasia.

The Resistant Ovary Syndrome

There is a rare patient with amenorrhea who has elevated gonadotropins despite the presence of ovarian follicles, and there is no evidence of autoimmune disease. Laparotomy is necessary to arrive at a correct diagnosis by obtaining adequate histological evaluation of the ovaries. This can demonstrate not only the presence of follicles but the absence of the lymphocytic infiltration seen with autoimmune disease. Because of the rarity of this condition and the very low chance of achieving pregnancy even with high doses of exogenous gonadotropins, we do not believe it is worthwhile to perform a laparotomy for the purpose of ovarian biopsy on every patient with amenorrhea, high gonadotropins, and a normal karyotype.

Premature Ovarian Failure

Premature ovarian failure (the early depletion of ovarian follicles) is surprisingly common. Approximately 1% of women will experience ovarian failure before the age of 40, and in women with primary amenorrhea, the prevalence ranges from 10% to 28%.[14,44] The etiology of premature ovarian failure is unknown in most cases. It is useful to explain to the patient that it is probably a genetic disorder with an increased rate of follicle disappearance. Often, specific sex chromosome anomalies can be identified.[45] The most common abnormalities are 45,X and 47,XXY, followed by mosaicism and specific structural abnormalities on the sex chromosomes. Accelerated atresia is most likely because even 45,X (Turner syndrome) patients begin with a full complement of germ cells. In addition, premature ovarian failure can be due to an autoimmune process, or perhaps to destruction of follicles by infections such as mumps oophoritis or a physical insult such as irradiation or chemotherapy.

The problem can present at varying ages depending upon the number of follicles left. It is useful to view the various presentations as representing a stage in the process of perimenopausal change, no matter what the chronological age of the patient. If loss of follicles has been rapid, then primary amenorrhea and lack of sexual development will be present. If loss of follicles takes place during or after puberty, then the extent of adult phenotypic development and the time of onset of secondary amenorrhea will vary accordingly.

In view of the increasing number of case reports documenting resumption of normal function, we cannot be certain that these patients will be sterile forever. On the other hand, laparotomy and full thickness ovarian biopsy surely are not necessary for all of these patients. We believe that a minimal approach, with a survey for autoimmune disease (recognizing that there is no practical clinical method to accurately diagnose autoimmune ovarian failure) and an assessment of ovarian-pituitary activity, is sufficient.

The Effect of Radiation and Chemotherapy

The effect of radiation is dependent upon age and the x-ray dose.[46,47] Steroid levels begin to fall and gonadotropins rise within 2 weeks after irradiation to the ovaries. The higher number of oocytes in younger age is responsible for the resistance to total castration in young women exposed to intense radiation. Function can resume after many years of amenorrhea. On the other hand, the damage may not appear until later in the form of premature ovarian failure. If pregnancy does occur, the risk of congenital abnormalities is no greater than normal. Gonads are not in danger in the kitchen; microwave ovens utilize wavelengths with low tissue penetrating power. The following table indicates the risk of sterilization according to dose:[48]

Ovarian Dose	Sterilization Effect
60 rads	No effect
150 rads	Some risk over age 40
250–500 rads	Ages 15–40: 60% sterilized
500–800 rads	Ages 15–40: 60–70% sterilized
over 800 rads	100% permanently sterilized

Alkylating agents are very toxic to the gonads. As with radiation, there is an inverse relationship between the dose required for ovarian failure and age at the start of therapy.[49] Other chemotherapeutic agents have the potential for ovarian damage, but they have been less well studied. The effect of combination chemotherapies is similar to those of the alkylating agents. Resumption of menses and pregnancy can occur, but there is no way to predict which patient will reacquire ovulatory function. As with radiotherapy, damage may present late with premature ovarian failure.

Compartment III: Disorders of the Anterior Pituitary

A consideration of the disorders of the hypothalamic-pituitary axis must first focus on the problem of the pituitary tumor. Through the appearance of amenorrhea, the patient with a slowly growing pituitary tumor can present years before the tumor becomes evident by standard radiologic techniques. Fortunately, malignant tumors are almost never encountered (through 1993, there were 6 reported cases of prolactin cell metastatic carcinomas and through 1989, no more than 40 cases of primary pituitary cancer in the world literature[50-52]), but growth of a benign tumor can cause problems because it expands in a confined space. The tumor grows upward, compressing the optic chiasm and producing the classic findings of bitemporal hemianopsia. With small tumors, however, abnormal visual fields are rarely encountered. In contrast, other tumors of this region (e.g., craniopharyngioma, usually marked by calcifications on x-ray) may be associated with the early development of blurring of vision and visual field defects because of their close proximity to the optic chiasm. Besides craniopharyngioma, other possible tumors include meningiomas, gliomas, metastatic tumors, and chordomas.

Sometimes the suspicion of a pituitary tumor is increased because of clinical signs of acromegaly caused by excessive secretion of growth hormone, or Cushing's disease due to excessive secretion of ACTH. Rarely, a TSH-secreting tumor will cause secondary hyperthyroidism. Amenorrhea and/or galactorrha may precede the eventual full clinical expression of a tumor that secretes ACTH or growth hormone. If clinical criteria suggest Cushing's disease, ACTH levels and the 24-hour urinary levels of free cortisol should be measured, and the rapid suppression test (Chapter 14) should be utilized. If acromegaly is suspected, growth hormone should be measured in the fasting state (less than 5 ng/mL [5 µg/L]) and during an oral glucose tolerance test (suppression of growth hormone levels), and the circulating level of IGF-I should be measured. Though usually a problem in adult life, prolactin secreting tumors can be seen in preadolescent and adolescent children, and thus can be a cause of failure of growth and development or of primary amenorrhea.

The majority of clinically nonfunctioning (null) adenomas are of gonadotroph origin and actively secrete FSH, free α-subunit, and rarely, LH (all of which do not exert clinical effects).[9] The α-subunit can be used as a tumor marke, however in postmenopausal women the situation can be confusing because increased free α-subunit secretion accompanies increased secretion of gonadotropins. In contrast to patients with normal pituitary glands, patients with pituitary adenomas usually fail to down-regulate gonadotropin secretion in response to GnRH agonist treatment, and repeated GnRH agonist administration is associated with persistent elevations in either FSH or α-subunit. Most patients with these tumors, however, have reduced secretion of gonadotropins (and amenorrhea) because of tumor compression of the pituitary stalk and interference with the delivery of hypothalamic GnRH. For this reason, these patients often present with modest elevations of prolactin (due to the inability of dopamine to reach the anterior pituitary).

Not all intrasellar masses are neoplastic. Gummas, tuberculomas, and fat deposits have been reported as causes of pituitary compression leading to hypogonadotropic amenorrhea. Nearby lesions such as internal carotid artery aneurysms and obstruction of the aqueduct of Sylvius can also cause amenorrhea. Pituitary insufficiency can be secondary to ischemia and infarction and appear as a late sequela to obstetrical hemorrhage — the well-known Sheehan's syndrome. These problems, as well as genetic disorders such as Laurence-Moon-Biedl and Prader-Willi syndromes, are so rarely encountered that consultation with textbooks and colleagues is necessary.

Treatment of Nonfunctioning Adenomas

If imaging discovers a microadenoma (less than 10 mm in diameter) in an asymptomatic patient, no treatment is necessary. These tumors are often incidental findings. A follow-up imaging is recommended in a year or two to be sure there is no growth. If a macroadenoma (greater than 10 mm in diameter) is present, surgery is usually necessary, especially since these tumors are commonly not detected until the onset of symptoms (headaches and visual disturbances). Because of their large size (residual tumor is often left after surgery) and the high risk of recurrence, adjunctive irradiation is recommended. Follow-up imaging is obtained every 6 months for 1 year, then yearly for 3–5 years. The radiation dose is high (4,500 rads), and the incidence of hypopituitarism may reach 50% over a 10-year period.[9] Ongoing surveillance of adrenal and thyroid function is necessary. Although a response to dopamine agonist therapy has been reported, in general, results are not satisfactory.

Pituitary Prolactin-Secreting Adenomas

Prolactin-secreting adenomas are the most common pituitary tumors, and they account for 50% of all pituitary adenomas identified at autopsy. Classically, pituitary adenomas have been grouped according to their staining ability as eosinophilic, basophilic, or chromophobic. This classification is misleading and of no clinical usefulness. Pituitary adenomas should be classified according to their function, e.g., prolactin-secreting adenoma.

With the utilization of the serum prolactin assay and the increased sensitivity of the new imaging techniques, the association of amenorrhea and small pituitary tumors has become recognized as a relatively common problem. This is not a new phenomenon, rather it reflects more sensitive diagnostic techniques. Attempts to link the problem to oral contraceptive use have proved negative.[53]

The exact incidence of this clinical problem is unknown. In autopsy series the number of pituitary glands found to contain adenomas ranged from 9% to 27%.[54–58] The age distribution ranged from 2 to 86, with the greatest incidence in the 6th decade of life. The sex distribution was equal. However, clinical manifestations, mainly a disruption of the reproductive mechanism, occur more commonly in women and are probably due to estrogen-induced activity of the pituitary lactotrophs.

A high prolactin level is encountered in about one-third of women with no obvious cause of amenorrhea.[59] Only one-third of women with high prolactin levels will have galactorrhea, probably because the low estrogen environment associated with the amenorrhea prevents a normal response to prolactin. Another possible explanation again focuses on the heterogeneity of peptide hormones. Prolactin circulates in various forms with structural modifications which are the result of glycosylation, phosphorylation, and deletions and additions. The various forms are associated with varying bioactivity (manifested by galactorrhea) and immunoactivity (recognition by immunoassay). The predominant variant is little prolactin (80–85%) which also has more biological activity compared to the larger sized variants. Therefore it is not surprising that big prolactins compose the major form of circulating prolactin in women with normal menses and minimal galactorrhea.[60] This is not always the case, however, because a high blood level (350–400 ng/mL [15,500–17,700 pmol/L]) of prolactin composed predominantly of high molecular weight prolactin has been reported in a woman with oligomenorrhea and galactorrhea but with no evidence of a pituitary tumor.[61] These high levels of relatively inactive prolactin in the absence of a tumor may be due to the creation of macromolecules of prolactin by antiprolactin autoantibodies.[62] Explanations for clinically illogical situations can be found in the variable molecular heterogeneity of the peptide hormones. At any one point in time, the bioactivity and the immunoactivity of prolactin represent the cumulative effect of the circulating family of structural variants.

Very high prolactin levels (greater than 1,000 ng/mL [44,400 pmol/L]) are associated with invasive tumors. These very rare tumors do not yield themselves to surgery, but fortunately they can be effectively treated and controlled with a dopamine agonist.

About one-third of women with galactorrhea have normal menses. As the prolactin concentration increases, a woman can progress sequentially from normal ovulation to an inadequate luteal phase to intermittent anovulation to total anovulation to complete suppression and amenorrhea.

Probably as many as one-third of patients with secondary amenorrhea will have a pituitary adenoma, and if galactorrhea is also present, half will have an abnormal sella turcica.[59] The clinical symptoms do not always correlate with the prolactin level, and patients with normal prolactins can have pituitary tumors.[63] The highest prolactin levels, however, are associated with amenorrhea, with or without galactorrhea.

The amenorrhea associated with elevated prolactin levels is due to prolactin inhibition of the pulsatile secretion of GnRH. The pituitary glands in these patients respond normally to GnRH, or in augmented fashion (perhaps due to increased stores of gonadotropins), thus indicating that the mechanism of the amenorrhea is a decrease in GnRH.[64,65] This inhibition is mediated by increased opioid activity.[66] Treatment that lowers the circulating levels of prolactin restores ovarian responsiveness and menstrual function. This is true whether the treatment consists of removal of a prolactin-secreting tumor or suppression of prolactin secretion.

The increased ability to detect pituitary tumors has been accompanied by the development of a surgical technique which effectively removes the small tumors with a high margin of safety. Utilizing the operating microscope, the transsphenoidal technique approaches via a sublabial incision (under the upper lip), with dissection under the nasal mucosa, removal of the nasal septum to expose the sphenoidal sinus, and resection of the floor of the sphenoid sinus to expose the sella turcica. Tumor tissue is usually distinguishable from the yellow-orange, firm tissue of the normal anterior pituitary. However, because pituitary adenomas do not have a capsule, the borderline between tumor and normal tissue is often vague. The ideal time for excision is when the adenoma is a small nodule. When enlarged it becomes more difficult to distinguish normal from pathological tissue. Once the adenoma grows beyond the sella, total removal is essentially impossible.

The development of transsphenoidal surgery was paralleled by the availability and clinical application of the drug, bromocriptine, that specifically suppresses prolactin secretion. Initially, appropriate decisions between the surgical approach and medical treatment were difficult to make. With increasing experience, clinical perspective has been achieved, and reasonable judgments are now possible. Let us first consider results with surgery, then examine dopamine agonist treatment.

Results with Surgery

Transsphenoidal neurosurgery achieves complete resolution of hyperprolactinemia with resumption of cyclic menses in about 40% of patients with macroadenomas and 80% of patients with microadenomas. Besides an inability to achieve a complete cure, surgery may be followed by recurrence of tumor (long-term cure rate is about 50% overall, ranging from as high as 70% for microadenomas to as low as 10% for macroadenomas) and a still unknown but significant percentage (perhaps as high as 10–30% after surgery for macroadenomas) of development of panhypopituitarism.[67,68] Other complications of surgery include cerebrospinal fluid leaks, an occasional case of meningitis, and the frequent postoperative problem of diabetes insipidus. The diabetes insipidus is usually a transient problem, rarely lasting as long as 6 months, but it can be permanent. While initial follow-up reports of the results of transsphenoidal adenomectomy were discouraging (high recurrence rates), other authors have argued that surgical techniques improved with time, and recurrent hyperprolactinemia is relatively low.[69] The best results are in patients with prolactin levels in the 150–500 ng/mL (6,660–22,200 pmol/L) range; the higher the prolactin the lower the cure rate.

There are 3 possible explanations for the recurrence or persistence of hyperprolactinemia after surgery.

1. The prolactin producing tumor looks like the surrounding normal pituitary, and it is difficult to resect completely.

2. The tumor may be multifocal in origin.

3. There may be a continuing abnormality of the hypothalamus giving rise to chronic stimulation of the lactotrophs. In other words, this is a problem of recurrent hyperplasia, not adenomas. However, molecular biology studies indicate that pituitary tumors are monoclonal.[70] If dysfunction were the etiologic factor, one would expect the tumors to be polyclonal.

We recommend the following surveillance for those patients who have had surgery:

1. If cyclic menses return: periodic evaluation for the problem of anovulation.

2. If amenorrhea or oligomenorrhea and hyperprolactinemia persist or recur: prolactin levels every 6 months and imaging yearly for 2 years, then a coned-down view every few years. If tumor growth becomes evident, control of growth should be achieved with dopamine agonist treatment. In addition, a dopamine agonist can be used to induce ovulation if pregnancy is desired.

Results with Radiation

Results with radiation therapy are less satisfactory than with surgery. In addition, response is very slow; prolactin concentrations may take several years to fall. After radiation, panhypopituitarism can occur as long as 10 years after treatment. Patients who have been treated with radiation should be followed for a long time, and any symptoms suggestive of pituitary failure require investigation. Irradiation should be reserved for controlling postoperative regrowth of large tumors and shrinking large tumors that are unresponsive to medical treatment.

Dopamine Agonist Treatment

Bromocriptine is a lysergic acid derivative with a bromine substitute at position 2.[71] It is available as the methane-sulfonate (mesylate) in 2.5 mg tablets. It is a dopamine agonist, binding to dopamine receptors and, therefore, directly mimicking dopamine inhibition of pituitary prolactin secretion. Absorption from the gastrointestinal tract is rapid but not complete; 28% is absorbed and 94% metabolized in the first-pass through the liver. Bromocriptine is metabolized into at least 30 excretory products. Excretion is mainly biliary, and more than 90% appears in the feces over 5 days after a single dose of 2.5 mg. A small part, 6–7%, is excreted unchanged or as metabolites in the urine.

The oral dose that suppresses prolactin is 10 times lower than that which improves the symptoms of Parkinson's disease. For some patients, one pill a day (or half a pill bid) will be effective. On the other hand, an occasional patient will require 7.5 mg or 10 mg daily in order to suppress adenoma secretion of prolactin.

Bromocriptine is also available in a long-acting form (depot-bromocriptine) for intramuscular injection and as a slow-release oral form. Depot-bromocriptine is administered in a dose of 50–75 mg monthly; the dose of the oral slow-release formulation is 5–15 mg daily. These forms are equally effective as the standard oral preparation and are associated with the same side effect severity and prevalence.[72] The response to the intramuscular form appears to be more rapid, and thus this preparation would offer an advantage in cases with large tumors with visual field impairment.[73,74]

Nausea, headache, and faintness are the usual initial problems. The faintness is due to orthostatic hypotension that can be attributed to relaxation of smooth muscle in the splanchnic and renal beds, as well as inhibition of transmitter release at noradrenergic nerve endings and central inhibition of sympathetic activity. Neuropsychiatric symptoms, occasionally with hallucinations, occur in less than 1% of patients. This may be due to hydrolysis of the lysergic acid part of the molecule. Other side effects include dizziness, fatigue, nasal congestion, vomiting, and abdominal cramps.

Side effects can be minimized by slowly building tolerance toward the usual dose, 2.5 mg bid. Treatment should be started with an initial dose of 2.5 mg given at bedtime. The peak level is achieved 2 hours after ingestion, and the biological half-life is about 3 hours. If intolerance occurs with this initial dose, then the tablet should be cut in half, and an even slower program should be followed. Usually a week after the initial dose, the second 2.5 mg dose can be added at breakfast or lunch. Patients who are extremely sensitive to the drug should be instructed to divide the tablets and to devise their own schedule of increasing dosage in order to achieve tolerance. A very small percentage of patients cannot tolerate any dosage.

Vaginal administration of bromocriptine is an excellent method to avoid side effects. One 2.5 mg tablet is inserted high into the vagina at bedtime. This dose will provide excellent clinical results and few side effects.[75] In contrast to oral bromocriptine which is not absorbed completely and that which is absorbed is largely metabolized in the first-pass through the liver, vaginal absorption is nearly complete, and avoidance of the liver first-pass effect (with longer maintenance of systemic levels) allows achievement of therapeutic results at a lower dose.

There are two bromocriptine treatment methods to follow in those patients seeking pregnancy. The first is simply daily administration of 2.5 mg bid until the patient is pregnant as judged by the basal body temperature chart. In the second method, bromocriptine is administered during the follicular phase, and the drug is stopped when a basal body temperature rise indicates that ovulation has occurred, thus avoiding high drug levels early in pregnancy. The drug is resumed at menses when it is apparent the patient is not pregnant. No comparative study has been performed to tell us whether the follicular phase only method is as effective as the daily method. Furthermore, there has been no evidence that bromocriptine ingestion during early pregnancy is harmful to the fetus.[76]

Results of Treatment

In 22 clinical trials, 80% of patients with amenorrhea/galactorrhea, associated with hyperprolactinemia but no demonstrable tumors, had menses restored.[77] The average treatment time to the initiation of menses was 5.7 weeks. Complete cessation of galactorrhea occurred in 50–60% of patients in an average time of 12.7 weeks, and a 75% reduction of breast secretions was achieved in 6.4 weeks. *It is important to advise patients that the loss of galactorrhea is a slower and less certain response compared to restoration of ovulation and menses.* Amenorrhea recurred in 41% of the patients within an average of 4.4 weeks of discontinuing treatment; galactorrhea recurred in 69% at an average of 6.0 weeks. About 5% of patients terminated treatment because of adverse reactions.

Regression of Tumors with Bromocriptine

There is no question that macroadenomas will regress with bromocriptine treatment.[71,78,79] In some there is prompt shrinkage with low dose treatment (5–7.5 mg daily); in others, prolonged treatment is required with higher doses. If a prolactin adenoma fails to shrink with 10 mg daily, further increases in dose are not useful. Visual improvement may be noted within several days. Reduction in tumor size can take place in several days to 6 weeks, but in some cases it is not observed until 6 months or more. In most cases, rapid shrinkage occurs during the first 3 months of therapy, followed by slower reduction.[80] Very high prolactin levels, greater than 2,000–3,000 ng/mL (88,800–133,200 pmol/L), are probably the result of invasion of the cavernous sinuses with release directly into the bloodstream. Levels greater than 1,000 ng/mL (44,400 pmol/L) are associated with locally invasive tumors. Even these cases show remarkable resolution with bromocriptine treatment. Indeed, surgical results with invasive tumors are so poor that long-term control with a dopamine agonist is recommended. While tumor shrinkage is always preceded by a decrease in prolactin levels, the overall response cannot be predicted by the basal prolactin level, the absolute or relative fall in prolactin, or even the attainment of normal prolactin levels. Visual impairment improves rapidly, but maximal effects may take several months.

The response of macroadenomas to bromocriptine is impressive, and a most compelling reason in favor of its use is that it has been successful when previous surgery or radiation has failed.[79] The problem, however, is that it probably must be taken indefinitely, because there is yet to be a convincing report of complete disappearance and resolution of tumor that can be attributed to drug therapy and not spontaneous resolution. Light and electron microscopic, immunohistochemical, and morphometric analyses all indicate that bromocriptine causes not only a reduction in the size of individual cells but also necrosis of the cells with replacement fibrosis.[80] Nevertheless, prolactin levels generally return to an elevated state after discontinuation of the drug. There are cases of improvement in sellar x-rays; however, the occurrence of spontaneous regression of prolactin-secreting tumors makes it impossible to attribute "cures" to bromocriptine. Recurrence of hyperprolactinemia has been observed following as many as 4–8 years of treatment.

New Drugs

Other ergoline derivatives with dopaminergic activity are available throughout the world. Pergolide is the most widely used. It is more potent, longer-lasting, and better tolerated by some patients than bromocriptine. Pergolide is given in a single daily dose of 50–150 μg, and it may be effective in bromocriptine-resistant patients.[81] Others are lysuride, terguride, and cabergoline. Cabergoline can be administered only once or twice weekly.[82] Quinagolide (CV 205-502) is a nonergot long-acting dopamine agonist given in a daily bedtime dose of 75–300 μg. Because CV205-502 has a higher affinity for the dopamine receptor, tumors resistant to bromocriptine have responded to this drug.[83] Side effects are reduced with CV205-502, and it appears to have antidepressive properties.[84] Side effects and intolerance with one of these drugs is often solved by utilizing another.

Summary: Therapy of Pituitary Prolactin-Secreting Adenomas

Macroadenomas

Currently bromocriptine treatment is advocated for the treatment of macroadenomas, utilizing as low a dose as possible. Shrinkage of a tumor may require 5–10 mg bromocriptine daily, but once shrinkage has occurred, the daily dose should be progressively reduced until the lowest maintenance dose is achieved. The serum prolactin level can be utilized as a marker. In many (but not all) patients, control of tumor growth correlates with maintenance of a baseline prolactin level and can be achieved in some patients with as little as one-half a tablet (0.625 mg) daily.[85] Withdrawal of the drug is usually associated with regrowth or re-expansion of the tumor, and therefore treatment must be long-term if not indefinite. Some patients will prefer surgery, and it is certainly a legitimate option. In view of better results claimed in more recent times, this choice should be presented to the patient. Transsphenoidal surgery is recommended when suprasellar extension persists after bromocriptine treatment of a macroadenoma. Because tumor recurrence is high, surgery should be followed by radiotherapy.[86] All patients receiving radiotherapy require on-going surveillance for the development of hypopituitarism. Surgery should be considered as a debulking procedure for very large tumors with or without invasion prior to long-term dopamine agonist therapy.

Short-term treatment (several weeks) with bromocriptine can make surgery easier due to a reduction in size (although not all neurosurgeons agree); however, long-term treatment (3 months or more) is associated with fibrosis that makes complete surgical removal more difficult and more likely to be associated with the sacrifice of other pituitary hormonal function. Even though prolactin levels usually increase when bromocriptine treatment is discontinued after several years, many tumors do not re-grow.[87] Pregnancy should be deferred until repeat imaging confirms shrinkage of the macroadenoma.

Approximately 10% of macroadenomas do not shrink with dopamine agonist therapy. *The failure of a tumor to shrink significantly in size despite a normalization of prolactin levels is consistent with a nonfunctioning tumor that is interrupting the supply of dopamine to the pituitary by stalk compression. Early surgery is indicated.*

Microadenomas

The treatment of microadenomas should be directed to alleviating one of two problems: infertility or breast discomfort. Bromocriptine is the method of choice. Again, some patients, deliberately and understandably, choose the surgical approach in hopes of achieving a cure and avoiding the worry and annoyance of continuing surveillance.

The major therapeutic dilemma can be expressed by the following question: should chronic bromocriptine treatment be utilized to retrieve ovarian function in those patients with hypoestrogenic amenorrhea, or should estrogen treatment be offered? Until a clear-cut benefit is demonstrated by clinical studies, we cannot advocate widespread bromocriptine therapy for those patients not interested in becoming pregnant. This conservative approach is supported by documentation of a benign clinical course with spontaneous resolution in many patients.[88,89] Patients with hypoestrogenic amenorrhea are encouraged to be on an estrogen therapy program to maintain the health of their bones and the vascular system. Low dose oral contraception is recommended for those patients who require contraception. *Estrogen-induced tumor expansion or growth has not been a problem in both our experience and in other's.*[90]

Long-Term Follow-Up

Because these tumors grow slowly, it is appropriate in the absence of symptoms to evaluate patients with microadenomas annually. The evaluation consists of a measure-ment of the prolactin level and a coned-down view of the sella turcica. If the course is unchanged, x-ray evaluation can be spaced out to every 2–3 years. More sophisticated sellar imaging is reserved for patients with a change in the coned-down x-ray view, an increasing prolactin, or the development of headaches and/or visual complaints. It should be noted that progressively increasing prolactin levels have been observed *without* associated tumor growth of a microadenoma.[91] Patients with macroadenomas deserve an initial period of follow-up every 6 months. If the adenoma appears to be clinically stable, yearly prolactin measurement and coned-down x-ray views are appro-priate. Again CT scanning or MRI is reserved for situations suggestive of tumor expansion. Tumor expansion and recurrent tumors after surgery or radiotherapy deserve a trial of treatment with a dopamine agonist.

Pregnancy and Prolactin Adenomas

Approximately 80% of hyperprolactinemic women achieve pregnancy with bromo-criptine treatment.[92] *Breastfeeding, if desired, can be carried out normally without fear of stimulating tumor growth.* Interestingly, some women resume cyclic menses after pregnancy. This spontaneous improvement may be due to tumor infarction brought about by the expansion and shrinkage during and after pregnancy, or there may be a correction of a hypothalamic dysfunction followed by a disappearance of the associated pituitary hyperplasia.

A very small percentage (less than 2%) of women with hyperprolactinemia and microadenomas will develop signs or symptoms suggestive of tumor growth during pregnancy.[92] About 5% of these patients will develop asymptomatic tumor enlargement (determined by radiologic techniques), and essentially none will ever require surgical intervention. The risk is higher with macroadenomas, approximately 15%. Headaches usually precede visual disturbances, and both may occur in any trimester. There is no characteristic headache; they are variable in intensity, location, and character. Bitemporal hemianopsia is the classic visual field finding, but other defects can occur. It has been argued in the past that a desire for pregnancy was a reason for the surgical approach. This argument hinged on the risk of tumor enlargement during pregnancy due to the well-known stimulatory effects of estrogen on the pituitary lactotrophs. As noted above, however, experience has indicated that very few patients develop problems.

It is impossible to identify which patient is at risk for symptomatic expansion during pregnancy. Other than a very large tumor, the size is not critical in that both microadenomas and macroadenomas can undergo uneventful pregnancies. There is no increase in abortions, or perinatal mortality or morbidity. It is virtually unheard of to develop a problem that results in perinatal damage or serious maternal sequelae. Nevertheless an occasional serious event can occur, e.g., hemorrhage of the tumor with diabetes insipidus and the potential for permanent visual impairment or life-threatening sequellae.[93]

Surveillance during pregnancy at first consisted of monthly visual field and prolactin measurements. With experience, this has proven to be unnecessary. The patient and the clinician can be guided by the development of symptoms. Assessment of visual fields, prolactin, and the sella turcica by imaging can await the onset of headaches or visual disturbances. Even macroprolactinomas with suprasellar extension can be followed closely; discontinuation of bromocriptine after conception is usually not associated with tumor growth during the pregnancy.[94] With repeated pregnancies, tumor regression often occurs with the development of an empty sella.

Definite evidence of tumor expansion, as well as the symptoms of headaches and visual changes, promptly regress with bromocriptine treatment.[79] Termination of pregnancy or neurosurgery, therefore, should rarely, if ever, be necessary. Although bromocriptine treatment profoundly lowers both maternal and fetal blood levels of prolactin, no adverse effects on the pregnancy or the newborn have been noted.[92,95–98] Fortunately, amniotic fluid prolactin (and its presumed action on regulation of amniotic fluid water and electrolytes) is derived from decidual tissue, and its secretion is controlled by estrogen and progesterone, not dopamine. Therefore, bromocriptine does not affect amniotic fluid levels of prolactin.

The Empty Sella Syndrome

A patient may have an abnormal sella turcica, but rather than a tumor, she may have the empty sella syndrome. In this condition there is a congenital incompleteness of the sellar diaphragm that allows an extension of the subarachnoid space into the pituitary fossa. The pituitary gland is separated from the hypothalamus and is flattened. The sella floor may be demineralized due to pressure from the cerebrospinal fluid, and the x-ray picture on coned-down views will be similar to a tumor. The empty sella syndrome can also occur secondary to surgery, radiotherapy, or infarction of a pituitary tumor.

An empty sella is found in approximately 5% of autopsies, and approximately 85% are in women, previously thought to be concentrated in middle-aged and obese women.[99] A closer look at the sella turcica, brought about by our pursuit of elevated prolactin levels, has revealed an incidence of empty sellas in 4–16% of patients who present with amenorrhea/galactorrhea.[59,63] Galactorrhea and elevated prolactins can be seen with an empty sella, and there may be a coexisting prolactin-secreting adenoma. This suggests that the empty sella in these patients may have arisen because of tumor infarction.

This condition is benign; it does not progress to pituitary failure. The chief hazard to the patient is inadvertent treatment for a pituitary tumor. Even though enlargement of the sella turcica with a normal shape is more likely associated with an empty sella than a tumor, all patients should have examination by imaging for confirmation.

Because of the possibility of a coexisting adenoma, patients with elevated prolactins or galactorrhea and an empty sella should undergo annual surveillance (prolactin assay and coned-down view) for a few years to detect tumor growth. It is totally safe and appropriate to offer hormone treatment or induction of ovulation.

Sheehan's Syndrome

Acute necrosis of the pituitary gland due to postpartum hemorrhage and shock is known as Sheehan's syndrome. The symptoms of hypopituitarism are usually seen early in the postpartum period, especially failure of lactation and loss of pubic and axillary hair. This can be a life-threatening condition, but fortunately, because of good obstetrical care, this syndrome is never encountered by most of us.

Compartment IV: Central Nervous System Disorders

Hypothalamic Amenorrhea

Patients with hypothalamic amenorrhea (hypogonadotropic hypogonadism) have a deficiency in GnRH pulsatile secretion. Hypothalamic problems are usually diagnosed by exclusion of pituitary lesions and are the most common category of hypogonadotropic amenorrhea. Frequently there is an association with a stressful situation, such as in business or in school. There is also a higher proportion of underweight women and a higher occurrence of previous menstrual irregularity. Nevertheless, the clinician is obliged to go through the process of exclusion prior to prescribing hormone therapy or attempting induction of ovulation to achieve pregnancy.

These patients are categorized by low or normal gonadotropins, normal prolactin levels, a normal x-ray evaluation of the sella turcica, and a failure to demonstrate withdrawal bleeding. A good practice is to evaluate such patients annually. This annual surveillance should include a prolactin assay and the coned-down view of the sella turcica. The x-ray is necessary only every 2–3 years after several years with no change. In the only long-term follow-up of a large group of women with secondary amenorrhea, it was noted that amenorrhea associated with psychological stress or weight loss demonstrated a spontaneous recovery after 6 years in 72% of the women.[100] This still leaves a significant percentage of women who require on-going surveillance.

Experimental evidence in the monkey indicates that corticotropin releasing hormone (CRH) inhibits gonadotropin secretion, probably by augmenting endogenous opioid secretion.[101] This could be the pathway by which stress interrupts reproductive function. Women with hypothalamic amenorrhea have reduced secretion of FSH, LH, and prolactin, but increased secretion of cortisol.[102] There is also evidence to indicate that some patients with hypothalamic amenorrhea have dopaminergic inhibition of GnRH pulse frequency.[103] The suppression of GnRH pulsatile secretion may be the result of increases in both endogenous opioids and dopamine. Thus far, abnormalities in the genes for GnRH and the beta-subunits for FSH and LH have not been detected in patients with hypothalamic amenorrhea.[104–106]

Even though a patient may not be currently interested in pursuing pregnancy, it is important to assure these patients that at the appropriate time treatment for the induction of ovulation will be available and that fertility can be achieved. Concern with potential fertility is often an unspoken fear, especially in the younger patients, even teenagers. On the other hand, induction of ovulation should be carried out only for the purpose of producing a pregnancy. There is no evidence that cyclic hormone administration or induction of ovulation will stimulate the return of normal function.

Weight Loss, Anorexia, Bulimia

St. Wilgefortis was the 7th daughter of the King of Portugal, living around the year 1000.[107] When confronted with an arranged marriage (she had made a vow of virginity to become a nun), she turned to intense prayer. The intensity of the prayer was marked by anorexia and the growth of body hair. Confronted with this new appearance, the King of Sicily changed his mind about the marriage, and Wilgefortis's father had her crucified. Around 1200, the legend of Wilgefortis spread throughout Europe. The fact that the cult developed around women with more than one name has suggested that many girls underwent an experience similar to that of Wilgefortis.

St. Wilgefortis became a symbol, a woman who liberated herself of female problems, and she became a protectress of women with sexual problems, including problems associated with childbirth. Indeed, women who wished to rid themselves of their husbands prayed to her, since she had successfully resisted both a father and a potential husband. In England, rather than St. Wilgefortis, she was known as St. Uncumber because women believed she could uncumber them of their husbands.

Thus emerged the medieval dark ages explanation (with ascendancy to sainthood) of a girl's response (anorexia nervosa) to her fears of marriage and sexuality. Our understanding of the reason for this extraordinary behavior continues today to focus on an inability to cope with the onset of adult sexuality, with a return to the prepubertal state. Both anorexia nervosa and bulimia nervosa (binge eating) are distinguished by a morbid fear of fatness.

Obesity can be associated with amenorrhea, but amenorrhea in an obese patient is usually due to anovulation, and a hypogonadotropic state is not encountered unless the patient also has a severe emotional disorder. Conversely, acute weight loss, in some unknown way, can lead to the hypogonadotropic state. Again, the clinician must pursue the presence of a pituitary tumor, and the diagnosis of hypothalamic amenorrhea is made by exclusion.

Clinically a spectrum is encountered that ranges from a limited period of amenorrhea associated with a crash diet, to the severely ill patient with the life-threatening attrition of anorexia nervosa. It is a common experience for a physician to be the first to recognize anorexia nervosa in a patient presenting with the complaint of amenorrhea. It is also not infrequent that a physician will evaluate and manage an infertility problem due to hypogonadotropism and not be aware of a developing case of anorexia. Because the mortality rate associated with this syndrome is significant (5–15%), it warrants close attention.[108]

Diagnosis of Anorexia Nervosa

1. Onset between ages 10 and 30.
2. Weight loss of 25% or weight 15% below normal for age and height.
3. Special attitudes:
   –Denial,
   –Distorted body image,
   –Unusual hoarding or handling of food.
4. At least one of the following:
   –Lanugo,
   –Bradycardia,
   –Overactivity,
   –Episodes of overeating (bulimia),
   –Vomiting, which may be self-induced.
5. Amenorrhea.
6. No known medical illness.
7. No other psychiatric disorder.
8. Other characteristics:
   –Constipation,
   –Low blood pressure,
   –Hypercarotenemia,
   –Diabetes insipidus.

Anorexia nervosa occurs frequently in young white middle to upper class females under age 25, but it is now recognized that this problem occurs at all socioeconomic levels. The families of anorectics are success-achievement-appearance oriented. Serious problems may be present within the family, but the parents make every effort to maintain an apparent marital harmony, glossing over or denying conflicts. In one psychiatric interpretation, each parent, in secret dissatisfaction with the other, expects affection from their "perfect" child. Anorexia begins when the role of the perfect child becomes too difficult. The pattern usually starts with a voluntary diet to control weight. This brings a sense of power and accomplishment, soon followed by a fear that weight cannot be controlled if discipline is allowed to relax. A reasonable view is to consider anorexia as a mechanism which identifies a generally disturbed family. The symptom pattern is the expression of the various psychological, familial, and cultural factors involved.

At puberty, the normal weight gain may be interpreted as excessive, and this can trip the teenager over into true anorexia nervosa. Excessive physical activity can be the earliest sign of incipient anorexia nervosa. The children are characteristically overachievers and strivers. They seldom give any trouble, but are judgmental and demand that others live up to their rigid value system, often resulting in social isolation.

The cultural value our society places on thinness definitely plays a role in eating disorders. Both occupational and recreational environments that stress thinness put women at greater risk for anorexia nervosa and bulimia. But basically, an eating disorder is a method being utilized to solve a psychological dilemma.

Besides amenorrhea, constipation is a common symptom, often severe and accompanied by abdominal pain. The preoccupation with food may manifest itself by large intakes of lettuce, raw vegetables, and low calorie foods. Hypotension, hypothermia, rough dry skin, soft lanugo-type hair on the back and buttocks, bradycardia, and edema are the most commonly encountered signs. Long-term diuretic and laxative abuse may produce significant hypokalemia. An elevation of the serum carotene is not always associated with a large intake of yellow vegetables, suggesting that a defect in vitamin A utilization is present. The yellowish coloration of the skin is usually seen on the palms.

Bulimia is a syndrome marked by episodic and secretive binge eating followed by self-induced vomiting, fasting, or the use of laxatives and diuretics.[109] It appears to be a growing problem among young women, however careful study indicates that while bulimic behaviors may be relatively common, clinically significant bulimia is not (approximately 1.0% of female students and 0.1% of male students in a college sample).[110,111] Bulimic behavior is frequently seen in patients with anorexia nervosa (about half), but not in all. Patients with bulimia have a high incidence of depressive symptoms, and a problem with shoplifting (usually food). Little is known about the long-term outcome. There is a growing tendency to divide patients with anorexia nervosa into bulimic anorectics and dieters. Bulimic anorectics are older, less isolated socially, and have a higher incidence of family problems. Body weight in a "pure" bulimic fluctuates, but it does not fall to the low levels seen in anorectics.

The serious case of anorexia nervosa is seen more often by an internist. However, the borderline anorectic frequently presents to a gynecologist, pediatrician, or family physician as a teenager who has low body weight, amenorrhea, and hyperactivity (excellent grades and many extracurricular activities). The amenorrhea can precede, follow, or appear coincidentally with the weight loss.

The various problems associated with anorexia represent dysfunction of the body mechanisms regulated by the hypothalamus: appetite, thirst and water conservation, temperature, sleep, autonomic balance, and endocrine secretion.[112] Endocrine studies can be summarized as follows: FSH and LH levels are low, cortisol levels are elevated, prolactin levels are normal, TSH and thyroxine (T_4) levels are normal, but the 3,5,3'-triiodothyronine (T_3) level is low and reverse T_3 is high. Indeed many of the symptoms can be explained by relative hypothyroidism (constipation, cold intolerance, bradycardia, hypotension, dry skin, low metabolic rates, hypercarotenemia). There appears to be a compensation to the state of undernourishment, with diversion from formation of the active T_3 to the inactive metabolite, reverse T_3. With weight gain, all of the metabolic changes revert to normal. Even though normal gonadotropin secretion may be restored with weight gain, 30% of patients remain amenorrheic.[111]

This is one of the rare conditions in which gonadotropins may be undetectable (large pituitary tumors and genetic deficiencies being the others). If necessary, a high plasma cortisol can differentiate this condition from pituitary insufficiency.

The central origin for the amenorrhea is suggested by the demonstration that the response to GnRH is regained at approximately 15% below the ideal weight, and this return to normal responsiveness occurs before the resumption of menses.[113] Patients with anorexia nervosa have persistent low levels of gonadotropins similar to prepubertal children. With weight gain, sleep-associated episodic secretion of LH appears, similar to the early pubertal child. With full recovery the 24-hour pattern is similar to that of an adult, marked by fluctuating peaks. This sequence of changes with increasing and decreasing weight is explained by increasing and decreasing pulsatile secretion of GnRH. Neuropeptide Y may be a link between the control of food intake and GnRH secretion.[114] Neuropeptide Y cell bodies are located in the arcuate nucleus of the hypothalamus. This peptide both stimulates feeding behavior and inhibits gonadotropin secretion (presumably by suppressing GnRH pulses, although a direct action on the pituitary is also possible). In response to food deprivation, the endogenous levels of neuropeptide Y increase, and elevated concentrations of neuropeptide Y can be measured in the cerebrospinal fluid of anorexic women.

Extensive laboratory testing in these patients is not necessary. Adherence to our scheme for the evaluation of amenorrhea is indicated to rule out other pathological processes. Further endocrine assessment, however, is not essential for patient management.

A careful and gentle revelation to the patient of the relationship between the amenorrhea and the low body weight is often all that is necessary to stimulate the patient to return to normal weight and normal menstrual function. Occasionally it is necessary to see the patient frequently and become involved in a program of daily calorie counting (a minimum intake of 2,600 calories) in order to break the patient's established eating habits. If progress is slow, hormone therapy should be initiated. In an adult weighing less than 100 pounds, continued weight loss requires psychiatric consultation. Some would argue that any patient with an eating disorder requires psychiatric intervention.

Going away to school or the development of a relationship with a male friend often are turning points for young women with mild to moderate anorexia. A failure to respond to these life changes is relatively ominous, predicting a severe problem with a protracted course.

It is disappointing that despite the impressive studies on anorexia there is no specific or new therapy available. This only serves to emphasize the need for early recognition to allow psychologic intervention before the syndrome is entrenched in its full severity.[115] Physicians (and parents) should pay particular attention to weight and diet in young women with amenorrhea.

Exercise and Amenorrhea

Soranus of Ephesus in the 1st century A.D. observed in his famous treatise "On the Diseases of Women," that amenorrhea is frequently observed in the youthful, the aged, the pregnant, in singers, and in those who take much exercise. In the 20th century, there has been a new awareness that competitive female athletes, as well as women engaged in strenuous recreational exercise and women engaged in other forms of demanding activity such as ballet and modern dance, have a significant incidence of menstrual irregularity and amenorrhea, in the pattern called hypothalamic suppression. The extent of this problem has perhaps been underestimated because of a lack of attention to anovulatory cycles. As many as two-thirds of runners who have menstrual periods have short luteal phases or are anovulatory.[116] When training starts before menarche, menarche can be delayed by as much as 3 years, and the subsequent incidence of menstrual irregularity is higher. In some individuals, secondary amenorrhea is associated with delayed menarche even though training did not begin until after menarche. It is suggested that some girls with these characteristics may be socially influenced to pursue athletic training. Contrary to the female situation, exercise has little effect on the timing of puberty in boys. Although changes in testicular function can be demonstrated in males, the changes are more subtle and less meaningful clinically.[117]

There appear to be two major influences: a critical level of body fat and the effect of stress itself. Young women who weigh less than 115 pounds and lose more than 10 pounds while exercising are the women most likely to develop the problem,[118] an association which supports the critical weight concept of Frisch.[119]

The critical weight hypothesis states that the onset and regularity of menstrual function necessitate maintaining weight above a critical level, and therefore, above a critical amount of body fat. In dealing with patients, it is helpful to use the nomogram derived from Frisch, which is based on the calculation of the amount of total body water as a percentage of body weight. This relates to the percentage of body fat and, therefore, is an index of fatness. The 10th percentile at age 16 is equivalent to about 22% body fat, the minimal weight for height necessary for sustaining menstruation, and the 10th percentile at age 13 is equivalent to 17% body fat, the minimum for initiating menarche. A loss of body weight in the range of 10–15% of normal weight for height represents a loss of about one-third of the body fat, which will result in a drop below the 22% line and may result in abnormal menstrual function.[120]

A Fatness Index Nomogram
modified from Frisch

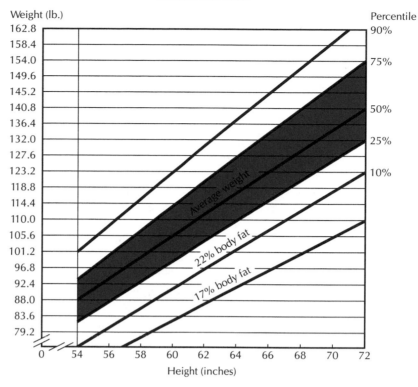

Although the nomogram is useful to show these relationships to patients, individual variation is such that the nomogram cannot be utilized to predict without fail the return of menses for an individual patient. Indeed, the accuracy of the nomogram has been challenged.[121] The fat criteria were derived from the indirect estimation of body fat from predicted total body water, using a regression equation that employs height and weight. There is no question that the most reliable and accurate method for estimating body fatness is hydrostatic weighing of body density (although dual energy x-ray absorptiometry [DEXA] is also excellent). But one can hardly maintain a small pool for this purpose in a clinical office. Granted that the nomogram and specifically the 22% body fat criterion are not absolutely accurate; nevertheless the concept is valid, and the nomogram remains useful to illustrate the concept to patients.

The competitive female athlete has about 50% less body fat than the noncompetitor, very much under the 10th percentile for secondary amenorrhea (the 22% body fat line). This change in body fat can occur with no discernible change in total body weight, because fat is converted to lean muscle mass.[122] A critical look at the critical weight hypothesis argues that there is not a cause and effect relationship between body fat and menstrual function, only a correlation.[123] For this reason, considerable variation is seen with many examples of normal and abnormal menstrual function at all levels of body fat content. On the other hand, the correlation does exist, and body fat content and body weight are useful guides to the relationship between menstrual function and the energy balance of the body.

In addition to the role of body fat, stress and energy expenditure appear to play an independent role. Warren has pointed out that dancers will have a return of menses during intervals of rest, despite no change in body weight or percent body fat.[124] High energy output and stress, therefore, can act independently, as well as additively, to low body fat in suppressing reproductive function. It is not surprising that a woman with low body weight who is engaged in competitive activity (athletic or aesthetic) is highly

439

susceptible to anovulation and amenorrhea.

Running in the dark is even more risky. Studies indicate that ovarian activity can be affected independently by strenuous activity and seasonal variation.[125] Decreased ovarian activity in Autumn could be related to a greater dark photoperiod with increased pineal secretion of melatonin. Indeed, the conception rate of women living in northern Scandinavia is higher during the Summer than in the Winter. The practical conclusion is that serious runners can expect to encounter more problems with menstrual function in Autumn and Winter.

This menstrual disruption is similar to the hypothalamic dysfunction which is more marked in the classic cases of anorexia nervosa. Acute exercise decreases gonadotropins and increases prolactin, growth hormone, testosterone, ACTH, the adrenal steroids, and endorphins as a result of both enhanced secretion and reduced clearance.[126] The prolactin increase is in contrast to the absence of prolactin changes in undernourished women. The prolactin increases are variable, small in amplitude, and exceedingly short in duration. Thus, it is unlikely that the prolactin increase is responsible for the suppression of the menstrual cycle. Most importantly, insignificant differences occur in prolactin when amenorrheic runners are compared to eumenorrheic runners or non-runners.[127] In addition, women athletes have elevated daytime melatonin levels, and amenorrheic athletes have an exaggerated nocturnal secretion of melatonin.[128] The nocturnal increase in melatonin is also seen in women with hypothalamic amenorrhea and appears to reflect suppression of GnRH pulsatile secretion.[129] Another contrast to undernourished women is found in the thyroid axis. Athletes have relatively low T_4 levels, but amenorrheic athletes have an overall suppression of all circulating thyroid hormones, including reverse T_3.[130]

It has been suggested that a suboptimal amount of body fat adversely affects estrogen metabolism, specifically leading to an increased conversion of biologically active estrogens to relatively inactive catecholestrogens.[131] The conversion of estradiol to its catecholestrogen rapidly yields 2-hydroxyestrone, an inactive metabolite. The extent of 2-hydroxylation correlates inversely with body fat, increasing with decreasing adiposity.[122,132] This could be a mechanism that interferes with the important feedback and local roles for estradiol in pituitary-ovarian interactions.

Among runners, there is frequent talk about the runner's "high," the feeling of euphoria and exhilaration after competition or an extensive workout. It is still not clear whether this is a psychologic reaction or whether it is due to an increase in endogenous opiates. The site of GnRH secretion, the arcuate nucleus area in the hypothalamus, is rich in opioid receptors and endorphin production. There is considerable evidence indicating that endogenous opiates inhibit gonadotropin secretion by suppressing hypothalamic GnRH. Women studied during a period of endurance conditioning demonstrated a steadily increasing endorphin output after exercise.[133–135] This link of endorphins to the menstrual suppression associated with exercise is very plausible, but yet unproven. Corticotropin-releasing hormone (CRH) directly inhibits hypothalamic GnRH secretion, probably by augmenting endogenous opioid secretion.[136,137] Women with hypothalamic amenorrhea (including exercisers and women with eating disorders) demonstrate hypercortisolism (due to increased CRH and ACTH), suggesting that this is the pathway by which stress interrupts reproductive function.[138,139] How this suppression is further intensified or activated by a state of low body fat is unknown. From a teliologic point of view, however, there is sense to these relationships; the responses which assist the body to withstand stress also inhibit menstrual function because a stressful period is not the ideal time for reproduction.

Whatever the mechanism, the final pathway is suppression of GnRH.[140] Even in runners with regular menstrual patterns, LH pulsatile frequency and amplitude are significantly reduced.[141,142] A central inhibition of GnRH can be discerned even before there is perceptible evidence of menstrual irregularity. The clinical presentation (inadequate luteal phase, anovulation, amenorrhea) will depend upon the degree of GnRH suppression.

The characteristics of women in the subculture of exercise and amenorrhea strikingly remind one of anorexia nervosa: significant physical exercise, a necessity for control of the body, striving for artistic and technical proficiency, and the consequent preoccupation with the body — combined with the stressful pressures of performing and competition.[143] Individuals in this lifestyle are prone to develop what can be called the anorectic reaction.[144] Fries has described four stages of dieting behavior which can form a continuum:[145]

1. Dieting for cosmetic reasons.

2. Dieting due to neurotic fixation on food intake and weight.

3. The anorectic reaction.

4. True anorexia nervosa.

There are several important distinctions between the anorectic reaction and true anorexia nervosa. Psychologically the patient with true anorexia nervosa has a misperception of reality and a lack of insight into the disease and her problem. She does not consider herself underweight and displays an impressive lack of concern over her dreadful physical condition and appearance. The doctor-patient relationship is difficult with no visible emotional involvement and a great deal of mistrust. Patients with the anorectic reaction have the capability for self-criticism. They can see the problem and describe it with insight and an absence of denial. The exercising woman and the competing athlete or dancer can develop an anorectic reaction. The anorectic reaction develops consciously and voluntarily, just as in anorexia nervosa, as the exercising woman deliberately makes an effort to decrease body weight. A clinician may be the first to be aware of the problem having encountered the patient because of the presenting complaint of either amenorrhea or now uncontrolled weight loss. Early recognition, concentrated counseling, and confidential support can intercept and prevent a progressive problem.

Prognosis is excellent with early recognition, and simple weight gain may reverse the state of amenorrhea. The degree of reversibility is unknown, although general experience indicates that the majority of women regain ovulation when stress and exercise diminish or cease.[146,147] However, these patients are often unwilling to give up their routines of exercise, and a sensitive clinician can perceive that the exercise is an important means for coping with daily life. Hormone therapy is therefore encouraged for these hypoestrogenic patients to provide protection against the loss of bone and cardiovascular changes. When pregnancy is desired, a reduction in the amount of exercise and a gain in weight should be recommended, or induction of ovulation must be pursued.

Eating Disorders and Pregnancy

It has been estimated that a typical pregnancy requires approximately 300 extra calories per day above that needed in the nonpregnant state.[148] With sufficient caloric intake, weight gain during pregnancy averages 10–12 kg (22–26 lb). Women who are underweight prior to pregnancy need to increase their energy intake and gain 12–15 kg (26–33 lb). Imagine the reaction of a patient with an eating disorder when confronted with these facts. This is fuel for the fire (the morbid fear of fatness).

Prior to the 1970s, obstetricians vigorously advised their patients to limit weight gain during pregnancy. This sadly misplaced advice could be traced to the false belief that excessive weight gain caused preeclampsia, made labor more difficult, and had a permanently detrimental impact on a woman's figure. More appropriate recommendations emerged in the 1970s, based upon a growing body of information derived from scientific studies. These studies documented the importance of prepregnancy weight as well as weight gain during pregnancy as two very important determinants for infant birth weight.

The critical issue is the relationship between the diet of the mother and the well-being of the fetus. There are three classic studies of acute famine in Leningrad, Holland, and Wuppertal during the dark days of World War II.[149–151] The mean birthweight during the siege of Leningrad declined 550 g to 2,789 g. During the Dutch famine, mean birth weight decreased by 300 g; there was no decrease in the birth weight of infants conceived during the famine whose mothers received adequate rations during the third trimester. In Wuppertal, mean birth weight was depressed by 170–227 g. These differences were proportional to the level of official rations, the conditions being the worst in Leningrad.

Studies of restriction of calories during pregnancy have indicated a ready achievement of lesser maternal weight gain, at the expense of lighter birth weights.[152] Women who gain less than 20 pounds compared to those who gain more than 20 pounds are 2.3 times more likely to deliver infants of low birth weight and 1.5 times more likely to have a fetal death.[153] These studies finally led to the abandonment of caloric limitation.

In general, studies of dietary supplementation have indicated increases in mean birth weights.[153] The Special Supplemental Food Program for Women, Infants, and Children (WIC) was begun in the U.S. in 1973. A review of this program finds a significant impact on decreasing preterm labor and delivery, an increase in mean birth weight, and a reduction in late fetal death.[154] These improvements are attributed to an improved maternal physiologic status, not upgraded health care. The head circumferences of infants of mothers who participated in WIC were significantly larger, presumably reflecting accelerated brain growth.

Gradually it came to be appreciated that there is a linear relationship between birth weight and maternal weight gain at all levels of prepregnancy weight.[155–159] However, as prepregnancy weight increases, the importance of maternal weight gain diminishes.[160] Thus, in underweight women, the importance of each factor, prepregnancy weight and the weight gain during pregnancy, is magnified.

Now that the many circumstances which influence infant birth weight are better recognized, a modern look at this subject is especially helpful. After adjusting for maternal age, race, parity, weight gain, socioeconomic status, cigarette consumption, and gestational age, there continues to be a statistically significant linear relationship between prepregnancy body mass and birth weight, as well as between prenatal weight gain and birth weight.[161,162] Furthermore, the fetal death rate increases exponentially as birth weight decreases at each gestational age.[163] Most importantly, a low prepregnancy weight can be overcome; weight gain during pregnancy (beginning in the first trimester) in underweight women can bring an infant into the normal range for birth weight.[164]

Low birth weight in an infant can be directly attributed mainly to two influencing factors: prematurity and fetal growth retardation. In developing countries, the major factor is intrauterine growth retardation, while in developed countries, prematurity is the predominant influence.[165] In patients with eating disorders, the outcome of pregnancy is significantly influenced by both of these factors.

In view of the well-recognized correlation between maternal weight (prepregnancy weight and pregnancy weight gain) and infant size, it is certainly logical to expect a problem with pregnancy outcome in patients with eating disorders. Older reports were anecdotal in nature and usually failed to provide birth weights, since our awareness of the importance of body weight to pregnancy outcome is a relatively recent development.[166–172]

More recent reports have documented problems with intrauterine growth retardation and preterm labor. The average weight gain in 7 pregnancies in patients with anorexia nervosa was 8 kg; all infants demonstrated intrauterine growth retardation in the third trimester, followed by accelerated growth after birth.[173] A review of 23 pregnancies in 74 women treated for anorexia or bulimia documented the importance of the severity of the disorder.[174] Women in remission gained more weight and had higher birth weights and 5-minute Apgar scores. Women with active disease had worsening symptoms and psychological problems during pregnancy. The smallest birth weights were born to those with anorexia and bulimia. All the women who were ill at conception continued to be ill. Nine of the 10 women who successfully breastfed for 6 months were in remission. The rate of preterm labor and delivery in patients with eating disorders is twice the normal incidence, and in a study of 50 Danish anorectic women, the perinatal mortality rate was 6 times the normal rate.[175] In an Australian review of 14 consecutive women who failed to respond to clomiphene, all the women had a history of an eating or exercise disorder, and one-third of the eventual live births weighed less than 2,500 g.[176]

While some patients with eating disorders do well during pregnancy, do not be lulled.[177] After the pregnancy rapid deterioration usually takes place. Expert help during the pregnancy is highly recommended. Some useful warning signs are the following:

1.   Unusual concern regarding body shape.

2.   Aversion to being weighed.

3.   Lack of weight gain.

About 25% of patients with amenorrhea are underweight due to self-imposed dietary restriction.[178] Because underweight women frequently are anovulatory, it is not surprising that they represent a significant population in whom ovulation is induced. Comparing the outcome of pregnancy in underweight women after spontaneous and induced ovulation, it is apparent that inadequate weight has serious consequences.[179] Underweight women who undergo induction of ovulation often fail to gain weight adequately during pregnancy despite care and counseling. As expected, intrauterine growth retardation and preterm labor are significant problems.

The seriousness of the problem is heightened because of its presence at conception and during the first trimester. A study of adolescent pregnancy concluded that inadequate weight gain before 24 weeks gestation was associated with a significantly increased risk of having a small for gestational age infant, *even when later weight gains brought the cumulative weight gain within normal adult standards.*[180] Later inadequate weight gain was associated with an increased risk of preterm delivery. These results suggest that prevention of preterm delivery and intrauterine growth retardation requires an effort encompassing the entire pregnancy, best beginning prior to conception. A rise in weight of more than 6 kg by the 28th week of pregnancy has predictive value, indicating with a high degree of probability that the rest of pregnancy will progress normally.[181]

In summary, dietary restriction decreases birth weight and can have as great an impact as a serious famine. The impact on perinatal morbidity and mortality has been poorly assessed, but there is reason to believe that preterm labor is increased and that children with intrauterine growth retardation have more problems later in life. An issue that has not been well studied is the impact of the eating disorder on parenting after the delivery.

Because intrauterine growth retardation before the third trimester is associated with significant long-term morbidity, physicians treating amenorrhea associated with weight loss should consider solving the dietary problem before subjecting a fetus to a struggle during intrauterine life. Patients with an active eating disorder should wait for remission before getting pregnant. These messages, therefore, especially apply to two groups of physicians: obstetricians and reproductive endocrinologists.

When encountering a patient who is pregnant and has an eating disorder, the obstetrician should seek expert consultation in order to achieve and maintain remission of the disorder during the pregnancy. Careful monitoring of maternal weight gain and fetal growth is essential. Consideration should be given to special dietary supplementation, especially when delayed fetal growth is demonstrated. Full exploitation of the pregnancy is warranted to provide·motivation for effective resolution of this psychodynamic disorder.

The best results can be achieved with stabilization of the disorder prior to pregnancy. The reproductive endocrinologist should hesitate before embarking on a program of ovulation induction. The reward of pregnancy should be offered as an inducement to reach a normal prepregnancy weight. Patients with an eating disorder who are considering pregnancy must be made aware of the potential adverse impact on fetal growth and development.

The timing of psychiatric intervention is important. The prospect of pregnancy should stimulate a preconceptual effort by the patient's physicians. At no other time will the patient's physicians have such a strong ally, the motivating force behind the desire for pregnancy.

Amenorrhea and Anosmia, Kallmann's Syndrome

A rare condition in females is the syndrome of congenital hypogonadotropic hypogonadism associated with anosmia or hyposmia, known as Kallmann's syndrome. There is a chronology of eponyms assigning credit for original descriptions of this syndrome, but with all due respect to the physicians who first recognized this association, it is far easier to remember it in a descriptive way, as a syndrome of amenorrhea and anosmia.[182–185] In the female, this problem is characterized by primary amenorrhea, infantile sexual development, low gonadotropins, a normal female karyotype, and the inability to perceive odors, e.g., coffee grounds or perfume. Often the affected individuals are not aware of their olfactory defect. The gonads can respond to gonadotropins; therefore induction of ovulation with exogenous gonadotropins is successful. However, clomiphene is ineffective.

Kallmann's syndrome is associated with a specific anatomic defect. Magnetic resonance imaging (as well as postmortem examination) demonstrates hypoplastic or absent olfactory sulci in the rhinencephalon.[186] This defect is a consequence of the failure of both olfactory axonal and GnRH neuronal migration from the olfactory placode in the nose. The cells that produce GnRH originate in the olfactory area and migrate during embryogenesis along cranial nerves which connect the nose and the forebrain. The mutations responsible for this syndrome involve a single gene on the short arm of the X chromosome that encodes a protein responsible for functions necessary for neuronal migration.[187,188] Location on the X chromosome explains why the syndrome occurs 5–7 times more frequently in males than in females. Other neurologic abnormalities (mirror movements, hearing loss, cerebellar ataxia) can be present, suggesting more widespread neurologic defects. Renal and bone abnormalities and cleft lip and palate also occur in affected individuals, probably reflecting the fact that the gene is expressed in tissues other than the hypothalamus.[189] The syndrome occurs as an inherited or sporadic defect. Three modes of transmission have been documented: X-linked, autosomal dominant, and autosomal recessive. The increased frequency in males indicates that X-linked transmission is the most common. X-linked Kallmann's syndrome can be associated with other disorders due to deletions or translocations of contiguous genes on the distal short arm of the X chromosome (such as X-linked short stature or ichthyosis and sulfatase deficiency).

It is possible that patients with hypothalamic amenorrhea due to isolated deficiency of GnRH secretion (and no other abnormalities) have a defect similar to that of Kallmann's syndrome. With a lesser penetrance, only the GnRH migratory defect is expressed. In some individuals with amenorrhea and a normal sense of smell, family members can be identified with anosmia.

Postpill Amenorrhea

In the past it was assumed that secondary amenorrhea reflected persistent suppressive effects of oral contraceptive medication or the use of the intramuscular depot form of medroxyprogesterone acetate (Depo-Provera). It is now recognized that the fertility rate is normal following discontinuance of either of these forms of contraception (Chapter 22), and attempts to identify a cause-effect relationship in case-control studies have failed. Therefore, amenorrhea following the use of steroids for contraception requires investigation as described in order to avoid missing a significant problem. This investigation should be pursued if a patient is amenorrheic 6 months after discontinuing oral contraception or 12 months after the last injection of Depo-Provera.

Hormone Therapy

The patient who is hypoestrogenic and who is not a candidate for induction of ovulation deserves hormone therapy. This includes patients appropriately evaluated and diagnosed as having gonadal failure, patients with hypothalamic amenorrhea, and postgonadectomy patients. The long-term impact of the hypoestrogenic state in terms of cardiovascular disease has long been recognized. The beneficial impact of exercise on the lipoprotein profile is reversed by estrogen deficiency.[190] The bone density in women is dependent upon normal reproductive age levels of estrogen and progesterone. Even the most strenuous of exercise does not balance the consequences of hypoestrogenism on the bones, especially in adolescents.[191–194] In the absence of estrogen, the normal response of bone to stress (to become stronger) is impaired.[195] The same arguments that apply to hormone treatment in older women (Chapter 18) can be convincingly used to encourage these younger women to replace the estrogen they are lacking. The amenorrheic exerciser should be made aware that the hypoestrogenic state is associated with a greater risk of stress fractures.[196–200] Ballet dancers with delayed menarche are more prone to scoliosis as well as stress fractures.[200] It is not certain, however, whether this greater risk of stress fractures is influenced solely by bone density changes in that some studies fail to correlate fractures with reductions in bone density.[201] It should be noted that bone loss in amenorrheic women shows the same pattern over time as seen in postmenopausal women.[202] The loss is most rapid in the first few years, emphasizing the need for early treatment.

In patients with eating disorders, bone density correlates with body weight.[203] The response to hormone therapy may be impaired as long as an abnormal weight is maintained. Furthermore, because the pubertal gain in bone density is so significant, individuals who fail to experience this adolescent increase may continue to have a deficit in bone mass despite hormone treatment. Reduced menstrual function for any reason early in life (even beyond adolescence) may leave a residual deficit in bone density which cannot be retrieved with resumption of menses or with hormone treatment.[204,205]

Several reports have indicated that patients with hyperprolactinemia are at risk for osteoporosis. At first this appeared not to be related to estrogen status, suggesting an independent effect of prolactin. Results have been confusing for several reasons. Controls in various studies were matched in different fashions, e.g., only for age, ignoring height and weight. Photon absorptiometry, the method of study in some reports, has a reduced sensitivity and significant variation when used to assess the axial skeleton. And finally, the estrogen status of the hyperprolactinemic patients was not always carefully quantified. It is now recognized that the bone density changes observed in hyperprolactinemic amenorrheic women are due to the hypoestrogenic state.[206-208]

The standard program for estrogen therapy should be used. A good schedule is the following: on days 1 through 25 of each month, take 0.625 mg conjugated estrogens; on days 16 through 25, add 10 mg medroxyprogesterone acetate. Beginning medication on the first of every month establishes an easily remembered routine. Another popular method is to administer the estrogen every day and the progestin the first 12 days of each month. If the progestational agent is responsible for side effects, the daily dose can be decreased to 5 mg. In a few individuals, the estrogen dosage may have to be increased to 1.25 mg in order to achieve menstrual bleeding. Whether a flow-provoking dose of estrogen is necessary for optimal protection of the bones has not been addressed in a clinical study. In patients who have not undergone pubertal development, a lower dose regimen should be used as outlined in Chapter 11.

Menstruation generally occurs 3 days after the last day of progestin medication. Bleeding that occurs at any time other than the usual expected time may be a sign that endogenous function has returned. The hormone treatment program should be discontinued and the patient monitored for the resumption of ovulation.

The importance of monthly menstruation to a young woman cannot be overemphasized. Regular and visible menstrual bleeding is often a gratifying experience in the young patient with gonadal dysgenesis and serves to reinforce her identification with the feminine gender role. On the other hand, serious exercisers (such as athletes and dancers) may wish to avoid menstrual bleeding. One can provide hormone therapy to these women utilizing the daily combination approach: 0.625 mg conjugated estrogens and 2.5 mg medroxyprogesterone acetate given together every day without a break.

If for some reason, a hypoestrogenic woman refuses hormone treatment, supplemental calcium (1,000–1,500 mg daily) should be strongly encouraged. High calcium intake when combined with a high level of exercise is more effective in protecting the vertebral bone density than either exercise or calcium alone.[209]

Patients with hypothalamic amenorrhea must be cautioned that hormone therapy will not protect against pregnancy in the event that normal function unknowingly returns. In the occasional patient who must have the most effective contraception possible, it is reasonable to utilize a low dose oral contraceptive to provide the missing estrogen. This is an excellent option in patients with premature ovarian failure because a spontaneous resumption of ovarian function can occur without warning. Athletes interested in avoiding menstruation can take oral contraceptives every day without a pill-free interval.

References

1. **Contreras P, Generini G, Michelson H, Pumarino H, Campino C,** Hyperprolactinemia and galactorrhea: spontaneous versus iatrogenic hypothyroidism, J Clin Endocrinol Metab 53:1036, 1981.

2. **Danziger J, Wallace S, Handel S, Samaan NG,** The sella turcica in primary end organ failure, Radiology 131:111, 1979.

3. **Poretsky L, Garber J, Kleefield J,** Primary amenorrhea and pseudoprolactinoma in a patient with primary hypothyroidism, Am J Med 81:180, 1986.

4. **Coulam CB, Annegers JF, Kraz JC,** Chronic anovulation syndrome and associated neoplasia, Obstet Gynecol 61:403, 1983.

5. **Lloyd RV, Chandler WF, Kovacs K, Ryan N,** Ectopic pituitary adenomas with normal anterior pituitary glands, Am J Surg Path 10:546, 1986.

6. **Palmer PE, Bogojavlensky S, Bhan AK, Scully RE,** Prolactinoma in wall of ovarian dermoid cyst with hyperprolactinemia, Obstet Gynecol 75:540, 1990.

7. **Comtois R, Bouchard J, Robert F,** Hypersecretion of gonadotropins by a pituitary adenoma: pituitary dynamic studies and treatment with bromocriptine in one patient, Fertil Steril 52:569, 1989.

8. **Katznelson L, Alexander JM, Bikkal HA, Jameson JL, Hsu DW, Klibanski A,** Imbalanced follicle-stimulating hormone β-subunit hormone biosynthesis in human pituitary adenomas, J Clin Endocrinol Metab 74:1343, 1992.

9. **Katznelson L, Alexander JM, Klibanski A,** Clinically nonfunctioning pituitary adenomas, J Clin Endocrinol Metab 76:1089, 1993.

10. **Daneshdoost L, Gennarelli TA, Bashey HM, Savino PJ, Sergott RC, Bosley TM, Snyder PJ,** Recognition of gonadotroph adenomas in women, New Engl J Med 324:589, 1991.

11. **Buckler HM, Evans A, Mamlora H, Burger HG, Anderson DC,** Gonadotropin, steroid and inhibin levels in women with incipient ovarian failure during anovulatory and ovulatory 'rebound' cycles, J Clin Endocrinol Metab 72:116, 1991.

12. **Talbert LM, Raj MHG, Hammond MG, Greer T,** Endocrine and immunologic studies in a patient with resistant ovary syndrome, Fertil Steril 442:741, 1984.

13. **Sutton C,** The limitations of laparoscopic ovarian biopsy, J Obstet Gynaecol Br Commonwlth 81:317, 1974.

14. **Alper MM, Garner PR,** Premature ovarian failure: its relationship to autoimmune disease, Obstet Gynecol 66:27, 1985.

15. **Cowchock FS, McCabe JL, Montgomery BB,** Pregnancy after corticosteroid administration in premature ovarian failure (polyglandular endocrinopathy syndrome), Am J Obstet Gynecol 158:118, 1988.

16. **Blumenfeld Z, Halachmi S, Peretz BA, Shmuel Z, Golan D, Makler A, Brandes JM,** Premature ovarian failure—the prognostic application of autoimmunity on conception after ovulation induction, Fertil Steril 59:750, 1993.

17. **Levy HL, Driscoll SG, Porensky RS, Wender DF,** Ovarian failure in galactosemia, New Engl J Med 310:50, 1984.

18. **Robinson ACR, Dockeray CJ, Cullen MJ, Sweeney EC,** Hypergonadotrophic hypogonadism in classical galactosaemia: evidence for defective oogenesis: case report, Br J Obstet Gynaecol 91:199, 1984.

19. **Manuel M, Katayama KP, Jones Jr HW,** The age of occurrence of gonadal tumors in intersex patients with a Y chromosome. Am J Obstet Gynecol 124:293, 1976.

20. **Aiman J, Smentek C,** Premature ovarian failure, Obstet Gynecol 66:9, 1985.

21. **Rebar RW, Connolly HV,** Clinical features of young women with hypergonadotropic amenorrhea, Fertil Steril 53:804, 1990.

22. **Axelrod L, Neer RM, Kliman B,** Hypogonadism in a male with immunologically active, biologically inactive luteinizing hormone: an exception to a venerable rule, J Clin Endocrinol Metab 48:279, 1979.

23. **Teasdale E, Teasdale G, Mohsen F, MacPherson P,** High-resolution computed tomography in pituitary microadenoma: is seeing believing? Clin Radiol 37:227, 1986.

24. **Stein AL, Levenick MN, Kletzky OA,** Computed tomography versus magnetic resonance imaging for the evaluation of suspected pituitary adenomas, Obstet Gynecol 73:996, 1989.

25. **Schlechte J, Dolan K, Sherman B, Chapler F, Luciano A,** The natural history of untreated hyperprolactinemia: a prospective analysis, J Clin Endocrinol Metab 68:412, 1989.

26. **Reincke M, Allolio B, Saeger W, Menzel J, Winkelmann W,** The 'incidentaloma' of the pituitary gland, JAMA 263:2772, 1990.

27. **Strebel PM, Zacur HA, Gold EB,** Headache, hyperprolactinemia, and prolactinomas, Obstet Gynecol 68:195, 1986.

28. **Reindollar RH, Novak M, Tho SPT, McDonough PG,** Adult-onset amenorrhea: a study of 262 patients, Am J Obstet Gynecol 155:531, 1986.

29. **Schenker JG, Margalioth EJ,** Intrauterine adhesions: an updated appraisal, Fertil Steril 37:593, 1982.

30. **Markham SM, Parmley TH, Murphy AA, Huggins GR, Rock JA,** Cervical agenesis combined with vaginal agenesis diagnosed by magnetic resonance imaging, Fertil Steril 48:143, 1987.

31. **Griffin JE, Edwards C, Ladden JD, Harrod MJ, Wilson JD,** Congenital absence of the vagina, Ann Intern Med 85:224, 1976.

32. **Letterie GS, Wilson J, Miyazawa K,** Magnetic resonance imaging of müllerian tract abnormalities, Fertil Steril 50: 365, 1988.

33. **Fedele L, Dorta M, Brioschi D, Giudici MN, Candiani GB,** Magnetic resonance imaging in Mayer-Rokitansky-Kuster-Hauser Syndrome, Obstet Gynecol 76:593, 1990.

34. **Frank RT,** Formation of artificial vagina without operation, Am J Obstet Gynecol 35:1053, 1938.

35. **Wabrek AJ, Millard PR, Wilson WB Jr, Pion RJ,** Creation of a neovagina by the Frank nonoperative method, Obstet Gynecol 37:408, 1971.

36. **Bates GW, Wiser WL,** A technique for uterine conservation in adolescents with vaginal agenesis and a functional uterus, Obstet Gynecol 66:290, 1985.

37. **Batzer FR, Corson SL, Gocial B, Daly DC, Go K, English ME,** Genetic offspring in patients with vaginal agenesis: specific medical and legal issues, Am J Obstet Gynecol 167:1288, 1992.

38. **Morris JM, Mahesh VB,** Further observations on the syndrome "testicular feminization," Am J Obstet Gynecol 87:731, 1963.

39. **Griffin JE,** Androgen resistance — the clinical and molecular spectrum, New Engl J Med 326:611, 1992.

40. **Simpson JL,** Genetics of sexual differentiation, in Rock JA, Carpenter SE, editors, *Pediatric and Adolescent Gynecology,* Raven Press, New York, 1992, pp 1-37.

41. **Gililland J, Cummings D, Hibbert ML, Crain T, Rozanski T,** Laparoscopic orchiectomy in a patient with complete androgen insensitivity, J Laparoendoscopic Surg 3:51, 1993.

42. **Simpson JL,** Genetic forms of gonadal dysgenesis in 46,XX and 46,XY individuals, Seminars Reprod Endocrinol 1:93, 1983.

43. **Medlej R, Lobaccaro JM, Berta P, Belon C, Leheup B, Toublanc JE, Weill J, Chevalier C, Dumas R, Sultan C,** Screening for Y-derived sex determining gene SRY in 40 patients with Turner syndrome, J Clin Endocrinol Metab 75:1289, 1992.

44. **Coulam CB, Adamsen SC, Annegers JF,** Incidence of premature ovarian failure, Obstet Gynecol 67:604, 1986.

45. **Dewald GW, Spurbeck JL,** Sex chromosome anomalies associated with premature gonadal failure, Seminars Reprod Endocrinol 1:79, 1983.

46. **Gradishar WJ, Schilsky RL,** Ovarian function following radiation and chemotherapy, Seminars Oncol 16:425, 1989.

47. **Wallace WH, Shalet SM, Crowne EC, Morris-Jones PH, Gattamanen HR,** Ovarian failure following abdominal irradiation in childhood: natural history and prognosis, Clin Oncol 1:75, 1989.

48. **Asch P,** The influence of radiation on fertility in man, Br J Radiol 53:271, 1980.

49. **Byrne J, Mulvihill JJ, Myers MH, Connelly RR, Naughton MD, Krauss MR, Steinhorn SC, Hassinger DD, Austin DF, Bragg K, et al,** Effects of treatment on fertility in long-term survivors of childhood cancer, New Engl J Med 317:1315, 1987.

50. **Schelthauer BW, Randall RV, Laws ER Jr, Kovacs KT, Horvath E, Whitaker MD,** Prolactin cell carcinoma of the pituitary, Cancer 55:598, 1985.

51. **Mountcastle RB, Roof BS, Mayflied RK, Mordes DB, Sage L J, Biggs PJ, Rawe SE,** Case report: pituitary adenocarcinoma in an acromegalic patient. Response to bromocriptine and pituitary testing: a review of the literature on 36 cases of pituitary carcinoma, Am J Med Sci 298:109, 1989.

52. **Walker JD, Grossman A, Anderson JV, Ur E, Trainer PJ, Benn J, Lowy C, Sonksen PH, Plowman PN, Lowe DG, Doniach I, Wass JAH, Besser GM,** Malignant prolactinoma with extracranial metastases: A report of three cases, Clin Endocrinol 38:411, 1993.

53. **Pituitary Adenoma Study Group,** Pituitary adenomas and oral contraceptives: a multicenter case-control study, Fertil Steril 39:753, 1983.

54. **Costello RT,** Subclinical adenoma of the pituitary gland, Am J Pathol 12:191, 1936.

55. **Kraus HE,** Neoplastic diseases of the human hypophysis, Arch Pathol 39:343, 1945.

56. **McCormick WF, Halmi NS,** Absence of chromophobe adenomas from a large series of pituitary tumors, Arch Pathol 92:231, 1971.

57. **Sheline GE,** Untreated and recurrent chromophobe adenomas of the pituitary, Radiology 112:768, 1971.

58. **Burrow GN, Wortzman G, Rewcastle NB, Holgate RC, Kovacs K,** Microadenomas of the pituitary and abnormal sellar tomograms in an unselected autopsy series, New Engl J Med 304:156, 1981.

59. **Schlechte J, Sherman B, Halmi N, Van Gilder J, Chapler FK, Dolan K, Granner D, Duello T, Harris C,** Prolactin-secreting pituitary tumors, Endocrin Rev 1:295, 1980.

60. **Jackson RD, Wortsman J, Malarkey WB,** Characterization of a large molecular weight prolactin in women with idiopathic hyperprolactinemia and normal menses, J Clin Endocrinol Metab 61:258, 1985.

61. **Jackson RD, Wortsman J, Malarkey WB,** Macroprolactinemia presenting like a pituitary tumor, Am J Med 78:346, 1985.

62. **Hattori N, Ishihara T, Ikekubo K, Moridera K, Hino M, Kurahachi H,** Autoantibody to human prolactin in patients with idiopathic hyperprolactinemia, J Clin Endocrinol Metab 75:1226, 1992.

63. **Speroff L, Levin RM, Haning RV Jr, Kase NG,** A practical approach for the evaluation of women with abnormal polytomography or elevated prolactin levels, Am J Obstet Gynecol 135:896, 1979.

64. **Monroe SE, Levine L, Chang RJ, Keye WR Jr, Yamamoto M, Jaffe RB,** Prolactin-secreting pituitary adenomas: V. Increased gonadotropin responsivity in hyperprolactinemic women with pituitary adenomas, J Clin Endocrinol Metab 52:1171, 1981.

65. **Sauder SE, Frager M, Case GD, Kelch RP, Marshall JC,** Abnormal patterns of pulsatile luteinizing hormone secretion in women with hyperprolactinemia and amenorrhea: responses to bromocriptine, J Clin Endocrinol Metab 59:941, 1984.

66. **Cook CB, Nippoldt TB, Kletter GB, Kelch RP, Marshall JC,** Naloxone increases the frequency of pulsatile luteinizing hormone secretion in women with hyperprolactinemia, J Clin Endocrinol Metab 73:1099, 1991.

67. **Schlechte JA, Sherman BM, Chapler FK, VanGilder J,** Long term follow-up of women with surgically treated prolactin-secreting pituitary tumors, J Clin Endocrinol Metab 62:1296, 1986.

68. **Parl FF, Cruz VE, Cobb CA, Bradley CA, Aleshire SL,** Late recurrence of surgically removed prolactinomas, Cancer 57:2422, 1986.

69. **Thomson JA, Teasdale GM, Gordon D, McCruden DC, Davies DL,** Treatment of presumed prolactinoma by transsphenoidal operation: early and late results, Br Med J 291:1550, 1985.

70. **Herman V, Fagin J, Gonsky R, Kovacs K, Melmed S,** Clonal origin of pituitary adenomas, J Clin Endocrinol Metab 71:1427, 1990.

71. **Vance ML, Evans WS, Thorner MO,** Bromocriptine, Ann Intern Med 100:78, 1984.

72. **Merola B, Colao A, Caruso E, Sarnacchiaro F, Briganti F, Lancranjan I, Lombardi G, Schettini G,** Oral and injectable long-lasting bromocriptine preparations in hyperprolactinemia: comparison of their prolactin lowering activity, tolerability, and safety, Gynecol Endocrinol 5:267, 1991.

73. **Beckers A, Petrossians P, Abs R, Flandroy P, Stadnik T, de Longueville M, Lancranjan I, Stevenaert A,** Treatment of macroprolactinomas with the long-acting and repeatable form of bromocriptine: a report on 29 cases, J Clin Endocrinol Metab 75:275, 1992.

74. **Brue T, Lancranjan I, Louvet J-P, Dewailly D, Roger P, Jaquet P,** A long-acting repeatable form of bromocriptine as long-term treatment of prolactin-secreting macroadenomas: a multicenter study, Fertil Steril 57:74, 1992.

75. **Ginsburg J, Hardiman P, Thomas M,** Vaginal bromocriptine — clinical and biochemical effects, Gynecol Endocrinol 6:119, 1992.

76. **Weil C,** The safety of bromocriptine in long-term use: a review of the literature, Curr Med Res Opin 10:25, 1986.

77. **Cuellar FG,** Bromocriptine mesylate (Parlodel) in the management of amenorrhea/galactorrhea associated with hyperprolactinemia, Obstet Gynecol 55:278, 1980.

78. **Sieck JO, Niles NL, Jinkins JR, Al-Mefty O, El-Akkad S, Woodhouse N,** Extrasellar prolactinomas: successful management of 24 patients using bromocriptine, Horm Res 23:167, 1986.

79. **Bevan JS, Webster J, Burke CW, Scanlon MF,** Dopamine agonists and pituitary tumor shrinkage, Endocrin Rev 13:220, 1992.

80. **Mori H, Mori S, Saitoh Y, Arita N, Aono T, Uozumi T, Mogami H, Matsumoto K,** Effects of bromocriptine on prolactin-secreting pituitary adenomas, Cancer 56:230, 1985.

81. **Lamberts SWJ, Quik RFP,** A comparison of the efficacy and safety of pergolide and bromocriptine in the treatment of hyperprolactinemia, J Clin Endocrinol Metab 72:635, 1991.

82. **Ciccarelli E, Giusti M, Miola C, Potenzoni F, Sghedoni D, Camanni F, Giordano G,** Effectiveness and tolerability of long term treatment with cabergoline, a new long-lasting ergoline derivative in hyperprolactinemic patients, J Clin Endocrinol Metab 69:725, 1989.

83. **Brue T, Pellegrini I, Gunz G, Morange I, Dewailly D, Brownell J, Enjalbert A, Jaquet P,** Effects of the dopamine agonist CV 205-502 in human prolactinomas resistant to bromocriptine, J Clin Endocrinol Metab 74:577, 1992.

84. **Lappohn RE, van de Wiel HBM, Brownell J,** The effect of two dopaminergic drugs on menstrual function and psychological state in hyperprolactinemia, Fertil Steril 58:321, 1992.

85. **Liuzzi A, Dallabonzana D, Oppizzi G, Verde GG, Cozzi R, Chiodini P, Luccarelli G,** Low doses of dopamine agonists in the long-term treatment of macroprolactinomas, New Engl J Med 313:656, 1985.

86. **Tsagarakis S, Grossman A, Plowman PN, et al,** Megavoltage pituitary irradiation in the management of prolactomas: long-term follow-up, Clin Endocrinol 34:399, 1991.

87. **Johnston DG, Hall K, Kendall-Taylor P, Patrick D, Watson MJ, Cook DB,** Effect of dopamine agonist withdrawal after long-term therapy in prolactinomas. Studies with high-definition computerized tomography, Lancet 2:187, 1984.

88. **Martin TL, Kim M, Malarkey WB,** The natural history of idiopathic hyperprolactinemia, J Clin Endocrinol Metab 60:855, 1985.

89. **Sluijmer AV, Lappohn RE,** Clinical history and outcome of 59 patients with idiopathic hyperprolactinemia, Fertil Steril 58:72, 1992.

90. **Corenblum B, Donovan L,** The safety of physiological estrogen plus progestin replacement therapy and oral contraceptive therapy in women with pathological hyperprolactinemia, Fertil Steril 59:671, 1993.

91. **Sisam DA, Sheehan JP, Schumacher OP,** Lack of demonstrable tumor growth in progressive hyperprolactinemia, Am J Med 80:279, 1986.

92. **Molitch ME,** Pregnancy and the hyperprolactinemic woman, New Engl J Med 312:1362, 1985.

93. **Freeman R, Wezenter B, Silverstein M, Kuo D, Weiss KL, Kantrowitz AB, Schubart UK,** Pregnancy-associated subacute hemorrhage into a prolactinoma resulting in diabetes insipidus, Fertil Steril 58:427, 1992.

94. **Ahmed M, Al-Dossary E, Woodhouse NJY,** Macroprolactinomas with suprasellar extension: effect of bromocriptine withdrawal during one or more pregnancies, Fertil Steril 58:492, 1992.

95. **Turkalj I, Braun P, Krupp P,** Surveillance of bromocriptine in pregnancy, JAMA 247:1589, 1982.

96. **De Wit W, Coelingh Bennink HJT, Gerards LJ,** Prophylactic bromocriptine treatment during pregnancy in women with macroprolactinomas: report of 13 pregnancies, Br J Obstet Gynaecol 91:1059, 1984.

97. **Ruiz-Velasco V, Tolis G,** Pregnancy in hyperprolactinemic women, Fertil Steril 41:793, 1984.

98. **Holmgren U, Bergstrand G, Hagenfeldt K, Werner S,** Women with prolactinoma—effect of pregnancy and lactation on serum prolactin and on tumour growth, Acta Endocrinol 111:452, 1986.

99. **Hodgson SF, Randall RV, Holman CB, MacCarty CS,** Empty sella syndrome, Med Clin North Am 56:897, 1972.

100. **Hirvonen E,** Etiology, clinical features and prognosis in secondary amenorrhea, Int J Fertil 22:69, 1977.

101. **Olster DH, Ferin M,** Corticotropin-releasing hormone inhibits gonadotropin secretion in the ovariectomized Rhesus monkey, J Clin Endocrinol Metab 65:262, 1987.

102. **Berga SL, Mortola JF, Suh GB, Laughlin G, Pham P, Yen SSC,** Neuroendocrine aberrations in women with functional hypothalamic amenorrhea, J Clin Endocrinol Metab 68:301, 1989.

103. **Berga SL, Loucks AB, Rossmanith WG, Kettel LM, Laughlin GA, Yen SSC,** Acceleration of luteinizing hormone pulse frequency in functional hypothalamic amenorrhea by dopaminergic blockade, J Clin Endocrinol Metab 72:151, 1991.

104. **Nakayama Y, Wondisford FE, Lash RW, Bale AE, Weintraub BD, Cutler GB Jr, Radovick S,** Analysis of gonadotropin-releasing hormone gene structure in families with familial central precocious puberty and idiopathic hypogonadotropic hypogonadism, J Clin Endocrinol Metab 70:1233, 1990.

105. **Weiss J, Adams E, Whitcomb RW, Crowley WF Jr, Jameson JL,** Normal sequence of the gonadotropin-releasing hormone gene in patients with idiopathic hypogonadotropic hypogonadism, Biol Reprod 45:743, 1991.

106. **Layman LC, Wilson JT, Huey LO, Lanclos KD, Plouffe L Jr, McDonough PG,** Gonadotropin-releasing hormone, follicle-stimulating hormone beta, luteinizing hormone beta gene structure in idiopathic hypogonadotropic hypogonadism, Fertil Steril 57:42, 1992.

107. **Lacey JH,** Anorexia nervosa and a bearded female saint, Br Med J 285:1816, 1982.

108. **Garner DM,** Pathogenesis of anorexia nervosa, Lancet 341:1631, 1993.

109. **Herzog DB, Coopeland PM,** Eating disorders, New Engl J Med 313:295, 1985.

110. **Schotte DE, Stunkard AJ,** Bulimia vs bulimic behaviors on a college campus, JAMA 258:1213, 1987.

111. **Kins MB,** Eating disorders in a general practice population. Prevalence, characteristics and follow-up at 12 to 18 months, Psychiatr Med (Suppl)14:1, 1989.

112. **Warren MP, Vande Wiele RL,** Clinical and metabolic features of anorexia nervosa, Am J Obstet Gynecol 117:435, 1973.

113. **Warren MP, Jewelewicz R, Dyrenfurth I, Ans R, Khalaf S, Vande Wiele RL,** The significance of weight loss in the evaluation of pituitary response to LH-RH in women with secondary amenorrhea, J Clin Endocrinol Metab 40:601, 1975.

114. **McShane TM, May T, Miner JL, Keisler DH,** Central actions of neuropeptide-Y may provide a neuromodulatory link between nutrition and reproduction, Biol Reprod 46:1151, 1992.

115. **Beumont PJV, Russell JD, Touyz SW,** Treatment of anorexia nervosa, Lancet 341:1635, 1993.

116. **Prior JC,** Luteal phase defects and anovulation: adaptive alterations occurring with conditioning exercise, Seminars Reprod Endocrinol 3:27, 1985.

117. **Cumming DC, Wheeler GD,** Exercise-associated changes in reproduction: a problem common to women and men, in Frisch RE, editor, *Adipose Tissue and Reproduction,* Prog Reprod Biol Med 14:125, 1990.

118. **Speroff L, Redwine DB,** Exercise and menstrual function, Physician Sport Med 8:42, 1980.

119. **Frisch RE,** Body fat, menarche, and reproductive ability, Seminars Reprod Endocrinol 3:45, 1985.

120. **Falsetti L, Pasinetti E, Mazzani MD, Gastaldi A,** Weight loss and menstrual cycle: clinical and endocrinological evaluation, Gynecol Endocrinol 6:49, 1992.

121. **Loucks AB, Horvath SM, Freedson PS,** Menstrual status and validation of body fat prediction in athletes, Hum Biol 56:383, 1984.

122. **Frisch RE, Snow RC, Johnson LA, Gerard B, Barbieri R, Rosen B,** Magnetic resonance imaging of overall and regional body fat, estrogen metabolism, and ovulation of athletes compared to controls, J Clin Endocrinol Metab 77:471, 1993.

123. **Bronson FH, Manning JM,** The energetic regulation of ovulation: a realistic role for body fat, Biol Reprod 44:945, 1991.

124. **Warren MP,** Effect of exercise and physical training on menarche, Seminars Reprod Endocrinol 3:17, 1985.

125. **Ronkainen H, Pakarinen A, Kirkinen P, Kauppila A,** Physical exercise-induced changes and season-associated differences in the pituitary-ovarian function of runners and joggers, J Clin Endocrinol Metab 60:416, 1985.

126. **Cumming DC, Rebar RW,** Hormonal changes with acute exercise and with training in women, Seminars Reprod Endocrinol 3:55, 1985.

127. **Chang FE, Richards SR, Kim MH, Malarkey WB,** Twenty-four prolactin profiles and prolactin responses to dopamine in long distance runners, J Clin Endocrinol Metab 59:631, 1984.

128. **Laughlin GA, Loucks AB, Yen SSC,** Marked augmentation of nocturnal melatonin secretion in amenorrheic athletes, but not in cycling athletes: unaltered by opioidergic or dopaminergic blockade, J Clin Endocrinol Metab 73:1321, 1991.

129. **Berga S, Mortola J, Yen SSC,** Amplification of nocturnal melatonin secretion in women with functional hypothalamic amenorrhea, J Clin Endocrinol Metab 66:242, 1988.

130. **Loucks AB, Laughlin GA, Mortola JF, Girton L, Nelson JC, Yen SSC,** Hypothalamic-pituitary-thyroidal function in eumenorrheic and amenorrheic athletes, J Clin Endocrinol Metab 75:514, 1992.

131. **Fishman J, Boyar RM, Hellman L,** Influence of body weight on estradiol metabolism in young women, J Clin Endocrinol Metab 41:989, 1975.

132. **Frisch RE, Snow R, Gerard E, Johnson L, Kennedy D, Barbieri R, Rosen BR,** Magnetic resonance imaging of body fat of athletes compared with controls, and the oxidative metabolism of estradiol, Metabolism 41:191, 1992.

133. **Howlett TA, Tomlin S, Hgahfoong L, Rees LH, Bullen BA, Skrinar GS, McArthur JW,** Release of beta-endorphin and met-enkephalin during exercise in normal women: response to training, Br Med J 288:1950, 1984.

134. **Russell JB, Mitchell DE, Musey PI, Collins DC,** The role of beta-endorphins and catechol estrogens on the hypothalamic-pituitary axis in female athletes, Fertil Steril 42:690, 1984.

135. **Laatikainen T, Virtanen T, Apter D,** Plasma immunoreactive beta-endorphin in exercise-associated amenorrhea, Am J Obstet Gynecol 154:94, 1986.

136. **Gindoff PR, Ferin M,** Endogenous peptides modulate the effect of corticotropin-releasing factor on gonadotropin release in the primate, Endocrinology 121:837, 1987.

137. **Barbarino A, de Marinis L, Tofani A, Della Casa S, D'Amico C, Mancini A, Corsello SM, Sciuto R, Barini A,** Corticotropin-releasing hormone inhibiton of gonadotropin release and the effect of opioid blockade, J Clin Endocrinol Metab 68:523, 1989.

138. **Biller BMK, Federoff HJ, Koenig JI, Klibanski A,** Abnormal cortisol secretion and responses to corticotropin-releasing hormone in women with hypothalamic amenorrhea, J Clin Endocrinol Metab 70:311, 1990.

139. **Chrousos GP, Gold PW,** The concepts of stress and stress system disorders, JAMA 267:1244, 1992.

140. **Veldhuis JD, Evans WS, Demers LM, Thorner MO, Wakat D, Rogol AD,** Altered neuroendocrine regulation of gonadotropin secretion in women distance runners, J Clin Endocrinol Metab 61:557, 1985.

141. **Cumming DC, Vickovic MM, Wall SR, Fluker MR,** Defects in pulsatile LH release in normally menstruating runners, J Clin Endocrinol Metab 60:810, 1985.

142. **Loucks AB, Mortola JF, Girton L, Yen SSC,** Alterations in the hypothalamic-pituitary-ovarian and the hypothalamic-pituitary-adrenal axes in athletic women, J Clin Endocrinol Metab 68:402, 1989.

143. **Smith NJ,** Excessive weight loss and food aversion in athletes simulating anorexia nervosa, Pediatrics 66:139, 1980.

144. **Gadpaille WJ, Sanborne CF, Wagner WW,** Athletic amenorrhea, major affective disorders and eating disorders, Am J Psychiatr 144:939, 1987.

145. **Fries H,** Secondary amenorrhea, self-induced weight reduction and anorexia nervosa, Acta Psychiatr Scand, Suppl 248, 1974.

146. **Bullen BA, Skriinar GS, Beitins IZ, von Mering G, Turnbull BA, McArthur JW,** Induction of menstrual disorders by strenuous exercise in untrained women, New Engl J Med 312:1349, 1985.

147. **Stager JM, Ritchie-Flanagan RB, Robertshaw D,** Reversibility of amenorrhea in athletes, New Eng J Med 310:51, 1984.

453

148. **Hytten FE, Chamberlain G,** editors, *Clinical Physiology in Obstetrics,* Blackwell, Oxford, 1980.

149. **Antonov AN,** Children born during the siege of Leningrad in 1942, J Pediatr 30:250, 1947.

150. **Smith CA,** The effect of wartime starvation in Holland upon pregnancy and its product, Am J Obstet Gynecol 53:599, 1947

151. **Dean RFA,** The size of the baby at birth and the yield of breast milk, in *Studies of Under-nutrition. Wuppertal 1946-49,* Medical Research Council Special Report Series, No. 275, Her Majesty's Stationery Office, London, 1951, pp 346-378.

152. **Campbell DM, MacGillivray I,** The effect of a low calorie diet or a thiazide diuretic on the incidence of pre-eclampsia and on birthweight, Br J Obstet Gynaecol 82:572, 1975.

153. **Rush D,** Effects of changes in protein and calorie intake during pregnancy on the growth of the human fetus, in Calmers I, Enkin M, Keirse MJNC, editors, *Effective Care in Pregnancy and Childbirth,* Oxford University Press, Oxford, 1989, pp 255-280.

154. **Taffel SM,** Maternal weight gain and the outcome of pregnancy: United States, 1980, National Center for Health Statistics, Series 21-No. 44, DHHS (PHS) 86 - Public Health Service, U.S. Government Printing Office, Washington, D.C., 1986.

155. **Peckham CH, Christianson RE,** The relationship between prepregnancy weight and certain obstetric factors, Am J Obstet Gynecol 111:1, 1971.

156. **Simpson JW, Lawless RW, Mitchell CA,** Responsiblity of the obstetrician to the fetus. II. Influence of prepregnancy weight gain on birthweight, Obstet Gynecol 45:481, 1975.

157. **Harrison GG, Udall JN, Morrow G,** Maternal obesity, weight gain in pregnancy, and infant birth weight, Am J Obstet Gynecol 136:411, 1980.

158. **Gormican A, Valentine J, Satter E,** Relationships of maternal weight gain, prepregnancy weight, and infant birth weight, J Am Diet Assoc 77:662, 1980.

159. **Arbuckle TE, Sherman GJ,** Comparison of the risk factors for pre-term delivery and intrauterine growth retardation, Paediatr Perinat Epidemiol 3:115, 1989.

160. **Winikoff B, Debrovner CH,** Anthropometric determinants of birth weight, Obstet Gynecol 58:678, 1981.

161. **Abrams BF, Laros RK,** Prepregnancy weight, weight gain, and birth weight, Am J Obstet Gynecol 154:503, 1986.

162. **Seidman DS, Ever-Hadani P, Gale R,** The effect of maternal weight gain in pregnancy on birth weight, Obstet Gynecol 74:240, 1989.

163. **Myers SA, Ferguson R,** A population study of the relationship between fetal death and altered fetal growth, Obstet Gynecol 74:325, 1989.

164. **Bruce L, Tchabo JG,** Nutrition intervention program in a prenatal clinic, Obstet Gynecol 74:310, 1989.

165. **Villar J, Belizan JM,** The relative contribution of prematurity and fetal growth retardation to low birth weight in developing and developed societies, Am J Obstet Gynecol 143:793, 1982.

166. **Kay DWK, Leigh D,** The natural history, treatment and prognosis of anorexia based on a study of 38 patients, J Ment Sci 100:411, 1954.

167. **Beck JC, Brockner-Mortensen K,** Observation on the prognosis in anorexia nervosa, Acta Med Scand 149:409, 1954.

168. **Dally P, Sargant W,** Treatment and outcome of anorexia nervosa, Br Med J 2:793, 1966.

169. **Farquharson RF, Hyland H,** Anorexia nervosa: the course of 15 patients treated from 20 to 30 years previously, J Can Med Assoc 94:411, 1969.

170. **Theander S,** Anorexia nervosa : a psychiatric investigation of 94 female patients, Acta Psychiatr Scand 214(Suppl):1, 1970.

171. **Hart T, Kase N, Kimball CP,** Induction of ovulation and pregnancy in patients with anorexia nervosa, Am J Obstet Gynecol 108:880, 1970.

172. **Willi J, Hagemann R,** Langzeitverlaufe von anorexia nervosa, Schweiz Med Wochenschr 106:1459, 1976.

173. **Treasure JL, Russell GFM,** Intrauterine growth and neonatal weight gain in babies of women with anorexia nervosa, Br Med J 296:1036, 1988.

174. **Stewart DE, Rasking J, Garfinkel PE, MacDonald OL, Robinson GE,** Anorexia nervosa, bulimia, and pregnancy, Am J Obstet Gynecol 157:1194, 1987.

175. **Brinch M, Isager T, Telstrup K,** Anorexia nervosa and motherhood: reproduction pattern and mothering behaviour of 50 women, Acta Psychiatr Scand 77:611, 1988.

176. **Abraham S, Mira M, Llewellyn-Jones D,** Should ovulation be induced in women recovering from an eating disorder or who are compulsive exercisers? Fertil Steril 53:566, 1990.

177. **Lacey JH, Smith G,** Bulimia nervosa. The impact of pregnancy on mother and baby, Br J Psychiatr 150:777, 1987.

178. **Knuth UA, Hull MGR, Jacobs HS,** Amenorrhoea and loss of weight, Br J Obstet Gynaecol 84:801, 1977.

179. **van der Spuy ZM, Steer PJ, McCusker M, Steele SJ, Jacobs HS,** Outcome of pregnancy in underweight women after spontaneous and induced ovulation, Br Med J 296:962, 1988.

180. **Hediger ML, Scholl TO, Belsky DH, Ances IG, Salmon RW,** Patterns of weight gain in adolescent pregnancy: effects on birth weight and preterm delivery, Obstet Gynecol 74:6, 1989.

181. **Lauckner A, Lauckner W,** Significance of initial weight and weight development for the course and outcome of pregnancy, Zentralbl Gynakol 110:1018, 1988.

182. **Maestre de San Juan A,** Falta total de los nervious olfaatorios con anosmia en un individuo en quien existia una atrofia congenita de los testiculos y meiembro viril, Siglo Medico 131:211, 1856.

183. **Kallmann FJ, Schoenfeld WA, Barrera SE,** The genetic aspects of primary eunuchoidism, Am J Ment Defic 48:203, 1944.

184. **De Morsier G, Gauthier G,** La dysplasie olfacto genitale, Pathol Biol 11:1267, 1963.

185. **Tagatz G, Fialkow PJ, Smith D, Spadoni L,** Hypogonadotropic hypogonadism associated with anosmia in the female, New Engl J Med 282:1326, 1970.

186. **Knorr JR, Ragland RL, Brown RS, Gelber N,** Kallmann's syndrome: MR findings, AJNR Am J Neuroradiol 14:845, 1993.

187. **Bick D, Franco B, Sherin RJ, Heye B, Pike L, Crawford J, Maddalena A, Incerti B, Pragliola A, Meitinger T, Ballabio A,** Brief report: intragenic deletion of the *KALIG-1* gene in Kallmann's syndrome, New Engl J Med 326:1752, 1992.

188. **Hardelin J-P, Levilliers J, Young J, Pholsena M, Legouis R, Kirk J, Boulooux P, Petit C, Schaison G,** Xp22.3 deletions in isolated familial Kallmann's syndrome, J Clin Endocrinol Metab 76:827, 1993.

189. **Franco B, Guioli S, Pragliola A, Incerti B, Bardoni B, Tonlorenzi R, Carrozzo R, Maestrini E, Pieretti M, Taillon-Miller P, Brown CJ, Willard HF, Lawrence C, Persico MG, Camerino G, Ballabio A,** A gene detected in Kallmann syndrome shares homology with neural cell adhesion and axonal path-finding molecules, Nature 353:529, 1991.

190. **Lamon-Fava S, Fisher EC, Nelson ME, Evans WJ, Millar JS, Ordovas JM, Schaefer EJ,** Effect of exercise and menstrual cycle status on plasma lipids, low density lipoprotein particle size, and apolipoproteins, J Clin Endocrinol Metab 68:17, 1989.

191. **Drinkwater BL, Nilson K, Chestnut CH, Bremner WJ, Shainholtz S, Southworth MB,** Bone mineral content of amenorrheic and eumenorrheic athletes, New Engl J Med 311:277, 1984.

192. **Drinkwater BL, Nilson K, Ott S, Chestnut CH III,** Bone mineral density after resumption of menses in amenorrheic athletes, JAMA 256:380, 1986.

193. **Myerson M, Gutin B, Warren MP, Wang J, Lichtman S, Pierson RN Jr,** Total bone density in amenorrheic runners, Obstet Gynecol 79:973, 1992.

194. **Baer JT, Taper LJ, Gwazdauskas GF, Walberg JL, Novascone M-A, Ritchey SJ, Thye FW,** Diet, hormonal, and metabolic factors affecting bone mineral density in adolescent amenorrheic and eumenorrheic female runners, J Sports Med Phys Fitness 32:51, 1992.

195. **Warren MP, Brooks-Gunn J, Fox RP, Lancelot C, Newman D, Hamilton WG,** Lack of bone accretion and amenorrhea: evidence for a relative osteopenia in weight-bearing bones, J Clin Endocrinol Metab 72:847, 1991.

196. **Lindberg JS, Fears WB, Hunt MM, Powell MR, Boll D, Wade CE,** Exercise-induced amenorrhea and bone density, Ann Intern Med 101:647, 1984.

197. **Marcus R, Cann C, Madvig P, Minkoff J, Goddard M, Bayer M, Martin M, Gaudiani L, Haskell W, Genant H,** Menstrual function and bone mass in elite women distance runners, Ann Intern Med 102:158, 1985.

198. **Lloyd T, Triantafyllou SJ, Baker ER, Houts PS, Whiteside JA, Kalenak A, Stumpf PG,** Women athletes with menstrual irregularity have increased musculoskeletal injuries, Med Sci Sports Exerc 18:374, 1986.

199. **Barrow GW, Subrata S,** Menstrual irregularity and stress fractures in collegiate female distance runners, Am J Sports Med 16:209, 1988.

200. **Warren MP, Brooks-Gunn J, Hamilton LH, Warren LF, Hamilton WG,** Scoliosis and fractures in young ballet dancers, New Engl J Med 314:1348, 1986.

201. **Carbon R, Sambrook PN, Deakin V, Fricker P, Eisman JA, Kelly P, Maguire K, Yeates MG,** Bone density of elite female athletes with stress fractures, Med J Aust 153:373, 1990.

202. **Cann CE, Martin MC, Jaffe RB,** Duration of amenorrhea affects rate of bone loss in women runners: implications of therapy, Med Sci Sports Exerc 17:214, 1985.

203. **Bachrach LK, Katzman DK, Litt IF, Guido D, Marcus R,** Recovery from osteopenia in adolescent girls with anorexia nervosa, J Clin Endocrinol Metab 72:602, 1991.

204. **Drinkwater BL, Bruemmer B, Chestnut CH III,** Menstrual history as a determinant of current bone density in young athletes, JAMA 263:545, 1990.

205. **Jonnavithula S, Warren MP, Fox RP, Lazaro MI,** Bone density is compromised in amenorrheic women despite return of menses: a 2-year study, Obstet Gynecol 81:669, 1993.

206. **Klibanski A, Biller BMK, Rosenthal DI, Schoenfeld DA, Saxe V,** Effects of prolactin and estrogen deficiency in amenorrheic bone loss, J Clin Endocrinol Metab 67:124, 1988.

207. **Biller BMK, Baum HBA, Rosenthal DI, Saxe VC, Charpie MP, Klibanski A,** Progressive trabecular osteopenia in women with hyperprolactinemic amenorrhea, J Clin Endocrinol Metab 75:692, 1992.

208. **Schlechte J, Walkner L, Kathol M,** A longitudinal analysis of premenopausal bone loss in healthy women and women with hyperprolactinemia, J Clin Endocrinol Metab 75:698, 1992.

209. **Kanders BS, Lindsay R,** The effect of physical activity and calcium intake on the bone density of young women age 24-35, Med Sci Sports Exerc 17:284, 1985.

13

Anovulation and the Polycystic Ovary

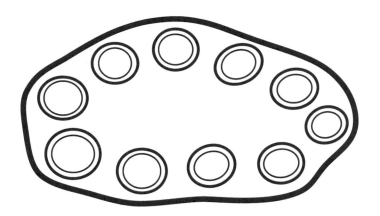

Anovulation is a very common problem that presents in a variety of clinical manifestations, including amenorrhea, irregular menses, and hirsutism. Serious consequences of chronic anovulation are infertility and a greater risk for developing carcinoma of the endometrium and perhaps the breast. The physician must appreciate the clinical impact of anovulation and undertake therapeutic management of all anovulatory patients to avoid these unwanted consequences.

Normal ovulation requires coordination of the menstrual system at all levels, the central hypothalamic-pituitary axis, the feedback signals, and local responses within the ovary. The loss of ovulation can be due to any one of an assortment of factors operating at each of these levels. The end result is a dysfunctional state: anovulation and the polycystic ovary. In this chapter, we will discuss the variety of mechanisms by which dysfunction of the ovulatory cycle can occur and how the clinical expressions of the resulting abnormal menstrual function are produced.

Pathogenesis of Anovulation	Just before and during menses, escape from the negative feedback of estrogen, progesterone, and inhibin results in increased follicle-stimulating hormone (FSH) secretion by the anterior pituitary. This initial increase in FSH is essential for follicular growth and steroidogenesis. With continued growth of the follicle, autocrine/paracrine factors produced within the follicle maintain follicular sensitivity to FSH allowing conversion from a microenvironment dominated by androgens to one dominated by estrogen, a change necessary for a complete and successful follicular lifespan. Continuing and combined action of FSH and activin leads to the appearance of luteinizing hormone (LH) receptors on the granulosa cells, a prerequisite for ovulation and luteinization. Ovulation is triggered by the rapid rise in circulating levels of estradiol. A positive feedback response at the level of the anterior pituitary (and perhaps at the hypothalamus as well) results in the midcycle surge of LH necessary for expulsion of the egg and formation of the corpus luteum. A rise in progesterone follows ovulation along with a second rise in estradiol, producing the 14-day luteal phase characterized by low FSH and LH levels. The demise of the corpus luteum, concomitant with a fall in hormone levels, allows FSH to increase again, thus initiating a new cycle.

In the early follicular phase, activin produced by granulosa in immature follicles enhances the action of FSH on aromatase activity and FSH and LH receptor formation, while simultaneously suppressing thecal androgen synthesis. In the late follicular phase, increased production of inhibin by the granulosa (and decreased activin) promotes androgen synthesis in the theca in response to LH and insulin-like growth factor-I (IGF-I) to provide substrate for even greater estrogen production in the granulosa. In the mature granulosa, activin serves to prevent premature luteinization and progesterone production.

The successful follicle is the one that acquires the highest level of aromatase activity and LH receptors in response to FSH. The successful follicle is characterized by the highest estrogen (for central feedback action) and the greatest inhibin production (for both local and central actions). This accomplishment occurs in synchrony with the appropriate activin and growth factor expression. The activin proteins (which enhance FSH activity) are produced in greatest amounts early in follicular development to enhance follicle receptivity to FSH.

The right concentration of androgens in granulosa cells promotes aromatase activity and inhibin production, and, in turn, inhibin promotes LH stimulation of thecal androgen synthesis. LH stimulation of androgen production in thecal cells is further enhanced by the autocrine activity of insulin-like growth factor-I (IGF-I). With development of the follicle, inhibin expression comes under control of LH. A key to successful ovulation and luteal function is conversion of the inhibin production to LH responsiveness, to maintain FSH suppression centrally and enhancement of LH action locally.

This recycling mechanism is regulated by substances functioning as classic hormones (FSH, LH, estradiol, inhibin) transmitting messages between the ovary and the hypothalamic-pituitary axis, and autocrine/paracrine factors (IGF-I, IGF-II, inhibin, and activin, among others) which coordinate sequential activities within the follicle destined to ovulate. The negative feedback relationship between corpus luteum products (estradiol, progesterone, and inhibin) and FSH results in the critical initial rise in FSH during menses, and the positive feedback relationship between estradiol and LH is the ovulatory stimulus. Within the ovary, IGF-I, IGF-II, inhibin, and activin modify follicular receptor responses necessary for growth and function. Dysfunction in the cycle can be due to an abnormality in one of the various roles for any one of these substances or an inability to respond to signals.

Central Defects

The hypothalamic-pituitary axis may be unable to respond, even if given adequate and appropriately timed feedback signals. A pituitary tumor represents an obvious example of a central defect in menstrual function and is discussed in Chapter 12, Amenorrhea.

Although difficult to demonstrate definitively, malfunction within the hypothalamus is both a likely, as well as a favorite, explanation for ovulatory failure. Normal pituitary ovulatory response to the follicle's steroid signals requires the presence of gonadotropin-releasing hormone (GnRH) pulsatile secretion within a critical range. The teenager between menarche and the onset of ovulation cannot generate a normal cycle until full GnRH pulsatile secretion is achieved. Increasing intensity of GnRH suppression is associated with increasing dysfunction and a changing clinical presentation. A variety of problems, such as stress and anxiety, borderline anorexia nervosa, and acute weight loss after a crash diet, is associated with an inhibition of normal GnRH pulsatile secretion. The gonadotropin surge is not possible, and only homeostatic pituitary-ovarian function is maintained.

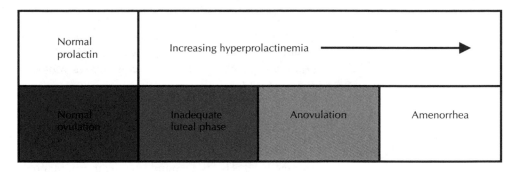

At least one specific clinical syndrome of central anovulatory dysfunction has been recognized: hyperprolactinemia. Increasing levels of prolactin can cause a woman to progress through a spectrum, beginning with an inadequate luteal phase to anovulation to the amenorrhea associated with complete GnRH suppression. *A search for galactorrhea and measurement of the prolactin level are important screening procedures for all women who are not ovulating normally.* The presence of galactorrhea or elevated prolactin levels dictates a choice of dopamine agonist treatment for the induction of ovulation.

Anovulatory women have a higher LH (and presumably GnRH) pulse frequency and amplitude when compared to the normal midfollicular phase.[1] Central opioid tone appears to be suppressed because there is no difference in response to naloxone.[2] Indeed, the enhanced pulsatile secretion of GnRH can be attributed to a reduction in hypothalamic opioid inhibition because of the chronic absence of progesterone.[3] Interaction at the dopamine-endorphin sites may be altered because pretreatment with a dopamine precursor leads to a naloxone-induced increase in LH in anovulatory women compared to controls.

Abnormal Feedback Signals

Abnormal cycles can be due to failures within the system or due to the introduction of confounding factors. In order to achieve the appropriate changes within the cycle, estradiol levels must rise and fall in synchrony with morphologic events. Therefore, two possible signal failures may occur: 1) estradiol levels may not fall low enough to allow sufficient FSH response for the initial growth stimulus, and 2) levels of estradiol may be inadequate to produce the positive stimulatory effects necessary to induce the ovulatory surge of LH.

Loss of FSH Stimulation

In order to achieve recycling, a nadir in blood sex steroid levels must occur so that the initial event in the cycle, the rise in FSH, can take place. Sustained estrogen at such a key moment would not permit FSH stimulation of follicular growth and maturation, and recycling would be thwarted. The necessary decline in blood estrogen requires reduction of secretion, appropriate clearance and metabolism, and the absence of a significant contribution of estrogen to the circulation by extragonadal sources.

Persistent Estrogen Secretion. The most common clinical example of anovulation associated with continued secretion of sex steroids is pregnancy. Persistent and elevated secretion of estrogen can be encountered rarely with an ovarian or adrenal tumor. In such a case, anovulation or amenorrhea may bring the patient to a physician's attention.

Abnormal Estrogen Clearance and Metabolism. The clearance and metabolism of estrogen can be impaired by other pathologic conditions, such as thyroid or hepatic disease. It is for this reason that a careful history and physical examination are important elements in the differential diagnosis of anovulation. Both hyperthyroidism and hypothyroidism can cause persistent anovulation by altering not only metabolic clearance but also the peripheral conversion rates among the various steroids. ***The subtle presence of hypothyroidism, which may be associated with elevated prolactin levels, demands screening of anovulatory and amenorrheic women with a thyroid-stimulating hormone (TSH) level.***

Extraglandular Estrogen Production. Extragonadal contribution to the blood estrogen level can reach significant proportions. Although the adrenal gland does not secrete appreciable amounts of estrogen into the circulation, it indirectly contributes to the total estrogen level. This is accomplished by the extragonadal peripheral conversion of C-19 androgenic precursors, mainly androstenedione, to estrogen. In this manner psychological or physical stress may increase the adrenal contribution of estrogenic precursor, and subsequent conversion to estrogen may sustain the blood level of estrogen at a time when a decline is necessary for successful recycling of the menstrual cycle. Adipose tissue is capable of converting androstenedione to estrogen; hence, the percent conversion increases with increasing body weight.[4] This is at least one mechanism for the well-known association between obesity and anovulation.

Loss of LH Stimulation

A failure in gonadal production of estrogen need not be absolute. Obviously the patient with gonadal dysgenesis and ovarian failure will present with amenorrhea and infertility because of a total lack of estrogen secretion. More commonly, the clinician is concerned with the patient who has gonadotropin and estrogen production but does not ovulate. The failure to achieve a critical midcycle level of estradiol necessary to trigger the gonadotropin surge may be due to a relative deficiency in steroid production. The perimenopausal woman undergoes a terminal period of anovulation which may represent a steroidogenic refractoriness within the remaining elderly follicles. This inadequacy may be due to intrinsic follicular weaknesses or an impairment in the follicular-gonadotropin interaction. In any case, the end result is the same — a failure to achieve critical signal levels of estradiol at the appropriate time in midcycle.

Local Ovarian Conditions

An understanding of the critical balances within the follicle indicates possible points of failure that may lead to anovulation. Local autocrine/paracrine factors prevent atresia despite declining FSH levels by enhancing the action of FSH in increasing the number of FSH receptors within the follicle, thus increasing follicular sensitivity to FSH. In addition, these factors enhance the induction of LH receptors by FSH, making it possible for the follicle to respond to the LH surge at midcycle. A follicle can fail to grow and ovulate because of inadequate expression or impaired function of any of the following local ovarian activities (described in detail in Chapter 6):

1. Selection of the dominant follicle is established during days 5–7, and consequently, peripheral levels of estradiol begin to rise significantly by cycle day 7.

2. Derived from the dominant follicle, estradiol levels increase steadily and, through negative feedback effects, exert a progressively greater suppressive influence on FSH release.

3. Insulin-like growth factor-I (IGF-I) is produced in theca cells in response to gonadotropin stimulation, and this response is enhanced by estradiol and growth hormone.

4. IGF-I stimulates granulosa cell proliferation, aromatase activity, and progesterone synthesis. Insulin-like growth factor-II may be especially important in the dominant follicle.

5. FSH inhibits IGF binding protein synthesis and thus maximizes growth factor availability.

6. FSH stimulates inhibin and activin production by granulosa cells.

7. Activin augments FSH activities: FSH receptor expression, aromatization, inhibin/activin production, and LH receptor expression.

8. Inhibin enhances LH stimulation of androgen synthesis in the theca to provide substrate for aromatization to estrogen in the granulosa.

9. While directing a decline in FSH levels, the midfollicular rise in estradiol exerts a positive feedback influence on LH secretion. LH levels rise steadily during the late follicular phase, stimulating androgen production in the theca.

10. The positive action of estrogen also includes modification of the gonadotropin molecule, increasing the quality (the bioactivity) as well as the quantity of LH at midcycle.

11. Inhibin and, less importantly, follistatin, secreted by the granulosa cells in response to FSH, directly suppress pituitary FSH secretion.

12. FSH induces the appearance of LH receptors on granulosa cells.

The factors that control follicular growth and development are now understood in terms of the two-cell explanation described in Chapter 2 and Chapter 6. A very precise coordination is necessary between morphologic development and hormone stimulation. Pertubations may arise from an infectious process, from the presence of endometriosis, or by abnormal qualitative or quantitative changes in tropic hormone receptors (ovarian insensitivity), or the necessary biologic effects may be blocked by an improper molecular constitution of the gonadotropins (heterogeneity of the glycopeptide hormones).

A Critical Role for the Concentration of Androgens in the Ovarian Follicle. Serving as substrate for FSH-induced aromatization, the androgens in low concentrations enhance aromatase activity and estrogen production. At higher concentrations, the granulosa cells favor the conversion of androgens to more potent 5α-reduced androgens, which cannot be converted to estrogen and, in addition, are capable of inhibiting aromatase activity and FSH induction of LH receptors (Chapter 6). Thus raising the local androgen concentration above a critical level inhibits the emergence of a dominant follicle and leads to follicular atresia. Whereas this action in the normal cycle may be important in ensuring that only one follicle reaches the point of ovulation, an excessive concentration of androgens (no matter what the source) can prevent normal cycling and cause chronic anovulation.

Excess Body Weight

Obesity is associated with three alterations that interfere with normal ovulation, and weight loss improves all three:

1. Increased peripheral aromatization of androgens to estrogens.

2. Decreased levels of sex hormone binding globulin (SHBG) resulting in increased levels of free estradiol and testosterone.

3. Increased insulin levels that can stimulate ovarian stromal tissue production of androgens.

Precise Etiology

The normal ovulatory function of the menstrual system relies on a dynamic coordination of complex actions. Abnormal function may represent discordance at all of the levels reviewed in the above paragraphs. Thus, a minor deficiency in the estradiol signal will be associated with a subnormal central response and an impaired or inappropriate degree of follicular growth and function. Dysfunction is sustained by the internal feedback mechanisms within the system, and anovulation can become a persistent problem.

It is usually impossible to reduce the issue of etiology to a single factor of abnormal menstrual function, except in severe states such as pituitary tumors, anorexia nervosa, gonadal dysgenesis, and perhaps hyperprolactinemia and obesity. Not only is it often impossible, but it is usually unnecessary to define the precise etiology. Regardless of the nature of the initial cause of the problem, the final clinical statement of the dysfunction is predictable, and easily diagnosed and managed. In patients who have abnormal or absent menstrual function, but are otherwise medically normal, the diagnosis will fall into one of three categories:

1. Ovarian Failure. Hypergonadotropic hypogonadism, the inability of the ovary to respond to any gonadotropic stimulation, usually due to the absence of follicular tissue on a genetic basis (discussed in Chapter 12).

2. Central Failure. Hypogonadotropic hypogonadism, hypothalamic or pituitary suppression as expressed in abnormal low or normal serum gonadotropins (discussed in Chapter 12).

3. Anovulatory Dysfunction. The patient who has asynchronous gonadotropin and estrogen production and does not ovulate presents with a variety of clinical manifestations. The associated clinical signs and symptoms depend upon the level of gonadal function preserved and are represented by the following principal problems:

   Amenorrhea (Chapter 12).
   Hirsutism (Chapter 14).
   Dysfunctional uterine bleeding (Chapter 16).
   Endometrial hyperplasia and cancer (Chapter 18).
   Breast disease (Chapter 17).
   Infertility and induction of ovulation (Chapter 30).
   The polycystic ovary (this chapter).

FSH &
LH   Estradiol   Progesterone
IU/L   pg/mL   17-OHP
                         ng/mL

20	500	10
18		9	Progesterone
16	400	8	LH
14		7	FSH
12	300	6
10		5
8	200	4
6		3
4	100	2
2		1	Estradiol
0	0	0	17-OH Progesterone

2 4 6 8 10 12 14 16 18 20 22 24 26 28

Menses   Ovulation

LH

FSH

Estradiol —
Progesterone

Steady state

Persistent anovulation

The Polycystic Ovary

In 1935, Stein and Leventhal first described a symptom complex associated with anovulation. Acceptance of this syndrome as a singular clinical entity led to a rather rigid approach to this problem for many years. Only those women qualified who had a history of oligomenorrhea, hirsutism, and obesity, together with a demonstration of enlarged, polycystic ovaries. It is far more useful clinically to avoid the use of eponyms and even the term polycystic ovary syndrome or disease. It is better to consider this problem as one of persistent anovulation with a spectrum of etiologies and clinical manifestations.

A question which has puzzled gynecologists and endocrinologists for many years is what causes polycystic ovaries. There is an answer that is appealing in its logic and clinical applicability. The characteristic polycystic ovary emerges when a state of anovulation persists for any length of time. Whether diagnosis is by ultrasonography or by the traditional clinical and biochemical criteria, a cross-section of anovulatory women at any one point of time will reveal that approximately 75% will have polycystic ovaries.[5,6] Because there are many causes of anovulation, there are many causes of polycystic ovaries. A similar clinical picture and ovarian condition can reflect any of the dysfunctional states discussed above. In other words, the polycystic ovary is the result of a functional derangement, not a specific central or local defect.

Insistence on a specific endocrine or clinical criterion for the diagnosis of the polycystic ovary syndrome results in the inclusion of a collection of patients that represents a focused segment isolated from the broad clinical spectrum in which these patients really belong. This especially applies to the use of ultrasonography to make the diagnosis of the polycystic ovarian syndrome (the presence of the necklace-like pattern of follicular cysts in the ovaries). Approximately 25% of normal women will demonstrate ultrasonographic findings typical of polycystic ovaries![7,8] Even 14% of women on oral contraceptives have been found to have this ultrasonographic picture.[8]

In contrast to the characteristic picture of fluctuating hormone levels in the normal cycle, a "steady state" of gonadotropins and sex steroids can be depicted in association with persistent anovulation. This steady state is only relative, and is being exaggerated here to present a concept of this clinical problem. In patients with persistent anovulation, the average daily production of estrogen and androgens is both increased and dependent upon LH stimulation.[9,10] This is reflected in higher circulating levels of testosterone, androstenedione, dehydroepiandrosterone (DHA), dehydroepiandrosterone sulfate (DHAS), 17-hydroxyprogesterone (17-OHP), and estrone.[11] The testosterone, andro-

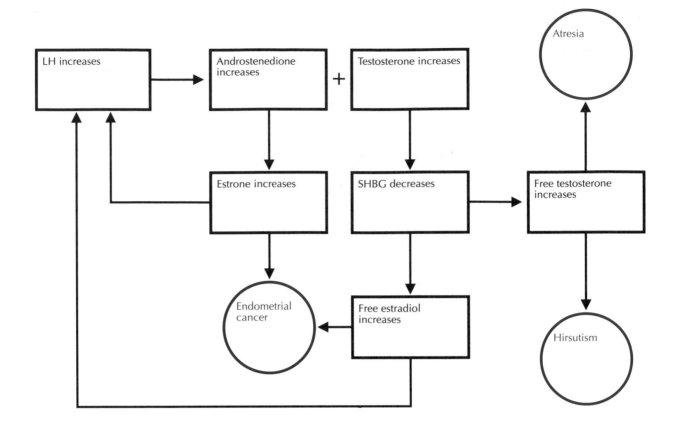

stenedione, and DHA are secreted directly by the ovary, while the DHAS is almost exclusively an adrenal contribution.

Treatment of women with polycystic ovaries with a GnRH agonist is associated with the following helpful observations:[9]

1. The increases in androstenedione and testosterone are almost exclusively from the ovary.

2. The increase in 17-OHP is also from the ovary.

3. Secretion of DHA, DHAS, and cortisol are not influenced by short-term GnRH agonist treatment; however, long-term treatment is associated with a decrease in DHAS when the circulating DHAS levels are increased (as they are in approximately 50% of patients with polycystic ovaries).[12] This suggests that an adrenal change is secondary to the ovarian hormonal steady state.

The ovary does not secrete increased amounts of estrogen, and estradiol levels are equivalent to early follicular phase concentrations. The increased total estrogen is due to peripheral conversion of the increased amounts of androstenedione to estrone. That is not to say that there is no ovarian secretion of estrogen. Both estrone and estradiol continue to be secreted in significant although low amounts.[13]

The levels of sex hormone binding globulin (SHBG) are controlled by a balance of hormonal influences on its synthesis in the liver; testosterone is inhibitory, estrogen and thyroxine are stimulatory. In anovulatory women with polycystic ovaries, there is an approximate 50% reduction in circulating levels of SHBG, a response to the increased testosterone, and in patients with hyperinsulinemia, due to a direct insulin effect on the liver (discussed later in this chapter).

When compared to levels found in normal women, patients with persistent anovulation have higher mean concentrations of LH, but low or low-normal levels of FSH.[14,15] The elevated LH levels are partly due to an increased sensitivity of the pituitary to releasing hormone stimulation, manifested by an increase in LH pulse amplitude and frequency.[16] This is consistent with the concepts discussed in Chapter 5, linking a high estrogen environment with anterior pituitary secretion of LH and suppression of FSH. It is noteworthy that this high level of LH is characterized by an increased level of LH bioactivity.[10,16]

The gonadotropin pattern (high LH and low FSH) can also be due to partial desensitization of the pituitary due to increased frequency of GnRH secretion.[17] This is associated with an increase in amplitude and frequency of LH secretion that is correlated with the level of circulating estrogen.[18] It is likely that this increased activity is taking place at both hypothalamic and pituitary sites.

The increased pituitary and hypothalamic sensitivity can be attributed to the increased estrone levels,[19] but a newly appreciated factor is the impact of the decreased SHBG concentration. Despite no increase in estradiol secretion, free estradiol levels are increased because of the significant decrease in SHBG. The increased LH secretion as expressed by the LH:FSH ratio is positively correlated with the increased free estradiol.[17,20] The lower FSH levels represent the sensitivity of the FSH negative feedback system to the elevated estrogen, both free estradiol and the estrone formed from peripheral conversion of androstenedione. In addition, the altered pattern of GnRH secretion can contribute to this characteristic LH:FSH ratio.[17] The clinical consequences of uninterrupted estrogen stimulation (endometrial and perhaps breast cancer) as well as the increased LH are the result of the two estrogenic influences, estrone and free estradiol.

Because the FSH levels are not totally depressed, new follicular growth is continuously stimulated, but not to the point of full maturation and ovulation. Despite the fact that full growth potential is not realized, follicular lifespan may extend several months in the form of multiple follicular cysts, 2–6 mm in diameter (some can be as large as 15 mm). These follicles are surrounded by hyperplastic theca cells, often luteinized in response to the high LH levels. The accumulation of follicular tissue in various stages of development allows an increased and relatively constant production of steroids in response to the gonadotropin stimulation. This condition is self-sustaining. As various follicles undergo atresia, they are immediately replaced by new follicles of similar limited growth potential.

The tissue derived from follicular atresia is also sustained by the steady state and now contributes to the stromal compartment of the ovary. In terms of the two-cell explanation of follicular steroidogenesis, atresia is associated with a degenerating granulosa, leaving the theca cells to contribute to the stromal compartment of the ovary. It is not surprising, therefore, that this functioning stromal tissue secretes significant amounts of androstenedione and testosterone, the usual products of theca cells. In response to the elevated LH levels, the androgen production rate is increased. In turn, in a vicious cycle, the elevated androgen levels compound the problem through the process of extraglandular conversion as well as the suppression of SHBG synthesis, resulting in elevated estrogen levels. In addition, the decrease in SHBG is associated with a two-fold increase in free testosterone.

The elevated androgens contribute to the morphologic effect within the ovary preventing normal follicular development and inducing premature atresia. Indeed, in another aspect of the vicious cycle, the local androgen block is a major obstacle which maintains the steady state of persistent anovulation. A sustained reduction in androgen levels following surgical wedge resection of the ovaries precedes the return of ovulatory cycles, indicating that the intraovarian androgen effect is a principal factor in preventing normal cycling.[21-24] In addition, testosterone can have a direct inhibitory action on the hypothalamic-pituitary axis.[25]

In this manner the classic picture of the polycystic ovary is attained, displaying numerous follicles in the early stages of development and atresia and dense stromal tissue. The loss of recycling has resulted in a hormonal steady state causing persistent anovulation that can be associated with an increased production of androgens.

The polycystic ovary is the result of a "vicious cycle" which can be initiated at any one of many entry points. Altered function at any point in the cycle leads to the same result: the polycystic ovary. Recent studies, in an effort to be accurate, have usually included only patients fulfilling strict criteria. Thus, only certain subgroups of a large heterogeneous clinical population have been characterized. ***Don't lose sight of the fact that the polycystic ovary is a sign, not a disease.***

The polycystic ovary is usually enlarged and is characterized by a smooth pearly white capsule. For years, it was erroneously believed that the thick sclerotic capsule acted as a mechanical barrier to ovulation. A more accurate concept is that the polycystic ovary is a consequence of the loss of ovulation and the achievement of the steady state of persistent anovulation. The characteristics of the ovary reflect this dysfunctional state:[26]

1. The surface area is doubled, giving an average volume increase of 2.8 times.

2. The same number of primordial follicles is present, but the number of growing and atretic follicles (up to the secondary follicle stage) is doubled. Each ovary may contain 20–100 cystic follicles.

3. The thickness of the tunica (outermost layer) is increased by 50%.

4. A one-third increase in cortical stromal thickness and a 5-fold increase in subcortical stroma are noted. The increased stroma is due both to hyperplasia of thecal cells and to increased formation subsequent to the excessive follicular maturation and atresia.

5. There are 4 times more ovarian hilus cell nests (hyperplasia).

Hyperthecosis refers to patches of luteinized theca-like cells scattered throughout the ovarian stroma. It is characterized by the same histologic findings as seen in polycystic ovaries.[27] The clinical picture of more intense androgenization is a result of greater androgen production. This condition is associated with lower LH levels, which is a possible consequence of the higher testosterone levels blocking estrogen action at the hypothalamic-pituitary level.[28,29] It seems appropriate to view hyperthecosis as a manifestation of the same process, persistent anovulation, but with greater intensity. A greater degree of insulin resistance is correlated with the degree of hyperthecosis.[29]

The typical histologic changes of the polycystic ovary can be encountered with any size ovary. There is a spectrum of time involved in the development of this condition, and it is useful to view the attainment of large ovaries as a stage of maximal effect of persistent anovulation. Increased size of the ovaries is not a critical feature, nor is it necessary for diagnosis. The key to understanding this clinical problem is an appreciation for the disruption in ovulatory recycling function.

There is no specific pathophysiologic defect. The hypothalamic-pituitary response is entirely appropriate, a response to chronically elevated estrogen feedback. The changes are a functional derangement brought about by accumulated and increased androgen due to a failure of ovulation, whatever the reason. Hence, the polycystic ovary may be associated with extragonadal sources of androgens[30,31] or with ovarian androgen-producing tumors.[32,33]

The functional problem can be understood in terms of the two-cell explanation of steroidogenesis (Chapter 6). The follicles are unable to successfully change their microenvironment from androgen dominance to estrogen dominance, the change that is essential for continued follicular growth and development.[34] Measurement of the insulin-like growth factor binding proteins in follicular fluid reveals that the profile in polycystic ovaries is the same as that found in atretic follicles, higher levels of IGFBP-2 and -4.[35,36] This is consistent with limitation of IGF-I and IGF-II activity, reducing the expression of aromatase action and allowing androgenic dominance in the microenvironment. However, there is a striking difference comparing polycystic granulosa cells to granulosa cells from atretic follicles. Granulosa cells from polycystic ovaries are very sensitive to FSH; granulosa cells from atretic follicles are not.[37]

The functional picture that emerges (unresponsive granulosa cells and very active theca cells) corresponds to the morphologic histology of underdeveloped granulosa and hyperplastic and luteinized theca. Granulosa cells obtained from the small follicles of polycystic ovaries produce negligible amounts of estradiol but show a dramatic increase in estrogen production when FSH or IGF-I is added and a synergistic action when FSH and IGF-I are added together.[38,39] In terms of the two-cell explanation, this behavior is consistent with a blockage of FSH response (probably through various growth factors), not an intrinsic steroid synthesis enzyme defect. Successful treatment depends, therefore, on altering the ratio of FSH to androgens; either increasing FSH (with clomiphene) or decreasing androgens (wedge resection) to overcome the androgen block at the granulosa level. This permits development of aromatization to bring about conversion of the microenvironment to estrogen dominance. Because anovulation with polycystic ovaries is a functional derangement, it is not surprising that these patients occasionally may ovulate spontaneously. Indeed, ovulation is unpredictable, and contraception may be necessary.

At least one group of patients with this condition inherits the disorder, possibly by means of an X-linked dominant transmission. There is a two-fold higher incidence of hirsutism and oligomenorrhea with paternal transmission but with marked variability of phenotypic expression.[40]

The adrenal gland is involved in this problem. Higher circulating levels of DHAS, almost exclusively an adrenal product, testify to adrenal participation. The mechanism and the clinical importance of this involvement will be discussed in Chapter 14, Hirsutism.

Insulin Resistance, Hyperinsulinemia, and Hyperandrogenism

The first recognition of an association between glucose intolerance and hyperandrogenism was the famous report of the bearded diabetic woman by Archard in 1921.[41] The association between increased insulin resistance and polycystic ovaries is now well-recognized. In addition, hyperandrogenism and insulin resistance are commonly associated with acanthosis nigricans.[42] Acanthosis nigricans is a gray-brown velvety, sometimes verrucous, discoloration of the skin, usually at the neck, groin, and axillae, which is a marker for insulin resistance. Hyperkeratosis and papillomatosis are the histological characteristics of acanthosis nigricans. The presence of acanthosis nigricans in hyperandrogenic women is dependent upon the presence and severity of hyperinsulinemia.[43] It is most highly correlated with the magnitude of peripheral insulin resistance and less well with the hyperinsulinemia measured by a glucose tolerance test. The mechanism responsible for the development of acanthosis nigricans is uncertain. Conflicting studies suggest mediation through various growth factor receptors, not just insulin or insulin-like growth factor-I. Because acanthosis nigricans can be present in normal women, its presence is not an absolute marker for hyperandrogenism.

Resistance to insulin-stimulated glucose uptake is a relatively common phenomenon.[44] The majority of patients with noninsulin-dependent diabetes mellitus have peripheral insulin resistance. The state of chronic hyperinsulinemia represents a compensatory response to the target tissue problem. These relationships involve changes in plasma free fatty acid concentrations. If the insulin levels necessary to suppress free fatty acid levels cannot be achieved then the increase in free fatty acids leads to increased hepatic glucose production and hyperglycemia.

There are several mechanisms for the state of insulin resistance: peripheral target tissue resistance, decreased hepatic clearance, or increased pancreatic sensitivity.[45] The euglycemic clamp technique establishes a steady state of normal glucose levels at which point the glucose infusion rate equals glucose utilization. Adding insulin will measure the glucose uptake rate (the more insulin required, the greater the peripheral resistance). Studies with this technique indicate that hyperandrogenic women with hyperinsulinemia have peripheral insulin resistance and, in addition, a reduction in the insulin clearance rate due to decreased hepatic insulin extraction.[45,46]

The clinical presentation of patients with insulin resistance (whether they have impaired glucose tolerance or diabetes mellitus) depends on the ability of the pancreas to compensate for the target tissue resistance to insulin. This compensatory response of hyperinsulinemia leads to hypertension; a direct relationship exists between plasma insulin levels and blood pressure. Resistance to insulin is further associated with increased triglycerides and decreased HDL-cholesterol levels.[47]

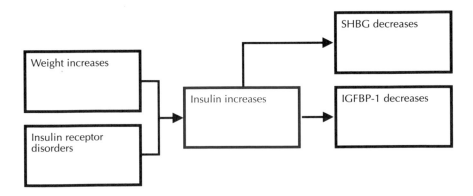

Peripheral insulin resistance associated with hyperandrogenism can be due to mutations of the insulin receptor gene (which leads to decreased numbers of insulin receptors in target tissue).[48] Leprechaunism is a rare syndrome in young girls with a mutation in the insulin receptor gene; it is associated with severe insulin resistance, polycystic ovaries, hyperandrogenism, and acanthosis nigricans. Another subgroup consists of patients with autoantibodies to insulin receptors. This leaves a large collection of women with neither reduced insulin receptors nor autoantibodies. Possible mechanisms include functional problems in the insulin receptor (which could also be a consequence of insulin receptor gene mutations) and inhibitors which can interfere with insulin-receptor function after binding.[49] Thus, there are at least 3 categories for peripheral target tissue insulin resistance: decreased insulin receptor numbers, decreased insulin binding, and post receptor failures.

There is some experimental evidence to indicate that in women with polycystic ovaries, the peripheral insulin resistance is due to a defect beyond activation of the receptor kinase.[50] This would suggest no abnormality in the number of receptors or in receptor function; the impaired insulin signal for glucose transport may be due to a post receptor problem. Of course, different patients with the same clinical presentation may have different reasons for the insulin resistance, a spectrum of etiologies with a common clinical expression.

Is the Link between Hyperinsulinemia and Hyperandrogenism Explained Solely by the Presence of Android Obesity in Hyperandrogenic Patients?

Android obesity is the result of fat deposited in the abdominal wall and visceral mesenteric locations. This fat is more sensitive to catecholamines and less sensitive to insulin, and thus more active metabolically. This fat distribution is associated with hyperinsulinemia, impaired glucose tolerance, diabetes mellitus, and an increase in androgen production rates resulting in decreased levels of sex hormone binding globulin and increased levels of free testosterone and estradiol.[51–53]

Central body (android) obesity is associated with cardiovascular risk factors, including hypertension and unfavorable cholesterol-lipoprotein profiles.[54] The waist:hip ratio is the variable most strongly and inversely associated with the level of HDL_2, the fraction of HDL-cholesterol most consistently linked with protection from cardiovascular disease.[55] A waist:hip ratio greater than 0.85 indicates android fat distribution (Chapter 19). The adverse impact of excess weight in adolescence can be explained by the fact that deposition of fat in adolescence is largely central in location.[56,57] Weight loss in women with lower body obesity is mainly cosmetic, whereas loss of central body weight is more important for general health in that an improvement in cardiovascular risk is associated with loss of central body fat.

There are at least three possible mechanisms for a link between android obesity and hyperinsulinemia:

1. Android obesity is more active metabolically, resulting in higher free fatty acid concentrations. Increasing free fatty acids lead to hyperglycemia.

2. Androgens may directly inhibit hepatic and peripheral insulin action.

3. Androgens plus increased free fatty acids inhibit hepatic insulin extraction.

Because obesity itself is associated with insulin resistance, it is important to note that this correlation of increased androgen secretion and insulin resistance has been reported in both obese and nonobese anovulatory women.[58–61] However, insulin levels are higher and LH, SHBG, and IGFBP-1 levels are lower in obese women with polycystic ovaries compared to nonobese women with polycystic ovaries.[62,63] For this reason, some have suggested that hyperandrogenic women with polycystic ovaries could be divided into two groups: those with obesity, insulin resistance, hyperinsulinemia, and normal or minimally elevated LH levels; and those with elevated LH, no insulin resistance, and normal insulin levels.[64,65] In our view, these two groups represent the ends of a spectrum, and division of this clinically broad spectrum of patients is artifactual and unhelpful.

Which Comes First, the Hyperinsulinemia or the Hyperandrogenism?

There are studies indicating that androgens can induce hyperinsulinemia. However, most of the evidence supports hyperinsulinemia as the primary factor, especially the experiments in which turning off the ovary with a GnRH agonist does not change the hyperinsulinemia or insulin resistance.[45,66–68] This indicates that disordered insulin action precedes the increase in androgens. Large doses of insulin were administered to a 16 year old female with insulin resistance secondary to insulin receptor autoantibodies; the increased insulin levels increased her circulating testosterone levels.[69] With resolution of her insulin resistance, her testosterone levels returned to normal, indicating that the hyperinsulinemia stimulates and increases testosterone and not vice-versa. Indeed, there are 6 reasons to believe that hyperinsulinism causes hyperandrogenism:

1. The administration of insulin to women with polycystic ovaries increases circulating androgen levels.[70]

2. The administration of glucose to hyperandrogenic women increases the circulating levels of both insulin and androgens.[71]

3. Weight loss decreases the levels of both insulin and androgens.[72]

4. In vitro, insulin stimulates thecal cell androgen production.[73,74]

5. The experimental reduction of insulin levels in women with polycystic ovaries reduces androgen levels.[75]

6. After normalization of androgens with GnRH agonist treatment, the hyperinsulin response to glucose tolerance testing remains abnormal in obese women with polycystic ovaries.[68,76]

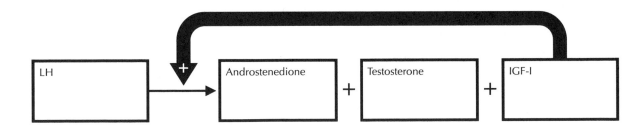

**How Does
Hyperinsulinemia Produce
Hyperandrogenism?**

There is an impressive correlation between the degree of hyperinsulinemia and hyperandrogenism.[58,60,61] At higher concentrations, insulin binds to the IGF-I receptors (which are similar in structure to insulin receptors). Thus, when insulin receptors are blocked or deficient in number, it is to be expected that insulin would bind to the IGF-I receptors.[77] In view of the known actions of IGF-I in augmenting the thecal androgen response to LH, activation of IGF-I receptors by insulin would lead to increased androgen production in thecal cells.[78] There are two other important actions of insulin which contribute to hyperandrogenism in the presence of hyperinsulinemia: inhibition of hepatic synthesis of sex hormone binding globulin and inhibition of hepatic production of insulin-like growth factor binding protein-1.

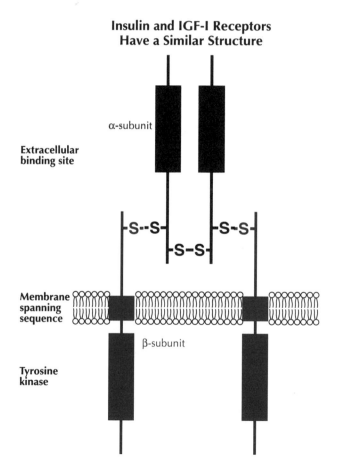

Independently of any effect on sex steroids, increased insulin will inhibit the hepatic synthesis of sex hormone binding globulin.[79] In vitro studies indicate that both insulin and IGF-I directly inhibit SHBG secretion by human hepatoma cells.[80,81] This is now known to be the mechanism for the inverse relationship between body weight and the circulating levels of SHBG. In addition, decreased SHBG levels in women represent an independent risk factor for noninsulin-dependent diabetes mellitus, regardless of body weight and fat distribution.[82]

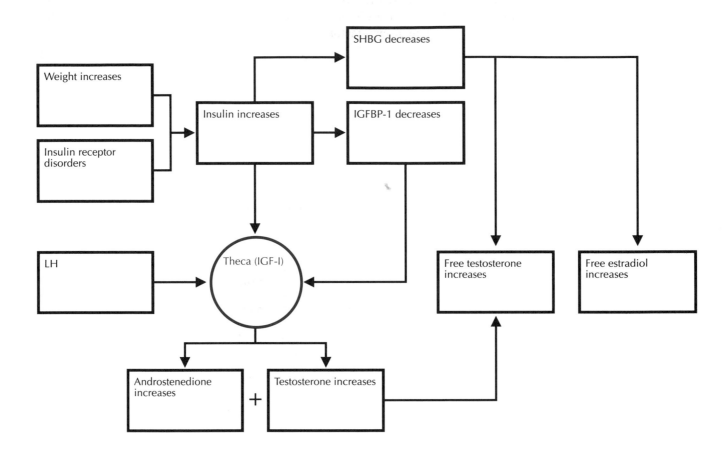

Nutritional intake decreases the circulating levels of insulin-like growth factor binding protein-1 (IGFBP-1) because of the increase in insulin which then directly inhibits IGFBP-1 production in the liver.[83] Obese individuals with increased insulin levels have lower circulating levels of IGFBP-1. This lower level of IGFBP-1 would allow greater local activity of IGF-I in the ovary. In addition, greater IGF-I activity in the endometrium due to reduced levels of IGFBP-1 and direct insulin activation of IGF-I receptors are possible mechanisms for endometrial growth (and the increased risk for endometrial cancer) in these patients.

The Clinical Consequences of Persistent Anovulation

Anovulation is the key feature of this condition and presents as amenorrhea in approximately 50% of cases and with irregular, heavy bleeding in 30%.[84,85] True virilization is rare, but 70% of anovulatory patients complain of cosmetically disturbing hirsutism. The development of hirsutism depends not only on the concentration of androgens in the blood but on the genetic sensitivity of hair follicles to androgens. Obesity has been classically regarded as an important feature, but in view of the concept of persistent anovulation arising from many causes, its presence is extremely variable and has no diagnostic value. However, the greater the body mass index, the higher the testosterone levels, and therefore hirsutism is more common in overweight anovulatory women. Alopecia and acne are also consequences of hyperandrogenism.[86,87]

While an elevated LH value in the presence of a low or low-normal FSH may be diagnostic, the diagnosis is easily made by the clinical presentation alone. About 20–40% of patients with this condition do not have elevated LH levels with reversal of the LH:FSH ratio.[88,89] We do not routinely measure FSH and LH levels in anovulatory patients.

The Clinical Consequences of Persistent Anovulation

1. **Infertility.**
2. **Menstrual bleeding problems, ranging from amenorrhea to dysfunctional uterine bleeding.**
3. **Hirsutism and acne.**
4. **An increased risk of endometrial cancer and, perhaps, breast cancer.**
5. **An increased risk of cardiovascular disease.**
6. **An increased risk of diabetes mellitus in patients with hyperinsulinemia.**

There are potentially severe clinical consequences of the steady state of hormone secretion. Besides the problems of bleeding, amenorrhea, hirsutism, and infertility, the effect of the unopposed and uninterrupted estrogen is to place the patient at considerable risk for cancer of the endometrium and, perhaps, cancer of the breast.[90–94] The risk of endometrial cancer is increased three-fold, while chronic anovulation during the reproductive years has been reported to be associated with a 3–4 times increased risk of breast cancer appearing in the postmenopausal years. However, the statistical power of these observational studies on breast cancer was limited by small numbers (all fewer than 15 cases). Others have failed to find a link between anovulation and the risk of breast cancer.[95,96]

If left unattended, patients with persistent anovulation develop clinical problems, and therefore appropriate therapeutic management is essential for all anovulatory patients. In a long-term follow-up of women with polycystic ovaries, the problems of android obesity, hyperinsulinemia, and hypertension were observed to persist into the postmenopausal years.[97]

The typical patient presents with anovulation and irregular menses or amenorrhea with withdrawal bleeding after a progestational challenge. If there is no hirsutism or virilism, evaluation of androgen production is not necessary. Documentation of anovulation is usually unnecessary, especially in view of menstrual irregularity with periods of amenorrhea. In the patient who has long-standing anovulation, an endometrial biopsy (with extensive sampling) is a wise precaution. The well-known association between this condition and abnormal endometrial changes must be kept in mind. ***The decision to perform an endometrial biopsy should not be influenced by the patient's age. It is the duration of exposure to unopposed estrogen that is critical.***

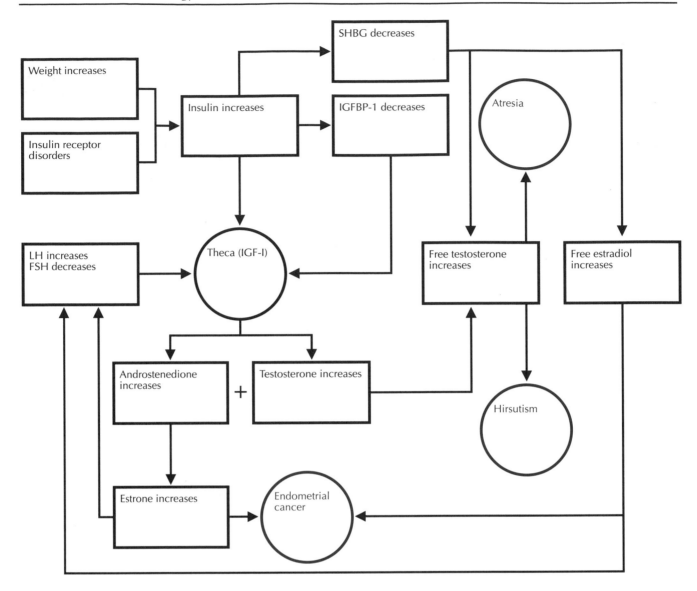

Therapy of most anovulatory patients can be planned at the first visit. If the patient desires pregnancy, she is a candidate for the medical induction of ovulation (Chapter 30). When pregnancy is achieved, patients with polycystic ovaries appear to have an increased risk of spontaneous abortion.[98–100] This has been attributed to elevated levels of LH which may produce an adverse environment for the oocyte, perhaps even inducing premature maturation and completion of the first meiotic division. For this reason, consideration should be given to pretreatment suppression prior to the induction of ovulation (Chapter 30).

If the patient presents with amenorrhea, an investigation must be pursued as outlined in Chapter 12. The management of significant dysfunctional uterine bleeding is discussed in Chapter 16 and hirsutism in Chapter 14.

For the patient who does not wish to become pregnant and does not complain of hirsutism, but is anovulatory and has irregular bleeding, therapy is directed toward interruption of the steady state effect on the endometrium and breast. The use of medroxyprogesterone acetate (10 mg daily for the first 10 days of every month) is favored to ensure complete withdrawal bleeding and to prevent endometrial hyperplasia and atypia. The monthly 10-day duration has been demonstrated to be essential to protect the endometrium from cancer in women on postmenopausal estrogen therapy. Until specific clinical data are available, it seems logical that young, anovulatory women also require 10 days of progestational exposure every month. The patient will be aware of the onset of ovulatory cycles because bleeding will occur at a time other than the expected withdrawal bleed. In our opinion, when reliable contraception is essential, the use of low dose combination oral contraception in the usual cyclic fashion is appropriate.

Besides contraception, there is another argument in favor of continuous suppression rather than periodic progestational interruption. The lipoprotein profile in androgenized women with polycystic ovaries is similar to the male pattern.[101–104] Although the elevated androgens associated with polycystic ovaries and anovulation offer some protection against osteoporosis, the adverse impact on the risk for cardiovascular disease is a more important consideration.[105] Monthly periodic treatment with a progestational agent has no significant effect on the androgen production by polycystic ovaries. Thus, if contraception is not required and hirsutism is not a complaint, assessment of the lipoprotein profile is a reasonable clinical response, and in the presence of a male pattern, serious consideration should be given to suppression with oral contraceptives. However, a major contributing factor to the abnormal lipid pattern in these patients is the hyperinsulinemia.[106] Therefore, a major effort must be directed to control of body weight.

Overweight, hyperandrogenic and hyperinsulinemic, anovulatory women must be cautioned regarding their increased risk of future diabetes mellitus. In addition, hyperinsulinemia contributes to the increased risk of cardiovascular disease both by means of a direct atherogenic action and indirectly by adversely affecting the lipoprotein profile. Indeed, insulin resistance may be a more significant factor than androgens in determining the abnormal lipoprotein profile in overweight, anovulatory women.[106] It has also been suggested that the increased insulin stimulation of IGF-I could produce bone changes similar to that seen in acromegaly.[107] Hyperinsulinemia may be a factor contributing to the higher risk of endometrial cancer in these patients by increasing IGF-I activity in the endometrium.[108]

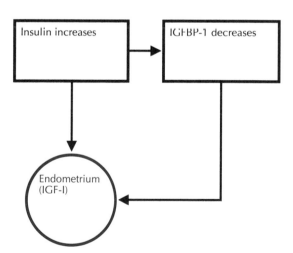

The only known effective therapy for these women is weight loss. Both the hyperinsulinemia and the hyperandrogenism can be reduced with weight loss which is at least more than 5% of the initial weight.[109,110] A goal for weight loss that correlates with a good chance of achieving pregnancy (improved menstrual function), a reduction in insulin levels, and a decrease in free testosterone levels is a body mass index of less than 27 (see the nomogram for calculating body mass index in Chapter 19). Insulin resistance is not detected with a body mass index less than 27.[111]

Who Should Be Tested for Hyperinsulinemia?

Do all anovulatory patients require testing for hyperinsulinemia? Both lean and obese women with polycystic ovaries can be found to have hyperinsulinemia, but not all women with polycystic ovaries (lean and obese) have hyperinsulinemia.[76,86] However, it is more common in overweight women and androgenic effects are more intense. Furthermore, lean women with hyperinsulinemia do not appear to have the same risk of future diabetes mellitus, although clinical follow-up may in time document an onset later in life of non-insulin dependent diabetes mellitus compared to an earlier onset in obese women.

It would be ideal if all patients with android obesity were tested for hyperinsulinemia. The waist:hip ratio is a means of estimating the degree of upper to lower body obesity. The waist measurement is the smallest circumference between the rib cage and the iliac crests. The hip measurement is the largest circumference between the waist and thighs. Interpretation is as follows:

> **Greater than 0.85 — Android Obesity**
> **Less than 0.75   — Gynoid Obesity**

Teenagers who present with persistent anovulation would also be good candidates for hyperinsulinemia testing. During puberty, insulin resistance develops, probably because of the increase in sex steroids and growth hormone, resulting in a secondary increase in insulin and IGF-I.[112] The increase in insulin leads to a decrease in SHBG that would allow greater sex steroid activity for pubertal development. There is reason to believe that some teenagers fail to normalize the hyperinsulinemia associated with the growth hormone increase in early puberty. It would be important to identify these teenagers who are at an increased risk for the development of diabetes mellitus.

Unfortunately, it is not certain what levels of insulin in the fasting state or in response to an oral glucose tolerance test are correlated with clinical outcome. A ratio of fasting glucose to fasting insulin less than 3.0 defines hyperinsulinemia, and we recommend the measurement of this ratio in order to provide evidence that lends credence and importance to counseling efforts. When all is said and done, however, concentration on weight loss in overweight, androgenized patients is the most effective therapeutic approach.

References

1. **Burger CW, Korsen T, van Kessel H, van Dop PA, Caron JM, Schoemaker J,** Pulsatile luteinizing hormone patterns in the follicular phase of the menstrual cycle, polycystic ovarian disease (PCOD) and non-PCOD secondary amenorrhea, J Clin Endocrinol Metab 61:1126, 1985.

2. **Barnes RB, Lobo RA,** Central opioid activity in polycystic ovary syndrome with and without dopaminergic modulation, J Clin Endocrinol Metab 61:779, 1985.

3. **Berga SL, Yen SSC,** Opioidergic regulation of LH pulsatility in women with polycystic ovary syndrome, Clin Endocrinol 30:177, 1989.

4. **Siiteri PK, MacDonald PC,** Role of extraglandular estrogen in human endocrinology, in Geyer SR, Astwood EB, Greep RO, editors, *Handbook of Physiology, Section 7, Endocrinology,* American Physiology Society, Washington DC, 1973, pp 615-629.

5. **Franks S,** Polycystic ovary syndrome: a changing perspective, Clin Endocrinol 31:87, 1989.

6. **Hull MGR,** Epidemiology of infertility and polycystic ovarian disease: endocrinological and demographic studies, Gynaecol Endocrinol 1:235:1987.

7. **Polson DW, Wadsworth J, Adams J, Franks S,** Polycystic ovaries: a common finding in normal women, Lancet 2:870, 1988.

8. **Clayton RN, Ogden V, Hodgkinson J, Worswick L, Rodin DA, Dyer S, Meade TW,** How common are polycystic ovaries in normal women and what is their significance for the fertility of the population? Clin Endocrinol 37:127, 1992.

9. **Chang RJ,** Ovarian steroid secretion in polycystic ovarian disease, Seminars Reprod Endocrinol 2:244, 1984.

10. **Calogero AE, Macchi M, Montanini V, Mongioi A, Maugeri G, Vicari E, Coniglione F, Sipione C, D'Agata R,** Dynamics of plasma gonadotropin and sex steroid release in polycystic ovarian disease after pituitary-ovarian inhibition with an analog of gonadotropin-releasing hormone, J Clin Endocrinol Metab 64:980, 1987.

11. **Laatikainen TJ, Apter DL, Paavonen JA, Wahlstrom TR,** Steroids in ovarian and peripheral venous blood in polycystic ovarian disease, Clin Endocrinol 13:125, 1980.

12. **Gonzalez F, Hatala DA, Speroff L,** Basal and dynamic hormonal responses to gonadotropin releasing hormone agonist treatment in women with polycystic ovaries with high and low dehydroepiandrosterone sulfate levels, Am J Obstet Gynecol 165:535, 1991.

13. **Wajchenberg BL, Achando SS, Mathor MM, Czeresnia CE, Neto DG, Kirschner MA,** The source(s) of estrogen production in hirsute women with polycystic ovarian disease as determined by simultaneous adrenal and ovarian venous catheterization, Fertil Steril 49:56, 1988.

14. **Kletzky OA, Davajan V, Nakamura RM, Thorneycroft IH, Mishell DR Jr,** Clinical categorization of patients with secondary amenorrhea using progesterone induced uterine bleeding and measurement of serum gonadotropin levels, Am J Obstet Gynecol 121:695, 1975.

15. **Rebar RW,** Gonadotropin secretion in polycystic ovary disease, Seminars Reprod Endocrinol 2:223, 1984.

16. **Imse V, Holzapfel G, Hinney B, Kuhn W, Wuttke W,** Comparison of luteinizing hormone pulsatility in the serum of women suffering from polycystic ovarian disease using a bioassay and five different immunoassays, J Clin Endocrinol Metab 74:1053, 1992.

17. **Waldstreicher J, Santoro NF, Hall JE, Filicori M, Crowley WF Jr,** Hyperfunction of the hypothalamic-pituitary axis in women with polycystic ovarian disease: indirect evidence for partial gonadotroph desensitizaiton, J Clin Endocrinol Metab 66:165, 1988.

18. **Schoemaker J,** Neuroendocrine control in polycystic ovary-like syndrome, Gynecol Endocrinol 5:277, 1991.

19. **Chang RJ, Mandel FP, Lu JK, Judd HL,** Enhanced disparity of gonadotropin secretion by estrone in women with polycystic ovarian disease, J Clin Endocrinol Metab 54:490, 1982.

20. **Lobo RA, Granger L, Goebelsmann U, Mishell DR Jr,** Elevations in unbound serum estradiol as a possible mechanism for inappropriate gonadotropin secretion in women with PCO, J Clin Endocrinol Metab 52:156, 1981.

21. **Judd HL, Rigg LA, Anderson DC, Yen SSC,** The effects of ovarian wedge resection on circulating gonadotropin and ovarian steroid levels in patients with polycystic ovary syndrome, J Clin Endocrinol Metab 43:347, 1976.

22. **Mahesh VB, Bratlid D, Lindabeck T,** Hormone levels following wedge resection in polycystic ovary syndrome, Obstet Gynecol 51:64, 1978.

23. **Katz M, Carr PJ, Cohen BM, Milhin RP,** Hormonal effects of wedge resection of polycystic ovaries, Obstet Gynecol 51:437, 1978.

24. **Casper RF, Greenblatt EM,** Laparoscopic ovarian cautery for induction of ovulation in women with polycystic ovarian disease, Seminars Reprod Endocrinol 8:208, 1990.

25. **Serafini P, Silva PD, Paulson RJ, Elind-Hirsch K, Hernandez M, Lobo RA,** Acute modulation of the hypothalamic-pituitary axis by intravenous testosterone in normal women, Am J Obstet Gynecol 155:1288, 1986.

26. **Hughesdon PE,** Morphology and morphogenesis of the Stein-Leventhal ovary and of so-called "hyperthecosis," Obstet Gynecol Survey 37:59, 1982.

27. **Judd HL, Scully RE, Herbst AL, Yen SSC, Ingersol FM, Kliman B,** Familial hyperthecosis: Comparison of endocrinologic and histologic findings with polycystic ovarian disease, Am J Obstet Gynecol 117:979, 1973.

28. **Nagamani M, Lingold JC, Gomez LG, Barza JR,** Clinical and hormonal studies in hyperthecosis of the ovaries, Fertil Steril 36:326, 1981.

29. **Nagamani M, Dinh TV, Kelver ME,** Hyperinsulinemia in hyperthecosis of the ovaries, Am J Obstet Gynecol 154:384, 1986.

30. **Kase N, Kowal J, Perloff W, Soffer LJ,** In vitro production of androgens by a virilizing adenoma and associated polycystic ovaries, Acta Endocrinol 44:15, 1963.

31. **Amerikia H, Savoy-Moore RT, Sundareson AS, Moghissi KS,** The effects of long-term androgen treatment on the ovary, Fertil Steril 45:202, 1986.

32. **Zourlas PA, Jones HW Jr,** Stein-Leventhal syndrome with masculinizing ovarian tumors, Obstet Gynecol 34:861, 1969.

33. **Dunaif A, Scully RE, Andersen RN, Chapin DS, Crowley WF Jr,** The effects of continuous androgen secretion on the hypothalamic-pituitary axis in women: evidence from a luteinized thecoma of the ovary, J Clin Endocrinol Metab 59:389, 1984.

34. **McNatty KP, Smith DM, Makris A, DeGrazia C, Tulchinsky D, Osathanondh R, Schiff I, Ryan KJ,** The intraovarian sites of androgen and estrogen formation in women with normal and hyperandrogenic ovaries as judged by in vitro experiments, J Clin Endocrinol Metab 50:755, 1980.

35. **Cataldo NA, Giudice LC,** Follicular fluid insulin-like growth factor binding protein profiles in polycystic ovary syndrome, J Clin Endocrinol Metab 74:695, 1992.

36. **San Roman GA, Magoffin DA,** Insulin-like growth factor binding proteins in ovarian follicles from women with polycystic ovarian disease: cellular source and levels in follicular fluid, J Clin Endocrinol Metab 75:1010, 1992.

37. **Erickson GF, Magoffin DA, Garzo VG, Cheung AP, Chang RJ,** Granulosa cells of polycystic ovaries: Are they normal or abnormal? Hum Reprod 7:293, 1992.

38. **Erickson GF, Hsueh AJN, Quigley ME, Rebar R, Yen SSC,** Functional studies of aromatase activity in human granulosa cells from normal and polycystic ovaries, J Clin Endocrinol Metab 49:514, 1979.

39. **Mason HD, Margara R, Winston RL, Seppala M, Koistinen R, Franks S,** Insulin-like growth factor-I (IGF-I) inhibits production of IGF-binding protein-1 while stimulating estradiol secretion in granulosa cells from normal and polycystic human ovaries, J Clin Endocrinol Metab 76:1275, 1993.

40. **Givens JR,** Hirsutism and hyperandrogenism, Adv Intern Med 21:221, 1976.

41. **Archard C, Thiers J,** Le virilisme pilaire et son association a l'insuffisance glycolytique (diabete des femmes a barbe), Bull Acad Natl Med 86:51, 1921.

42. **Barbieri RL, Ryan KJ,** Hyperandrogenism, insulin resistance and acanthosis nigricans: a common endocrinopathy with distinct pathophysiologic features, Am J Obstet Gynecol 147:90, 1983.

43. **Dunaif A, Green G, Phelps RG, Lebwohl M, Futterweit W, Lewy L,** Acanthosis nigricans, insulin action, and hyperandrogenism: clinical, histological, and biochemical findings, J Clin Endocrinol Metab 73:590, 1991.

44. **Reavens GM,** Role of insulin resistance in human disease, Diabetes 37:1595, 1988.

45. **Poretsky L,** On the paradox of insulin-induced hyperandrogenism in insulin-resistant states, Endocrin Rev 12:3, 1991.

46. **O'Meara NM, Blackman JD, Ehrman DA, Barnes RB, Jaspan JB, Rosenfeld RL, Polonsky KS,** Defects in β-cell function in functional ovarian hyperandrogenism, J Clin Endocrinol Metab 76:1241, 1993.

47. **Haffner SM, Valdez RA, Hazuda HP, Mitchell BD, Morales PH, Stern MP,** Prospective analysis of the insulin-resistance syndrome (syndrome X), Diabetes 41:715, 1992.

48. **Imano E, Kadowaki H, Kadowaki T, Iwama N, Watarai T, Kawamori R, Kamada T, Taylor SI,** Two patients with insulin resistance due to decreased levels of insulin-receptor mRNA, Diabetes 40:548, 1991.

49. **Kadowaki T, Kadowaki H, Rechler MM, Serrrano-Rios M, Roth J, Gorden P, Taylor SI,** Five mutant alleles of the insulin receptor gene in patients with genetic forms of insulin resistance, J Clin Invest 86:254, 1990.

50. **Ciaraldi TP, El-Roeiy A, Madar Z, Reichart D, Olefsky JM, Yen SSC,** Cellular mechanisms of insulin resistance in polycystic ovarian syndrome, J Clin Endocrinol Metab 75:577, 1992.

51. **Peiris AN, Sothmann MS, Aiman EJ, Kissebah AH,** The relationship of insulin to sex hormone-binding globulin: role of adiposity, Fertil Steril 52:69, 1989.

52. **Kirschner MA, Samojlik E, Drejka M, Szmal E, Schneider G, Ertel N,** Androgen-estrogen metabolism in women with upper body *versus* lower body obesity, J Clin Endocrinol Metab 70:473, 1990.

53. **Pasquali R, Casimirri F, Balestra V, Flamia R, Melchionda N, Fabbri R, Barbara L,** The relative contribution of androgens and insulin in determining abdominal fat distribution in premenopausal women, J Endocrinol Invest 14:839, 1991.

54. **Lapidus L, Bengtsson C, Larsson B, Pennert K, Rybo E, Sjostrom L,** Distribution of adipose tissue and risk of cardiovascular disease and death: a 12 year follow up of participants in the population study of women in Gothenburg, Sweden, Br Med J 289:1257, 1984.

55. **Ostlund RE Jr, Staten M, Kohrt W, Schultz J, Malley M,** The ratio of waist-to-hip circumference, plasma insulin level, and glucose intolerance as independent predictors for the HDL_2 cholesterol level in older adults, New Engl J Med 322:229, 1990.

56. **Deutsch MI, Mueller WH, Malina RM,** Androgyny in fat patterning is associated with obesity in adolescents and young adults, Ann Hum Biol 12:275, 1985.

57. **Must A, Jacques PF, Dallal GE, Bajema CJ, Dietz WH,** Long-term morbidity and mortality of overweight adolescents: a follow-up of the Harvard Growth Study of 1922 to 1935, New Engl J Med 327:1350, 1992.

58. **Chang RJ, Nakamura RM, Judd HL, Kaplan SA,** Insulin resistance in non-obese patients with polycystic ovarian disease, J Clin Endocrinol Metab 57:356, 1983.

59. **Jialal I, Naiker P, Reddi K, Moodley J, Joubert SM,** Evidence for insulin resistance in nonobese patients with polycystic ovarian disease, J Clin Endocrinol Metab 64:1066, 1987.

60. **Dunaif A, Segal K, Futterweit W, Dobrjansky A,** Profound peripheral resistance independent of obesity in polycystic ovary syndrome, Diabetes 38:1165, 1989.

61. **Buyalos RP, Geffner ME, Bersch N, Judd HL, Watanabe RM, Bergman RN, Golde DW,** Insulin and insulin-like growth factor-I responsiveness in polycystic ovarian syndrome, Fertil Steril 57:796, 1992.

62. **Anttila L, Ding Y-Q, Ruutiainen K, Erkkola R, Irjala K, Huhtaniemi I,** Clinical features and circulating gonadotropin, insulin, and androgen interactions in women with polycystic ovarian disease, Fertil Steril 55:1057, 1991.

63. **Insler V, Shoham Z, Barash A, Koistinen R, Seppala M, Hen M, Lunenfeld B, Zadik Z,** Polycystic ovaries in non-obese and obese patients: possible pathophysiological mechanism based on new interpretation of facts and findings, Hum Reprod 8:379, 1993.

64. **Dale PO, Tanbo T, Vaaler S, Abyholm T,** Body weight, hyperinsulinemia, and gonadotropin levels in the polycystic ovarian syndrome: evidence of two distinct populations, Fertil Steril 58:487, 1992.

65. **Homburg R, Pariente C, Lunenfeld B, Jacobs HS,** The role of insulin-like growth factor-I (IGF-I) and IGF binding protein-1 (IGFBP-1) in the pathogenesis of polycystic ovary syndrome, Hum Reprod 7:1379, 1992.

66. **Geffner ME, Kaplan SA, Bersch N, Golde DW, Landaw EM, Chang RJ,** Persistence of insulin resistance in polycystic ovarian disease after inhibition of ovarian steroid secretion, Fertil Steril 45:327, 1986.

67. **Grainger D, Thornton K, Rossi G, Connoly-Diamond M, DeFronzo R, Sherwin R, Diamond MP,** Influence of basal androgen levels in euandrogenic women on glucose homeostasis, Fertil Steril 58:1113, 1992.

68. **Dunaif A, Green G, Futterweit W, Dobrjansky A,** Suppression of hyperandrogenism does not improve peripheral or hepatic insulin resistance in the polycystic ovary syndrome, J Clin Endocrinol Metab 70:699, 1990.

69. **DeClue TJ, Shah SC, Marchese M, Malone JI,** Insulin resistance and hyperinsulinemia induce hyperandrogenism in a young type B insulin-resistant female, J Clin Endocrinol Metab 72:1308, 1991.

70. **Elkind-Hirsch KE, Valdes CT, McConnell TG, Malinak LR,** Androgen responses to acutely increased endogenous insulin levels in hyperandrogenic and normal cycling women, Fertil Steril 55:486, 1991.

71. **Smith S, Ravnikar VA, Barbieri RL,** Androgen and insulin response to an oral glucose challenge in hyperandrogenic women, Fertil Steril 48:72, 1987.

72. **Kiddy DS, Hamilton-Fairley D, Seppala M, Koistinen R, James VHT, Reed MJ, Franks S,** Diet-induced changes in sex hormone binding globulin and free testosterone in women with normal or polycystic ovaries: correlation with serum insulin and insulin-like growth factor-I, Clin Endocrinol 31:757, 1989.

73. **Barbieri RL, Makris A, Ryan KJ,** Insulin stimulates androgen accumulation in incubations of human ovarian stroma and theca, Obstet Gynecol 64:73S, 1984.

74. **Barbieri RL, Makris A, Randall RW, Daniels G, Kistner RW, Ryan KJ,** Insulin stimulates androgen accumulation in incubations of ovarian stroma obtained from women with hyperandrogenism, J Clin Endocrinol Metab 62:904, 1986.

75. **Nestler JC, Barlascini CO, Matt DW, Steingold KA, Plymate SR, Clore JN, Blackard WG,** Suppression of serum insulin by diazoxide reduces serum testosterone levels in obese women with polycystic ovary syndrome, J Clin Endocrinol Metab 68:1027, 1989.

76. **Dale PO, Tanbo T, Djoseland O, Jervell J, Abyholm T,** Persistence of hyperinsulinemia in polycystic ovary syndrome after ovarian suppression by gonadotropin-releasing hormone agonist, Acta Endocrinol 126:132, 1992.

77. **Fradkin JE, Eastman RC, Lesniak MA, Roth J,** Specificity spillover at the hormone receptor: exploring its role in human disease, New Engl J Med 320:640, 1989.

78. **Bergh C, Carlsson B, Olsson J-H, Selleskog U, Hillensjo T,** Regulation of androgen production in cultured human thecal cells by insulin-like growth factor I and insulin, Fertil Steril 59:323, 1993.

79. **Nestler JE, Powers LP, Matt DW, Steingold KA, Plymate SR, Rittmaster RS, Clore JN, Blackard WG,** A direct effect of hyperinsulinemia on serum sex hormone-binding globulin levels in obese women with the polycystic ovary syndrome, J Clin Endocrinol Metab 72:83, 1991.

80. **Plymate SR, Matej LA, Jones RE, Friedl KE,** Inhibition of sex hormone binding globulin production in human hepatoma (hep G2) cell line by insulin and prolactin, J Clin Endocrinol Metab 67:460, 1988.

81. **Singh A, Hamilton-Fairley D, Koistinen R, Seppala M, James VHT, Franks S, Reed MJ,** Effect of insulin-like growth factor-I (IGF-I) and insulin on the secretion of sex hormone-binding globulin and IGF-binding protein (IGFBP-1) by human hepatoma cells, J Endocrinol 124:R1, 1990.

82. **Haffner SM, Valdez RA, Morales PA, Hazuda HP, Stern MP,** Decreased sex hormone-binding globulin predicts noninsulin-dependent diabetes mellitus in women but not in men, J Clin Endocrinol Metab 77:56, 1993.

83. **Conover CA, Lee PDK, Kanaley JA, Clarkson JT, Jensen MD,** Insulin regulation of insulin-like growth factor binding protein-1 in obese and nonobese humans, J Clin Endocrinol Metab 74:1355, 1992.

84. **Goldzieher JW, Axelrod LR,** Clinical and biochemical features of polycystic ovarian disease, Fertil Steril 14:631, 1963.

85. **Prunty FTG,** Hirsutism, virilism, and appparent virilism, and their gonadal relationships, J Endocrinol 38:203, 1967.

86. **Conway GS, Honour JW, Jacobs HS,** Heterogeneity of the polycystic ovary syndrome: clinical endocrine and ultrasound features in 556 patients, Clin Endocrinol 30:459, 1989.

87. **Futterweit W, Dunaif A, Yeh HC, Kingsley P,** The prevalence of hyperandrogenism in 109 consecutive female patients with diffuse alopecia, J Am Acad Dermatol 19:831, 1988.

88. **Fauser BCJM, Pache TD, Hop WCJ, de Jong FH, Dahl KD,** The significance of a single LH measurement in women with cycle disturbances: discrepancaies between immunoreactive and bioactive hormone estimates, Clin Endocrinol 37:445, 1992.

89. **Pache TD, de Jong FH, Hop WC, Fauser BCJM,** Association between ovarian changes assessed by transvaginal sonography and clinical and endocrine signs of the polycystic ovary syndrome, Fertil Steril 59:544, 1993.

90. **Coulam CB, Annegers JF,** Breast cancer and chronic anovulation syndrome, Surg Forum 33:474, 1982.

91. **Coulam CB, Annegers JF, Krans JS,** Chronic anovulation sydrome and associated neoplasia, Obstet Gynecol 61:403, 1983.

92. **Cowan LD, Gordis L, Tonascia JA, Jones GS,** Breast cancer incidence in women with a history of progesterone deficiency, Am J Epidemiol 114:209, 1981.

93. **Ron E, Lunenfeld B, Menczer J, Blumstein T, Katz L, Oelsner G, Serr D,** Cancer incidence in a cohort of infertile women, Am J Epidemiol 125:780, 1987.

94. **Escobedo LG, Lee NC, Peterson HB, Wingo PA,** Infertility-associated endometrial cancer risk may be limited to specific subgroups of infertile women, Obstet Gynecol 77:124, 1991.

95. **Gammon MD, Thompson WD,** Infertility and breast cancer: a population-based case-control study, Am J Epidemiol 132:708, 1990.

96. **Gammon MD, Thompson WD,** Polycystic ovaries and the risk of breast cancer, Am J Epidemiol 134:818, 1991.

97. **Dahlgren E, Johansson S, Lindstedt G, Knutsson F, Oden A, Janson PO, Mattson L-A, Crona N, Lundberg P-A,** Women with polycystic ovary syndrome wedge resected in 1956 to 1965: a long-term follow-up focusing on natural history and circulating hormones, Fertil Steril 57:505, 1992.

98. **Sagle M, Bishop K, Ridley N, Alexander FM, Michel M, Bonney RC, Beard RW, Franks S,** Recurrent early miscarriage and polycystic ovaries, Br Med J 297:1027, 1988.

99. **Regan L, Owen EJ, Jacobs HS,** Hypersecretion of luteinising hormone, infertility, and miscarriage, Lancet 336:1141, 1990.

100. **Tulppala M, Stenman U-H, Cacciatore B, Ylikorkala O,** Polycystic ovaries and levels of gonadotrophins and androgens in recurrent miscarriage: prospective study in 50 women, Br J Obstet Gynaecol 100:348, 1993.

101. **Wild RA, Painter PC, Coulson PB, Carruth KB, Ranney GB,** Lipoprotein lipid concentrations and cardiovascular risk in women with polycystic ovary syndrome, J Clin Endocrinol Metab 61:946, 1985.

102. **Wild RA, Van Nort JJ, Grubb B, Bachman W, Hartz A, Bartholomew M,** Clinical signs of androgen excess as risk factors for coronary artery disease, Fertil Steril 54:255, 1990.

103. **Conway GS, Agrawal R, Betteridge DJ, Jacobs HS,** Risk factors for coronary artery disease in lean and obese women with polycystic ovary syndrome, Clin Endocrinol 37:119, 1992.

104. **Graf MJ, Richards CJ, Brown V, Meissner L, Dunaif A,** The independent effects of hyperandrogenaemia, hyperinsulinemaemia, and obesity on lipid and lipoprotein profiles in women, Clin Endocrinol 33:119, 1990.

105. **Di Carlo C, Shoham Z, MacDougall J, Patel A, Hall ML, Jacobs HS,** Polycystic ovaries as a relative protective factor for bone mineral loss in young women with amenorrhea, Fertil Steril 57:314, 1992.

106. **Wild RA, Alaupovic P, Parker IJ,** Lipid and apolipoprotein abnormalities in hirsute women. I. The association with insulin resistance, Am J Obstet Gynecol 166:1191, 1992.

107. **Fox R, Wardle PG, Clarke L, Hull MGR,** Acromegaloid bone changes in severe polycystic ovarian disease: an effect of hyperinsulinaemia? Br J Obstet Gynaecol 98:410, 1991.

108. **Giudice LC, Dsupin BA, Jin IH, Vu TH, Hoffman AR,** Differential expression of messenger ribonucleic acids encoding insulin-like growth factors and their receptors in human uterine endometrium and decidua, J Clin Endocrinol Metab 76:1115, 1993.

109. **Pasquali R, Antenucci D, Casimirri F, Venturoli S, Paradisi R, Fabbri R, Balestra V, Melchiondra N, Barbara L,** Clinical and hormonal characteristics of obese amenorrheic hyperandrogenic women before and after weight loss, J Clin Endocrinol Metab 68:173, 1989.

110. **Kiddy DS, Hamilton-Fairley D, Bush A, Short F, Anyaoku V, Reed MJ, Franks S,** Improvement in endocrine and ovarian function during dietary treatment of obese women with polycystic ovary syndrome, Clin Endocrinol 36:105, 1992.

111. **Campbell PJ, Gerich JE,** Impact of obesity on insulin action in volunteers with normal glucose tolerance: demonstration of a threshold for the adverse effect of obesity, J Clin Endocrinol Metab 70:1114, 1990.

112. **Bloch CA, Clemons P, Sperling MA,** Puberty decreased insulin sensitivity, J Pediatr 110:481, 1987.

14 Hirsutism

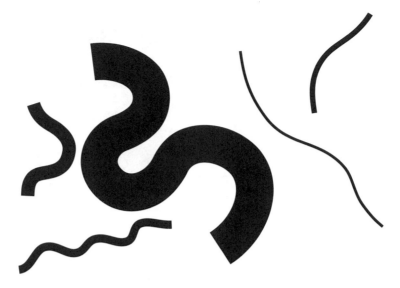

Excessive facial and body hair caused by excess androgen production is usually associated with anovulatory ovaries and loss of cyclic menstrual function. The more severe states of virilism (clitoromegaly, deepening of the voice, balding, and changes in body habitus) are rarely seen and usually are secondary to adrenal hyperplasia or androgen-producing tumors of adrenal or ovarian origin. Although these are rare, diagnostic evaluation is required.

A concerned and sympathetic approach must be offered to women who complain of hirsutism. The responsible clinician must view hirsutism both as an endocrine problem and as a cosmetic problem. To the affected woman, hair growth over the face, abdomen, or breasts is disturbing on several levels: Is there disease? Is sexuality changing? Is social acceptance altered? Is fertility impaired?

This chapter reviews the biology of hair growth[1] and the endocrine causes that can yield hirsutism. An uncomplicated, effective program for diagnostic evaluation and therapeutic management is presented.

The Biology of Hair Growth

Embryology

Each hair follicle develops at about 8–10 weeks of gestation as a derivative of the epidermis. It is composed initially of a solid column of cells that proliferates from the basal layers of the epidermis and protrudes downward into the dermis. As the column elongates it encounters a cluster of mesodermal cells (the dermal papilla) which it envelops at its bulbous tip (bulb). The solid epithelial column then hollows out to form a hair canal, and the pilosebaceous apparatus (a hair follicle, sebaceous glands, and arrector pili muscles) is laid down.

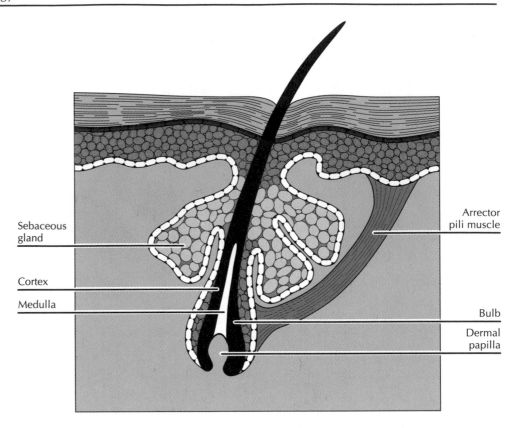

Hair growth begins with proliferation of the epithelial cells at the base of the column in contact with the dermal papilla. The ***lanugo hair*** that covers the fetus is lightly pigmented, thin in diameter, short in length, and fragile in attachment. Important to note is the fact that the total endowment of hair follicles is made at an early gestational stage (by 22 weeks) and that no new hair follicles will be produced de novo. The concentration of hair follicles laid down per unit area of facial skin does not differ materially between sexes but does differ between races and ethnic groups (Caucasian > Oriental; Mediterranean > Nordic). In addition, hair growth differences between races probably reflect hair follicle differences in 5α-reductase activity (the production of the active androgen, dihydrotestosterone).[2] The pattern of hair growth is genetically predetermined.

Structure and Growth

Hair does not grow continuously but rather in a cyclic fashion with alternating phases of activity and inactivity. The cycles are referred to by the following terms:

> **Anagen** — **the growing phase.**
> **Catagen** — **rapid involution phase.**
> **Telogen** — **quiescent phase.**

In the resting phase (telogen), the hair is short and loosely attached to the base (the bulb) of the epithelial canal. As growth begins (anagen), epithelial matrix cells at the base begin to proliferate and extend downward into the dermis. The epithelial column elongates some 4–6 times from the resting state. Once downward extension is completed, continued rapid growth of the matrix cells pushes upward to the skin surface. The tenuous contact of the previous hair is broken, and that hair is shed. The superficial matrix cells differentiate forming a keratinized column. Growth continues as long as active mitoses persist in the basal matrix cells. When finished (catagen), the column shrinks, the bulb shrivels, and the resting state is reachieved (telogen).

The length of hair is primarily determined by duration of the growth phase (anagen). Scalp hair remains in anagen for 3 years and has only a relatively short resting phase. Elsewhere (forearm) a short anagen and long telogen will lead to short hair of stable nongrowing length. The appearance of continuous growth (or periodic shedding) is determined by the degree to which individual hair follicles act asynchronously with their neighbors. Scalp hair is asynchronous and therefore always seems to be growing. The resting phase that some hairs (10–15%) are in is not apparent. If marked synchrony is achieved, then all hairs may undergo telogen at the same time leading to the appearance of shedding. Occasionally, women will complain of marked hair loss from the scalp, but this time period of shedding is usually limited (6–8 months), and growth resumes when asynchrony is re-established.

Hypertrichosis is a generalized increase in hair of the fetal lanugo type, associated with the use of drugs or malignancy. *Vellus hair* is the downy hair associated with the prepubertal years. *Terminal hair* is the coarse hair that grows on various parts of the body during the adult years. Hirsutism implies a vellus to terminal hair transformation.

Factors Which Influence Hair Growth

The dermal papilla is the director of the events that control hair growth. Despite major injury to the epithelial component of the follicle (such as freezing, x-rays, or a skin graft), if the dermal papilla survives, the hair follicle will regenerate and regrow hair. Injury to, or degeneration of, the dermal papilla is the crucial factor in permanent hair loss.

Sexual hair is defined as that hair which responds to the sex steroids. Sexual hair grows on the face, lower abdomen, anterior thighs, the chest, the breasts, the pubic area, and in the axillae. Once androgen influences hair follicles in sexual areas and larger, longer, more pigmented hair is induced, these final hair characteristics recur in typical cycles of activity and inactivity, even in the absence of sustaining androgen.

From animal studies and human disease patterns, the following list of hormonal effects can be compiled:

1. Androgens, particularly testosterone, initiate growth, increase the diameter and pigmentation of the keratin column, and probably increase the rate of matrix cell mitoses in all but scalp hair.

2. Estrogens act essentially opposite from androgens, retarding the rate and initiation of growth, and leading to finer, less pigmented and slower growing hair.

3. Progestins have minimal direct effect on hair.

4. Pregnancy (high estrogen and progesterone) can increase the synchrony of hair growth, leading to periods of growth or shedding.

An important clinical characteristic of hair growth can be understood from studies of the effects of castration. If castration occurs before puberty, the male will not grow a beard. If castration occurs after puberty with beard and sexual hair distribution fully developed, then these hairs continue to grow albeit more slowly and with finer caliber. Androgen stimulates sexual hair follicle conversion from lanugo to terminal adult hair growth patterns, but *once established, these patterns persist despite withdrawal of androgen.*

Sexual and nonsexual hair growth can be affected by endocrine problems. In hypopituitarism, there is marked reduction of hair growth. Acromegaly will be associated with hirsutism in 10–15% of patients. While the impact of thyroid hormone is not clear, hypothyroid individuals sometimes display less axillary, pubic, and, curiously, lateral eyebrow hair. 5α-Reductase activity is stimulated by insulin-like growth factor-I (IGF-I).[3] Increased IGF-I activity in anovulatory patients with insulin resistance and hyperinsulinemia can intensify the hirsute response in these hyperandrogenic patients.

Hair growth can be influenced by nonhormonal factors, such as local skin temperature, blood flow, and edema. Hair grows faster in the summer than in the winter. Hair growth can be seen with central nervous system (CNS) problems such as encephalitis, cranial trauma, multiple sclerosis, and with certain drugs.

Androgen Production

The production rate of testosterone in the normal female is 0.2 to 0.3 mg/day. Approximately 50% of testosterone is derived from peripheral conversion of androstenedione, while the adrenal gland and ovary contribute approximately equal amounts (25%) to the circulating levels of testosterone, except at midcycle when the ovarian contribution increases by 10–15%. Dehydroepiandrosterone sulfate (DHAS) arises almost exclusively from the adrenal gland, while 90% of dehydroepiandrosterone (DHA) is from the adrenal.

About 80% of circulating testosterone is bound to a beta-globulin known as sex steroid hormone binding globulin (SHBG). In women, approximately 19% is loosely bound to albumin, leaving about 1% unbound. Androgenicity is dependent mainly upon the unbound fraction and partly upon the fraction associated with albumin. DHA, DHAS, and androstenedione are not significantly protein bound, and routine immunoassay reflects their biologically available hormone activity. This is not the case with testosterone because routine assays measure the total testosterone concentration, bound and unbound.

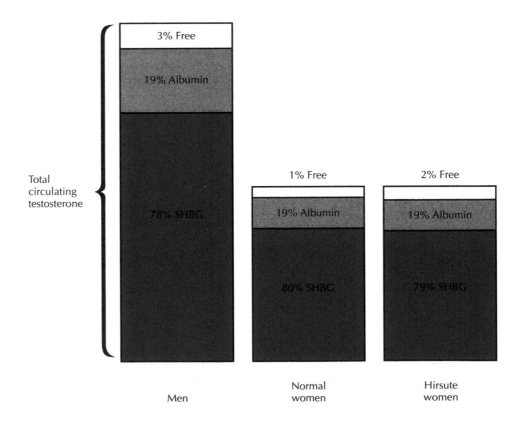

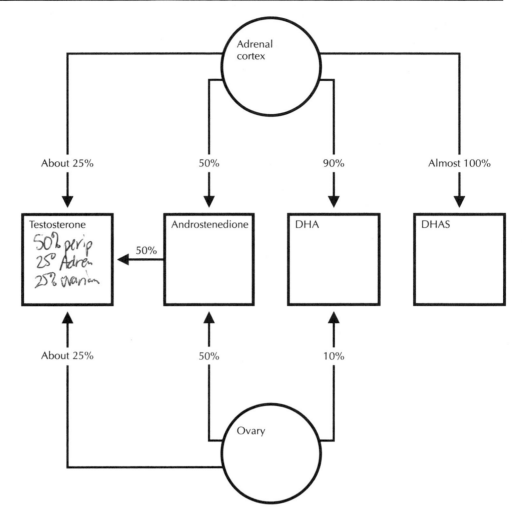

SHBG production in the liver is decreased by androgens. Hence, the binding capacity in men is lower than in normal women, and 2–3% of testosterone circulates in the free, active form in men. SHBG is decreased by insulin, and increased by estrogens and thyroid hormone. Therefore, binding capacity is increased in women with hyperthyroidism, in pregnancy, and by estrogen-containing medication. In a hirsute woman, the SHBG level is depressed by the excess androgen (and, when present, by hyperinsulinemia), and the percent free and active testosterone is elevated as is the metabolic clearance rate of testosterone. The total testosterone concentration, therefore, can be in the normal range in a woman who is hirsute. However, there is no clinical need for a specific assay for the free portion of testosterone. The very presence of hirsutism or masculinization indicates increased androgen effects. One can reliably interpret a normal total testosterone level in these circumstances as being compatible with decreased binding capacity and increased free testosterone.

In hirsute women, only 25% of the circulating testosterone arises from peripheral conversion, and most is due to direct tissue secretion. Indeed, data overwhelmingly indicate that the ovary is the major source of increased testosterone and androstenedione in hirsute women.[4] The most common cause of hirsutism in women is anovulation and excessive androgen production by the ovaries. Adrenal causes are most uncommon.

3α-Androstanediol Glucuronide

While testosterone is the major circulating androgen, dihydrotestosterone (DHT) is the major nuclear androgen in many sensitive tissues, including hair follicles and the pilosebaceous unit in skin. 3α-Androstanediol is the peripheral tissue metabolite of DHT, and its glucuronide, 3α-androstanediol glucuronide (3α-AG) has been utilized as a marker of target tissue cellular action.[5,6] There is an excellent correlation between the serum levels of 3α-AG and the clinical manifestations of androgens. Specifically, 3α-AG correlates with the level of 5α-reductase activity (testosterone and androstenedione to dihydrotestosterone) in the skin.

Thus, there are 3 principal laboratory measurements of *potential* clinical use for the evaluation of androgen excess:

1. Testosterone — a measure of ovarian and adrenal activity.

2. DHAS — a measure of adrenal activity.

3. 3α-AG — a measure of peripheral target tissue activity.

Hirsutism is not a disorder of hair, rather it reflects increased 5α-reductase activity which produces more DHT, leading to the stimulation of hair growth. This enzyme activity is increased by an increased availability of precursor (the circulating level of testosterone, therefore, is a primary factor) or by still unknown local tissue mechanisms. Measurement of 3α-AG has revealed that true idiopathic hirsutism may not exist (or at least it is very rare). In the presence of other laboratory measurements which are normal, increased levels of 3α-AG indicate an increased activity of 5α-reductase in the peripheral compartment.[7] However, 3α-AG also reflects hepatic conjugation activity and the impact of major precursors which are derived from the adrenal gland and not from peripheral sources.[8] Therefore 3α-AG is not solely a measure of cutaneous androgen metabolism.

There are 2 reasons why the measurement of 3α-AG is not part of the routine clinical approach to the problem of hirsutism. First, it is not an absolute measurement. Values in hirsute women overlap the normal range by about 20%. Second, and most importantly, the ultimate diagnosis and therapy of the problem are not affected by this test.

Evaluation of Hirsutism

Cosmetically disfiguring hirsutism is the end result of a number of factors:

1. The number of hair follicles present (Japanese women bearing androgen-producing tumors rarely are hirsute because of the low concentration of hair follicles per unit skin area).

2. The degree to which androgen has converted resting vellus hair to terminal adult hair.

3. The ratio of the growth to resting phases in affected hair follicles.

4. The asynchrony of growth cycles in aggregates of hair follicles.

5. The thickness and degree of pigmentation of individual hairs.

The primary factor in hirsutism is an increase in androgen levels (usually testosterone) which produces an initial growth stimulus and then acts to sustain continued growth.

Essentially every woman with hirsutism will be found to have an increased production rate of testosterone and androstenedione.[9]

The most sensitive marker for increased androgen production is hirsutism. This is followed in order by acne and increased oiliness of the skin, increased libido, clitoromegaly, and, finally, masculinization. Masculinization and virilization are terms reserved for extreme androgen effects (usually, but not always, associated with a tumor) leading to the development of a male hair pattern, clitoromegaly, deepening of the voice, increased muscle mass, and general male body habitus.

Alopecia can be a vexing problem for patient and physician. In many instances, alopecia is a temporary phenomenon, a response of the scalp hair to some change which has induced a period of synchronous hair growth and loss. Often, this is a response to acute, stressful events. With time, usually 6 months to a year, the scalp hair becomes asynchronous again and the hair thickens. In a series of consecutive patients presenting with diffuse alopecia, the majority had no evidence of hirsutism or menstrual dysfunction; however, anovulation with polycystic ovaries was the most common problem, and nearly 40% demonstrated hyperandrogenism.[10] Patients complaining of alopecia deserve evaluation for hyperandrogenism because a significant number of them can be appropriately treated. In addition, a laboratory survey is indicated for thyroid dysfunction or chronic illness. Hair loss is also a consequence of aging, beginning in both sexes about the age of 50.[11]

Acne is another sign of increased androgen activity. Up to 60% of women with acne who have normal circulating levels of androgens display evidence of increased 5α-reductase activity in the pilosebaceous unit.[12] These are the women who benefit from anti-androgenic treatment.

Acanthosis nigricans in an overweight patient with hirsutism is a reliable clinical marker of insulin resistance and hyperinsulinemia. This gray-brown velvety discoloration of the skin is usually present at the neck, groin, and axillae; however, the vulva is a very common site in hirsute women.[13] Acanthosis nigricans indicates the need to determine the state of glucose metabolism, as discussed in Chapter 13. Serious consideration should be given to the presence of hyperinsulinemia in hyperandrogenic women.

The most common clinical problem is the hirsute woman with irregular menses, with the onset of hirsutism during teenage years or in the early 20s, and long, gradual worsening of the condition. About 70% of anovulatory women develop hirsutism. The picture is so characteristic that a careful history may be sufficient for the diagnosis.

A good history can reveal some of the rare causes of hirsutism: environmental factors producing chronic irritation or reactive hyperemia of the skin, the use of drugs, changes associated with Cushing's syndrome or acromegaly, or even the presence of pregnancy (indicating the possibility of a luteoma). Hair-stimulating drugs include methyltestosterone, anabolic agents such as Nilevar or Anavar, phenytoin, diazoxide, and danazol. The 19-nortestosterones in the current low dosage oral contraceptives rarely (if ever) cause acne or hirsutism. ***Especially important in the history is the rapidity of development.*** A woman who develops hirsutism after the age of 25 and demonstrates very rapid progression of masculinization over several months usually has an androgen-producing tumor.

Adrenal hyperplasia caused by an enzymatic deficiency presenting in adult life is rare. Congenital adrenal hyperplasia which can lead to hirsutism is usually diagnosed and treated prior to puberty. Hirsutism in childhood is usually caused by congenital adrenal hyperplasia or androgen-producing tumors. Genetic problems, such as Y-containing mosaics or incomplete androgen sensitivity, will produce signs of androgen stimulation at puberty.

Virilization during pregnancy raises the suspicion of a luteoma which is not a true tumor but an exaggerated reaction of the ovarian stroma to chorionic gonadotropin.[14] The solid luteoma is unilateral in 45% of cases and associated with a normal pregnancy. Theca-lutein cysts seen with trophoblastic disease are virtually always bilateral. Virilization due to theca-lutein cysts can also be seen with the high human chorionic gonadotropin (HCG) titers associated with multiple gestation. Since a luteoma regresses postpartum, the only risk is masculinization of a female fetus; a risk not reported with theca-lutein cysts. Subsequent pregnancies are usually normal, but maternal virilization is occasionally recurrent.[15] Androgen-secreting ovarian tumors are very rarely encountered during pregnancy, probably because the excess androgen usually suppresses ovulation.[16] Ultrasonographic evaluation of the pelvis in women experiencing virilization in pregnancy is very helpful. Malignancy is frequently encountered when a unilateral ovarian lesion is present.

Hirsutism, therefore, is usually associated with persistent anovulation (Chapter 13). Although anovulatory ovaries are usually the source for excess androgens, a minimal workup is necessary, dedicated to ruling out the adrenal sources and tumors. It should be emphasized that hospitalization for extensive evaluation of hirsutism is required only rarely.

The Diagnostic Workup

The initial laboratory evaluation of hirsutism consists of immunoassays for the blood levels of testosterone, DHAS, and 17-hydroxyprogesterone (17-OHP). As part of the evaluation for anovulation, prolactin levels and thyroid function should be assessed, careful examination of the breasts for the presence of galactorrhea is important, and an aspiration endometrial biopsy should be considered. In addition, consideration should be directed to the possible presence of hyperinsulinemia. ***Patients with intense androgen action may be amenorrheic due to endometrial suppression (with a decidual response) and may not demonstrate withdrawal bleeding after a progestational challenge.***

Cushing's syndrome can present with hirsutism, and later, masculinization. Remember that one of the most common referral diagnoses is Cushing's syndrome, but this is one of the least common final diagnoses. When clinical suspicion is high, a screen for Cushing's syndrome is indicated.

The Screen for Cushing's Syndrome

Cushing's syndrome is the persistent oversecretion of cortisol. It can develop in 5 different ways: pituitary ACTH overproduction (Cushing's disease), ectopic ACTH overproduction by tumors, autonomous cortisol-secreting adrenal or, very rarely, ovarian tumors, or a fifth extremely rare possibility, the secretion of corticotropin releasing hormone (CRH) by a tumor. A clinician must first make the diagnosis of Cushing's syndrome (excessive cortisol secretion) before determining the etiology.

The most useful measurements in the basal state to detect Cushing's syndrome are the 24-hour urinary free cortisol excretion (10–90 µg [28–250 nmol]) and the late evening plasma cortisol level (< 15 µg/dL [420 nmol/L]). The urinary excretion of 17-ketosteroids and 17-hydroxysteroids and measurement of morning and afternoon plasma cortisol levels are less reliable because of a significant overlap between normal and abnormal patients.

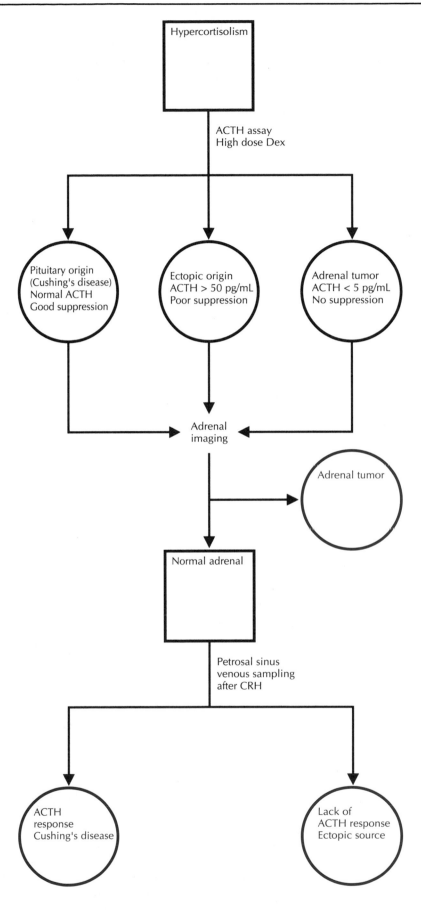

The single dose overnight dexamethasone test is excellent because of the very low incidence of false results. Dexamethasone (1 mg) is given orally at bedtime, and a plasma cortisol is drawn at 8:00 the next morning. A value less than 5 μg/dL (140 nmol/L) rules out Cushing's syndrome. Cushing's syndrome is unlikely with intermediate values between 5 (140 nmol/L) and 10 μg/dL (280 nmol/L), while a value higher than 10 μg/L (280 nmol/L) is diagnostic of adrenal hyperfunction. The number of patients with Cushing's syndrome who show a normal suppression in the single dose overnight test is negligible (less than 1%).[17] Obese patients, however, have a false positive rate up to 13%.

If the single dose overnight test is abnormal, go to the low dose suppression test. Dexamethasone (0.5 mg every 6 hours) is administered for 2 consecutive days after 2 days of baseline 24-hour urinary 17-hydroxysteroid and cortisol measurements. Patients with Cushing's will not lower their urine 17-hydroxysteroids below 4.0 mg/day and the cortisol below 20 μg (55 nmol) on the second day of dexamethasone suppression. Combining the low dose test with the 24-hour urinary free cortisol should definitely provide the diagnosis of Cushing's syndrome. A 24-hour urinary free cortisol greater than 250 μg (700 nmol) is virtually diagnostic of Cushing's syndrome, and a urinary free cortisol greater than 200 μg/day provides 90% diagnostic accuracy.

Pseudo-Cushing's states exist in patients with mild hypercortisolism due to conditions such as alcoholism, response to stress, anorexia and bulimia nervosa, severe obesity, and depression. Combining the low dose dexamethasone suppression test with CRH stimulation is an accurate method to distinguish the real syndrome from the hypercortisolism associated with these other conditions.[18] After two days of low dose dexamethasone suppression, a single plasma cortisol level is obtained 15 minutes after administering CRH (1 μg/kg) intravenously. A 15 minute cortisol level greater than 1.4 μg/dL (40 nmol/L) requires further evaluation.

The etiology of Cushing's syndrome can be established by combining a high dose dexamethasone suppression test with measurement of the basal state blood ACTH level. Dexamethasone (2 mg every 6 hours) is administered for 2 days, and the urinary 17-hydroxysteroid and cortisol levels on the second day are compared with basal levels. If basal ACTH is less than 5 pg/mL (1.0 pmol/L), and the urinary steroids do not decrease by at least 40%, an adrenal tumor is likely. When ACTII is measurable in the blood (above 20 pg/mL [4.5 pmol/L]), an ectopic ACTH-producing tumor is unlikely if the urinary steroids decrease by at least 40%. Cushing's disease is present when the blood ACTH level is in the normal range, a chest x-ray is normal, and imaging detects an abnormal sella turcica. A level of plasma ACTH greater than 50 pg/mL (10 pmol/L) suggests ectopic ACTH release; a level less than 5 pg/mL (1.0 pmol/L) suggests an autonomous cortisol-secreting tumor.

Imaging is very accurate and reliable in detecting adrenal tumors.[19] In addition, imaging reliably predicts which patients have ectopic ACTH-producing tumors by detecting bilateral adrenal enlargement in such patients.

The evaluation of a patient with Cushing's syndrome can yield inconclusive results, and a failure to recognize an occult, ectopic ACTH-secreting neoplasm can lead to unnecessary pituitary or adrenal surgery. Bilateral venous sampling from the inferior petrosal sinus (sampling the blood draining from the pituitary gland) for the measurement of ACTH before and after CRH stimulation is an effective means to achieve accurate diagnosis of a pituitary origin for the ACTH.[20,21] Approximately 15% of patients with ACTH-dependent Cushing's syndrome will have an occult, ectopic source for the ACTH. Most of these ACTH-secreting lesions are in the thorax, some in the abdomen.[22]

Petrosal sinus sampling is recommended in all patients with ACTH-dependent Cushing's syndrome who do not have an obvious adrenal tumor on imaging.[23]

A very rare cause of Cushing's syndrome is the autonomous production of cortisol by an ovarian tumor.[24] Chest and abdominal imaging is recommended for all atypical presentations.

Assessment of Insulin Secretion

Hyperandrogenism and hyperinsulinemia are commonly associated, as discussed in detail with complete references in Chapter 13. In many patients, a disorder in insulin action precedes the increase in androgens. Because of similarity between the receptors for insulin and insulin-like growth factor-I (IGF-I), hyperinsulinemia can augment thecal cell androgen production in the ovary. In addition, hyperinsulinemia contributes to the hyperandrogenism by inhibiting hepatic synthesis of sex hormone binding globulin and insulin-like growth factor binding protein-1, actions which increase free testosterone levels and augment IGF-I stimulation of thecal androgen synthesis, respectively.

The only effective treatment for the hyperinsulinemia is weight loss. In addition, hyperandrogenic and hyperinsulinemic women must be counseled regarding the risk of future diabetes mellitus and cardiovascular disease. The mechanism of hyper-androgenism can be attributed to hyperinsulinemia in an occasional case where the circumstances are hard to understand, for example, the onset of hirsutism in an elderly woman who is found to have hyperthecosis in the ovaries. For these reasons, we recommend that testing for hyperinsulinemia be considered in all patients with android obesity (see Chapters 13 and 19 for the waist:hip ratio diagnosis of obesity), as well as in individuals who remain anovulatory from their teenage years.

Unfortunately, testing for hyperinsulinemia is not straightforward. Clinical guidelines for the interpretation of insulin levels and insulin response to glucose loading have not been established. A ratio of fasting glucose to fasting insulin less than 3.0 can be utilized to identify those patients with significant hyperinsulinemia. However, because weight loss is currently the only effective treatment for hyperinsulinemia, this laboratory assessment adds little to clinical management. Future clinical studies may indicate the value of treating hyperinsulinemia medically (e.g., with metformin, an antihyper-glycemic agent used to treat noninsulin-dependent diabetes mellitus), and in that case laboratory diagnosis of hyperinsulinemia would be of greater value.

The DHAS Level

A random sample of DHAS is sufficient for the evaluation of hirsutism, needing no corrections for body weight, creatinine excretion, or episodic variation. Variations are minimized because of its high circulating concentration and its long half-life. A slow turnover rate results in a large and stable pool in the blood with insignificant variation. Elevated levels of DHAS contribute to the clinical problem of hirsutism because DHAS serves as a prehormone in hair follicles, providing substrate for the hair follicle synthesis of androgens.[25]

DHAS circulates in higher concentration than any other steroid and is derived almost exclusively from the adrenal gland. It is, therefore, a direct measure of adrenal androgen activity, correlating clinically with the urinary 17-ketosteroids.[26] The upper limit of normal in most laboratories is 350 µg/dL (9.5 µmol/L), but because of laboratory variation, attention must be paid to the local range of normal.

Aging is associated with a decrease in the blood concentration of DHAS. The decrease accelerates after menopause, and DHAS is almost undetectable after age 70.[27] This decline is 4 times greater than the age-related decline in cortisol, which is further support for the contention that cortisol and DHAS secretion are separately controlled.

Both 17-ketosteroids and circulating levels of DHAS are elevated in association with hyperprolactinemia.[28,29] The levels return to normal with prolactin suppression by dopamine agonist treatment. In addition, free testosterone levels associated with decreased SHBG are often found in hyperprolactinemic women.[30,31] This underscores the need to search for galactorrhea and to obtain a prolactin measurement in all anovulatory women. The androgen changes are probably secondary to the persistent anovulatory state induced by the elevated prolactin, although direct prolactin effects on the adrenal, ovary, or SHBG are possible.

When the DHAS level is normal, adrenal disease is most unlikely, and the diagnosis of excess androgen production by the ovaries is likely. There are only rare cases of adrenal tumors with normal DHAS levels, and further evaluation of such cases would be indicated by the presence of markedly elevated blood levels of testosterone.[32] These rare tumors are responsive to luteinizing hormone (LH), suggesting that they are derived from embryonic rest cells. Late-onset adrenal hyperplasia commonly is not associated with an increased level of DHAS; the diagnosis of this condition relies on the measurement of 17-OHP for screening.

The clinical problem with DHAS measurements in the evaluation of hirsutism is the frequent finding of a moderately elevated DHAS level in anovulatory patients with polycystic ovaries. This is similar to the moderate elevations of 17-ketosteroids encountered in these patients. If the 17-OHP level is normal, we believe that it is not worthwhile to subject these patients to a search for an adrenal enzyme defect. Clinical experience has established that moderate elevations of DHAS are associated with anovulation; suppression of ovarian function restores the DHAS level to normal.

 A DHAS level of 700 μg/dL (20 μmol/L) or greater has been accepted as a marker for abnormal adrenal function. But how often is a DHAS of this level encountered? ***DHAS levels of 700 μg/dL or more are confronted so rarely that we must now question the clinical usefulness of measuring DHAS. We cannot identify a single case in our experience in which the DHAS level changed patient management. We believe that adrenal secretion of extremely high levels of DHAS will be associated with high levels of testosterone, either by direct secretion or by peripheral conversion of the DHAS.*** Therefore, in the absence of Cushing's syndrome, we believe that measurement of testosterone will suffice to screen for adrenal abnormalities. An imaging assessment of the adrenal glands whenever an elevated testosterone is encountered will be more cost-effective than measuring DHAS in all hirsute women.

Late-Onset Adrenal Hyperplasia

Congenital adrenal hyperplasia is due to an enzyme defect leading to excessive androgen production. This severe condition, with its prenatal onset, is inherited in an autosomal recessive fashion (discussed in Chapter 10). A more mild form of the disease, appearing later in life, has been designated by a variety of adjectives, including late-onset, partial, nonclassical, attenuated, and acquired adrenal hyperplasia.[33] An asymptomatic form, cryptic adrenal hyperplasia, is revealed only with biochemical testing.

Although each of the enzymatic steps from cholesterol to cortisol can be expressed in specific clinical disease, the most common enzymes to be deficient are 21-hydroxylase (p450c21), 11β-hydroxylase (p450c11), and 3β-hydroxysteroid dehydrogenase.

The 21-Hydroxylase Defect

Women with late-onset adrenal hyperplasia due to a 21-hydroxylase deficiency respond to ACTH stimulation in a moderate fashion, between the classical homozygote response and the mild heterozygote reaction (see the 17-OHP nomogram). The severity of the clinical presentation is explained by a concept of allelic variants.[34] It is proposed that there are 3 alleles for 21-hydroxylase deficiency:

1. 21-hydroxylase deficiency[normal]

2. 21-hydroxylase deficiency[mild]

3. 21-hydroxylase deficiency[severe]

Classical disease results when an individual is homozygous for the severe allele. Late-onset, attenuated, acquired, nonclassical (including the cryptic form) refer to individuals who are either homozygous for the mild allele or carry one mild and one severe allele.

This condition is now recognized to be the most common autosomal recessive disorder, surpassing cystic fibrosis and sickle cell anemia.[35] The clinical presentation is extremely variable, and the symptoms may appear and disappear over time. Therefore the diagnosis requires laboratory evaluation as discussed under "The 17-OHP Level."

There are at least 3 reasons that make it worthwhile to seek the correct diagnosis:

1. Therapy should be accurately applied because it must be long-term.

2. Pregnant couples with this condition require genetic counseling for the prenatal diagnosis and possible treatment of the congenital form of the disease, as well as the assessment of asymptomatic offspring. However, without knowing the father's carrier status an accurate estimate of risk is impossible. Although the risk of having a child with congenital adrenal hyperplasia is very low, the couple should consider paternal testing for heterozygosity. If the father tests positively, prenatal diagnosis and treatment would be reasonable.

3. Theoretically, these patients might be subject to cortisol deficiency during severe stress; however, to our knowledge this has not been a clinical problem.

Other Enzyme Defects

The 3β-hydroxysteroid dehydrogenase deficiency exists in both the ovaries and adrenals. This defect precludes significant androgen production; however, this enzyme activity appears to remain intact in peripheral tissues. Therefore, hirsutism seen with this deficiency is probably due to target tissue conversion of the increased secretion of precursors.[36] Unlike 21-hydroxylase deficiency, no genetic markers are currently available; diagnosis requires ACTH stimulation and demonstration of an altered 17-hydroxypregnenolone to 17-OHP ratio. Some argue that late-onset 3β-hydroxysteroid dehydrogenase deficiency is encountered more frequently than 21-hydroxylase deficiency.[37] However, although an exaggerated 17-hydroxypregnenolone response to ACTH stimulation is common in women with hyperandrogenism, the response is consistent with adrenal hyperactivity and not an enzyme deficiency.[38] We believe that this deficiency is so subtle that accurate diagnosis is not essential. Our usual therapeutic approach to hirsutism will be effective. The 11β-hydroxylase deficiency is quite rare, and it is usually diagnosed at a younger age (Chapter 10). It is not worth measuring the 11-deoxycortisol response to ACTH stimulation in adult hirsute women in an effort to detect this rare deficiency.[39]

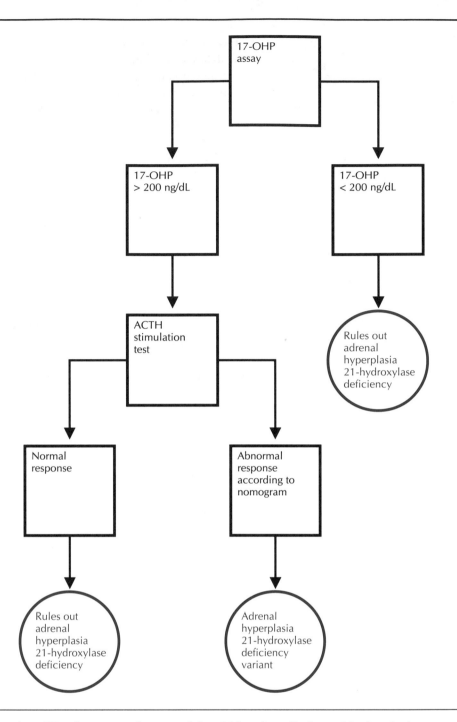

The 17-OHP Level

From 1 to 5% of women who complain of hirsutism display a biochemical response which is consistent with the less severe form of adrenal hyperplasia.[40–42] This relative frequency of late-onset adrenal hyperplasia dictates routine 17-OHP screening of women who complain of hirsutism. On the other hand, the routine use of the ACTH stimulation test is not warranted.[40,43]

Besides using the 17-OHP screen to make a cost-effective decision regarding ACTH stimulation, one can be swayed by pertinent clinical findings.[44] A strong family history of androgen excess suggests the presence of an inherited disorder. Hirsutism due to an adrenal enzyme defect usually is more severe and begins at a young age, typically at puberty. Short stature and very high blood levels of androgens also signify a more severe problem. Finally, it is worth considering the following: *With normal baseline steroid levels, even if a woman has a subtle enzyme defect, the management of the problem does not require its discovery.*

17-OHP must be measured first thing in the morning to avoid later elevations due to the diurnal pattern of ACTH secretion. The baseline 17-OHP level should be less than 200 ng/dL (6 nmol/L).[43] Levels greater than 200 ng/dL, but less than 800 ng/dL (24 nmol/L), require ACTH testing. Levels over 800 ng/dL are virtually diagnostic of the 21-hydroxylase deficiency. The DHAS level is usually normal. The hallmarks of late-onset adrenal hyperplasia are elevated levels of 17-OHP and a dramatic increase after ACTH stimulation.[41] However, the elevated baseline levels of 17-OHP are often not impressive (e.g., overlapping with those found in women with polycystic ovaries due to anovulation), and a simple ACTH stimulation test must be utilized.

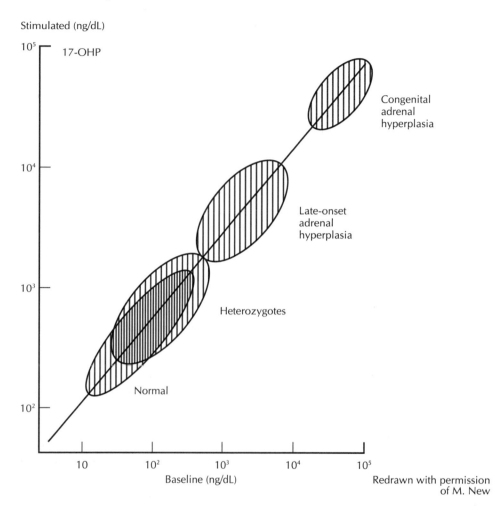

The ACTH Stimulation Test

Synthetic ACTH (Cortrosyn) is administered intravenously in a dose of 250 μg. Blood samples for the measurement of 17-OHP are obtained at time 0 and again at 1 hour. The testing must be performed in the morning (8 A.M.), but it can be scheduled at any time during the menstrual cycle. The 1 hour value is plotted on the nomogram which predicts the genotype of homozygote and heterozygote forms of the 21-hydroxylase deficiency.[45] Dexamethasone pretreatment the night before is not necessary.[46] Heterozygote carriers for 21-hydroxylase deficiency have ACTH-stimulated levels of 17-OHP up to 1,000 ng/dL (30 nmol/L); patients with late-onset deficiency have stimulated levels above 1,200 ng/dL (36 nmol/L).

For the diagnosis of the 3β-hydroxysteroid dehydrogenase deficiency, the same ACTH stimulation test is utilized, measuring 17-OHP and 17-hydroxypregnenolone. An abnormal 17-hydroxypregnenolone/17-OHP ratio is usually greater than 6.0.[36] This deficiency is also usually marked by a significant elevation of DHAS in the face of normal or mildly elevated testosterone levels. In the 11β-hydroxylase deficiency, the level of 11-deoxycortisol will be increased; it is normal with the 21-hydroxylase defect.

The Adrenal Gland and Anovulation

Adrenal involvement in the syndrome of anovulation and hirsutism has long been recognized. Adrenal suppression, for example, will induce regular menses and ovulation in some patients, and empiric treatment with glucocorticoids has been advocated in the past.

Late-onset adrenal hyperplasia does not explain every anovulatory woman encountered with a moderate elevation in DHAS. The important clinical question is the following: is excessive androgen secretion by the adrenal gland a primary disorder in these women, or is it a secondary reaction to the hormonal milieu associated with anovulation?

One possibility is that the adrenal hyperactivity (as indicated by elevated DHAS levels) is due to an estrogen-induced 3β-hydroxysteroid dehydrogenase insufficiency. Considerable effort has been devoted to demonstrating an estrogen influence on adrenal androgen secretion. Unfortunately there is no clear-cut conclusion, with both positive[47–51] and negative[52–56] results reported.

This picture is similar to that of the fetal adrenal gland. Studies have demonstrated that the low level of 3β-hydroxysteroid dehydrogenase activity and high secretion of DHAS by the fetal adrenal cortex are due to estrogen.[57] Inconsistent with this explanation is the fact that ACTH levels in adult anovulatory women are not elevated.[58] The activity of 3β-hydroxysteroid dehydrogenase is inhibited by both androgens and estrogens in concentrations to be expected within the adrenal gland but difficult to achieve with exogenous administration; changes in adrenal secretion, therefore, can reflect varying action of steroids, especially estrogen, in different layers of the adrenal cortex without changes in ACTH.[59] The failure to affect adrenal steroidogenesis with the exogenous administration of androgens is consistent with this hypothesis.[60] Thus, it remains attractive to explain adrenal hyperactivity seen in anovulatory women as a secondary reaction induced and maintained by the constant estrogen state associated with persistent anovulation. This action, however, may be the result of mechanisms other than inhibition of 3β-hydroxysteroid dehydrogenase (see discussion of the fetal adrenal gland in Chapter 8).

Suppression of ovarian function by treatment with a GnRH agonist has been utilized in hopes of bringing clarity to this puzzle by assessing adrenal function after elimination of ovarian steroid production. Short-term suppression (3–6 months) has been reported to have no impact on adrenal androgen production.[61,62] However, these studies did not include women with high levels of DHAS. When anovulatory women with levels of DHAS greater than normal are treated with a GnRH agonist for at least 3 months, the elevated DHAS levels are suppressed, supporting the contention that an adrenal change is secondary to the ovarian hormonal steady state.[63]

Regardless of differences in weight, diet, race, and environmental factors, excess adrenal androgen activity is present in one-half to two-thirds of anovulatory women and hyperinsulinemia in approximately 70%.[64] It makes sense that similar growth factor modulation takes place in adrenal steroid-producing cells as in the ovary. Women with polycystic ovaries (both obese and nonobese) and hyperinsulinemia have a greater steroidogenic response to ACTH than anovulatory patients with normal insulin levels.[65]

Insulin and IGF-I receptors are present on adrenal cells. The infusion of insulin into women causes a decrease in DHAS, and hyperinsulinemia inhibits adrenal 17,20 lyase (p450c17) activity, suggesting that insulin decreases the production of this adrenal androgen.[66,67] It is further suggested that the age-related decline in DHAS may be related to increasing insulin resistance.[68] How do these changes relate to DHAS levels in anovulatory women, levels that range from normal to moderately elevated? A simple inverse relationship between insulin and adrenal androgen levels in anovulatory women does not exist.[69]

An ovulatory response following the treatment of anovulatory women with dexamethasone can be explained in part by a contribution made to ovarian androgen production by circulating DHAS. A significant percentage of testosterone production by the ovarian follicle can be attributed to circulating DHAS serving as a substrate or prehormone.[70] Thus, dexamethasone suppression cannot separate adrenal and ovarian testosterone secretion in that the two glands are involved in a complex interaction, with DHAS providing at least one mechanism for this interaction.

The inconclusiveness of this situation and the rarity of a true adrenal enzyme deficiency in adult women make a cost-effective argument against routine endocrine testing. Accordingly, we have adopted a blood DHAS level of 700 µg/dL (20 µmol/L) and a 17-OHP level of 200 ng/dL (6 nmol/L), below which we do not pursue the possibility of a primary adrenal enzyme problem, and we now find little use for DHAS measurements. Mild adrenal enzyme defects can be treated by our usual methods and do not require glucocorticoid administration.

The Testosterone Level

Plasma testosterone levels (normal 20–80 ng/dL [0.7–3.0 nmol/L]) are elevated in the majority of women (70%) with anovulation and hirsutism. Individual variation is great, however, largely because of the changes in the testosterone binding capacity of the sex hormone binding globulin in the blood. Because the binding globulin levels are depressed by androgen and insulin, the total testosterone concentration can be in the normal range in a woman who is hirsute even though the percent unbound and active testosterone is elevated. Indeed, the unbound or free testosterone is approximately twice normal (an increase from 1% to 2%) in women with anovulation and polycystic ovaries.[71] Therefore a normal total testosterone level in hirsute women is still consistent with elevated androgen production rates.

It is not necessary to measure the free testosterone (a technically difficult and expensive assay) because a routine total testosterone assay adequately serves the purpose of screening for testosterone-secreting tumors. Such tumors are associated with testosterone levels that are usually in the male range, and therefore the fine discrimination of the free testosterone level is unnecessary.[72,73] *If the testosterone level exceeds 200 ng/dL (7 nmol/L), an androgen-producing tumor must be suspected.*

The arbitrary cut off point has been challenged because variations in secretion can yield misleading values, and not all androgen-producing tumors will be this active, and some women with polycystic ovaries (especially hyperthecosis) will have testosterone levels greater than 200 ng/dL.[74,75] Nevertheless, the combination of the patient's historical chronology of the development of hirsutism, the pelvic examination, and the 200 ng/dL (7 nmol/L) testosterone level will provide accurate diagnosis in virtually all cases. *A patient with an acute, rapid course of virilizing symptoms requires a full evaluation for the presence of an androgen-producing tumor even if the testosterone and DHAS concentrations are less than the cut off levels.*

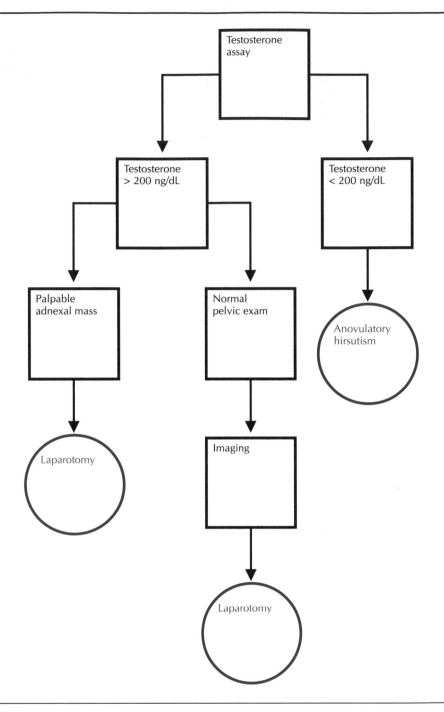

Androgen-Producing Tumors

There are two findings that should stimulate the clinician to suspect the presence of an androgen-producing tumor. One is a history of rapidly progressive masculinization. Hirsutism associated with anovulation is generally slow to develop, usually covering a time period of at least several years. Tumors are associated with a short time course, measured in months. The second finding that should arouse suspicion is a testosterone level greater than 200 ng/dL (7 nmol/L).

In our view, androgen-producing tumors are one of medicine's vastly overrated problems. First, they are incredibly rare, yet they attract an inordinate amount of attention at our meetings and a disproportionate number of printed pages in texts and journals. Second, there is an endocrine mystique surrounding the functioning tumor. Actually it is a straightforward problem.

Functioning ovarian tumors are almost all palpable, and like any ovarian mass, rapid laparotomy and surgical removal are in order. It is well recognized, however, that very small ovarian tumors (usually in the hilus of the ovary) can secrete testosterone. Occasionally, virilization is encountered with a nonfunctional tumor due to tumor stimulation of androgen secretion in the surrounding stromal tissue.[76]

The only diagnostic dilemma is when to explore the patient in whom a mass is not palpable. Suppression and stimulation tests are known to falsely lead to oophorectomy in the presence of a virilizing adrenal adenoma.[73] In addition, suppression and stimulation methods do not specifically isolate ovarian or adrenal function.[77,78] Ovarian androgen-producing tumors are usually responsive to LH and, therefore, will respond to ovarian suppression and stimulation.[79,80]

Selective angiography with venous sampling and measurement of adrenal and ovarian steroids is not without problems. It is technically difficult to achieve bilateral catheterization of the ovaries, steroid secretion is episodic (especially by the adrenal glands), and the technique is not without risk. Selective retrograde catheterization of ovarian and adrenal veins by an expert should be reserved for those few patients who have been imaged with negative findings. Surgical exploration and bivalving of the ovaries may be necessary if the catheterization studies are negative.

In postmenopausal women with hyperandrogenism, it is usually appropriate to be more aggressive surgically; however, keep in mind that hyperinsulinemia in the postmenopausal years can stimulate hyperthecosis which would simulate the presentation of a tumor.[81] GnRH agonist treatment can avoid surgery in these patients because insulin-induced steroidogenic activity in the ovary is still LH-dependent.

When an androgen-producing tumor is suspected and an adnexal mass is not palpable, imaging of the adrenal glands and ovaries should be obtained. Imaging of the adrenal is a sensitive diagnostic technique for small tumors which produce Cushing's syndrome as well as for virilizing adrenal adenomas.[19,73]

The Incidental Adrenal Mass

Adrenal masses will be discovered incidentally in approximately 2% of patients undergoing abdominal imaging.[82] Bilateral lesions are more serious. Common causes of bilateral lesions are metastatic cancer, infection (tuberculous and fungal), and adrenal hyperplasia; hence, surgery is rarely indicated. A primary malignancy of the adrenal is usually associated with excess secretion of glucocorticoids and androgens. The size of a lesion is significant.[83,84] The probability of malignancy roughly parallels the diameter of the lesion; a 2 cm lesion has a 20% chance of being malignant, an 8 cm lesion has an 80% probability. Bilateral lesions less than 3 cm usually are due to metastatic disease. Thus, the current recommendation is to excise unilateral masses if they are greater than 3 cm in diameter. Fine needle aspiration is also recommended for all unilateral adrenal lesions.[83] When following a mass, imaging should be performed at 3, 9, and 18 months. Any mass which is stable after 18 months can be left in place.

Incidental adrenal masses require evaluation for biochemical function. The presence of hypertension raises the suspicion of Cushing's syndrome, hyperaldosteronism, or pheochromocytoma. The evaluation should include a screening test for pheochromocytoma (plasma catecholamines after clonidine), electrolyte and renin activity assessment for aldosteronism, a 24-hour urinary free cortisol, and a testosterone level. A relatively high incidence of cortisol-secreting tumors in the presence of normal 24-hour urinary free cortisol excretion indicates the need to perform an overnight dexamethasone suppression test in patients with asymptomatic incidental adrenal masses.[85] There appears to be a high incidence of adrenal masses in patients with adrenal hyperplasia. These need not be removed surgically, but a laboratory evaluation for adrenal hyperplasia is, therefore, indicated in patients with incidental adrenal masses.[86]

Treatment of Hirsutism

Almost all patients presenting with hirsutism represent excess androgen production in association with the steady state of persistent anovulation. Treatment is directed toward interruption of the steady state. In those patients who wish to become pregnant, ovulation can be induced as discussed in Chapter 30. In patients in whom pregnancy is not desired, the steady state can be interrupted by suppression of ovarian steroidogenesis by utilizing the potent inhibitory action of progestational agents on LH.

Androgen production in hirsute women is usually an LH-dependent process. Suppression of ovarian steroidogenesis depends upon adequate LH suppression. In addition to the inhibitory action of the progestational component, oral contraceptives provide a further benefit because of the increase in SHBG levels induced by the estrogen component. The increase in SHBG results in a greater androgen binding capacity with a decrease in free testosterone levels. The progestins in oral contraceptives also inhibit 5α-reductase activity in skin, further contributing to the clinical impact of oral contraceptives on hirsutism.[87]

The low dose oral contraceptives are effective in treating acne and hirsutism. Suppression of free testosterone levels is comparable to that achieved with higher dosage.[88,89] Multiphasic formulations appear to be equally effective. The beneficial clinical effect is the same with low dose preparations containing levonorgestrel, previously recognized to cause acne at high dosage. Formulations with desogestrel, gestodene, and norgestimate are associated with greater increases in sex hormone binding globulin and decreases in free testosterone levels. Theoretically these products would be more effective in the treatment of acne and hirsutism; however, this is yet to be documented by clinical studies.

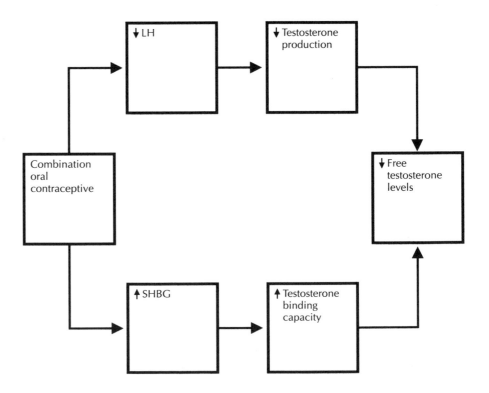

In the patient in whom oral contraceptives are contraindicated or unwanted, good results can be achieved with the use of medroxyprogesterone acetate, either 150 mg intramuscularly every 3 months or 30 mg orally per day. The mechanism of action of medroxyprogesterone acetate is slightly different from that of the combination oral contraceptive. Suppression of gonadotropins is less intense, hence ovarian follicular activity continues. LH suppression is significant, however, and testosterone production is decreased, although to a lesser degree than with combined oral contraceptives. In addition, testosterone clearance from the circulation is increased.[90] This latter effect is due to an induction of liver enzyme activity. Medroxyprogesterone acetate also decreases SHBG so that less testosterone is bound; however, suppression of total testosterone production is so great that the actual amount of free testosterone decreases.[91] The overall effect yields a clinical result comparable to that achieved with the combination oral contraceptive.

A noteworthy feature of hirsutism is the slow response to treatment. Because of the hair growth cycle, change takes time. The patient should be cautioned that treatment with hormonal suppression will be necessary for at least 6 months before an observable diminution in hair growth occurs. Combined treatment with electrolysis is not recommended, therefore, until hormonal suppression has been used at least 6 months.

New hair follicles will no longer be stimulated to grow but hair growth which has been previously established will not disappear with hormone treatment alone. This can be affected temporarily by shaving, tweezing, waxing, or the use of depilatories.[92] None of these tactics alters the inherent growth of the hair; therefore, they must be reapplied at frequent intervals. Permanent removal of hair can be accomplished only by electrocoagulation of dermal papillae.

Some patients return after a period of treatment expressing disappointment because hair is still present. The effect of the treatment (prevention of new hair growth) may not be apparent unless the previously established hair is removed. The combination of ovarian suppression preventing new hair growth, and electrolysis removing the old hair, yields the most complete and effective treatment of hirsutism.

How long should treatment be continued? After 1–2 years it is worthwhile to stop the medication and observe the patient for a return of ovulatory cycles. Even in those patients who continue to be anovulatory, testosterone suppression continues for 6 months to 2 years after discontinuing treatment. Of course, if anovulation is still present, one can expect the eventual return of hirsutism.

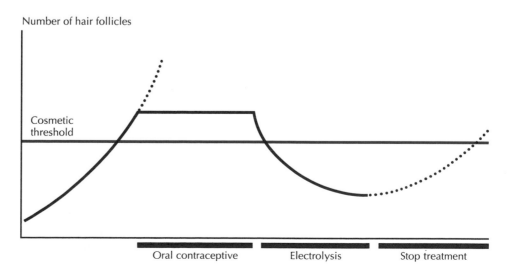

The really resistant patient deserves further consideration. Combination therapy with one of the alternative approaches discussed below is worthwhile.

In most patients, DHAS levels are suppressed by progestational treatment.[93,94] The mechanism is not definitely known, but there are several possible explanations. If the original stimulus for the increased DHAS secretion is the steady estrogen state of anovulation, then the change in the endocrine milieu of the adrenal gland brought about by the suppression of ovarian steroidogenesis will restore a normal adrenal secretory pattern. Oral contraceptives may also produce subtle but significant alterations in ACTH secretion or response in the adrenal gland.

The effectiveness of adrenal suppression in inducing ovulatory cycles in some anovulatory patients can be attributed to a lowering of circulating androgen levels due to a decrease in the adrenal contribution as well as a reduction in the amount of DHAS available for conversion to testosterone within the ovarian follicle. The intraovarian androgen level is decreased, therefore lowering the inhibitory action of androgens on follicular growth and development. In terms of ovulation, the frequency of successful response with this type of treatment does not match that of the first drug of choice, clomiphene. In terms of treatment of hirsutism, progestin suppression of ovarian steroidogenesis is more effective and should remain the first therapeutic approach. Adrenal suppression should be reserved for patients with a clearly established diagnosis of an adrenal enzyme deficiency.

In an older woman who has no further desire for fertility, and in the woman for whom continued use of steroid medication is disturbing because of increasing risks with increasing age, serious consideration should be given to a surgical solution. A persistent problem of hirsutism, especially if it is progressive in severity, is a reasonable indication for hysterectomy and bilateral salpingo-oophorectomy. Patients with hyperthecosis respond poorly to suppression and are usually older. Surgical treatment for these patients is often very appropriate. Of course, a hormonal program is recommended for these patients postoperatively.

Keep in mind the strong association between hyperandrogenism and hyperinsulinemia as discussed in Chapter 13. Treating the problem of hirsutism by suppression of androgen production and action will not restore glucose metabolism to normal; these patients will continue to demonstrate insulin resistance. In overweight, hyperandrogenic patients, a weight control program is essential to reduce the risks of diabetes mellitus and cardiovascular disease.

Alternative Approaches

Spironolactone

Spironolactone is an aldosterone-antagonist diuretic. In the treatment of hirsutism, spironolactone has multiple actions, inhibiting the ovarian and adrenal biosynthesis of androgens, competing for the androgen receptor in the hair follicle, and directly inhibiting 5α-reductase activity. The inhibition of steroidogenesis is achieved through an effect on the cytochrome p450 system, but the steroid suppressive effects are so variable that the receptor-blocking action is the most important mechanism.[95] It is probably for this reason that cortisol, DHA, and DHAS levels are not significantly changed with spironolactone treatment, even though androstenedione levels are decreased.[96]

The impact of spironolactone treatment on hirsutism is related to dosage, and a better effect is seen with a dose of 200 mg daily.[97–99] After a period of time, one can attempt lowering spironolactone to a maintenance dose of 25–50 mg daily. As with progestational agents, the response is relatively slow, and a maximal effect can be demonstrated

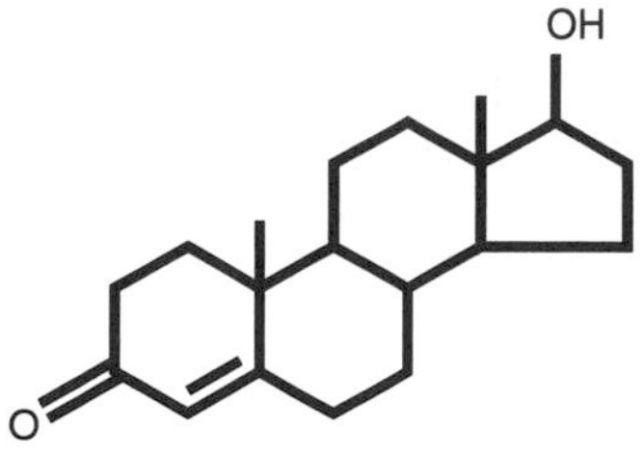

Testosterone

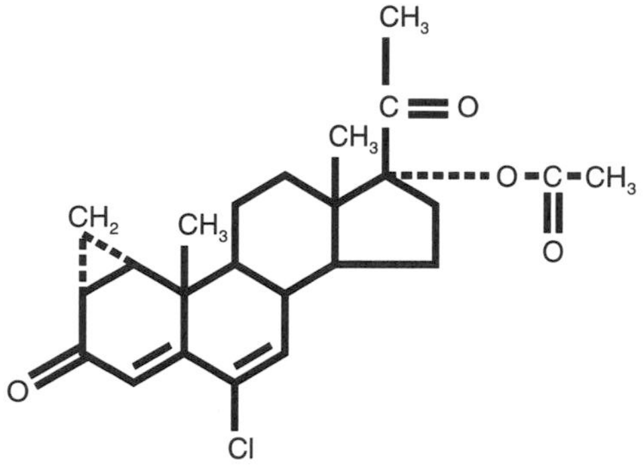

Cyproterone acetate

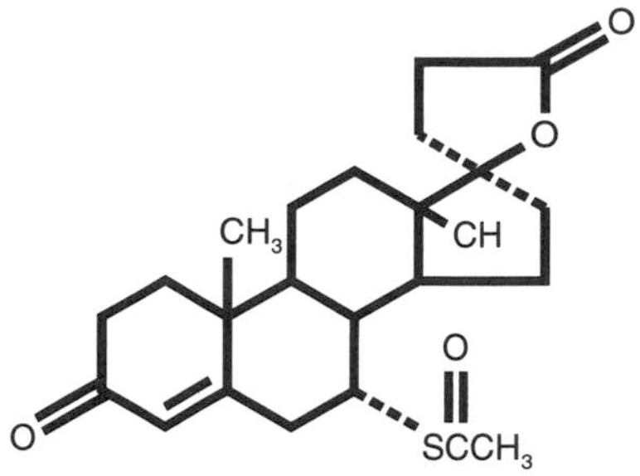

Spironolactone

only after 6 months of treatment. Side effects are minimal, including diuresis in the first few days of use, occasional complaints of fatigue, and dysfunctional uterine bleeding. Remember that the anovulatory state requires progestational management in order to avoid abnormal uterine bleeding (and endometrial hyperplasia).

We use spironolactone when patients find oral contraceptives unacceptable or the response is disappointing. Indeed, it makes sense to combine the peripheral tissue action of spironolactone with oral contraceptives to achieve a more dramatic result.[100] Acne has been effectively treated with the local application of a cream containing 2–5% spironolactone.[101] Systemic absorption does not occur, and there are no side effects.

One word of caution: with inhibition of androgen secretion, ovulation can occur. In view of the unknown impact of spironolactone on a fetus, effective contraception is important. Theoretically, spironolactone interference with testosterone action could result in the feminization of a male fetus. Combined treatment with an oral contraceptive may produce a better clinical effect and, at the same time, prevent menstrual irregularity and provide contraception.

Cyproterone Acetate

Cyproterone is a potent progestational agent that both inhibits gonadotropin secretion and blocks androgen action by binding to the androgen receptor. In many parts of the world, it has been used in an oral contraceptive agent called "Diane" (2 mg cyproterone acetate and 50 µg ethinyl estradiol). "Dianette" contains 2 mg cyproterone acetate and 35 µg ethinyl estradiol. In a method for the treatment of hirsutism called the reversed sequential regimen, cyproterone acetate is given in a dose of 100 mg daily on days 5–14, with 30 or 50 µg of ethinyl estradiol daily on days 5–25.[102] In a comparison of Diane with the high dose (100 mg) cyproterone acetate treatment, the therapeutic effect was greater (but probably not of clinical significance) with the higher dose, and there was a similar incidence of side effects at both doses.[103] In a comparison of Dianette with higher doses of cyproterone acetate (20 and 100 mg), the clinical response with the 2 mg dose of cyproterone was equal to that of the higher doses.[104] The most common reactions include fatigue, edema, loss of libido, weight gain, and mastalgia. Significant improvement in facial hirsutism is seen by the 3rd month of treatment. A high relapse note has been noted unless the 100 mg dose is maintained.[105] The effect of this potent progestational agent on carbohydrate metabolism and the lipoprotein profile is similar to the adverse impact of the older high dose oral contraceptives. In comparisons of spironolactone and cyproterone acetate, a monophasic low dose oral contraceptive combined with spironolactone 100 mg daily was as effective as cyproterone acetate, and spironolactone 100 mg daily combined with a multiphasic low dose oral contraceptive was as effective as the reversed sequential regimen of cyproterone and estrogen.[106,107]

Dexamethasone

Dexamethasone suppression of endogenous ACTH secretion is used in women who have an adrenal enzyme deficiency. Dexamethasone is given nightly (to achieve maximal suppression of the central nervous system (CNS)-adrenal axis which peaks during sleep) in a dose of 0.5 mg. An equivalent dose of prednisone is 5–7.5 mg. If this treatment suppresses the morning plasma cortisol level below 2.0 μg/dL (60 nmol/L), the dose should be reduced to avoid an inability to react to stress. Fortunately, adrenal androgen secretion is more sensitive to suppression by dexamethasone than is cortisol secretion.[108] Patients with adrenal hyperplasia may require higher doses to normalize the steroid blood levels. With higher doses, alternate day therapy can still accomplish significant adrenal androgen suppression without affecting cortisol secretion.[109] It should be emphasized that moderate elevations of DHAS do not indicate patients who will benefit from dexamethasone treatment.[110]

Treatment with GnRH Agonists

Because ovarian androgen production is LH-dependent, suppression of the pituitary with chronic GnRH agonist treatment improves hirsutism. However, inconsistent results in the literature attest to the fact that sufficient dosage must be administered to achieve effective suppression and clinical response. Therefore, monitoring dosage and response is recommended. A greater dose of GnRH agonist is required to suppress ovarian androgen secretion compared to estradiol secretion.[111] Therefore we recommend monitoring treatment with testosterone levels. Leuprolide in a dose of 3.75 mg monthly is effective. To avoid the problems associated with estrogen deficiency, estrogen-progestin add back should be initiated after the maintenance dose of a long-acting GnRH agonist has been established. We recommend the daily administration of 0.625 mg conjugated estrogens or 1.0 mg estradiol combined with 2.5 mg medroxyprogesterone acetate or 0.35 mg norethindrone, or, even better, an oral contraceptive. This method of treatment is relatively complicated and expensive and should be reserved for the severe case of ovarian hyperandrogenism which is usually due to significant hyperthecosis and marked hyperinsulinemia (a condition that responds poorly to the usual methods of treatment).

Flutamide

Flutamide is a nonsteroidal antiandrogen that can be administered in a dose of 250 mg tid.[112] Flutamide directly inhibits hair growth without significant side effects. Comparison studies with other treatments for hirsutism are not available. Treatment with flutamide should be combined with a method of contraception.

Other Agents

Cimetidine (300 mg qid) has been used to treat hirsutism, but it is the least potent of the androgen receptor blockers, and the clinical response is disappointing.[113] The use of a skin cream containing progesterone is effective, but it must be applied frequently (because of rapid metabolic clearance) and its action is very concentrated at the point of application.[114] Minoxidil has unknown direct stimulatory actions on hair follicles; it has not been studied in women with alopecia. Ketoconazole in a dose of 400 mg daily blocks androgen synthesis by inhibiting the cytochrome P450 system. While the impact on hirsutism is significant, there is a high incidence of side effects as well as changes in liver enzymes.[115] Ketoconazole, at best, should be a last resort, requiring frequent monitoring of liver function.

End Organ Hypersensitivity (Idiopathic Hirsutism)

There are some patients who present with hirsutism, but ovulate regularly. This category of patients has in the past been labeled idiopathic or familial hirsutism and is more pronounced in certain geographic areas and among certain ethnic groups. The only satisfactory explanation for this distressing problem is hypersensitivity of the skin's hair apparatus to normal levels of androgens, probably due to increased 5α-reductase activity.[116] Because of this excessive sensitivity, normal levels of androgen stimulate hair growth. Even in these cases, hirsutism responds to ovarian suppression with a combination oral contraceptive. Suppression of normal female androgen levels to subnormal concentrations diminishes the stimulus to the hair follicles, yielding the same stabilizing results seen in other hirsute women. Spironolactone is also effective for this group of patients. Clinical response to pharmacologic treatment correlates with the circulating levels of 3α-AG, supporting the diagnosis of a target tissue (hair follicle) locus for this problem.[117] While hirsutism due to an endocrine disorder requires control, end organ hypersensitivity is treated only for the purpose of cosmetic improvement. Electrolysis is a useful adjunct in this group of patients.

Limitations and Pitfalls

We have outlined a simple, straightforward approach for the evaluation of the hirsute woman; however, as in all of medicine, exceptions occur.

1. Occasionally testosterone levels may be extremely elevated with anovulation, leading to very heavy hair growth and even masculinization. A testosterone level over 200 ng/dL (7 nmol/L) does not absolutely indicate the presence of a tumor.

2. Enlarged ovaries are not necessary for the clinical syndrome of anovulation and excessive androgen production. On the other hand, the presence of enlarged, polycystic ovaries does not assure the diagnosis of anovulation and excess ovarian production of androgen. They can be associated with adrenal disease or exogenous androgen ingestion.

3. Laparoscopy and ovarian biopsy are not indicated procedures in the evaluation of hirsutism.

4. The association of elevated testosterone production and hirsutism with normal ovulatory cycles should make the clinician suspicious of an adrenal problem.

5. Suppression of elevated androgens by progestin treatment does not rule out the presence of an ovarian tumor. Functional ovarian tumors are usually gonadotropin-dependent and responsive.

6. Failure of progestin treatment to suppress hair growth and testosterone levels after 6–12 months raises the suspicion of adrenal disease or a very small ovarian tumor.

7. Androgen levels in postmenopausal women are lower. A testosterone level greater than 100 ng/dL (4 nmol/L) and a DHAS level greater than 400 μg/dL (11 μmol/L) are suspicious for a tumor.

References

1. **Montagna W, Ellis RA,** editors, *The Biology of Hair Growth,* Academic Press, New York, 1958.

2. **Lookingbill DP, Demers LM, Wang C, Leung A, Rittmaster RS, Santen RJ,** Clinical and biochemical parameters of androgen action in normal and healthy caucasian *versus* Chinese subjects, J Clin Endocrinol Metab 72:1242, 1991.

3. **Horton R,** Dihydrotestosterone is a peripheral paracrine hormone, J Androl 13:23, 1992.

4. **Chang RJ,** Ovarian steroid secretion in polycystic ovarian disease, Seminars Reprod Endocrinol 2:244, 1984.

5. **Serafini P, Lobo R,** Increased 5α-reductase activity in idiopathic hirsutism, Fertil Steril 43:74, 1985.

6. **Serafini P, Ablan F, Lobo RA,** 5α-Reductase activity in the genital skin of hirsute women, J Clin Endocrinol Metab 60:349, 1985.

7. **Greep N, Hoopes M, Horton R,** Androstanediol glucuronide plasma clearance and production rates in normal and hirsute women, J Clin Endocrinol Metab 62:22, 1986.

8. **Rittmaster RS,** Androgen conjugates: physiology and clinical significance, Endocrin Rev 14:121, 1993.

9. **Bardin CW, Lipsett M,** Testosterone and androstenedione blood production rates in normal women and women with idiopathic hirsutism and polycystic ovaries, J Clin Invest 46:891, 1967.

10. **Futterweit W, Dunaif A, Yeh HC, Kingsley P,** The prevalence of hyperandrogenism in 109 consecutive female patients with diffuse alopecia, J Am Acad Dermatol 19:831, 1988.

11. **Reid RL, Van Vugt DA,** Hair loss in the female, Obstet Gynecol Survey 43:135, 1988.

12. **Carmina E, Lobo RA,** Evidence for increased androsterone metabolism in some normo-androgenic women with acne, J Clin Endocrinol Metab 76:1111, 1993.

13. **Grassinger CC, Wild RA, Parker IJ,** Vulvar acanthosis nigricans: a marker for insulin resistance in hirsute women, Fertil Steril 59:583, 1993.

14. **Garcia-Bunuel R, Berek JS, Woodruff JD,** Luteomas of pregnancy, Obstet Gynecol 45:407, 1975.

15. **VanSlooten AJ, Rechner SF, Dodds WG,** Recurrent maternal virilization during pregnancy caused by benign androgen-producing ovarian lesions, Am J Obstet Gynecol 167:1342, 1992.

16. **McClamrock HD, Adashi EY,** Gestational hyperandrogenism, Fertil Steril 57:257, 1992.

17. **Meikle AW,** A diagnostic approach to Cushing's syndrome, Endocrinologist 3:311, 1993.

18. **Yanovski JA, Cutler GB Jr, Chrousos GP, Nieman LK,** Corticotropin-releasing hormone stimulation following low-dose dexamethasone administration, JAMA 269:2232, 1993.

19. **White FE, White MC, Drury PL, Fry IK, Besser GM,** Value of computed tomography of the abdomen and chest in investigation of Cushing's syndrome, Br Med J 284:771, 1982.

20. **Findling JW, Kehoe ME, Shaker JL, Raff H,** Routine inferior petrosal sinus sampling in the differential diagnosis of adrenocorticotropin (ACTH)-dependent Cushing's syndrome: early recognition of the occult ectopic ACTH syndrome, J Clin Endocrinol Metab 73:408, 1991.

21. **Oldfield EH, Doppman JL, Nieman LK, Chrousos GP, Miller DL, Katz DA, Cutler GB Jr, Loriaux DL,** Petrosal sinus sampling with and without corticotropin-releasing hormone for the differential diagnosis of Cushing's syndrome, New Engl J Med 325:897, 1991.

22. **Findling JW, Tyrrell JB,** Occult ectopic secretion of corticotropin, Arch Intern Med 146:929, 1986.

23. **Yanovski JA, Cutler GB Jr, Doppman JL, Miller DL, Chrousos GP, Oldfield EH, Nieman LK,** The limited ability of inferior petrosal sinus sampling with corticotropin-releasing hormone to distinguish Cushing's disease from pseudo-Cushing states or normal physiology, J Clin Endocrinol Metab 77:503, 1993.

24. **Chetkowski RJ, Judd HL, Jagger PI, Nieberg RK, Chang RJ,** Autonomous cortisol secretion by a lipoid cell tumor of the ovary, JAMA 254:2628, 1985.

25. **Haning RV Jr, Flood CA, Hackett RJ, Loughlin JS, McClure N, Longcope C,** Metabolic clearance rate of dehydroepiandrosterone sulfate, its metabolism to testosterone, and its intrafollicular metabolism to dehydroepiandrosterone, androstenedione, testosterone, and dihydrotestosterone *in vivo,* J Clin Endocrinol Metab 72:1088, 1991.

26. **Lobo RA, Paul WL, Goebelsmann U,** Dehydroepiandrosterone sulfate as an indicator of adrenal androgen function, Obstet Gynecol 57:69, 1981.

27. **Cumming DC, Rebar RW, Hopper BR, Yen SSC,** Evidence for an influence of the ovary on circulating dehydroepiandrosterone sulfate levels, J Clin Endocrinol Metab 54:1069, 1982.

28. **Lobo RA, Kletsky OA, Kaptein EM, Goebelsmann U,** Prolactin modulation of dehydro-epiandrosterone sulfate secretion, Am J Obstet Gynecol 138:632, 1980.

29. **Schiebinger RJ, Chrousos GP, Cutler GB Jr, Loriaux DL,** The effect of serum prolactin on plasma adrenal androgens and the production and metabolic clearance rate of dehydro-epiandrosterone sulfate in normal and hyperprolactinemic subjects, J Clin Endocrinol Metab 62:202, 1986.

30. **Vermeulen A, Ando S, Verdonck L,** Prolactinomas, testosterone-binding globulin and androgen metabolism, J Clin Endocrinol Metab 54:409, 1982.

31. **Glickman SP, Rosenfield RL, Bergenstal RM, Helke J,** Multiple androgenic abnormalities, including elevated free testosterone, in hyperprolactinemic women, J Clin Endocrinol Metab 55:251, 1982.

32. **Kamilaris TC, DeBold CR, Manolas KJ, Hoursanidis A, Panageas S, Yiannatos J,** Testosterone-secreting adrenal adenoma in a peripubertal girl, JAMA 258:2558, 1987.

33. **White PC, New MI, Dupont B,** Congenital adrenal hyperplasia, New Engl J Med 316:1519, 1580, 1987.

34. **Kohn B, Levine LS, Pollack MS, Pang S, Lorenzen F, Levy DJ, Lerner AJ, Gian FR, Dupont B, New MI,** Late-onset steroid 21-hydroxylase deficiency: a variant of classical congenital adrenal hyperplasia, J Clin Endocrinol Metab 55:817, 1982.

35. **Speiser PW, Dupont B, Rubenstein P, Piazza A, Kastelan A, New MI,** High frequency of non-classical steroid 21-hydroxylase deficiency, Am J Hum Genet 37:650, 1985.

36. **Pang S, Lerner AJ, Stoner E, Levine LS, Oberfield SE, Engel I, New MI,** Late-onset adrenal steroid 3β-hydroxysteroid dehydrogenase deficiency. I. A cause of hirsutism in pubertal and postpubertal women, J Clin Endocrinol Metab 60:428, 1985.

37. **Schram P, Zerah M, Mani P, Jewelewicz R, Jaffe S, New MI,** Nonclassical 3β-hydroxysteroid dehydrogenase deficiency: a review of our experience with 25 female patients, Fertil Steril 58:129, 1992.

38. **Azziz R, Bradley EL Jr, Potter HD, Boots LR,** 3β-Hydroxysteroid dehydrogenase deficiency in hyperandrogenism, Am J Obstet Gynecol 168:889, 1993.

39. **Azziz R, Boots LR, Parker CR Jr, Bradley E, Zacur HA,** 11β-Hydroxylase deficiency in hyperandrogenism, Fertil Steril 55:733, 1991.

40. **Cobin RH, Futterweit W, Fiedler RP, Thornton JC,** Adrenocorticotropic hormone testing in idiopathic hirsutism and polycystic ovarian disease: a test of limited usefulness, Fertil Steril 44:224, 1985.

41. **Kuttenn F, Couillin P, Girard F, Billaud L, Vincens M, Boucekkine C, Thalabarad J-C, Maudelonde T, Spritzer P, Mowszowicz I, Boue A, Mauvais-Jarvis P,** Late-onset adrenal hyperplasia in hirsutism, New Engl J Med 313:224, 1985.

42. **Benjamin F, Deutsch S, Saperstein H, Seltzer BVL,** Prevalence of and markers for the attenuated form of congenital adrenal hyperplasia and hyperprolactinemia masquarading as polycystic ovarian disease, Fertil Steril 46:215, 1986.

43. **Azziz R, Zacur H,** 21-Hydroxylase deficiency in female hyperandrogenism: screening and diagnosis, J Clin Endocrinol Metab 69:577, 1989.

44. **Lobo RA,** The role of the adrenal in polycystic ovary syndrome, Seminars Reprod Endocrinol 2:251, 1984.

45. **New MI, Lorenzen F, Lerner AJ, Kohn B, Oberfield SE, Pollack MS, Dupont B, Stoner E, Levy DJ, Pang S, Levine LS,** Genotyping steroid 21-hydroxylase deficiency: hormonal reference data, J Clin Endocrinol Metab 57:320, 1983.

46. **Rosenfield RL, Helke J, Lucky AW,** Dexamethasone preparation does not alter corticoid and androgen responses to adrenocorticotropin, J Clin Endocrinol Metab 60:585, 1985.

47. **Sobrino L, Kase N, Grunt J,** Changes in adrenocortical function in patients with gonadal dysgenesis after treatment with estrogen, J Clin Endocrinol Metab 33:110, 1971.

48. **Abraham G, Maroulis G,** Effect of exogenous estrogen on serum pregnenolone, cortisol and androgens in postmenopausal women, Obstet Gynecol 45:271, 1975.

49. **Lucky AW, Marynick SP, Rebar RW, Cutler GB, Glen M, Johnsonbaugh E, Loriaux DL,** Replacement oral ethinyloestradiol therapy for gonadal dysgenesis: growth and adrenal androgen studies, Acta Endocrinol 91:519, 1979.

50. **Lobo RA, March CM, Goebelsmann U, Mishell DR Jr,** The modulating role of obesity and of 17β-estradiol (E$_2$) on bound and unbound E$_2$ and adrenal androgens in oophorectomized women, J Clin Endocrinol Metab 54:320, 1982.

51. **Lobo RA, Goebelsmann U, Brenner PF, Mishell DR Jr,** The effects of estrogen on adrenal androgens in oophorectomized women, Am J Obstet Gynecol 142:471, 1982.

52. **Rosenfield RL, Famg IS,** The effects of prolonged physiologic estradiol therapy on the maturation of hypogonadal teenagers, J Pediatr 85:830, 1974.

53. **Anderson D, Yen SSC,** Effects of estrogens on adrenal 3β-hydroxysteroid dehydrogenase in ovariectomized women, J Clin Endocrinol Metab 43:561, 1976.

54. **Rose DP, Fern M, Liskowski L, Milbrath JR,** Effect of treatment with estrogen conjugates on endogenous plasma steroids, Obstet Gynecol 49:80, 1977.

55. **Steingold K, de Ziegler D, Cedars M, Meldrum DR, Lu JKH, Judd HL, Chang RJ,** Clinical and hormonal effects of chronic gonadotropin-releasing hormone agonist treatment in polycystic ovarian disease, J Clin Endocrinol Metab 65:773, 1987.

56. **Tazuke S, Khaw K-T, Barrett-Connor E,** Exogenous estrogen and endogenous sex hormones, Medicine 71:44, 1992.

57. **Fujieda K, Faiman C, Reyes FI, Winter JSD,** The control of steroidogenesis by human fetal adrenal cells in tissue culture: IV. The effects of exposure to placental steroids, J Clin Endocrinol Metab 54:89, 1982.

58. **Chang RJ, Mandel FP, Wolfren AR, Judd HL,** Circulating levels of plasma adrenocorticotropin in polycystic ovary disease, J Clin Endocrinol Metab 54:1265, 1982.

59. **Byrne GC, Perry YS, Winter JSD,** Steroid inhibitory effects upon human adrenal 3β-hydroxysteroid dehydrogenase activity, J Clin Endocrinol Metab 62:413, 1986.

60. **Futterweit W, Green G, Tarlin N, Dunaif A,** Chronic high-dosage androgen administration to ovulatory women does not alter adrenocortical steroidogenesis, Fertil Steril 58:124, 1992.

61. **Dunaif A, Green G, Futterweit W, Dobrjansky A,** Suppression of hyperandrogenism does not improve peripheral or hepatic insulin resistance in the polycystic ovary syndrome, J Clin Endocrinol Metab 70:699, 1990.

62. **Wild RA, Alaupovic P, Parker IJ,** Lipid and apolipoprotein abnormalities in hirsute women. I. The association with insulin resistance, Am J Obstet Gynecol 166:1191, 1992.

63. **Gonzalez F, Hatala DA, Speroff L,** Basal and dynamic hormonal responses to gonadotropin releasing hormone agonist treatment in women with polycystic ovaries with high and low dehydroepiandrosterone sulfate levels, Am J Obstet Gynecol 165:535, 1991.

64. **Carmina E, Koyama T, Chang L, Stanczyk FZ, Lobo RA,** Does ethnicity influence the prevalence of adrenal hyperandrogenism and insulin resistance in polycystic ovary syndrome? Am J Obstet Gynecol 167:1807, 1992.

65. **Lanzone A, Fulghesu AM, Guido M, Fortini A, Caruso A, Mancuso S,** Differential androgen response to adrenocorticotropic hormone stimulation in polycystic ovarian syndrome: relationship with insulin secretion, Fertil Steril 58:296, 1992.

66. **Nestler JE, Clore JN, Strauss JF III, Blackard WG,** Effects of hyperinsulinemia on serum testosterone, progesterone, dehydroepiandrosterone sulfate, and cortisol levels in normal women and in a woman with hyperandrogenism, insulin resistance and acanthosis nigricans, J Clin Endocrinol Metab 64:180, 1987.

67. **Nestler JE, McClanahan MA, Clore JN, Blackard WG,** Insulin inhibits adrenal 17,20-lyase activity in man, J Clin Endocrinol Metab 74:362, 1992.

68. **Liu CH, Laughlin GA, Fischer UG, Yen SSC,** Marked attenuation of ultradian and circadian rhythms of dehydroepiandrosterone in postmenopausal women: evidence for a reduced 17,20-desmolase enzymatic activity, J Clin Endocrinol Metab 71:900, 1990.

69. **Alper MM, Garner PR,** Elevated serum dehydroepiandrosterone sulfate levels in patients with insulin resistance, hirsutism, and acanthosis nigricans, Fertil Steril 47:255, 1987.

70. **Haning RV Jr, Hackett RJ, Flood CA, Loughlin JS, Zhao QY, Longcope C,** Plasma dehydroepiandrosterone sulfate serves as a prehormone for 48% of follicular fluid testosterone during treatment with menotropins, J Clin Endocrinol Metab 76:1301, 1993.

71. **Easterling WE Jr, Talbert LM, Potter HD,** Serum testosterone levels in the polycystic ovary syndrome, Am J Obstet Gynecol 120:385, 1974.

72. **Meldrum DR, Abraham GE,** Peripheral and ovarian venous concentrations of various steroid hormones in virilizing ovarian tumors, Obstet Gynecol 53:36, 1979.

73. **Gabrilove JL, Seman AT, Sabet R, Mitty HA, Nicolis GL,** Virilizing adrenal adenoma with studies on the steroid content of the adrenal venous effluent and a review of the literature, Endocrin Rev 2:462, 1981.

74. **Friedman CI, Schmidt GE, Kim MH, Powell J,** Serum testosterone concentrations in the evaluation of androgen-producing tumors, Am J Obstet Gynecol 153:44, 1985.

75. **Surrey ES, de Ziegler D, Gambone JC, Judd HL,** Preoperative localization of androgen-secreting tumors: clinical, endocrinologic, and radiologic evaluation of ten patients, Am J Obstet Gynecol 158:1313, 1988.

76. **Caron P, Roche H, Gorguet B, Martel P, Bennet A, Carton M,** Mammary ovarian metastases with stroma cell hyperplasia and postmenopausal virilization, Cancer 66:1221, 1990.

77. **Moltz L, Schwartz U,** Gonadal and adrenal androgen secretion in hirsute females, Clin Endocrinol Metab 15:229, 1986.

78. **Brumsted JR, Chapitis J, Riddick D, Gibson M,** Norethindrone inhibition of testosterone secretion by an ovarian Sertoli-Leydig cell tumor, J Clin Endocrinol Metab 65:194, 1987.

79. **Kennedy L, Trasub AI, Atkinson AB, Sheridan B,** Short-term administration of gonadotropin-releasing hormone analog to a patient with a testosterone-secreting ovarian tumor, J Clin Endocrinol Metab 64:1320, 1987.

80. **Cohen I, Shapira M, Cuperman S, Goldberger S, Siegal A, Altaras M, Beyth Y,** Direct in-vivo detection of atypical hormonal expression of a Sertoli-Leydig cell tumour following stimulation with human chorionic gonadotropin, Clin Endocrinol, in press.

81. **Leedman PJ, Bierre AR, Martin FIR,** Virlizing nodular ovarian stromal hyperthecosis, diabetes mellitus and insulin resistance in a postmenopausal woman. Case report, Br J Obstet Gynaecol 96:1095, 1989.

82. **Ross NS, Aron DC,** Hormonal evaluation of the patient with an incidentally discovered adrenal mass, New Engl J Med 323:1401, 1990.

83. **Katz RL, Shobhana P, Mackay B, Zornoza J,** Fine needle aspiration cytology of the adrenal gland, Acta Cytol 28:269, 1984.

84. **Copeland PM,** The incidentally discovered adrenal mass, Ann Surg 199:116, 1984.

85. **Reincke M, Nieke J, Krestin GP, Saeger W, Allolio B, Winkelmann W,** Preclinical Cushing's syndrome in adrenal "incidentalomas:" comparison with adrenal Cushing's syndrome, J Clin Endocrinol Metab 75:826, 1992.

86. **Jaresch S, Kornely E, Kley H-K, Schlaghecke R,** Adrenal incidentaloma and patients with homozygous or heterozygous congenital adrenal hyperplasia, J Clin Endocrinol Metab 74:685, 1992.

87. **Cassidenti DL, Paulson RJ, Serafini P, Stanczyk FZ, Lobo RA,** Effects of sex steroids on skin 5α-reductase activity in vitro, Obstet Gynecol 78:103, 1991.

88. **Jung-Hoffman C, Kuhl H,** Divergent effects of two low-dose oral contraceptives on sex hormone-binding globulin and free testosterone, Am J Obstet Gynecol 156:199, 1987.

89. **van der Vange N, Blankenstein MA, Kloosterboer HJ, Haspels AA, Thijssen JHH,** Effects of seven low-dose combined oral contraceptives on sex hormone binding globulin, corticosteroid binding globulin, total and free testsosterone, Contraception 41:345, 1990.

90. **Gordon GG, Southern AL, Tochimoto S, Olivo J, Altman K, Rand J, Lemberger L,** Effect of medroxyprogesteorne acetate (Provera) on the metabolism and biological activity of testosterone, J Clin Endocrinol Metab 30:449, 1970.

91. **Wortsman J, Khan MS, Rosner W,** Suppression of testosterone-estradiol binding globulin by medroxyprogesterone acetate in polycystic ovary syndrome, Obstet Gynecol 67:705, 1986.

92. **Richards RN, Uy M, Meharg G,** Temporary hair removal in patients with hirsutism: a clinical study, Cutis 45:199, 1990.

93. **Wild RA, Umstot ES, Andersen RN, Givens JR,** Adrenal function in hirsutism: II. Effect of an oral contraceptive, J Clin Endocrinol Metab 54:676, 1982.

94. **Wiebe RH, Morris CV,** Effect of an oral contraceptive on adrenal and ovarian androgenic steroids, Obstet Gynecol 63:12, 1984.

95. **Young RL, Goldzieher JW, Elkind-Hirsch K,** The endocrine effects of spironolactone used as an antiandrogen, Fertil Steril 48:223, 1987.

96. **Serafini P, Lobo RA,** The effects of spironolactone on adrenal steroidogenesis in hirsute women, Fertil Steril 44:595, 1985.

97. **Lobo RA, Shoupe D, Serafini P, Brinton D, Horton R,** The effects of two doses of spironolactone on serum androgens and anagen hair in hirsute women, Fertil Steril 43:200, 1985.

98. **Evans DJ, Burke CW,** Spironolactone in the treatment of idiopathic hirsutism and the polycystic ovary syndrome, J R Soc Med 79:453, 1986.

99. **Barth JH, Cherry CA, Wojnarowaka F, Dawber RP,** Spironolactone is an effective and well tolerated systemic anti-androgen therapy for hirsute women, J Clin Endocrinol Metab 68:966, 1989.

100. **Pittaway DE, Maxson WS, Wentz AC,** Spironolactone in combination drug therapy for unresponsive hirsutism, Fertil Steril 43:878, 1985.

101. **Messina M, Manieri C, Rizzi G, Gentile L, Milani P,** Treating acne with antiandrogens: the confirmation of the validity of a percutaneous treatment with spironolactone, Curr Ther Res Clin Exp 38:269, 1985.

102. **Miller JA, Jacobs HS,** Treatment of hirsutism and acne with cyproterone acetate, Clin Endocrinol Metab 15:373, 1986.

103. **Belisle S, Love EJ,** Clinical efficacy and safety of cyproterone acetate in severe hirsutism: results in a multicentered Canadian study, Fertil Steril 46:1015, 1986.

104. **Barth JH, Cherry CA, Wojnarowska F, Dawber RPR,** Cyproterone acetate for severe hirsutism: results of a double-blind dose-ranging study, Clin Endocrinol 35:5, 1991.

105. **Holdaway IM, Croxson MS, Ibbertson HK, Sheehan A, Knox B, France J,** Cyproterone acetate as initial treatment and maintenance therapy for hirsutism, Acta Endocrinol 109:522, 1985.

106. **Chapman MG, Dowsett M, Dewhurst CJ, Jeffcoate SL,** Spironolactone in combination with an oral contraceptive: an alternative treatment for hirsutism, Br J Obstet Gynaecol 92:983, 1985.

107. **O'Brien RC, Cooper ME, Murray RML, Seeman E, Thomas AK, Jerums G,** Comparison of sequential cyproterone acetate/estrogen *versus* spironolactone/oral contraceptive in the treatment of hirsutism, J Clin Endocrinol Metab 72:1008, 1991.

108. **Rittmaster RS, Loriaux DL, Cutler GB Jr,** Sensitivity of cortisol and adrenal androgens to dexamethasone suppression in hirsute women, J Clin Endocrinol Metab 61:462, 1985.

109. **Avgerinos PC, Cutler GB Jr, Tsokos GC, Gold PW, Feuillan P, Galucci WT, Pillemer SR, Loriaux DL, Chraousos GP,** Dissociation between cortisol and adrenal androgen secretion in patients receiving alternate day prednisone therapy, J Clin Endocrinol Metab 65:24, 1987.

110. **Steinberger E, Smith KD, Rodriguez-Rigau J,** Testosterone, dehydroepiandrosterone, and dehydroepiandrosterone sulfate in hyperandrogenic women, J Clin Endocrinol Metab 59:471, 1984.

111. **Rittmaster RS,** Differential suppression of testosterone and estradiol in hirsute women with the superactive gonadotropin-releasing hormone agonist leuprolide, J Clin Endocrinol Metab 67:651, 1988.

112. **Marcondes JAM, Minnani SL, Luthold WW, Wajchenberg BL, Samojlik E, Kirschner MA,** Treatment of hirsutism in women with flutamide, Fertil Steril 57:543, 1992.

113. **Golditch IM, Price VH,** Treatment of hirsutism with cimetidine, Obstet Gynecol 75:911, 1990.

114. **Rowe TC, Mezei M, Hilchie J,** Treatment of hirsutism with liposomal progesterone, Prostate 5:346, 1984.

115. **Venturoli S, Fabbri R, Dal Prato L, Mantovani B, Capelli M, Magrini O, Flamigni C,** Ketoconazole therapy for women with acne and/or hirsutism, J Clin Endocrinol Metab 71:335, 1990.

116. **Paulson RJ, Serafini PC, Catalino JA, Lobo RA,** Measurements of 3α-, 17β-androstenediol glucuronide in serum and urine and the correlation with skin 5α-reductase activity, Fertil Steril 46:222, 1986.

117. **Kirschner MA, Samojlik E, Szmal E,** Clinical usefulness of plasma androstanediol glucuronide measurements in women with idiopathic hirsutism, J Clin Endocrinol Metab 65:597, 1987.

15 Menstrual Disorders

	1	2	3	4	5	6
7	8	9	10	11	12	13
14	15	16	17	18	19	20
21	22	23	24	25	26	27
28	29	30	31			

Since antiquity, the appearance of menses in correlation with lunar phases has inspired names for menses such as a period or the monthly time. The regularity of this appearance was easily appreciated; more difficult was understanding the purpose of the bleeding. Ancient physicians viewed menstruation as a process of detoxification, and throughout history myths and attitudes toward menstruation have kept alive negative connotations that range from magic to danger and poison.[1]

The health care profession has an obligation to promote menstrual education. This must start with ourselves. We must have an understanding of reproductive physiology in order to impart it to our patients, and we must be sensitive to the need to present a positive attitude regarding sexual and reproductive functions. An educated understanding of these normal events is a powerful mechanism for dealing with perceived discomforts and disorders of menstruation.

Unfortunately, some menstrual disorders are still not well understood (such as the premenstrual syndrome), although others, such as dysmenorrhea, can be physiologically explained in a framework that provides for appropriate pharmacologic treatment. In this chapter we will consider several common medical problems which are linked to menstruation and do our best to provide an objective point of view based on physiology.

The Premenstrual Syndrome

The simplest definition of the premenstrual syndrome (PMS) is a commonsense one: the cyclic appearance of one or more of a large constellation of symptoms (over 100) just prior to menses, occurring to such a degree that lifestyle or work is affected, followed by a period of time entirely free of symptoms. The most frequently encountered symptoms include the following: abdominal bloating, anxiety, breast tenderness, crying spells, depression, fatigue, irritability, thirst and appetite changes, and variable degrees of edema of the extremities — usually occurring in the last 7 to 10 days of the cycle. The exact collection of symptoms in an individual is irrelevant; the diagnosis is made by prospectively and accurately charting the cyclic nature of the symptoms. However, the symptoms are not to be underrated; the various symptoms of premenstrual syndrome have been recounted time and time again in clinicians' offices in poignant detail.

When women's daily moods are prospectively charted, a subgroup emerges in which mood changes demonstrate a cyclic pattern with increasing symptoms during the luteal phase and an elimination of symptoms at or soon after menses. Fewer than 50% of women who complain of premenstrual syndrome can be demonstrated to have a pattern of mood changes with a cyclic pattern.[2]

There are two established guidelines for the diagnosis of PMS. The first is from the American Psychiatric Association (APA) and consists of the criteria for what the APA has designated as the luteal phase dysphoric disorder.[3] These criteria (which correspond to our simple definition above) are as follows:

A. Symptoms are temporally related to the menstrual cycle, beginning during the last week of the luteal phase and remitting after the onset of menses.

B. The diagnosis requires at least 5 of the following, and one of the symptoms must be either one of the first 4:

1. Affective lability, e.g., sudden onset of being sad, tearful, irritable, or angry.
2. Persistent and marked anger or irritability.
3. Marked anxiety or tension.
4. Markedly depressed mood, feelings of hopelessness.
5. Decreased interest in usual activities.
6. Easy fatigability or marked lack of energy.
7. Subjective sense of difficulty in concentrating.
8. Marked change in appetite, overeating, or food craving.
9. Hyersomnia or insomnia.
10. Physical symptoms such as breast tenderness, headaches, edema, joint or muscle pain, weight gain.

C. The symptoms interfere with work or usual activities or relationships.

D. The symptoms are not an exacerbation of another psychiatric disorder.

The guidelines from the National Institute of Mental Health (NIMH) state that the diagnosis of PMS requires the documentation of at least a 30% increase in severity of symptoms in the 5 days prior to menses compared with the 5 days following menses. Using the NIMH and APA criteria, it is estimated that about 5% of women of reproductive age can be diagnosed with PMS.[2]

Approximately 40% of women report significant problems related to their cycles, and about 2–10% report a degree of impact on work or lifestyle.[4] The exact prevalence, however, is difficult to ascertain. The symptoms are variable and difficult to quantitate. A further problem which complicates the evaluation of published studies as well as dealing with individual cases, is that behavior is usually related to menstruation in a retrospective fashion. This is prone to considerable subjective bias.[5] For example, studies in the literature point out that some women do not actually experience problems in relation to menstruation but believe that they do.[6] It is argued, rather convincingly, that men and women in our culture have been conditioned to expect symptoms in a woman's premenstrual phase and have been taught to expect fluid retention, pain, and emotional reactions. These sterotypic expectations are precisely what are reported when retrospective charting is utilized. Most importantly, carefully constructed studies (prospective with appropriate statistical analyses) show no significant variation associated with the cycle for cognitive, motor, or social behavior.[7]

Is PMS due to an individual pathologic problem or is it due to cultural beliefs, beliefs that lead to the menstrual cycle being associated with a variety of negative reactions, or a combination of both? There is a significant correlation between menstrual symptoms in daughters and mothers, and between sisters, suggesting that these are responses that can be learned.[8,9] Throughout our recorded history, we find evidence of menstrual taboos. What if our societies and cultures had celebrated menstruation as a time of pleasure (and even public joy) rather than something private (to be hidden) and negative? Would we have PMS today? The answer may lie in the unraveling of the role of our shared beliefs about menstruation in society, rather than the functioning of those beliefs in individuals.

It is generally recognized that R. T. Frank, an American gynecologist, first defined premenstrual syndrome in 1931. His description still stands as a graphic and vivid statement. He wrote the following:[10]

> The group of women to whom I refer especially complain of a feeling of indescribable tension from 10 to 7 days preceding menstruation which in most instances continues until the time that the menstrual flow occurs. The patients complain of unrest, irritability, like jumping out of their skin and a desire to find relief by foolish and ill considered actions. Their personal suffering is intense and manifests itself in many reckless and sometimes reprehensible actions. Not only do they realize their own suffering, but they feel conscience-stricken toward their husbands and families, knowing well that they are unbearable in their attitude and reactions. Within an hour or two after the onset of the menstrual flow complete relief from both physical and mental tension occurs.

Frank went on to summarize 15 cases. He reported that he could obtain relief by withdrawing blood from his patients, and therefore theorized that the problem was inadequate excretion of female sex hormones. Accordingly he used treatments to enhance excretion such as calcium lactate, caffeine, and laxatives. For severe cases, he produced ovarian failure by irradiation. S. Leon Israel, in the 1930s, was the first to propose that the syndrome was due to defective luteinization resulting in a progesterone deficiency and a relative hyperestrogenic state.[11] The phrase, "Premenstrual Syndrome," was first used in 1953 by Dalton in a report of 84 cases with Greene.[12]

Despite a vast literature, we are still handicapped by a lack of knowledge as to what the premenstrual syndrome really is, how to establish a diagnosis, and how best to treat the condition. A brief look backwards into history finds reason enough to conclude that we are limited in our reactions to menses, limited by what has been provided by our culture throughout history.

Historical Myths

Recorded beliefs, many of them truly ancient, include magical beliefs, superstitions regarding the milk supply from cows, and beliefs about crops and animals.[13] It was held, almost universally, that the menstrual woman was possessed by an evil spirit.

Pliny, born in 23 A.D., consulted approximately 2,000 available books by physicians in writing his *Historia Naturalis*. Pliny's treatise was a resource throughout the Dark Ages, and there are still more than 100 copies of it, all 37 volumes. The oft-quoted Pliny, who clearly was unencumbered with the burden of objectivity, wrote almost exhaustively on menstruation.[14]

> Contact with it turns new wine sour, crops touched by it become barren, grafts die, seeds in gardens are dried up, the fruit of trees falls off, the edge of steel and the gleam of ivory are dulled, hives of bees die, even bronze and iron are at once seized by rust, and a horrible smell fills the air; to taste it drives dogs mad and infects their bites with an

incurable poison. If a woman strips herself naked while she is menstruating and walks around a field of wheat, the caterpillars, worms, beetles, and other vermin will fall off from the ears of corn. All plants will turn of a yellow complexion on the approach of a woman who has the menstrual discharge upon her. Bees will forsake their hives at her touch, for they have a special aversion to a thief and a menstrous woman, and a glance of her eyes suffices to kill a swarm of bees.

Household articles were not immune. Aristotle said that a menstrous woman could dull a mirror with a look, and the next person to look into it would be bewitched. There were numerous tales of women breaking things at the time of menses — needles snapping, glasses breaking, and clocks stopping. In general there has been a universal horror of blood throughout early history. It is not surprising, therefore, that this (probably) instinctive horror led to taboos on blood and all that came in contact with it. This led in turn to prohibition and seclusion. Almost universally, menstruating women were isolated and prevented from handling food. Most primitive peoples regarded women as unclean during menstruation and subjected menstruating women to segregation and special rituals. Ultimately, with growing sophistication, this led to a generally negative attitude.

The scientific study of menstruation has been hampered by the overpowering influence of traditions and social and cultural beliefs. We have all, men and women, been conditioned to view menstruation in a negative way. Perhaps it is time to look at menstruation from another point of view. How many fine novels have been finished in a burst of creativity in the premenstrual period? How many great ideas have been born premenstrually? If PMS reflects socially mediated expectations, the answer may lie in social re-education.

The Social Consequences of PMS

It was a common view in Europe in the 19th and early 20th centuries that menstruation was associated with antisocial behavior.[15] A domestic servant who murdered one of her employer's children in 1845 was acquitted on the grounds of insanity due to obstructed menstruation. In 1851, a woman was acquitted of murdering her baby niece on the grounds of insanity due to disordered menstruation. Acquittals for shoplifting because of suppression of menses date back to 1845. When we consider the fact that PMS (although not known by this specific phrase) has been recognized throughout recorded history, it is not unexpected that it has been utilized as a defense in the courts before modern times.

Dalton has argued that PMS is responsible for an increased incidence of crime, jailing for alcoholism, school misdemeanors, sickness in industry, hospitalization for accidents, and general hospital admissions.[16] However studies on premenstrual symptoms which have appropriate controls and statistical treatment find no significant variation associated with the menstrual cycle for cognitive or motor behavior.[7,17] Social behavior (including crime and suicide) reveals effects similar to all others seen in self-report studies. When social or psychological expectations are altered, the effect disappears. PMS is likely to be accepted by courts in the same manner that factors related to social and psychological stress or physical illness are accepted, and such factors do not absolve the accused of criminal responsibility.

Unfortunately, PMS is still used to explain apparently motiveless and impulsive acts, as well as poor academic performance. In contrast to Dalton's contention that schoolgirls have impaired academic performance during the premenstrual phase, the results of 244 female medical and paramedical students in all examinations taken during one year did not reveal any significant menstrual cycle effects on examination performance.[18]

One of the biggest problems with the studies which have sought to link behavior with the cycles is an underlying assumption that the premenstrual phase is the crucial variable, ignoring the fact that any phase of the cycle is vulnerable to life stresses. In other words, the premenstrual phase must be controlled for all life stresses in order to conclude that that phase of the cycle has an etiologic influence on some life event.

Etiologies and Treatments

Where scientists have failed to provide proof, practitioners have seldom failed to provide theories. The list of biological theories is impressive:

> Low progesterone levels.
> High estrogen levels.
> Falling estrogen levels.
> Changes in estrogen:progesterone ratios.
> Increased aldosterone activity.
> Increased renin-angiotensin activity.
> Increased adrenal activity.
> Endogenous endorphin withdrawal.
> Subclinical hypoglycemia.
> Central changes in catecholamines.
> Response to prostaglandins.
> Vitamin deficiencies.
> Excess prolactin secretion.

Studies prior to 1983 did not incorporate appropriate diagnostic criteria and, therefore, suffer from inaccuracy and heterogeneity. Since 1983, efforts to isolate a specific pathophysiologic mechanism have failed to demonstrate differences between women with and without symptoms for all hormone levels throughout the menstrual cycle (including estrogens, progesterone, testosterone, follicle-stimulating hormone [FSH], luteinizing hormone [LH], prolactin, and sex hormone binding globulin) or weight gain and measurements of substances involved in fluid regulation, such as aldosterone.[19] This further includes both the circulating levels as well as the pattern of secretion over the menstrual cycle. Dynamic testing has revealed no abnormalities in the hypothalamic-pituitary axis and its relationships with the adrenal glands, the thyroid gland, and the ovaries. No differences can be detected in magnesium, zinc, vitamin A, vitamin E, thiamin, or vitamin B_6.[20] Some have argued for a greater change in endorphins, proposing that the luteal phase symptom complex is due to a greater withdrawal from endogenous opioids (in effect, an autoaddiction and withdrawal), but others have been unable to detect a difference in circulating endorphins in symptomatic patients.[21-23]

There have been reported differences in various biologic factors, but these differences are not always confined to the luteal phases. Some of these factors, besides the endorphins, include the response to thyrotropin releasing hormone (TRH), melatonin secretion, red blood cell magnesium levels, growth hormone and cortisol responses to tryptophan, cortisol response to corticotropin releasing hormone, free cortisol secretion, and cortisol secretion patterns. The strongest argument against a luteal phase hormonal change is derived from experiments at the National Institute of Mental Health.[24] These experiments utilized the progesterone antagonist, RU486, in combination with human chorionic gonadotropin (HCG) or placebo to induce bleeding at various times during the cycle. Altering the menstrual cycle had no effect on the timing or severity of the PMS symptoms; thus, the neuroendocrine and endocrine events during the luteal phase should not be involved.

In general, thyroid function is normal in patients with PMS. About 10% of women with PMS have abnormal thyroid function, but this compares to the prevalence rate of subclinical hypothyroidism. Although there are no differences in thyroid-stimulating horomone (TSH) response to TRH, PMS patients do demonstrate more abnormal responses, both exaggerated and blunted (which would balance out in group comparisons).[25] However, these abnormal responses occur just as often in the follicular phase as in the luteal phase. Furthermore, there is no evidence of a therapeutic response to thyroxine compared to placebo, even in patients with abnormal responses to TRH.

Various methods of treatment have been proposed, each championing a presumed etiology. All of the following have failed to demonstrate any clear-cut benefits over placebo: oral contraceptives, vitamin B_6, bromocriptine, monoamine oxidase inhibitors, and synthetic progestational agents. The use of spironolactone has many advocates, especially for women with a major complaint of bloating; however, appropriate double-blind, placebo-controlled trials have failed to demonstrate a clinical impact greater than placebo.[26,27] It has been argued that patients with PMS have a deficiency in fatty acid metabolism, and evening of primrose oil has been advocated for therapy. Evening of primrose oil is extracted from the seed of the evening primrose; it provides linoleic and gamma-linoleic acids (precursors of prostaglandin E). Appropriately blinded and controlled studies failed to find a difference comparing primrose oil to placebo.[28,29] The one positive study used retrospective assessment of symptoms, a method known to be inaccurrate.[30] Significant improvement has been noted with the use of prostaglandin synthesis inhibitors, but it is difficult to know if this is influenced by a positive impact on dysmenorrhea.[31]

There has been significant publicity given to the use of progesterone treatment by injection or vaginal suppository, long proposed and promoted by Dalton.[16] Four early studies that failed to detect a positive effect of progesterone were criticized for study size and progesterone dosage.[32–35] A very well-designed study attempted to remove a placebo effect by providing no contact with the investigators or any health care providers during the course of the study; both progesterone and placebo failed to achieve an improvement in symptoms.[36] The criticism of study size and progesterone dose was effectively answered in a randomized placebo-controlled, double-blind, clinical crossover trial of 168 women.[37] Progesterone in doses of 400 mg and 800 mg (doses used by Dalton) did not differ from placebo. Only one study has reported beneficial effects with progesterone, a study of only 23 highly motivated women, and the major effect occurred only in the first month of treatment.[38]

Medical and surgical oophorectomy has been described to have dramatic success. A lasting response to surgical hysterectomy and oophorectomy was reported in women unresponsive to medical therapy.[39,40] Gonadotropin-releasing hormone (GnRH) agonist treatment can produce hypogonadotropic hypogonadism, in effect, a medical oophorectomy. GnRH agonist treatment has been effective; adding estrogen-progestin to avoid the side effects of the GnRH agonist diminished somewhat the improvement in symptoms. However, the beneficial impact was still considerable.[41,42] While medical and surgical oophorectomy is undoubtedly effective, it is impossible to blind such treatment, and the mechanism is therefore uncertain. In the GnRH agonist-steroid addback study, patients receiving a placebo instead of estrogen-progestin had a return of symptoms (despite continued GnRH agonist treatment), probably in anticipation of a negative reaction to estrogen-progestin. This experience is a strong statement of the power of the placebo response (in this case, a negative response).

The only randomized trials, double-blinded and placebo-controlled, which have had consistent, excellent results are those with the antidepressents, fluoxetine (Prozac) and alprazolam (Xanax). A dose (20–60 mg daily) of fluoxetine (which inhibits neuronal uptake of serotonin) effectively abolished symptoms without side effects.[43–45] Alprazolam is a short acting benzodiazepine with anxiolytic, antidepressant, and smooth muscle relaxant properties. A dose of 0.25 mg bid-tid during the luteal phase is very effective.[46,47] In contrast, lithium has no effect.

Problems and Questions

The problems and questions are many:

1. The clinical symptoms are variable, difficult to quantitate, and enormous in number. The symptoms cover emotions, sexual feelings, mood states, behavioral changes, and somatic complaints. Despite multiple questionnaires, we are still not convinced that there exists a reliable, objective method for observing and measuring symptoms that are experienced internally, rather than manifested via external behavior.[6]

2. The discrepancy between retrospective and prospective accounts regarding cyclic changes is now well-documented and recognized.[48] Women use menses as a marker of time, and unpleasant, easily remembered experiences are attributed to an easily recognized signpost. If women in our culture have been conditioned to expect symptoms in the premenstrual phase and have been taught to expect fluid retention, pain, and emotional reactions, that is precisely what will be reported.[48] Our lives are rhythmical. Day alternates with night. There are sleeping and waking, being hungry and being full, the circadian rhythms of our glands, and the ultimate rhythm: the sexual cycle. It is the most natural thing to seek a rhythm for our behavior.

   The Ruble study is now a classic.[49] In this study, 44 undergraduates at Princeton University were deliberately deceived about which phase of the menstrual cycle they were experiencing. A bogus electroencephalogram, complete with electrodes attached to the head, was heralded as a new technique capable of predicting the date of menstruation. Subjects were told they were either premenstrual (due in 1–2 days) or intermenstrual (due in 7–10 days). Only those women who were led to believe that their period would begin in 2 days reported significantly higher symptom ratings on pain, water retention, and eating habit changes. This was interpreted as a reflection of stereotypic expectations.

3. Is there a specific syndrome? A syndrome must have a specific pathophysiology; specific signs and symptoms can be documented; and a specific treatment achieves a beneficial response. Not a single one of these criteria can be met. One of the basic problems is that we have lumped everything into PMS, including behavioral changes, somatic complaints, and psychological problems, implying the existence of a specific syndrome. Part of the problem is that all the tools of research reflect the way the author of the tool conceptualizes PMS, which in turn is based upon the background and training of the author.[50]

4. The experimenter expectancy effect has to be properly controlled. Subjects tend to comply with what they deem to be the experimenter's hypothesis. This has been studied in regard to PMS, and no significant difference in PMS symptomatology can be demonstrated when the purpose of the study is disguised, and in addition the responses can be influenced by positive or negative manipulations.[51–53] This relates to findings of negative mood changes when subjects are asked to assess their menstrual distress retrospectively.

5. Studies are complicated by high placebo responses. Clinical studies of premenstrual syndrome typically demonstrate a 30–50% response to placebo and, if a positive effect is anticipated by the subjects, up to 80%. Only well-designed, double-blind, placebo-controlled, randomized trials yield reliable data.

The Placebo Response

The strange sounding word, placebo, comes from the Latin verb meaning "I shall please." Physicians and patients have been educated to observe a prescription ritual. Most people seem to feel that their complaints are not taken seriously unless they are in possession of a prescription. But the placebo is not so much a pill as a process.[54]

The process begins with patient confidence in the clinician and extends through to the full functioning of the patient's own healing system. Interaction with the clinician provides a better understanding of what's going on (at least some elimination of unfounded fears) and provides some hope. Many of the treatment modalities for PMS, if not all, provide a woman with a greater sense of control over life; thus, minimal interaction, such as focusing on diet or lifestyle, can yield a positive result. In the process of making detailed, prospective observations of one's own life, a patient can experience an increase in self-control, which is in itself a therapeutic process.

Leon Eisenberg has written the following insightful and helpful thoughts on the placebo:[55]

> So emphatically does the phrase "placebo response" discredit the psychosocial aspects of the therapeutic encounter that it may be time to eradicate it from our language. Let us replace it by some such term as "the response to care," "the response to the doctor," or "the healing response" in order to emphasize that it is (a). powerful, (b). no less "real" than drug actions, and (c). embedded in every therapeutic transaction. . . Its mechanisms are some compound of the arousal of hope, the comfort of reassurance, taking an active rather than a passive role in managing the illness experience, and reinterpreting the meaning of the illness. . . It is perverse that "placebo" has almost become an epithet implying charlatanism rather than a descriptor of a fundamental characteristic of medical practice. . . We ought equally to seek an understanding of the healing response rather than disdaining it, as the "hard" scientist does, or being deceived by it, as practitioners often are.

Until PMS is better understood, the placebo response will continue to play an important role in therapy. There is a psychosocial subjective component of medicine that makes the placebo process a legitimate part of every patient-physician interaction.

Treatment of Premenstrual Syndrome

The first step is to be convinced (both patient and physician) that the problem is cyclic. The only instrument of diagnosis available at the present time is the menstrual calendar. At least 3 months of prospective recording, aided if possible by other observers (such as family members), are necessary in order to document a recurring problem in the luteal phase of the cycle, interfering with work or lifestyle, and followed by a period entirely free of symptoms. This time period should be utilized to develop a solid patient-physician relationship and, in so doing, to provide as much education as possible for the patient.

We offer our perspective on this syndrome, suggesting that it is not a single disorder, but rather a collection of different problems. We believe that PMS is basically psychological in origin, but tied to the menstrual cycle, either biologically, psychologically, or sociologically. This can be a learned response or it can be a response triggered by normal neuroendocrine and hormonal changes. The hormonal changes of the menstrual cycle are not an etiologic factor, but they can operate to produce a susceptibility to mood changes or a destabilization of mood. This may be the reason that elimination of menses with drugs or oophorectomy appears to be effective.

Often patients present to the clinician totally focused on complaints that occur premenstrually. With exploration of lifestyle, relationships, and interactions, the focus on a premenstrual syndrome can be shifted to the underlying issues that are producing conflict and lack of control. Helping a patient to come to grips with the subtle nature of this problem, the fundamental psychologic response involved, and the need to take charge of one's life represent the type of broad involvement required of a clinician. Without this type of broad involvement, only a short-term reponse can be achieved with little hope for long-term success.

Any changes that allow individuals to exert greater control over their lives will produce a positive impact. It is for this reason that lifestyle changes are effective in the treatment of PMS. Changes in diet, changes in exercise, changes in work or recreation — all are examples of exerting control over life rather than having life's circumstances control the individual.

If the practitioner is convinced of the cyclic nature of a problem (by a prospective record of at least 3 months duration), try to isolate the specific symptoms and treat with a specific therapy. If fluid retention is perceived by the patient as a principal problem, offer diuretic therapy with spironolactone. If dysmenorrhea is a component of the symptom complex, try one of the inhibitors of prostaglandin synthetase or oral contraceptives.

A failure to identify a specific disorder with a specific mechanism suggests that premenstrual syndrome represents a variety of psychological manifestations triggered by normal, physiologic hormonal changes. This latter process can be either physiologic in nature or psychosocial and deeply rooted in our cultural history. For that reason, it makes some sense to completely eliminate endogenous sex steroid variability. This can be achieved with medroxyprogesterone acetate, 10–30 mg daily, or depot medroxyprogesterone acetate, 150 mg every 3 months. On occasion, we have induced beneficial and gratifying results in patients with incapacitating emotional swings. But in view of the vague and subjective nature of this syndrome, any such empiric therapeutic treatment must be pursued in a fully informed fashion. If a patient is willing to undergo an empiric trial, we are willing. In doing so, however, neither partner in this contract should be deceived; we must remember that the placebo response may be the underlying basis for any positive response. But keep in mind that the placebo response is another example of an individual exerting control. In this case it represents the subtle effort of the body at a subconscious level to exert self-healing.

Last resort treatments, in our view, are the expensive and complicated medical oophorectomy by GnRH agonist combined with estrogen-progestin addback, and the use of fluoxetine and alprazolam. The clinical studies with these methods are very convincing, but this serious medical therapy does not diminish the important contribution to be made by the clinician in an ongoing relationship and interaction with the patient.

Dysmenorrhea

Dysmenorrhea is pain with menstruation, usually cramping in nature and centered in the lower abdomen. Studies on the prevalence of dysmenorrhea are few. In a random sample of 19 year old women in Gothenburg, Sweden, 72% reported dysmenorrhea, 15% had to limit their daily activity and the severity was unimproved by analgesics, 8% missed school or work at every menses, and 38.2% regularly used medical treatment.[56] Oral contraceptive use and previous vaginal deliveries were associated with less dysmenorrhea. The severity of dysmenorrhea was directly related to the duration and amount of menstrual flow. In another older but good prevalence study, 45% of surveyed women had moderate or severe dysmenorrhea.[57] Most adolescents experience dysmenorrhea in the first 3 years after menarche. In the U.S., about 60% of menstruating adolescents have dysmenorrhea, and 14% regularly miss school.[58]

Primary dysmenorrhea, a condition associated with ovulatory cycles, is due to myometrial contractions induced by prostaglandins originating in secretory endometrium, while secondary dysmenorrhea is associated with a variety of pathological conditons.[59] Other symptoms associated with menstrual flow, such as headache, nausea and vomiting, backache, and diarrhea, can be explained by entry of the prostaglandins and prostaglandin metabolites into the systemic circulation. There is a 3-fold increase in prostaglandin levels in the endometrium from the follicular phase to the luteal phase, with a further increase during menstruation. Women with primary dysmenorrhea have greater endometrial production of prostaglandins compared to asymptomatic women. Most of the release of prostaglandins during menstruation occurs during the first 48 hours, which coincides with the greatest intensity of the symptoms.

Prostaglandin $F_{2\alpha}$ ($PGF_{2\alpha}$) is the agent responsible for dysmenorrhea. It always stimulates uterine contractions, while the E prostaglandins inhibit contractions in the nonpregnant uterus. Uterine muscle from both normal and dysmenorrheic women is sensitive to $PGF_{2\alpha}$, but the amount of $PGF_{2\alpha}$ produced is the major differentiating factor.

The clinical benefit derived from the pharmacologic use of inhibitors of prostaglandin synthesis depends upon a significant decrease in prostaglandin production in the endometrium. An additional role may be attributed to decreased prostaglandins from the platelets participating in the clotting of menstrual blood. The explanation for the benefit seen with oral contraceptives is decreased prostaglandin synthesis associated with the atrophic decidualized endometrium. Oral contraception is a good choice for therapy, combining contraception with a beneficial impact on dysmenorrhea, menstrual flow, and menstrual irregularity. In women who do not desire hormonal contraception, the best therapy is one of the agents that inhibit prostaglandin synthesis.

There are several families of nonsteroidal anti-inflammatory agents. The acetic acid group is associated with more side effects, and these agents are not the drugs of choice for dysmenorrhea; indomethacin belongs to this group. The propionic acid derivatives (ibuprofen, naproxen, ketoprofen) and the fenamates (mefenamic acid, meclofenamate, flufenamic acid) are very effective for the treatment of dysmenorrhea.

The findings in 51 clinical trials of prostaglandin synthetase inhibitors indicate that the fenamates are most effective for relieving pain.[60] The fenamates, in addition to inhibiting prostaglandin synthesis, also have an antagonistic action, competing for prostaglandin binding sites. Side effects associated with these agents are minimal, but can include blurred vision, headaches, dizziness, and gastrointestinal discomfort. The latter can be reduced by taking the medication with milk or food. All of these agents are more potent than aspirin, because the uterus is relatively insensitive to aspirin. The major contraindications to the use of these agents include gastrointestinal ulcers and hypersensitivity to aspirin and similar agents.

About 80% of dysmenorrheic women are relieved by prostaglandin inhibitors. Improvement is noted in the symptoms associated with menses, specifically cramping, backache, nausea, vomiting, dizziness, leg pain, insomnia, and headache. A trial of up to 6 months is warranted, with necessary changes in dosage and inhibitors, before abandoning this therapy. Initially it was felt that better relief was achieved if treatment was started 2–3 days before menses in order to lower the tissue level of prostaglandins before breakdown of the endometrium. Fortunately, studies have indicated that treatment is just as effective if begun at the sign of first bleeding, thus decreasing the possibility of taking one of these agents early in pregnancy. Another benefit of prostaglandin inhibition is a reduction in the amount of blood lost with periods. Indeed the agents may be used to treat idiopathic menorrhagia, or the excess flow associated with an intrauterine device (IUD). Most women do not need to take the medication more than 2–3 days.

If dysmenorrhea is not relieved by one of the nonsteroidal, anti-inflammatory analgesics, laparoscopy should be seriously considered to determine the cause of the symptoms. Conditions associated with dysmenorrhea include müllerian duct anomalies, endometriosis, and pelvic inflammatory disease. We should especially be aware that endometriosis occurs in adolescents; dysmenorrhea caused by endometriosis in adolescents usually begins 3 or more years after menarche.

Menstrual Headache

Headaches are very common, but it is rare when the cause of the headache is a serious problem. Most headaches are due to vasodilatation, muscle contraction, or psychologic stress. Menstrual headaches include all headaches related in temporal fashion to menses, beginning before or during menstrual flow.[61] For many women with premenstrual syndrome, headache is part of the constellation of PMS symptoms. Here we are considering the occurrence of headache as a single, solitary symptom associated with menses.

Migraine headaches have a peak incidence of first occurrence at age 15–19, and they are rare after menopause.[62] An association with menses is observed by 60% of women with migraine headaches. In 14% of women with migraine, headaches occur exclusively with menses. Because menstrual migraine improves in two-thirds of migraineurs with pregnancy, this type of migraine seems to be due to falling levels of estrogen and progesterone.

Vascular Headaches

Acute and throbbing headaches are due to abnormal vasodilatation. The vasodilatation associated with migraine headaches is believed to follow a period of vasoconstriction. Migraine headaches are usually, but not always, preceded by prodromal symptoms (which may reflect the period of vasoconstriction). Significant vascular headaches can be precipitated by stress, alcohol, or tyramine and tryptophan rich foods (red wine, chocolate, ripe cheeses). Vascular headaches can accompany other problems, such as systemic viral infections, fever, or hypertension. Common migraine headaches are known as "migraine without aura."[62] Classic migraine is referred to as "migraine with aura."

Tension Headaches

The common tension headache is due to prolonged and excessive muscle contraction. The pain is dull, steady, bilateral, and worsens throughout the day.

Secondary Headaches

This type of headache is due to underlying organic disease. The pain is usually due to pressure or pulling of structures. Headaches associated with brain tumors are usually accompanied by neurologic abnormalities. Other causes are brain abscesses, subdural hematomas, hypertension, drug-use, and concussions. The main cause of inflammatory headaches is meningitis.

Evaluation

The acute onset of severe headache pain deserves attention. The following signs suggest the presence of a serious problem: neck stiffness, altered mental status, focal neurologic abnormalities, visual impairment, and fever. Any patient with meningeal signs requires hospitalization. Keep carbon monoxide exposure and drug withdrawal in mind as etiologic agents.

Chronic headaches should be characterized according to location, quality, and course over time. Head trauma in the past is an important piece of information, raising the suspicion of a subdural hematoma. When the headache is cyclic, with periodic complete resolution, one can comfortably ascribe the headache to a vascular origin. Tension headaches are either variable or relatively constant without relentless progression. Any recurrent or chronic headache that gets worse with time deserves a neurologic evaluation.

Management

Menstrually related migraines are more refractory to the battery of therapy used by neurologists.[62] Early studies of menstrual migraine indicated that administration of estrogen could delay the onset of migraine even if menses were not delayed.[63] Progesterone administration delayed menses, but not the onset of headache. Others have claimed effective treatment of menstrual migraine with maintenance of estrogen levels.[64] Still others have reported success with tamoxifen or danazol treatment. Unfortunately this field suffers from a lack of well-designed, double-blind, placebo-controlled studies, and we must make our judgments based upon experience.

We have had personal success (anecdotal to be sure) alleviating headaches by eliminating the menstrual cycle, either with the use of *daily* oral contraceptives or the daily administration of a progestational agent (such as 10 mg medroxyprogesterone acetate). Some women with migraine headaches have extremely gratifying responses.

If menstrual headaches are a reaction to cyclic changes in circulating levels of the sex steroids, it makes sense to avoid cyclicity and maintain a relatively steady state with daily administration of exogenous hormones. This same approach can be applied to postmenopausal women who experience exacerbation or onset of headaches on a sequential hormone regimen. The maintenance of daily, relatively constant hormone levels with the daily, continuous program of combined estrogen-progestin has been effective in our experience.

The run of the mill headache is treated with mild analgesics such as aspirin, acetaminophen, or the nonsteroidal anti-inflammatory agents. A problem of severe headaches on oral contraception requires an immediate response. The conservative reaction is to discontinue the oral contraceptives. On the other hand, the headache can be due to stress or some other reversible condition. We would argue that automatic discontinuation of oral contraception is not necessary with the low dose preparations. It would be better to evaluate the patient and find out if the patient can continue her contraceptive protection, by discovering an explanation for the headaches. Case-control studies with the old higher dose oral contraceptives indicated that migraine headaches were linked to a risk of stroke. Strokes are essentially no longer seen with low dose oral contraception. This probably reflects both lower dosage as well as the reluctance of clinicians to prescribe oral contraception to women with severe headaches.

True severe vascular headaches (migraine with aura) are an indication to discontinue oral contraception. The symptom complex that deserves serious consideration includes headaches that last a long time; dizziness, nausea, or vomiting with headaches; scotomata or blurred vision; episodes of blindness; unilateral, unremitting headaches; and headaches that continue despite medication.

Concern over headaches with oral contraception should be limited to the use of combined oral contraceptives. The progestin-only methods are not associated with problems with headaches. Therefore, the sustained release progestin-only methods are also free of headache concern.

Catamenial Seizures

Catemenial epilepsy in ancient times was attributed to the moon, giving rise to the word, "lunatic."[65] Epileptic seizures increase in frequency during menstruation and decrease during the luteal phase.[66,67] Exacerbation of seizure activity with menses occurs in 50% of epileptic women.[68] In addition, seizure frequency increases at the time of the midcycle peak in estrogen and during anovulatory cycles. In animal experiments, estrogen increases seizure activity and progesterone is antiepileptic. These observations suggest an antiepileptic effect of progesterone.

Progestational hormones are known to have a sedative effect on the central nervous system. This pharmacologic effect combined with the observations indicating increased seizure activity at times when circulating levels of progesterone are low indicated that treatment with a progestin would have a beneficial impact on seizures.

The administration of oral medroxyprogesterone acetate has little impact, but intramuscular injections of depot-medroxyprogesterone acetate can improve seizure control. Depot-medroxyprogesterone acetate, 150 mg im every 1–2 months, can decrease seizure frequency by approximately 50%.[69] In a case report of an 8 year old girl, 150 mg administered every 2 weeks abolished seizure activity.[68] Intravenous progesterone (producing luteal phase levels) can produce a significant decrease in spike frequency.[70]

Antiepileptic drugs enhance hepatic metabolic activity, and therefore doses must be relatively high. Oral medroxyprogesterone acetate is relatively ineffective, probably because it is difficult to achieve high blood levels.

References

1. **Golub S,** *Periods, from Menarche to Menopause,* Sage Publications, Newbury Park, California, 1992

2. **Rubinow DR,** The premenstrual syndrome: new views, JAMA 268:1908, 1992.

3. **American Psychiatric Association,** *Diagnostic and Statistical Manual of Mental Disorders,* Third edition revised, Washington DC, American Psychiatric Association, 1987.

4. **Logue CM, Moos RH,** Perimenstrual symptoms: prevalence and risk factors, Psychosom Med 48:388, 1986.

5. **Endicott J, Halbreich U,** Retrospective report of premenstrual depressive changes: factors affecting confirmation by daily ratings, Psychopharm Bull 18:109, 1983.

6. **Rubinow DR, Roy-Byrne P,** Premenstrual syndromes: overview from a methodologic perspective, Am J Psychiatr 141:2, 1984.

7. **Sommer B,** The effect of menstruation on cognitive and perceptual-motor behavior: a review, Psychosom Med 35:515, 1973.

8. **Freeman EW, Sondheimer SJ, Rickels K,** Effects of medical history factors on symptom severity in women meeting criteria for premenstrual syndrome, Obstet Gynecol 72:236, 1988.

9. **Wilson CA, Turner CW, Keye WR,** Firstborn adolsescent daughters and mothers with and without premenstrual sydnrome: a comparison, J Adolesc Health 12:130, 1991.

10. **Frank RT,** The hormonal causes of premenstrual tension, Arch Neurol Psychiatr 26:1052, 1931.

11. **Israel SL,** Premenstrual tension, JAMA 110:1721, 1934.

12. **Greene R, Dalton K,** The premenstrual syndrome, Br Med J 1:1007, 1953.

13. **Crawford R,** Superstitions of menstruation, Lancet 2:1331, 1915.

14. **Secundus Plinius C,** *Historia Naturalis,* Translated by Carbondale HP, Southern Illinois Press, 1962.

15. **d'Orban PT,** Medicolegal aspects of the premenstrual syndrome, Br J Hosp Med, December, 1983.

16. **Dalton K,** *The Premenstrual Syndrome and Progesterone Therapy,* 2nd edition, Yearbook Medical Publishers, Inc., Chicago, 1984.

17. **Gannon FL,** Evidence for a psychological etiology of menstrual disorders: a critical review, Psychol Rep 48:287, 1981.

18. **Walsh RM, Budtz-Olsen I, Leader C, Cummins RA,** The menstrual cycle, personality, and academic performance, Arch Gen Psychiatr 38:219, 1981.

19. **Rubinow DR, Schmidt PJ,** Premenstrual sydnrome: a review of endocrine studies, Endocrinologist 2:47, 1992.

20. **Mira M, Stewart PM, Abraham SF,** Vitamin and trace element status in premenstrual syndrome, Am J Clin Nutr 47:636, 1988.

21. **Chuong CJ, Coulam CB, Bergstralh EJ, O'Fallon WM, Steinmetz GI,** Clinical trial of naltrexone in premenstrual syndrome, Obstet Gynecol 72:332, 1988.

22. **Facchinetti F, Martignoni E, Petraglia F, Sances MG, Nappi G, Genazzani AR,** Premenstrual fall of plasma β-endorphin in patients with premenstrual syndrome, Fertil Steril 47:570, 1987.

23. **Tulenheimo A, Laatikainen T, Salminen K,** Plasma β-endorphin immunoreactivity in premenstrual tension, Br J Obstet Gynaecol 94:26, 1987.

24. **Schmidt PJ, Nieman LK, Grover GN, Muller KL, Merriam GR, Rubinow DR,** Lack of effect of induced menses on symptoms in women with premenstrual syndrome, New Engl J Med 324:1174, 1991.

25. **Schmidt PJ, Grover GN, Roy-Byrne PP, Rubinow DR,** Thyroid function in women with premenstrual sydnrome, J Clin Endocrinol Metab 76:671, 1993.

26. **Vellacott ID, Shroff NE, Pearce MY, Stratford ME, Akbar FA,** A double-blind, placebo-controlled evaluation of spironolactone in the premenstrual syndrome, Curr Med Res Opin 10:450, 1987.

27. **Burnet RB, Radden HS, Easterbrook EG, McKinnon RA,** Premenstrual syndrome and spironolactone, Aust NZ J Obstet Gynaecol 31:366, 1991.

28. **Khoo SK, Munro C, Battistutta D,** Evening primrose oil and treatment of premenstrual syndrome, Med J Aust 153:189, 1990.

29. **Collins A, Cerin A, Coleman G, Landgren B-M,** Essential fatty acids in the treatment of premenstrual syndrome, Obstet Gynecol 81:93, 1993.

30. **Puolakka J, Makarainen L, Viinikka L, Ylikorkola O,** Biochemical and clinical effects of treating the premenstrual sydnrome with prostaglandin synthesis precursors, J Reprod Med 30:149, 1985.

31. **Mira M, McNeil D, Fraser IS, Vizzard J, Abraham S,** Mefenamic acid in the treatment of premenstrual syndrome, Obstet Gynecol 68:395, 1986.

32. **Sampson GA,** Premenstrual syndrome: a double-blind controlled trial of progesterone and placebo, Br J Psychiatr 135:209, 1979.

33. **Van der Meer YG, Benedek-Jaszmann LJ, Van Loenen AC,** Effects of high-dose progesterone on the premenstrual sydnrome: a double-blind cross-over trial, J Psychosom Obstet Gynecol 2:220, 1983.

34. **Andersch B, Hahn L,** Progesterone treatment of premenstrual tension — a double blind study, J Psychosom Res 29:489, 1985.

35. **Richter MA, Haltvick R, Shapiro SS,** Progesterone treatment of premenstrual syndrome, Curr Ther Res 36:840, 1984.

36. **Maddocks S, Hahn P, Moller F, Reid RL,** A double-blind placebo-controlled trial of progesterone vaginal suppositories in the treatment of premenstrual syndrome, Am J Obstet Gynecol 154:573, 1986.

37. **Freeman E, Rickels K, Sondheimer SJ, Plansky M,** Ineffectiveness of progesterone suppository treatment for premenstrual syndrome, JAMA 264:349, 1990.

38. **Dennerstein L, Spencer-Gardner C, Gotts G, Brown JB, Smith MA, Burrows GD,** Progesterone and the premenstrual syndrome: a double blind cross-over trial, Br Med J 290:1617, 1985.

39. **Casson P, Hahn PM, Van Vugt DA, Reid RL,** Lasting response to ovariectomy in severe intractable premenstrual syndrome, Am J Obstet Gynecol 162:99, 1990.

40. **Casper RF, Hearn MT,** The effect of hysterectomy and bilateral oophorectomy in women with severe premenstrual syndrome, Am J Obstet Gynecol 162:105, 1990.

41. **Hussain SY, Massil JH, Matta WH, Shaw RW, O'Brien PMS,** Buserelin in premenstrual syndrome, Gynecol Endocrinol 6:57, 1992.

42. **Mortola JF, Girton L, Fischer U,** Successful treatment of severe premenstrual syndrome by combined use of gonadotropin-releasing hormone agonist and estrogen/progestin, J Clin Endocrinol Metab 71:252, 1991.

43. **Stone AB, Pearlstein TB, Brown WA,** Fluoxetine in the treatment of late luteal phase dysphoric disorder, J Clin Psychiatr 52:290, 1991.

44. **Wood SH, Mortola JF, Chan Y-F, Moossazadeh F, Yen SSC,** Treatment of premenstrual sydnrome with fluoxetine: a double-blind, placebo-controlled, crossover study, Obstet Gynecol 80:339, 1992.

45. **Menkes DB, Taghavi E, Mason PA, Spears GFS, Howard RC,** Fluoxetine treatment of severe premenstrual syndrome, Br Med J 305:346, 1992.

46. **Smith S, Rinehart JS, Ruddock VE, Schiff I,** Treatment of premenstrual syndrome with alprazolam: results of a double-blind, placebo-controlled, randomized crossover clinical trial, Obstet Gynecol 70:37, 1987.

47. **Harrison WM, Endicott J, Nee J,** Treatment of premenstrual dysphoria with alprazolam, Arch Gen Psychiatr 47:270, 1990.

48. **Brooks J, Ruble D, Clark A,** College women's attitudes and expectations concerning menstrual-related changes, Psychosom Med 39:288, 1977.

49. **Ruble DN,** Premenstrual symptoms: a reinterpretation, Science 197:291, 1977.

50. **Halbreich U, Endicott J,** Methodological issues in studies of premenstrual changes, Psychoneuroendocrinology 10:15, 1985.

51. **Vila J, Breech HR,** Premenstrual symptomatology: an interaction hypothesis, Br J Soc Clin Psychol 19:73, 1980.

52. **AuBuchon PG, Calhoun KS,** Menstrual cycle symptomatology: the role of social expectancy and experimental demand characteristics, Psychosom Med 47:35, 1985.

53. **Olasov B, Jackson J,** Effects of expectancies on women's reports of moods during the menstrual cycle, Psychosom Med 49:65, 1987.

54. **Cousins N,** *Anatomy of an Illness,* Bantam Books, New York, 1979.

55. **Eisenberg L,** The subjective in medicine, Perspectives Biol Med 27:48, 1983.

56. **Andersch B, Milsom I,** An epidemiologic study of young women with dysmenorrhea, Am J Obstet Gynecol 144:655, 1982.

57. **Coppen A, Kessel N,** Menstruation and personality, Br J Psychiatr 109:771, 1963.

58. **Klein JR, Litt IF,** Epidemiology of adolescent dysmenorrhea, Pediatrics 68:661, 1981.

59. **Dawood MY,** editor, *Dysmenorrhea,* Williams & Wilkins, Baltimore, 1981.

60. **Owens PR,** Prostaglandin synthetase inhibitors in the treatment of primary dysmenorrhea: outcome trials reviewed, Am J Obstet Gynecol 148:96, 1984.

61. **Nattero G,** Menstrual headache, Adv Neurol 33:215, 1982.

62. **Sheftell FD, Silberstein SD, Rapoport AM, Rossum RW,** Migraine and women: diagnosis, pathophysiology, and treatment, J Women's Health 1:5, 1992.

63. **Somerville BW,** Estrogen-withdrawal migraine. II. Attempted prophylaxis by continuous estradiol administration, Neurology 25:245, 1975.

64. **DeLignieres B, Vincens M, Mauvais-Jarvis P, Mas JL, Touboul PJ, Bousser MG,** Prevention of menstrual migraine by percutaneous oestradiol, Br Med J 193:1540, 1986.

65. **Newmark ME, Penry JK,** Catamenial epilepsy: a review, Epilepsia 21:281, 1980.

66. **Backstrom T,** Epileptic seizures in women related to plasma estrogen and progesterone during the menstrual cycle, Acta Neurol Scand 54:321, 1976.

67. **Mattson RH, Kamer JA, Cramer JA, Caldwell BV,** Seizure frequency and the menstrual cycle: a clinical study, Epilepsia 22:242, 1981.

68. **Zimmerman AW, Holden KR, Reiter EO, Dekaban AS,** Medroxyprogesterone acetate in the treatment of seizures associated with menstruation, J Pediatr 83:959, 1973.

69. **Mattson RH, Cramer JA, Caldwell BV, Siconolfi BC,** Treatment of seizures with medroxyprogesterone aceate: preliminary report, Neurology 34:1255, 1984.

70. **Backstrom T, Zetterlund B, Blom S, Romano M,** Effects of intravenous progesterone infusions on the epileptic discharge frequency in women with partial epilepsy, Acta Neurol Scand 69:240, 1984.

16 Dysfunctional Uterine Bleeding

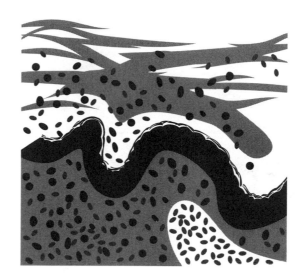

Dysfunctional uterine bleeding is defined as a variety of bleeding manifestations of anovulatory cycles (in the absence of pathology or medical illness). It can be confidently managed without surgical intervention by therapeutic regimens founded on sound physiologic principles. Our formulation is based on knowledge of how the postovulatory menstrual function is naturally controlled, and utilizes pharmacologic application of sex steroids to reverse the abnormal tissue factors that lead to the excessive and prolonged flow typical of anovulatory cycles.

Three major categories of dysfunctional endometrial bleeding are dealt with:

1. Estrogen breakthrough bleeding,

2. Estrogen withdrawal bleeding, and

3. Progestin breakthrough bleeding.

In each instance, the manner in which the endometrium deviates from the norm is characterized, and specific steroid therapy is recommended to counter the difficulties each situation presents.

This mode of clinical management has been in regular use for many years, and failure to control vaginal bleeding with this therapy, despite appropriate application and utilization, excludes the diagnosis of dysfunctional uterine bleeding. If this occurs, attention is directed to a pathologic entity within the reproductive tract as the cause of abnormal bleeding.

Length of Menstrual Cycles

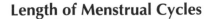
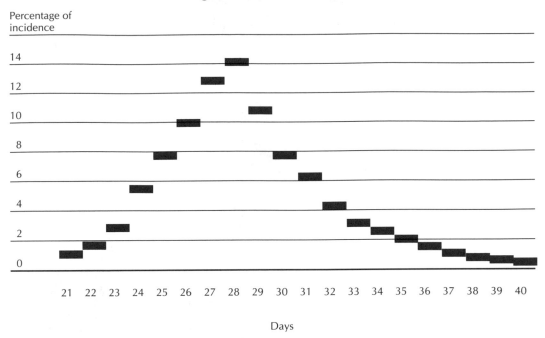

Days

Normal Withdrawal (Menstrual) Bleeding

Of all the types of hormonal-endometrial relationships, the most stable endometrium and the most reproducible menstrual function in terms of quantity and duration occurs with postovulatory estrogen-progesterone withdrawal bleeding. It is so controlling that many women over the years come to expect a certain characteristic flow pattern. Any slight deviations, such as plus or minus 1 day in duration or minor deviation from expected napkin or tampon utilization, are causes for major concern in the patient. So ingrained is the expected flow that considerable physician reassurance may be required in some instances of minor variability. The usual duration of flow is 4–6 days, but many women flow as little as 2 days, and as much as 8 days. The normal volume of menstrual blood loss is 30 mL.[1] Greater than 80 mL is abnormal. Most of the blood loss occurs during the first 3 days of a period, so excessive flow may exist without prolongation of flow.[2,3]

While the postovulatory phase averages 14 days, greater variability in the proliferative phase produces a distribution in the duration of a menstrual cycle. Based on the normal experience, menstrual bleeding more often than every 24 days or less often than every 35 days deserves evaluation. Flow which lasts 7 or more days also deserves evaluation. A flow that totals more than 80 mL per month usually leads to anemia and should be treated.[4,5] In general, however, an effort to quantitate menstrual flow beyond historical information is not necessary because evaluation and treatment are responses to a patient's own perceptions regarding duration, amount, and timing of her menstrual bleeding. Midcycle bleeding can be a consequence of the preovulatory fall in estrogen; however, intermenstrual bleeding is often due to pathology.

The histologic changes in the endometrium of a normal, ovulatory menstrual cycle have been detailed in Chapter 4. An understanding of these events provides the foundation and framework to understand abnormal endometrial bleeding. There are three reasons for the self-limited character of estrogen-progesterone withdrawal bleeding.

1. *It is a universal endometrial event.* Because the onset and conclusion of menses are related to a precise sequence of hormonal events, menstrual changes occur almost simultaneously in all segments of the endometrium.

2. ***The endometrial tissue which has responded to an appropriate sequence of estrogen and progesterone is structurally stable, and random breakdown of tissue due to fragility is avoided.*** The events leading to ischemic disintegration of the endometrium are orderly and progressive, being related to rhythmic waves of vasoconstriction of increasing duration.

3. ***Inherent in the events that start menstrual function following estrogen-progesterone are the factors involved in stopping menstrual flow.*** Just as waves of vasoconstriction initiate the ischemic events, prolonged vasoconstriction abetted by the stasis associated with endometrial collapse enables clotting factors to seal off the exposed bleeding sites. Additional and significant effects are obtained by resumed estrogen activity.

Platelets and fibrin play a direct part in the hemostasis achieved in a bleeding menstrual endometrium. Deficiencies in these constituents cause the increased blood loss seen in von Willebrand's disease and in thrombocytopenia. The blood loss at menses in afibrinogenemia indicates the importance of fibrin-generating and fibrinolytic factors in the menstrual process. Intravascular thrombi are observed in the functional layers and are localized to the shedding surface of the tissue. These are known as impeding "plugs" in that blood may flow past these only partially occlusive barriers. Therefore, thrombi continue to develop within the menstrual blood, accounting for the platelets and large amounts of fibrin found in this effluent. Fibrinolysis occurs in the endometrial tissue, limiting fibrin deposition in the proximal, still unshed layer. Despite large holes in vessel walls, with blood exposed to collagen surfaces, no occlusive surface thrombus is formed. After early dependence on thrombin plugs to restrain blood loss, later generalized vasoconstrictive hemostasis without thrombin plugs occur. The healing endometrium is pale, collapsed, and disorderly, but no thrombi and no fibrin deposits are seen.

The mechanisms of tissue breakdown, as well as clearance of debris and restructuring of the endometrium, are thought to proceed via sex steroid effects on the endometrial cell lysosomes. With reduced steroids, lysosomal membrane destabilization and leakage of lysosomal prostaglandin synthetase enzymes, proteases, and collagenases occur. These cause breakdown of endometrial structures, dissolution of ground substance and cell walls, and vasoconstriction. Further "liquefaction" permits efficient absorption and possible recycling of protein components.

Traditional Definitions

Oligomenorrhea — Intervals greater than 35 days.
Polymenorrhea — Intervals less than 21 days.
Menorrhagia — Regular normal intervals, excessive flow and duration.
Metrorrhagia — Irregular intervals, excessive flow and duration.

Endometrial Responses to Steroid Hormones: Physiologic and Pharmacologic

Obviously estrogen and progesterone withdrawal is not the only type of endometrial bleeding provoked by the presence of sex steroids and their effects on the endometrium. There are clinical examples for estrogen withdrawal bleeding and estrogen breakthrough bleeding, as well as for progesterone withdrawal and breakthrough bleeding.

Estrogen Withdrawal Bleeding

This category of uterine bleeding can occur after bilateral oophorectomy, radiation of mature follicles, or administration of estrogen to a castrate and then discontinuation of therapy. Similarly, the bleeding that occurs postcastration can be delayed by concomitant estrogen therapy. Flow will occur on discontinuation of exogenous estrogen. Midcycle bleeding can occur secondary to the decrease in estrogen which immediately precedes ovulation.

Estrogen Breakthrough Bleeding

Here a semiquantitative relationship exists between the amount of estrogen stimulating the endometrium and the type of bleeding that can ensue. Relatively low doses of estrogen yield intermittent spotting that may be prolonged, but is generally light in quantity of flow. On the other hand, high levels of estrogen and sustained availability lead to prolonged periods of amenorrhea followed by acute, often profuse bleeds with excessive loss of blood.

Progesterone Withdrawal Bleeding

Removal of the corpus luteum will lead to endometrial desquamation. Pharmacologically, a similar event can be achieved by administration and discontinuation of progesterone or a nonestrogenic synthetic progestin. Progesterone withdrawal bleeding occurs only if the endometrium is initially proliferated by endogenous or exogenous estrogen. If estrogen therapy is continued as progesterone is withdrawn, the progesterone withdrawal bleeding still occurs. Only if estrogen levels are increased 10–20-fold will progesterone withdrawal bleeding be delayed.[6]

Progesterone Breakthrough Bleeding

Progesterone breakthrough bleeding occurs only in the presence of an unfavorably high ratio of progesterone to estrogen. In the absence of sufficient estrogen, continuous progesterone therapy will yield intermittent bleeding of variable duration, similar to low dose estrogen breakthrough bleeding noted above. This is the type of bleeding associated with the long-acting progestin-only contraceptive methods, Norplant and Depo-Provera.

Hyperplasia vs. Neoplasia

Ferenczy argues that there are two separate and biologically unrelated diseases: hyperplasia and neoplasia.[7] He suggests that all hyperplasia without atypia be referred to as *endometrial hyperplasia*, and this is usually not a precursor of carcinoma. He further proposes that lesions with cytologic atypia be referred to as *endometrial intraepithelial neoplasia (EIN)*. In these cases, persistence after multiple curettings or high dose progestin therapy is approximately 75%. EIN would replace the following terms: atypical adenomatous hyperplasia and carcinoma in situ of the endometrium. This lesion is characterized by nuclear atypia of the cells lining the endometrial glands (enlargement, rounding, and pleomorphism of the nuclei with aneuploid DNA content). Invasive carcinoma is distinguished from EIN by stromal invasion.

EIN is best treated surgically! If future pregnancy is desired, daily progestin therapy (30 mg medroxyprogesterone acetate daily) should be followed by repeat endometrial aspiration curettage in 3–4 months. If EIN is still present, the choice is between surgery and high dose progestin (200 mg medroxyprogesterone acetate daily, 500 mg megestrol acetate biweekly, or depot medroxyprogesterone acetate 1,000 mg weekly) with repeat biopsy surveillance.

The benign lesions include all of the following traditional interpretations: anovulatory, proliferative, cystic glandular hyperplasia, simple hyperplasia, adenomatous hyperplasia without atypia. These lesions are basically the same (perhaps exaggerations at most) as preovulatory, proliferative endometrium. This hyperplasia regresses spontaneously, after curettage, or with hormonal treatment.[8,9] *This argument is an important one: benign lesions can be treated hormonally. With one exception, only the presence of cytonuclear atypia should raise immediate and serious concern for progression to cancer. The exception is the patient with an apparently benign lesion which does not respond to progestin therapy. Was the diagnosis accurate? Will clinical data eventually indicate that this type of patient is also at higher risk for progression?*

Suggestions for Why Anovulatory Bleeding Is Excessive

Most instances of anovulatory bleeding are examples of estrogen withdrawal or estrogen breakthrough bleeding. The heaviest bleeding is secondary to high sustained levels of estrogen associated with polycystic ovaries, obesity, immaturity of the hypothalamic-pituitary-ovarian axis as in postpubertal teenagers, and late anovulation, usually involving women in their late 30s and early 40s. In the absence of growth limiting progesterone and periodic desquamation, the endometrium attains an abnormal height without concomitant structural support. The tissue increasingly displays intense vascularity, back to back glandularity, but without an intervening stromal support matrix. This tissue is fragile and will suffer spontaneous superficial breakage and bleeding. As one site heals, another, and yet another new site of breakdown will appear. The typical clinical picture is that of a pale frightened teenager who has bled for weeks. Also frequently encountered is the older woman with prolonged bleeding who is deeply concerned over this experience as a manifestation of cancer.

In these instances the usual endometrial control mechanisms are missing. This bleeding is not a universal event, but rather it involves random portions of the endometrium at variable times and in asynchronous sequences. The fragility of the vascular adenomatous hyperplastic tissue is responsible for this experience, in part because of excessive growth, but mostly because of irregular stimulation in which the structural rigidity of a well-developed stroma or stratum compactum does not occur. Finally, the flow is prolonged and excessive not only because there is a large quantity of tissue available for bleeding, but more importantly because there is a disorderly, abrupt, random, breakdown of tissue with consequent opening of multiple vascular channels. There is no vasoconstrictive rhythmicity, no tight coiling of spiral vessels, no orderly collapse to induce stasis. The anovulatory tissue can only rely on the "healing" effects of endogenous estrogen to stop local bleeds. However, this is a vicious cycle in that this healing is only temporary. As quickly as it rebuilds, tissue fragility and breakdown recur at other endometrial sites.

Alternate Hypothesis

Another explanation for the control of postovulatory endometrial bleeding and regeneration has been presented.[10] Based on light and scanning electron microscopy of hysterectomy specimens, this thesis favors nonhormone-related regeneration of surface epithelium from basal glands and cornual area residual tissue with restoration of the continuous binding membrane as the critical events in cessation of blood flow. Endometrial regeneration is viewed as a response to tissue loss, not hormonal changes. By this account, estrogen withdrawal or breakthrough bleeding is uncontrolled because there is insufficient stimulus (loss of tissue) for binding surface restoration to occur. Furthermore, curettage is effective in this condition by reachieving sufficient basal glandular denudation (as is seen also in combined estrogen and progestin withdrawal) which stimulates regeneration of surface integrity and thus controls blood flow.

Additional studies are needed to clarify the difference of opinion concerning the pathophysiology of dysfunctional uterine bleeding. Our therapeutic approach favored in this book utilizes hormonal control of endometrial events and rarely finds it necessary to resort to surgery.

Differential Diagnosis

Dysfunctional uterine bleeding is a diagnosis made by exclusion. A very common cause of abnormal uterine bleeding is pregnancy and pregnancy-related problems such as ectopic pregnancy or spontaneous abortion. This category of problems should always receive diagnostic consideration. Patients may be using medications unknowingly with an impact on the endometrium. For example, the use of ginseng, an herbal root, has been associated with estrogenic activity and abnormal bleeding.[11] Pathology of the menstrual outflow tract includes cancers of the cervix and endometrium, endometrial polyps, and leiomyomata uteri. While uterine bleeding is a common problem with various contraceptive methods and postmenopausal hormonal therapy, the clinician should always be confident no pathology is present. Abnormal menstrual cycles are occasionally the first sign of either hypothyroidism or hyperthyroidism. One should keep in mind that as many as 20% of adolescents with dysfunctional uterine bleeding will have a coagulation defect, although the most common cause is anovulation.[12] Bleeding secondary to a blood dyscrasia is usually a heavy flow with regular, cyclic menses (menorrhagia), and this same pattern can be seen in patients being treated with anticoagulants.[13] Irregular, serious bleeding is often associated with severe organ disease, such as renal failure and liver failure. Finally, careful examination is worthwhile to discover genital injury or a foreign object.

The effects of tubal ligation are still not certain. The first well-controlled studies of this issue demonstrated no change in menstrual patterns, volume, or pain.[14,15] Subsequently, these same authors reported an increase in dysmenorrhea and changes in menstrual bleeding.[16,17] However, these authors failed to agree in their findings (a change found by one group was not confirmed by the other). Adding to the confusion, the incidence of hysterectomy for bleeding disorders in women after tubal sterilization was reported to be increased by some,[18] but not by others.[19] In a large cohort of women in a group health plan, hospitalization for menstrual disorders was significantly increased; however, the authors believed this reflected bias by patient and physician preference for surgical treatment.[20] It is possible that extensive electrocoagulation of the fallopian tubes can change ovarian steroid production. Perhaps this is why menstrual changes have been detected with longer (4 years) follow-up, while no changes have been noted with the use of rings or clips.[17,21,22] However, attempts to relate poststerilization menstrual changes with extent of tissue destruction fail to find a correlation, and an increase in hospitalization for menstrual disorders after unipolar cautery cannot be documented.[20,22] Still another long-term follow-up study (3–4.5 years) failed to document any significant changes in menstrual cycles.[23] This inconsistency can reflect differences in sterilization techniques, as well as the fact that a surgical solution is more likely to be chosen if continuing fertility is no longer an issue. The best answer for now is that some women experience menstrual changes, but most do not.

Treatment Program for Anovulatory Bleeding

The immediate objective of medical therapy in anovulatory bleeding is to retrieve the natural controlling influences missing in this tissue: universal, synchronous endometrial events, structural stability, and vasomotor rhythmicity.

Progestin Therapy

Most women will, at sometime during their reproductive years, either fail to ovulate or not sustain adequate corpus luteum function or duration. But this occurs with increased frequency in adolescence and in the decade prior to menopause. The usual clinical presentation is oligomenorrhea with bouts of heavy bleeding. Women correctly seek medical advice promptly because these menstrual aberrations suggest unplanned pregnancy or uterine pathology. Therefore, it is uncommon to find significant blood loss or excessive tissue proliferation in these women. Under most circumstances, progestin therapy will suffice to control the abnormality once uterine pathology is ruled out.

Progesterone and progestins are powerful antiestrogens when given in pharmacologic doses. Progestins stimulate 17β-hydroxysteroid dehydrogenase and sulfotransferase activity, which convert estradiol to estrone sulfate (which is rapidly excreted from the cell).[24] Progestins also diminish estrogen effects on target cells by inhibiting the augmentation of estrogen receptors that ordinarily accompanies estrogen action (receptor replenishment inhibition). In addition, progestins suppress estrogen-mediated transcription of oncogenes.[25] These influences account for the antimitotic, antigrowth impact of progestins on the endometrium (prevention and reversal of hyperplasia, limitation of growth postovulation, and the marked atrophy during pregnancy or in response to combined oral contraceptives).

In the treatment of oligomenorrhea, orderly limited withdrawal bleeding can be accomplished by administration of a progestin such as medroxyprogesterone acetate, 10 mg daily for 10 days every month. Absence of induced bleeding requires workup. In the treatment of dysfunctional menometrorrhagia or polymenorrhea, progestins are prescribed for 10 days to 2 weeks (to induce stabilizing predecidual stromal changes) followed by a withdrawal flow — the so-called "medical curettage." Thereafter, repeat progestin is offered cyclically the first 10 days of each month to ensure therapeutic effect. Failure of progestin to correct irregular bleeding requires diagnostic reevaluation. ***If contraception is desired, the use of an oral contraceptive is a better choice.***

Oral Contraceptive Therapy

In young women, anovulatory bleeding may be associated with prolonged endometrial buildup, delayed diagnosis, and heavy blood loss. In these cases, combined estrogen-progestin therapy is used in the form of oral contraceptives. Any of the low dose oral combination monophasic tablets are useful. Whatever formulation is available or chosen, therapy is administered as one pill twice a day for 5–7 days. This therapy is maintained despite cessation of flow within 12–24 hours. If flow does not abate, other diagnostic possibilities (polyps, incomplete abortion, and neoplasia) should be reevaluated.

If flow does diminish rapidly, the remainder of the week of treatment can be given over to the evaluation of causes of anovulation, investigation of hemorrhagic tendencies, and blood replacement or initiation of iron therapy. In addition, the week provides time to prepare the patient for the estrogen-progestin withdrawal flow that will soon be induced. For the moment, therapy has produced the structural rigidity intrinsic to the compact pseudodecidual reaction. Continued random breakdown of formerly fragile tissue is avoided and blood loss stopped. However, a large amount of tissue remains to react to estrogen-progestin withdrawal. The patient must be warned to anticipate a heavy and severely cramping flow 2–4 days after stopping therapy. If not prepared in this way, it

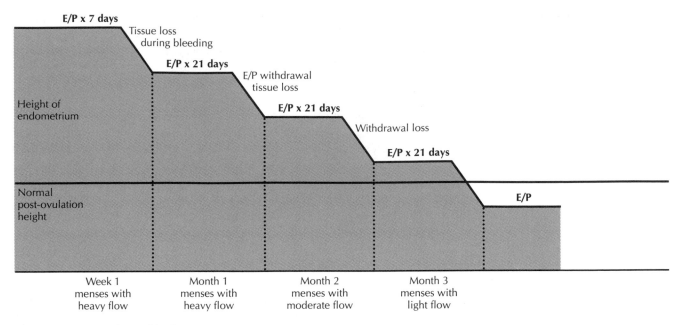

E/P = Estrogen-Progestin combination

is certain that the patient will view the problem as recurrent disease or failure of hormonal therapy.

In successful therapy, on the 5th day of flow, a low dose combination oral contraceptive medication (one pill a day) is started. This will be repeated for several (usually three) 3-week treatments, punctuated by 1-week withdrawal flow intervals. A decrease in volume and pain with each successive cycle is reassuring. Birth control pills reduce menstrual flow by at least 60% in normal uteri.[26] Early application of the estrogen-progestin combination limits growth and allows orderly regression of excessive endometrial height to normal controllable levels. If the estrogen-progestin combination is not applied, abnormal endometrial height and persistent excessive flow will recur.

In the patient not requiring contraception, in whom cyclic estrogen-progestin for 3 months has reduced endometrial tissue to normal height, the oral contraceptive can be discontinued and unopposed endogenous estrogen permitted to reactivate the endometrium. In the absence of spontaneous menses, the recurrence of the anovulatory state is suspected, and a brief preemptive course of an orally active progestin is administered to counter endometrial proliferation. Once pregnancy is ruled out, medroxyprogesterone acetate, 10 mg orally daily for 10 days, is given monthly. Reasonable flow (progestin withdrawal flow) will occur 2–7 days after the last pill. With this therapy, excessive endometrial buildup is avoided, and an increased risk of endometrial and possibly breast cancer is avoided. If contraception is desired, routine use of oral contraception is warranted and will also be of prophylactic value.

Estrogen Therapy

Intermittent vaginal spotting is frequently associated with minimal (low) estrogen stimulation (estrogen breakthrough bleeding). In this circumstance, where minimal endometrium exists, the beneficial effect of progestin treatment is not achieved, because there is insufficient tissue on which the progestin can exert action. A similar circumstance also exists in the younger anovulatory patient in whom prolonged hemorrhagic desquamation leaves little residual tissue.

In these circumstances, when bleeding is acute and heavy, high dose estrogen therapy is applied using as much as 25 mg conjugated estrogens intravenously every 4 hours until bleeding abates or for 12 hours.[27] Decreased bleeding is the sign that the "healing" events are initiated to a sufficient degree. The mechanism of action for estrogen is believed to be a stimulus to clotting at the capillary level.[28] Progestin treatment (usually an oral contraceptive) is started at the same time. Where bleeding is less, lower oral doses of estrogen (1.25 mg of conjugated estrogens or 2.0 mg estradiol daily for 7–10 days) can be prescribed initially. When bleeding is moderately heavy, a more intensive oral program can be utilized, 1.25 mg conjugated estrogens or 2 mg estradiol every 4 hours for 24 hours, followed by the single daily dose for 7–10 days. All estrogen therapy must be followed by progestin coverage and a withdrawal bleed; continuing treatment with a low dose oral contraceptive is recommended.

Estrogen therapy is also useful in two examples of problems associated with progestin breakthrough bleeding. These are the breakthrough bleeding episodes occurring with use of oral contraception or with depot forms of progestational agents. In the absence of sufficient endogenous and exogenous estrogen, the endometrium shrinks by pharmacologically induced pseudoatrophy. Furthermore, it is composed almost exclusively of pseudodecidual stroma and blood vessels with minimal glands. Peculiarly, experience has shown that this type of endometrium also leads to the fragility bleeding more typical of pure estrogen stimulation.

The usual clinical story is a patient on long-standing oral contraception who, after experiencing marked diminution or absence of withdrawal flow in the pill free interval, begins to see breakthrough bleeding while on medication. Conjugated estrogens 1.25 mg or estradiol 2.0 mg daily for 7 days during, and in addition to, the usual birth control pill administration is useful. This rejuvenates the endometrium and intermenstrual flow stops. Another frequently encountered problem is the progestin breakthrough bleeding experienced with chronic depot administration of progestin (Depo-Provera). This therapy is used not only for contraception, but also in the treatment of endometriosis and the prevention of menses during chemotherapy. In 75% of recipients, continuous therapy is not associated with abnormal menstrual bleeding. In the remainder, breakthrough progestin bleeding occurs. Judicious use of estrogen is the appropriate and effective therapy in these instances.

Bleeding problems are common with Norplant, another example of the effect of persistent progestational influence on the endometium. Patients who can no longer tolerate prolonged bleeding will benefit from a short course of oral estrogen as above.[29]

The Risk Associated with Estrogen Therapy
There is concern that high doses of estrogen could precipitate a thrombotic event. More than one oral contraceptive per day and multiple doses of oral or intravenous estrogen in a 24-hour period certainly should be regarded as high doses. There are no data available, however, to verify or quantitate any risk associated with this use of hormonal therapy. This treatment must be chosen by clinician and patient after weighing the risk-benefit considerations which surround the uterine bleeding problem. As a matter of clinical judgment and prudent practice, lower doses can be used in patients with lifestyle or medical history consistent with an increased risk of vascular complications.

The Use of Antiprostaglandins

There seems little doubt that prostaglandins (PG) have important actions on the endometrial vasculature and presumably on endometrial hemostasis. The concentrations of PGE_2 and $PGF_{2\alpha}$ increase progressively in human endometrium during the menstrual cycle, and nonsteroidal eicosanoid synthesis inhibitors decrease menstrual blood loss perhaps by also altering the balance between the platelet proaggregating vasoconstrictor thromboxane A_2 (TXA_2) and the antiaggregating vasodilator prostacyclin (PGI_2).[30] Excessive bleeding in women with menorrhagia can be reduced by approximately 40–

50%.[31] In a comparison study of ovulating women with menorrhagia, treatment during menses with a prostaglandin synthetase inhibitor was no more effective than high dose progestin supplementation during the 7 days preceding menstruation, but both treatments were effective.[32] Occasionally a woman will demonstrate, for unknown reasons, an anomalous response to this treatment, with an increase in menstrual bleeding.[33] A study of postoperative surgical specimens after mefenamic acid treatment revealed evidence of vasoconstriction and improved platelet aggregation.[34]

Whatever the exact mechanism, prostaglandin synthetase inhibitors diminish menstrual bleeding in normal women as well as in the bleeding secondary to intrauterine device (IUD) use. This approach should be considered as a first line of defense in the absence of pathology in those women who are ovulatory but bleed heavily. Side effects are unusual because treatment is limited, usually beginning with the onset of bleeding and continuing for 3–4 days. This treatment will also relieve the other symptoms of menstrual molimina.

Treatment with a Progestin IUD

The delivery of a progestational agent directly to the endometrium in a local fashion is possible with an intrauterine device which releases progesterone or levonorgestrel.[35,36] In a comparison trial with a prostaglandin synthetase inhibitor and an antifibrinolytic agent, the levonorgestrel-releasing IUD outperformed the medical treatment dramatically.[36] The reduction in menstrual flow reached 96% after 12 months, and some patients even become amenorrheic. This is an attractive option in patients with intractable bleeding associated with chronic illnesses (such as renal failure).

Treatment with GnRH Agonists

Treatment with a GnRH agonist can achieve short-term relief from a bleeding problem, for example, in a patient with renal failure or a blood dyscrasia. This choice is a good one for patients who experience menstrual bleeding problems after organ transplantation (especially after liver transplantation) where the toxicity of immunosuppressive drugs makes the use of sex steroids less desirable. However, the expense and long-term side effects make this an unlikely choice for chronic therapy. If long-term GnRH agonist therapy is chosen, after gonadal suppression is achieved (2–4 weeks), we recommend add-back treatment with a daily combination of 0.625 mg conjugated estrogens or 1.0 mg estradiol and 2.5 mg medroxyprogesterone acetate or 0.35 mg norethindrone.

Treatment with Desmopressin

Desmopressin is a synthetic analog of arginine vasopressin. It has been used to treat abnormal uterine bleeding in patients with coagulation disorders.[37] It can be administered intranasally, but the intravenous route (0.3 μg/kg diluted in 50 mL saline and administered over 15–30 minutes) is more effective. Treatment is followed by a rapid increase in coagulation factor VIII which lasts approximately 6 hours. This treatment should be regarded as a last resort for selected patients with coagulation problems.

Ablation of the Endometrium

Persistent bleeding despite treatment is both aggravating and concerning. Hysterectomy is an appropriate choice for some of these patients. Others would prefer to avoid a major operation, and still others have conditions that make major surgery a high risk procedure. Patients and clinicians should consider the option of endometrial ablation. Ablation of the endometrium can be accomplished with either a laser, a resectoscope with a loop or rolling ball electrode, or radio frequency-induced thermal destruction. Success with these methods is not 100%. Approximately 90% of women with menorrhagia will have an improvement following an ablation procedure; only 50% will become amenorrheic.[38,39] The best results are obtained if the endometrium is first suppressed for 4–6 weeks with either a high dose of a progestin, GnRH agonist treatment, or danazol. Caution must be exercised regarding the possiblity of excessive absorption of irrigating fluid with subsequent fluid overload.

There is concern that obliteration of segments of the uterine cavity can allow isolated, residual endometrium to progress to carcinoma without recognition. Long-term follow-up will be necessary before we know if this is a real risk.

Summary of Key Points in Therapy of Anovulatory (Dysfunctional) Bleeding

Teenager	Adult
Preliminary:	*Preliminary:*
Pelvic or rectal examination	Pelvic examination
	PAP smear
	Endometrial biopsy

1. Intense estrogen-progestin therapy for 7 days.

2. Cyclic low dose oral contraceptive for 3 months.

3. If contraception is desired, continue oral contraception.

4. If contraception is not desired, medroxyprogesterone acetate, 10 mg daily for 10 days every month.

If bleeding has been prolonged, if biopsy yields minimal tissue, if the patient is on progestin medication, if follow-up is uncertain:

Conjugated estrogens (1.25 mg) or estradiol (2.0 mg) daily for 7–10 days, followed by the daily estrogen combined with 10 mg medroxyprogesterone acetate for 7 days. If acute bleeding is moderately heavy, the oral estrogen dose can be administered every 4 hours during the first 24 hours. For very heavy, acute bleeding, conjugated estrogens, 25 mg intravenously every 4 hours until bleeding stops or significantly slows, then proceed to Step 1 above. If no response in 12–24 hours, proceed to D and C.

The clinical problem of dysfunctional bleeding is associated with either anovulation and estrogen withdrawal or breakthrough bleeding, or with anovulation caused by exogenous progestin medication and bleeding due to progestational endometrial breakthrough. These categories of bleeding lack the three important characteristics of normal estrogen-progesterone withdrawal bleeding:

1. Universal, simultaneous change in all segments of the endometrium.

2. An orderly progression of events involving a rigid, compact structure.

3. Vasomotor rhythmicity with vasoconstriction, structural collapse, and clotting.

Questioning should be directed by the differential diagnosis of abnormal uterine bleeding. Clues to the diagnosis may be apparent on physical examination, such as hirsutism, acne, galactorrhea, thyroid enlargement, evidence of an eating disorder, bruises, and, of course, abnormalities on examination of the pelvis. Brown, dark colored bleeding is often secondary to obstruction in a müllerian anomaly. Laboratory tests which are often helpful (but not always necessary) are coagulation studies (prothrombin time, partial thromboplastin time, platelet count, bleeding time), quantitative human chorionic gonadotropin (HCG), prolactin, thyroid function tests, liver function tests, and appropriate cervical cultures.

Office aspiration biopsy of the endometrium should always be performed in patients considered to be at high risk for endometrial hyperplasia and cancer. Texts and review articles continue to emphasize that endometrial biopsy is in order if the patient is older; e.g., greater than 35 or 40 years old. *It is not the age of the patient that is critical; it is the duration of exposure to unopposed estrogen. Women in their 20s and even teenagers can develop endometrial cancer.*[40] The small flexible suction cannulas are preferred for greater patient comfort, and results are comparable to the older, traditional methods.[41–43] Office hysteroscopy is also useful for the direction of biopsies and the detection of polyps and submucous myomas.

Therapy involves an initial choice between intensive estrogen-progestin combination medication or relatively high doses of estrogen. The estrogen-progestin combination will be ineffective unless endometrium of sufficient quantity and responsiveness to allow the formation of pseudodecidual tissue is present. Therefore, the initial choice of therapy should be estrogen in the following situations:

1. When bleeding has been heavy for many days and it is likely that the uterine cavity is now lined only by a raw basalis layer.

2. When the endometrial curet yields minimal tissue.

3. When the patient has been on progestin medication (oral contraceptives, intramuscular progestins) and the endometrium is shallow and atrophic.

4. When follow-up is uncertain, because estrogen therapy will temporarily stop all categories of dysfunctional bleeding.

If estrogen therapy does not significantly abate flow within 12–24 hours, reevaluation is mandatory, and the need for curettage is likely. It is believed that patients with coagulation disorders respond better if the uterine cavity is first evacuated with a suction curet.

Once the acute bleeding episode in an anovulatory patient is under control, the patient should not be forgotten. With persistent anovulation, recurrent hemorrhage is a common pattern, and, more importantly, chronic unopposed estrogen stimulation to the endometrium can eventually lead to atypical tissue changes. It is absolutely necessary that the patient undergo periodic progestational withdrawal either with a routine oral contraceptive regimen or if contraception is not desired, a progestational agent (medroxyprogesterone acetate, 10 mg daily for 10 days) should be administered every month.

Curettage is *not* the first line of defense, but rather the last. The utilization of appropriate steroids for the clinical management of dysfunctional bleeding is based upon a physiologic understanding of the endometrium and its responses to hormones. Adherence to this program will avoid D and C except in a rare case of dysfunctional bleeding and except in those cases where bleeding is due to a pathologic entity within the reproductive tract where D and C is truly indicated and necessary.

If a patient has recurrent bleeding despite repeated medical therapy, submucous myomas or endometrial polyps must be suspected. Thorough curettage can miss such pathology, and further diagnostic study can be helpful. Either hysterosalpingography with slow instillation of dye and careful fluoroscopic examination or hysteroscopy may reveal a myoma or polyp; hysteroscopy can also direct a more accurate biopsy of the endometrium.[44,45] A pathologic problem such as this should especially be suspected in the puzzling case of the patient who has abnormal bleeding and ovulatory cycles.

Patients who are ovulating but have a heavy menstrual flow (menorrhagia) can be effectively treated with prostaglandin inhibitors, progestins administered daily for the 7 days preceding menses, or oral contraceptives in the routine manner. If contraception is not required, we prefer the use of one of the fenamate prostaglandin inhibitors (which block both synthesis and prostaglandin receptors). The IUD which releases progesterone or a progestin should be considered in patients with chronic illnesses.

References

1. **Hallberg L, Hogdahl A, Nilsson L, Rybo G,** Menstrual blood loss — a population study, Acta Obstet Gynecol Scand 45:320, 1966.

2. **Rybo G,** Menstrual blood loss in relation to parity and menstrual pattern, Acta Obstet Gynecol Scand 45:119, 1966.

3. **Haynes PJ, Hodgson H, Anderson ABM, Turnbull AC,** Measurement of menstrual blood loss in patients complaining of menorrhagia, Br J Obstet Gynaecol 84:763, 1977.

4. **Higham JM, O'Brien PMS, Shaw RM,** Assessment of menstrual blood loss using a pictorial chart, Br J Obstet Gynaecol 97:734, 1990.

5. **Cohen BJB, Gibor J,** Anemia and menstrual blood loss, Obstet Gynecol Survey 35:597, 1980.

6. **de Ziegler D, Bergeron C, Cornel C, Medalie A, Massai MR, Milgrom E, Frydman R, Bouchard P,** Effects of luteal estradiol on the secretory transformation of human endometrium and plasma gonadotropins, J Clin Endocrinol Metab 74:322, 1992.

7. **Ferenczy A, Gelfand MM, Tzipris F,** The cytodynamics of endometrial hyperplasia and carcinoma, a review, Ann Pathol 3:189, 1983.

8. **Kurman RJ, Kaminski PT, Norris HJ,** The behavior of endometrial hyperplasia. A long-term study of "untreated" hyperplasia in 170 patients, Cancer 56:403, 1985.

9. **Ferenczy A, Gelfand M,** The biologic significance of cytologic atypia in progestogen-treated endometrial hyperplasia, Am J Obstet Gynecol 160:126, 1989.

10. **Ferenczy A,** Studies on the cytodynamics of human endometrial regeneration. I. Scanning electron microscopy, Am J Obstet Gynecol 124:64, 1976.

11. **Hopkins MP, Androff L, Benninghoff AS,** Ginseng face cream and unexplained vaginal bleeding, Am J Obstet Gynecol 159:1121, 1988.

12. **Claessens EA, Cowell CL,** Acute adolescent menorrhagia, Am J Obstet Gynecol 139:377, 1981.

13. **van Eijkeren MA, Christiaens GCML, Haspels AA, Sixma JJ,** Measured menstrual blood loss in women with a bleeding disorder or using oral anticoagulant therapy, Am J Obstet Gynecol 162:1261, 1990.

14. **Rulin MC, Turner JH, Dunworth R, Thompson D,** Post tubal sterilization syndrome: a misnomer, Am J Obstet Gynecol 151:13, 1985.

15. **DeStafano F, Huezo CM, Peterson HB, et al,** Menstrual changes after tubal sterilization, Obstet Gynecol 62:673, 1983.

16. **Rulin MC, Davidson AR, Philliber SG, Graves WL, Cushman LF,** Changes in menstrual symptoms among sterilized and comparison women: a prospective study, Obstet Gynecol 79:749, 1989.

17. **DeStafano F, Perlman J, Peterson HB, Diamond E,** Long-term risk of menstrual disturbances after tubal sterilization, Am J Obstet Gynecol 152:835, 1985.

18. **Kjer J, Knudsen L,** Hysterectomy subsequent to laparoscopic sterilization, Eur J Obstet Gynecol 35:63, 1990.

19. **Stergachis A, Shy KK, Gouthaus LC, Wagner EH, Hecht JA, Anderson G, Normand EH, Raboud J,** Tubal sterilization and the long-term risk of hysterectomy, JAMA 264:2893, 1990.

20. **Shy KK, Stergachis A, Grothaus LG, Wagner EH, Hecth J, Anderson G,** Tubal sterilization and risk of subsequent hospital admission for menstrual disorders, Am J Obstet Gynecol 166:1698, 1992.

21. **Thranov I, Hertz JB, Kjer JJ, Andresen A, Micic S, Nielsen J, Hancke S,** Hormonal and menstrual changes after laparoscopic sterilizatin by Falope-rings or Filshie-clips, Fertil Steril 57:751, 1992.

22. **Wilcox LS, Martinez-Schnell B, Peterson HB, Ware JH, Hughes JM,** Menstrual function after tubal sterilization, Am J Epidemiol 135:1368, 1992.

23. **Rulin MC, Davidson AR, Philliber SG, Graves WL, Cushman LF,** Long-term effect of tubal sterilization on menstrual indices and pelvic pain, Obstet Gynecol 82:118, 1993.

24. **Gurpide E, Gusberg S, Tseng L,** Estradiol binding and metabolism in human endometrial hyperplasia and adenocarcinoma, J Steroid Biochem 7:891, 1976.

25. **Kirkland JL, Murthy L, Stancel GM,** Progesterone inhibits the estrogen-induced expression of *c-fos* messenger ribonucleic acid in the uterus, Endocrinology 130:3223, 1992.

26. **Nelson L, Rybo G,** Treatment of menorrhagia, Am J Obstet Gynecol 110:713, 1971.

27. **DeVore GR, Owens O, Kase N,** Use of intravenous premarin in the treatment of dysfunctional uterine bleeding - a double-blind randomized control study, Obstet Gynecol 59:285, 1982.

28. **Livio M, Mannucci PM, Vigano G, Mingardi G, Lombardi R, Mecca G, Remuzzi G,** Conjugated estrogens for the management of bleeding associated with renal failure, New Engl J Med 315:731, 1986.

29. **Diaz S, Croxatto HB, Pavez M, Belhadj H, Stern J, Sivin I,** Clinical assessment of treatments for prolonged bleeding in users of Norplant implants, Contraception 42:97, 1990.

30. **Fraser IS,** Prostaglandin inhibitors in gynaecology, Aust NZ J Obstet Gynecol 25:114, 1985.

31. **Hall P, Maclachlan N, Thorn N, Nudd MWE, Taylor CG, Garrioch DB,** Control of menorrhagia by the cyclo-oxygenase inhibitors naproxen sodium and mefenamic acid, Br J Obstet Gynaecol 94:554, 1987.

32. **Cameron IT, Haining R, Lumsden M-A, Thomas VR, Smith SK,** The effects of mefenamic acid and norethisterone on measured menstrual blood loss, Obstet Gynecol 76:85, 1990.

33. **Fraser IS, McCarron G,** Randomized trial of 2 hormonal and 2 prostaglandin-inhibiting agents in women with a complaint of menorrhagia, Aust NZ J Obstet Gynecol 31:66, 1991.

34. **van Eijkeren MA, Christianes GCML, Geuze JH, Haspels AA, Sixma JJ,** Effects of mefenamic acid on menstrual hemostasis in essental menorrhagia, Am J Obstet Gynecol 166:1419, 1992.

35. **Bergqvist A, Rybo G,** Treatment of menorrhagia with intrauterine release of progesterone, Br J Obstet Gynaecol 90:255, 1983.

36. **Milsom I, Andersson K, Andersch B, Rybo G,** A comparison of flurbiprogen, tranexamic acid, and a levonorgestrel-releasing intrauterine contraceptive device in the treatment of idiopathic menorrhagia, Am J Obstet Gynecol 164:879, 1991.

37. **Kubrinsky NL, Tulloch H,** Treatment of refractory thrombocytopenic bleeding with desamino-8-D-arginine vasopressin (desmopressin), J Pediatr 112:993, 1988.

38. **Townsend DE, Richart RM, Paskowitz RA, Woolfork RE,** Rollerball coagulation of the endometrium, Obstet Gynecol 76:310, 1990.

39. **Phipps JH, Lewis BV, Prior MF, Roberts T,** Experimental and clinical studies with radio frequency-induced thermal endometrial ablation for functional menorrhagia, Obstet Gynecol 76:876, 1990.

40. **Farhi B, Nosanchuk J, Silverberg S,** Endometrial adenocarcinoma in women under 25 years of age, Obstet Gynecol 68:741, 1986.

41. **Silver MM, Miles P, Rosa C,** Comparison of Novak and Pipelle endometrial biopsy instruments, Obstet Gynecol 78:828, 1991.

42. **Eddowes HA, Read MD, Codling BW,** Pipelle: a more acceptable technique for outpatient endometrial biopsy, Br J Obstet Gynaecol 97:961, 1990.

43. **Fothergill DJ, Brown VA, Hill AS,** Histological sampling of the endometrium-A comparison between formal curettage and the Pipelle sampler, Br J Obstet Gynaecol 99:779, 1992.

44. **Gimpelson RJ, Rappold HD,** A comparative study between panoramic hysteroscopy with directed biopsies and dilatation and curettage, Am J Obstet Gynecol 158:489, 1988.

45. **Loffer FD,** Hysteroscopy with selective endometrial sampling compared with D&C for abnormal uterine bleeding: the value of a negative hysteroscopic view, Obstet Gynecol 73:16, 1989.

17   The Breast

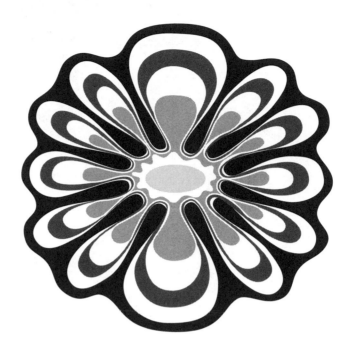

The form, function, and pathology of the human female breast are major concerns of medicine and society. As mammals, we define our biologic class by the function of the breast in nourishing our young. Breast contours occupy our attention. As obstetricians, we seek to enhance or diminish function, and as gynecologists, the appearance of inappropriate lactation (galactorrhea) may signify serious disease. Cancer of the breast is the most frequent cancer in women, an issue of growing magnitude.

In this chapter, the factors involved in normal growth and development of the breast will be reviewed, including the physiology of normal lactation. A description of the numerous factors leading to inappropriate lactation will follow, and finally, the endocrine aspects of breast cancer will be considered.

Growth and Development

The basic component of the breast lobule is the hollow alveolus or milk gland lined by a single layer of milk-secreting epithelial cells, derived from an ingrowth of epidermis into the underlying mesenchyme at 10–12 weeks of gestation. Each alveolus is encased in a crisscrossing mantle of contractile myoepithelial strands. Also surrounding the milk gland is a rich capillary network.

The lumen of the alveolus connects to a collecting intralobular duct by means of a thin nonmuscular duct. Contractile muscle cells line the intralobular ducts that eventually reach the exterior via 15–20 collecting ducts in a radial arrangement, corresponding to the 15–20 distinct mammary lobules in the breast, each of which contains many alveoli.

Growth of this milk-producing system is dependent on numerous hormonal factors that occur in two sequences, first at puberty and then in pregnancy. Although there is considerable overlapping of hormonal influences, the differences in quantities of the stimuli in each circumstance and the availability of entirely unique inciting factors

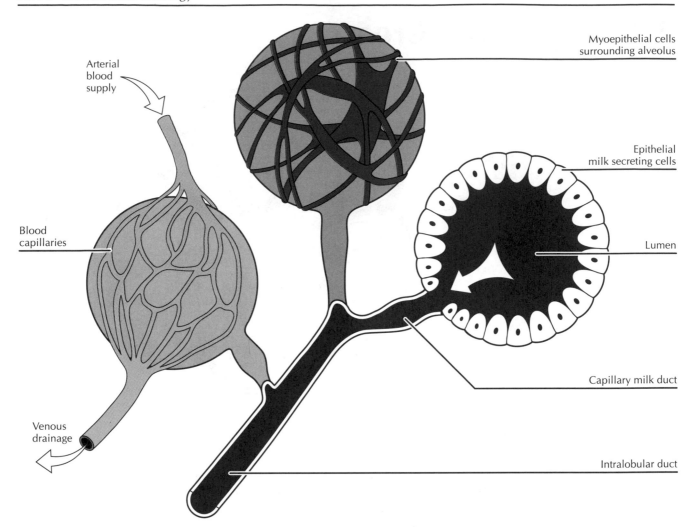

Myoepithelial cells
surrounding alveolus

Arterial
blood
supply

Blood
capillaries

Epithelial
milk secreting cells

Lumen

Venous
drainage

Capillary milk duct

Intralobular duct

(human placental lactogen and prolactin) during pregnancy permit this chronologic distinction. The strength of the hormonal stimulus to breast tissue during pregnancy is responsible for the fact that nearly half of male and female newborns have breast secretions.

The major influence on breast growth at puberty is estrogen. In most girls, the first response to the increasing levels of estrogen is an increase in size and pigmentation of the areola and the formation of a mass of breast tissue just underneath the areola. Breast tissue binds estrogen in a manner similar to the uterus and vagina. The development of estrogen receptors in the breast does not occur in the absence of prolactin. The primary effect of estrogen in subprimate mammals is to stimulate growth of the ductal portion of the gland system. Progesterone in these animals influences growth of the alveolar components of the lobule. However, neither hormone alone, or in combination, is capable of yielding optimal breast growth and development. Full differentiation of the gland requires insulin, cortisol, thyroxine, prolactin, and growth hormone.[1,2]

The pubertal response is a manifestation of closely synchronized central (hypothalamus-pituitary) and peripheral (ovary-breast) events. For example, gonadotropin releasing hormone (GnRH) is known to stimulate prolactin release, and this action is potentiated by estrogen.[3] This suggests a paracrine interaction between gonadotrophs and lacto-trophs, linked by estrogen, ultimately with an impact on the breast.

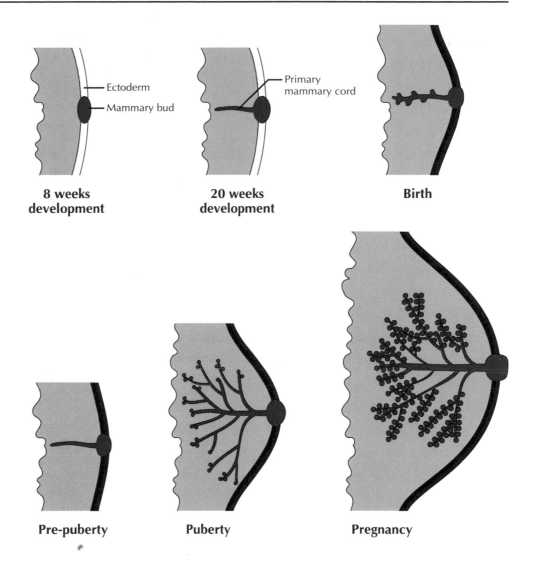

Changes occur routinely in response to the estrogen-progesterone sequence of a normal menstrual cycle. Maximal size of the breast occurs late in the luteal phase. Fluid secretion, mitotic activity, and DNA production of nonglandular tissue and glandular epithelium peak during the luteal phase.[4–6] This accounts for cystic and tender premenstrual changes.

Final differentiation of the alveolar epithelial cell into a mature milk cell is accomplished in the presence of prolactin, but only after prior exposure to cortisol and insulin. The complete reaction depends on the availability of minimal quantities of thyroid hormone. Thus, the endocrinologically intact individual in whom estrogen, progesterone, thyroxine, cortisol, insulin, prolactin, and growth hormone are available can have appropriate breast growth and function. Mild deficiencies in any of the hormones, short of severe restrictions or total absence, can be compensated for by excess prolactin. Furthermore, the growth of the breast and breast function can be incited by an excess of prolactin.

Abnormal Shapes and Sizes

Early differentiation of the mammary gland anlage is under fetal hormonal control. Abnormalities in adult size or shape may reflect the impact of hormones (especially the presence or absence of testosterone) during this early period of development. This prenatal hormonal influence programs the breast development that will occur in response to the increase in hormones at puberty. Occasionally, the breast bud will begin to develop on one side first. Similarly, one breast may grow faster than the other. These inequalities usually disappear by the time development is complete. However, exact equivalence in size usually is never attained. Significant asymmetry is correctable only by the plastic surgeon. Likewise hypoplasia and hypertrophy can be treated only by corrective surgery. With one exception, hormone therapy is totally ineffective in producing a permanent change in breast shape or size. Of course in patients with primary amenorrhea secondary to deficient ovarian function, estrogen treatment will induce significant and gratifying breast growth.

Accessory nipples can be found anywhere from the groin to the neck, remnants of the mammary line that extends early in embryonic life (6th week) along the ventral, lateral body wall. They occur in approximately 1% of women and require no therapy.

Pregnancy and Milk Secretion

During pregnancy, prolactin levels rise from the normal level of 10–25 ng/mL (440–1,100 pmol/L) to high concentrations, beginning about 8 weeks and reaching a peak of 200–400 ng/mL (8,800–17,600 pmol/L) at term.[7,8] The increase in prolactin parallels the increase in estrogen beginning at 7–8 weeks gestation, and the mechanism for increasing prolactin secretion (discussed in Chapter 5) is believed to be estrogen suppression of the hypothalamic prolactin inhibiting factor, dopamine, and direct stimulation of prolactin gene transcription in the pituitary.[9,10] There is marked variability in maternal prolactin levels in pregnancy, with a diurnal variation similar to that found in nonpregnant persons. The peak level occurs 4–5 hours after the onset of sleep.[11]

Made by the placenta and actively secreted into the maternal circulation from the 6th week of pregnancy, human placental lactogen (HPL) rises progressively reaching a level of approximately 6,000 ng/mL at term. HPL, though displaying less activity than prolactin, is produced in such large amounts that it may exert a lactogenic effect.

Although prolactin stimulates significant breast growth, and is available for lactation, only colostrum (composed of desquamated epithelial cells and transudate) is produced during gestation. Full lactation is inhibited by progesterone which interferes with prolactin action at the alveolar cell prolactin receptor level. Both estrogen and progesterone are necessary for the expression of the lactogenic receptor, but progesterone antagonizes the positive action of prolactin on its own receptor while progesterone and pharmacologic amounts of androgens reduce prolactin binding.[12–14] The effective use of high doses of estrogen to suppress postpartum lactation suggests that pharmacologic amounts of estrogen also block prolactin action.

Prolactin receptors exist in more than one form, all containing an extracellular region, a single transmembrane region, and a relatively long cytoplasmic domain. The amino acid identity between prolactin and growth hormone receptors is approximately 30%, with certain regions having up to 70% homology.[14] The prolactin and growth hormone receptors are each encoded by a single gene, both located on chromosome 5. Prolactin receptors are expressed in many tissues throughout the body. Because of the various forms and functions of prolactin, it is likely that multiple signal mechanisms are involved, and for that reason, no single second messenger for prolactin's intracellular action has been identified.

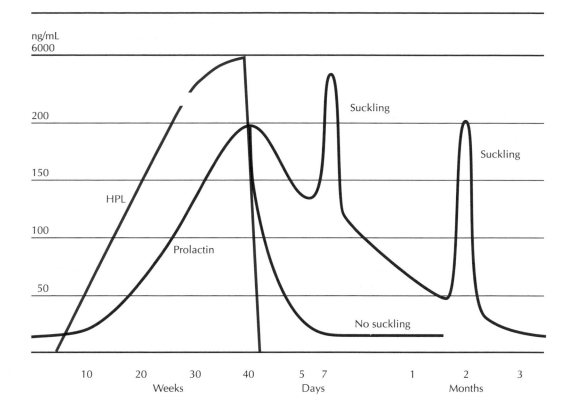

Amniotic fluid concentrations of prolactin parallel maternal serum concentration until the 10th week of pregnancy, rise markedly until the 20th week, and then decrease. Maternal prolactin does not pass to the fetus in significant amounts. Indeed the source of amniotic fluid prolactin is neither the maternal pituitary nor the fetal pituitary. The failure of dopamine agonist treatment to suppress amniotic fluid prolactin levels, and studies with in vitro culture systems, indicate a primary decidual source with transfer via amnion receptors to the amniotic fluid, requiring the intactness of amnion, chorion, and adherent decidua. This decidual synthesis of prolactin is initiated by progesterone, but once decidualization is established, prolactin secretion continues in the absence of both progesterone and estradiol.[15] Various decidual factors regulate prolactin synthesis and release, including relaxin, insulin, and insulin-like growth factor-I. It is hypothesized that amniotic fluid prolactin plays a role similar to its regulation of sodium transport and water movement across the gills in fish (allowing the ocean dwelling salmon and steelhead to return to freshwater streams for reproduction). Thus prolactin would protect the human fetus from dehydration by control of salt and water transport across the amnion. Prolactin reduces the permeability of the human amnion in the fetal to maternal direction by a receptor-mediated action on the epithelium lining the fetal surface.[16]

Prolactin is involved in many biochemical events during pregnancy. Surfactant synthesis in the fetal lung is influenced by prolactin, and decidual prolactin modulates prostaglandin-mediated uterine muscle contractility.[17,18] Prolactin also contributes to the prevention of the immunologic rejection of the conceptus by suppressing the maternal immune response.

The principal hormone involved in milk biosynthesis is prolactin. Without prolactin, synthesis of the primary protein, casein, will not occur, and true milk secretion will be impossible. The hormonal trigger for initiation of milk production within the alveolar cell and its secretion into the lumen of the gland is the rapid disappearance of estrogen and progesterone from the circulation after delivery. The clearance of prolactin is much slower, requiring 7 days to reach nonpregnant levels in a nonbreastfeeding woman.

These discordant hormonal events result in removal of the estrogen and progesterone inhibition of prolactin action on the breast. Breast engorgement and milk secretion begin 3–4 days postpartum when steroids have been sufficiently cleared. Maintenance of steroidal inhibition or rapid reduction of prolactin secretion (bromocriptine, 2.5 mg bid for 2 weeks) are effective in preventing postpartum milk synthesis and secretion. Augmentation of prolactin (by thyrotropin releasing hormone or sulpiride, a dopamine receptor blocker) results in increased milk yield.

In the first postpartum week, prolactin levels in breastfeeding women decline approximately 50% (to about 100 ng/mL [4,400 pmol/L]). Suckling elicits increases in prolactin, which are important in initiating milk production. Until 2–3 months postpartum, basal levels are approximately 40–50 ng/mL (1,760–2,200 pmol/L), and there are large (about 10–20-fold) increases after suckling. Throughout breastfeeding baseline prolactin levels remain elevated, and suckling produces a two-fold increase that is essential for continuing milk production.[19,20] The failure to lactate within the first 7 days postpartum may be the first sign of Sheehan's syndrome (hypopituitarism following intrapartum infarction of the pituitary gland).

Maintenance of milk production at high levels is dependent on the joint action of both anterior and posterior pituitary factors. By mechanisms to be described in detail shortly, suckling causes the release of both prolactin and oxytocin as well as thyroid-stimulating hormone (TSH).[21,22] Prolactin sustains the secretion of casein, fatty acids, lactose, and the volume of secretion, while oxytocin contracts myoepithelial cells and empties the alveolar lumen, thus enhancing further milk secretion and alveolar refilling. The increase in TSH with suckling suggests that thyrotropin releasing hormone (TRH) may play a role in the prolactin response to suckling (see "Prolactin Releasing Factor"). The optimal quantity and quality of milk are dependent upon the availability of thyroid, insulin, cortisol, and the dietary intake of nutrients and fluids.

Secretion of calcium into the milk of lactating women approximately doubles the daily loss of calcium.[23] In women who breastfeed for 6 months or more, this is accompanied by significant bone loss even in the presence of a high calcium intake.[24] However, bone density rapidly returns to baseline levels in the 6 months after weaning. The bone loss is due to increased bone resorption, probably secondary to the relatively low estrogen levels associated with lactation. It is possible that recovery is impaired in women with inadequate calcium intake; total calcium intake during lactation should be at least 1,500 mg per day.

Antibodies are present in breast milk and contribute to the health of an infant. Human milk prevents infections in infants both by transmission of immunoglobulins and by modifying the bacterial flora of the infant's gastrointestinal tract. Viruses are transmitted in breast milk, and although the actual risks are unknown, women infected with cytomegalovirus, hepatitis B, or human immunodeficiency virus are advised not to breastfeed. Vitamin A, vitamin B_{12}, and folic acid are significantly reduced in the breast milk of women with poor dietary intake. As a general rule approximately 1% of any drug ingested by the mother appears in breast milk.

Frequent emptying of the lumen is important for maintaining an adequate level of secretion. Indeed, after the 4th postpartum month, suckling appears to be the only stimulant required; however, environmental and emotional states also are important for continued alveolar activity.

The ejection of milk from the breast does not occur as the result of a mechanically induced negative pressure produced by suckling. Tactile sensors concentrated in the areola activate, via thoracic sensory nerve roots 4, 5, and 6, an afferent sensory neural arc which stimulates the paraventricular and supraoptic nuclei of the hypothalamus to synthesize and transport oxytocin to the posterior pituitary. The efferent arc (oxytocin) is blood-borne to the breast alveolus-ductal systems to contract myoepithelial cells and empty the alveolar lumen. Milk contained in major ductal repositories is ejected from openings in the nipple. This rapid release of milk is called "letdown." In many instances, the activation of oxytocin release leading to letdown does not require initiation by tactile stimuli. The central nervous system can be conditioned to respond to the presence of the infant, or to the sound of the infant's cry, by inducing activation of the efferent arc. These messages are the result of many stimulating and inhibiting neurotransmitters. The release of oxytrocin is also important for uterine contractions that contribute to involution of the uterus.

The oxytocin effect is a release phenomenon acting on secreted and stored milk. Prolactin must be available in sufficient quantities for continued secretory replacement of ejected milk. This requires the transient increase in prolactin associated with suckling. The amount of milk produced correlates with the amount removed by suckling. The breast can store milk for a maximum of 48 hours before production diminishes.

Breastfeeding by Adopting Mothers

Adopting mothers occasionally request assistance in initiating lactation.[25] Successful breastfeeding can be achieved by approximately half of the women by ingestion of 25 mg chlorpromazine tid together with vigorous nipple stimulation every 1–3 hours. Milk production will not appear for several weeks. This preparation ideally should be practiced for several months.

Prolactin Inhibiting Factor

Suckling suppresses the formation of a hypothalamic substance, prolactin inhibiting factor (PIF). This intrahypothalamic effect is either mediated by dopamine, or most likely, in contrast to the peptide nature of other hypothalamic hormones, PIF is dopamine itself.[26] Dopamine is secreted by the basal hypothalamus into the portal system and conducted to the anterior pituitary. Dopamine binds specifically to lactotroph cells and suppresses the secretion of prolactin into the general circulation; in its absence, prolactin is secreted. Suckling, therefore, acts to refill the breast by activating both portions of the pituitary (anterior and posterior) causing the breast to produce new milk and to eject milk.

Prolactin Releasing Factor

Prolactin may also be influenced by a positive hypothalamic factor (prolactin-releasing factor [PRF]). PRF does exist in various fowl (e.g., pigeon, chicken, duck, turkey, and the tricolored blackbird). While the identity of this material has not been elucidated, or its function substantiated in normal human physiology, it is possible that TRH is a potent stimulant of prolactin secretion in humans. The smallest doses of TRH which are capable of producing an increase in TSH also increase prolactin levels, a finding which supports a physiologic role for TRH in the control of prolactin secretion, at least in response to suckling.[27] However, except in hypothyroidism, normal physiologic changes as well as abnormal prolactin secretion are best explained and understood in terms of variations in the inhibiting factor, PIF. A large collection of peptides has been reported to stimulate the release of prolactin in vitro. These include growth factors, angiotensin II, GnRH, vasopressin, and others. But it is unknown whether these peptides participate in the normal physiologic regulation of prolactin secretion.

Cessation of Lactation

Lactation can be terminated by discontinuing suckling. The primary effect of this cessation is loss of milk letdown via the neural evocation of oxytocin. With passage of a few days, the swollen alveoli depress milk formation probably via a local pressure effect. With resorption of fluid and solute, the swollen engorged breast diminishes in size in a few days. In addition to the loss of milk letdown the absence of suckling reactivates dopamine (PIF) production so that there is less prolactin stimulation of milk secretion. Routine use of a dopamine agonist for suppression of lactation is not recommended because of reports of hypertension, seizure, myocardial infarctions, and strokes associated with its postpartum use.

Contraceptive Effect of Lactation

A moderate contraceptive effect accompanies lactation and produces child-spacing, which is very important in the developing world as a means of limiting family size. The contraceptive effectiveness of lactation, i.e., the length of the interval between births, depends on the level of nutrition of the mother (if low, the longer the contraceptive interval), the intensity of suckling, and the extent to which supplemental food is added to the infant diet. If suckling intensity and/or frequency is diminished, contraceptive effect is reduced. Only amenorrheic women who exclusively breastfeed at regular intervals, including nighttime, during the first 6 months have the contraceptive protection equivalent to that provided by oral contraception; with menstruation or after 6 months, the chance of ovulation increases.[28] Supplemental feeding increases the chance of ovulation (and pregnancy) even in amenorrheic women.[29] Total protection is achieved by the exclusively breastfeeding woman for a duration of only 10 weeks. Half of women studied ovulate before the 6th week, the time of the traditional postpartum visit; a visit during the 3rd postpartum week is strongly recommended for contraceptive counseling.

Rule of 3's for Postpartum Initiation of Contraception

Full breastfeeding: *Begin in 3rd postpartum month.*
Partial or no breastfeeding: *Begin in 3rd postpartum week.*

In nonbreastfeeding women, gonadotropin levels remain low during the early puerperium and return to normal concentrations during the 3rd to 5th week when prolactin levels have returned to normal. In an assessment of this important physiologic event (in terms of the need for contraception), the mean delay before first ovulation was found to be approximately 45 days, while no woman ovulated before 25 days after delivery.[28] Of the 22 women, however, 11 ovulated before the 6th postpartum week, underscoring the need to move the traditional postpartum medical visit to the 3rd week after delivery. In women who do receive dopamine agonist treatment at or immediately after delivery, return of ovulation is slightly accelerated, and contraception is required a week earlier, in the 2nd week postpartum.[30,31]

The mechanism of the contraceptive effect is of interest because a similar interference with normal pituitary-gonadal function is seen with elevated prolactin levels in nonpregnant women, the syndrome of galactorrhea and amenorrhea. Prolactin concentrations are increased in response to the repeated suckling stimulus of breastfeeding. Given sufficient intensity and frequency, prolactin levels will remain elevated. Under these conditions, follicle-stimulating hormone (FSH) concentrations are in the normal range (having risen from extremely low concentrations at delivery to follicular range in the 3 weeks postpartum) and luteinizing hormone (LH) values are in the low normal range. Despite the presence of gonadotropin, the ovary during lactational hyperprolactinemia does not display follicular development and does not secrete estrogen.

Earlier experimental evidence suggested that the ovaries might be refractory to gonadotropin stimulation during lactation, and, in addition, the anterior pituitary might be less responsive to GnRH stimulation. Other studies, done later in the course of lactation, indicated, however, that the ovaries as well as the pituitary were responsive to adequate tropic hormone stimulation.[32]

These observations suggest that high concentrations of prolactin work at both central and ovarian sites to produce lactational amenorrhea and anovulation. Prolactin appears to affect granulosa cell function in vitro by inhibiting synthesis of progesterone. It also may change the testosterone:dihydrotestosterone ratio, thereby reducing aromatizable substrate and increasing local antiestrogen concentrations. Nevertheless, a direct effect of prolactin on ovarian follicular development does not appear to be a major factor. The central action predominates.

Elevated levels of prolactin inhibit the pulsatile secretion of GnRH.[33,34] Prolactin excess has short loop positive feedback effects on dopamine. Increased dopamine reduces GnRH by suppressing arcuate nucleus function, perhaps in a mechanism mediated by endogenous opioid activity.[35,36] However, blockade of dopamine receptors with a dopamine antagonist or the administration of an opioid antagonist in breastfeeding women does not always affect gonadotropin secretion.[37] The exact mechansim for the suppression of gonadotropin secretion remains to be unraveled.

At weaning, as prolactin concentrations fall to normal, gonadotropin concentrations increase and estradiol secretion rises. This prompt resumption of ovarian function is also indicated by the occurrence of ovulation within 14–30 days of weaning.

Inappropriate Lactation — Galactorrheic Syndromes

Galactorrhea refers to the mammary secretion of a milky fluid which is nonphysiologic in that it is inappropriate (not immediately related to pregnancy or the needs of a child), persistent, and sometimes excessive. Although usually white or clear, the color may be yellow or even green. In the latter circumstance, local breast disease should be considered. To elicit breast secretion, pressure should be applied to all sections of the breast beginning at the base of the breast and working up toward the nipple. *Hormonal secretions usually come from multiple duct openings in contrast to pathologic discharge that usually comes from a single duct.* The quantity of secretion is not an important criterion. Any galactorrhea demands evaluation in a nulliparous woman and if at least 12 months have elapsed since the last pregnancy or weaning in a parous woman. Galactorrhea can involve both breasts or just one breast. Amenorrhea does not necessarily accompany galactorrhea, even in the most serious provocative disorders.

Differential Diagnosis of Galactorrhea

The differential diagnosis of galactorrhea is a difficult and complex clinical challenge. The difficulty arises from the multiple factors involved in the control of prolactin release. In most pathophysiologic states the final common pathway leading to galactorrhea is an inappropriate augmentation of prolactin release. The following considerations are important:

1. Excessive estrogen (e.g., oral contraceptives) can lead to milk secretion via hypothalamic suppression, causing reduction of PIF and release of pituitary prolactin and direct stimulation of the pituitary lactotrophs. Galactorrhea developing during oral contraceptive administration may be most noticeable during the days free of medication (when the steroids are cleared from the body and the prolactin interfering action of the estrogen and progestin on the breast wanes). Galactorrhea caused by excessive estrogen disappears within 3–6 months after discontinuing medication. This is now a rare occurrence with the lower dose pills. A longitudinal study of 126 women did demonstrate a 22% increase in prolactin values over mean control levels, but the response to low dose oral contraceptives was not out of the normal range.[38]

2. Prolonged intensive suckling can also release prolactin, via hypothalamic reduction of PIF. Similarly, thoracotomy scars, cervical spinal lesions, and herpes zoster can induce prolactin release by activating the afferent sensory neural arc, thereby simulating suckling.

3. A variety of drugs can inhibit hypothalamic PIF.[39] There are nearly 100 phenothiazine derivatives with indirect mammotropic activity. In addition, there are many phenothiazine-like compounds, reserpine derivatives, amphetamines, and an unknown variety of other drugs (opiates, diazepams, butyrophenones, α-methyldopa, and tricyclic antidepressants) which can initiate galactorrhea via hypothalamic suppression. The final action of these compounds is either to deplete dopamine levels or to block dopamine receptors. Chemical features common to many of these drugs are an aromatic ring with a polar substituent as in estrogen and at least two additional rings or structural attributes making spatial arrangements similar to estrogen. Thus, these compounds may act in a manner similar to estrogens to decrease PIF or to act directly on the pituitary. In support of this conclusion, it has been demonstrated that estrogen and phenothiazine derivatives compete for the same receptors in the median eminence. Prolactin is uniformly elevated in patients on therapeutic amounts of phenothiazines, but essentially never as high as 100 ng/mL (4,400 pmol/L). Approximately 30–50% will exhibit galactorrhea that should not persist beyond 3–6 months after drug treatment is discontinued.

4. Stresses can inhibit hypothalamic PIF, thereby inducing prolactin secretion and galactorrhea. Trauma, surgical procedures, and anesthesia can be seen in temporal relation to the onset of galactorrhea.

5. Hypothalamic lesions, stalk lesions, or stalk compression (events that physically reduce production or delivery of PIF to the pituitary) allow release of excess prolactin leading to galactorrhea.

6. Hypothyroidism (juvenile or adult) can be associated with galactorrhea. With diminished circulating levels of thyroid hormone, hypothalamic TRH is produced in excess and acts as a PRF to release prolactin from the pituitary. Reversal with thyroid hormone is strong circumstantial evidence to support the conclusion that TRH stimulates prolactin.

7. Increased prolactin release may be a consequence of prolactin elaboration and secretion from pituitary tumors which function independently of the otherwise appropriate restraints exerted by PIF from a normally functioning hypothalamus. This infrequent but potentially dangerous tumor, which has endocrine, neurologic, and ophthalmologic liabilities that can be disabling, makes the differential diagnosis of persistent galactorrhea a major clinical challenge. Beyond producing prolactin, the tumor may also suppress pituitary parenchyma by expansion and compression, interfering with the secretion of other tropic hormones. Other pituitary tumors may be associated with lactotroph hyperplasia and present with the characteristic syndrome of hyperprolactinemia and amenorrhea.

8. Increased prolactin concentrations can result from nonpituitary sources such as lung and renal tumors and even a uterine leiomyoma. Severe renal disease requiring hemodialysis is associated with elevated prolactin levels due to the decreased glomerular filtration rate.

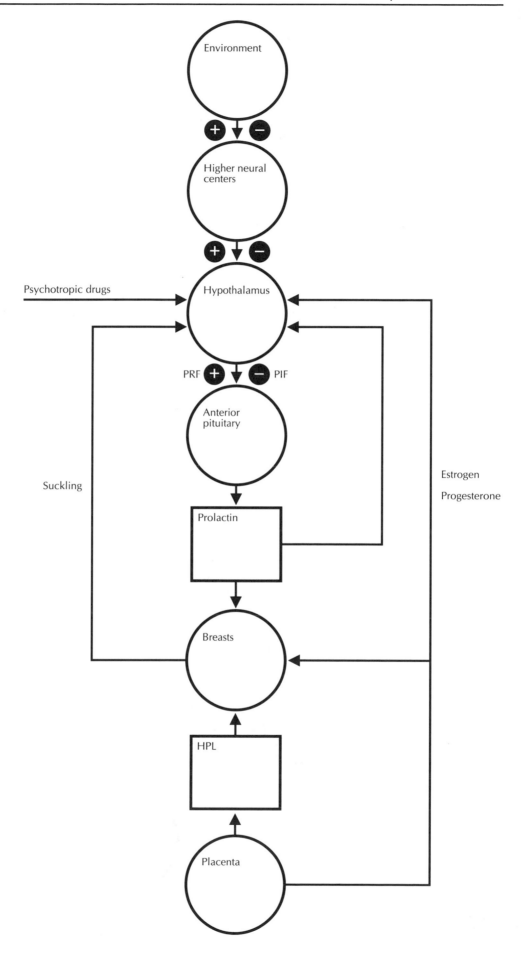

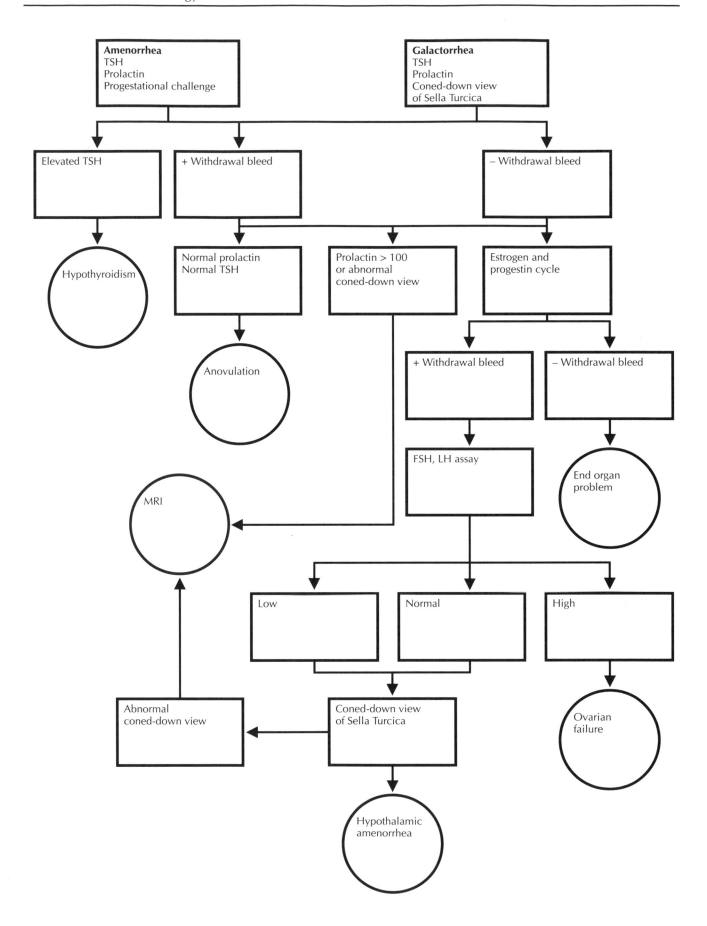

**The Clinical Problem
of Galactorrhea**

A variety of eponymic designations have been applied to variants of the lactation syndromes. These are based on the association of galactorrhea with intrasellar tumor (Forbes, Henneman, Griswold, and Albright, 1951), antecedent pregnancy with inappropriate persistence of galactorrhea (Chiari and Frommel, 1852), and in the absence of previous pregnancy (Argonz and del Castillo, 1953). In all, the association of galactorrhea with eventual amenorrhea was noted.

On the basis of currently available information, categorization of individual cases according to these eponymic guidelines is neither helpful nor does it permit discrimination of patients who have serious intrasellar or suprasellar pathology.

Hyperprolactinemia may be associated with a variety of menstrual cycle disturbances: oligoovulation, corpus luteum insufficiency, as well as amenorrhea. About one-third of women with secondary amenorrhea will have elevated prolactin concentrations. Pathologic hyperprolactinemia inhibits the pulsatile secretion of GnRH, and the reduction of circulating prolactin levels restores menstrual function.

Mild hirsutism may accompany ovulatory dysfunction caused by hyperprolactinemia. Whether excess androgen is stimulated by a direct prolactin effect on adrenal cortex synthesis of DHA (dehydroepiandrosterone) and its sulfate (DHAS) or is primarily related to the chronic anovulation of these patients (and hence ovarian androgen secretion) is not settled.

Not all patients with hyperprolactinemia display galactorrhea. The reported incidence is about 33% (Chapter 12). The disparity may not be due entirely to the variable zeal with which the presence of nipple milk secretion is sought during physical examination. The absence of galactorrhea may be due to the usual accompanying hypoestrogenic state. A more attractive explanation focuses on the concept of heterogeneity of tropic hormones (Chapter 2). The immunoassay for prolactin may not discriminate among heterogeneous molecules of prolactin. A high circulating level of prolactin may not represent material capable of interacting with breast prolactin receptors. On the other hand, galactorrhea can be seen in women with normal prolactin serum concentrations. Episodic fluctuations and sleep increments may account for this clinical discordance, or, in this case, bioactive prolactin may be present that is immunoactively not detectable. Remember that at any one point in time, the bioactivity (galactorrhea) and the immunoactivity (immunoassay result) of prolactin represent the cumulative effect of the family of structural, molecular variants present in the circulation.

In the pathophysiology of male hypogonadism, hyperprolactinemia is much less common, and the incidence of actual galactorrhea quite rare. Hyperprolactinemia in men usually presents with decreased libido and potency.

If galactorrhea has been present for 6 months to 1 year, or hyperprolactinemia is noted in the process of working up menstrual disturbances, infertility, or hirsutism, the probability of a pituitary tumor must be recognized. The workup of hyperprolactinemia is presented in detail in Chapter 12, "Amenorrhea." It is worth reemphasizing the salient clinical issues here.

With the current diagnostic techniques there is no difficulty in discovering and monitoring the size and function of a pituitary prolactin secreting "tumor." With few exceptions the combination of elevation in basal levels of prolactin and radiographic imaging offers complete confidence in diagnosing sellar pathology. The major concern remains in determining management — medical, surgical, or expectant? The considerations that influence management include:

1. Microadenomas, if exclusively prolactin producing, rarely progress to macroadenoma size. Most are exceedingly slow growing or stable.

2. The histology of many so-called tumors is not one of neoplasia. Most contain nodular or diffuse hyperplasia of basically normal lactotrophs. It is possible that a primary hypothalamic dysfunction which drives the lactotroph to hyperfunction and hyperplasia is the fundamental factor in the genesis of these "tumors." Thus, uncertain long-term cures, recurrence and new tumor formation remain possibilities.

3. Some tumors regress spontaneously. Medical therapy with dopamine agonists shrinks tumors and can prevent growth, although complete elimination of a tumor by dopamine agonist treatment does not occur, and rapid regrowth usually follows discontinuation of the drug.

4. Transsphenoidal microsurgery is a very safe procedure, but there is a high recurrence rate.

As a result of these considerations, many patients can be observed, others treated medically, and rarely some treated with surgery, with or without prior medically induced tumor reduction (see Chapter 12).

Treatment of Galactorrhea

Galactorrhea as an isolated symptom of hypothalamic dysfunction existing in an otherwise healthy woman does not require treatment. Periodic prolactin levels will, if within normal range, confirm the stability of the underlying process. However, some patients find the presence or amount of galactorrhea sexually, cosmetically, and emotionally burdensome. Treatment with a combined oral contraceptive, androgens, danazol and progestins has met with minimal success. Dopamine agonist treatment, therefore, is the therapy of choice. Even with normal prolactin concentrations and a normal skull x-ray, treatment with a dopamine agonist can eliminate galactorrhea.

We have adopted a conservative approach of close surveillance for pituitary prolactin-secreting adenomas, recommending surgery only for those tumors that display rapid growth or those tumors that are already large and do not shrink in response to dopamine agonists. If the prolactin level is greater than 100 ng/mL (4,400 pmol/L), or if the coned-down view of the sella turcica is abnormal, we recommend magnetic resonance imaging (MRI) evaluation. If the MRI rules out an empty sella syndrome or a suprasellar problem, surgical intervention after preoperative dopamine agonist treatment is then dictated by the patient's desires, the size of the tumor, and the response of the tumor to a dopamine agonist. Patients with prolactin levels less than 100 ng/mL (4,400 pmol/L) and with normal coned-down views of the sella turcica are offered a choice between dopamine agonist therapy and surveillance. An annual prolactin level and periodic coned-down views are indicated for continued observation to detect a growing tumor. Dopamine agonist therapy is recommended for patients wishing to achieve pregnancy, and for those patients who have galactorrhea to the point of discomfort.

The Management of Mastalgia

The cyclic occurrence of breast discomfort is a common problem and is usually associated with dysplastic, benign histologic changes in the breast. Medical treatment of mastalgia has historically included a bewildering array of options. Several are of questionable value. Diuretics have little impact, and thyroid hormone replacement is indicated only when hypothyroidism is documented. Steroid hormone treatment has been tried in many combinations, mostly unsupported by controlled studies. An old favorite, with many years of clinical experience testifying to its effectiveness, is testosterone. One must be careful, however, to avoid virilizing doses. A good practice is to start with small doses, such as 5 mg methyltestosterone every other day during the time of discomfort. In recent years, however, these methods have been supplanted by several new approaches.

Danazol in a dose of 200 mg/day is effective in relieving discomfort as well as decreasing nodularity of the breast.[40] A daily dose is recommended for a period of 6 months. This treatment may achieve long-term resolution of the histologic changes in addition to the clinical improvement. Doses below 400 mg daily do not assure inhibition of ovulation, and a method of effective contraception is necessary because of possible teratologic effects of the drug. Significant improvement has been noted with vitamin E, 600 units/day of the synthetic tocopheral acetate. No side effects have been noted, and the mechanism of action is unknown. Bromocriptine (2.5–5.0 mg/day) and antiestrogens such as tamoxifen (20 mg daily) are also effective for treating mammary discomfort and benign disease.[40,41]

Clinical observations had suggested that abstinence from methylxanthines leads to resolution of symptoms. Methylxanthines are present in coffee, tea, chocolate, and cola drinks. In controlled studies, however, a significant placebo response rate (30–40%) has been observed. Careful assessments of this relationship have failed to demonstrate a link between methylxanthine use and mastalgia, mammographic changes, or atypia (premalignant tissue changes).[42–44]

Cancer Site Incidence in U.S. Women [45]

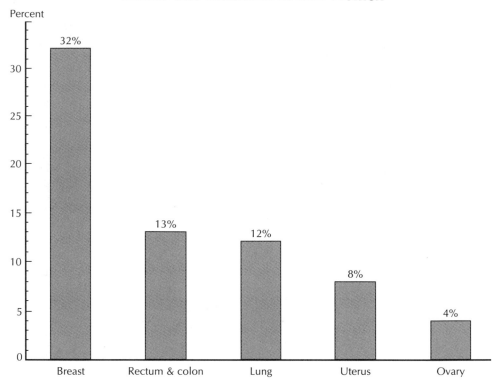

Cancer of the Breast

Scope of the Problem

One of every 9 American women who will live to age 85 will develop breast cancer.[45] The incidence has increased over the past 2 decades but plateaued in 1987 (about 182,000 new cases per year). Mortality rates have remained disappointingly constant (46,000 deaths per year). However, in view of an increasing incidence, this indicates an improvement. The 5-year survival rate for localized breast cancer has risen from 78% in the 1940s to 93% in 1993.[45] This is attributed to earlier diagnosis because of the greater

Cancer Deaths in U.S. Women [45]

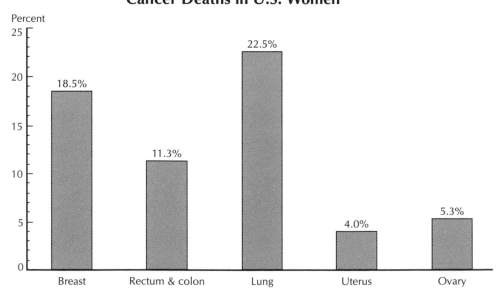

Mortality rate per 100,000 female population[45]

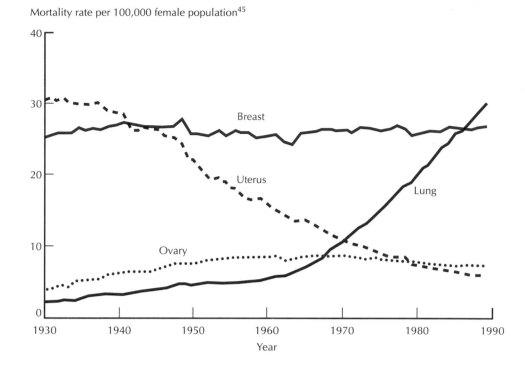

utilization of screening mammography. The breast is the leading site of cancer in women (32% of all cancers) and is now unfortunately (because smoking is obviously the reason) only exceeded by lung cancer as the the leading cause of death from cancer in women. With regional spread, the 5-year survival rate for breast cancer is 71%; with distant metastases, the rate is 18%.

Breast cancer has an increasing frequency with age. A woman at age 70 has almost 10 times the risk as a 40-year-old woman. About one-half of all breast cancers in the U.S. occur in women over age 65. However, after menopause, although the incidence rate continues to increase, it is less dramatic than the rise before menopause.

Over the years breast cancer has continued this deadly impact despite advances in surgical and diagnostic techniques. Classically, the single most useful prognostic information in women with operable breast cancer has been the histologic status of the axillary lymph nodes.[46] At 10 years only 25% of patients with positive nodes are free of disease compared to 75% of patients with negative nodes. If more than 3 nodes are involved, the 10-year survival rate drops from about 38% to 13%. Because of this recognition for the importance of the axillary nodes, the traditional approach to breast cancer (the Halsted surgical approach) was based on the concept that breast cancer is a disease of stepwise progression. ***There is an important change in concept. Breast cancer is now viewed as a systemic disease, with spread to local and distant sites at the same time. Breast cancer is best viewed as occultly metastatic at the time of presentation.*** Therefore, dissemination of tumor cells has occurred by the time of surgery in many patients.

Because we have been dealing with a disease which has already reached the point of dissemination in most patients, we must move the diagnosis forward several years in order to have an impact on breast cancer mortality. Earlier diagnosis requires that we be aware of what it is that makes a high risk patient. However, keep in mind that the great majority of women who develop breast cancer do not have an identifiable risk factor other than age.

Risk Factors

A constellation of factors influences the risk for breast cancer.[46] These include reproductive experience, ovarian activity, benign breast disease, familial tendency, genetic differences, dietary considerations, and specific endocrine factors.

Reproductive Experience

The risk of breast cancer increases with the increase in age at which a woman bears her first full-term child. A woman pregnant before the age of 18 has about one-third the risk of one who first delivers after the age of 35. To be protective, pregnancy must occur before the age of 30. In fact, women over the age of 30 years at the time of their first birth have a greater risk than women who never become pregnant.[47] There is, however, a significant protective effect with increasing parity, present even when adjusted for age at first birth and other risk factors.[48] Delayed childbearing in modern society probably has contributed significantly to the increased incidence of breast cancer observed over the last decades.

The fact that pregnancy early in life is associated with reduced breast cancer implies that etiologic factors are operating during that period of life. The protection afforded only by the first pregnancy suggests that the first full-term pregnancy has a trigger effect which either produces a permanent change in the factors responsible for breast cancer, or changes the breast tissue and makes it less susceptible to malignant transformation. There is evidence for a lasting impact of a first pregnancy on a woman's hormonal milieu. A small but significant elevation of estriol, a decrease in DHA and DHAS, and lower prolactin levels all persist for many years after delivery.[49,50] These changes take on great significance when viewed in terms of the endocrine factors considered below.

Lactation may offer a weak to moderate protective effect (20% reduced risk) only for premenopausal breast cancer.[51-54] There is a unique and helpful study of the Chinese Tanka, who are boat people living on the coast of southern China.[55] The women of the Chinese Tanka wear clothing with an opening only on the right side, and they breastfeed only with the right breast. All breast cancers were in postmenopausal women, and the cancers were equally distributed between the two sides, suggesting a protective effect only for premenopausal breast cancer. The Nurses' Health Study could not detect a protective effect of lactation, and a Norwegian prospective study, including a high percentage of women with long durations of breastfeeding, found no benefit on either premenopausal or postmenopausal breast cancer incidence.[56,57] The impact of lactation, if significant, must be small.

Ovarian Activity

Women who have an oophorectomy have a lower risk of breast cancer, and the lowered risk is greater the younger a woman is when ovariectomized. There is a 70% risk reduction in women who have oophorectomy before age 35. There is a small decrease in risk with late menarche and a moderate increase in risk with late natural menopause, indicating that ovarian activity plays a continuing role throughout reproductive life.[58] Obese women have earlier menarche and later menopause, higher estrone production rates and free estradiol levels (lower sex hormone binding globulin), and greater risk for breast cancer.[59]

Benign Breast Disease

With obstruction of ducts (probably by stromal fibrosis), ductule-alveolar secretion persists, the secretory material is retained, and cysts form from the dilatation of terminal ducts (duct ectasia) and alveoli. Women with cystic mastitis have about 4 times the breast cancer rate of comparable normal women. Despite their risk, women with prior benign breast disease form only a small proportion of breast cancer patients, approximately 5%.

There is strong support to eliminate the phrase "fibrocystic disease of the breast." In a review of over 10,000 breast biopsies in Nashville, Tennessee, 70% of the women were found to not have a lesion associated with an increased risk for cancer.[60] The most important variable on biopsies is the degree and character of the epithelial proliferation. Women with atypical hyperplasia had a relative risk of 5.3, while women with atypia and a family history of breast cancer had a relative risk of 11. In the Nurses' Health Study, biopsies with proliferative disease had a relative risk of breast cancer of 1.6, and with atypical hyperplasia, the relative risk was 3.7.[61] Only 4–10% of benign biopsies have atypical hyperplasia. The point is that we needlessly frighten patients with the use of the phrase fibrocystic disease. For most women, this is not a disease, but a physiologic change brought about by cyclic hormonal activity. **Let's call this problem *Fibrocystic change or condition*.**

The College of American Pathologists supports this position and has offered this classification:[62]

> **Classification of Breast Biopsy Tissue According to Risk for Breast Cancer**
> **No increased risk:**
> **Adenosis**
> **Duct ectasia**
> **Fibroadenoma**
> **Fibrosis**
> **Mild hyperplasia (3–4 cells deep)**
> **Mastitis**
> **Periductal mastitis**
> **Squamous metaplasia**
>
> **Slightly increased risk (1.5–2.0 times):**
> **Moderate or florid hyperplasia**
> **Papilloma**
>
> **Risk Increased 3–5 times:**
> **Atypical hyperplasia**

Familial Tendency

Female relatives of women with breast cancer have 2–3 times the rate of the general population. There is an excess of bilateral disease among patients with a family history of breast cancer. Relatives of women with bilateral disease have about a 45% lifetime chance of developing breast cancer. In data from the Centers for Disease Control and Prevention (CDC), these relative risks were observed:[63]

Affected mother or sister:	**2.3 relative risk.**
Affected aunt or grandmother:	**1.5 relative risk.**
Affected mother and sister:	**14.0 relative risk**

Results from the Nurses' Health Study indicate that the magnitude of risk associations with a positive family history is smaller than previously believed, comparable to the CDC data above, except for a relative risk of only 2.3 when both mother and sister had breast cancer.[64] In general the size of the increased risk with a positive family history is approximately 2 times the normal incidence. In the Nurses' Health data, there was no interaction between family history and alcohol intake.

In some families, breast and ovarian cancers are inherited; however, only 5–10% of all breast and ovarian cancer can be attributed to the inheritance of a gene associated with high risk.[65,66] Cancer is genetic in the sense that normal cells are transformed to malignant cells; consequently most cancer is not inherited. Nevertheless, genetic alterations have been identified in familial cancers. The breast and ovarian cancer gene (*BRCA1*) associated with familial cancer is on the long arm of chromosome 17, but other genetic alterations have also been observed in breast tumors. It is estimated that approximately 1 in 200 women in the U.S. have an inherited susceptibility to breast cancer, which tends to occur earlier in life in these patients.[66] This risk reaches 50% by age 50 and 80% by age 65. The risk of ovarian cancer is also increased in these women but to a lesser degree, perhaps by 10% by age 60. When the gene sequences are identified, high risk women will be able to be identified. In the meantime, women with a family history of multiple breast and ovarian cancers require earlier and more intensive surveillance. These women will also require counseling regarding prophylactic mastectomy and oophorectomy. The choices are not easy. Prophylactic surgery does not totally eliminate the risk. The rate of malignancies of the peritoneum after oophorectomy is about 2%, and the incidence of breast cancer after mastectomy is less than 1%.

Fat in the Diet

The geographical variation in incidence rates of breast cancer is considerable (the United States has the highest rates and Japan the lowest), and it has been correlated with the amount of animal fat in the diet.[67] Lean women, however, have been found to have an increased incidence of breast cancer, although this increase is limited to small, localized, and well-differentiated tumors.[68] Furthermore, studies have failed to find evidence for a positive relationship between breast cancer and dietary total or saturated fat or cholesterol intake.[69,70] On the other hand, there is evidence that dietary fat is a stronger risk factor for postmenopausal breast cancer than for premenopausal breast cancer.[71] Although a cohort study concluded that dietary fat is a determinant of postmenopausal breast cancer, the association did not achieve statistical significance.[72] Thus, the epidemiologic literature provides little support for a major contribution of dietary fat to the risk of breast cancer.

Alcohol in the Diet

There is a 60% increase in the risk for breast cancer with the consumption of one or more alcoholic drinks of all forms per day.[73] Almost all of many studies conclude that even moderate drinking increases the risk by 40–60%.

Specific Endocrine Factors

Adrenal Steroids

Subnormal levels of etiocholanolone (a urinary excretion product of androstenedione) have been found from 5 months to 9 years before the diagnosis of breast cancer in women living on the island of Guernsey, off the English coast.[74] A subnormal excretion of this 17-ketosteroid was also found in sisters of patients with breast cancer. A 6-fold increase in the incidence of breast cancer was found between women excreting less than 0.4 mg of etiocholanolone and those excreting over 1 mg/24 hours. Measurement of this 17-ketosteroid might be a useful screening procedure to detect a high risk group of patients because approximately 25% of the population excretes less than 1 mg/24 hours.

Endogenous Estrogen

Epidemiologic and other information continue to suggest some estrogen-related promoter function. These include the following: 1) the condition is 100 times more common in women than in men; 2) breast cancer invariably occurs after puberty; 3) untreated gonadal dysgenesis and breast cancer are mutually exclusive; 4) a 65% excess rate of breast cancer has been observed among women who have had an endometrial cancer; and 5) breast tumors contain estrogen receptors which are biologically active as indicated by the presence of progesterone receptors in tumor tissue. Taken together, these data suggest an element of estrogen dependence, if not provocation, in many breast cancers.

Estriol generally has failed to produce breast cancer in rodents, and in fact, estriol protects the rat against breast tumors induced by various chemical carcinogens. The hypothesis is that a higher estriol level protects against the more potent effects of estrone and estradiol. This might explain the protective effect of early pregnancies. Women having had an early pregnancy continue to excrete more estriol than nulliparous women. Premenopausal healthy Asiatic women have a lower breast cancer risk than Caucasians and also have a higher rate of urinary estriol excretion.[75] When Asiatic women migrate to the United States, however, the risk of breast cancer increases, and their urinary excretion of estriol decreases.

Stanley G. Korenman has promulgated a most interesting hypothesis concerning the endocrinology of breast cancer.[76,77] Recognizing that the endocrine changes thought to be related to the promotion or provocation of breast cancer were small, inconsistent, and could hardly account for the differential risk of breast cancer among populations, Korenman concluded that endocrine status is related to breast cancer by influencing the patient's susceptibility to environmental carcinogens. Called the "Open Window Hypothesis," Korenman argued that unopposed estrogen stimulation is the most favorable state for tumor induction (the "open" window). Susceptibility to breast cancer declines with the establishment of normal luteal phase progesterone secretion and becomes very low during pregnancy; the open window is closed.

The two main open window periods are the pubertal years prior to the establishment of regular ovulatory menstrual cycles and the perimenopausal period of waning follicle maturation and ovulation. The prolongation of these open windows by obesity, infertility, delayed pregnancy, earlier menarche, and later menopause would be associated with greater susceptibility. This argument is supported by observational studies indicating that anovulatory and infertile women (exposed to less progesterone) have an increased risk of breast cancer later in life.[78–81] However, the statistical power of these observational studies was limited by small numbers (all fewer than 15 cases).

Although theoretically appealing on the basis of presumed correlation with epidemiologic risks (infertility, late menopause) clinical research has not always confirmed the thesis. Young women at high genetic risk for breast cancer had normal luteal phases, and a group of premenopausal women with breast cancer also had normal luteal phases.[82] Others have failed to find a link between anovulation and the risk of breast cancer.[83,84] Another attempt to link the risk of breast cancer to the endogenous estrogen level focused on prenatal exposure. A reduced risk for breast cancer is observed for women born to mothers with pregnancy-induced hypertension, suggesting that this finding is due to the lower estrogen levels associated with preeclampsia.[85,86]

The logic and epidemiologic support for an estrogen link are impressive arguments. Whether the important factor is the total amount of estrogen, the amount of estrogen unopposed by progesterone, or some other combination is not known. Biologically available estrogen may be the more important factor. Women who develop breast cancer have higher levels of nonbound estradiol and lower levels of sex hormone binding globulin (SHBG).[87] Perhaps SHBG measurements should be added to our screening efforts.

Endogenous Progesterone

Because mitotic activity in the breast reaches its peak during the progesterone dominant luteal phase of the menstrual cycle, it can be argued that progesterone is the key to influencing the risk of breast cancer. Both proliferation and inhibition of proliferation have been observed with various progestational agents with in vitro studies of human breast cancer cells.[88] However, in vitro studies of normal breast epithelial cells reveal that progestins inhibit proliferation.[89] Several clinical observations would argue against progesterone as a key factor. The high levels of estrogen and progesterone during pregnancy have no adverse impact on the course of breast cancer diagnosed during pregnancy or when pregnancy occurs subsequent to diagnosis and treatment. Medroxy-progesterone acetate is not associated with an increased risk of breast cancer when used for contraception over long durations (Chapter 22). The hormonal sensitivity of breast cancer appears to be unquestionable, but whether estrogen or progesterone plays a key role in the risk of breast cancer continues to be uncertain.

Exogenous Estrogen and Progestin

The relationship between the use of exogeneous estrogens and the risk of breast cancer has been intensively studied (reviewed with complete references in Chapter 18). At the present time there is no conclusive evidence that estrogen doses known to protect against osteoporosis and cardiovascular disease (0.625 mg conjugated estrogens and 1.0 mg estradiol) increase the risk of breast cancer. Some have concluded that a slight increase is noted with long durations of use. However, notable studies (e.g., the Nurses' Health study and the CDC study) have failed to document such an increase. There certainly is no evidence that women who have used estrogen have an increased mortality rate from breast cancer.

The use of regimens that combine estrogen with a progestin is relatively recent (in the time frame of epidemiology), and thus far neither a protective effect nor a detrimental effect has been demonstrated with the addition of a progestational agent.

Thyroid, Prolactin, Various Nonestrogen Drugs

Despite isolated suggestions of increased risk, hypothyroidism, reserpine, and prolactin excess, whether spontaneous or drug induced, are not related to an enhanced risk of breast cancer.

Oral Contraception and Breast Cancer

The large number of women taking or having taken oral contraceptive steroids, combined with the belief that steroids provoke or promote abnormal breast growth and possibly cancer, has provided a source of major concern for years. The Royal College of General Practitioners, Oxford Family Planning Association, and Walnut Creek studies have indicated no significant differences in breast cancer rates between users and nonusers. However, patients were enrolled in these studies at a time when oral contraceptives were used primarily by married couples spacing out their children. Because this population may not reflect use by younger women for long durations to delay their first pregnancy, case-control studies have focused on the use of oral contraceptives at a younger age. This subject is reviewed in detail with complete references in Chapter 22. Long-term use of oral contraception during the reproductive years is not associated with a significant increase in the risk of breast cancer which occurs later in life, after age 45. There is the possibility that a subgroup of young women who use oral contraceptives early and for more than 4 years has a slightly increased risk (a relative risk less than 1.5) of breast cancer that occurs earlier in life, before age 45. It takes considerable statistical power to demonstrate a risk of this magnitude; only time and greater statistical power will verify if this is a real relationship. The use of oral contraception does not further increase the risk of breast cancer in women with positive family histories of breast cancer or in women with proven benign breast diseases.

Higher dose oral contraception, used for 2 or more years, protects against benign breast disease, but this protection is limited to current and recent users. It is unknown whether this same protection is provided by the current low dose formulations.

Breast Cancer in Diethylstilbestrol (DES)-exposed Women

Exposure to DES occurred in association with 2 million live births; therefore, the risk for induction of breast cancer during a period of breast differentiation could be significant if DES were a true breast carcinogen. The first study on this subject reported on the follow-up of women who participated in a controlled trial of DES in pregnancy between 1950 and 1952 at the University of Chicago. In this study, an increase which did not reach significance was observed between breast cancer risk and DES exposure.[90] A large collaborative study, involving approximately 6,000 women, concluded that there is a small but significant increase in the risk of breast cancer many years later in life in women exposed to DES during pregnancy.[91] A longer follow-up (more than 30 years) of this large cohort of DES-exposed women is now available. Exposure to DES is associated with a significant, but modest (less than two-fold), increase in the risk of breast cancer.[92] Importantly, the relative risk did not increase with duration of follow-up and remained stable over time. Certainly it is wise to recommend to DES-exposed women that they adhere religiously to screening for breast cancer, including mammography as discussed below.

Receptors and Clinical Prognosis

There is an excellent correlation between the presence of estrogen receptors and certain clinical characteristics of breast cancer, including response to endocrine therapy. Premenopausal and younger patients are more frequently receptor negative. Patients with receptor positive tumors survive longer and have longer disease-free intervals after mastectomy than those with receptor negative tumors. The presence of estrogen receptors correlates with increased disease-free interval regardless of the presence of axillary nodes or the size and location of the tumors. Similarly, patients without axillary lymph node metastases, but with estradiol receptor negative tumors, have the same high rate of recurrence as do patients with axillary lymph node metastases. Patients with tumors that are positive for estrogen receptors are more likely to respond to endocrine treatment.

It appears that patients with estrogen receptors are those with the more slowly growing tumors. Several reports indicate that estrogen receptor status correlates with the degree of differentiation of the primary tumor. A large proportion of highly differentiated Grade I carcinomas are receptor positive, while the reverse is true of Grade III tumors.

Remember that it takes estrogen to make progesterone receptors. Therefore the presence of progesterone receptors proves that the estrogen receptor in the tumor is biologically active. Thus, the presence of progesterone receptors has a correlation with disease free survival of patients only second to the number of positive nodes.[93] The best prognosis is seen in patients with positive progesterone receptors, even with subsequent disease if the recurrent disease is still progesterone receptor positive. The loss of progesterone receptors is an ominous sign.

Adjuvant Treatment of Breast Cancer

We have available a remarkable world-wide overview of 133 randomized trials which include a total of 75,000 women treated for breast cancer and 30,000 women involved in tamoxifen trials.[94] Adjuvant treatment with the antiestrogen, tamoxifen, achieves highly significant reductions in recurrence and increases in survival. The beneficial effect of tamoxifen is evident no matter what the age of the patient, in both premenopausal and postmenopausal women, in node positive and node negative disease, and in both estrogen receptor positive and negative tumors. The benefit of tamoxifen is of course more concentrated in estrogen receptor positive disease. The impact on recurrence occurs in the first 5 years, but continued impact on survival occurs throughout 10 years (and this was achieved with a median duration of treatment of only 2 years). The 10-year survival difference is even greater than that at 5 years. Adjuvant treatment (which is either tamoxifen, chemotherapy, or ovarian ablation) yields world-wide an extra 100,000 10-year survivors.

The conclusion is that tamoxifen therapy is definitely justified for postmenopausal women with estrogen receptor positive disease, and a benefit with tamoxifen alone can be demonstrated with early breast cancer regardless of receptor status.[95] The disease-free interval is consistently prolonged with postsurgical tamoxifen treatment of early breast cancer. In addition, there is a reduced rate of recurrence. The ideal duration of therapy remains unsettled. Certainly the data support a duration of at least 5 years, but there is reason to believe that longer treatment with tamoxifen will be worthwhile.[94,96,97] Longer, even lifelong, durations are now being studied. Dose-response studies with tamoxifen have failed to demonstrate an increase in activity with doses larger than the standard, 20 mg daily.[98]

After the publication of the 10-year data from the worldwide collaborative group, an international conference was held in St. Gallen, Switzerland, in February, 1992. This conference brought together experts from all over the world, and resulted in an updated consensus for treatment.[99]

For premenopausal women, chemotherapy is the first line of therapy, with tamoxifen added as an option to receptor positive patients. For postmenopausal women, tamoxifen is favored for receptor positive disease and chemotherapy for receptor negative tumors. The combination and the sequence with chemotherapy need further study, but there appears to be a benefit.

The clinical response to tamoxifen in premenopausal patients occurs despite the maintenance of normal, even higher, estrogen levels. The rate of response, 30%, is similar to that of bilateral oophorectomy.[100] The response rate reaches 50% for patients with estrogen receptor positive tumors. The probability of response to tamoxifen in postmenopausal patients with estrogen receptor positive disease is 50% or better, while estrogen receptor negative tumors have a response rate of less than 10%.[99] Patients unresponsive to other endocrine treatment seldom respond to tamoxifen. Tamoxifen, therefore, is recommended for all postmenopausal women with estrogen receptor positive breast cancer which has spread to the axillary lymph nodes. It is believed that tamoxifen treatment must be continued for at least 2 years, preferably longer. The role in premenopausal women is not well-defined.[101] The delayed recurrence in premenopausal women observed in some trials was not associated with improved survival.[95,102] Nevertheless, tamoxifen has replaced ovarian ablation as the initial choice of treatment for premenopausal women with estrogen receptor positive metastatic breast cancer.

About two-thirds of the new cases of breast cancer each year do not involve the axillary lymph nodes and thus require decisions regarding adjuvant therapy. Because 70% of node negative patients are cured without adjuvant therapy, this is not an easy decision for patients and physicians.[93] A reasonable approach is to focus on high risk patients grouped according to known prognostic factors.

The most favorable prognosis is associated with ductal ca-in-situ, a tumor size less than 1 cm, and a nuclear grade of 1 (nuclear grade 1 is well-differentiated, which is about 10% of node negative patients); 25% of patients have small tumors and favorable histologic subtypes (a recurrence rate of less than 10%); 25% of patients have large tumors with poor prognostic features (a recurrence rate greater than 50%), but fully half of patients are in between (with an average recurrence rate of 30%).

Summary of Current Treatment Recommendations

1992 Consensus for Treating Node-Negative Breast Cancer[99]

	Low Risk	Good Risk
Premenopausal	Observation vs tamoxifen	Tamoxifen
Postmenopausal	Observation vs tamoxifen	Tamoxifen
Over age 70	No treatment	Tamoxifen

Definition of Low Risk (Less than a 10% chance of recurrence at 10 years):
   Noninvasive tumors (ductal ca-in-situ).
   Pure (not mixed) tubular, papillary, or medullary types of cancer.
   Tumor size less than 1 cm.
   Diploid tumor (normal amount of DNA) with low S-phase fractions (low
      proliferation).
   Nuclear grade 1 (score according to nuclear size and shape, mitotic figures, and
      other histologic characteristics).

Definition of Good Risk (85–90% chance of being disease free at 5 years):
   Estrogen receptor positive tumors 1–2 cm in size.
   No high risk histologic features.
   Low nuclear grade.

1992 Consensus for Treating Node-Negative High Risk Patients[99]

Premenopausal:	Receptor positive	Chemotherapy, ? tamoxifen
	Receptor negative	Chemotherapy
Postmenopausal:	Receptor positive	Tamoxifen, ? chemotherapy
	Receptor negative	Chemotherapy, ? tamoxifen
Over age 70		Tamoxifen

Definition of High Risk:
   Receptor negative tumors that are 1 cm or greater in size or receptor positive
      tumors greater than 2 cm and with poor nuclear grade.
   Aneuploid tumor (abnormal amount of DNA).
   High S-phase fractions (high proliferation).
   High cathepsin D levels (a lysomal enzyme oversecreted in invasive and
      metastatic breast cancers).

1992 Consensus for Treating Node-Positive Breast Cancer[99]

	Receptor Positive	Receptor Negative
Premenopausal	Chemotherapy, ? tamoxifen	Chemotherapy
Postmenopausal	Tamoxifen, ? chemotherapy	Chemotherapy, ? tamoxifen
Over age 70	Tamoxifen	Chemotherapy

Problems with Tamoxifen

Tamoxifen is both an estrogen antagonist and an estrogen agonist (Chapter 2). There have been many reports of endometrial hyperplasia, endometrial polyps, rapid and symptomatic growth of endometriosis, and endometrial cancer occurring in women receiving tamoxifen treatment. A tissue that is highly sensitive to estrogen, the endometrium, responds to the weak estrogenic action of tamoxifen, which is present in high doses for long durations in women receiving adjuvant treatment for breast cancer. The development of endometrial cancer in women receiving tamoxifen should not be so surprising. We know that duration of exposure to estrogen is more important than the dose of estrogen in influencing progression from proliferative endometrium through hyperplasia to cancer. The proper surveillance and management of women being treated with tamoxifen are critical problems.

It is inappropriate to advocate progestational treatment to prevent the endometrial response to tamoxifen. The progestational impact (at the low doses currently used for endometrial protection) on the risk of breast cancer recurrence and the interaction with tamoxifen are not known. Periodic endometrial aspiration biopsy, of course, would be sufficient, but this procedure carries with it the potential for a very significant negative effect on patient compliance (with her tamoxifen and with her clinician).

We recommend the following program for monitoring women on long-term tamoxifen treatment:

All women:	**Careful pelvic examination every 6 months to detect the emergence of endometriosis.**
Postmenopausal women:	**Annual measurement of endometrial thickness by transvaginal ultrasonography. Endometrial biopsy of all women with a thickness of 5 mm or greater.**
Premenopausal women:	**Periodic assessment for ovulation; if ovulatory, no further intervention is necessary; however, contraceptive counseling should not be ignored. If anovulatory, an annual endometrial aspiration biopsy.**
	Consider the use of the progesterone-releasing IUD for both contraception and protection against endometrial change. Measureable amounts of progesterone do not reach the circulation. For this purpose, replacement is necessary only every 18–24 months.

A woman being treated for breast cancer will naturally focus her attention and energy on the cancer itself, especially in the early years of treatment. The same can be said for the specialist who is monitoring the treatment. It falls to the patient's health care manager, her primary physician, to look at the broader picture. A clinician interacting with patients being treated for breast cancer has an obligation to consider the impact of the patient's treatment on other body systems and functions. Tamoxifen offers the hope of adding many years to a woman's life. Medical intervention by a clinician can help make those years better with good preventive health care.

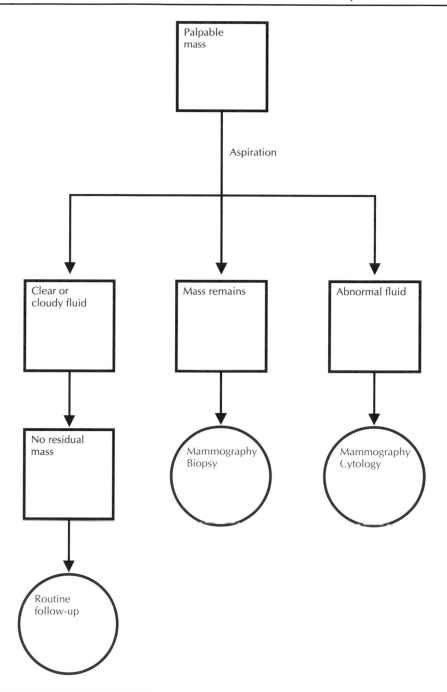

Needle Aspiration

Needle aspiration of breast lumps should be part of the practice of everyone who cares for women.[103] The technique is easy. A small infiltrate of xylocaine is placed in the skin (many clinicans believe that local anesthesia is unnecessary). Holding the lesion between thumb and index fingers with one hand, the other hand passes a 22-gauge needle attached to a 3-finger control syringe into the lesion. Aspiration will reveal the presence of cystic fluid from a cyst. If the mass is solid, the needle should be passed at least 10 times back and forth through the lesion with continuous suction on the syringe. Air is forcibly ejected through the needle on to a cytology slide for smearing and fixing. The usual Pap smear fixative can be used.

The procedure is very cost-effective. When aspiration yields clear or yellow fluid and the mass disappears, the procedure is both diagnostic and therapeutic. Fluid of any other nature requires cytologic assessment.[104] Failure to obtain material for cytologic evaluation or the persistence of a mass requires biopsy. Locally recurrent cysts should be surgically removed.

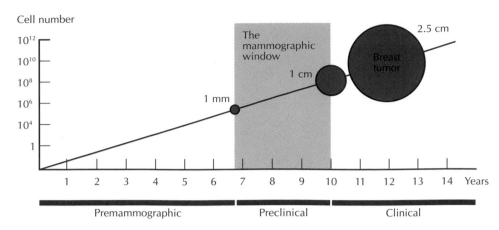

Cell number

After Wertheimer, et al.[106]

| Premammographic | Preclinical | Clinical |

Screening Mammography

Mammography is a means of detecting the nonpalpable cancer. Technical advancements have significantly improved the mammographic image and reduced the radiation dose.[105] The doubling time of breast cancer is very variable, but, in general, a tumor doubles in size every 100 days. Thus, it takes a single malignant cell approximately 10 years to grow to a clinically detectable 1 cm mass, but by this time a tumor of 1 cm has already progressed through 30 of the 40 doublings in size which is estimated to be fatal.[106] Furthermore, the average size at which a tumor is detected (70–75% of tumors are found by patients themselves) is 2.5 cm, a size which has a 50% incidence of lymph node involvement. To decrease the mortality from breast cancer, we must utilize a technique to find the tumors when they are smaller. Mammography is the answer.

Mammography is the technique of choice. Thermography has a high rate of false positive findings, and, at best, should be considered experimental. Ultrasound can rarely reveal malignant lesions smaller than 1 cm in size. It is useful, however, to guide the aspiration of lesions. CT scanning has 2 serious limitations. The x-ray dose is large, and the slices are too thick to detect early lesions. Finally, magnetic resonance imaging is not practical because of the expense and the long scan times that are necessary.

Mammography is the only method that detects clustered microcalcifications. These calcifications are less than 1 mm in diameter and are frequently associated with malignant lesions. More than 5 calcifications in a cluster are associated with cancer 25% of the time and require biopsy.

Mammography has a false negative rate of 5–10%. This means that masses are palpable but not visible. Mammography cannot and should not replace examination by patient and physician. Cancer commonly presents as a solitary, solid, painless (but not always), hard, unilateral, irregular nonmobile mass. A mass requires biopsy regardless of the mammographic picture.

A pattern of dysplasia on the mammogram carries with it an increased risk (2.0–3.5 times normal) of breast cancer. The risk is similar to that seen with the other known risk factors.[107]

The Effectiveness of Mammography

Mammography can reduce the mortality of breast cancer. In Nijmegan, the breast cancer mortality rate in women 35 and over was reduced by 50% by annual mammographic screening.[108] In Utrecht, the relative risk of dying from breast cancer among screened women was reduced by 70%.[109] The first randomized, controlled trials of mammography were begun in Sweden in 1977. Results have demonstrated a 24% reduction in mortality, 29% in women aged 50–69.[110] Most impressively, the results in Sweden were obtained with a screening only every 2–3 years and with only a single mediolateral oblique view. A greater impact is to be expected with an increased and regular frequency of use combined with state-of-the-art technology.

It has been questioned whether mammography screening is effective for women under 50.[111,112] The American Breast Cancer Detection Demonstration Project has demonstrated that screening is just as effective for women in their 40s as in women over 50.[113] This program that was organized by the American Cancer Society and the National Cancer Institute began operating in 1973 in 27 locations throughout the United States, enrolling more than 280,000 women. Despite the fact that this is not an organized research study with a control group, the massive database permits many valuable conclusions. From 1977 to 1982, similar high survival rates (87%) for women in their 40s compared with women in their 50s verify that screening was just as effective in the younger women. A 5-year survival rate for patients under 50 with breast cancers detected by examination was 77% compared to 95% in those patients with breast cancers detected by mammography.[114] However, the combined results from randomized controlled clinical trials have indicated no reduction in mortality in women screened under the age of 50.[115] It is more difficult to reach a conclusion regarding mammography in younger women because breast cancer is less common at lower ages (longer follow-up is required), and mammographic imaging is less sensitive in younger women. Only in recent years has mammography become sensitive enough to be effective in younger women.

There is a special problem with elderly women. Old women are less likely to be screened with mammography, probably due to both patient misconceptions and erroneous physician beliefs. The effectiveness of mammography for women over age 75 has not been established; however, decision-analysis of available data predicts a major benefit for elderly women as well.[116] Older women need to be reminded that risk continues to increase with increasing age.

There are problems to be anticipated with extensive mammography screening. Small nonpalpable lesions have less than a 5% chance of being malignant, and overall only about 20–30% of biopsy specimens contain carcinoma. That means there will be a large number of biopsies and mammograms performed (including the treatment of clinically irrelevant lesions), which involves costs to the health care system and cost to the individual in terms of stress and anxiety. Indeed, one analysis of risks and benefits concludes that because breast cancer is relatively infrequent under the age of 50, it is not cost-effective to screen all asymptomatic women aged 40–49.[111] Nevertheless mammography is the most potent weapon we possess in the battle against breast cancer. Mammography not only lowers mortality, but it also decreases morbidity because less radical surgery is necessary for smaller lesions.

Every woman should be regarded as at risk. Health care professionals who interact with women have the opportunity to initiate an aggressive program of preventive health care. The major deterrent to patient use of mammography is the absence of a strong clinician recommendation. We urge you to follow these suggested guidelines:

Screening for Breast Cancer

All women should be taught self-breast examination by age 20. Because of the changes which occur routinely in response to the hormonal sequence of a normal menstrual cycle, breast examination is most effective during the follicular phase of the cycle and should be performed monthly.

All women over the age of 35 should have an annual breast examination.

A baseline mammogram should be obtained by age 40, or earlier if high risk factors are present.

From ages 40 to 50, mammography should be performed every 2 years in low risk women and every year in women with significant risk factors.

Annual mammography should be performed in all women over age 50.

References

1. **Topper YL, Freeman C,** Multiple hormone interactions in the developmental biology of the mammary gland, Physiol Rev 60:1049, 1980.

2. **Klineberg DL, Niemann W, Flamm E, Cooper P, Babitsky G,** Primate mammary development, J Clin Invest 75:1943, 1985.

3. **Christiansen E, Veldhuis JD, Rogol AD, Stumpf P, Evan WS,** Modulating actions of estradiol on gonadotropin-releasing hormone-stimulated prolactin secretion in postmenopausal individuals, Am J Obstet Gynecol 157:320, 1987.

4. **Ferguson DP, Anderson TJ,** Morphological evaluation of cell turnover in relation to menstrual cycle in the "resting" human breast, Br J Cancer 44:177, 1988.

5. **Longacre TA, Bartow SA,** A correlative morphologic study of human breast and endometrium in the menstrual cycle, Am J Surg Path 10:382, 1986.

6. **Going JJ, Anderson TJ, Battersby S, MacIntyre CC,** Proliferative and secretory activity in human breast during natural and artificial menstrual cycles, Am J Path 130:193, 1988.

7. **Tyson JE, Hwang P, Guyda H, Friesen HG,** Studies of prolactin secretion in human pregnancy, Am J Obstet Gynecol 113:14, 1972.

8. **Kletzky OA, Marrs RP, Howard WF, McCormick W, Mishell DR Jr,** Prolactin synthesis release during pregnancy and puerperium, Am J Obstet Gynecol 136:545, 1980.

9. **Tyson JE, Friesen HG,** Factors influencing the secretion of human prolactin and growth hormone in menstrual and gestational women, Am J Obstet Gynecol 116:377, 1973.

10. **Barberia JM, Abu-Fadil S, Kletzky OA, Nakamura RM, Mishell DR Jr,** Serum prolactin patterns in early human gestation, Am J Obstet Gynecol 121:1107, 1975.

11. **Ehara Y, Siler TM, Yen SSC,** Effects of large doses of estrogen on prolactin and growth hormone release, Am J Obstet Gynecol 125:455, 1976.

12. **Murphy LJ, Murphy LC, Stead B, Sutherland RL, Lazarus L,** Modulation of lactogenic receptors by progestins in cultured human breast cancer cells, J Clin Endocrinol Metab 62:280, 1986.

13. **Simon WE, Pahnke VG, Holzel F,** In vitro modulation of prolactin binding to human mammary carcinoma cells by steroid hormones and prolactin, J Clin Endcrinol Metab 60:1243, 1985.

14. **Kelly PA, Kjiane J, Postel-Vinay M-C, Edery M,** The prolactin/growth hormone receptor family, Endocrin Rev 12:235, 1991.

15. **Daly DC, Kuslis S, Riddick DH,** Evidence of short-loop inhibition of decidual prolactin synthesis by decidual proteins, Part I, Am J Obstet Gynecol 155:358, 1986.

16. **Raabe MA, McCoshen JA,** Epithelial regulation of prolactin effect on amnionic permeability, Am J Obstet Gynecol 154:130, 1986.

17. **Snyder JM, Dekowski SA,** The role of prolactin in fetal lung maturation, Seminars Reprod Endocrinol 10:287, 1992.

18. **McCoshen JA, Bose R, Embree JE,** Uterine prolactin and labor: modulation by human chorionic gonadotropin affects prostaglandin (PG) E_2 and $PGF_{2\alpha}$ production, Seminars Reprod Endocrinol 10:294, 1992.

19. **Battin DA, Marrs RP, Fleiss PM, Mishell DR Jr,** Effect of suckling on serum prolactin, luteinizing hormone, follicle-stimulating hormone, and estradiol during prolonged lactation, Obstet Gynecol 65:785, 1985.

20. **Stern JM, Konner M, Herman TN, Reichlin S,** Nursing behaviour, prolactin, and postpartum amenorrhoea during prolonged lactation in American and !Kung mothers, Clin Endocrinol 25:247, 1986.

21. **Dawood MY, Khan-Dawood FS, Wahl RS, Fuchs F,** Oxytocin release and plasma anterior pituitary and gonadal hormones in women during lactation, J Clin Endocrinol Metab 52:678, 1981.

22. **McNeilly AS, Robinson KA, Houston MJ, Howe PW,** Release of oxytocin and prolactin in response to suckling, Br Med J 286:257, 1983.

23. **Kumar R, Cohen WR, Epstein FH,** Vitamin D and calcium hormones in pregnancy, New Engl J Med 302:1143, 1980.

24. **Sowers M, Corton G, Shapiro B, Jannausch ML, Crutchfield M, Smith ML, Randolph JF, Hollis B,** Changes in bone density with lactation, JAMA 269:3130, 1993.

25. **Auerbach KG, Avery JL,** Induced lactation, Am J Dis Child 135:340, 1981.

26. **Ben-Jonathan N,** Dopamine: a prolactin-inhibiting hormone, Endocrin Rev 6:564, 1985.

27. **de Greef WJ, Voogt JL, Visser TJ, Lamberts SWJ, van der Schoot P,** Control of prolactin release induced by suckling, Endocirnology 121:316, 1987.

28. **Campbell OM, Gray RH,** Characteristics and determinants of postpartum ovarian function in women in the United States, Am J Obstet Gynecol 169:55, 1993.

29. **Diaz S, Aravena R, Cardenas H, Casado ME, Miranda P, Schiappacasse V, Croxatto HB,** Contraceptive efficacy of lactational amenorrhea in urban Chilean women, Contraception 43:335, 1991.

30. **Kremer JAM, Thomas CMG, Rolland R, van der Heijden PF, Thomas CM, Lancranjan I,** Return of gonadotropic function in postpartum women during bromocriptine treatment, Fertil Steril 51:622, 1989.

31. **Haartsen JE, Heineman MJ, Elings M, Evers JLH, Lancranjan I,** Resumption of pituitary and ovarian activity post-partum: endocrine and ultrasonic observations in bromocriptine-treated women, Hum Reprod 7:746, 1992.

32. **Tyson JE, Carter JN, Andreassen B, Huth J, Smith B,** Nursing mediated prolactin and luteinizing hormone secretion during puerperal lactation, Fertil Steril 30:154, 1978.

33. **Sauder SE, Frager M, Case GD, Kelch RP, Marshall JC,** Abnormal patterns of pulsatile luteinizing hormone secretion in women with hyperprolactinemia and amenorrhea: responses to bromocriptine, J Clin Endocrinol Metab 59:941, 1984.

34. **Tay CCK, Glasier A, McNeilly AS,** Twenty-four hour secretory profiles of gonadotropins and prolactin in breastfeeding women, Hum Reprod 7:951, 1992.

35. **Ishizuka B, Quigley ME, Yen SSC,** Postpartum hypogonadotrophinism: evidence for increased opioid inhibition, Clin Endocrinol 20:573, 1984.

36. **Petraglia F, De Leo V, Nappi C, Facchinetti F, Montemagno U, Brambilla F, Genazzani AR,** Differences in the opioid control of luteinizing hormone secretion between pathological and iatrogenic hyperprolactinemic states, J Clin Endocrinol Metab 64:508, 1987.

37. **Tay CCK, Glasier AF, McNeilly AS,** Effect of antagonists of dopamine and opiates on the basal and GnRH-induced secretion of luteinizing hormone, follicle stimulating hormone and prolactin during lactational amenorrhea in breastfeeding women, Hum Reprod 8:532, 1993.

38. **Hwang PLH, Ng CSA, Cheong ST,** Effect of oral contraceptives on serum prolactin: A longitudinal study in 126 normal premenopausal women, Clin Endocrinol 24:127, 1986.

39. **Sherman L, Fisher A, Klass E, Markowitz S,** Pharmacologic causes of hyperprolactinemia, Seminars Reprod Endocrinol 2:31, 1984.

40. **Pye JK, Mansel RE, Hughes LE,** Clinical experience of drug treatments for mastalgia, Lancet 2:373, 1985.

41. **Fentiman IS, Brame K, Caleffi M, Chaudary MA, Hayward JL,** Double-blind controlled trial of tamoxifen therapy for mastalgia, Lancet 1:287, 1986.

42. **Ernster VL, Mason L, Goodson WH III, Sickles EA, Sacks ST, Selvin S, Dupuy ME, Hawkinson J, Hunt TK,** Effects of caffeine-free diet on benign breast disease: a randomized trial, Surgery 91:263, 1982.

43. **Lubin F, Ron E, Wax Y, Black M, Funaro M, Shitrit A,** A case-control study of caffeine and methylxanthines in benign breast disease, JAMA 253:2388, 1985.

44. **Schairer C, Brinton LA, Hoover RN,** Methylxanthines and benign breast disease, Am J Epidemiol 124:603, 1986.

45. **American Cancer Society,** Cancer facts & figures — 1993.

46. **Harris JR, Lippman ME, Veronesi U, Willett W,** Breast cancer, New Engl J Med 327:319,390,473, 1992.

47. **Ewertz M, Duffy SW, Adami H-O, et al,** Age at first birth, parity and risk of breast cancer: a meta-analysis of 8 studies from the Nordic countries, Int J Cancer 46:597, 1990.

48. **Pathak DR, Speizer FE, Willett WC, Rosner B, Lipnick RJ,** Parity and breast cancer risk: possible effect on age at diagnosis, Int J Cancer 37:21, 1986.

49. **Musey VC, Collins DC, Brogan DR, Santos VR, Musey PI, Martino-Saltzman D, Preedy JRK,** Long term effects of a first pregnancy on the hormonal environment: estrogens and androgens, J Clin Endocrinol Metab 64:111, 1987.

50. **Musey VC, Collins DC, Musey PI, Martino-Saltzman D, Preedy JRK,** Long-term effects of a first pregnancy on the secretion of prolactin, New Engl J Med 316:229, 1987.

51. **McTiernan A, Thomas DB,** Evidence for a protective effect of lactation on risk of breast cancer in young women: results from a case-control study, Am J Epidemiol 124:353, 1986.

52. **Layde PM, Webster LA, Baughman L, et al,** The independent associations of parity, age at first full term pregnancy, and duration of breastfeeding with the risk of breast cancer, J Clin Epidemiol 42:963, 1989.

53. **United Kingdom National Case-Control Study Group,** Breast feeding and risk of breast cancer in young women, Br Med J 307:17, 1993.

54. **Newcomb PA, Storer BE, Longnecker MP, Mittendorf R, Greenberg ER, Clapp RW, Burke KP, Willett WC, MacMahon B,** Lactation and a reduced risk of premenopausal breast cancer, New Engl J Med 330:81, 1994.

55. **Ing R, Ho JHC, Petrakis NL,** Unilateral breast-feeding and breast cancer, Lancet 2:124, 1977.

56. **London SJ, Colditz GA, Stampfer MJ, Willett WC, Rosner BA, Corsano K, Speizer FE,** Lactation and the risk of breast cancer in a cohort of US women, Am J Epidemiol 132:17, 1990.

57. **Kvåle G, Heuch I,** Lactation and cancer risk: is there a relation specific to breast cancer? J Epidemiol Comm Health 42:30, 1987.

58. **La Vecchia C, Negri E, Bruzzi P, Dardanoni G, Decarli A, Franceschi S, Palli D, Talamini R,** The role of age at menarche and at menopause on breast cancer risk: combined evidence from four case-control studies, Ann Oncol 3:625, 1992.

59. **Sherman B, Wallace R, Beam J, Schlabaugh L,** Relationship of body weight to menarchial and menopausal age: implication for breast cancer risk, J Clin Endocrinol Metab 52:488, 1981.

60. **Dupont WD, Page DL,** Risk factors for breast cancer in women with proliferative breast disease, New Engl J Med 312:146, 1985.

61. **London SJ, Connolly JL, Schnitt SJ, Colditz GA,** A prospective study of benign breast disease and the risk of breast cancer, JAMA 267:941, 1992.

62. **Cancer Committee, College of American Pathologists,** Is 'fibrocystic disease' of the breast precancerous? Arch Path Lab Med 110:171, 1986.

63. **Sattin RW, Rubin GL, Webster LA, Huezo CM, Wingo PA, Ory HW, Layde PM,** Family history and the risk of breast cancer, JAMA 253:1908, 1985.

64. **Colditz GA, Willett WC, Hunter DJ, Stampfer MJ, Manson JE, Hennekens CH, Rosner BA, Speizer FE,** Family history, age, and risk of breast cancer, JAMA 270:338, 1993.

65. **Biesecker BB, Boehnke M, Calzone K, Markel DS, Garber JE, Collins FS, Weber BL,** Genetic counseling for families with inherited susceptibility to breast and ovarian cancer, JAMA 269:1970, 1993.

66. **King M-C, Rowell S, Love SM,** Inherited breast and ovarian cancer: what are the risks? what are the choices? JAMA 269:1975, 1993.

67. **Carroll KK,** Experimental studies on dietary fat and cancer in relation to epidemiological data, Prog Clin Biol Res 222:231, 1986.

68. **Willett WC, Browne ML, Bain C, Lipnick RJ, Stampfer MJ, Rosner B, Colditz GA, Hennekens CH, Speizer FE,** Relative weight and risk of breast cancer among premenopausal women, Am J Epidemiol 122:731, 1985.

69. **Willett WC, Hunter DJ, Stampfer MJ, Colditz G, Manson JE, Spiegelman D, Rosner B, Hennekens CH, Speizer FE,** Dietary fat and fiber in relation to risk of breast cancer: an 8-year follow-up, JAMA 268:2037, 1992.

70. **Jones DY, Schatzkin A, Green SB, Block G, Brinton LA, Ziegler RG, Hoover R, Taylor PR,** Dietary fat and breast cancer in the National Health and Nutrition Examination Survey Epidemiologic Follow-up Study, J Natl Cancer Inst 79:465, 1987.

71. **Howe GR, Hirohata R, Hislop TG, et al,** Dietary factors and risk of breast cancer: Combined analysis of 12 case-control studies, J Natl Cancer Inst 82561, 1990.

72. **Kushi LH, Sellers TA, Potter JD, Nelson CL, Munger RG, Kaye SA, Folsom AR,** Dietary fat and postmenopausal breast cancer, J Natl Cancer Inst 84:1092, 1992.

73. **Willett WC, Stampfer MJ, Colditz GA, Rosner BA, Hennekens CH, Speizer FE,** Moderate alcohol consumption and the risk of breast cancer, New Engl J Med 316:1174, 1987.

74. **Bulbrook RD,** Urinary androgen excretion and the etiology of breast cancer, J Natl Cancer Inst 48:1039, 1972.

75. **Dickinson LE, MacMahon B, Cole P, Brown JB,** Estrogen profiles of Oriental and Caucasian women in Hawaii, N Engl J Med 291:1211, 1974.

76. **Korenman SG,** The endocrinology of breast cancer, Cancer 46:874, 1980.

77. **Korenman SG,** Estrogen window hypothesis of the etiology of breast cancer, Lancet 1:700, 1980.

78. **Coulam CB, Annegers JF,** Breast cancer and chronic anovulation syndrome, Surgical Forum 33:474, 1982.

79. **Coulam CB, Annegers JF, Krans JS,** Chronic anovulation syndrome and associated neoplasia, Obstet Gynecol 61:403, 1983.

80. **Cowan LD, Gordis L, Tonascia JA, Jones GS,** Breast cancer incidence in women with a history of progesterone deficiency, Am J Epidemiol 114:209, 1981.

81. **Ron E, Lunenfeld B, Menczer J, Blumstein T, Katz L, Oelsner G, et al,** Cancer incidence in a cohort of infertile women, Am J Epidemiol 1987;125:780.

82. **McFayden IJ, Forrest APM, Prescott RJ, Golder MP, Groom GV, Fahmy DR,** Circulating hormone concentrations in women with breast cancer, Lancet 1:1000, 1976.

83. **Gammon MD, Thompson WD,** Infertility and breast cancer: a population-based case-control study, Am J Epidemiol 132:708, 1990.

84. **Gammon MD, Thompson WD,** Polycystic ovaries and the risk of breast cancer, Am J Epidemiol 134:818, 1991.

85. **Thompson WD, Jacobson HI, Negrini B, Janerich DT,** Hypertension, pregnancy, and risk of breast cancer, J Natl Cancer Inst 81:1571, 1989.

86. **Ekbom A, Trichopoulos D, Adami H-O, Hsieh C-C, Lan S-J,** Evidence of prenatal influences on breast cancer risk, Lancet 340:1015, 1992.

87. **Cuzick J, Wang DY, Bulbrook RD,** The prevention of breast cancer, Lancet 1:83, 1986.

88. **Clarke CL, Sutherland RL,** Progestin regulation of cellular proliferation, Endocrin Rev 11:266, 1990.

89. **Gompel A, Malet C, Spritzer P, Lalardrie J-P, Kuttenn F, Mauvais-Jarvis P**, Progestin effect on cell proliferation and 17β-hydroxysteroid dehydrogenase activity in normal human breast cells in culture, J Clin Endocrinol Metab 63:1174, 1986.

90. **Bibbo M, Haenszel W, Wied GL, Hubby M, Herbst AL,** A twenty-five year follow-up study of women exposed to DES during pregnancy, New Engl J Med 298:763, 1978.

91. **Greenburg ER, Barnes AB, Resseguie L, Barrett JA, Burnside S, Lanza LL, Neff RK, Stevens M, Young RH, Colton T,** Breast cancer in mothers given diethylstilbestrol in pregnancy, New Engl J Med 311:1393, 1984.

92. **Colton T, Greenberg ER, Noller K, Resseguie L, Van Bennekom C, Heeren T, Zhang Y,** Breast cancer in mothers prescribed diethylstilbestrol in pregnancy, JAMA 269:2096, 1993.

93. **McGuire WL, Clark GM,** Prognostic factors and treatment decisions in axillary-node-negative breast cancer, New Engl J Med 326:1756, 1992.

94. **Early Breast Cancer Trialists' Collaborative Group,** Systemic treatment of early breast cancer by hormonal, cytotoxic, or immune therapy, Lancet 339:1,71, 1992.

95. **Nolvadex Adjuvant Trial Organization,** Controlled trial of tamoxifen as single adjuvant agent in management of early breast cancer, Lancet 1:836, 1985.

96. **Tormey DC, Rasmussen P, Jordan VC,** Long-term adjuvant tamoxifen study: clinical update, Breast Cancer Res Treat 9:157, 1989.

97. **Fisher B, Brown A, Wolmark N, Redmond C, Wickerham DL, Nittliff J, Dimitrov N, Legault-Poisson S, Schipper H, Prager D,** Prolonging tamoxifen therapy for primary breast cancer, Ann Intern Med 106:649, 1987.

98. **Rose C, Theilade K, Boesen E, et al,** Treatment of advanced breast cancer with tamoxifen: Evaluation of the dose response relationship at 2 dose levels, Breast Cancer Res Treat 2:295, 1982.

99. **Glick JH, Gelber RD, Goldhirsch A, Senn H-J,** Meeting highlights: adjuvant therapy for primary breast cancer, J Natl Cancer Inst 84:1479, 1992.

100. **Buckley MM-T, Goa KL,** Tamoxifen: a reappraisal of its pharmacodynamic and pharmacokinetic properties, and therapeutic use, Drugs 37:451, 1989.

101. **Sunderland MC, Osborne CK,** Tamoxifen in premenopausal patients with metastatic breast cancer: a review, J Clin Oncol 9:1283, 1991.

102. **Breast Cancer Trials Committee, Scottish Cancer Trials Office,** Adjuvant tamoxifen in the management of operable breast cancer: the Scottish Trial, Lancet 2:171, 1987.

103. **Hindle WH,** Fine needle aspiration, in Hindle WH, editor, *Breast Disease for Gynecologists,* Appleton & Lange, Norwalk, Connecticut, 1990, pp 67-120.

104. **Donegan WL,** Evaluation of a palpable breast mass, New Engl J Med 327:937, 1992.

105. **Kopans LDB, Meyer JE, Sadowsky N,** Breast imaging, New Engl J Med 310:960, 1984.

106. **Wertheimer MD, Costanza ME, Dodson TF, D'Orsi C, Pastides H, Zapka JG,** Increasing the effort toward breast cancer detection, JAMA 255:1311, 1986.

107. **Carlile T, Kopecky KJ, Thompson DJ, Whitehead JR, Gilbert FI Jr, Present AJ, Threatt BA, Krook P, Hadaway E,** Breast cancer prediction and the Wolfe classification on mammograms, JAMA 254:1050, 1985.

108. **Verbeek ALM, Holland R, Sturmans F, Hendriks JHCL, Miravunac M, Day NE,** Reduction of breast cancer mortality through mass screening with modern mammography, Lancet 1:1222, 1984.

109. **Collette HJA, Rombach JJ, Day NE, De Waard F,** Evaluation of screening for breast cancer in non-randomized study (the DOM project by means of a case-control study), Lancet 1:124, 1984.

110. **Nystrom L, Rutqvist LE, Wall S, Lindgren A, Lindqvist M, Ryden S, Andersson I, Bjurstam N, Fagerberg G, Frisell J, Tabar L, Larsson L-G,** Breast cancer screening with mammography: overview of Swedish randomised trials, Lancet 341:973, 1993.

111. **Eddy DM, Hasselblad V, McGivney W, Hendee W,** The value of mammography screening in women under age 50 years, JAMA 259:1512, 1988.

112. **Miller AB, Baines CJ, To T, Wall C,** Canadian National Breast Screening Study: 1. Breast cancer detection and death rates among women aged 40 to 49 years, Can Med Assoc J 147:1459, 1992.

113. **Seidman H, Gelb SK, Silverberg E, LaVerda N, Lubera JA,** Survival experience in the breast cancer detection demonstration project, CA 37:258, 1987.

114. **Stacey-Clear A, McCarthy KA, Hall DA, Pile-Spellman E, White G, Hulka G, Whitman GJ, Mahoney E, Kopans DB,** Breast cancer survival among women under age 50: is mammography detrimental? Lancet 340:991, 1992.

115. **Elwood JM, Cox B, Richardson AK,** The effectiveness of breast cancer screening in young women, Curr Clin Trials 2:227, 1993.

116. **Mandelblatt JS, Wheat ME, Monane M, Moshief RD, Hollenberg JP, Tang J**, Breast cancer screening for elderly women with and without comorbid conditions: a decision analysis model, Ann Intern Med 116:722, 1992.

18

Menopause and Postmenopausal Hormone Therapy

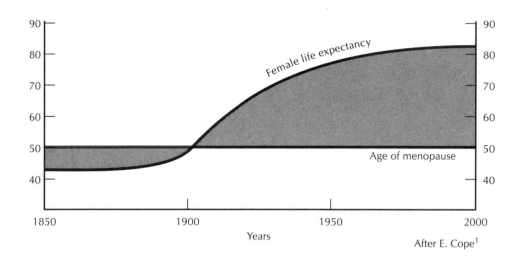

After E. Cope[1]

Throughout recorded history, multiple physical and mental conditions have been attributed to the menopause. While medical writers often wrote colorfully in the past, unfortunately they were also less than accurate, unencumbered by scientific information and data. A good example of the stereotypical, inaccurate thinking promulgated over the years is the following written in 1887:[2]

> The ovaries, after long years of service, have not the ability of retiring in graceful old age, but become irritated, transmit their irritation to the abdominal ganglia, which in turn transmit the irritation to the brain, producing disturbances in the cerebral tissue exhibiting themselves in extreme nervousness or in an outburst of actual insanity.

The belief that behavioral disturbances are related to manifestations of the female reproductive system, although an ancient one, has persisted to contemporary times. This belief is not totally illogical; there is reason to associate the middle years of life with negative experiences. The events that come to mind are impressive: onset of a major illness or disability (and even death) in a spouse, relative, or friend; retirement from employment; financial insecurity; the need to provide care for very old parents and relatives; and separation from children. And thus, it is not surprising that a middle age event, the menopause, shares in this negative outlook.

The scientific study of all aspects of menstruation has been hampered by the overpowering influence of social and cultural beliefs and traditions. Problems arising from life circumstances have often been erroneously attributed to the menopause. But data (especially more reliable longitudinal data) now indicate that the increase in most symptoms and problems in middle-aged women reflects social and personal circumstances, not the endocrine events of the menopause.[3–5]

The Massachusetts Women's Health Study, the largest and most comprehensive prospective, longitudinal study of middle-aged women, provides a powerful argument that the menopause is not and should not be viewed as a negative experience by the vast majority of women.[6] The cessation of menses was perceived by these women to have almost no impact on subsequent physical and mental health. This is reflected by women expressing either positive or neutral feelings about menopause. An exception is the group of women who experienced surgical menopause, but here there is good reason to believe that the reasons for the surgical procedure are more important than the cessation of menses.

Although many of the behavioral complaints at the time of the menopause can be explained by psychological and sociocultural influences, that is not to say that important interactions between biology, psychology, and culture do not occur. However, it is time to stress the normalcy of this life event. Menopausal women do not suffer from a disease (specifically a hormone deficiency disease), and postmenopausal hormone therapy should be viewed as specific treatment for symptoms in the short term and preventive pharmacology in the long term.

The variability in menopausal reactions makes the cross-sectional study design particularly unsuitable. More and larger longitudinal studies are needed to document what is normal and the variations around normal. Changes in menstrual function are not symbols of some ominous "change." There are good physiologic reasons for changing menstrual function, and understanding the physiology will do much to reinforce a healthy, normal attitude.

It can be further argued that physicians have had a biased (negative) point of view, because the majority of women, being healthy and happy, do not seek contact with physicians. It is important, therefore, that clinicians not only are familiar with the facts relative to the menopause but also have an appropriate attitude and philosophy regarding this period of life. Medical intervention at this point of life should be regarded as an opportunity to provide and reinforce a program of preventive health care. The issues of preventive health care for women are familiar ones. They include family planning, cessation of smoking, control of body weight and alcohol consumption, prevention of heart disease and osteoporosis, maintenance of mental well-being (including sexuality), cancer screening, and treatment of urologic problems.

The menopause serves a useful purpose. This physiologic event brings clinicians and patients together, providing the opportunity to enroll patients in a preventive health care program. Contrary to popular opinion, the menopause is not a signal of impending decline but rather a phenomenon that can signal the start of something positive, a good health program. ***Rather than being a lightning rod for social and personal problems, the menopause can be a signal for the future.***

Growth of the Older Population

Since 1960, the older segment of the U.S. population has been growing in size faster than the younger segment. By the year 2050, more than one out of five of us will be elderly. This is a world-wide development, not limited to affluent societies.[7] The population of the earth will continue to grow until the year 2100 or 2150, when it is expected to stabilize at approximately 11 billion; 95% of this growth will occur in developing countries, and the number of women over age 45 will exceed 700 million by the year 2000. The poorest countries today (located in Africa and Asia) account for about half of the global population, but by 2000, 87% of the world's population will be living in what are now called developing countries.

The decline in mortality has been greatest in the young. The reproduction of this increased younger population ultimately yields more old people. Another contribution

Projected Size of World Population Age 60 and Older[7]

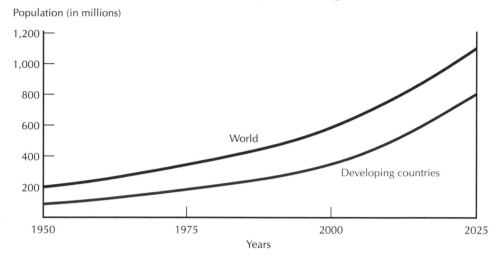

to aging of a national population is control of fertility; a decrease in fertility results in a decrease in the proportion of the younger population. Thus, control of fertility has an impact, but paradoxically, undeveloped countries with high fertility rates also develop a growing elderly population.

In developed countries, mortality rates in the young are near nadir levels; thus the main contribution to population aging in America in recent years has come from reduction in mortality in older ages (38% overall). The countries of northwestern Europe have reached a point of nearly stationary population; a population in which mortality and fertility rates are constant and there is no population growth. At this point about 18% of the total population is 65 or older.

In addition to the growing numbers of elderly people in the U.S., the older population itself is getting older.[8] For example, in 1984, the 65–74 age group was over 7 times larger than in 1900, but the 75–84 group was 11 times larger, and the 85 and older group was 21 times larger. The most rapid increase is expected between 2010 and 2030 when the post World War II baby boom generation hits 65. In the next century, the only age groups in the U.S. expected to experience significant growth will be those past age 55.

The death rate is higher for men at all ages. Coronary heart disease accounts for 40% of the mortality difference between men and women.[9] Another one-third is from lung cancer, emphysema, cirrhosis, accidents, and suicides. It is interesting to note that in our society the mortality difference between men and women is largely a difference in lifestyle. Smoking, drinking, coronary prone behavior, and accidents account for most of the higher male mortality rate over age 65. It has been estimated that perhaps two-thirds of the difference has been due to cigarettes alone.[9] Women lag behind men in the incidence of coronary heart disease by 10 years, and for myocardial infarction and sudden death, women have had a 20-year advantage.[10]

Men per 100 U.S. Women[11]

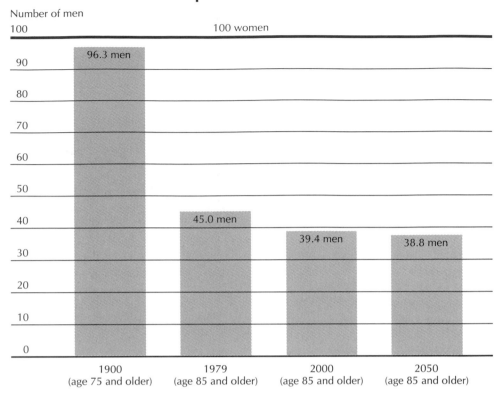

Number of men

In 1900 in the U.S., older men outnumbered women 102 to 100. In the 1980s, there were only 68 men for every 100 women over the age 65.[11] By age 85, only 45 men were alive for every 100 women. In 1985, 40% of American white women reached age 85 compared to only 20% of white men. Men and women, therefore, reach old age with different prospects for older age, a sex differential which (it can be argued) is due in part to the sex hormone-induced differences in the cholesterol-lipoprotein profile and thus the greater incidence of atherosclerosis and earlier death in men.[12] Therefore, the use of postmenopausal estrogen therapy, with its protective effect on atherosclerosis, may in fact exaggerate the sex differential in mortality. From a public health point of view, the greatest impact on the sex differential in mortality would be gained by concentrating on lifestyle changes designed to diminish atherosclerosis in men: low cholesterol diet, no smoking, optimal body weight, and active exercise.

Unmarried women will be an increasing proportion of the elderly. By 1983, 50% of American women ages 65–74 were unmarried (partly divorced, but mostly widowed), and after age 75, 77%![13] Because the unmarried tend to be more disadvantaged, there will be a need for more services for this segment of the elderly population. Older

The Older U.S. Female Population[11]

Age	1990		2000		2010		2020	
55–64	10.8 mill.	(8.6%)	12.1 mill.	(9.0%)	17.1 mill.	(12.1%)	19.3 mill.	(12.9%)
65–74	10.1	(8.1%)	9.8	(7.3%)	11.0	(7.8%)	15.6	(10.4%)
>75	7.8	(6.2%)	9.3	(7.0%)	9.8	(6.9%)	11.0	(7.3%)
Total	28.7		31.2		37.9		45.9	

unmarried people are more vulnerable, demonstrating higher mortality rates and lower life satisfaction.

Perhaps because more women are smoking, drinking, and working, the mortality sex difference has begun to lessen. The U.S. Census Bureau projects that the difference in life expectancy between men and women will increase until the year 2050, then level off.[11] In 2050, life expectancy for women will be 81 years and for men, 71.8 years. There will be 33.4 million women 65 and older compared to 22.1 million men. Today, women can expect to live nearly one-third of their lives after the menopause. The problems of the postmenopausal period, by virtue of the older population size alone, have achieved the status of a major public health concern.

There is concern at the individual level as well. For some women, menopause signals the beginning of an era of aging with its connotations of diminishing abilities and competence. The menopause, however, should and can mark the beginning of a new and promising period of life, relatively free from previous obligations, ready for new career choices, more education, and new ventures. Good medical practice dictates that the concerned clinician should support patients in a positive outlook for this period of time, a period of time which is growing in length and should be increasingly productive and rewarding.

The Age of Menopause

The *menopause* is that point in time when permanent cessation of menstruation occurs following the loss of ovarian activity. The *perimenopause* is the period immediately before and after the menopause. The *climacteric* is a more encompassing word, indicating the period of time when a woman passes through a transition from the reproductive stage of life to the postmenopausal years, a period marked by waning ovarian function.

Designating the average age of menopause has been somewhat difficult. Based upon cross-sectional studies, the median age has been estimated to be somewhere between 50 and 52.[14] These studies relied upon retrospective memories and the subjective vagaries of the individual being interviewed. Prospective studies with longitudinal follow-up to observe women and record their experiences as they pass through menopause have been hampered by relatively small numbers. The Massachusetts Women's Health Study now provides us with data from 2,570 women.[15]

In the Massachusetts Study, women who reported the onset of menstrual irregularity were considered to be perimenopausal. The median age for the onset of the perimenopause was 47.5 years. Only 10% of women ceased menstruating abruptly with no period of prolonged irregularity. The perimenopausal transition was, for most women, approximately 4 years in duration.

The median age for menopause in the Massachusetts Study was 51.3 years. Only current smoking could be identified as a cause of earlier menopause, a shift of approximately 1.5 years. Those factors that did not affect the age of menopause included the use of oral contraception, socioeconomic status, and marital status. Keep in mind that a median age of menopause means that only half the women have reached menopause at this age. Thus, it is more useful clinically to remember the range for the age of menopause, approximately age 48 to age 55.

Although clinical impression has suggested that mothers and daughters tend to experience menopause at the same age, what little data that exist are derived from retrospective, cross-sectional studies. The existence of a familial (inherited) effect must await longitudinal data. Ethnic differences suffer from the same methodologic problems. There is sufficient evidence to believe that undernourished women experience an earlier menopause.[16] There is no correlation between age of menarche and age of menopause.[17] Because of the contribution of body fat to estrogen production, thinner women experience a slightly earlier menopause.[18] Race, parity, and height have no influence on the age of menopause.[15,18]

An earlier menopause is associated with living at high altitudes and, as mentioned previously, with cigarette smoking. There is a dose-response relationship with the number of cigarettes smoked and the duration of smoking.[19] Even former smokers show evidence of an impact. There is reason to believe that premature ovarian failure can occur in women who have previously undergone abdominal hysterectomy, presumably because ovarian vasculature has been compromised.[20] About 1% of women will experience menopause before the age of 40.[21]

Unlike the decline in age of menarche that occurred with an improvement in health and living conditions, most historical investigation indicates that the age of menopause has changed little since early Greek times.[22,23] Others (a minority) have disagreed, concluding that the age of menopause did undergo a change, starting with an average age of about 40 years in ancient times.[24,25] If there has been a change, however, history indicates it has been minimal. Even in ancient writings, an age of 50 is usually cited as the age of menopause.

Sexuality and Menopause

Sexuality is a lifelong behavior with evolving change and development. It begins with birth (maybe before) and ends with death. The notion that it ends with aging is inherently illogical. The need for closeness, caring, and companionship is lifelong. Old people today live longer, are healthier, have more education and leisure time, and have had their consciousness raised in regard to sexuality.

Younger people, especially physicians, underrate the extent of sexual interest in older people. In a random sample of women aged 50 to 82 in Madison, Wisconsin, nearly one-half of the women reported an on-going sexual relationship.[26] In the Duke longitudinal study on aging, 70% of men in the 67 to 77 age group were sexually active, and 80% reported continuing sexual interest, while 50% of all older women were still interested in sex.[27]

There are two main sexual changes in the aging woman. There is a reduction in the rate of production and volume of vaginal lubricating fluid, and there is some loss of vaginal elasticity. The dyspareunia associated with postmenopausal urogenital atrophy includes a feeling of dryness and tightness, vaginal irritation and burning with coitus, and postcoital spotting and soreness. Less vaginal atrophy is noted in sexually active women compared to inactive women; presumably the activity maintains vaginal vasculature and circulation.

The decline in sexual activity with aging is influenced more by culture and attitudes than by nature and physiology (or hormones). The two most important influences on older sexual interaction are the strength of a relationship and the physical condition of each partner. The single most significant determinant of sexual activity for older women, therefore, is the unavailability of partners due to divorce and the fact that women are outliving men. Given the availability of a partner, the same general high or low rate of sexual activity can be maintained throughout life.[3,28] Longitudinal studies indicate that the level of sexual activity is more stable over time than previously suggested.[29–31] Individuals who are sexually active earlier in life continue to be sexually active into old age.

Hormone Production after Menopause

When women are in their forties, anovulation becomes more prevalent, and prior to anovulation, menstrual cycle length increases, beginning 2 to 8 years before menopause.[32] At the same time fewer follicles grow during each cycle until eventually the supply of follicles is depleted.[33]

The duration of the follicular phase is the major determinant of cycle length.[34] This menstrual cycle change prior to menopause is marked by elevated follicle-stimulating hormone (FSH) levels and decreased levels of inhibin, but normal levels of estradiol and luteinizing hormone (LH).[35] We now know that estradiol levels do not gradually wane in the years before menopause, but remain in the normal range until follicular growth and development cease. The FSH and inhibin change and inverse relationship indicate that inhibin is a more sensitive marker of ovarian follicular competence and, in turn, that FSH measurement is a clinical assessment of inhibin. Thus, the changes in the later reproductive years (the decline in inhibin allowing a rise in FSH) reflect lesser follicular competence because the better follicles respond early in life, leaving the lesser follicles for later.[36] The decrease in inhibin secretion by the ovarian follicles begins early (around age 35), but accelerates after 40 years of age. This is reflected in the decrease in fecundability that occurs with aging. Furthermore, the ineffective ability to suppress gonadotropins with postmenopausal hormone therapy is a consequence of the loss of inhibin, and for this reason ***FSH cannot be used clinically to titer estrogen dosage.***

The premenopausal years are a time period during which postmenopausal levels of FSH (greater than 30 IU/L) can be seen despite continued menstrual bleeding, while LH levels still remain in the normal range. Occasionally corpus luteum formation and function occur, and the perimenopausal woman is not totally safe from the threat of an unplanned and unexpected pregnancy until elevated levels of both FSH and LH can be demonstrated. According to the the Guinness Book of World Records, a woman from Portland, Oregon, holds the modern record for the oldest spontaneous pregnancy, conceiving when 57 years and 120 days old.

As cycles become irregular, vaginal bleeding occurs at the end of an inadequate luteal phase or after a peak of estradiol without subsequent ovulation or corpus luteum formation. But shortly after the menopause, one can safely say that there are no remaining ovarian follicles.[37] Eventually there is a 10–20-fold increase in FSH and approximately a 3-fold increase in LH, reaching a maximal level 1–3 years after menopause, after which there is a gradual, but slight, decline in both gonadotropins. Elevated levels of both FSH and LH at this time in life are conclusive evidence of ovarian failure. FSH levels are higher than LH because LH is cleared from the blood so much faster (half-lives are about 30 minutes for LH and 4 hours for FSH).

After menopause, the circulating level of androstenedione is about one half that seen prior to menopause.[38] Most of this postmenopausal androstenedione is derived from the adrenal gland, with only a small amount secreted from the ovary. Testosterone levels do not fall appreciably, and, in fact, the postmenopausal ovary in most women, but not all, secretes more testosterone than the premenopausal ovary. With the disappearance of follicles and estrogen, the elevated gonadotropins drive the remaining stromal tissue in the ovary to a level of increased testosterone secretion. Suppression of gonadotropins with gonadotropin releasing hormone (GnRH) agonist or antagonist treatment of postmenopausal women results in a significant decrease in circulating levels of testosterone, indicating the gonadotropin-dependent postmenopausal ovarian origin.[39,40] The total amount of testosterone produced after menopause, however, is decreased because the amount of the primary source, peripheral conversion of androstenedione, is reduced.

Blood Production Rates of Steroids[43]

	Reproductive age	Postmenopausal	Oophorectomized
Androstenedione	2–3 mg/day	0.5–1.0 mg/day	0.4–0.8 mg/day
Dehydroepiandrosterone	6–8	1.5–4.0	1.5–4.0
Dehydroepiandrosterone sulfate	8–16	4–9	4–9
Testosterone	0.2–0.25	0.05–0.1	0.02–0.07
Estrogen	0.350	0.045	0.045

The circulating estradiol level after menopause is approximately 10–20 pg/mL (40–70 pmol/L), most of which is derived from peripheral conversion of estrone.[38,41,42] The circulating level of estrone in postmenopausal women is higher than that of estradiol, the mean level being approximately 30–70 pg/mL (110–260 pmol/L). The average post-menopausal production rate of estrogen is approximately 45 μg/24 hours, almost all, if not all, being estrogen derived from the peripheral conversion of androstenedione. The androgen:estrogen ratio changes drastically after menopause because of the more marked decline in estrogen, and an onset of mild hirstism is common, reflecting this marked shift in the sex hormone ratio. With increasing age, a decrease can be measured in the circulating levels of dehydroepiandrosterone (DHA) and its sulfate (DHAS), whereas the circulating postmenopausal levels of androstenedione, testosterone, and estrogen remain relatively constant.

Estrogen production by the ovaries does not continue beyond the menopause; however, estrogen levels in postmenopausal women can be significant, principally due to the extraglandular conversion of androstenedione and testosterone to estrogen. The clinical impact of this estrogen will vary from one postmenopausal woman to another, depending upon the degree of extraglandular production, modified by a variety of factors.

The percent conversion of androstenedione to estrogen correlates with body weight. Increased production of estrogen from androstenedione with increasing body weight is probably due to the ability of fat to aromatize androgens. This fact and a decrease in the levels of sex hormone binding globulin (which results in increased free estrogen concentrations) contribute to the well-known association between obesity and the development of endometrial cancer. Body weight, therefore, has a positive correlation with the circulating levels of estrone and estradiol. Aromatization of androgens to estrogens is not limited to adipose tissue, however, because almost every tissue tested has this activity.

Eventually, the ovarian stroma is exhausted and, despite huge reactive increments in FSH and LH, no further steroidogenesis of importance results from gonadal activity. With increasing age, the adrenal contribution of precursors for estrogen production proves inadequate. In this final stage of estrogen availability, levels are insufficient to sustain secondary sex tissues.

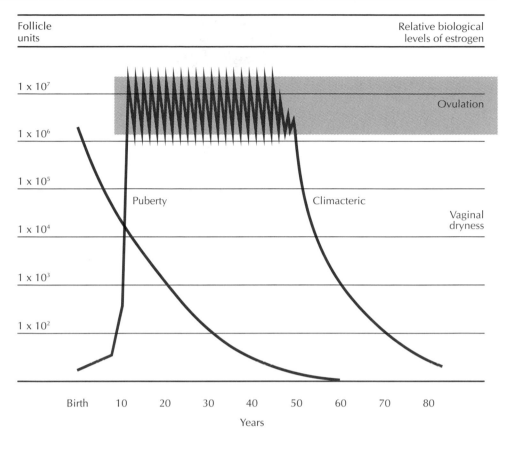

Follicle
units

Relative biological
levels of estrogen

The symptoms frequently seen and related to decreasing ovarian follicular competence and then estrogen loss in this protracted climacteric are:

1. Disturbances in menstrual pattern, including anovulation and reduced fertility, decreased flow or hypermenorrhea, and irregular frequency of menses.

2. Vasomotor instability (hot flushes and sweats).

3. Psychological symptoms, including anxiety, increased tension, mood depression, and irritability, although a direct cause and effect relationship between these symptoms and estrogen is hard to establish.

4. Atrophic conditions: atrophy of vaginal epithelium, formation of urethral caruncles, dyspareunia and pruritus due to vulvar, introital, and vaginal atrophy, general skin atrophy, urinary difficulties such as urgency and abacterial urethritis and cystitis.

5. Health problems secondary to long-term deprivation of estrogen: the consequences of osteoporosis and cardiovascular disease.

A precise understanding of the symptom complex the individual patient may display is often difficult to achieve. Some patients will experience severe multiple reactions that may be disabling. Others will show no reactions, or minimal reactions, which go unnoticed until careful medical evaluation.

It is helpful to classify the hormonal problems in 3 categories:

1. Those associated with relative *estrogen excess* such as dysfunctional uterine bleeding, edometrial hyperplasia, and endometrial cancer.

2. Those associated with *estrogen deprivation* such as flushes, atrophic vaginitis, urethritis, and osteoporosis.

3. Those associated with *estrogen-progestin therapy*.

Problems of Estrogen Excess

Not all climacteric women experience symptoms or signs of estrogen deprivation. Some actually manifest estrogen excess via the presence of uterine bleeding (dysfunctional uterine bleeding).

Throughout the usual period of life identified with perimenopause (ages 45–55), there is a significant incidence of dysfunctional uterine bleeding. Although the greatest concern provoked by this symptom is endometrial neoplasia, the usual finding is non-neoplastic tissue displaying estrogen effects unopposed by progesterone. This results from anovulation in premenopausal women and from extragonadal endogenous estrogen production or estrogen administration in the postmenopausal woman.

There are 4 mechanisms which could result in increased endogenous estrogen levels:

1. Increased precursor androgen (functional and nonfunctional endocrine tumors, liver disease, stress).

2. Increased aromatization (obesity, hyperthyroidism, liver disease).

3. Increased direct secretion of estrogen (ovarian tumors).

4. Decreased levels of SHBG (sex hormone binding globulin) leading to increased levels of free estrogen.

In all women, whether premenopausal or postmenopausal, whether on or off hormone therapy, specific organic causes (neoplasia, complications of unexpected pregnancy, or bleeding from extrauterine sites) must be ruled out. In addition to careful history and physical examination, dysfunctional uterine bleeding should be evaluated by aspiration endometrial biopsy. If the uterus is normal on examination, for reasons of both accuracy and cost effectiveness, the method of biopsy should be an office aspiration curettage, *NOT* the traditional, more costly and risky, in-hospital dilatation and curettage (D and C).[44]

We recommend the use of the plastic endometrial suction device. It is easy to use, requires no cervical dilatation (3 mm diameter), and is frequently painless. This device is as efficacious as older more painful techniques.[45] Insertion should first be attempted without the use of a tenaculum. In many patients, this is feasible and avoids the sensation of the tenaculum grasping the cervix. Once the suction is applied, the endometrial cavity should be thoroughly curetted in all directions, just as one would with a sharp curette during a D and C. If the cannula fills up with tissue, a second and even a third cannula should be inserted until tissue is no longer obtained. Although most patients report no problems with cramps or pain, the application of suction in some patients stimulates cramping that usually passes within 5–10 minutes. Because cramping occurs in such a small minority of patients, it is not our practice to routinely give an inhibitor of prostaglandin synthesis. For repeat biopsies, in patients known to cramp, it would be helpful to use such an agent at least 20 minutes before the procedure.

Less than 10% of postmenopausal women cannot be adequately evaluated by office biopsy. Most commonly, the reason is the inability to enter the uterine cavity. In such instances, an in-hospital D and C is in order. *Furthermore, if the uterus is not normal on pelvic examination, the office endometrial biopsy must yield to an in-hospital D and C in order to achieve accuracy of diagnosis.*

If vulva, vagina, and cervix appear normal on inspection, perimenopausal bleeding can be assumed to be intrauterine in origin. Confirmation requires the absence of abnormal cytology on the Pap smear. The principal symptom of endometrial cancer is abnormal vaginal bleeding, but carcinoma will be encountered in only about 2% of postmenopausal endometrial biopsies.[46] Normal endometrium is found over half the time, polyps in about 3%, and endometrial hyperplasia about 15% of the time. Postmenopausal bleeding should always be taken seriously.

Additional procedures include the following:

Colposcopy and cervical biopsy for abnormal cytology or obvious lesions.

Endocervical assessment by curettage for abnormal cytology (the endocervix must always be kept in mind as a source for abnormal cytology).

Hysterogram or hysteroscopy if bleeding persists to determine the presence of endometrial polyps or submucosal fibroids.

Keep in mind that the pathology reading, "tissue insufficient for diagnosis," when a patient is on estrogen-progestin treatment, represents atrophic, decidualized endometrium that yields little to the exploring curet. The clinician must be confident in his or her technique, knowing that a full investigation of the intrauterine cavity has been accomplished, then this reading can be interpreted as comforting and benign, the absence of pathology.

In postmenopausal women, one must view any adnexal mass as cancer until proven otherwise. Surgical intervention is usually necessary, and appropriate consultation must be obtained not only for the surgical procedure but also for suitable preoperative evaluation and preparation. Cysts which are less than 5 cm in diameter and without septations or solid components have a very low potential for malignant disease and may be managed with serial ultrasound surveillance.[47]

In the absence of organic disease, appropriate management of uterine bleeding is dependent upon the age of the woman and endometrial tissue findings. In the perimenopausal woman with dysfunctional uterine bleeding associated with proliferative or hyperplastic endometrium (uncomplicated by atypia or dysplastic constituents), periodic oral progestin therapy is mandatory, such as 10 mg medroxyprogesterone acetate given daily the first 10 days of each month. If hyperplasia is present, follow-up aspiration curettage after 3–4 months is required, and if progestin is ineffective and histological regression is not observed, formal curettage is an essential preliminary to alternate therapeutic surgical choices.

When monthly progestin therapy reverses hyperplastic changes (which it does in 95–98% of cases) and controls irregular bleeding, treatment should be continued until withdrawal bleeding ceases. This is a reliable sign (in effect, a bioassay) indicating the onset of estrogen deprivation and the need for the addition of estrogen. If vasomotor disturbances begin before the cessation of menstrual bleeding, the combined estrogen-progestin program can be initiated as needed to control the flushes.

If contraception is required, the clinician and the healthy, nonsmoking patient should seriously consider the use of oral contraception. The anovulatory woman cannot be guaranteed that spontaneous ovulation and pregnancy will not occur. The use of a low dose oral contraceptive will at the same time provide contraception and prophylaxis against irregular, heavy anovulatory bleeding and the risk of endometrial hyperplasia and neoplasia.

Clinicians have been made so wary of providing oral contraceptives to older women that a traditional hormone regimen is often utilized to treat a woman with the kind of irregular cycles usually experienced in the perimenopausal years. This addition of exogenous estrogen when a woman is not amenorrheic or experiencing menopausal symptoms is inappropriate and even risky (exposing the endometrium to excessively high levels of estrogen). The appropriate response is to regulate anovulatory cycles with monthly progestational treatment or to utilize low dose oral contraception.

A common clinical dilemma is when to change from oral contraception to postmenopausal hormone therapy. It is important to change because even with the lowest estrogen dose oral contraceptive available, the estrogen dose is four-fold greater than the standard postmenopausal dose, and with increasing age, the dose-related risks with estrogen become significant. One approach to establish the onset of the postmenopausal years is to measure the FSH level, beginning at age 50, on an annual basis, being careful to obtain the blood sample on day 5–7 of the pill-free week (when steroid levels have declined sufficiently to allow FSH to rise). Friday afternoon of the pill-free week works for patients on Sunday start schedules. When FSH is greater than 30 IU/L, it is time to change to a postmenopausal hormone program.

The Impact of Postmenopausal Estrogen Deprivation

During the menopausal years, some women will experience severe multiple symptoms, while others will show no reactions or minimal reactions that can go unnoticed. The differences in menopausal reactions in symptoms across different cultures is poorly documented, and indeed, it is difficult to do so. Individual reporting is so conditioned by sociocultural factors that it is hard to determine what is due to biological vs cultural variability. Nevertheless, there is reason to believe that the nature and prevalence of menopausal symptoms are common to all women.[48]

Vasomotor Symptoms

The vasomotor flush is viewed as the hallmark of the female climacteric, experienced to some degree by most postmenopausal women. The term "hot flush" is descriptive of a sudden onset of reddening of the skin over the head, neck, and chest, accompanied by a feeling of intense body heat and concluded by sometimes profuse perspiration. The duration varies from a few seconds to several minutes and rarely for an hour. The frequency may be rare to recurrent every few minutes. Flushes are more frequent and severe at night (when a woman is often awakened from sleep) or during times of stress. In a cool environment, hot flushes are fewer, less intense, and shorter in duration compared to a warm environment.[49]

In the Massachusetts Women's Health Study, the incidence of hot flushes increased from 10% during the perimenopausal period to about 50% just after cessation of menses.[14] By approximately 4 years after menopause, the rate of hot flushes declined to 20%. Although the flush can occur in the premenopause, it is a major feature of postmenopause, lasting in most women for 1–2 years but, in some (as many as 25–50%) for longer than 5 years.

The physiology of the hot flush is still not understood, but it apparently originates in the hypothalamus and is brought about by a decline in estrogen. However, not all hot flushes are due to estrogen deficiency. In a massive review of hot flushes, it was concluded that exact estimates on prevalence are hampered by inconsistencies and differences in methodologies, cultures, and definitions.[50] In the longitudinal follow-up of a large number of American women, fully 10% of the women experienced hot flushes before menopause, while in other studies as many as 15–25% of premenopausal women report hot flushes.[14,51,52] Unfortunately, the hot flush is a relatively common psychosomatic symptom, and women often are unnecessarily treated with estrogen. ***When the clinical situation is not clear and obvious, estrogen deficiency as the cause of hot flushes should be documented by elevated levels of FSH.***

Although the hot flush is the most common problem of the postmenopause, it presents no inherent health hazard. The flush is accompanied by a discrete and reliable pattern of physiologic changes.[53] The flush coincides with a surge of LH (not FSH) and is preceded by a subjective prodromal awareness that a flush is beginning. This aura is followed by measurable increased heat over the entire body surface. The body surface experiences an increase in temperature, accompanied by changes in skin conductance, and followed by a fall in core temperature — all of which can be objectively measured. In short, the flush is not a release of accumulated body heat but is a sudden inappropriate excitation of heat release mechanisms. Its relationship to the LH surge and temperature change within the brain is not understood. The observation that flushes occur after hypophysectomy indicates that the mechanism is not dependent on or due directly to LH release. In other words, the same hypothalamic event that causes flushes also stimulates gonadotropin releasing hormone (GnRH) secretion and elevates LH.

The correlation between the onset of flushes and estrogen reduction is clinically supported by the effectiveness of estrogen therapy and the absence of flushes in hypoestrogen states, such as gonadal dysgenesis. Only after estrogen is administered and withdrawn do hypogonadal women experience the hot flush. Although the clinical impression that premenopausal surgical castrates suffer more severe vasomotor reactions is widely held, this is not borne out in objective study.[54]

Atrophic Changes

With extremely low estrogen production in the late postmenopausal age, or many years after castration, atrophy of mucosal surfaces takes place, accompanied by vaginitis, pruritus, dyspareunia, and stenosis. Genitourinary atrophy leads to a variety of symptoms which affect the ease and quality of living. Urethritis with dysuria, urgency incontinence, and urinary frequency are further results of mucosal thinning, in this instance, of the urethra and bladder. Recurrent urinary tract infections are effectively prevented by postmenopausal estrogen treatment.[55] Vaginal relaxation with cystocele, rectocele, and uterine prolapse, and vulvar dystrophies are not a consequence of estrogen deprivation. Although it is argued that genuine stress incontinence will not be affected by treatment with estrogen, others contend that estrogen treatment improves or cures genuine stress incontinence in over 50% of patients due to a direct effect on the urethral mucosa.[56,57] Most cases of urinary incontinence in elderly women are a mixed problem with a significant component of urge incontinence that definitely can be improved by estrogen therapy.

Unless dermatologic conditions exist masquerading as menopausal atrophy, estrogen therapy is invariably successful in reversing these atrophic problems. Relief from these problems often results in significant improvements in general well-being. There is a general clinical consensus that certain physical changes (redistribution of fat deposits and loss of elastic tissue in the skin with wrinkling) are due to aging rather than to estrogen deprivation. Nevertheless, the decline in skin collagen content and skin thickness which occurs with aging can be considerably avoided by postmenopausal estrogen therapy; whether this makes a difference in physical appearance is uncertain.[58]

Dyspareunia seldom brings older women to our offices. A basic reluctance to discuss sexual behavior still permeates our society, especially among older patients and physicians. Gentle questioning may lead to estrogen treatment of atrophy and enhancement of sexual enjoyment. Objective measurements have demonstrated that vaginal factors which influence the enjoyment of sexual intercourse can be maintained by appropriate doses of estrogen.[59] Both patient and clinician should be aware that a significant response can be expected by one month, but it takes a long time to fully restore the genitourinary tract (6–12 months), and clinicians and patients should not be discouraged by an apparent lack of immediate response. Furthermore, sexual activity by itself supports the circulatory response of the vaginal tissues and enhances the therapeutic effects of estrogen. Therefore sexually active older women will have less atrophy of the vagina even without estrogen.

One of the features of aging in men and women is a steady reduction in muscular strength. Many factors affect this decline, including height, weight, and level of physical activity. However, women currently using estrogen do not demonstrate this age-related decline in muscular competence (as measured by handgrip strength).[60] This can be viewed as another substantial benefit of estrogen, with potential protective consequences against fractures, as well as a benefit due to the ability to maintain vigorous physical exercise. In addition, there is some evidence that estrogen treatment before the onset of joint disease is associated with protection against rheumatoid arthritis, however this protective effect is debatable.[61]

Psychophysiologic Effects

The view that menopause has a deleterious effect on mental health is not supported in the psychiatric literature, or in surveys of the general population.[62,63] The concept of a specific psychiatric disorder (involutional melancholia) has been abandoned. Indeed, depression is less common, not more common, among middle-aged women.[5,64–66] A negative view of mental health at the time of the menopause is not justified; many of the problems reported at the menopause are due to the vicissitudes of life. Thus, there are problems encountered in the early postmenopause that are seen frequently, but their causal relation with estrogen is uncertain. These problems include fatigue, nervousness, headaches, insomnia, depression, irritability, joint and muscle pain, dizziness, and palpitations.

Attempts to study the effects of estrogen on these problems have been hampered by the subjectivity of the complaints (high placebo responses) and the "domino effect" of what reduction of hot flushes does to the frequency of the symptoms. Using a double-blind crossover prospective study format, Campbell and Whitehead[67] concluded that many symptomatic "improvements" ascribed to estrogen therapy result from relief of hot flushes — a domino effect. Improvement in memory and reduction of anxiety were also noted in these observations. Another short-term study failed to document an objective improvement in memory, although a slight improvement in mood was recorded.[68] On the other hand, estrogen treatment of women immediately after bilateral oophorectomy was associated with improvement in certain, but not all, specific tests of memory.[69] Perhaps this lack of agreement is due to the variability in test vehicles and the specific aspects of memory function studied. Fatigue, irritability, headache, and depression are not thought to be estrogen-related phenomena.

Emotional stability during the perimenopausal period can be disrupted by poor sleep patterns. Estrogen therapy improves the quality of sleep, decreasing the time to onset of sleep and increasing the rapid eye movement (REM) sleep time.[70,71] Perhaps flushing may be insufficient to awaken a woman but sufficient to affect the quality of sleep, thereby diminishing the ability to handle the next day's problems and stresses.

It is still uncertain whether estrogen treatment has a direct antidepressant effect or whether the mood response is an indirect benefit of relief from physical symptoms and, consequently, improved sleep. Utilizing various assessment tools for measuring depression, improvements with estrogen treatment have been recorded in oophorectomized women.[72,73] In a large cross-sectional study of the Rancho Bernardo retirement community, no benefit could be detected in measures of depression in current users of postmenopausal estrogen compared to untreated women.[74] Indeed, treated women had higher depressive symptom scores, presumably reflecting treatment selection bias; symptomatic and depressed women seek hormone therapy.

Tests of cognitive function in a prospective, but cross-sectional study of the Rancho Bernardo retirement community failed to support a positive impact of postmenopausal estrogen on mental function in old age.[75] The Rancho Bernardo study has the attribute of being large in size (800 women), which also allowed for testing of duration of use (there was no benefit that resulted from long duration of use). There were too few patients in the Rancho Bernardo cohort with dementia to assess the impact of estrogen on Alzheimer's disease.

Important early findings in the Leisure World cohort indicate that Alzheimer's disease and related dementia occurred less frequently in estrogen users, and the effect was greater with increasing dose and duration of use.[76] Furthermore, the administration of estrogen to patients with Alzheimer's disease has improved cognitive performance.[77] If this effect of estrogen can be verified, the potential impact on this dreadful condition which is more prevalent in women cannot be underrated. This would be another argument in favor of long-term treatment.

Osteoporosis

Osteoporosis is epidemic in the United States, presently affecting more than 20 million individuals.[78] The increase in osteoporotic fractures in the developed world is partly due to an increase in the elderly population, but not totally. This is a major global public health problem. A comparison of bone densities in proximal femur bones in specimens from a period of over 200 years suggested that women lose more bone today, perhaps due to less physical activity and less parity.[79] Other contributing factors include a dietary decrease in dairy products and an earlier and greater loss of bone because of the impact of smoking.

Osteoporosis is characterized by microarchitectural deterioration of bone tissue, leading to enhanced bone fragility and a consequent increase in the risk of fractures. The skeleton consists of two bone types. Cortical bone is responsible for 80% of total bone, while trabecular bone, the bone of the spinal column, constitutes a honeycomb structure providing greater surface area per unit volume. The onset of spinal bone loss begins in the 20s, but the overall change is small until menopause. Bone density in the femur peaks in the mid to late 20s and begins to decrease around age 30. In general, trabecular bone resorption and formation occur four to eight times as fast as cortical bone. Beyond age 40 resorption begins to exceed formation by about 0.5% per year. This adverse relationship accelerates after menopause and up to 5% of trabecular bone and 1–1.5% of total bone mass loss will occur per year after menopause. This accelerated loss will continue for 10–15 years, after which bone loss is considerably diminished but continues as the aging-related loss. For the first 20 years following cessation of menses, menopause-related bone loss results in a 50% reduction in trabecular bone and a 30% reduction in cortical bone.[80,81] The process is slower in blacks.

The change in trabecular bone in postmenopausal women is attributed to estrogen deficiency; 75% or more of the bone loss that occurs in women during the first 15 years after menopause is attributable to estrogen deficiency rather than to aging itself.[82,83] A study of the premenopausal daughters of women with osteoporosis revealed a reduction in bone mass, suggesting either a genetic influence or the sharing of a lifestyle which produces a relatively low peak bone mass.[84]

The subsequent risk of fracture from osteoporosis will depend upon bone mass at the time of menopause and the rate of bone loss following menopause. In general, bone mass is increased in black and obese women and decreased in white, Asian, thin and sedentary women. Vertebral bone is especially vulnerable, with a bone density threshold for fracture only slightly below the lower limit of normal for premenopausal women. It is no surprise that vertebral fractures account for 50% of all fractures. Indeed 25% of individuals over 70 years of age show radiographic evidence of these crush type fractures that lead to dorsal kyphosis (dowager's hump). The average nontreated postmenopausal white woman can expect to shrink 2.5 inches (6.4 cm).

Hip fractures begin to occur in the 10–15 years following menopause such that by age 90, 20% of all white women will have developed hip fractures, of which one-sixth will be fatal within three months. Hip fractures alone occur in about 250,000 women per year in the U.S. with a mortality of 40,000 annually and an associated cost of billions of dollars. In addition, the survivors are frequently severely disabled and may become permanent invalids.

Estrogen therapy will stabilize the process of osteoporosis or prevent it from occurring. *The critical blood level of estradiol that is necessary to maintain bone is 40–50 pg/mL (150–180 pmol/L).* With estrogen therapy one can expect a 50–60% decrease in fractures of the arm and hip,[85–87] and when estrogen is supplemented with calcium, an 80% reduction in vertebral compression fractures can be observed.[88] This reduction is seen primarily in patients who have taken estrogen for more than 5 years.[89] If bone loss can be delayed with estrogen therapy for 8 years, fracture incidence can be reduced by 75%.

The positive impact of hormone therapy on bone has been demonstrated to take place even in women over age 65.[89–91] This is a strong argument in favor of treating very old women who have never been on estrogen. Estrogen use between the ages of 65 and 74 has been documented to protect against fractures.[87] *However, protection against fractures wanes with age, and long-term estrogen use is necessary to reduce the risk of fracture after age 75.*[90]

Studies have demonstrated that a dose of 0.625 mg of conjugated estrogens is necessary to preserve bone density.[92] A lower dose of 0.3 mg daily of conjugated estrogens or 0.5 mg estradiol prevented loss of vertebral trabecular bone when combined with calcium supplementation (to achieve a total intake of 1,500 mg daily).[93,94] A study of women randomized to treatment either with continuous transdermal delivery of estradiol 50 μg or oral estrogen demonstrated that both equally prevented postmenopausal bone loss.[95] The positive impact of estrogen increases with increasing dose; thus, whether fracture protection with either the lower oral dose regimens or via a transdermal route of administration is equal to the standard oral program awaits further epidemiologic study. Furthermore, some decrease in cardiovascular protection occurs with the use of lower doses of estrogen.

The precise mechanism of action for sex steroid protection of bones remains unknown; however a growing body of knowledge indicates complex interactions at the molecular level. Increased efficiency of calcium absorption (probably secondary to estrogen-induced enhancement of the availability of the active metabolite of vitamin D, 1,25-dihydroxyvitamin D) and a direct role for the estrogen receptors in the osteoblasts are likely important factors. Many estrogen-dependent growth factors and cytokines are involved in bone remodeling.[96] Estrogen modulates the production of bone resorbing cytokines such as interleukin-1 and -6, bone stimulating factors such as insulin-like growth factors I and II, and transforming growth factor-β. Estrogen also promotes the synthesis of calcitonin (which inhibits bone resorption).[97] Estrogen increases vitamin D receptors in osteoblasts, and this may be a method by which estrogen modulates 1,25-dihydroxyvitamin D activity in bone.[98]

While progestational agents are considered antiestrogenic, they have been known to act independently, in a manner similar to estrogen, to reduce bone resorption. However, this effect may be limited to cortical bone.[97] When added to estrogen, progestins actually lead to a synergistic increase in bone formation associated with a positive balance of calcium.[99–103] The daily, continuous combination of estrogen-progestin is equally efficacious in maintaining bone density as the standard sequential regimens.[104]

There has been considerable confusion over whether calcium supplementation by itself can offer protection against postmenopausal osteoporosis. This is partly due to the fact that calcium studies have been performed in women who were in the very early postmenopausal years, in the midst of the rapid loss of calcium associated with estrogen deficiency. Studies that involve women beyond this early stage of the postmenopausal period definitely indicate a positive impact of calcium supplementation.

Calcium absorption decreases with age and becomes significantly impaired after menopause. A positive calcium balance is mandatory to achieve adequate prevention against osteoporosis. Calcium supplementation (1,000 mg per day) reduces bone loss and decreases fractures, especially in individuals with low daily intakes.[105] However, estro-

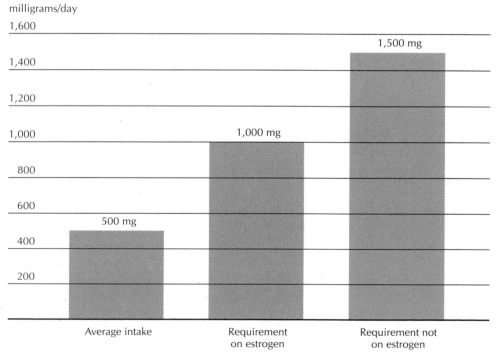

Calcium Requirement for Zero Balance[106]

milligrams/day

599

gen acts to improve calcium absorption and makes it possible to utilize effective supplemental calcium in lower doses. In order to remain in zero calcium balance, women on estrogen therapy require a total of 1,000 mg elemental calcium per day.[106,107] Since the average woman receives only 500 mg of calcium in her diet, the minimal daily supplement equals an additional 500 mg. Women not on estrogen require a daily supplement of at least 1,000 mg calcium. Even with the commonly used therapeutic doses of calcium, nearly 40% of postmenopausal women will have inefficient absorption.[108] Therefore estrogen improves calcium absorption and makes it possible to utilize supplemental calcium in effective doses without the side effects associated with higher doses (constipation and flatulence) that diminish compliance. Nevertheless, the calcium supplementation should be administered in divided doses with meals. We must emphasize that although calcium supplementation is important, it cannot provide the same degree of protection against osteoporosis as that achieved by hormonal therapy.[109]

The addition of vitamin D or its active metabolite in some studies has no impact on the osteoporosis fracture rate and may cause hypercalcemia and renal stone formation.[110] However, elderly people in nursing homes are usually deficient in vitamin D, and it is now recommended that individuals over age 70 should add 800 units of vitamin D to calcium supplementation.[80] A large randomized trial in Finland has documented a reduced rate of fractures in elderly women receiving supplementation of vitamin D (by an annual intramuscular injection), and in France, supplementation of calcium and vitamin D reduced the number of hip fractures by 43%.[111,112] Because adequate vitamin D depends upon cutaneous generation mediated by sun exposure, women who live in cloudy areas during the winter months are relatively vitamin D deficient and lose bone.[113] Vitamin D supplementation is recommended for these women as well but at a lower level, 400 units daily. If uncertain regarding vitamin D supplementation, the serum level of the active metabolite, 1,25-dihydroxyvitamin D, can be measured; the normal range is 19–57 ng/L (45–140 pmol/L).

The addition of fluoride, a potent stimulator of bone formation, does offer some benefit but with a high rate of side effects (which may be greatly reduced with slow release preparations). A further concern is that this therapy may lead to more brittle bones subject to fracture.[114]

Calcitonin will act to prevent bone resorption and eventually might be used in patients for whom hormone therapy is contraindicated. Given by injection in a dose of 100 IU daily to women early after menopause it has the same effectiveness as estrogen in conserving bone density.[115] Studies with intranasal delivery of calcitonin (200 IU daily) suggest it may be similarly effective.[116]

Etidronate disodium is an oral biphosphonate compound known to reduce bone resorption through the inhibition of osteoclastic activity. In postmenopausal women with osteoporosis randomized to intermittent cyclical etidronate (400 mg daily for 2 weeks followed by a 12-week drug free interval during which 1500 mg/day of calcium is administered) or placebo, a significant increase in vertebral bone mineral content and a significant decrease in fracture rate was observed in the treatment group.[117] Newer biphosphates are more active than etidronate. Alendronate given in various doses to postmenopausal women for only 6 weeks increased bone density with a lack of side effects.[118] Biphosphates may prove to be an effective addition to osteoporotic prevention because they are well tolerated and have no discernible side effects. However, unlike estrogens, biphosphates have no effect on cardiovascular disease, hot flushes, or the atrophic changes seen in menopause. At the present time further studies must be performed to evaluate the efficacy and value of biphosphates for prevention of osteoporosis.

Lifestyle can have a beneficial effect on bone density. Physical activity (weight bearing), as little as 30 minutes a day for 3 days a week, will increase the mineral content of bone in older women.[119] The exercise need not be extreme. Walking 1.5 miles and ordinary calisthenics will suffice. The impact of exercise on bone is significantly less, however, than that achieved by hormone therapy.[109] Women require the full combination of hormone therapy, calcium supplementation, and exercise in order to fully minimize the risk of fractures.

Adverse habits such as cigarette smoking or excessive alcohol consumption are associated with an increased risk of osteoporosis. The lower blood levels of estrogen in smokers have been correlated with an earlier menopause and a reduced bone density, and therefore estrogen therapy will not totally counteract the predisposition of smoking toward osteoporosis.[120] The titration of estrogen dosage with circulating blood estradiol levels in smokers makes clinical sense, allowing the use of higher hormonal doses to maintain bone density. Clinicians should always remember that exposure to excessive thyroid and glucocorticoid hormones is associated with osteoporosis and an increased rate of fractures.

The protection of estrogen is maintained only while women are maintained on the hormone. In the 3 to 5 year period following loss of estrogen, whether after menopause or after cessation of estrogen therapy, there is an accelerated loss of bone.[121–123] For the greatest impact on the risk of fractures, it is vital that hormone therapy be initiated as close to the menopause as possible, and it must be maintained long-term, if not life long.

Patients with osteoporosis or with a history of osteoporotic fracture should be treated more vigorously. While hormone therapy will significantly increase bone mass, agents such as fluoride, calcitonin and perhaps etidronate should also be considered.

Patients with osteoporosis should be screened for other conditions that lead to osteoporosis:

1.   Serum parathyroid hormone, calcium, phosphorus, and alkaline phosphatase: for primary hyperparathyroidism.

2.   Renal function tests: for secondary hyperparathyroidism with chronic renal failure.

3.   Blood count and smear, sedimentation rate, protein electrophoresis: for multiple myeloma, leukemia, or lymphoma.

4.   Thyroid function tests: for hyperthyroidism.

5.   Careful history and, when indicated, appropriate laboratory studies to rule out hypercortisolism, alcohol abuse, and metastatic cancer.

Measuring Bone Density

There is a 50–100% increase in fracture risk for each standard deviation decline in bone mass.[124] Measurement of lower bone mass in the hip is even more predictive; a one standard deviation is associated with nearly a 3-fold increase in risk of fracture.[125] This impressive correlation between fracture risk and bone density has raised the question whether it is of value to screen for osteoporosis. It is not cost-effective to attempt to screen all postmenopausal women, especially since hormonal treatment is advised for nearly all. However, bone density measurements are useful when an individual woman requires the information in order to make an informed decision regarding hormone therapy. Indeed, better compliance with a hormone program is correlated with patients' knowledge of an increased risk of fracture. Because smokers have lower estrogen levels on estrogen therapy, it might be worthwhile to document the impact of treatment on bone density in order to consider whether dosage is adequate. Patients who have received long-term corticosteroid or thyroxine treatment deserve bone mass assessment.

There is a percentage of postmenopausal women on hormone therapy (about 10–20%) who continue to lose bone. It is likely that this reflects poor compliance, and consideration should be given to an occasional measurement of bone density as an effective method of assessment and to motivate compliance.

Summary of Reasons to Measure Bone Mass
1. **To help patients to make decisions regarding hormone therapy.**
2. **To assess response to therapy in selected patients, e.g., smokers.**
3. **To confirm the diagnosis and assess the severity of osteoporosis to aid in treatment decisions.**

Standard x-rays do not provide an early assessment of fracture risk; 30–40% of bone must be lost before radiographic changes become apparent. Photon absorptiometry measures the transmission of photons through bone. Single photon absorptiometry uses an ^{125}I source of energy or, more recently, miniature x-ray tubes. This method measures bone density in the radius and the calcaneus. These measurements correlate with vertebral bone density but not very accurately. Dual energy absorptiometry employs photons from two energy sources. Dual energy x-ray absorptiometry (DEXA) provides good precision for all sites of osteoporotic fractures. Whole body scans by DEXA can measure total body calcium, lean body mass, and fat mass. Quantitative computed tomography for bone density measurements can be performed on most commercial computed tomography (CT) systems; however, radiation exposure is higher than with DEXA, and measurements of the femur are not available. The most accurate information is provided by the DEXA technique, measuring the three sites of greatest interest, the radius, the hip, and the spine. Serial measurements are usually at least one year apart.

Prevention of Osteoporosis
The risk of osteoporosis is significantly influenced by the amount of bone accumulation during growth and maturation, followed by the rate of bone loss thereafter. The preventive health efforts of clinicians should be directed to those factors that influence accumulation and loss of bone throughout life.[126] Improved calcium intake in adolescents results in significant increases in bone density and skeletal mass, providing protection against osteoporosis later in life.[127] As always, counseling should be provided regarding diet, exercise, avoidance of smoking and alcohol abuse, and maintenance of normal menstrual function. The primary care clinician should always keep in mind the necessity to monitor thyroid hormone dosage with periodic measurements of thyroid-stimulating hormone (TSH). Postmenopausal women receiving long-term treatment with corticosteroids should be urged to use estrogen-progestin therapy and calcium supplementation.

Cardiovascular Disease

It wasn't until results from randomized clinical trials were available that clinicians began to treat hypertension seriously, and the cholesterol crusade was initiated. There have been no significant clinical trials addressing the question whether postmenopausal hormonal treatment reduces the risk of cardiovascular disease in women. Such scientific proof will be hard and expensive to come by. In the meantime, patients and colleagues are asking for a strong medical judgment on this issue. This is not as difficult as it sounds. A consideration of all available data allows a firm conclusion that is clinically useful.

Cardiovascular Disease in Women

Cardiovascular disease is the most common cause of death in the United States. It includes coronary heart disease, cerebral vascular disease, hypertension, and peripheral vascular disease. Diseases of the heart are the leading cause of death for women in the United States, followed by malignant neoplasms, cerebrovascular disease, and motor vehicle accidents. In the U.S., 500,000 women die each year of cardiovascular disease.[128]

Most cardiovascular disease results from atherosclerosis in major vessels. The risk factors are the same for men and women: high blood pressure, smoking, diabetes mellitus, and obesity. When controlling for these risk factors, men have a risk of developing coronary heart disease over 3.5 times that of women. Even taking into consideration the changing lifestyle of women (e.g., employment outside the home), women still maintain their advantage in terms of risk for coronary heart disease.

Prior to the 1960s, there was an epidemic rise in mortality from coronary heart disease. Now the death rate is declining in most industrialized countries.[129] The male:female ratios of the rates vary from 3:1 to 6:1 among 27 countries, with a rather consistent incidence around the world. Despite the favorable male:female ratio and the decline in disease, this is an expensive health care problem for women.

In the last 30 years, stroke mortality has declined by 60% and mortality from coronary heart disease by 30% in the U.S. Improvements in medical and surgical care can account for some of this decline, but 60–70% of the improvement is due to preventive measures.[130] Excellent data from epidemiologic studies and clinical trials demonstrate a decline in morbidity and mortality from smoking cessation, blood pressure reduction, and lowering of cholesterol. We can now recognize that there is a strong and growing scientific basis for preventive medicine and health promotion efforts in clinical practice.

Most research involving the prevention of cardiovascular disease has been performed with male subjects. Although there is some skepticism regarding whether results can be extrapolated from men to women, most of the recommendations for risk intervention are the same for men and women. Evidence that risk factor modification in women makes a difference can be derived from the 43% decline in cardiovascular death rates in women in the U.S. from 1963 to 1983.[130]

We now have another opportunity. Postmenopausal hormone therapy deserves consideration as a legitimate component of preventive health care for older women. One can argue convincingly that protection against cardiovascular disease is the major benefit of postmenopausal estrogen treatment, and the magnitude of this benefit is considerable. There is a sound rationale for this protection in the link between cardiovascular disease and the sex hormones.

The Difference between Men and Women

During the reproductive years, women are "protected" from coronary heart disease. For this reason women lag behind men in the incidence of coronary heart disease by 10 years, and for myocardial infarction and sudden death, women have had a 20-year advantage.[10] The reasons for this are complex, but a significant contribution to this protection can be assigned to the higher high-density lipoprotein (HDL) levels in younger women, an effect of estrogen. Throughout adulthood, the blood HDL-cholesterol level is about 10 mg/dL higher in women, and this difference continues through the postmenopausal years. Total and low-density (LDL)-cholesterol levels are lower in premenopausal women than in men, but after menopause they rise rapidly. After menopause, the risk of coronary heart disease doubles for women as the atherogenic lipids rise to about age 60, and then decline. At all ages, however, HDL-cholesterol values in women are 10 mg/dL higher than in men.

The higher HDL levels in women compared to men represent the net effect of estrogen (HDL elevating) in women and androgens (HDL lowering) in men. While the exact mechanism of protection provided by HDL is not totally understood, it is fair to say that HDL promotes the efflux of cholesterol from macrophages and the intimal wall of the arteries. At roughly the age of menopause (48–55) the average cholesterol level in women rises higher than the average level in men as the HDL declines and LDL increases.[131] In women, data from two large prospective studies indicate that HDL-cholesterol is more closely related to cardiovascular disease than is LDL-cholesterol.[132,133]

Cross-sectional examination of mortality statistics has revealed a steady increase in the death rate from heart disease with increasing age in both men and women. This smooth linear increase fails to show an impact of menopause on death from heart disease. However, cross-sectional studies do indicate a shift to an atherogenic lipid and lipoprotein profile after menopause.[134] This is confirmed by longitudinal surveillance which reveals during menopause a decline in HDL and an increase in LDL which exceed that caused by aging alone.[131] This is then reflected by the increasing incidence of cardiovascular disease in the years after menopause.

Another newly appreciated factor is the connection between hormones and fat. Adiposity of the trunk is a risk factor for coronary heart disease in women and is associated with a relatively androgenic hormonal state, hypertension, and disorders of lipid and carbohydrate metabolism.[135] Central fat distribution in women is positively correlated with increases in total cholesterol, triglycerides, and LDL and negatively correlated with HDL.[136] The atherogenic lipid profile associated with abdominal adiposity is at least partly mediated through an interplay with insulin and estrogen.[137]

The pharmacologic effects of estrogen as used postmenopausally are just beginning to be understood. Estrogen increases triglyceride levels and increases LDL catabolism as well as lipoprotein receptor activity, resulting in decreasing LDL levels and increasing HDL levels.[138–140] LDL particle size gets smaller (an adverse effect) with estrogen treatment, however it is not certain to what degree this change is related to dose, nor is the clinical significance understood.[140] Furthermore this change in LDL particle size may be compensated by the antioxidant activity of estrogen which protects against atherosclerosis by inhibiting lipoprotein oxidation.[141]

Animal studies have indicated that estrogen inhibits the development of atherosclerotic lesions by means of one or more mechanisms independently of any effects on lipids and lipoproteins. This is supported by the significant presence of estrogen and progesterone receptors in the endothelium and smooth muscles of human arterial vessels.[142] Many studies indicate that these receptors are physiologically active, affecting cholesterol changes, platelet aggregation, smooth muscle cell proliferation, and changes in the prostaglandin system.

Thus there is a biologic and plausible rationale which supports a protective role for estrogen against cardiovascular disease.

The Evidence for Estrogen A review of the literature finds overwhelming support for a reduced risk of - cardiovascular disease in estrogen users.[143–155] A population-based case-control study in Rochester, Minnesota, concluded that if all eligible women utilized estrogen, myocardial infarctions could be reduced as much as 45%, an impact comparable to the elimination of smoking or the prevention of hypertension.[155]

One important and large cross-sectional study (1,444 cases and 744 controls) compared postmenopausal women undergoing coronary arteriography and therefore utilized an objective endpoint for coronary disease.[151] The relative risk of coronary disease was decreased 56% in estrogen users after adjustment for age, cigarette smoking, diabetes, cholesterol, and hypertension. Even women over age 70 demonstrated a 44% reduction in risk. Two other observations were especially noteworthy. Estrogen protection was increased at high cholesterol levels, and while smokers were protected, the degree of protection was less compared to nonsmokers.

In three other studies of women undergoing angiography a comparison of coronary artery occlusion in users and nonusers of estrogen indicated a significant protective effect of postmenopausal estrogen.[152–154] A higher rate of myocardial infarction was also noted in the nonusers of estrogen. The only significant lipid difference between users and nonusers consisted of elevated HDL-cholesterol levels in users of estrogen. Notably, there were no differences in LDL-cholesterol or triglycerides.

In cohort studies, only two produced conflicting data.[156–166] The Walnut Creek Study, one initially with conflicting data, had, in its first report, only 26 women with infarctions, and only 9 were estrogen users.[159] An update of the Walnut Creek data now documents a 50% reduction in death from diseases of the circulatory system when adjusted for all other factors.[167]

The Framingham Heart Study presented data in 1978, and in 1985, which argued that there was a 50% increased risk for cardiovascular disease among estrogen users, although there was no difference in fatality rates between users and nonusers.[157,161] Because of the respect the Framingham Heart Study carries, its impact was significant. There are, however, major criticisms of the Framingham report. First, the patient numbers were relatively small (302 postmenopausal women on estrogen) in comparison to the patient numbers in other studies on this particular issue. Furthermore, the effect of dose and duration of treatment could not be ascertained; they were not recorded. Finally and most conclusively, a subsequent reanalysis of the Framingham data (eliminating angina as a consideration) by the authors of the study reversed their conclusion.[168] The early reports from the Framingham Heart Study, therefore, stand in lonely opposition to overwhelming evidence that appropriately low doses of estrogen protect postmenopausal women against cardiovascular disease.

The Leisure World Study (a prospective, longitudinal study in a large retirement community under relatively controlled and accurate conditions) has documented a reduced risk of death due to myocardial infarction in current and past users of estrogen.[165]

The Nurses' Health Study has reached 10 years of follow-up; 48,470 postmenopausal women were free of coronary heart disease when initially evaluated, and subsequently 629 had either nonfatal or fatal disease.[162] The age-adjusted relative risk of coronary disease in current users showed approximately a 50% reduction. No association between use and stroke was observed. It was suggested that higher doses might be harmful in that there was an apparent increase in the risk of coronary disease among women taking more than 1.25 mg conjugated estrogens per day.

The Lipid Research Clinics Follow-up Study (a prospective 8.5-year follow-up of 2,270 women) has demonstrated a 63% reduction in the relative risk of fatal cardiovascular disease in current estrogen users, including a protective effect in current and exsmokers.[163]

A report is available from the National Health and Nutrition Examination Survey Epidemiologic Follow-up Study.[166] This is a longitudinal study of a cohort derived from the first National Health and Nutrition Examination Survey (NHANES I) conducted from 1971 to 1975. Within this study were 2,575 women who were aged 55 and menopausal at the time of the baseline examination. During the follow-up period (through 1986) there were 816 total deaths, 444 of which were due to cardiovascular disease. The use of estrogen significantly reduced (40% to 60%) the risk of cardiovascular disease regardless of the age of menopause.

There is one randomized, clinical trial.[169] Although the numbers were very small, limiting the power of the study, the results indicated protection against cardiovascular disease in the estrogen users.

An important question has been raised, asking whether estrogen treatment is a marker for variables (such as better diet and better health care) that place postmenopausal estrogen users in a low risk group for cardiovascular disease. This question has been directly addressed by the Lipid Research Clinics study, as well as the Nurses' Health Study.[162,163] Both groups of epidemiologists have concluded that their evidence strongly indicates that women receiving estrogen treatment have the same risk factors for cardiovascular disease as those not receiving treatment.

One case-control study has found no evidence for a protective effect of estrogen against stroke.[170] However, only 16% of the women in the study had filled more than one prescription, only 1% were current users, and average use was for only 15 months. In a prospective cohort study, estrogen therapy was associated with a 46% overall reduction in the risk of death from stroke, with a 79% reduction in recent users.[171] This protection was present in both women with hypertension and those without and in both smokers and nonsmokers. This level of protection was similar to that observed in this same Leisure World population for estrogen protection against deaths due to myocardial infarction.[165] The failure to observe protection against stroke in the Nurses' Health Study cohort is in striking contrast to the Leisure World cohort. This difference is probably due to the fact that the population in the Leisure World cohort is older than that in the Nurses' Health Study. Perhaps an effect against stroke will be demonstrated in the Nurses' Health Study when the cohort reaches older age, the age when stroke is more common. The population-based cohort study in Uppsala, Sweden, has documented a reduced incidence of stroke in postmenopausal users of estrogen, and, importantly, women prescribed an estrogen-progestin combination, containing a significant dose of the potent androgenic agent levonorgestrel, also experienced a reduced incidence of stroke.[172]

Studies that have assessed the impact of estrogen use on the risk of death from stroke have consistently indicated a beneficial impact. The National Health and Nutrition Examination Survey (NHANES) recruited a very large cohort of women in 1971–1975 for epidemiologic analysis. The follow-up longitudinal study of this cohort yielded a U.S. national sample of 1,910 white postmenopausal women. Postmenopausal hormone use in this cohort provided a 31% reduction in stroke incidence (confidence interval 0.47–1.0) and a strongly significant 63% reduction in stroke mortality.[173] These relative risks were present even after adjusting for age, hypertension, diabetes, body weight, smoking, socioeconomic status, and previous cardiovascular disease. This study specifically addressed the criticism that one should expect less disease in estrogen users because they are healthier. After adjusting for physical activity as a marker of general health status, the risk estimates remained identical. By virtue of the size of the cohort and the magnitude of the hormone effect, the results of this study provide impressive evidence of the beneficial impact of postmenopausal estrogen on the risk of stroke.

The protective effect of estrogen is achieved by specific pharmacologic consequences. Approximately 75% of the overall reduction in mortality in estrogen ever-users is due to protection against heart disease. The mechanism of this protection is due in part to a pharmacologic effect of estrogen on lipoprotein levels. In the Walnut Creek Study, 0.625 mg conjugated estrogens produced the following average changes: an increase in HDL of 9%, a decrease in LDL of 4%, and an increase in the HDL:Cholesterol ratio of 7%.

The impact of estrogen therapy on the lipid profile is maintained as long as women remain on the estrogen. A higher HDL-cholesterol and lower LDL-cholesterol have been documented to persist through at least 10 years of postmenopausal treatment. However, the degree of protection is greater than what can be attributed statistically to the impact on the lipoprotein profile.[163] Thus, the protection not mediated by lipoproteins is growing in importance.

Hypertension

Hypertension is both a risk factor for cardiovascular mortality and a common problem in older people. It is important, therefore, to know that no relationship has been established between hypertension and the doses of estrogen used for postmenopausal therapy. Studies have either shown no effect or a small, but statistically significant, decrease in blood pressure due to estrogen treatment.[174–178] This has been the case in both normotensive and hypertensive women. The very rare cases of increased blood pressure due to oral estrogen therapy truly represent idiosyncratic reactions. Because of the protective impact of appropriate estrogen treatment on the risk of cardiovascular disease, it can be argued that a woman with controlled hypertension is in need of that specific benefit of estrogen.

Protection Not Mediated by Lipids and Lipoproteins

An important study in monkeys has supported the protective action of estrogen against atherosclerosis, but by a mechanism independent of the cholesterol profile. Oral administration of a combination of estrogen and a high dose of progestin to monkeys fed a high cholesterol diet decreased the extent of coronary atherosclerosis despite a reduction in HDL-cholesterol levels.[179–181] In somewhat similar experiments, estrogen treatment has markedly prevented arterial lesion development in rabbits, and this effect was not reduced by adding progestin to the treatment regimen.[182–185] This suggests that women with already favorable cholesterol profiles may benefit through this additional action. And, in considering the impact of progestational agents, lowering of HDL is not necessarily atherogenic if accompanied by an increased estrogen impact.

The monkey colony studies have been extended to a postmenopausal model (ovariectomized monkeys). Compared to no hormone treatment, treatment with either estrogen alone or estrogen with progesterone in a sequential manner, significantly reduced atherosclerosis, once again independently of the circulating lipid and lipoprotein profile.[186] A direct inhibition of LDL accumulation and an increase in LDL metabolism in arterial vessels could be demonstrated in these monkeys being fed a highly atherogenic diet.[187]

Thus, estrogen exerts a protective effect directly on the arterial wall independent of its effects on circulating lipoproteins. The presence of sex steroid receptors in arterial endothelium and smooth muscle lends support for the importance of this direct action; however, the mechanisms involved remain unknown. Endothelium modulates the degree of contraction and function of the surrounding smooth muscle, primarily by the release of endothelium-derived relaxing and contracting factors (EDRFS and EDCFs). In hypertension and other cardiovascular diseases, the release of EDRFs (which is probably one factor, nitric oxide) is blunted, and the release of EDCFs (the most important being endothelin-1) is augmented.[188] Nitric oxide (and estrogen) also inhibits the adhesion and aggregation of platelets in a synergistic manner with prostacyclin (also a potent vasodilator derived from the endothelium).[189] These local actions are a likely site for sex steroid involvement; the vasodilating and antiplatelet action of estrogen, especially in the coronary arteries, is probably a consequence of endothelial response. Finally postmenopausal women experience greater stress-induced blood pressure responses that are ameliorated by estrogen treatment.[190]

Another action of estrogen (with or without progestin) is to prevent the tendency to increase central body fat with aging.[191,192] This would inhibit the interaction among abdominal adiposity, hormones, insulin resistance, hyperinsulinemia, and an atherogenic lipid profile. Hyperinsulinemia also has a direct atherogenic effect on blood vessels. Postmenopausal women being treated with oral estrogen have lower fasting insulin levels and a lesser insulin response to glucose, indicating another mechanism for the protection against cardiovascular disease.[193–195] Consistent with this salutary impact of estrogen, the Nurses' Health Study has documented a 20% decreased risk of non-insulin dependent diabetes mellitus in current users of estrogen.[196] The addition of a progestational agent attenuates this beneficial response to oral estrogen, but the clinical impact is unknown.[195,197] Nonoral administration of estrogen has little effect on insulin metabolism.

Estrogen treatment increases left ventricular diastolic filling and stroke volume.[198,199] This effect is probably a direct inotropic action of estrogen which delays the age-related change in compliance that impairs cardiac relaxation.

Therefore, the possible beneficial actions of estrogens on cardiovascular disease include all of the following:

1. **A favorable impact on the circulating lipid and lipoprotein profile, specifically a decrease in total cholesterol and LDL-cholesterol and an increase in HDL-cholesterol.**

2. **A direct antiatherosclerotic effect in arteries.**

3. **Augmentation of vasodilating and antiplatelet aggregation factors, especially nitric oxide and prostacyclin (endothelium-dependent mechanisms), and vasodilatation by means of endothelium-independent mechanisms.**

4. **Direct inotropic actions on the heart.**

5. **Improvement of peripheral glucose metabolism with a subsequent decrease in circulating insulin levels.**

6. **Inhibition of lipoprotein oxidation.**

Cardiovascular Disease and Progestins

Because the public health benefit of estrogen therapy on cardiovascular disease is of such enormous impact, it is vital that we know whether the addition of progestin has an adverse effect on the lipid profile and ultimately on cardiovascular disease. A review of the literature on this question suggests a dose-response relationship.[200–208]

A decrease in HDL-cholesterol has been noted with 10-day monthly treatment with norethindrone (5 mg), megestrol acetate (5 mg), levonorgestrel (250 µg), and even medroxyprogesterone acetate (10 mg). No significant change was noted with micronized progesterone (200 mg). The lack of an effect noted with micronized progesterone was observed with a dose (200 mg daily) which yields a normal luteal phase blood level of progesterone. A similar "physiologic" dose of synthetic progestins may be free of an adverse impact on HDL-cholesterol. Barrett-Connor and colleagues have been studying the adult residents of Rancho Bernardo, California. The women using both estrogen and progestin demonstrated the same favorable impact on cardiovascular risk factors as estrogen-only users when compared to the nonusers.[209] On the other hand, a well-designed study has indicated that although the sequential estrogen plus progestin program had a favorable impact on lipids and the lipoprotein profile, the impact was less than that achieved by estrogen alone.[210]

Conclusions regarding the impact of progestational agents on cardiovascular disease are very much influenced by dose and duration of administration of the progestational agent involved. While short-term studies suggest a negative impact of progestin (i.e., subtracting from the beneficial effect of estrogen), long-term studies indicate that this short-term effect disappears.

Studies with the combination of an estrogen and a low dose of a progestational agent administered continuously (every day without a break) are emerging and documenting a favorable impact on lipids and lipoproteins. The various formulations include estradiol and levonorgestrel,[211] estradiol and 1 mg norethindrone acetate,[212] estradiol valerate and levonorgestrel or cyproterone acetate,[213] ethinyl estradiol and 0.5–1.0 mg norethindrone acetate,[214] and 0.625 conjugated estrogens and 2.5–5.0 mg medroxyprogesterone acetate.[215] Christiansen has documented the maintenance of a favorable lipid profile over a period of 5 years of treatment with continuous, combined estradiol and 1 mg norethindrone acetate.[212]

A large, prospective, randomized clinical trial compared sequential and combined regimens of conjugated estrogens and medroxyprogesterone acetate to unopposed estrogen.[195] Although the increase in HDL-cholesterol, HDL_2, and apoprotein A-1 levels was greater with unopposed estrogen, there was still a significant increase with combined estrogen-progestin treatment. Importantly, the decrease in total cholesterol, LDL-cholesterol, apoprotein B, and Lp(a) was equivalent, comparing unopposed estrogen to either sequential or daily, combined estrogen-progestin. Fasting glucose and insulin levels were improved in all treatment groups. In a large cross-sectional study of 4,958 postmenopausal women, the same favorable impact on the lipoprotein profile and fasting insulin levels was observed in users of unopposed estrogen and combined estrogen-progestin compared to nonusers.[193]

In Spain, 8 months of uninterrupted treatment with a daily dose of 2.5 mg medroxyprogesterone acetate in a combined estrogen-progestin program produced a favorable effect on the lipoprotein profile not substantially different from that achieved with estrogen alone.[216] A large multicenter trial in the United States produced a favorable lipoprotein profile over a 12-month period of time in women receiving daily 0.625 mg conjugated estrogens and 2.5 mg medroxyprogesterone acetate (and the positive effect was more pronounced in women with lower baseline HDL levels).[217]

A report from the on-going cohort study from Uppsala, Sweden, provides information from the follow-up of approximately 23,000 women who were prescribed hormone therapy.[218] Overall there is a 30% reduction in myocardial infarction in women prescribed estradiol valerate or conjugated estrogens. What is especially noteworthy is a 50% reduced risk of myocardial infarction in women exposed to a sequential estrogen-progestin regimen consisting of 2 mg estradiol valerate and 10 days each month of levonorgestrel (250 µg). These data do not support the contention that exposure to a progestin (even the most androgenic of progestins) counteracts the cardiovascular benefit of estrogen.

Studies in women of arterial vascular resistance by Doppler ultrasound flow patterns have indicated no detrimental effects of exogenous progesterone to the beneficial decrease in resistance produced by estrogen administration.[219]

Protection Against Cardiovascular Disease Is the Major Benefit of Hormone Therapy

More than 30 published studies have addressed postmenopausal estrogen use and cardiovascular disease. Only a handful of studies have failed to find evidence for a protective effect of estrogens, most noteworthy the 1978 and 1985 reports from the Framingham study, the only prospective cohort study to report an increased risk among estrogen users. However, the Framingham reports adjusted the data for total and HDL cholesterol levels, an inappropriate adjustment since an impact on these variables is a major effect of estrogen. Reanalysis of the Framingham data (excluding angina as an endpoint) indicated a protective effect among women 50–59 years old, with too few estrogen users to estimate risk among older women. Because this analysis still adjusted for HDL, it probably underestimated the benefit of postmenopausal use of estrogen.

Most impressive, therefore, are the uniformity and consistency of the literature on this subject. All the population-based case-control studies and (with the reanalysis of the Framingham Heart Study) all of the prospective studies conclude that postmenopausal use of estrogens protects against cardiovascular disease. Indeed, the studies probably all underestimate the protective effect because of the high percentage of postmenopausal women who discontinue their treatment. Sophisticated assessment and analysis (using the methods of information synthesis and meta-analysis) indicate that the effect of estrogen on heart disease is not controversial or ambiguous, but there clearly exists a protective benefit.[220,221] We have such uniformity and consistency among the epidemiologic studies that the argument is very convincing. There remains, therefore, the important question of the nature and degree of impact due to the addition of progestational agents.

Evidence is accumulating to indicate that a progestational dose that protects the endometrium is available that avoids a significant impact on lipids and the lipoprotein profile. Furthermore, the growing appreciation for an impact of estrogen on mechanisms independent of lipids and the lipoprotein profile makes the presence of the progestin less concerning. With growing confidence we can offer and support hormone therapy as an important contribution to good health for postmenopausal women.

The Problems of Estrogen-Progestin Therapy

General and Metabolic

The increased incidence of thromboembolic disease, hypertension, and altered carbohydrate metabolism during older, high dose oral contraceptive usage is well documented. Because of the lower dosage in a postmenopausal hormone program, these metabolic effects are not seen in postmenopausal therapy.

Clinical data on the association between postmenopausal estrogen therapy and the risk of venous thrombosis are limited. Older case-control studies failed to find a link between postmenopausal doses of estrogen and venous thrombosis.[222,223] However, these studies excluded cases with pre-existing risk factors for thrombosis. A well-designed case-control study of older women unselected for other thrombotic risk factors indicated that postmenopausal doses of estrogen did not increase the risk of venous thrombosis.[224] Because venous thrombosis occurs later in life and is relatively infrequent in younger women, the cohort studies have had insufficient experience with this clinical problem to provide us with data; however, it is helpful to note that the Nurses' Health Study has failed to find an increased risk of pulmonary embolism in estrogen users.[225] It is also worth noting that postmenopausal doses of estrogen do not cause significant alterations in clotting factors, e.g., antithrombin III.[226]

These reports are especially useful in considering whether to provide hormone therapy to women who have previously had thrombotic episodes. When a venous thrombotic episode was clearly related to trauma, the decision to prescribe postmenopausal estrogen is relatively easy. If a patient presents with a history of venous thrombosis related to oral contraceptive use, the issue becomes difficult, especially from a medical-legal point of view. Careful informed consent documentation is essential. The risk in women with a past history of thromboembolism is not known, and a careful assessment of the risk-benefit balance may justify treatment of such patients.

As with oral contraception, estrogen therapy may carry a 1.5–2.0-fold increased risk of gallbladder disease.[227] However, at least two case-control studies concluded that estrogen use is not a risk factor for gallstone disease in postmenopausal women.[228,229] The routine, periodic use of blood chemistries is not cost-effective, and careful monitoring for the appearance of the symptoms and signs of biliary tract disease will suffice.

Patients with high risk factors need special attention when estrogen therapy is being considered. Metabolic contraindications to estrogen therapy include: chronically impaired liver function, acute vascular thrombosis (with or without emboli), and neurophthalmologic vascular disease. Estrogens may have adverse effects on some patients with seizure disorders, familial hyperlipidemias (very high triglycerides), and migraine headaches.

Endometrial Neoplasia

Estrogen normally promotes mitotic growth of the endometrium. Abnormal progression of growth through simple hyperplasia, complex hyperplasia, atypia, and early carcinoma has been associated with unopposed estrogen activity, administered either continuously or in cyclic fashion. Only one year of treatment with unopposed estrogen (0.625 mg conjugated estrogens or the equivalent) will produce a 20% incidence of hyperplasia.[230] Some 10% of women with complex hyperplasia progress to frank cancer, and complex hyperplasia is observed to antedate adenocarcinoma in 25–30% of cases. If atypia is present, 20–25% of cases will progress to carcinoma within a year.[231] The average time required for progression from hyperplasia to carcinoma is approximately 5 years, and atypia is expected to appear prior to the malignant change. Retrospective studies have estimated that the risk of endometrial cancer in women on estrogen therapy (unopposed by a progestational agent) is increased by a factor of somewhere from 2 to 10 times the normal incidence of 1 per 1,000 postmenopausal women per year. The risk increases with duration of exposure and dose of estrogen, lingers for up to 10 years after estrogen is discontinued, and the risk of cancer that has already spread beyond the uterus is increased 3-fold in women who have used estrogen a year or longer.[232,233]

It is now apparent, however, that this risk can be reduced by the addition of a progestational agent to the program. Whereas estrogen promotes the growth of endometrium, progestins inhibit that growth. This countereffect is accomplished by progestin reduction in cellular receptors for estrogen, and by induction of target cell enzymes that convert estradiol to an excreted metabolite, estrone sulfate. As a result, the number of estrogen receptor complexes that are retained in the endometrial nuclei are decreased in number, as is the overall intracellular availability of the powerful estradiol. In addition, progestational agents suppress estrogen-mediated transcription of oncogenes.

Reports of the clinical impact of adding progestin in sequence with estrogen include both the reversal of hyperplasia and a diminished incidence of endometrial cancer.[234–238] The protective action of progestational agents operates via a mechanism that requires time in order to reach its maximal effect. For that reason, the duration of exposure to the progestin each month is critical. While one standard method has incorporated the addition of a progestational agent for the last 10 days of estrogen exposure, some have argued in favor of 12 or 14 days. Studies indicate that the minimal requirement is a monthly exposure of at least 10 days duration.[239,240] About 2–3% of women develop endometrial hyperplasia when the progestin is administered for less than 10 days monthly.

It is likely that the daily dose of the progestational agent is associated with a threshold level below which endometrial protection can be insufficient. Currently, the sequential program utilizes 10 mg medroxyprogesterone acetate and the combined daily method uses 2.5 mg. Although lower doses of progestational agents are effective in achieving target tissue responses (such as reducing the nuclear concentration of estrogen receptors), the long-term impact on endometrial histology has not yet been firmly established. The question of dose is an issue of major importance, especially in terms of the cardiovascular system and compliance because of progestin-induced side effects. While the protective effect of progestin is considerable and predictable, it is unwise to expect all patients on estrogen-progestin therapy to never develop endometrial cancer. Appropriate monitoring of patients cannot be disregarded. Atlthough routine assessments are not cost-effective, interventions directed by clinical responses are prudent and necessary.

Breast Cancer

The possibility that estrogen use increases the risk of breast cancer must be intensively scrutinized. The American epidemiologic data on the scope of human female breast cancer are astonishing: 1 of every 9 women will develop breast cancer in her lifetime (assuming an 85-year life expectancy). In America, breast cancer is the leading type of cancer in women (32%) and now second to lung cancer as the leading cause of cancer death in women (18%), about 10 times the number of deaths from endometrial cancer.[241]

Sufficient evidence exists to indicate the possibility of a slightly increased risk of breast cancer associated with long durations (10 or more years) of postmenopausal estrogen use. However, the epidemiologic data on this relationship are by no means consistent and uniform. A review of the epidemiologic studies on postmenopausal hormone therapy and the risk of breast cancer fails to provide definitive evidence regarding this issue. Nevertheless, we believe that patients must consider this possibility in their informed decision-making.

A significant study from Uppsala, Sweden, concluded that estrogen use was associated with a slight increase in the risk of breast cancer (relative risk 1.1), and that there was a relationship with duration of use; the relative risk reaching 1.7 after 9 years.[242,243] This increased risk was associated only with the use of estradiol (56% of the women) at a dose approximately equivalent to 1.25 mg conjugated estrogens; no increase in risk was found with the use of conjugated estrogens (22% of the women) or other types of estrogen (22%). These conclusions have influenced many reviewers over the last several years. However, there are many reasons why the conclusions of this investigation are tenuous and at best only suggestive. The authors indicate that this investigation is a case-cohort type of epidemiologic study, prospective in the nature of its follow-up. The impression, strongly given, is that the cohort is large, consisting of 23,244 women. Actually the cohort consisted of the 653 women who answered the questionnaire sent to 1 in 30 of the 23,244 women. One should note immediately that 11% did not return the questionnaire, introducing the question of selection bias. The results in this subgroup were *extrapolated* to the large group of women. Furthermore, the case component, consisting of the 253 women who developed breast cancer through December, 1983, also contained an element of possible selection bias. A significant number of the women with breast cancer did not return the questionnaire and 6 gave incomplete answers, which means that 23% of the cases represented incomplete data. The authors correctly indicated that there was a *trend* toward increasing relative risk with duration of use (in other words, it was not statistically significant).

Another conclusion of this study, given great weight by others, was the indication of increased risk with combined treatment with estrogen-progestin. This conclusion was not statistically significant, based on only 10 women with breast cancer, and the confidence interval (CI) was impressively wide: 0.9–22.4.

There is another case-control study which utilized questionnaires to obtain information from both the cases and controls and which also indicated a slightly increased risk of breast cancer associated with postmenopausal hormone therapy.[244] Interestingly this report indicated an increased risk only with sequential estrogen and progestin and not with the daily administration of combined estrogen and progestin (however, these conclusions are very limited by the small numbers involved). This study contains statistical problems similar to the Uppsala study (e.g., the relative risk associated with estrogen-progestin use was 1.41 but the confidence interval included 1.0 and was not statistically significant).

Recent Studies
Early studies on estrogen use and breast cancer indicated higher risks in special subcategories, such as women with benign breast disease, long duration of use, or natural vs. surgical menopause.[245–256] These studies were all limited by a lack of control groups or by numbers too small to provide statistical significance.

The CASH (Cancer and Sex Hormone) Study of the Centers for Disease Control and Prevention (CDC) has not detected an overall increased risk of breast cancer with postmenopausal estrogen use and no relationship with duration of use up to 20 years or longer.[255] An absence of an effect was evident in all of the following: parity, age at first pregnancy, early or late menopause, menopause by hysterectomy or oophorectomy, family history of breast cancer, presence of benign breast disease, use for many years (20 years or longer), and use of high doses.

The latest report from the Nurses' Health Study represents 12 years of follow-up (1976–1988).[256] During that period, 1,050 cases of breast cancer were identified among more than 20,000 women. The analysis revealed that women who had used estrogen in the past (even for 10 or more years) were not at increased risk of breast cancer. However, the relative risk for current users was 1.33 (CI, 1.12–1.57). Compared with never users, current users were slightly more likely to have certain risk factors (history of benign breast disease, nulliparity, use of alcohol). However, adjustment for several of these risk factors only minimally reduced the relative risk for current use. The one confounding variable that appeared to play a prominent role was alcohol intake. Among women who did not consume alcohol, the risk of breast cancer was not increased by current use of postmenopausal estrogen.

By virtue of the large numbers in the Nurses' Health Study and the careful analyses by the investigators, reports from this study must be given great credibility. The 12-year follow-up report is disturbing with its finding of an increased risk in current users. Because estrogen users may be examined more frequently, detection bias is a major concern. The investigators analyzed factors that might be affected by detection bias (tumor size and lymph node metastasis at diagnosis) and found no difference between current users and never users. It is noteworthy, however, that a higher percentage of current users had a mammogram during the previous year. It is also of note that current users had a lower odds ratio for death from breast cancer (0.82) compared with never users. The Nurses' Health epidemiologists suggest that the lack of association between duration of estrogen use and increased risk of breast cancer among past users suggests that estrogen treatment can promote or accelerate development of a breast cancer that was present during the early years of use. However, the finding of an increased relative risk in current users is not definitive and not free of all confounding variables. Both the reduced odds ratio for death from breast cancer in current users and the absence of a statistically significant increased overall risk of fatal breast cancer among estrogen users in the total cohort support the possibility of surveillance and detection bias. The size of the statistical risk is not outside the range of influence by this bias.

A case-control study from Australia which attempted to control for secular trends in estrogen use, type of menopause, and duration of estrogen use concluded that that there was no evidence for an association between estrogen use and the risk of breast cancer in postmenopausal women.[257]

There is a very helpful study that specifically addressed the relationship between the use of estrogen and benign breast disease.[258] This study is impressive in that it is based upon 10,366 consecutive breast biopsy specimens with follow-up information on 4,227 biopsy specimens in 3,303 women (a mean duration of follow-up of 17 years). Analysis indicated that the use of estrogen was associated with a reduced risk of developing breast cancer. Most importantly, in patients with atypical hyperplasia in their biopsies, the use of estrogen lowered the risk of breast cancer. While the protective effect may indicate surveillance bias, certainly this is strong evidence that estrogen use does not increase the risk of breast cancer in women with surgically proven benign breast disease, even with atypia.

In a study of 1,686 cases and 2,077 controls in the eastern U.S., the relative risk for current use was 1.1 (CI, 0.7–1.6), for a duration of use of 15 or more years, the relative risk was 0.9 (CI, 0.4–1.9).[259] As in the eastern U.S., a study from Toronto found no evidence for an increased risk in either current or recent users or in users for up to 15 years.[260] These two large case-control studies failed to support the conclusion of the Nurses' Health Study that current users are associated with an increased risk. In addition and importantly, these more recent studies have consistently failed to demonstrate a link between increased risk and duration of estrogen use. On the other hand, a case-control study (of smaller size and limited statistical power) did find an increased risk of breast cancer in current users and long-term users.[261]

Meta-Analysis

Meta-analysis is an increasingly popular statistical method in which many studies are combined and undergo rigorous analysis. Simply put, the purpose of a meta-analysis is to gain the statistical power that is lacking in individual studies.

An Australian meta-analysis of 23 studies of estrogen use and breast cancer concluded "unequivocally" that estrogen use did not alter the risk of breast cancer.[262] In the meta-analysis by Dupont and Page (Nashville, Tennessee), the authors concluded that "considerable and consistent" evidence exists that a daily dose of 0.625 mg conjugated estrogens taken for several years does not appreciably increase the risk of breast cancer.[263] They found no evidence of an association between the duration of treatment and the risk of breast cancer at this dosage. On the other hand, the bulk of the data suggests that a daily dose of at least 1.25 mg conjugated estrogens may increase the risk of breast cancer. This analysis failed to reveal an increased risk in patients with a history of benign breast disease.

A third meta-analysis is from the CDC.[264] This meta-analysis was conducted using what the authors called a "dose-response curve" for duration of use. The curve for each study analyzed was calculated by plotting breast cancer risk against duration of estrogen use. The combined dose-response slope represented the average change in risk associated with estrogen use over time. The analysis concluded that duration of estrogen use was associated with an increased risk of breast cancer, regardless of whether menopause was natural or surgical. No increase in risk was noted in the first 5 years of use, but after 15 years of use, the risk was increased by 30%. The effect was present irrespective of other risk factors, such as family history, parity, or history of benign breast disease. The effect of estrogen therapy on risk of breast cancer was enhanced in women with a positive family history of breast cancer.

A fourth meta-analysis, from Spain, concluded that estrogen is associated with a very small, but statistically significant, increased relative risk of breast cancer and that the increased risk is higher among current users.[265] Confining their analysis to a dose of 0.625 mg conjugated estrogens; however, the Spanish epidemiologists could not detect a statistically significant increased risk. Indeed, this meta-analysis concludes that an estrogen dose of 0.625 mg conjugated estrogens is safe.

A fifth meta-analysis from the epidemiologists associated with the Nurses' Health Study concluded that although there is no increased risk of breast cancer in ever users of estrogen, current use is associated with an increased risk and a slight increase with more than 10 years of use (but there was no linear trend with increasing duration of use).[266] This observation in long-term users could be influenced by an increased proportion of current users in this group, and the increased risk in current users could be a consequence of detection bias. This meta-analysis could not detect a link between risk of breast cancer and dosage. Nevertheless, we continue to be concerned with a possible effect of higher doses. The Australia, Nashville, and Spain meta-analyses indicated an increased risk with a daily dose of conjugated estrogens greater than 0.625 mg (or its equivalent).

The Nashville, CDC, and Nurses' Health analyses did not find an enhanced risk in women with a history of benign breast disease. In contrast to the CDC report, the Australia and Nurses' Health analyses found no link between positive family history and estrogen use. The Nashville and Spain investigators did not consider family history.

In a major overview and assessment (yet another meta-analysis) of the world's literature on postmenopausal hormone therapy, commissioned by the American College of Physicians, the authors concluded that long-term use of estrogen was associated with a relative risk of breast cancer of 1.25 (CI, 1.04–1.51).[267] This conclusion, in our view, was not appropriately critical and represents a judgment that extends beyond the statistical power available from the many heterogeneic studies. The heterogeneity of the many studies is an important issue: different drugs, different doses, different methods of diagnosis, different comparison and control groups. The Spanish meta-analysis is the only one to raise the question: perhaps the heterogeneity is too great to allow an accurate meta-analysis of this literature. The results of a meta-analysis should not be accepted in a sacrosanct fashion. A meta-analysis can have the same problems encountered by individual epidemiologic studies. Selection bias is a major confounding variable.

It is relevant to note that all of the studies that have examined the mortality rates of women who were taking estrogen at the time of breast cancer diagnosis have documented improved survival rates. However, this undoubtedly reflects earlier diagnosis in users because the greater survival rate in current users is associated with a lower frequency of late stage disease.[243,268]

Where does that leave clinicians and patients? The positive conclusions are strongly influenced by statistical limitations or by dose. The largest case-control study (from the CDC), the largest cohort follow-up study (the Nurses' Health Study), and the most recent case-control studies failed to find a link between breast cancer and use of estrogen for up to 20 years. If estrogen use were associated with an increased risk of breast cancer, wouldn't one expect to see an impact on mortality? In the latest report from the Leisure World follow-up study in California, the risk of breast cancer mortality was 0.81.[269] This lower relative risk probably is influenced by surveillance bias, but certainly there is no evidence that women using estrogen for a long time are dying of breast cancer at a greater rate.

In a very recent and impressive review of breast cancer, the authors concluded that "estrogenic stimulation increases the risk; the elevated risk among users of estrogen supplements supports this mechanism most directly." They further stated, "widespread use of estrogen-replacement therapy has almost certainly contributed to the higher incidence among postmenopausal women."[241] In our view, these definitive conclusions cannot be made. Doses of estrogen known to protect against osteoporosis and cardiovascular disease (0.625 mg conjugated estrogens and 1.0 mg estradiol) are, at the present time, not known to be associated with any clear-cut increased risk of breast cancer. However, because of the concern raised by some studies and reviews that there is a slightly increased risk of breast cancer associated with long-term use of postmenopausal estrogen, this issue requires discussion during the clinician-patient dialogue regarding postmenopausal hormone therapy.

The Risk of Breast Cancer and Estrogen-Progestin Therapy

The addition of a progestational agent to postmenopausal estrogen therapy is now accepted as a standard part of the treatment program. The obvious reason for this combined estrogen-progestin approach is the need to prevent the increased risk of endometrial cancer associated with exposure to unopposed estrogen. Even though this endometrial cancer is not frequently encountered and survival rates are excellent with early disease, the fear of this cancer is a major force in patient compliance, and therefore the combined approach is warranted. Clinicians and patients have rapidly turned to the method of a daily combination of estrogen and a progestin, in order to overcome bleeding which is the second major compliance problem.

Only two reports have claimed that the addition of a progestational agent protects against breast cancer; the first (the Nachtigall study), although it is the only randomized, placebo-controlled trial, was hampered by small numbers, and the second was limited by bias in treatment selection (the breast cancer risk factor profiles were not matched in the treated and untreated groups).[270,271]

The Nachtigall study deserves comment because it is the only long-term randomized clinical trial with postmenopausal hormone therapy thus far reported.[271] In 1965–1966, 84 matched pairs were selected from more than 400 chronically hospitalized postmenopausal women. For the first 10 years of the study, patients received either estrogen-progestin given in a sequential manner with a relatively high dose of conjugated estrogens, 2.5 mg per day, and 10 mg medroxyprogesterone acetate for 7 days each month, or a placebo. After the first 10 years, patients were allowed to choose whether to continue or stop treatment. In addition, the subjects could choose to begin hormone treatment. At this point in time, however, the dose of estrogen was lowered to 0.625 mg per day, and the duration of the progestational treatment was increased to 10 days each month. These patients were then followed for the subsequent 12 years. After 22 years of surveillance, there were available 116 patients on hormone treatment and 52 control patients. In the original 10 year study, 4 cases of breast cancer were found in the placebo group and none in the hormone treatment group. During the subsequent 12 years of surveillance, two new breast cancers were diagnosed in the control group. Therefore during the entire 22 years, 6 cases of breast cancer were diagnosed in the 52 women who had never received hormone treatment, and there were no cases in the 116 women who were receiving hormone treatment, a statistically significant difference.

For a randomized clinical trial, the numbers in the Nachtigall study are relatively small. Thus, even though one can find statistical significance, is it biologically real? When numbers are this small, confounding variables are even more important. For example, there is a major difference in parity between the placebo group and the treatment group, which may explain the low rate of breast cancer in the treated group. If an increased risk is influenced by estrogen dose, however, then the Nachtigall results are even more meaningful since the dose of estrogen in the initial 10 years of treatment was very high.

At the present time, the available epidemiologic evidence on the impact of combined estrogen-progestin treatment on the risk of breast cancer is still too limited. Neither a protective nor a detrimental effect has yet to be convincingly demonstrated; the Nurses' Health Study group finds that the addition of a progestin does not change the findings with estrogen alone.[266] Balancing the information available involving all of the health issues affected by hormone therapy, a combined estrogen-progestin program in appropriate doses continues to offer significant benefits for postmenopausal women. As time goes on, more studies and greater duration of use should provide us with better answers to many of our questions. By virtue of the magnitude of the postmenopausal female population, these questions deserve continuing biologic and epidemiologic research from both the public health and individual points of view.

Postmenopausal Hormone Therapy

In view of the above considerations, our opinion is as follows: there is little question that women who suffer from hot flushes or atrophy of reproductive tract tissues can be relieved of their problems by use of estrogens. It also is now definite that the long-term disabilities of osteoporosis can be largely prevented by therapy with estrogen and progestin. It is very probable that appropriate doses of estrogen have a beneficial impact on the risk of cardiovascular disease. We suggest treatment with estrogen for all women showing any stigmata of hormone deprivation and advocate hormonal prophylaxis against osteoporosis and cardiovascular disease. The decision to use or not to use estrogen belongs to the patient, and it should be based upon the information available in this chapter. The recommendation that hormone therapy be given for the shortest period of time appears to be shortsighted in view of the impressive evidence that therapy has a profound impact on osteoporosis and cardiovascular disease and that there are more beneficial than potentially harmful effects.

Women Under the Age of 40 (Castrates and Women with Gonadal Dysgenesis)

In these women, the duration of estrogen deprivation is prolonged and the loss of estrogen acute. The cyclic use of estrogen is recommended for short-term reduction of vasomotor symptoms and for long-term prophylaxis against cardiovascular disease, osteoporosis, and target organ atrophy. In some young patients, the equivalent of 0.625 mg conjugated estrogens is insufficient to allow menstrual bleeding. Because women of this age ordinarily are exposed to estrogen levels which stimulate endometrial growth and withdrawal bleeding, and for psychological reasons, a higher dose should be used, if necessary, to maintain withdrawal bleeding until the menopausal time of life. The standard sequential program is utilized. In those patients castrated because of endometriosis, recurrence of endometriosis has very rarely been a problem with estrogen therapy, but because endometrial cancer has been reported to occur in remaining endometriosis exposed to unopposed estrogen, the estrogen and progestin daily combination is recommended.

The Perimenopause

After exclusion of other gynecologic causes, dysfunctional bleeding is treated by progestin or oral contraceptive therapy and, if necessary, biopsy surveillance. Vasomotor reactions appearing in women despite the presence of menstrual bleeding should receive careful evaluation. Abnormal thyroid function should be ruled out. If an FSH level is not greater than 30 IU/mL, serious consideration should be directed toward psychosocial reasons for the flushing response.

Perimenopausal bone loss which is secondary to a decrease in estrogen is limited to those women with fluctuating hormonal and menstrual function, irregular bursts of follicular function alternating with no ovarian response to gonadotropins, so that these women are exposed to low estrogen over significant periods of time. The bone loss that begins in the 20s is due to a mechanism that is independent of hormones, and longitudinal studies have documented that trivial amounts of bone are lost prior to menopause.

The Early Postmenopause

The long-term postmenopausal use of hormone therapy depends heavily upon a woman's own informed assessment, a process which should occur at this point in life. An understanding of hormone therapy is an important component in any preventive health program directed toward the postmenopausal years. As a result of immediate responses in early climacteric symptoms, the patient enters the climacteric more confident of herself emotionally, sexually, and physically. In our view, this establishes or cements good patient-physician interchange and relations. The follow-up of the patient on effective estrogen-progestin therapy is more secure and certain. The practitioner offering estrogen-progestin treatment has a better and more reliable opportunity to act as primary physician for these aging women. All monitoring of health systems will be improved as a result of this single involvement.

The Late Postmenopause

Atrophic conditions can be effectively treated with local or oral therapy in low maintenance doses. If there is no apparent basis for osteoporosis other than aging and ovarian failure, estrogen-progestin therapy and calcium supplementation are advisable even for very old women. Further loss of bone can be slowed and the risk of fractures reduced. In these older women, an assessment of progress can be obtained by measuring bone density. The impact of initiating hormone therapy in elderly women on the risk of cardiovascular disease has not been ascertained. However, it makes sense that elderly women would benefit from estrogen's dynamic protective mechanisms.

Method of Management

Which Hormonal Agent or Route of Administration Should Be Used?

There currently is no evidence that one form of estrogen is superior to another. The specific estrogen is not as important as the duration, dose, and the presence or absence of a progestin. Which estrogen is administered is not as important as the method with which it is used.

The dose of estrogen that is effective in maintaining the axial and peripheral bone mass is equivalent to 0.625 mg conjugated estrogens.[92,272] The relative potencies of commercially available estrogens become of great importance when prescribing estrogen.

The dose-response effect of ethinyl estradiol on bone has not been sufficiently studied, and it is probable that the dose equivalent to 0.625 mg conjugated estrogens approximates 5–10 μg. The 17α-ethinyl group of ethinyl estradiol appears to be responsible for a specific hepatic effect, for no matter by which route it is administered, liver metabolism is affected.[276] The same is true for conjugated equine estrogens. Contrary to the case with estradiol, the liver appears to preferentially extract ethinyl estradiol and conjugated equine estrogens no matter what the route of administration. Thus, the route of administration appears to influence the metabolic responses only in the case of specific estrogens, most notably estradiol.

The effect of steroids on lipids and lipoproteins is determined by the type of steroid, the dose, and the route of administration. An obstacle to the utilization of transdermal hormone therapy has been the lack of data indicating a beneficial impact on the lipoprotein profile. There has been concern that delivery of estrogen through the skin yields a blood level that might be too low to provide this important benefit. English data are now available indicating that the transdermal administration of 50 μg estradiol twice

Relative Estrogen Potencies [272–275]

Estrogen	FSH levels	Liver proteins	Bone density
Piperazine estrone sulfate	1.0 mg	2.0 mg	0.625 mg
Micronized estradiol	1.0 mg	1.0 mg	1.0 mg
Conjugated estrogens	1.0 mg	0.625 mg	0.625 mg
Ethinyl estradiol	5.0 µg	2–10 µg	5–10 µg
Transdermal estradiol	—	—	50 µg

a week is as effective as 0.625 mg oral conjugated estrogens on bone density and lipids over a year's time.[277,278] The transdermal administration of 100 µg estradiol combined with a progestin will not only increase bone density, but also reduce the fracture rate in older women who already have significant osteoporosis.[279] However, 100 µg estradiol administered transdermally produces estrogen blood levels approximately twice that of the usual postmenopausal regimens.

The concentration of estrogen in the portal system after oral administration is 4–5 times higher than that in the periphery.[280] Furthermore, the estradiol/estrone ratio differs in the portal system. Thus, the first pass effect is either significant for the lipoprotein effects, or it is important only in the short-term. For example, a short-term study (6 weeks) could document increased catabolism of LDL with oral estrogen, but no effect with transdermal estrogen.[281] And a 2-year study in Los Angeles with a transdermal dose (100 µg) twice the standard dose detected no significant change in HDL-cholesterol levels.[282]

Until data are available documenting the degree of impact of the various routes of administration on actual clinical events (fractures and cardiovascular disease), the prudent clinical decision is to select the method (an oral program) that has epidemiologic support. The argument that the transdermal route is safer is specious. Because the proper oral dose of estrogen has no impact on hypertension or the clotting cascade, how can a method be safer than safe?

Because estrogen increases triglyceride levels, women with elevated triglycerides should be treated with an estrogen-progestin combination (progestins lower triglycerides) and the triclyceride level should be monitored. If fasting triglyceride levels increase to 250 mg/dL (2.8 mmol/L) or higher, a nonoral route of administration should be tried.

Estradiol Implants

Estradiol pellets are available in doses of 25, 50, and 75 mg for subcutaneous administration twice yearly. The 25 mg pellet provides blood levels in the range of 40–60 pg/mL (150–220 pmol/L), levels which are comparable to those obtained with the standard oral dose.[283] However, the effect is cumulative, and after several years the blood levels are 2–3 times higher. Significant blood levels of estradiol will perist for up to 2 years after the last insertion. Progestational treatment is necessary, and because of the higher blood levels, a minimal duration of 14 days each month is advised. We believe that the estradiol pellets confer no advantages over the usual treatment regimens. We further recommend that women receiving pellets be monitored with blood estradiol levels, and levels greater than 200 pg/mL (and preferably, 100 pg/mL) should be avoided.

Percutaneous Estrogen

Estradiol delivery can be accomplished by the application of an ointment to the skin, usually over the abdomen or thighs. The preparation which contains 1.5 mg estradiol produces blood levels of estradiol of approximately 95–125 pg/mL (350–450 pmol/L), levels which are both higher and more variable than the standard oral regimens.[284] As with pellets, we recommend that blood estradiol levels be monitored and maintained at a level below 100–200 pg/mL (370–740 pmol/L).

Monitoring Estrogen Dosage with Estradiol Blood Levels

Monitoring the estradiol blood level in postmenopausal women receiving hormone therapy is not as straightforward as it would seem. There are two primary difficulties. First, the clinical assays available differ considerably in their technqiue and quality (laboratory and antibody variations). Second, the various commercial products represent a diverse collection of estrogenic compounds, ranging from estradiol to unique equine estrogens. Although the body interconverts various estrogens into estrone and estradiol, is this process relatively consistent within and between individuals? For example, a highly specific assay for estradiol will detect very low levels of estradiol in women receiving conjugated equine estrogens; however, most clinical assays will report a level of 40–100 pg/mL (150–370 pmol/L) in these women. We find measurement of blood estradiol levels very useful in selected patients, such as the patient who requests ever-increasing doses of estrogen for the treatment of symptoms which in the presence of very high blood levels of estradiol can be confidently diagnosed as psychosomatic. What each clinician must do is learn what blood level of estradiol as performed by the local laboratory is associated with the standard doses of hormone therapy (0.625 conjugated estrogens, 1 mg estradiol, 50 μg transdermal estradiol). In our laboratory this range is 40–100 pg/mL (150–370 pmol/L) estradiol. *Remember that because FSH is regulated by factors other than estrogen (e.g., inhibin), FSH levels cannot be used to monitor estrogen dosage.*

Which Regimen Is Best: Sequential or Continuous?

Several regimens for oral administration are currently used. The two most common sequential methods involve estrogen administration with 0.625 mg conjugated estrogens or 1.0 mg micronized estradiol either daily or from the 1st through the 25th of each month. A daily dose of 10 mg medroxyprogesterone acetate (MPA) is added for the first 14 days of the month or for the last 10 days of estrogen administration, respectively. Problems with this sequential regimen include adverse symptoms related to the dose of progestin such as breast tenderness, bloating, fluid retention and depression. A lower dose (5 mg) usually resolves these complaints. However, the lowest effective dose of medroxyprogesterone acetate required for endometrial protection in a sequential program has not been established, and the standard dose remains 10 mg. Unfortunately, progestin withdrawal bleeding occurs in 80–90% of women on a sequential regimen.[285]

The continuous/combined method of treatment evolved to improve patient compliance in the presence of bleeding and other symptoms. The continuous presence of progestin allows the use of lower doses. This approach involves the continuous daily use of the following estrogen-progestin combinations:

Daily estrogen: *0.625 mg conjugated estrogens, or*
    0.625 mg estrone sulfate, or
    1.0 mg micronized estradiol

Daily progestin: *2.5 mg medroxyprogesterone acetate, or*
    0.35 mg norethindrone

Combined with calcium supplementation (250 mg bid with meals), and Vitamin D (400 IU in cloudy winter months and 800 IU for elderly women).

In our own experience, this continuous approach maintains a beneficial lipoprotein pattern and increases the bone density in the spinal column in the first year of use to a level which is then maintained, while others have noted an increasing bone density for at least 18 months. Also of note, no adverse effects on blood pressure are encountered.

Compliance with hormone therapy programs is notoriously poor.[286] The two most common reasons why women discontinue or do not start hormone treatment are fear of cancer and vaginal bleeding.[287] The current data on breast cancer are reassuring, and the addition of a progestational agent has effectively prevented endometrial cancer. But the persistence of bleeding with the traditional sequential regimen continues to be a barrier to good compliance. To go from 80–90% withdrawal bleeding to 80% no bleeding represents a major accomplishment, and thus, the continuous approach has a significant advantage.

Breakthrough Bleeding with Continuous Therapy

The single most aggravating and worrisome problem with daily, continuous therapy is breakthrough bleeding. One can expect 40–60% of patients to experience breakthrough bleeding during the first 6 months of treatment; however, this percentage decreases to approximately 20% after one year.[288] While this percentage of amenorrhea is a gratifying accomplishment, the number of women who experience breakthrough bleeding is considerable and it is a difficult management problem.

This breakthrough bleeding is similar to that seen with oral contraceptives. It originates from an endometrium dominated by progestational influence; hence the endometrium is usually atrophic and yields little, if anything, to the exploring biopsy instrument. It takes confidence and experience with this method to withstand the urge to biopsy. The endometrial biopsy in this circumstance, no matter what the instrument or method, is not cost-effective. Patients require constant support through the early months of continuous therapy. If bleeding persists for 6 months, consider an office hysteroscopy; an impressive number of polyps and intrauterine fibroids will be discovered.

There is no effective method of drug alteration or substitution to manage this breakthrough bleeding. The breakthrough bleeding rate is not much better with a higher dose of progestin (5.0 mg medroxyprogesterone acetate) compared to the lower dose (2.5 mg).[288] Therefore, there is no reason to use the higher dose, thus minimizing side effects. The best approach is to gain time, as most patients will cease bleeding. This means good educational preparation of the patient beforehand and frequent telephone contact to allay anxiety and encourage persistence. It is appropriate to perform an endometrial aspiration biopsy when the patient's anxiety over the possibility of pathology requires this response. It is also appropriate to perform a biopsy when the physician is concerned; with increasing experience with this method, it takes more and more to be concerned.

That leaves a hard core of patients who continue to bleed. The closer a patient is to having been bleeding (either to her premenopausal state or to having been on a sequential method with withdrawal bleeding), the more likely that patient will experience breakthrough bleeding. Some clinicians, therefore, prefer to start patients near the menopause on the sequential method and convert to the continuous method some years later. For the small number of patients who persist in having breakthrough bleeding, it is better to return to the sequential program in order to have expected and orderly withdrawal bleeding instead of the irregularity of breakthrough bleeding.

Some patients may choose to undergo endometrial ablation in order to overcome the problem of breakthrough bleeding. But remember that concern still exists regarding the potential for isolated, residual endometrium to progress to carcinoma without recognition. Another option deserving of consideration is the progestin intrauterine device

(IUD). The local release of progestin is effective in suppressing endometrial response and preventing bleeding.[289]

When To Biopsy?

It is not essential to perform endometrial biopsies prior to treatment. Endometrial abnormalities in asymptomatic postmenopausal women are very rare.[290] A reasonable economic moderation would be to limit pretreatment biopsies (using the plastic endometrial suction device in the office) to patients at higher risk for endometrial changes: those women with conditions associated with chronic estrogen exposure (obesity, dysfunctional uterine bleeding, anovulation and infertility, hirsutism, high alcohol intake, hepatic disease, metabolic problems such as diabetes mellitus and hypothyroidism) and those women in whom irregular bleeding occurs while on estrogen-progestin therapy. In the absence of abnormal bleeding, a certain amount of trust in the protective effects of the progestin is justified, and routine, periodic biopsies are not necessary. *Abnormal endometrium is more frequently encountered in patients on combination estrogen-progestin when the patients have previously been treated for a period of time with unopposed estrogen. Breakthrough bleeding in these patients requires endometrial sampling because an increased risk for endometrial cancer persists beyond the period of exposure to unopposed estrogen, and it is unknown how effective the subsequent protective exposure to a progestin will be.*[291,292]

The timing of withdrawal bleeding in women on a sequential estrogen-progestin program has been suggested as a screening method for biopsy decision-making. In women taking a variety of progestins for 12 days each month, bleeding on or before day 10 after the addition of the progestin was associated with proliferative endometrium.[293] Bleeding beginning on day 11 or later was associated with secretory endometrium, presumably indicating less need for biopsy. Whether this truly correlates with the risk of hyperplasia and cancer is not known.

Women who elect to be treated with unopposed estrogen require endometrial surveillance at least once a year.

Measurement of Endometrial Thickness by Transvaginal Ultrasound

The thickness of the postmenopausal endometrium as measured by transvaginal ultrasonography correlates with the presence or absence of pathology in women not receiving hormonal therapy. Endometrial thickness (the two layers of the anterior and posterior walls in the longitudinal axis) under 5 mm is reassuring and allows conservative management.[294] Endometrial thickness greater than 5 mm requires biopsy; it is estimated that only 15% of patients will require biopsy.[295] Experience with women on hormone therapy is less extensive; however, it appears that an endometrial thickness less than 5 mm in women receiving a combination of estrogen-progestin is also reassuring with these patients.

The Progestin Challenge Test

The administration of a progestational agent (e.g., 10 mg medroxyprogesterone acetate for 10 days) has been promoted as a means of detecting the presence of estrogen-dependent endometrium in menopausal women. A withdrawal bleed would indicate that an endometrial response has occurred to the progestin, a response that requires previous endometrial stimulation by estrogen. Is there a false negative and a false positive response? Can this method be combined with transvaginal measurement of endometrial thickness to reliably indicate those patients who require histologic diagnosis?[296] We cannot recommend this approach because the validity of this test has not been established by appropriate clinical studies.

Progestational Side Effects

Many women do not tolerate treatment with progestational hormones. Typical side effects include breast tenderness, bloating, and depression. These reactions are significant detrimental factors with compliance.

Can the progestational agent be administered less frequently? We are secure in our position, supported by clinical data, that a monthly estrogen-progestin sequential or a daily combination program effectively prevents endometrial hyperplasia. Experience with other regimens is very limited. The administration of medroxyprogesterone acetate every 3 months is associated with an incidence of hyperplasia that would require more intensive monitoring. Indeed, any program that differs from the standard regimen is untested by clinical studies and, therefore, requires periodic surveillance of the endometrium.

Some patients are very sensitive to medroxyprogesterone acetate. In our experience, these patients are relieved of their symptoms by switching to norethindrone. In a sequential regimen, the dose of norethindrone is 0.7 mg (available in the progestin-only, minipill oral contraceptive; each pill contains 0.35 mg norethindrone). In the continuous, combined regimen, the dose of norethindrone is 0.35 mg daily.

Should Progestins Be Administered to Hysterectomized Women?

There are at least 5 special conditions that warrant the use of a combined estrogen-progestin regimen in hysterectomized women.

1. It has been demonstrated that patients who have had Stage I adeno-carcinoma of the endometrium can take estrogen without fear of recurrence,[297–299] but the combination of estrogen-progestin is recommended in view of the potential protective action of the progestational agent.

2. The combined estrogen-progestin approach makes sense for patients previously treated for endometriid tumors of the ovary.

3. Because adenocarcinoma has been reported in patients with pelvic endometriosis being treated with unopposed estrogen,[300,301] the combined estrogen-progestin program is advised in patients with a past history of endometriosis.

4. There is evidence that the combination of estrogen and progestin has a greater positive impact on bone density than estrogen alone. Thus, in hysterectomized women at high risk for osteoporosis, the combined estrogen-progestin program offers an important potential advantage.

5. In women with elevated triglyceride levels, the addition of a progestin will attenuate a further estrogen-induced increase.

Is It Appropriate to Add Androgens to the Hormone Regimen?

After menopause, the circulating level of androstenedione is about one half that seen prior to menopause.[38] Most of this postmenopausal androstenedione is derived from the adrenal gland, with only a small amount secreted from the ovary. Testosterone levels do not fall appreciably, and in most women, the postmenopausal ovary, for a few years, actually secretes more testosterone than the premenopausal ovary. The remaining active stromal tissue in the ovary is stimulated by the elevated gonadotropins to this level of increased testosterone secretion. The total amount of testosterone produced, however, is decreased because the primary source, the peripheral conversion of androstenedione, is reduced. Because of this decrease, some argue that androgen treatment is indicated in the postmenopausal period.

The potential benefits of androgen treatment include improvement in psychological well-being and an increase in sexually motivated behavior. These effects, however, follow the administration of relatively large doses of androgen.[302] In a well-designed, placebo-controlled study, lower doses of androgen contributed little to actual sexual behavior, although an increase in sexual fantasies and masturbation could be documented.[303]

Any benefit must be balanced by the unwanted effects, in particular, a negative impact on the cholesterol-lipoprotein profile. Unfortunately, data are scanty on this issue. In a short-term study comparing a product with estrogen and a relatively low dose of testosterone (1.25 mg methyltestosterone) to estrogen alone, a negative impact on the lipid profile was apparent within 3 months.[304] It should also be remembered that the addition of androgen does not protect the endometrium, and the addition of a progestin is still necessary. It is uncertain (and unstudied) how much aromatization of the administered testosterone increases the estrogen impact and whether this might further increase the risk of endometrial and/or breast cancer. The addition of testosterone to an estrogen therapy program provides no additional beneficial impact on bone.[305]

There is no doubt that pharmacologic amounts of androgen can increase libido, but these same doses produce unwanted effects.[306] In addition, patients on high doses of androgens often are somewhat addicted to this therapy. Small amounts of androgen supplementation can be provided in situations where the patient and clinician are convinced a depressed libido cannot be explained by psychosocial circumstances. In these cases, the lipid profile should be carefully monitored. Any positive clinical response may well be a placebo effect. After some months or a few years, conversion to a standard program is recommended.

Should Very Old Women Be Started on Hormone Therapy?

The positive impact of hormone therapy on bone has been demonstrated to take place even in women over age 65.[89] This is a strong argument in favor of treating very old women who have never been on estrogen. Estrogen use between the ages of 65 and 74 has been documented to protect against hip fractures.[87] Whether estrogen's cardiovascular protection has anything significant to contribute in the elderly has not been addressed. It makes clinical sense, however, that some positive contribution can be expected. Adding a pharmacologic regimen to an old woman's daily life is not a trivial consideration. This judgment requires the conclusion that a relatively youthful and vigorous elderly woman has something to gain from the treatment. Patients with osteoporosis and/or unfavorable lipoprotein profiles would certainly qualify.

If postmenopausal hormone therapy is demonstrated to have a beneficial effect on the risk and severity of Alzheimer's disease, this would become a powerful reason to recommend treatment for very old women.

Contraindications to Postmenopausal Hormone Therapy

Estrogen sensitive cancer stands out as the most logical and convincing contraindication to hormone therapy. However, ethical, as well as logistical, considerations prevent the proper study of this issue. Therefore, decisions regarding the two major cancers sensitive to estrogen, breast cancer and endometrial cancer, must be based upon medical-legal fears and the knowledge reviewed in this chapter.

Endometrial Cancer, Endometrioid Tumors, and Endometriosis

It has been demonstrated that patients who have had Stage I, low grade adenocarcinoma of the endometrium can take estrogen without fear of recurrence.[297–299] Nothing is known about the risk in patients with more advanced disease. If a high risk tumor is estrogen and progesterone receptor negative, it seems reasonable to allow immediate hormone therapy. Because the latent period with endometrial cancer is relatively short, a period of time (5 years) without evidence of recurrence would increase the likelihood of safety on an estrogen program. We recommend that hormone therapy be avoided in patients with high risk tumors that are receptor positive until 5 years have elapsed. The combination of estrogen-progestin is recommended in view of the potential protective action of the progestational agent. A similar approach makes sense for patients previously treated for endometrioid tumors of the ovary. In view of the fact that adenocarcinoma has been reported in patients with pelvic endometriosis and on unopposed estrogen, the combined estrogen-progestin program is advised in patients with a past history of endometriosis.[300,301]

Should a Woman Who Has Had Breast Cancer Use Postmenopausal Hormones?

A decision regarding hormone therapy is even more difficult in women with a previous history of breast cancer.

The increasing incidence of breast cancer, together with earlier detection and treatment, is producing a growing pool of patients for whom the question of estrogen treatment is important and at the same time difficult. The problem is easy to articulate: we have no data. There are absolutely no published studies of sufficient size and scope in which the impact of estrogen treatment has been documented when given to women with previously treated breast cancer.

Because there is good reason to believe that breast cancer is hormonally influenced, it is not hard to understand the breast surgeon or medical oncologist who believes that estrogen treatment is foolish and dangerous. Yet that position is just as unencumbered by data as the position of the gynecologist who believes that appropriate patients stand to benefit more from estrogen compared to the unknown risk of breast cancer recurrence.

The single most useful prognostic information in women with operable breast cancer has been the histologic status of the axillary lymph nodes.[241] At 10 years only 25% of patients with positive nodes are free of disease compared to 75% of patients with negative nodes. If more than 3 nodes are involved, the 10-year survival rate drops to 13%. Because of this recognition for the importance of the axillary nodes, the traditional approach to breast cancer (the Halsted surgical approach) was based on the concept that breast cancer is a disease of stepwise progression. There has been an important change in concept. Breast cancer is now viewed as a systemic disease, with spread to local and distant sites at the same time. Breast cancer is best viewed as occultly metastatic (microscopically disseminated) at the time of presentation. Dissemination of tumor cells has occurred by the time of surgery in many patients, and it is concern over the possible response of these cells that fires the debate over this question: should women who have had breast cancer take postmenopausal hormones?

There are two opposing hypotheses that link breast cancer to a hormonal influence: one assigns the critical role to estrogen; the other, to progesterone.

Is Estrogen the Important Influence?

When one reviews the various factors associated with breast cancer, many of the factors support a role for increased exposure to estrogen, specifically the importance of age of menarche, age of menopause, obesity, the effect of pregnancy and, added to this list is the therapeutic effect of an antiestrogen, tamoxifen.

Stanley Korenman, therefore, suggested that the endocrine environment does not cause the disease but influences the susceptibility to carcinogens — the so-called estrogen window hypothesis.[307,308] The two periods of life when the estrogen window is open (this means long periods of unopposed estrogen) are after menarche before ovulation is established and the perimenopausal years. Estrogen shows a significant increase at about Tanner stage 2, ages 8 to 10. Since ovulation occurs on the average 1.5 years after menarche, this window can last 4 to 5 years. It is well-recognized that anovulation is common in the perimenopausal years because of the lesser capabilities of the remaining ovarian follicles. The window is closed by exposure to progesterone after ovulation and during pregnancy.

In Korenman's analysis of atom bomb survivors, he found the inducibility of breast cancer was most evident during the pubertal open window. No breast cancer was seen in those irradiated under the age of 10, and no increased risk was noted with irradiation between 30 and 49 years of age. He also examined data from women with tuberculosis receiving repeated fluoroscopies. Again, the greatest increase in risk occurred with exposures in the 15 to 20-year age group, with no increase after age 30. This argument is supported by observational studies indicating that anovulatory and infertile women (exposed to less progesterone) have an increased risk of breast cancer later in life.[309–311] However, the statistical power of these studies was limited by small numbers (all fewer than 15 cases), and others have failed to find a link between anovulation and the risk of breast cancer.[312,313] In summary, factors that would be associated with an increased risk of breast cancer are those that would prolong the duration of the open window: obesity, infertility due to anovulation, delayed pregnancy, early menarche, late menopause.

Is Progesterone the Important Influence?

Some argue that progesterone is the key to influencing the risk of breast cancer because mitotic activity in the breast reaches its peak during the progesterone dominant luteal phase of the menstrual cycle.[314–316] An earlier age of menarche is sometimes used to buttress the progesterone hypothesis because earlier menarche means an earlier onset of ovulatory cycles. The interaction of estrogen and progesterone on target tissue has been studied mostly in the endometrium, where estrogen clearly stimulates cell growth and progesterone inhibits this estrogen effect. Unfortunately, in vitro studies with normal and malignant breast cells have yielded confusing results. There are studies with normal breast cells that are in agreement with the protective action of progesterone against estrogen stimulation.[317] With human breast cancer cells, both proliferation and inhibition of proliferation have been observed with various progestational agents.[318]

Which Hypothesis Is Correct?

The hormonal sensitivity of breast cancer appears to be unquestionable, but whether estrogen or progesterone plays a key role is not certain. And perhaps, it is a unique exposure to a combination of factors that is pivotal. Both the estrogen hypothesis and the progesterone hypothesis continue to fuel the debate over these issues. There are specific areas in our clinical experience, however, which are relevant to this consideration.

**Clinical Observations
of Relevance**

Pregnancy and Breast Cancer

At one point in time, it was believed that pregnancy (and its impressive levels of estrogens and progesterone) had an adverse impact on the prognosis of breast cancer diagnosed during the pregnancy. It is now apparent that there is no difference in survival when pregnant women with breast cancer are matched to nonpregnant women by age and stage of disease, and termination of pregnancy is not associated with improved survival.[319] Pregnant women do have a 2.5-fold higher risk of metastatic disease, but the reason is later diagnosis because the breast changes associated with pregnancy make diagnosis difficult. Because of diagnosis at a more advanced stage of disease, pregnant women with breast cancer usually have less well-differentiated (receptor negative) tumors.[320] Thus, it can be argued, the intense hormonal stimulation of pregnancy (both estrogen and progesterone) has no adverse impact on the course of breast cancer.

Breast Cancer and Subsequent Pregnancy

As with breast cancer diagnosed in already pregnant women, subsequent pregnancy, after diagnosis and treatment, has no negative impact on prognosis.[321] This, too, would argue against an impact of hormonal stimulation on the risk of recurrent or new disease.

Oral Contraception and the Risk of Breast Cancer

The experience with oral contraceptives over the last 30 years has provided neither definitive evidence that exogenous estrogen and progestin increase the risk of breast cancer, nor evidence that exposure to these exogenous hormones offers major protection against breast cancer (Chapter 22). The lack of a major detrimental effect is an effective argument against a major link between breast cancer and exogenous hormone treatment.

Depo-Provera and the Risk of Breast Cancer

Medroxyprogesterone acetate, in large continuous doses, produced breast tumors in beagle dogs. This is an effect unique to the beagle dog and has not appeared in other animals or in women after years of use. A very large, hospital-based case-control World Health Organization study conducted over 9 years in 3 developing countries has indicated that exposure to Depo-Provera very slightly increased the risk of breast cancer in the first 4 years of use, but there was no evidence for an increase in risk with increased duration of use.[322] The results were interpreted to suggest that growth of already existing tumors is enhanced. The number of cases was not large, and the confidence intervals reflected this. For example, the relative risk for recent users (based on a total of 19 cases) was 1.21, but the confidence interval included 1.0 and thus was not statistically significant.

Two earlier population-based case-control studies indicated a possible association between breast cancer and Depo-Provera. One, from Costa Rica, was subject to several biases.[323] The other, from New Zealand, did not find an increased relative risk in ever users but did find an indication of increased risk shortly after initiating use in early age.[324] These studies have been all limited by very small numbers and thus have been inconclusive.

Certainly the risk, if real, is very slight, and it is equally possible that the suggestions of increased risk have not been free of confounding variables. It is more appropriate to emphasize that these studies did not find evidence for an increased risk of breast cancer with long durations of use. Thus, experience with exposure to a pure progestational agent does not support the argument that progestational influence will increase the risk of breast cancer.

Postmenopausal Hormone Therapy and the Risk of Recurrent Breast Cancer

The argument that postmenopausal hormone therapy should not be given to women who have had breast cancer is a reasonable one. It is based on the recognition of a large body of evidence that indicates that breast cancer is a hormone responsive tumor. The overriding fear of many clinicians (and patients) is that metastatic cells are present (perhaps being controlled by various host defense factors) that will be susceptible to stimulation by exogenous hormones.[325] However, many women who have had breast cancer are aware of the benefits of postmenopausal hormone treatment (especially protection against cardiovascular disease and osteoporosis) and are asking clinicians to help make this risk-benefit decision. In addition, some women suffer from such severe hot flushing and vaginal dryness that they are willing to consider hormonal treatment.

Sitting on the other side of this debate is the clinician who has a positive response to the observational studies reviewed above. Recognizing that the prognosis of breast cancer is not influenced by the high hormone levels of pregnancy removes some of the fear of exogenous hormone treatment. The lack of a clear-cut impact of oral contraceptives and postmenopausal hormone treatment on the risk of breast cancer is further reassuring. There is one small series in which a combination of 0.625 conjugated estrogens and 0.15 mg norgestrel was given continuously for a short period of time (a maximum of 6 months) to women who had been previously treated for breast cancer.[326] Over the next two years, no patients developed recurrence. Another small series (25 women with breast cancer ranging from in situ to stage III disease) received estrogen-progestin therapy for 24 to 82 months; the recurrence rate was not greater than that expected.[327]

Because of the current lack of epidemiologic data, both sides of this debate are strongly influenced by theoretical considerations and clinical experiences, which, unfortunately, often become an obstacle to the patient's own informed choice.

Can the decision be assisted by any of the following: status of the axillary nodes, negative or positive receptors, size or type of tumor, or time elapsed since diagnosis and treatment? Postmenopausal women who are 5–10 years from diagnosis of breast cancer have an excellent prognosis, but every patient cannot be considered cured. Besides the presence or absence of positive axillary nodes (70% of node negative patients are cured without adjuvant therapy), there are other factors that indicate a low risk of recurrence.[328]

> Factors associated with low risk of recurrence:
> Ductal Ca-in-situ
> Pure (not mixed) tubular, papillary, or medullary types of cancer
> Tumor size less than 1 cm
> Diploid tumor (normal amount of DNA) with low S phase fractions (low proliferation)
> Nuclear grade 1
> Tumor 1–3 cm, without high risk features
>
> High risk factors:
> Aneuploid tumor
> High S phase fractions
> High cathepsin D levels (a lysosomal enzyme oversecreted in invasive and metastatic breast cancers)
> Absent estrogen receptors
> Tumor size greater than 3 cm

The most favorable prognosis is associated with ductal ca-in-situ, a tumor size less than 1 cm, and a nuclear grade of 1 (nuclear grade 1 is well-differentiated, which is about 10% of node negative patients).[329] About 25% of patients have small tumors and favorable histologic subtypes (a recurrence rate of less than 10%); 25% of patients have large tumors with poor prognostic features (a recurrence rate greater than 50%), but fully half of patients are in between (with an average recurrence rate of 30%).

Because of better treatment and earlier diagnosis, 50–75% of women diagnosed with breast cancer are now cured.[329] Of 100 patients with breast cancer, about 60 will be cured by mastectomy or lumpectomy with radiotherapy and would receive no benefit from adjuvant treatment. Is this group safe for hormone therapy? Of the remaining 40, some will live longer (an average of 2–3 years) because of adjuvant treatment, but only a few. Is the unknown risk with exogenous hormone treatment worth it in this group? Although intuitively it seems that the risk:benefit ratio would be more favorable in the presence of negative nodes, negative receptors, and small tumors, are negative estrogen and progesterone receptor assessments sufficient to conclude that the cancer is not sensitive to hormones? And if the patient is in the high cure category, does it make any difference what the receptor status is? The answers to all of these questions are obviously not known. Receptor status is not absolute; it is always a relative measure.

Patients and clinicians have to incorporate all of the above considerations into this medical decision. But when all is said and done, patients have to take an unknown risk if they want the benefits of estrogen treatment, and clinicians have to take an unknown medical-legal risk. Some patients will choose to take estrogen, judging the benefits to be worth the unknown risk. Physicians should support patients in this decision. Other patients will prefer to avoid any unknown risks. These patients, too, deserve support in their decision.

Tamoxifen, it has been argued, is a better choice for women who have had breast cancer.[325] This argument stresses that the agonistic, estrogenic actions of tamoxifen on bone and lipids will offer protection against osteoporosis and cardiovascular disease, while tamoxifen's antagonism of estrogen at the breast will prevent recurrence and contralateral disease. An important assumption is that tamoxifen and estrogen provide equal protection against osteoporosis and cardiovascular disease.

In general, thus far, the studies indicate that the estrogenic, agonistic actions of tamoxifen do prevail upon the cholesterol profile and bone density. Bone density studies demonstrate no loss of bone, indicating an estrogen agonistic action of tamoxifen to maintain bone in comparison to the loss usually encountered after menopause.[330–333] In a two-year randomized study tamoxifen had a positive impact on trabecular bone in the lumbar spine.[333] At the end of two years, the difference between tamoxifen and the placebo group was 3%, identical to the difference observed with the use of etidronate. This difference is less than the usual 5–10% difference comparing women who use calcitonin or estrogen to placebo. Thus, the bone density data (still limited) suggest that the degree of protection is not equivalent to that of estrogen. Furthermore, in premenopausal women, tamoxifen may, in the presence of higher levels of estrogen, exert an antagonistic action on the bone, resulting in bone loss (clinical data in premenopausal women are not yet available).

Tamoxifen is associated with an estrogen-like decrease in total cholesterol and LDL-cholesterol, with an increase in triglycerides and HDL-cholesterol (although some studies do not find a significant impact on HDL).[334–338] In a report from the Scottish cancer trial, 10 myocardial infarctions were observed in the tamoxifen arm and 25 in the placebo group, a statistically significant difference.[339]

Postmenopausal patients can be reassured that the antagonistic actions of tamoxifen do not prevail in regard to osteoporosis and cardiovascular disease; however, to what extent the agonistic effect protects against clinical events and how it compares to the benefits of a hormone treatment program will require future epidemiologic studies. At this point in time, one cannot assume that tamoxifen protects against cardiovascular disease and osteoporosis with an impact equal to that of hormone treatment.

The problem of hot flushing should not be underrated. About 25% of women have vasomotor symptoms on tamoxifen, and those that already had flushing have worse flushing.[333] Alternative treatments are available (see below).

The Vaginal Administration of Estrogen

The common belief is that estrogen administered intravaginally is not absorbed, and systemic effects can be avoided. However, estrogen is absorbed very readily from a vagina with immature, atrophic mucosa.[340] Indeed the initial absorption is rapid, and relatively high circulating levels of estrogen are easily reached. As the vaginal mucosa cornifies, absorption decreases. This decline takes approximately 3–4 months, after which lesser, but still significant absorption takes place. European studies have demonstrated that vaginal maturation can be achieved with incredibly small doses (10–25 µg estradiol) of intravaginal estrogen, without significant systemic absorption.[341] In fact, after an initial period (several weeks) of daily treatment, the vaginal mucosa could be maintained with treatment twice a week. This would be an acceptable treatment to relieve atrophic vaginal symptoms in women with contraindications to estrogen treatment, but unfortunately these low dose preparations are unavailable in the United States. Clinician and patient can try to match this experience by titrating small amounts of commercially available vaginal estrogen formulations with circulating blood estradiol levels.

Women with Cardiovascular Disease

Another area that is difficult is the problem case of a woman who wishes to use hormone therapy, but there is a previous history of a cardiovascular event, such as a myocardial infarction, stroke, or embolism. While it is known that the doses of estrogen used for postmenopausal treatment have no significant impact on the clotting mechanism and no increased risks for thrombotic clinical events have been demonstrated, these findings are derived from women without previous events. Does the woman with a previous event represent a different risk? On the other hand, the woman with a previous event may be the very woman who needs the protection of estrogen against cardiovascular disease. There is evidence to support this contention. In the Leisure World study, estrogen users with previous myocardial infarctions, strokes, or hypertension had a 50% reduction in risk for death from a subsequent stroke or myocardial infarction. In the Lipids Research Clinics study, the cardiovascular mortality in women with previous cardiovascular disease was reduced 85%. And finally, and most impressively, in women with severe coronary disease (documented by arteriography), estrogen users had a 97% survival rate at 5 years compared to a significantly different 81% rate in nonusers.[342] In women with mild to moderate disease, there was no difference at 5 years, but at 10 years, estrogen users had a 96% survival rate compared to 85% in nonusers. In our opinion, estrogen treatment is indicated for these patients.

Other Conditions

Metabolic contraindications to estrogen include impaired liver function and acute vascular disease (including embolus and thrombosis). Close surveillance is indicated for some patients with seizure disorders, familial hyperlipidemias (elevated triglycerides), and migraine headaches. Patients with migraine headaches often improve if a daily, continuous method of treatment is used, eliminating a cyclic change in hormone levels that can serve to trigger headaches.

Conditions that do not represent contraindications include controlled hypertension, diabetes mellitus, and varicose veins. The belief that estrogen is potentially harmful with each of these clinical situations is derived from old studies of high dose birth control pills. Estrogen in appropriate doses is acceptable in the presence of these conditions.

Fibroid tumors of the uterus almost always are not stimulated to grow by postmenopausal doses of estrogen. Nevertheless, pelvic examination surveillance is a wise course. No other cancers (besides those mentioned above) are known to be adversely affected by hormone therapy. Postmenopausal hormone therapy can be administered to all patients with cervical, ovarian, or vulvar malignancies. Interestingly, the Nurses' Health Study reported a marginally significant reduced risk of colorectal cancer in past users of postmenopausal estrogen.[343]

Unusual anecdotal reports include the following:

1. Provocation of chorea by estrogen therapy in a woman with a history of Sydenham's chorea.[344]

2. Exacerbation of pulmonary leiomyomatosis by estrogen therapy.[345]

Estrogen Therapy and Rheumatic Diseases

No clear conclusion is apparent from the studies of estrogen's effect on rheumatic diseases, especially rheumatoid arthritis.[61] There is no benefit in osteoarthritis, but some alleviation has been observed with carpal tunnel syndrome and fibromyalgia. There have been anecdotal case reports of serious flares in patients with systemic lupus erythematosis given estrogen, but the cardiovascular benefit warrants use with close monitoring.

General Considerations

A striking and consistent finding in most studies dealing with menopause and hormonal therapy is a marked placebo response in a variety of symptoms including flushing. A significant clinical problem encountered in our referral practice is the following scenario: a woman will occasionally undergo an apparent beneficial response to estrogen, only to have the response wear off in several months. This leads to a sequence of periodic visits to the physician and ever-increasing doses of estrogen therapy. When a patient reaches a point of requiring large doses of estrogen, a careful inquiry must be undertaken to search for a basic psychoneurotic or psychosocial problem.

Assessing vaginal cytology is not useful. The vaginal mucosa is too sensitive to estrogen to allow dose-response titering.

High dose calcium supplementation can unmask asymptomatic hyperparathyroidism. Women receiving calcium supplementation in excess of 500 mg daily should have their blood levels of calcium and phosphorous measured yearly for the first 2 years. If normal, no further surveillance is necessary.

Assessment of the cholesterol-lipoprotein profile should follow the guidelines for general preventive care. No further measurements are required in women on postmenopausal hormone therapy, neither before nor during treatment. The one exception is the patient with previous evidence of elevated triglycerides. After 6 months of hormone treatment, the triglyceride level should be measured to make sure the patient is not the rare individual who responds to estrogen with excessively high triglyceride levels. Although the risk associated with a high triglyceride is uncertain, levels greater than 500 mg/dL should be avoided.

Alternate Treatments for Hot Flushes

Clonidine, bromocriptine, and naloxone given orally are only partially effective for the relief of hot flushes and require high doses with a high rate of side effects. Bellergal treatment is no better than a placebo. Veralipride, a dopamine antagonist that is active in the hypothalamus, is relatively effective in inhibiting flushing at a dose of 100 mg daily.[346,347] Mastodynia and galactorrhea are the major side effects. Medroxyprogesterone acetate is also effective, but concerns regarding exogenous steroids would apply to progestins as well.[348] Methyldopa, in doses of 250–500 mg/day, is said to be effective, but there have been no properly controlled studies with this agent. Propranolol and similar agents are ineffective.

We recommend transdermal clonidine, applied with the 100 μg dose once weekly.[349] Side effects are minimal, and the treatment is twice as effective as a placebo.

The Menopause as a Signal for the Future

The menopause should serve to remind patients and clinicians that this is a time for education. Certainly preventive health care education is important throughout life, but at the time of the menopause, a review of the major health issues can be especially rewarding. Besides the general issues of good health, attention should be focused (because of their relationship to hormone therapy) on cardiovascular disease and osteoporosis.

Postmenopausal hormone therapy deserves consideration as a legitimate component of preventive health care for older women. One can argue convincingly that protection against cardiovascular disease is the major benefit of postmenopausal estrogen treatment, and the magnitude of this benefit is considerable. Estrogen therapy will stabilize the process of osteoporosis or prevent it from occurring. Postmenopausal hormone therapy is an option that should be offered to most women as they consider their paths for successful aging.

References

1. **Cope E,** Physical changes associated with the post-menopausal years, in Campbell S, editor, *The Management of the Menopause & Post-Menopausal Years,* University Park Press, Baltimore, 1976, p 33.

2. **Farnham AM,** Uterine disease as a factor in the production of insanity, Alienst Neurologist 8:532, 1887.

3. **Matthews KA, Wing RR, Kuller LH, Meilahn EN, Kelsey SF, Costello EJ, Caggiula AW,** Influences of natural menopause on psychological characteristics and symptoms of middle-aged healthy women, J Consulting Clin Psychiatr 58:345, 1990.

4. **Koster A,** Change-of-life anticipations, attitudes, and experiences among middle-aged Danish women, Health Care Women 12:1, 1991.

5. **Kaufert PA, Gilbert P, Tate R,** The Manitoba Project: a re-examination of the link between menopause and depression, Maturitas 14:143, 1992.

6. **McKinlay SM, McKinlay JB,** The impact of menopause and social factors on health, in Hammond CB, Haseltine FP, Schiff I, editors, *Menopause: Evaluation, Treatment, and Health Concerns,* Alan R. Liss, New York, 1989, pp 137–161.

7. **Diczfalusy E,** Menopause, developing countries and the 21st century, Acta Obstet Gynecol Scand (Suppl) 134:45, 1986.

8. **Manton KG, Soldo BJ,** Dynamics of health changes in the oldest old: new perspectives and evidence, Health and Soc 63:206, 1985.

9. **Hazzard WR,** Biological basis of the sex differential in longevity, J Am Geriatr Soc 34:455, 1986.

10. **Kannel WB,** Metabolic risk factors for coronary heart disease in women: perspective from the Framingham Study, Am Heart J 114:413, 1987.

11. **U.S. Bureau of the Census,** Projections of the population of the United States: 1977 to 2050, Current Population Reports, Series P-25, No. 704.

12. **Eaker ED, Packard B, Wenger NK,** editors, *Coronary Heart Disease in Women,* New York, Haymarket Doyma, 1987.

13. **Keith PM,** The social context and resources of the unmarried in old age, Intl J Aging Hum Dev 23:81, 1986.

14. **McKinlay SM, Bigano NL, Mckinlay JB,** Smoking and age at menopause, Ann Intern Med 103:350, 1985.

15. **McKinlay SM, Brambilla DJ, Posner JG,** The normal menopause transition, Maturitas 14:103, 1992.

16. **Weg RB,** Demography, in Mishell DR Jr, editor, *Menopause: Physiology and Pharmacology,* Year Book Medical Publishers, Chicago, 1987, pp 23–40.

17. **Treolar AE,** Menarche, menopause and intervening fecundability, Hum Biol 46:89, 1974.

18. **MacMahon B, Worcester J,** Age at menopause U.S. 1960–62, Vital Health Stat 19:1, 1966.

19. **Midgette AS, Baron JA,** Cigarette smoking and the risk of natural menopause, Epidemiology 1:474, 1990.

20. **Siddle N, Sarrel P, Whitehead M,** The effect of hysterectomy on the age at ovarian failure: identification of a subgroup of women with premature loss of ovarian function and literature review, Fertil Steril 47:94, 1987.

21. **Coulam CB, Adamson SC, Annaegers JF,** Incidence of premature ovarian failure, Obstet Gynecol 67,604, 1986.

22. **Amundsen DW, Diers CJ,** The age of menopause in classical Greece and Rome, Hum Biol 42:79, 1970.

23. **Amundsen DW, Diers CJ,** The age of menopause in medieval Europe, Hum Biol 45:605, 1973

24. **Backman von G,** Die beschlanigte entwicklund der jugend, Acta Anat 4:421, 1948.

25. **Frommer DJ,** Changing age at menopause, Br Med J 2:349, 1964.

26. **Traupman J, Eckels E, Hatfield E,** Intimacy in older women's lives, Gerontologist 2:493, 1982.

27. **Pfeiffer E, Verwoerdt A, Davis GC,** Sexual behavior in middle life, Am J Psychiatr 128:1262, 1972.

28. **Martin CE,** Factors affecting sexual functioning in 60–79 year-old married males, Arch Sex Behav 10:399, 1981.

29. **George LK, Weiler SJ,** Sexuality in middle and late life, Arch Gen Psychiatr 38:919, 1981.

30. **White CB,** Sexual interest, attitudes, knowledge, and sexual history in relation to sexual behavior in the institutionalized aged, Arch Sex Behav 11:11, 1982.

31. **Renshaw DC,** Sex, intimacy, and the older woman, Women Health 8:43, 1983.

32. **Treloar AE, Boynton RE, Borghild GB, Brown BW,** Variation of the human menstrual cycle through reproductive life, Int J Fertil 12:77, 1967.

33. **Richardson SJ, Senikas V, Nelson JF,** Follicular depletion during the menopausal transition — evidence for accelerated loss and ultimate exhaustion, J Clin Endocrinol Metab 65:1231, 1987.

34. **Sherman BM, West JH, Korenman SG,** The menopausal transition: analysis of LH, FSH, estradiol, and progesterone concentrations during menstrual cycles of older women, J Clin Endocrinol Metab 42:629, 1976.

35. **Buckler HM, Evans A, Mamlora H, Burger HG, Anderson DC,** Gonadotropin, steroid and inhibin levels in women with incipient ovarian failure duirng anovulatory and ovulatory 'rebound' cycles, J Clin Endocrinol Metab 72:116, 1991.

36. **MacNaughton J, Banah M, McCloud P, Hee J, Burger H,** Age related changes in follicle stimulating hormone, luteinizing hormone, oestradiol and immunoreactive inhibin in women of reproductive age, Clin Endocrinol 36:339, 1992.

37. **Gosden RG,** Follicular status at menopause, Hum Reprod 2:617, 1987

38. **Meldrum DR, Davidson BJ, Tataryn IV, Judd HL,** Changes in circulating steroids with aging in postmenopausal women, Obstet Gynecol 57:624, 1981.

39. **Dowsett M, Cantwell B, Anshumala L, Jeffcoate SL, Harris SL,** Suppression of postmenopausal ovarian steroidogenesis with the luteinizing hormone-releasing hormone agonist Goserelin, J Clin Endocrinol Metab 66:672, 1988.

40. **Andreyko JL, Monroe SE, Marshall LA, Fluker MR, Nerenberg CA, Jaffe RB,** Concordant suppression of serum immunoreactive luteinizing hormone (LH), follicle-stimulating hormone, α subunit, bioactive LH, and testosterone in postmenopausal women by a potent gonadotropin releasing hormone antagonist (Detirelix), J Clin Endocrinol Metab 74:399, 1992.

41. **Judd HL, Judd GE, Lucas WE, Yen SSC,** Endocrine function of the postmenopausal ovary; concentration of androgens and estrogens in ovarian and peripheral vein blood, J Clin Endocrinol Metab 39:1020, 1974.

42. **Judd HL, Shamonki IM, Frumar AM, Lagasse LD,** Origin of serum estradiol in postmenopausal women, Obstet Gynecol 59:680, 1982.

43. **Longcope C, Jaffe W, Griffing G,** Production rates of androgens and oestrogens in postmenopausal women, Maturitas 3:215, 1981.

44. **Grimes DA,** Diagnostic dilation and curettage: a reappraisal, Am J Obstet Gynecol 142:1, 1982.

45. **Stovall TG, Ling FW, Morgan PL,** A prospective, randomized comparison of the Pipelle endometrial sampling device with the Novak curette, Am J Obstet Gynecol 165:1287, 1991.

46. **Einerth Y,** Vacuum curettage by the Vabra method. A simple procedure for endometrial diagnosis, Acta Obstet Gynecol Scand 61:373, 1982.

47. **Goldstein SR, Subramanyam B, Snyder JR, Beller U, Raghavendra BN, Beckman EM,** The postmenopausal cystic adnexal mass: the potential role of ultrasound in conservative management, Obstet Gynecol 73:8, 1989.

48. **Moore B, Kombe H,** Climacteric symptoms in a Tanzanian community, Maturitas 13:229, 1991.

49. **Kronnenberg F, Barnard RM,** Modulation of menopausal hot flashes by ambient temerature, J Therm Biol 17:43, 1992.

50. **Kronnenberg F,** Hot flashes: epidemiology and physiology, Ann NY Acad Sci 592:52, 1990.

51. **Hunter M,** The South-East England longitudinal study of the climacteric and postmenopause, Maturitas 14:117, 1992.

52. **Oldenhave A, Jaszmann LJB, Haspels AA, Everaerd WThAM,** Impact of climacteric on well-being, Am J Obstet Gynecol 168:772, 1993.

53. **Swartzman LC, Edelberg R, Kemmann E,** The menopausal hot flush: symptom reports and concomitant physiological changes, J Behav Med 13:15, 1990.

54. **Aksel S, Schomberg DW, Tyrey L, Hammond CB,** Vasomotor symptoms, serum estrogens and gonadotropin levels in surgical menopause, Am J Obstet Gynecol 126:165, 1976.

55. **Raz R, Stamm WE,** A controlled trial of intravaginal estriol in postmenopausal women with recurrent urinary tract infection, New Engl J Med 329:753, 1993.

56. **Wilson PD, Faragher B, Butler B, Bullock D, Robinson EL, Brown ADG,** Treatment with oral piperazine oestrone sulphate for genuine stress incontinence in postmenopausal women, Br J Obstet Gynaecol 94:568, 1987.

57. **Bhatia NN, Bergman A, Karram MM,** Effects of estrogen on urethral function in women with urinary incontinence, Obstet Gynecol 160:176, 1989.

58. **Castelo-Branco C, Duran M, Gonzalez-Merlo J,** Skin collagen changes related to age and hormone replacement therapy, Maturitas 15:113, 1992.

59. **Semmens JP, Wagner G,** Effects of estrogen therapy on vaginal physiology during menopause, Obstet Gynecol 66:15, 1985.

60. **Cauley JA, Petrini AM, LaPorte RE, Sandler RB, Bayles CM, Robertson RJ, Slemenda CW,** The decline of grip strength in the menopause: relationship to physical activity, estrogen use and anthropometric factors, J Chron Dis 40:115, 1987.

61. **Vandenbroucke JP, Witteman JCM, Valkenburg HA, Boersma JW, Cats A, Festen JJM, Hartman AP, Huber-Bruning O, Rasker JJ, Weber J,** Noncontraceptive hormones and rheumatoid arthritis in perimenopausal and postmenopausal women, JAMA 255:1299, 1986.

62. **Ballinger CB,** Psychiatric aspects of the menopause, Br J Psychiatr 156:773, 1990.

63. **Schmidt PJ, Rubinow DR,** Menopause-related affective disorders: a justification for further study, Am J Psychiat 148:844, 1991.

64. **Hallstrom T, Samuelsson S,** Mental health in the climacteric. The longitudinal study of women in Gothenburg, Acta Obstet Gynecol Scand (Suppl) 130:13, 1985.

65. **Gath D, Osborn M, Bungay G, Iles S, Day A, Bond A, Passingham C,** Psychiatric disorder and gynaecological symptoms in middle aged women: a community survey, Br Med J 294:213, 1987.

66. **McKinlay JB, McKinlay SM, Brambila D,** The relative contributions of endocrine changes and social circumstances to depression in middle-aged women, J Health Soc Behav 28:345, 1987

67. **Campbell S, Whitehead M,** Estrogen therapy and the menopausal syndrome, Clin Obstet Gynecol 4:31, 1977.

68. **Ditkoff EC, Crary WG, Cristo M, Lobo RA,** Estrogen improves psychological function in asymptomatic postmenopausal women, Obstet Gynecol 78:991, 1991.

69. **Phillips SM, Sherwin BB,** Effects of estrogen on memory function in surgically menopausal women, Psychoneuroendocrinology 17:485, 1992.

70. **Schiff I, Regestein Q, Tulchinsky D, Ryan KJ,** Effects of estrogens on sleep and psychological state of hypogonadal women, JAMA 242:2405, 1979.

71. **Wiklund I, Karlberg J, Mattsson L-A,** Quality of life of postmenopausal women on a regimen of transdermal estradiol therapy: a double-blind placebo-controlled study, Am J Obstet Gynecol 168:824, 1993.

72. **Denerstein L, Burrows GD, Hyman GJ, Wood C,** Hormone therapy and affect, Maturitas 1:247, 1979.

73. **Sherwin BB,** Affective changes with estrogen and androgen replacment therapy in surgically menopausal women, J Affective Disord 14:177, 1988.

74. **Palinkas LA, Barrett-Connor E,** Estrogen use and depressive symptoms in postmenopausal women, Obstet Gynecol 80:30, 1992.

75. **Barrett-Connor E, Kritz-Silverstein D,** Estrogen replacement therapy and cognitive function in older women, JAMA 269:2637, 1993.

76. **Pagnini-Hill A,** in press.

77. **Henderson V,** in press.

78. **Dempster DW, Lindsay R,** Pathogenesis of osteoporosis, Lancet 341:797, 1993.

79. **Lees B, Molleson T, Arnett TR, Stevenson JC,** Differences in proximal femur bone density over two centuries, Lancet 341:673, 1993.

80. **Lindsay R,** Prevention and treatment of osteoporosis, Lancet 341:801, 1993.

81. **Ettinger B,** Prevention of osteoporosis: treatment of estradiol deficiency, Obstet Gynecol 72:125, 1988.

82. **Richelson LS, Wahner HW, Melton LJ III, Riggs BL,** Relative contributions of aging and estrogen deficiency to postmenopausal bone loss, New Engl J Med 311:1273, 1984.

83. **Nilas L, Christiansen C,** Bone mass and its relationship to age and the menopause, J Clin Endocrinol Metab 65:697, 1987.

84. **Seeman E, Hopper JL, Bach LA, Cooper ME, Parkinson E, McKay J, Jerums G,** Reduced bone mass in daughters of women with osteoporosis, New Engl J Med 320:554, 1989.

85. **Weiss NC, Ure CL, Ballard JH, Williams AR, Daling JR,** Estimated incidence of fractures of the lower forearm and hip in postmenopausal women, New Engl J Med 303:1195, 1980.

86. **Ettinger B, Genant HK, Cann CE,** Long-term estrogen replacement therapy prevents bone loss and fractures, Ann Intern Med 102:319, 1985.

87. **Kiel DP, Felson DT, Anderson JJ, Wilson PWF, Moskowitz MA,** Hip fracture and the use of estrogen in postmenopausal women: the Framingham Study, New Engl J Med 317:1169, 1987.

88. **Riggs BL, Seeman E, Hodgson SF, Taves DR, O'Fallon WM,** Effect of the fluoride/calcium regimen on vertebral fracture occurrence in postmenopausal osteoporosis, New Engl J Med 306:446, 1982.

89. **Quigley MET, Martin PL, Burnier AM, Brooks P,** Estrogen therapy arrests bone loss in elderly women, Am J Obstet Gynecol 156:1516, 1987.

90. **Felson DT, Zhang Y, Hannan MT, Kiel DP, Wilson PWF, Anderson JJ,** The effect of postmenopausal estrogen therpay on bone density in elderly women, New Engl J Med 329:1141, 1993.

91. **Naessén T, Persson I, Thor L, Mallmin H, Ljunghall S, Bergstrom R,** Maintained bone density at advanced ages after long-term treatment with low-dose estradiol implants, Br J Obstet Gynaecol 100:454, 1993.

92. **Lindsay R, Hart DM, Clark DM,** The minimum effective dose of estrogen for postmenopausal bone loss, Obstet Gynecol 63:759, 1984.

93. **Ettinger B, Gerrant HK, Cann CE,** Postmenopausal bone loss is prevented by treatment with low-dosage estrogen with calcium, Ann Intern Med 106:40, 1987.

94. **Ettinger B, Genant HK, Steiger P, Madvig P,** Low-dosage micronized 17β-estradiol prevents bone loss in postmenopausal women, Am J Obstet Gynecol 166:479, 1992.

95. **Stevenson, JC, Cust MP, Gangar KF, Hillard TC, Lees B, Whitehead MI,** Effects of transdermal versus oral hormone replacement therapy on bone density in spine and proximal femur in postmenopausal women, Lancet 336:1327, 1990.

96. **Horowitz M,** Cytokines and estrogen in bone: anti-osteoporotic effects, Science 260:626, 1993.

97. **Tiegs RD, Body JJ, Wahner HW, Barta J, Riggs BL, Heath H,** Calcitonin secretion in postmenopausal osteoporosis, New Engl J Med 312:1097, 1985.

98. **Liel Y, Kraus S, Levy J, Shany S,** Evidence that estrogens modulate activity and increase the number of 1,25-dihydroxyvitamin D receptors in osteoblast-like cells (ROS 17/2.8), Endocrinology 130:2597, 1992.

99. **Gallagher JC, Kable WT, Goldgar D,** Effect of progestin therapy on cortical and trabecular bone: comparison with estrogen, Am J Med 90:171, 1991.

100. **Abdalla HI, Hart DM, Lindsay R, Leggate I, Hooke A,** Prevention of bone mineral loss in postmenopausal women by norethisterone, Obstet Gynecol 66:789, 1985.

101. **Selby PL, Peacock M, Barkworth SA, Brown WB, Taylor GA,** Early effects of ethinyl oestradiol and norethisterone treatment in postmenopausal women on bone resorption and calcium regulating hormones, Clin Sci 69:265, 1985.

102. **Christiansen C, Nilas L, Riis BJ, Rodbro P, Deftos L,** Uncoupling of bone formation and resorption by combined oestrogen and progestagen therapy in postmenopausal osteoporosis, Lancet 2:800, 1985.

103. **Munk-Jensen N, Nielsen SP, Obel EB, Eriksen PB,** Reversal of postmenopausal vertebral bone loss by oestrogen and progestogen: a double blind placebo controlled study, Br Med J 296:1150, 1988.

104. **Fuleihan GE, Brown EM, Curtis K, Berger MJ, Berger BM, Gleason R, LeBoff MS,** Effect of sequential and daily continous hormone replacement therapy on indexes of mineral metabolism, Arch Intern Med 152:1904, 1992.

105. **Reid IR, Ames RW, Evans MC, Gamble GD, Sharpe SJ,** Effect of calcium supplementation on bone loss in postmenopausal women, New Engl J Med 328:460, 1993.

106. **Heaney RP, Recker RR, Saville PD,** Menopausal changes in calcium balance performance, Lab Clin Med 92:953, 1978.

107. **Hasling C, Charles P, Jensen FT, Mosekilde L,** Calcium metabolism in postmenopausal osteoporosis: the influence of dietary calcium and net absorbed calcium, J Bone Min Res 5:939, 1990.

108. **Heaney RP, Recker RR,** Distribution of calcium absorption in middle-aged women, Am J Clin Nutrition 43:299, 1986.

109. **Prince RL, Smith M, Dick IM, Price RI, Webb PG, Henderson NK, Harris MM,** Prevention of postmenopausal osteoporosis: a comparative study of exercise, calcium supplementation, and hormone-replacement therapy, New Engl J Med 325:1189, 1991.

110. **Jensen GF, Christiansen C, Transbol I,** Treatment of postmenopausal osteoporosis. A controlled therapeutic trial comparing oestrogen/gestagen, 1,25-dihydroxy-vitamin D3, and calcium, Clin Endocrinol 16:515, 1982.

111. **Heikinheimo RJ, Inkovaara JA, Harju EJ, Haavisto MV, Kaarela RH, Kataja JM, Kokko AM, Kolho LA, Rajala S,** Annual injection of vitamin D and fractures of aged bones, Calcif Tissue Int 51:105, 1992.

112. **Chapuy MC, Arlot ME, Duboeuf F, Brun J, Crouzet B, Arnaud S, Delmas PD, Meunier PJ,** Vitamin D_3 and calcium to prevent hip fractures in elderly women, New Engl J Med 327:1637, 1992.

113. **Dawson-Hughes B, Dallal GE, Krall EA, Harris S, Sokoll LJ, Falconer G,** Effect of vitamin D supplementation on wintertime and overall bone loss in healthy postmenopausal women, Ann Intern Med 115:505, 1991.

114. **Hedlund LR, Gallagher JC,** Increased incidence of hip fracture in osteoporotic women treated with sodium fluoride, J Bone Min Res 4:223, 1989.

115. **MacIntyre I, Stevenson JC, Whitehead MI, Wimalawansa SJ, Banks LM, Healy MJ,** Calcitonin for prevention of postmenopausal bone loss, Lancet 1:900, 1988.

116. **Fioretti P, Gambacciani M, Taponeco F, Melis GB, Capelli N, Spinetti,** Effects of continuous and cyclic nasal calcitonin administration in ovariectomized women, Maturitas 15:225, 1992.

117. **Storm T, Thamsborg G, Steiniche T, Genant HK, Sorenson OH,** Effect of intermittent cyclical etidronate therapy on bone mass and fracture rate in women with postmenopausal osteoporosis, New Engl J Med 322:1265, 1990.

118. **Harris ST, Gertz BJ, Genant HK, Eyre DR, Survill TT, Ventura JN, DeBrock J, Ricerca E, Chesnut CH III,** The effect of short term treatment with alendronate on vertebral density and biochemical markers of bone remodeling in early postmenopausal women, J Clin Endocrinol Metab 76:1399, 1993.

119. **Chow RK, Harrison JE, Brown CF, Hajek V,** Physical fitness effect on bone mass in postmenopausal women, Arch Phys Med Rehabil 67:231, 1986.

120. **Jensen J, Christiansen C, Rodbro P,** Cigarette smoking, serum estrogens, and bone loss during hormone replacement therapy early after menopause, New Engl J Med 313:973, 1985.

121. **Lindsay R, MacLean A, Kraszewski A, Clark AC, Garwood J,** Bone response to termination of estrogen treatment, Lancet 1:1325, 1978.

122. **Horsman A, Nordin BEC, Crilly RG,** Effect on bone of withdrawal of estrogen therapy, Lancet 2:33, 1979.

123. **Christiansen C, Christiansen MS, Transbol IB,** Bone mass in postmenopausal women after withdrawal of oestrogen/gestagen replacement therapy, Lancet 1:459, 1981.

124. **Johnston CC Jr, Slemenda CW, Melton LJ III,** Clinical use of bone densitometry, New Engl J Med 324:1105, 1991.

125. **Cummings SR, Black DM, Nevitt MC, Browner W, Cauley J, Ensrud K, Genant KH, Palermo L, Scott J, Vogt TM,** Bone density at various sites for prediction of hip fractures, Lancet 341:72, 1993.

126. **Paganini-Hill A, Chao A, Ross RK, Henderson BE,** Exercise and other factors in the prevention of hip fracture: the Leisure World Study, Epidemiology 2:16, 1991.

127. **Lloyd T, Andon MB, Rollings N, Martel JK, Landis JR, Demers LM, Eggli DF, Kiesselhorst K, Kulin HE,** Calcium supplementation and bone mineral density in adolescent girls, JAMA 270:841, 1993.

128. **Wenger NK, Speroff L, Packard B,** Cardiovascular health and disease in women, New Engl J Med 329:247, 1993.

129. **Thom TJ,** International mortality from heart disease: rates and trends, Int J Epidemiol 18:S20, 1989.

130. **Levy RL, Moskowitz J,** Cardiovascular research: decades of progress, decade of promise, Science 217:121, 1982.

131. **Matthews KA, Meilahn E, Kuller LH, Kelsey SF, Caggiula AW, Wing RR,** Menopause and risk factors for coronary heart disease, New Engl J Med 321:641, 1989.

132. **Jacobs DR Jr, Mebane IL, Bangdiwala SI, Criqui MH, Tyroler HA,** High density lipoprotein cholesterol as a predictor of cardiovascular disease mortality in men and women: the follow-up study of the Lipid Research Clinics Prevalence Study, Am J Epidemiol 131:32, 1990.

133. **Wilson PW, Garrison RJ, Castelli WP, Feinleib M, McNamara PM, Kannel WB,** Prevalence of coronary heart disease in the Framingham offspring study: role of lipoprotein cholesterols, Am J Cardiol 46:649, 1980.

134. **Campos H, McNamara JR, Wilson PW, Ordovas JM, Schaefer EJ,** Differences in low density lipoprotein subfractions and apolipoproteins in premenopausal and postmenopausal women, J Clin Endocrinol Metab 67:30, 1988.

135. **Lapidus L, Bengtsson C, Larsson B, Pennert K, Rybo E, Sjostrom L,** Distribution of adipose tissue and risk of cardiovascular disease and death: a 12 year follow up of participants in the population study of women in Gothenburg, Sweden, Br Med J 289:1257, 1984.

136. **Haarbo J, Hassager C, Riis BJ, Christiansen C,** Relation of body fat distribution to serum lipids and lipoproteins in elderly women, Atherosclerosis 80:57, 1989.

137. **Soler JT, Folsom AR, Kaye SA, Prineas RJ,** Associations of abdominal adiposity, fasting insulin, sex hormone binding globulin and estrogen with lipids and lipoproteins in post-menopausal women, Atherosclerosis 79:21, 1989.

138. **Eriksson M, Berglund L, Rudling M, Henriksson P, Angelin B,** Effects of estrogen on low density lipoprotein metabolism in males. Short-term and long-term studies during hormonal treatment of prostatic carcinoma, J Clin Invest 84:802, 1989.

139. **Walsh BW, Schiff I, Rosner B, Greenberg L, Ravnikar V, Sacks FM,** Effects of postmenopausal estrogen replacement on the concentrations and metabolism of plasma lipoproteins, New Engl J Med 325:1196, 1991.

140. **Granfone A, Campos H, McNamara JR, Schaefer MM, Lemon-Fava S, Ordovas JM, Schaefer EJ,** Effects of estrogen replacement on plasma lipoproteins and apolipoproteins in postmenopausal dyslipidemic women, Metabolism 41:1193, 1992.

141. **Rifici VA, Khachadurian AK,** The inhibition of low-density lipoprotein oxidation by 17-beta estradiol, Metabolism 41:1110, 1992.

142. **Ingegno MD, Money SR, Thelmo W, Greene GL, Davidian M, Jaffe BM, Pertschuk LP,** Progesterone receptors in the human heart and great vessels, Lab Invest 59:353, 1988.

143. **Rosenberg L, Armstrong B, Jick H,** Myocardial infarction and estrogen therapy in postmenopausal women, New Engl J Med 294:1256, 1976.

144. **Pfeffer RI, Whipple GH, Kurosake TT, Chapman JM,** Coronary risk and estrogen use in postmenopausal women, Am J Epidemiol 107:479, 1978.

145. **Jick H, Dinan B, Rothman KJ,** Noncontraceptive estrogens and non-fatal myocardial infarction, JAMA 239:1407, 1978.

146. **Rosenberg L, Sloane D, Shapiro S, Kaufman D, Stolley PD, Miethinen OS,** Noncontraceptive estrogens and myocardial infarction in young women, JAMA 224:339, 1980.

147. **Ross RK, Paganini-Hill A, Mack TM, Arthur M, Henderson BE,** Menopausal oestrogen therapy and protection from death from ischaemic heart disease, Lancet 1:585, 1981.

148. **Bain C, Willett W, Hennekens CH, Rosner B, Belanger C, Speizer FE,** Use of postmenopausal hormones and risk of myocardial infarction, Circulation 64:42, 1981.

149. **Adam S, Williams V, Vessey MP,** Cardiovascular disease and hormone replacement treatment: a pilot case-control study, Br Med J 282:1277, 1981.

150. **Szklo M, Tonascia J, Gordis L, Bloom I,** Estrogen use and myocardial infarction risk: a case-control study, Prev Med 13:510, 1984.

151. **Sullivan JM, Vander Zwaag R, Lemp GF, Hughes JP, Maddock V, Kroetz FW, Ramanathan KB, Mirvis DM,** Postmenopausal estrogen use and coronary atherosclerosis, Ann Intern Med 108:358, 1988.

152. **Gruchow HW, Anderson AJ, Barboriak JJ, Sobocinski KA,** Postmenopausal use of estrogen and occlusion of coronary arteries, Am Heart J 115:954, 1988.

153. **McFarland KF, Boniface ME, Hornung CA, Earnhardt W, Humphries JO,** Risk factors and noncontraceptive estrogen use in women with and without coronary disease, Am Heart J 117:1209, 1989.

154. **Hong MG, Romm PA, Reagan K, Green CE, Rackley CE,** Effects of estrogen replacement therapy on serum lipid values and angiographically defined coronary artery disease in postmenopausal women, Am J Cardiol 69:176, 1992.

155. **Beard CM, Kottke TE, Annegers JF, Ballard DJ,** The Rochester Coronary Heart Disease Project: effect of cigarette smoking, hypertension, diabetes, and steroidal estrogen use on coronary heart disease among 40- to 59-year-old women, 1960 through 1982, Mayo Clin Proc 64:1471, 1989.

156. **Burch JC, Byrd BF, Vaughn WK,** The effects of long-term estrogen on hysterectomized women, Am J Obstet Gynecol 118:778, 1974.

157. **Gordon T, Kannel WB, Hjortland MC, McNamara PM,** Menopause and coronary heart disease: the Framingham Study, Ann Intern Med 89:157, 1978.

158. **Hammond CB, Jelovsek FR, Lee KL, Creasman WT, Parker RT,** Effects of long-term estrogen replacement therapy: I. Metabolic effects, Am J Obstet Gynecol 133:525, 1979.

159. **Petitti DB, Wingerd J, Pellegrin F, Ramcharan S,** Risk of vascular disease in women: smoking, oral contraceptives, non-contraceptive estrogens, and other factors, JAMA 242:1150, 1979.

160. **Lafferty FW, Helmuth DO,** Postmenopausal estrogen replacement: the prevention of osteoporosis and systemic effects, Maturitas 7:147, 1985.

161. **Wilson PWF, Garrison RJ, Castelli WP,** Postmenopausal estrogen use, cigarette smoking, and cardiovascular morbidity in women over 50. The Framingham Study, New Engl J Med 313:1038, 1985.

162. **Stampfer MJ, Colditz GA, Willett WC, Manson JE, Rosner B, Speizer FE, Hennekens CH,** Postmenopausal estrogen therapy and cardiovascular disease: ten-year follow-up from the Nurses' Health Study, New Engl J Med 325:756, 1991.

163. **Bush TL, Barrett-Connor E, Cowan DK, Criqui MH, Wallace RB, Suchindran CM, Tyroler HA, Rifkind BM,** Cardiovascular mortality and noncontraceptive use of estrogen in women: results from the Lipid Research Clinics Program Follow-up Study, Circulation 75:1102, 1987.

164. **Criqui MH, Suarez L, Barrett-Connor E, McPhillips J, Wingard DL, Garland C,** Postmenopausal estrogen use and mortality, Am J Epidemiol 128:606, 1988.

165. **Henderson BE, Paganini-Hill A, Ross RK,** Estrogen replacment therapy and protection from acute myocardial infarction, Am J Obstet Gynecol 159:312, 1988.

166. **Perlman J, Wolf P, Finucane F, Madans J,** Menopause and the epidemiology of cardiovascular disease in women, Prog Clin Biol Res 320:283, 1989.

167. **Petitti DB, Perlman JA, Sidney S,** Noncontraceptive estrogens and mortality: long-term follow-up of women in the Walnut Creek study, Obstet Gynecol 70:289, 1987.

168. **Eaker ED, Castelli WP,** Coronary heart disease and its risk factors among women in the Framingham Study, in Eaker ED, Packard B, Wenger NG, editors, *Coronary Heart Disease in Women,* Haymarket Doyma, New York, 1987, pp 122-130.

169. **Nachtigall LE , Nachtigall RH, Nachtigall RD, Beckman EM,** Estrogen replacment therapy II: a prospective study in the relationship to carcinoma and cardiovascular and metabolic problems, Obstet Gynecol 54:74, 1979.

170. **Thompson SG, Meade TW, Greenberg G,** The use of hormonal replacement therapy and the risk of stroke and myocardial infarction in women, J Epidemiol Comm Health 43:173, 1989.

171. **Paganini-Hill A, Ross RK, Henderson BE,** Postmenopausal oestrogen treatment and stroke: a prospective study, Br Med J 297:519, 1988.

172. **Falkeborn M, Persson I, Terent A, Adami HO, Lithell H, Bergstrom R,** Hormone replacement therapy and the risk of stroke. Follow-up of a population-based cohort in Sweden, Arch Intern Med 153:1201, 1993.

173. **Finucane FF, Madans JH, Bush TL, Wolf PH, Kleinman JC,** Decreased risk of stroke among postmenopausal hormone users, Arch Intern Med 153:73, 1993.

174. **Lind T, Cameron EC, Hunter WM, Leon C, Moran PF, Oxley A, Gerrard J, Lind UCG,** A prospective, controlled trial of six forms of hormone replacement therapy given to postmenopausal women, Br J Obstet Gynaecol (Suppl 3) 86:1, 1979.

175. **Pfeffer RI, Kurosaki TT, Charlton SK,** Estrogen use and blood pressure in later life, Am J Epidemiol 110:469, 1979.

176. **Lutola H,** Blood pressure and hemodynamics in postmenopausal women during estradiol-17β substitution, Ann Clin Res (Suppl 38) 15:9, 1983.

177. **Wren BG, Routledge AD,** The effect of type and dose of oestrogen on the blood pressure of postmenopausal women, Maturitas 5:135, 1983.

178. **Hassager C, Christiansen C,** Blood pressure during oestrogen/progestogen substitution therapy in healthy post-menopausal women, Maturitas 9:315, 1988.

179. **Adams MR, Clarkson TB, Koritnik DR, Nash HA,** Contraceptive steroids and coronary artery atherosclerosis in cynomolgus macaques, Fertil Steril 47:1010, 1987.

180. **Clarkson TB, Adams MR, Kaplan JR, Shively CA, Koritnik DR,** From menarche to menopause: coronary artery atherosclerosis and protection in cyanomolgus monkeys, Am J Obstet Gynecol 160:1280, 1989.

181. **Clarkson TB, Shively CA, Morgan TM, Koritnik DR, Adams MR, Kaplan JR,** Oral contraceptives and coronary artery atherosclerosis of cynomolgus monkeys, Obstet Gynecol 75:217, 1990.

182. **Kushwaha RS, Hazzard WR,** Exogenous estrogens attenuate dietary hypercholesterolemia and atherosclerosis in the rabbit, Metabolism 30:57, 1981.

183. **Hough JL, Zilversmit DB,** Effect of 17 beta estradiol on aortic cholesterol content and metabolism in cholesterol-fed rabbits, Arteriosclerosis 6:57, 1986.

184. **Henriksson P, Stamberger M, Eriksson M, Rudling M, Diczfalusy U, Berglund L, Angelin B,** Oestrogen-induced changes in lipoprotein metabolism: role in prevention of atherosclerosis in the cholesterol-fed rabbit, Europ J Clin Invest 19:395, 1989.

185. **Haarbo J, Leth-Espensen P, Stender S, Christiansen C,** Estrogen monotherapy and combined estrogen-progestogen replacement therapy attenuate aortic accumulation of cholesterol in ovariectomized cholesterol-fed rabbits, J Clin Invest 87:1274, 1991.

186. **Adams MP, Kaplan JR, Manuck SB, Koritnik DR, Parks JS, Wolfe MS, Clarkson TB,** Inhibition of coronary artery atherosclerosis by 17-beta estradiol in ovariectomized monkeys. Lack of an effect of added progesterone, Arteriosclerosis 10:151, 1990.

187. **Wagner JD, St Clair RW, Schwenke DC, Shively CA, Adams MR, Clarkson TB,** Regional differences in arterial low density lipoprotein metabolism in surgically postmenopausal Cynomolgus monkeys: effects of estrogen and progesterone replacement therapy, Arteriosclerosis Thrombo 12:717, 1992.

188. **Vanhoutte PM,** Endothelium-derived relaxing and contracting factors, Adv Nephrol 19:3, 1990.

189. **Bar J, Tepper R, Fuchs J, Pardo Y, Goldberger S, Ovadia J,** The effect of estrogen replacement therapy on platelet aggregation and adenosine triphosphate release in postmenopausal women, Obstet Gynecol 81:261, 1993.

190. **Lindheim SR, Legro RS, Bernstein L, Stanczyk FZ, Vijod MA, Presser SC, Lobo RA,** Behavioral stress responses in premenopausal and postmenopausal women and the effects of estrogen, Am J Obstet Gynecol 167:1831, 1992.

191. **Haarbo J, Marslew U, Gotfredsen A, Christiansen C,** Postmenopausal hormone replacement therapy prevents central distribution of body fat after menopause, Metabolism 40:1323, 1991.

192. **Ley CJ, Lees B, Stevenson JC,** Sex- and menopause-associated changes in body-fat distribution, Am J Clin Nutr 55:950, 1992.

193. **Nabulsi AA, Folsom AR, White A, Patsch W, Heiss G, Wu KK, Szklo M,** Association of hormone-replacement therapy with various cardiovascular risk factors in postmenopausal women, New Engl J Med 328:1069, 1993.

194. **Cagnacci A, Soldani R, Carriero PL, Paoletti AM, Fioretti P, Melis GB,** Effects of low doses of transdermal 17 beta-estradiol on carbohydrate metabolism in postmenopausal women, J Clin Endocrinol Metab 74:1396, 1992.

195. **Lobo R, Pickar JH, Wild RA, Walsh B, Hirvonen E, for The Menopause Study Group,** Metabolic impact of adding medroxyprogesterone acetate to conjugated estrogen therapy in postmenopausal women, in press.

196. **Manson JE, Rimm EB, Colditz GA, Willett WC, Nathan DM, Arky RA, Rosner B, Hennekens CH, Speizer FE, Stampfer MJ,** A prospective study of postmenopausal estrogen therapy and subsequent incidence of non-insulin dependent diabetes mellitus, Ann Epidemiol 2:665, 1992.

197. **Godsland IF, Ganger K, Walton C, Cust MP, Whitehead MI, Wynn V, Stevenson JC,** Insulin resistance, secretion, and elimination in postmenopausal women receiving oral or transdermal hormone replacement therapy, Metabolism 42:846, 1993.

198. **Pines A, Fishman EZ, Levo Y, Auerbuch M, Lidor A, Drory Y, Finkelstein A, Hetman-Peri M, Moshkowitz M, Ben-Ari E, Ayalon D,** The effects of hormone replacement therapy in normal postmenopausal women: measurements of Doppler-derived parameters of aortic flow, Am J Obstet Gynecol 164:806, 1991.

199. **Voutilainen S, Hippelainen M, Hulkko S, Karppinen K,** Ventila M, Kupari M, Left ventricular diastolic function by Doppler echocardiography in relation to hormone replacement therapy in healthy postmenopausal women, Am J Cardiol 71:614, 1993.

200. **Hirvonen E, Malkonen M, Manninen V,** Effects of different progestogens on lipoproteins during postmenopausal therapy, New Engl J Med 304:560, 1981.

201. **Mattsson L, Cullberg LG, Samsioe G,** Influence of esterified estrogens and medroxy-progesterone on lipid metabolism and sex steroids. A study in oophorectomized women, Horm Metab Res 14:602, 1982.

202. **Silferstolpe G, Gustafsson A, Samsioe G, Syanborg A,** Lipid metabolic studies in oophorec-tomized women: effects on serum lipids and lipoproteins of three synthetic progestogens, Maturitas 4:103, 1983.

203. **Ylostalo P, Kauppila A, Kivinen S, Tuimala R, Vihkoo R,** Endocrine and metabolic effects of low-dose estrogen-progestin treatment in climacteric women, Obstet Gynecol 62:682, 1983.

204. **Mattsson L, Cullberg G, Samsioe G,** A continuous estrogen-progestogen regimen for climac-teric complaints, Acta Obstet Gynecol Scand 63:673, 1984.

205. **Ottosson UB, Carlstrom K, Damber JE, von Schoultz B,** Serum levels of progesterone and some of its metabolites including deoxycorticosterone after oral and parenteral administration, Br J Obstet Gynaecol 91:1111, 1984.

206. **Wren B, Garrett D,** The effect of low-dose piperazine oestrogen sulphate and low-dose levo-norgestrel on blood lipid levels in postmenopausal women, Maturitas 7:141, 1985.

207. **Ottosson UB, Johansson BG, von Schoultz B,** Subfractions of high-density lipoprotein choles-terol during estrogen replacement therapy: a comparison between progestogens and natural progesterone, Am J Obstet Gynecol 151:746, 1985.

208. **Obel EB, Munk-Jensen N, Svenstrup B, Bennett P, Micic S, Henrik-Nielsen R, Nielsen SP, Gydesen H, Jensen, BM,** A two-year double-blind controlled study of the clinical effect of combined and sequential postmenopausal replacement therapy and steroid metabolism during treatment, Maturitas 16:13, 1993.

209. **Barrett-Connor E, Wingard DL, Criqui MH,** Postmenopausal estrogen use and heart disease risk factors in the 1980s, JAMA 261:2095, 1989.

210. **Sherwin BB, Gelfand MM,** A prospective one-year study of estrogen and progestin in postmenopausal women: effects on clinical symptoms and lipoprotein lipids, Obstet Gynecol 73:759, 1989.

211. **Wolfe BM, Huff MW,** Effects of combined estrogen and progestin administration on plasma lipoprotein metabolism in postmenopausal women, J Clin Invest 83:40, 1989.

212. **Christiansen C, Riis BJ,** Five years with continous combined oestrogen/progestogen therapy. Effects on calcium metabolism, lipoproteins, and bleeding pattern, Br J Obstet Gynaecol 97:1087, 1990.

213. **Marslew U, Overgaard K, Riis BJ, Christiansen C,** Two new combinations of estrogen and progestogen for prevention of postmenopausal bone loss: long-term effects on bone, calcium and lipid metabolism, climacteric symptoms, and bleeding, Obstet Gynecol 79:202, 1992.

214. **Williams SR, Frenchek B, Speroff T, Speroff L,** A study of combined continuous ethinyl estradiol and norethindrone acetate for postmenopausal hormone replacement, Am J Obstet Gynecol 162:438, 1990.

215. **Weinstein L, Bewtra C, Gallagher JC,** Evaluation of a continuous combined low-dose regimen of estrogen-progestin for treatment of the menopausal patient, Am J Obstet Gynecol 162:1534, 1990.

216. **Cano A, Fernandes H, Serrano S, Mahiques P,** Effect of continuous oestradiol-medroxy-progesterone administration on plasma lipids and lipoproteins, Maturitas 13:35, 1991.

217. **Gibbons WE, Judd HL, Luciano AA, et al,** Comparison of sequential versus continuous estrogen/progestin replacement therapy on serum lipid patterns, Abstract 491, Society for Gynecological Investigation, Annual Meeting, 1991.

218. **Falkeborn M, Persson I, Adami HO, Bergstrom R, Eaker E, Lithell H, Mohsen R, Taessen T,** The risk of acute myocardial infarction after oestrogen and oestrogen-progestogen replacement, Br J Obstet Gynecol 99:821, 1992.

219. **de Ziegler D, Bessis R, Frydman R,** Vascular resistance of uterine arteries: physiological effects of estradiol and progesterone, Fertil Steril 55:775, 1991.

220. **Speroff T, Dawson N, Speroff L,** Is postmenopausal estrogen use risky? Results from a methodologic review and information synthesis, Clin Res 35:362A, 1987.

221. **Stampfer MJ, Colditz GA,** Estrogen replacement therapy and coronary heart disease: a quantitative assessment of the epidemiological evidence, Prev Med 20:47, 1991.

222. **Boston Collaborative Drug Surveillance Program,** Surgically confirmed gallbladder disease, venous thromboembolism, and breast tumors in relation to postmenopausal estrogen therapy, New Engl J Med 290:15, 1974.

223. **Pettiti DB, Wingerd J, Pellegrin F, Ramcharan S,** Risk of vascular disease in women, JAMA 242:1150, 1979.

224. **Devor M, Barrett-Connor E, Renvall M, Feigal D Jr, Ramsdell J,** Estrogen replacement therapy and the risk of venous thrombosis, Am J Med 92:275, 1992.

225. **Nurses' Health Study,** in press.

226. **Enzelsberger H, Heytmanek H, Kurz Ch, Metka M,** Zum enfluss einer hormonsubstitutionstherapie auf AT III bei frauen im klimakterium, Zentralbl Gynakol 113:639, 1991.

227. **Grodstein F, Colditz GA, Stampfer MJ,** Postmenopausal hormone use and cholecystectomy in a large prospective study, Obstet Gynecol 83:5, 1994.

228. **Scagg RKR, McMichael AJ, Seamark RF,** Oral contraceptive, pregnancy and endogenous estrogen in gallstone disease - a case-control study, Br Med J 288:1795, 1984.

229. **Kakar F, Weiss NS, Strite SA,** Non-contraceptive estrogen use and the risk of gallstone disease in women, Am J Public Health 78:564, 1988.

230. **Woodruff JD, PickarJH, for The Menopause Study Group,** Incidence of endometrial hyperplasia in postmenopausal women taking premarin with medroxyprogesterone acetate or premarin alone, in press.

231. **Kurman RJ, Kalminski PF, Norris HJ,** The behavior of endometrial hyperplasia: a long term study of "untreated" hyperplasia in 170 patients, Cancer 56:403, 1985.

232. **Shapiro S, Kelly JP, Rosenberg L, Kaufman DW, Helmrich SP, Rosenshein NB, Lewis JL Jr, Knapp RC, Stolley PD, Schottenfeld D,** Risk of localized and widespread endometrial cancer in relation to recent and discontinued use of conjugated estrogens, New Engl J Med 313:969, 1985.

233. **Paganini-Hill, Ross RK, Henderson BE,** Endometrial cancer and patterns of use of oestrogen replacement therapy: a cohort study, Br J Cancer 59:445, 1989.

234. **Thom MH, White PJ, Williams RM, Sturdee PW, Paterson MEL, Wade-Evans T, Studd JWW,** Prevention and treatment of endometrial disease in climacteric women receiving estrogen, Lancet 2:455, 1979.

235. **Whitehead MI, Townsend PT, Pryse-Davies J, Ryder TA, King RJB,** Effects of estrogen and progestins on the biochemistry and morphology of the postmenopausal endometrium, New Engl J Med 305:1599, 1981.

236. **Gambrell RD Jr, Babgnell CA, Greenblatt RB,** Role of estrogens and progesterone in the etiology and prevention of endometrial cancer: a review, Am J Obstet Gynecol 146:696, 1983.

237. **Persson I, Adami H-O, Bergkvist L, Lindgren A, Pettersson, Hoover R, Schairer C,** Risk of endometrial cancer after treatment with oestrogens alone or in conjunction with progestogens: results of a prospective study, Br Med J 298:147, 1989.

238. **Voigt LF, Weiss NS, Chu JR, Daling J, McKnight B, van Belle G,** Progestagen supplementation of exogenous oestrogens and risk of endometrial cancer, Lancet 338:274, 1991.

239. **Varma TR,** Effect of long-term therapy with estrogen and progesterone on the endometrium of postmenopausal women, Acta Obstet Gynecol Scand 64:41, 1985.

240. **Weiss N,** in press.

241. **Harris JR, Lippman ME, Veronesi U, Willett W,** Breast cancer, New Engl J Med 327:319,390,473, 1992.

242. **Bergkvist L, Adami H-O, Persson I, Hoover R, Schairer C,** The risk of breast cancer after estrogen and estrogen-progestin replacment, New Engl J Med 321:293. 1989.

243. **Bergkvist L, Adami H-O, Persson I, Bergstrom R, Krusemo UB,** Prognosis after breast cancer diagnosis in women exposed to estrogen and estrogen-progestogen replacement therapy, Am J Epidemiol 130:221, 1989.

244. **Ewertz M,** Influence of non-contraceptive exogenous and endogenous sex hormones on breast cancer risk in Denmark, Int J Cancer 42:832, 1988.

245. **Brinton LA, Hoover R, Fraumeni JF Jr,** Menopausal oestrogens and breast cancer risk: an expanded case-control study, Br J Cancer 54:825, 1986.

246. **Hiatt RA, Bawol R, Friedman GD, Hoover R,** Exogenous estrogen and breast cancer after bilateral oophorectomy, Cancer 54:139, 1984.

247. **Hoover R, Gray LA Sr, Cole P, MacMahon B,** Menopausal estrogens and breast cancer, New Engl J Med 295:401, 1976.

248. **Hoover R, Glass A, Finkle WE, Azevedo D, Milne K,** Conjugated estrogens and breast cancer risk in women, J Natl Ca Inst 67:815, 1981.

249. **Hulka BS, Chambless LE, Deubner DC, Wilkinson WE,** Breast cancer and estrogen replacement therapy, Am J Obstet Gynecol 143:638, 1982.

250. **Jick H, Walker AM, Watkins RN, D'Ewart DC, Hunter JR, Danford A, Madsen S, Dinan BJ, Rothman KJ,** Replacement estrogens and breast cancer, Am J Epidemiol 112:586, 1980.

251. **Kaufman DW, Miller DR, Rosenberg L, Helmrich SP, Stolley P, Schottenfeld D, Shapiro S,** Noncontraceptive estrogen use and the risk of breast cancer, JAMA 252:63, 1984.

252. **Kelsey JL, Fischer DB, Holford TR, Livoisi VA, Mostowed D, Goldenberg IS, et al,** Exogenous estrogens and other factors in the epidemiology of breast cancer, J Natl Ca Inst 67:327, 1981.

253. **Lawson DH, Jick H, Hunter JR, Madsen S,** Exogenous estrogens and breast cancer, Am J Epidemiol 114:710, 1981.

254. **Ross RK, Paganini-Hill A, Gerkins VR, Mack TM, Pfeffer R, Arthur M, et al,** A case-control study of menopausal estrogen therapy and breast cancer, JAMA 243:1635, 1980.

255. **Wingo PA, Layde PM, Lee NC, Rubin G, Ory HW,** The risk of breast cancer in postmenopausal women who have used estrogen replacement therapy, JAMA 257:209, 1987.

256. **Colditz GA, Stampfer MJ, Willett WC, Hunter DJ, Manson JE, Hennekens CH, Rosner BA, Speizer FE,** Type of postmenopausal hormone use and risk of breast cancer: 12-year follow-up from the Nurses' Health Study, Cancer Causes Control 3:433, 1992.

257. **Rohan TE, McMichael AJ,** Non-contraceptive exogenous oestrogen therapy and breast cancer, Med J Aust 148:217, 1988.

258. **Dupont WD, Page DL, Rogers LW, Parl FF,** Influence of exogenous estrogens, proliferative breast disease, and other variables on breast cancer risk, Cancer 63:948, 1989.

259. **Kaufman DW, Palmer JR, De Mouzon J, Rosenberg L, Stolley PD, Warshaver ME, Shapiro S,** Estrogen replacement therapy and the risk of breast cancer: results from the case-control surveillance study, Am J Epidemiol 134:1375, 1991.

260. **Palmer JR, Rosenberg L, Clarke EA, Miller DR, Shapiro S,** Breast cancer risk after estrogen replacement therapy: results from the Toronto Breast Cancer Study, Am J Epidemiol 134:1386, 1991.

261. **Yang CP, Daling JR, Band PR, Gallagher RP, White E, Weiss NS,** Noncontraceptive hormone use and risk of breast cancer, Cancer Causes Control 3:475, 1992.

262. **Armstrong BK,** Oestrogen therapy after the menopause — boon or bane? Med J Aust 148:213, 1988.

263. **Dupont WD, Page DL,** Menopausal estrogen replacement therapy and breast cancer, Arch Intern Med 151:67, 1991.

264. **Steinberg KK, Thacker SB, Smith SJ, Stroup DF, Zack MM, Flanders WD, Berkelman RL,** A meta-analysis of the effect of estrogen replacement therapy on the risk of breast cancer, JAMA 265:1985, 1991.

265. **Sillero-Arenas M, Delgado-Rodriguez M, Rodigues-Canteras R, Bueno-Cavanillas A, Galvez-Vargas R,** Menopausal hormone replacement therapy and breast cancer: a meta-analysis, Obstet Gynecol 79:286, 1992.

266. **Colditz GA, Egan KM, Stampfer MJ,** Hormone replacement therapy and risk of breast cancer: results from epidemiologic studies, Am J Obstet Gynecol 168:1473, 1993.

267. **Grady D, Rubin SM, Petitti DB, Fox CS, Black D, Ettinger B, Ernster VL, Cummings SR,** Hormone therapy to prevent disease and prolong life in postmenopausal women, Ann Intern Med 117:1016, 1992.

268. **Strickland DM, Gambrell RD Jr, Butzin CA, Strickland K,** The relationship between breast cancer survival and prior postmenopausal estrogen use, Obstet Gynecol 80:400, 1992.

269. **Henderson BE, Paganini-Hill A, Ross RK,** Decreased mortality in users of estrogen replacement therapy, Arch Intern Med 151:75, 1991.

270. **Gambrell RD Jr, Maier RC, Sanders BI,** Decreased incidence of breast cancer in postmenopausal estrogen-progestogen users, Obstet Gynecol 62:435, 1983.

271. **Nachtigall MJ, Smilen SW, Nachtigall RAD, Nachtigall RH, Nachtigall LI,** Incidence of breast cancer in a 22-year study of women receiving estrogen-progestin replacement therapy, Obstet Gynecol 80:827, 1992.

272. **Genant HK, Cann CE, Ettinger B, Gordan GS,** Quantitative computed tomography of vertebral spongiosa: a sensitive method for detecting early bone loss after oophorectomy, Ann Intern Med 97:699, 1982.

273. **Mashchak CA, Lobo RA, Dozono-Takano R, Eggena P, Nakamura RM, Brenner PF, Mishell DR Jr,** Comparison of pharmacodynamic properties of various estrogen formulations, Am J Obstet Gynecol 144:511, 1982.

274. **Horsman A, Jones M, Francis R, Nordin C,** The effect of estrogen dose on postmenopausal bone loss, New Engl J Med 309:1405, 1983.

275. **Field CS, Ory SJ, Wahner HW, Herrmann RR, Judd HL, Riggs BL,** Preventive effects of transdermal 17β-estradiol on osteoporotic changes after surgical menopause: a two-year placebo-controlled trial, Am J Obstet Gynecol 168:114, 1993.

276. **Goebelsmann U, Mashchak CA, Mishell DR Jr,** Comparison of hepatic impact of oral and vaginal administration of ethinyl estradiol, Am J Obstet Gynecol 151:868, 1985.

277. **Stevenson, JC, Cust MP, Gangar KF, Hillard TC, Lees B, Whitehead MI,** Effects of transdermal versus oral hormone replacement therapy on bone density in spine and proximal femur in postmenopausal women, Lancet 336:1327, 1990.

278. **Crook D, Cust MP, Gangar KF, Worthington M, Hillard TC, Stevenson JC, Whitehead MI, Wynn V,** Comparison of transdermal and oral estrogen-progestin replacement therapy: effects on serum lipids and lipoproteins, Am J Obstet Gynecol 166:950, 1992.

279. **Lufkin EG, Wahner HW, O'Fallon WM, Hodgson SF, Kotowicz MA, Lane AW, Judd HL, Caplan RH, Riggs BL,** Treatment of postmenopausal osteoporosis with transdermal estrogen, Ann Intern Med 117:1, 1992.

280. **Pasetto N, Piccione E, Pasetto, et al,** Treatment of patients at risk. Cross-over study betwen natural estrogens, in Pasetto N, editor, *The Menopause and Postmenopause,* MTP Press, Lancaster, England, 1980, pp 141-151.

281. **Colvin PL Jr, Auerbach BJ, Koritnik DR, Hazzard WR, Applebaum-Bowden D,** Differential effects of oral estrogen versus 17β-estradiol on lipoproteins in postmenopausal women, J Clin Endocrinol Metab 70:1568, 1990.

282. **Pang SC, Greendale GA, Cedars MI, Gambone JC, Lozano K, Eggena P, Judd HL,** Long-term effects of transdermal estradiol with and without medroxyprogesterone acetate, Fertil Steril 59:76, 1993.

283. **Lobo R, March CM, Goebelsmann U, Krauss RM, Mishell DR Jr,** Subdermal estradiol pellets following hysterectomy and oophorectomy, Am J Obstet Gynecol 138:714, 1980.

284. **Dupont A, Dupont P, Cusan L, Tremblay M, Rioux J, Cloutier D, Mailloux J, De Lignieres B, Gutkowska J, Boucher H, Belanger A, Moyer DL, Moorjani S, Labrie F,** Comparative endocrinological and clinical effects of percutaneous estadiol and oral conjugated estrogens as replacement therapy in menopausal women, Maturitas 13:297, 1991.

285. **Strickland DM, Hammond TL,** Postmenopausal estrogen replacement in a large gynecologic practice, Am J Gynecol Health 2:33, 1988.

286. **Speroff T, Dawson NV, Speroff L, Harber RJ,** A risk-benefit analysis of elective bilateral oophorectomy: effect of changes in compliance with estrogen therapy on outcome, Am J Obstet Gynecol 164:165, 1991.

287. **Ravnikar, VA,** Compliance with hormonal therapy, Am J Obstet Gynecol 156:1332, 1987.

288. **Archer DF, Pickar JH, Bottiglioni F, for The Menopause Study Group,** Bleeding patterns in postmenopausal women taking continuous combined or sequential regimens of conjugated estrogens with medroxyprogesterone acetate, in press.

289. **Andersson K, Mattsson L, Rybo G, Stadberg E,** Intrauterine release of levonorgestrel—a new way of adding progestogen in hormone replacement therapy, Obstet Gynecol 79:963, 1992.

290. **Archer DF, McIntyre-Seltman K, Wilborn WH, Dowling EA, Cone F, Creasy GW, Kafrissen ME,** Endometrial morphology in asymptomatic postmenopausal women, Am J Obstet Gynecol 165:317, 1991.

291. **Weiss N,** in press.

292. **Judd HL,** in press.

293. **Padwick ML, Psryse-Davies J, Whitehead MI,** A simple method for determining the optimal dosage of progestin in postmenopausal women receiving estrogens, New Engl J Med 315:930, 1986.

294. **Wikland M, Granberg S, Karlsson B,** Assessment of the endometrium in the postmenopausal woman by vaginal sonography, Ultrasound Q 10:15, 1992.

295. **Botsis D, Kassanos D, Pyrgiotis E, Zourlas PA,** Vaginal sonography of the endometrium in postmenopausal women, Clin Exp Obstet Gynecol 19:189, 1992.

296. **Pansini F, DePaoli D, Serra MM, et al,** Combined use of progesterone challenge test and endometrium thickness evaluated by transvaginal ultrasonography in the preventive management of postmenopausal women, Gynecol Obstet Invest 34:237, 1992.

297. **Creasman WT,** Estrogen replacement therapy: Is previously treated cancer a contraindication? Obstet Gynecol 77:308, 1991.

298. **Lee RB, Burke TW, Park RC,** Estrogen replacement therapy following treatment for stage 1 endometrial carcinoma, Gynecol Oncol 36:189, 1990.

299. **Baker DP,** Estrogen-replacement therapy in patients with previous endometrial carcinoma, Compr Ther 16:28, 1990.

300. **Heaps JM, Nieberg RK, Berek JS,** Malignant neoplasms arising in endometriosis, Obstet Gynecol 75:1023, 1990.

301. **Reimnitz C, Brand E, Nieberg RK, Hacker NF,** Malignancy arising in endometriosis associated with unopposed estrogen replacement, Obstet Gynecol 71:444, 1988.

302. **Sherwin BB, Gelfand MM,** The role of androgen in the maintenance of sexual functioning in oophorectomized women, Psychosom Med 49:397, 1987.

303. **Myers LS, Dixen J, Morrissette D, Carmichael M, Davidson JM,** Effects of estrogen, androgen, and progestin on sexual psychophysiology and behavior in postmenopausal women, J Clin Endocrinol Metab 70:1124, 1990.

304. **Hickok LR, Toomey C, Speroff L,** A comparison of esterified estrogens with and without methyltestosterone: effects on endometrial histology and serum lipoproteins in postmenopausal women, Obstet Gynecol 82:919, 1993..

305. **Garnett T, Studd J, Watson N, Savvas M, Leather A,** The effects of plasma estradiol levels on increases in vertebral and femoral bone density following therapy with estradiol and estradiol with testosterone implants, Obstet Gynecol 79:968, 1992.

306. **Urman B, Pride SM, Ho Yuen B,** Elevated serum testosterone, hirsutism, and virilism associated with combined androgen-estrogen hormone replacement therapy, Obstet Gynecol 77:595, 1991.

307. **Korenman SG,** The endocrinology of breast cancer, Cancer 46:874, 1980.

308. **Korenman SG,** Estrogen window hypothesis of the etiology of breast cancer, Lancet 1:700, 1980.

309. **Coulam CB, Annegers JF, Kranz JS,** Chronic anovulation syndrome and associated neoplasia Obstet Gynecol 61:403, 1983.

310. **Cowan LD, Gordis L, Tonascia JA, Jones GS,** Breast cancer incidence in women with a history of progesterone deficiency, Am J Epidemiol 114:209, 1981.

311. **Ron E, Lunenfeld B, Menczer J, Blumstein T, Katz L, Oelsner G, et al,** Cancer incidence in a cohort of infertile women, Am J Epidemiol 125:780, 1987.

312. **Gammon MD, Thompson WD,** Infertility and breast cancer: a population-based case-control study, Am J Epidemiol 132:708, 1990.

313. **Gammon MD, Thompson WD,** Polycystic ovaries and the risk of breast cancer, Am J Epidemiol 134:818, 1991.

314. **Key TJA, Pike MC,** The role of oestrogens and progestogens in the epidemiology and prevention of breast cancer, Eur J Cancer Clin Oncol 24:29, 1988.

315. **Henderson BE, Ross RK, Judd HL, Krailo MD, Pike MC,** Do regular ovualtory cycles increase breast cancer risk? Cancer 56:1206, 1985.

316. **Anderson TJ, Ferguson DJP, Raab GM,** Cell turnover in the "resting" human breast: influence of parity, contraceptive pill, age and laterality, Br J Cancer 46:376, 1982.

317. **Gompel A, Malet C, Spritzer P, Lalardrie J-P, Kuttenn F, Mauvais-Jarvis P,** Progestin effect on cell proliferation and 17β-hydroxysteroid dehydrogenase activity in normal human breast cells in culture, J Clin Endocrinol Metab 63:1174, 1986.

318. **Clarke CL, Sutherland RL,** Progestin regulation of cellular proliferation, Endocrin Rev 11:266, 1990.

319. **Zemlickis D, Lishner M, Degendorfer P, Panzarella T, Burke B, Sutcliffe SB, Koren G,** Maternal and fetal outcome after breast cancer in pregnancy, Am J Obstet Gynecol 166:781, 1992.

320. **Nugent P, O'Connell TX,** Breast cancer and pregnancy, Arch Surg 120:1221, 1985.

321. **Ribeiro G, Jones DA, Jones M,** Carcinoma of the breast associated with pregnancy, Br J Surg 73:607, 1986.

322. **WHO Collaborative Study of Neoplasia and Steroid Contraceptives,** Breast cancer and depot-medroxyprogesterone acetate: a multinational study, Lancet 338:833, 1991.

323. **Lee NC, Rosero-Bixby L, Oberle MW, Grimaldo C, Whatley AS, Rovira EZ,** A case-control study of breast cancer and hormonal contraception in Costa Rica, J Natl Ca Inst 79:1247, 1987.

324. **Paul C, Skegg DCG, Spears GFS,** Depot medroxyprogesterone (Depo-Provera) and risk of breast cancer, Br Med J 299:7591, 1989.

325. **Spicer D, Pike MC, Henderson BE,** The question of estrogen replacement therapy in patients with a prior diagnosis of breast cancer, Oncology 4:49, 1990.

326. **Stoll BA, Parbhoo S,** Treatment of menopausal symptoms in breast cancer patients, Lancet 1:1278, 1988.

327. **Wile AG, Opfell RW, Margileth DA,** Hormone replacement therapy in previously treated breast cancer patients, Am J Surg 165:372, 1993.

328. **McGuire WL, Clark GM,** Prognostic factors and treatment decisions in axillary-node-negative breast cancer, New Engl J Med 326:1756, 1992.

329. **Henderson IC,** Breast cancer therapy — The price of success, New Engl J Med 326:1774, 1992.

330. **Love RR, Mazess RB, Tormey DC, et al,** Bone mineral density in women with breast cancer treated with adjuvant tamoxifen for at least two years, Breast Cancer Res Treat 12:297, 1988.

331. **Fornander T, Rutquist LE, Sjoberg HE, Blomqvist L, Mattsson A, Glas U,** Long-term adjuvant tamoxifen in early breast cancer: effect on bone mineral density in postmenopausal women, J Clin Oncol 8:1019, 1990.

332. **Turken S, Siris E, Seldin D, Flaster E, Hyman G, Lindsay R,** Effects of tamoxifen on spinal bone density in women with breast cancer, J Natl Ca Inst 81:1086, 1989.

333. **Love RR, Mazess RB, Barden HS, Epstein S, Newcomb PA, Jordan VC, Carbone PP, DeMets DL,** Effects of tamoxifen on bone mineral density in postmenopausal women with breast cancer, New Engl J Med 326:852, 1992.

334. **Wolter J, Ryan WG, Subbiah JD,** Apparent beneficial effects of tamoxifen on serum lipoprotein subfractions and bone mineral content in patients with breast cancer, Proc Am Soc Clin Oncol 7:10, 1988.

335. **Bertellie G, Pronzato P, Amoroso D, et al,** Adjuvant tamoxifen in primary breast cancer: influence on plasma lipids and antithrombin III levels, Breast Cancer Res Treat 52:339, 1988.

336. **Love RR. Newcombe PA, Wiebe DA, Surawicz TS, Jordan VC, Carbone PP, DeMets DL,** Effects of tamoxifen therapy on lipid and lipoprotein levels in postmenopausal patients with node-negative breast cancer, J Natl Ca Inst 82:1327, 1990.

337. **Bagdade JD, Wolter J, Subbaiah PV, Ryan W,** Effects of tamoxifen treatment on plasma lipids and lipoprotein composition, J Clin Endocrinol Metab 70:1132, 1990.

338. **Dewar JA, Horobin JM, Preece PE, Tavendale R, Tunstall-Pedoe H, Wood RAB,** Longterm effects of tamoxifen on blood lipid values in breast cancer, Br Med J 305:225, 1992.

339. **McDonald CC, Stewart HG,** Fatal myocardial infarction in the Scottish adjuvant tamoxifen trial, Br Med J 303:435, 1991.

340. **Rigg LA, Hermann H, Yen SSC,** Absorption of estrogens from vaginal creams, New Engl J Med 298:195, 1978.

341. **Nilsson K, Heimer G,** Low-dose oestradiol in the treatment of urogenital oestrogen deficiency — a pharmacokinetic and pharmacodynamic study, Maturitas 15:121, 1992.

342. **Sullivan JM, Vander Zwaag R, Hughes JP, Maddock V, Kroetz FW, Ramanathan KB, Mirvis DM,** Estrogen replacement and coronary artery disease: effect on survival in postmenopausal women, Arch Intern Med 150:2557, 1990.

343. **Chute CG, Willett WC, Colditz GA, Stampfer MJ, Rosner B, Speizer FE,** A prospective study of reproductive history and exogenous estrogens on the risk of colorectal cancer in women, Epidemiology 2:201, 1991.

344. **Steiger MJ, Quinn NP,** Hormone replacement therapy induced chorea, Br Med J 302:762, 1991.

345. **Thomas JM,** Hormone-replacement therapy and pulmonary leiomyomatosis, New Engl J Med 327:1956, 1992 (letter).

346. **Melis GB, Bambacciani M , Cagnacci A, Paoletti AM, Mais V, Fioretti P,** Effects of the dopamine antagonist veralipride on hot flushes and luteinizing horomone secretion in postmenopausal women, Obstet Gynecol 72:688, 1988.

347. **David A, Don R, Tajchner G, Weissglas L,** Veralipride: alternative antidopaminergic treatment for menopausal symptoms, Am J Obstet Gynecol 158:1107, 1988.

348. **Lobo RA, McCormick W, Singer F., Roy S,** Depo-medroxyprogesterone acetate compared with conjugated estrogens for the treatment of postmenopausal women, Am J Obstet Gynecol 63:105, 1984.

349. **Nagamani M, Kelver ME, Smith ER,** Treatment of menopausal hot flushes with transdermal administration of clonidine, Am J Obstet Gynecol 156:561, 1987.

19 Obesity

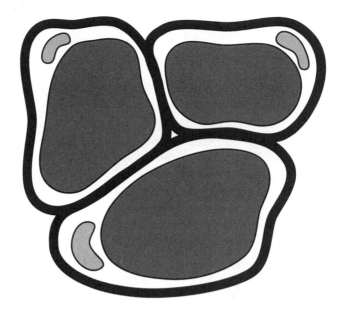

Because at least 20% of American adults (20–30% of women) older than 30 years old are more than 20% overweight, the unrewarding fight against obesity is all too common, not only with our patients but also with ourselves. Unfortunately, for over 100 years the incidence of obesity has been increasing in the United States, a reflection of an increasingly sedentary life in an affluent society.[1]

The lack of success in treating obesity is not due to an unawareness of the implications of obesity; there is a clear-cut relationship between mortality and weight.[2] The death rate from diabetes mellitus, for example, is approximately 4 times higher among obese diabetics than among those who control their weight. Also higher among obese individuals is the incidence of gallbladder disease, cardiovascular disease, renal disease, and cirrhosis of the liver. The death rate from appendicitis is double, presumably from anesthetic and surgical complications. Even the rate of accidents is higher, perhaps because fat people are awkward or because their view of the ground or floor is obstructed. Being overweight in adolescence is a more powerful predictor of cardiovascular adverse health effects than being overweight as an adult.[3] The incidence of heart disease, noninsulin dependent diabetes mellitus, gout, colorectal cancer, and arthritis is elevated in overweight people. When the personal and social problems encountered by obese persons are also considered, it is no wonder that a physician without a weight problem cannot comprehend why fat individuals remain overweight.

The frequency with which a practitioner encounters the obese patient whose weight does not decrease despite a sworn adherence to a limited-calorie diet makes one question if there is something physiologically different about this patient. Is the problem due to lack of discipline and cheating on a diet, or does it also involve a pathophysiologic factor? Is the physiology of obese people unusual, or are they simply gluttons?

Definition of Obesity

Obesity is an excess storage of triglycerides in adipose cells. There is a difference between obesity and overweight.[4] Obesity is an excess of body fat. Overweight is a body weight in excess of some standard or ideal weight. The ideal weight for any adult is believed to correspond to his or her ideal weight from age 20 to 30. The following formulas give ideal weight in pounds:

Women: **100 + (4 x (height in inches minus 60))**
Men: **120 + (4 x (height in inches minus 60))**

At a weight close to ideal weight, individuals may be overweight, but not over fat. This is especially true of individuals engaged in regular exercise. An estimate of body fat, therefore, rather than a measurement of height and weight is significant.

The most accurate method of determining body fat is to determine the density of the body by underwater measurement. It certainly is not practical to measure density by submerging individuals in water in our offices; therefore skinfold measurements with calipers have become popular as an index of body fat. The skinfold measurement is also not necessary for clinical practice. It is far simpler to utilize the body mass index nomogram, a method which has been found to correspond closely to densitometry measurements.[5]

The body mass index (the Quetelet index) is the ratio of weight divided by the height squared (in metric units):

Quetelet Index = kilograms/meters^2

To use the nomogram for body mass index, read the central scale by aligning a straight edge between height and body weight. The average adult has a body mass index of 25. A body mass index of 28 or more warrants treatment. A body mass index of about 30 is roughly equivalent to 30% excess body weight, the point at which excess mortality begins (approximately 10–12% of people in the U.S. have a body mass index of 30 or greater). Above 40, the risk from obesity itself is comparable to that associated with major health problems such as hypertension and heavy smoking.

A person is obese when the amount of adipose tissue is sufficiently high (20% or more over ideal weight) to detrimentally alter biochemical and physiologic functions and to shorten life expectancy. Obesity is associated with four major risk factors for atherosclerosis: hypertension, diabetes, hypercholesterolemia, and hypertriglyceridemia. Overweight individuals have a higher prevalence of hypertension at every age, and the risk of developing hypertension is related to the amount of weight gain after age 25.[6] The two in combination (hypertension and obesity) increase the risk of heart disease, cerebrovascular disease, and death.

It is well recognized that women have a greater prevalence of obesity compared to men. One reason may be the fact that women have a lower metabolic rate than men, even when adjusted for differences in body composition and level of activity.[7] Another reason that more women gain weight with age is the postmenopausal loss of the increase in metabolic rate that is associated with the luteal phase of the menstrual cycle.[7] The difference between men and women is even greater in older age. Unfortunately the basal metabolic rate decreases with age. After age 18, the resting metabolic rate declines about 2% per decade. A 30-year-old individual will inevitably gain weight if there is no change in caloric intake or exercise level over the years. The middle-age spread is both a biologic and a psychosociologic phenomenon. It is therefore important for both our patients and ourselves to understand adipose tissue and the problem of obesity.

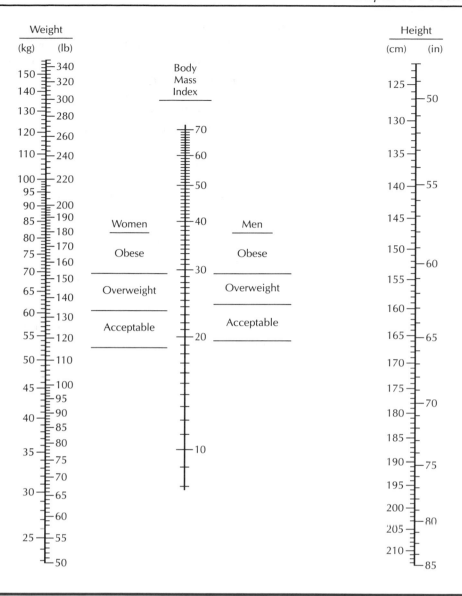

Physiology of Adipose Tissue

Adipose tissue serves three general functions:

1. Adipose tissue is a storehouse of energy.

2. Fat serves as a cushion from trauma.

3. Adipose tissue plays a role in the regulation of body heat.

Each cell of adipose tissue can be regarded as a package of triglyceride, the most concentrated form of stored energy. There are 8 calories per gram of triglyceride as opposed to 1 calorie per gram of glycogen. The total store of tissue and fluid carbohydrate in adults (about 300 calories) is inadequate to meet between-meal demands. The storage of energy in fat tissue allows us to do other things beside eating. Our energy balance, therefore, is essentially equivalent to our fat balance. Thus, obesity is a consequence of the fat imbalance inherent in high-fat diets.

The mechanism for mobilizing energy from fat involves various enzymes and neurohormonal agents. Following ingestion of fat and its breakdown by gastric and pancreatic lipases, absorption of long-chain triglycerides and free fatty acids takes place in the small bowel. Chylomicrons (microscopic particles of fat) transferred through lymph channels into the systemic venous circulation are normally removed by hepatic paren-chymal cells where a new lipoprotein is released into the circulation. When this lipoprotein is exposed to adipose tissue, lipolysis takes place through the action of lipoprotein lipase, an enzyme derived from the fat cells themselves. The fatty acids that are released then enter the fat cells where they are reesterified with glycerophosphate into triglycerides. Because alcohol diverts fat from oxidation to storage, body weight is directly correlated with the level of alcohol consumption.[8]

Glucose serves three important functions:

1.   Glucose supplies carbon atoms in the form of acetyl coenzyme A (acetyl CoA).

2.   Glucose provides hydrogen for reductive steps.

3.   Glucose is the main source of glycerophosphate.

The production and availability of glycerophosphate (required for reesterification of fatty acids and their storage as triglycerides) are considered rate-limiting in lipogenesis, and this process depends on the presence of glucose.

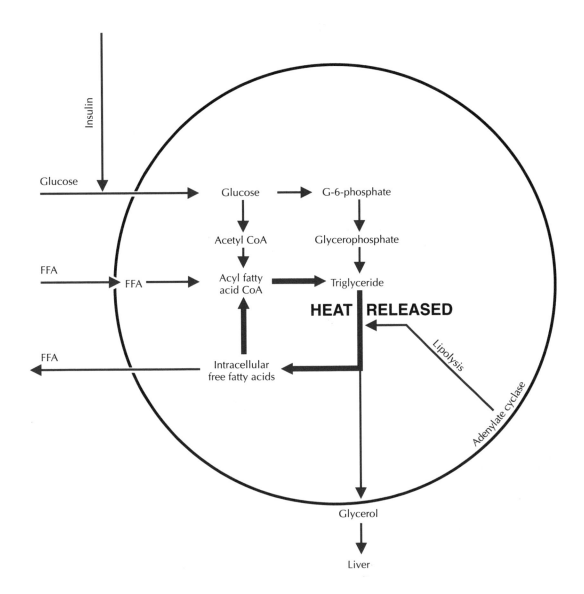

After esterification, subsequent lipolysis results in the release of fatty acids and glycerol. In the cycle of lipolysis and reesterification, energy is freed as heat. A low variable level of lipolysis takes place continuously; its basic function may be to provide body heat.

The chief metabolic products produced from fat are the circulating free fatty acids. Their availability is controlled by adipose tissue cells. When carbohydrate is in short supply, a flood of free fatty acids can be released. The free fatty acids in the peripheral circulation are almost wholly derived from endogenous triglyceride that undergoes rapid hydrolysis to yield free fatty acid and glycerol. The glycerol is returned to the liver for resynthesis of glycogen.

Free fatty acid release from adipose tissue is stimulated by physical exercise, fasting, exposure to cold, nervous tension, and anxiety. The release of fatty acids by lipolysis varies from one anatomic site to another. Omental, mesenteric, and subcutaneous fat are more labile and easily mobilized than fat from other sources. Areas from which energy is not easily mobilized are retrobulbar and perirenal fat where the tissue serves a structural function. Adipose tissue lipase is sensitive to stimulation by both epinephrine and norepinephrine. Other hormones that activate lipase are ACTH, thyroid-stimulating hormone (TSH), growth hormone, thyroxine (T_4), 3,5,3'-triiodothyronine (T_3), cortisol, glucagon, as well as vasopressin and human placental lactogen (HPL).

Lipase enzyme activity is inhibited by insulin, which appears to be alone as the major physiologic antagonist to the array of stimulating agents. When both glucose and insulin are abundant, transport of glucose into fat cells is high, and glycerophosphate production increases to esterify fatty acids.

The carbohydrate and fat composition of the fuel supply is constantly changing, depending upon stresses and demands. Since the central nervous system and some other tissues can utilize only glucose for energy, a homeostatic mechanism for conserving carbohydrate is essential. When glucose is abundant and easily available, it is utilized in adipose tissue for producing glycerophosphate to immobilize fatty acids as triglycerides. The circulating level of free fatty acids in muscle will, therefore, be low, and glucose will be used by all of the tissues.

Glucose abundant

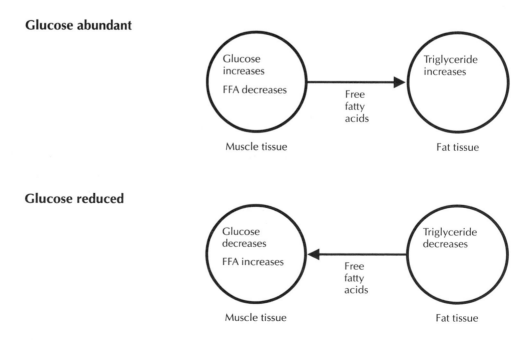

Glucose reduced

When carbohydrate is scarce, the amount of glucose reaching the fat cells declines and glycerophosphate production is reduced. The fat cell releases fatty acids, and their circulating levels rise to a point where glycolysis is inhibited. Thus, carbohydrate is spared in those tissues capable of using lipid substrates. If the rise of fatty acids is great enough, the liver is flooded with acetyl CoA. This is converted into ketone bodies, and clinical ketosis results.

In the simplest terms, when a person eats, glucose is available, insulin is secreted, and fat is stored. In starvation, the glucose level falls, insulin secretion decreases, and fat is mobilized.

If only single large meals are consumed, the body learns to convert carbohydrate to fat very quickly. Epidemiologic studies on school children demonstrate a positive correlation between fewer meals and a greater tendency toward obesity.[9] The person who does not eat all day and then stocks up at night is perhaps doing the worst possible thing.

Clinical Obesity

Obesity and the Brain

The hypothalamic location of the appetite center was established in 1940 by the demonstration that bilateral lesions of the ventromedial nucleus produce experimental obesity in rats. Such lesions lead to hyperphagia and decreased physical activity. Interestingly, this pattern is similar to that seen in human beings — the pressure to eat is reinforced by the desire to be physically inactive. The ventromedial nucleus was thought to represent an integrating center for appetite and hunger information. Destruction of the ventromedial nucleus was believed to result in a loss of satiety signals, leading to hyperphagia.

Overeating and obesity, however, may not be due to ventromedial nucleus damage but rather to destruction of the nearby ventral noradrenergic bundle.[10] Hypothalamic noradrenergic terminals are derived from long fibers ascending from hindbrain cell bodies. Lesions of the ventromedial nucleus produced by radiofrequency current fail to cause obesity. These lesions lead to overeating and obesity only when they extend beyond the ventromedial nucleus. Selective destruction of the ventral noradrenergic bundle results in hyperphagia. The lesions that produce hyperphagia also reduce the potency of amphetamine as an appetite suppressant. This noradrenergic bundle may function as a satiety system and be the site of amphetamine action. A sudden onset of hyperphagia can be due to a hypothalamic lesion. Possible causes include tumors, trauma, inflammatory processes, and aneurysms.

Signals arriving at these centers originate in peripheral tissues. Opiates, substance P, and cholecystokinin play a role in mediating taste, the gatekeeper for feeding, while peptides released from the stomach and intestine act as satiety signals.[11] Neuropeptides that inhibit appetite include corticotropin releasing hormone, neurotensin, and cyclo(HisPro), a peptide derived by proteolysis of thyrotropin releasing hormone.[12] The concentrations of cyclo(HisPro) rise and fall in the hypothalamus in response to fasting and eating.

Neuropeptide Y acts within the hypothalamus and stimulates feeding.[13] Because neuropeptide Y cell bodies are located in the arcuate nucleus (the primary location of gonadotropin releasing hormone neurons) and neuropeptide Y affects GnRH secretion, this peptide may be a link between appetite and reproductive function. Growth hormone releasing hormone, the primary stimulating signal for growth hormone secretion, is influenced by metabolic regulation and also may affect feeding behavior through its hormonal activities throughout the body. These peptides may be involved in aberrant appetite regulation.

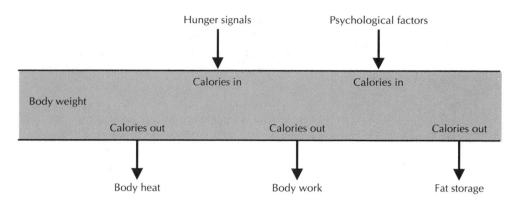

There may be two kinds of obesity: obesity stemming from a central nervous system (CNS) regulatory defect, or obesity due to a metabolic problem occurring despite a normal central mechanism.

Psychologic Factors

Obese and lean people respond differently to their environments. Obese people appear to regulate their desire for food through external signals. Lean people, on the other hand, regulate their intake by endogenous signals of hunger and satiety.

Fear does not inhibit gastrointestinal activity and dull the appetite in obese persons as it does in others. Fat people eat because it is mealtime, and food looks, smells, and tastes good. They also eat because other people are eating but not necessarily because they themselves are hungry.

Obese people are also less physically active than are people of normal weight. The obese person will drive a car around the block repeatedly until a parking space is available, rather than walk a few blocks. Time-lapse photography studies show that obese people when in a swimming pool spend most of their time floating; lean people move around actively.[14] An obese baby is more willing than is a normal baby to take formula after it has been sweetened, but will take less formula, even though it is sweetened if the work of eating is increased by a nipple with a smaller hole.

There may be two classes of obesity: one class may include those individuals who clearly eat too much. The other class would be composed of individuals who eat relatively normal diets but who are extremely inactive.

Fat Cells

Fat cells develop from connective tissue early in fetal life. An important question is whether new fat cells are produced by metaplasia in the adult, or whether an individual achieves a total complement during a certain period of life. In other words is excess fat stored by increasing the size of the fat cell, or by increasing the number of cells? The possibility arises that there is an increase in the total number of fat cells, which just wait to be packed full of storage fat. Furthermore, the total number of fat cells may depend upon an infant's nutritional state during the neonatal period and perhaps in utero as well.

Studies of fat obtained at surgery indicate that the mean fat cell volume is increased 3-fold in obese people, but an increase in the number of fat cells is seen only in the grossly obese. When patients diet, the fat cells decrease in size but not in number. Hypercellular obesity may be a more difficult problem to overcome, since an individual may be saddled with a permanent increase in fat cells.

Some researchers think that, at some period in a person's life, a fixed number of fat cells is obtained. Adolescence, infancy, and intrauterine life seem particularly critical.[15,16]

This premise is not solidly established, because there is no certain way to identify an empty fat cell, and potential fat cells cannot be recognized. Nevertheless, a hyperplastic type of obesity (more fat cells) may be associated with childhood and have a poor prognosis; a hypertrophic type (enlarged fat cells) that is responsive to dieting may occur in adults.

There certainly appears to be a genetic component. The weights of adopted children in Denmark correlated with the body weights of their biologic parents but not with their adoptive parents.[17] This would suggest that the genetic influence is even more important in childhood than environmental factors. Other work suggests that the familial occurrence of obesity can be attributed in part to a genetically related reduced rate of energy expenditure.[18] In studies of identical and fraternal twins reared apart, approximately 70% of the variance in the body mass index could be assigned to genetic influences and the remaining 30% to environmental effects.[19]

Some argue that each individual has a setpoint, a level regulated by signals between the fat cells and the brain. According to this argument, previously obese people who have successfully lost weight have to maintain themselves in a state of starvation (at least as far as their fat cells are concerned).

Genetics and biochemistry are against many obese people. It is best to recognize that an obese individual who has suffered with the problem lifelong does have a disorder, a disorder which is not well understood. However, for each individual, the extent to which the genetic predisposition is expressed depends upon environmental influences. The prevalence of obesity is inversely related to the level of physical activity and education and directly related to parity.[20] Thus, socioeconomic and behavioral factors are important determinants of body weight, and surely each individual will reflect varying impacts of genetics and environment.

Endocrine Changes

The most important endocrine change in obesity is elevation of the basal blood insulin level. Increases in body fat change the body's secretion and sensitivity to insulin. There is a decrease in the number of insulin receptor sites at a cellular level, most significantly in fat, liver, and muscle tissue. The key factors which affect insulin resistance are the amount of fat tissue in the body, the caloric intake per day, the amount of carbohydrates in the diet, and the amount of daily exercise. At least one mechanism for the increased resistance to insulin observed with increasing weight is down-regulation of insulin receptors brought about by the increase in insulin secretion. The increase in insulin resistance affects the metabolism of carbohydrate, fat and protein. Circulating levels of free fatty acids increase as a result of inadequate insulin suppression of the fat cell. Insulin resistance results in decreased catabolism of triglycerides, yielding a decrease in HDL-cholesterol and an increase in LDL-cholesterol. This, of course, is a major mechanism for the development of atherosclerosis. Hyperinsulinemia is also directly associated with hypertension. The hyperinsulinemia associated with obesity is reversible with weight loss.

The simplest way to assess insulin resistance is to measure the ratio of fasting glucose to fasting insulin. A ratio lower than 3.0 is characteristic of obesity. This method has limitations, the most notable being the variation due to assay precision and pulsatile secretion of insulin. However, if a patient is obese, one can assume the patient is insulin resistant.

Genetics plays a greater role in the development of maturity onset diabetes than juvenile onset.[21] It is impossible to predict exactly who eventually will develop diabetes because the tendency is recessive and it will not develop in every generation in a family. But weight is a good tip-off. As weight increases, the frequency of occurrence of diabetes increases. Both gestational diabetes and insulin-dependent diabetes are more common in overweight pregnant patients.

Contrary to popular misconception, hypothyroidism does not cause obesity. Weight gain due to hypothyroidism is confined to the fluid accumulation of myxedema. There is no place, therefore, for thyroid hormone administration in the treatment of obesity when the patient is euthyroid.

Obese people are relatively unable to excrete both salt and water, especially while dieting. During dieting this seems to be mediated by increased output of aldosterone and vasopressin. Since water produced from fat outweighs the fat, people on diets often show little initial weight loss. The early use of a diuretic may encourage a patient to persist with dieting.

The basic question is whether metabolic changes observed in obesity represent adaptive responses to a markedly enlarged fat organ or whether they are representative of a metabolic or hormonal defect. The former is true. These changes are secondary responses; they are totally reversible with weight loss. Four-year follow-up in a group of patients who did not regain their weight after dieting revealed persistently normal insulin and glucose responses; patients who regained their weight showed further deterioration in these metabolic factors.[22]

Anatomic Obesity

Gynoid obesity (the pear shape) refers to fat distribution in the lower body (femoral and gluteal regions), while android obesity (the apple shape) refers to central body distribution. Gynoid fat is more resistant to catecholamines and more sensitive to insulin than abdominal fat; thus extraction and storage of fatty acids easily occur, and fat is accumulated more readily in the thighs and buttocks. This fat is associated with minimal fatty acid flux, and therefore the negative consequences of fatty acid metabolism are less. Gynoid fat is principally stored fat. The clinical meaning of all this is that women with gynoid obesity are less likely than women with android obesity to develop diabetes mellitus and coronary heart disease.[23]

During pregnancy, lipoprotein lipase activity increases in gynoid fat, further promoting fat storage and explaining the tendency for women to gain thigh and hip weight during pregnancy. Also because this fat is more resistant to mobilization, it is harder to get rid of. This difficulty is related to the adrenergic receptor concentration in the fat cells, the regulation of which remains a mystery.

Android obesity refers to fat located in the abdominal wall and visceral-mesenteric locations. This fat is more sensitive to catecholamines and less sensitive to insulin and thus more active metabolically. It more easily delivers triglyceride to other tissues to meet energy requirements. This fat distribution is associated with hyperinsulinemia, impaired glucose tolerance, diabetes mellitus, an increase in androgen production rates, decreased levels of sex hormone binding globulin, and increased levels of free testosterone and estradiol.[24,25] In addition, women with central obesity have greater adrenal activity with increases in ACTH and cortisol secretion.[26]

It is central body obesity that is associated with cardiovascular risk factors, including hypertension and adverse cholesterol-lipoprotein profiles.[27] The waist:hip ratio is the variable most strongly and inversely associated with the level of HDL_2, the fraction of HDL-cholesterol most consistently linked with protection from cardiovascular disease.[28] The adverse impact of excess weight in adolescence can be explained by the fact that deposition of fat in adolescence is largely central in location.[3,29] Weight loss in women with lower body obesity is mainly cosmetic, whereas loss of central body weight is more important for general health in that an improvement in cardiovascular risk is associated with loss of central body fat.

The waist:hip ratio is a means of estimating the degree of upper to lower body obesity; the ratio accurately predicts the amount of intra-abdominal fat (which is greater with android obesity).[30,31] The waist measurement is measured as the smallest circumference (girth) between the rib cage and iliac crests. The hip measurement is the largest circumference between the waist and thighs. Interpretation is as follows:

Greater than 0.85 — **Android Obesity**
Less than 0.75 — **Gynoid Obesity**

Management of Obesity

Aside from not smoking cigarettes, weight reduction is the most important health measure available for reducing the risk of cardiovascular disease.[32] After adjusting for age and smoking, the Nurses' Health Study documented a 3-fold increase in risk for coronary disease among women with a body mass index of 29 or greater.[33] Even women who are mildly or moderately overweight have a substantial increase in coronary risk. In the Nurses' Health Study, 40% of coronary events could be attributed to excessive body weight, and in the heaviest women, 70%.

For most patients, after a routine evaluation to rule out pathology such as diabetes mellitus, the physician is left with the frustrating task of prescribing a diet. But it is not enough to just prescribe a diet or prescribe an anorectic drug. An effective weight loss program requires commitment from both patient and physician.

Physician and patient should agree on the goal of a diet program. While the physician may wish the patient to reach ideal weight, the patient may be satisfied with less. Motivation is improved when the goals meet both personal and medical objectives. It is realistic to lose 4–5 pounds in the first month and 20–30 pounds in 4–5 months. To achieve a respectable rate of weight loss, intake must be 500–1,000 calories below energy expenditure.[34] But as weight is lost, energy requirements decrease; therefore unless energy intake decreases, the rate of weight loss will slow.

Despite various fads and diet books, the best diet continues to be a limitation of calories to between 900 and 1200 calories per day, the actual amount depending on what the individual patient will accept and pursue. When energy intake is less than this, it is very difficult to obtain the recommended levels of vitamins and minerals.

Ideal Diet: Carbohydrates —   50%
              Protein   —   15–20%
              Fat   —   <30%

The discouraging aspect is that to lose a pound of fat, the equivalent to a 3,500 calorie intake must be expended. Dieting has to be slow and steady to be effective. Successful programs include behavior modification, frequent visits to the physician, and involvement of family members. Behavior modification starts with daily recording of activity and behavior related to food intake, followed by the elimination of inappropriate cues (other than hunger) that lead to eating.

Careful studies (performed in hospitalized subjects on metabolic wards) have indicated that the carbohydrate and fat composition of the diet has no effect on the rate of weight loss.[35] Restriction of calories remains the important principle, recognizing that reduction in fat intake is the most effective method of weight loss. Substituting one of the liquid formulas for meals has been successful in many individuals. Unbalanced formulations, however, have the same side effects as seen with total starvation (carbohydrate-deprived regimens). Adequate carbohydrate is necessary for utilization of amino acids. In addition, electrolyte problems have been encountered, and there is an initial diuretic phase that can lead to postural hypotension.

The protein sparing modified fast is a ketogenic regimen providing approximately 800 calories per day. Unsupplemented liquid protein diets have been associated with deaths due to cardiac arrhythmias. The low-calorie diets which utilize protein and carbohydrate supplemented with minerals and vitamins as the sole source of nutrition are safer but should be used only for severe obesity and under medical supervision.[36] These diets are still potentially dangerous. The other disadvantage to the semistarvation diet is that short-term success does not guarantee long-term weight maintenance. It is reported that at best only one-fourth to one-third of individuals who lose weight by a semistarvation ketogenic regimen plus behavior modification therapy will have significant long-term weight reduction.[37] On the other hand, for that one-fourth to one-third, this represents a major accomplishment and is worth doing. Unfortunately, repeated dieting and recidivism have a negative impact. With each episode, the body learns to become more efficient, so that with each diet, weight comes off more slowly and is regained more rapidly.

It is not unusual to encounter patients who claim to be unable to lose weight despite following a diet with less than 1200 calories per day. In a study of such patients, it was discovered that underreporting of actual food intake and overreporting of physical activity are both common.[38] While it may not be true for all patients, certainly some individuals do eat more than they think and exercise less than they report to their physicians. This is not a deliberate conscious attempt to deceive the physician. These patients truly believe their resistance to weight loss is genetic and not due to their own personal behavior. They are astonished and distressed to learn the results of accurate recording of dietary intake and physical exercise. The use of a dietitian to record a typical week's worth of eating and exercise is worthwhile. This kind of knowledge proves to be a powerful lever in providing the motivation to make the changes in lifestyle that can yield loss of weight.

As an index of the general lack of success with diets, a summary of 10 studies (approximately 1200 patients) revealed that only 30% lose 20 pounds or more, and only 4% lose 40 pounds or more.[39] Commercial organizations are no more successful than physician-directed programs or nonprofit self-help groups.[40] Thus, it is obvious why gimmicks abound in this area of patient management.

Anorectics are useful as short-term therapy to control hunger, especially at the beginning of a diet and at a plateau or relapse stage. Compared to amphetamines, there is less abuse associated with the catecholamine congeners that are serotonin agonists (diethylpropion, fenfluramine, methamphetamine, and phentermine). Other non-amphetamine anorectics are phendimetrazine and mazindol. All of these agents act on the central nervous system to depress appetite. The most widely used anorectic is fenfluramine (fluoxetine, 15 mg bid).[41]

Over-the-counter products contain phenylpropanolamine as the active ingredient. This drug is a sympathomimetic derived from ephedrine and can act synergistically with caffeine to produce amphetamine-like reactions. ***It should be noted that phenylpropanolamine taken in combination with bromocriptine or a monoamine oxidase inhibitor can precipitate a hypertensive crisis.***

Surgical treatment and starvation should be reserved for patients who are morbidly obese. Both methods involve many potential problems and require close monitoring.

Controlled studies have not demonstrated the effectiveness of thyroid preparations or human chorionic gonadotropin.[42] Indeed, adding thyroid hormone increases the loss of lean body mass rather than fat tissue. It is clear that adjunctive drug measures are not successful unless the patient is also motivated either to limit caloric intake or to increase the exercise level in what will be a lifelong battle.

A regular pattern of physical exercise reduces the risk of myocardial infarction in all people.[43] Both weight loss and increased physical activity, through an unknown mechanism, lower the level of low density lipoprotein (LDL), and increase the level of high density lipoprotein (HDL).[44] A further benefit of strenuous or prolonged exercise is an inhibition of appetite that lasts many hours and that is associated with an increase in the resting metabolic rate for 2–48 hours. There is one study, however, that indicates a rebound increase in appetite 1–2 days after exercise.[45] The optimal program includes, therefore, a *daily* period of exercise. The best time for exercise is before meals or about 2 hours after eating. It is probably wise to take a day off at least once a week to give muscles and joints a rest.

Unfortunately one cannot burn up significant calories quickly; it takes 18 minutes of running to compensate for the average hamburger.[46]

Activity	Calories per Hour
Sleeping	90
Office work	240
Walking	240
Golf	300
Housework	300
Bicycling	360
Swimming	360
Tennis	480
Bowling	510
Running slowly	750 (ca. 120/mile)
Cross country skiing	840
Running fast	960 (ca. 160/mile)

Most frustrating is the problem of some patients who limit caloric intake yet do not lose weight. In fact, as the weights of certain patients increase, the number of calories required to remain in equilibrium decreases, probably due to a combination of reduced activity and a change in metabolism. The Vermont study demonstrated that the normal person with induced obesity requires 2,700 calories to remain in equilibrium; spontaneously obese patients require only about 1,300 calories.[47] Others argue that virtually everyone can lose weight on a diet of 1,000 calories per day in that the maintenance requirement for a sedentary adult is about 1.5 times the resting metabolic rate (about 1,000–1,500 calories per day).[48] The physician must be careful to avoid a condemning or punitive attitude and understand that it is possible to significantly restrict caloric intake and not lose weight.

Patients appear doomed to frustration and despair unless the physician can motivate them to increase physical activity. In all individuals dieting is more effective when combined with physical exercise, but this is especially true in chronically obese patients. In other words, the lifestyle of an obese person must be changed to overcome the desire to be inactive (walk instead of riding). Only by significantly increasing caloric expenditure will the input-output equilibrium be disturbed.

The obese person feels trapped. Obesity leads to characteristic behavioral manifestations, including passive personality, frequent periods of depression, decreased self-respect, and a sense of being hopelessly overwhelmed by problems. But just as the endocrine and metabolic changes are secondary to obesity, many of the psychosocial attributes surrounding obesity are also secondary.[49]

Maintenance of a newly gained lower weight requires constant preventive attention. Motivation to change and emotional support during the change are important. They can be provided by friends, relatives, physicians, or self-help organizations. If the vicious circle of failed diets, resignation to fate, guilt, and shame can be broken, a more effective, happier person will emerge.

References

1. **Harlan WR, Landis JR, Flegal KM, Davis CS, Miller ME,** Secular trends in body mass in the United States, 1960–1980, Am J Epidemiol 128:1065, 1988.

2. **Foster WR, Burton BT,** Health implications of obesity, Ann Intern Med 103:1024, 1985.

3. **Must A, Jacques PF, Dallal GE, Bajema CJ, Dietz WH,** Long-term morbidity and mortality of overweight adolescents: a follow-up of the Harvard Growth Study of 1922 to 1935, New Engl J Med 327:1350, 1992.

4. **Ravussin E, Swinburn BA,** Pathophysiology of obesity, Lancet 340:404, 1992.

5. **Thomas AE, McKay DA, Cutlip MB,** A nomograph method for assessing body weight, Am J Clin Nutr 29:302, 1976.

6. **Stamler R, Stamler J, Riedlinger WF, Algera G, Roberts RH,** Weight and blood pressure: findings in hypertension screening of 1 million Americans, JAMA 240:1607, 1978.

7. **Ferraro R, Lillioja S, Fontvieille A-M, Rising R, Bogardus C, Ravussin E,** Lower sedentary metabolic rate in women compared with men, J Clin Invest 90:780, 1992.

8. **Suter PM, Schutz Y, Jequier E,** The effect of ethanol on fat storage in healthy subjects, New Engl J Med 326:983, 1992.

9. **Fabry P, Hejda S, Cerny K,** Effects of meal frequency in school children. Changes in weight-height proportion and skinfold thickness, Am J Clin Nutr 18:358, 1966.

10. **Gold RM,** Hypothalamic obesity: the myth of the ventromedial nucleus, Science 182:488, 1973.

11. **Morley JE,** Neuropeptide regulation of appetite and weight, Endocrin Rev 8:256, 1987.

12. **Wilber JF,** Neuropeptides, appetite regulation, and human obesity, JAMA 266:257, 1991.

13. **Berelowitz M, Bruno JF, White JD,** Regulation of hypothalamic neuropeptide expression by peripheral metabolism, Trends Endocrinol Metab 3:127, 1992.

14. **Mayer J,** Inactivity as a major factor in adolescent obesity, Ann NY Acad Sci 131:502, 1965.

15. **Charney E, Goodman HC, McBride M, Lyon B, Pratt R,** Childhood antecedents of adult obesity, New Engl J Med 295:6, 1976.

16. **Garn SM, LaVelle M, Rosenberg KR, Hawthorne VM,** Maturational timing as a factor in female fatness and obesity, Am J Clin Nutr 43:879, 1986.

17. **Stunkard AJ, Sorensen TIA, Teasdale TW, Chakraborty R, Schull WJ, Schulsinger F,** An adoptive study of human obesity, New Engl J Med 314:193, 1986.

18. **Ravussin E, Lillioja S, Knowler WC, Christin L, Freymond D, Abbott WGH, Boyce V, Howard BV, Bogardus C,** Reduced rate of energy expenditure as a risk factor for body-weight gain, New Engl J Med 318:467, 1988.

19. **Stunkard AJ, Harris JR, Pederson NL, McClearn GE,** The body-mass index of twins who have been reared apart, New Engl J Med 322:1483, 1990.

20. **Rissanen AM, Heliovaara M, Knekt P, Reunanen A, Aromaa A,** Determinants of weight gain and overweight in adult Finns, Eur J Clin Nutr 45:419, 1991.

21. **Fanda OP, Soeldner SS,** Genetic, acquired, and related factors in the etiology of diabetes mellitus, Arch Intern Med 137:461, 1977.

22. **Hewing R, Liebermeister H, Daweke H, Gries FA, Gruneklee D,** Weight regain after low calorie diet: long term pattern of blood sugar, serum lipids, ketone bodies, and serum insulin levels, Diabetologia 9:197, 1973.

23. **Stern MP, Haffner SM,** Body fat distribution and hyperinsulinemia as risk factors for diabetes and cardiovascular disease, Arteriosclerosis 6:123, 1986.

24. **Peiris AN, Sothmann MS, Aiman EJ, Kissebah AH,** The relationship of insulin to sex hormone-binding globulin: role of adiposity, Fertil Steril 52:69, 1989.

25. **Kirschner MA, Samojlik E, Drejka M, Szmal E, Schneider G, Ertel N,** Androgen-estrogen metabolism in women with upper body *versus* lower body obesity, J Clin Endocrinol Metab 70:473, 1990.

26. **Pasquali R, Cantobelli S, Casimirri F, Capelli M, Bortoluzzi L, Flamia R, Labate AMM, Barbara L,** The hypothalamic-pituitary-adrenal axis in obese women with different patterns of body fat distribution, J Clin Endocrinol Metab 77:341, 1993.

27. **Lapidus L, Bengtsson C, Larsson B, Pennert K, Rybo E, Sjostrom L,** Distribution of adipose tissue and risk of cardiovascular disease and death: a 12 year follow up of participants in the population study of women in Gothenburg, Sweden, Br Med J 289:1257, 1984.

28. **Ostlund RE Jr, Staten M, Kohrt W, Schultz J, Malley M,** The ratio of waist-to-hip circumference, plasma insulin level, and glucose intolerance as independent predictors fo the HDL_2 cholesterol level in older adults, New Engl J Med 322:229, 1990.

29. **Deutsch MI, Mueller WH, Malina RM,** Androgyny in fat patterning is associated with obesity in adolescents and young adults, Ann Hum Biol 12:275, 1985.

30. **Ashwell M, Chinn S, Stalley S, Garrow JS,** Female fat distribution — a simple classification based on two circumference measurements, Int J Obesity 6:143, 1982.

31. **Ashwell M, Cole TJ, Dixon AK,** Obesity: new insight into the anthropometric classification of fat distribution shown by computed tomography, Br Med J 290:1692, 1985.

32. **Gordon T, Kannel WB,** Obesity and cardiovascular disease: the Framingham study, Clin Endocrinol Metab 5:367, 1976.

33. **Manson JE, Colditz GA, Stampfer MJ, Willett WC, Rosner B, Monson RR, Speizer FE, Hennekens CH,** A prospective study of obesity and risk of coronary heart disease in women, New Engl J Med 322:882, 1990.

34. **Garrow JS,** Treatment of obesity, Lancet 340:409, 1992.

35. **Gordon ES,** Metabolic aspects of obesity, Adv Metab Disord 4:229, 1970.

36. **Council on Scientific Affairs, AMA,** Treatment of obesity in adults, JAMA 260:2547, 1988.

37. **Wadden TA, Stunkard AJ, Brownell KD,** Very low calorie diets: their efficacy, safety, and future, Ann Intern Med 99:675, 1983.

38. **Lichtman SW, Pisarska K, Berman ER, Pestone M, Dowling H, Offenbacher E, Weisel H, Heshka S, Matthews DE, Heymsfield SB,** Discrepancy between self-reported and actual caloric intake and exercise in obese subjects, New Engl J Med 327:1893, 1992.

39. **Bray GA, Davidson MB, Drenick EJ,** Obesity: a serious symptom, Ann Intern Med 77:787, 1972.

40. **Volkmar FR, Stunkard AJ, Woolston J, Bailey RA,** High attrition rates in commercial weight reduction programs, Arch Intern Med 141:426, 1981.

41. **Darga LL, Carroll-Michals L, Borsford SJ, Lucas CP,** Fluoxetine's effect on weight loss in obese subjects, Am J Clin Nutr 54:321, 1991.

42. **Rivlin RS,** Drug therapy: therapy of obesity with hormones, New Engl J Med 292:26, 1975.

43. **Paffenbarger RS Jr, Wing AL, Hyde RT,** Physcial activity as an index of heart attack risk in college alumni, Am J Epidemiol 108:161, 1978.

44. **Weisweiler P,** Plasma lipoproteins and lipase and lecithin: cholesterol acyltransferase activities in obese subjects before and after weight reduction, J Clin Endocrinol Metab 65:969, 1987.

45. **Edholm OG, Fletcher JG, Widdowson EM, McCance RA,** The energy expenditure and food intake of individual men, Br J Nutr 9:286, 1955.

46. **Konishi F,** Food energy equivalents of various activities, J Am Diet Assoc 46:186, 1965.

47. **Sims EAH, Danforth E Jr, Horton ES, Bray GA, Glennon JA, Salans LB,** Endocrine and metabolic effects of experimental obesity in man, Recent Prog Horm Res 29:457, 1973.

48. **Welle SL, Amatruda JM, Forbes GB, Lockwood DH,** Resting metabolic rates of obese women after rapid weight loss, J Clin Endocrinol Metab 59:41, 1984.

49. **Solow C, Siberfarb PM, Swift K,** Psychosocial effects of intestinal bypass surgery for severe obesity, New Engl J Med 290:300, 1974.

20   Reproduction and the Thyroid

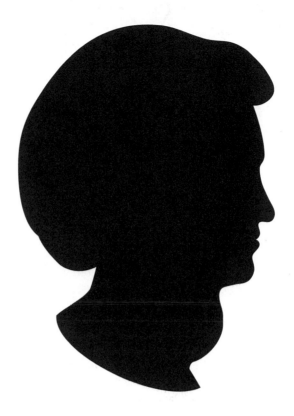

Thomas Wharton, in 1656, gave the thyroid gland its modern name (meaning oblong shield) because he believed the function of the thyroid was to fill vacant spaces and contribute to the shape and beauty of the neck, especially in women.[1] For unknown reasons, thyroid disease is more common in women than in men. Because most thyroid disease is autoimmune in nature, an increased susceptibility to autoimmune diseases, perhaps secondary to the female endocrine environment, is a likely contributing factor.

The objective is to detect and treat thyroid disease before the clinical signs are significant and intense. Subtle thyroid disease is easily diagnosed by the sensitive laboratory assessments now available. Therefore the key to early diagnosis is to maintain a high index of suspicion and to readily screen for the presence of abnormal thryoid function.

Normal Thyroid Physiology

Thyroid hormone synthesis depends in large part upon an adequate supply of iodine in the diet. In the small intestine iodine is absorbed as iodide that is then transported to the thyroid gland. Plasma iodide enters the thyroid under the influence of thyroid-stimulating hormone (TSH), the anterior pituitary thyrotropin hormone. Within the thyroid gland, iodide is oxidized to elemental iodine which is then bound to tyrosine. Mono-iodotyrosine and diiodotyrosine combine to form thyroxine (T_4) and triiodothyronine (T_3). These iodinated compounds are part of the thyroglobulin molecule, the colloid that serves as a storage depot for thyroid hormone. TSH induces a proteolytic process that results in the release of iodothyronines into the bloodstream as thyroid hormone.

$$T_4$$

$$T_3 \qquad\qquad\qquad Reverse\ T_3$$

Removal of one iodine from the phenolic ring of T_4 yields T_3, while removal of an iodine from the nonphenolic ring yields reverse T_3 (RT_3) which is biologically inactive. In a normal adult, about one-third of the T_4 secreted each day is converted in peripheral tissues, largely liver and kidney, to T_3, and about 40% is converted to the inactive, reverse T_3 (RT_3). About 80% of the T_3 generated is derived outside the thyroid gland, chiefly in the liver and kidney. T_3 is 3–5 times more potent than T_4, and virtually all the biologic activity of T_4 can be attributed to the T_3 generated from it. Although T_4 is secreted at 20 times the rate of T_3, it is T_3 which is responsible for most if not all the thyroid action in the body. T_3 is more potent than T_4 because the nuclear thyroid receptor has a ten-fold greater affinity for T_3 compared to T_4. While T_4 may have some intrinsic activity of its own, it serves mainly as a prohormone of T_3. It is hard to think of a body process or function that doesn't require thyroid hormone for its normal operation, not only metabolism but also development, steroidogenesis, and most specific tissue activities.

Carbohydrate calories appear to be the primary determinant of T_3 levels in adults. A reciprocal relationship exists between T_3 and RT_3. Low T_3 and elevated RT_3 are seen in a variety of illnesses such as febrile diseases, burn injuries, malnutrition, and anorexia nervosa. The metabolic rate is determined to a large degree by the relative production of T_3 and RT_3. During periods of stress, when a decrease in metabolic rate would conserve energy, the body produces more RT_3 and less T_3, and metabolism slows. Upon recovery, this process reverses and metabolic rate increases.

Circulating thyroid hormones are present in the circulation mainly bound to proteins. Approximately 75–80% of thyroid hormones are bound to thyroxine-binding globulin (TBG), which therefore, is the major determining factor in the total thyroid hormone concentration in the circulation. The remaining 20–25% is bound to thyroxine-binding prealbumin and albumin. The binding proteins have a greater affinity for T_4 and thus allow T_3 to have greater entry into cells. TBG is synthesized in the liver, and this synthesis is increased by estrogens.

The nuclear receptor for thyroid hormone is a member of the super family that includes the steroid hormone receptors (Chapter 2). The thyroid hormone receptor exists in several forms, the products of 2 genes located on different chromosomes. The α receptor is on chromosome 17, and the β receptor is on chromosome 3. The nuclear T_3 receptor is truly ubiquitous, indicating the widespread actions of thyroid hormone throughout the body. Mutations in the gene for the thyroid receptor lead to the synthesis of a receptor that actually antagonizes normal receptors, a syndrome of thyroid resistance characterized by elevated thyroid hormone levels. TSH is elevated as well because of the impairment in thyroid hormone action.

The thyroid axis is stimulated by the hypothalamic factor, thyrotropin releasing hormone (TRH) and inhibited by somatostatin and dopamine. Thyroid hormones regulate TSH by suppressing TRH secretion, but primarily affecting the pituitary sensitivity to TRH (by reducing the number of TRH receptors). Pituitary secretion of TSH is very sensitive to changes in the circulating levels of thyroid hormone; a slight change in the circulating level of T_4 will produce a many-fold greater response in TSH. TSH-secreting cells are regulated by T_4, but only after the T_4 is converted to T_3 in the pituitary cells. Although modulation of thyroid hormone occurs at the pituitary level, this function is permitted by the hypothalamic releasing hormone, TRH. Although some tissues depend mainly on the blood T_3 for their intracellular T_3, the brain and the pituitary depend on their own intracellular conversion of T_4. The measurement of T_4 and TSH, therefore, provides the most accurate assessment of thyroid function.

The TSH response to TRH is influenced mainly by the thyroid hormone concentration in the circulation; however, lesser effects are associated with dopamine agonists (inhibition), glucocorticoids (inhibition), and dopamine antagonists (stimulation). Estrogen increases the TRH receptor content of the pituitary; hence the TSH response to TRH is greater in women compared to men, and greater in women taking combined oral contraceptives.

TRH also stimulates prolactin secretion by the pituitary. The smallest doses of TRH that are capable of producing an increase in TSH, also increase prolactin levels, indicating a physiologic role for TRH in the control of prolactin secretion. However, except in hypothyroidism, normal physiologic changes as well as abnormal prolactin secretion can be understood in terms of dopaminergic inhibitory control, and TRH need not be considered.

Functional Changes with Aging

Thyroxine metabolism and clearance decrease in older people, and thyroxine secretion decreases in compensation to maintain normal serum thyroxine concentrations.[2] With aging, conversion of T_4 to T_3 decreases, and TSH levels increase. The TSH response to TRH is normal in older women. TBG concentrations decrease slightly in postmenopausal women but not enough to alter measurements in serum.

Thyroid Function Tests

Free Thyroxine (FT$_4$)

Assays are now available to measure free T_4. These are usually displacement assays using an antibody to T_4. The result is not affected by changes in TBG and binding. The free T_4 level has a different range of normal values from laboratory to laboratory.

Total Thyroxine (TT$_4$)

The total thyroxine, both the bound portion to TBG and the free unbound portion, is measured by displacement assays, and in the absence of hormone therapy or other illnesses, estimates the thyroxine concentration in the blood. However, the free thyroxine assay is now available and preferred.

Free Thyroxine Index (FTI or T7)

The free thyroxine index is calculated from the TT_4 and the T_3 resin uptake measurements. This test too has been replaced by the free T_4 assay.

Total T_3 and Reverse T_3

Both of these thyronines can be measured by sensitive immunoassays. However, in most clinical circumstances they add little to what is learned by the free T_4 and TSH measurements. The clinical situations where measurement will be useful will be discussed under the specific diseases and indicated on the algorithm.

Thyroid-Stimulating Hormone (TSH)

TSH can now be measured by highly sensitive assays utilizing monoclonal antibodies, usually in a technique that uses two antibodies, one directed at the α-subunit and one directed at the β-subunit of TSH. The normal levels vary from laboratory to laboratory. TSH is a very sensitive indicator of thyroid hormone action at the tissue level because it is dependent upon the pituitary exposure to T_4. In the absence of hypothalamic or pituitary disease, the sensitive TSH assays will provide the best indication of excess or deficient thyroxine; slight changes in T_4 are reflected in a many-fold greater response in TSH. Nearly all women with elevated TSH levels have hypothyroidism. Transient changes in TSH can be caused by systemic illnesses, major psychiatric disturbances, and pharmacologic treatment with glucocorticoid agents or dopamine.

Radioactive Iodine Uptake

Because the thyroid gland is the only tissue that utilizes iodine, radioisotopes of iodine can be used as a measure of thyroid gland activity and to localize activity within the gland.

The Laboratory Evaluation. The algorithm represents a cost-effective and accurate clinical strategy.[3] For screening purposes, or when there is a relatively low clinical suspicion of thyroid disease, the initial step is to measure the TSH by a sensitive assay. A normal TSH essentially excludes hypothyroidism or hyperthyroidism. A high TSH requires the measurement of free T_4 to confirm the diagnosis of hypothyroidism.

If the initial TSH is low, especially less than 0.08 μU/mL, then measurement of a high T_4 will confirm the diagnosis of hyperthyroidism. If the T_4 is normal, the T_3 level is measured, since some patients with hyperthyroidism will have predominantly T_3 toxicosis. If the T_3 is normal, it implies that thyroxine secretion is autonomous from TSH, and this is called subclinical hyperthyroidism. Some of these patients will eventually have increased T_4 or T_3 levels with true hyperthyroidism.

Hypothyroidism

In most cases of hypothyroidism, a specific cause is not apparent. It is believed that the hypothyroidism is secondary to an autoimmune reaction, and when goiter formation is present, it is called Hashimoto's thyroiditis. Unless abnormal thyroid function can be documented by specific laboratory assessment, empiric treatment with thyroid hormone is not indicated, and it is especially worth emphasizing that thyroid hormone treatment does not help infertility in euthyroid women. It is uncertain whether hypothyroidism can be a cause of recurrent abortions, but an assessment of thyroid function is worthwhile in these patients.

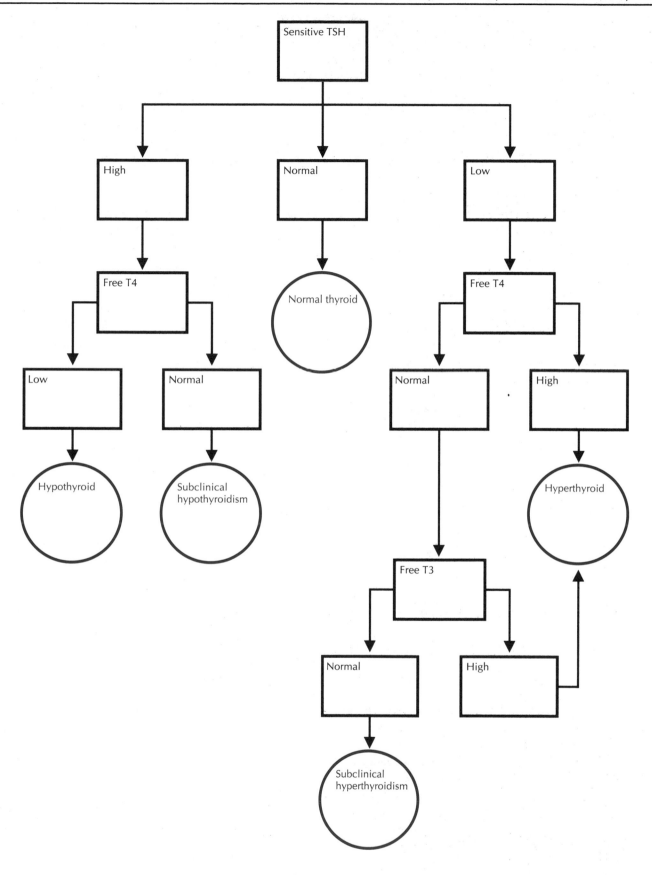

Hypothyroidism increases with aging and is more common in women.[4] Up to 45% of thyroid glands from women over age 60 show evidence of thyroiditis.[5] The incidence of antithyroglobulin antibodies is 7.4% in women over age 75 years, while 16.9% of women age 60 and 17.4% of women over age 75 have elevated TSH levels. In women admitted to geriatric wards, 2–4% have clinically apparent hypothyroidism. *Therefore, hypothyroidism is frequent enough to warrant consideration in most older women, justifying screening even in asymptomatic older women. We recommend that older women be screened with the highly sensitive TSH assay at age 45, then every 2 years beginning at age 60, or with the appearance of any symptoms suggesting hypothyroidism.*

Menstrual irregularites and bleeding problems are common in hypothyroid women. Amenorrhea can be a consequence of hypothyroidism, either with TRH-induced increases in prolactin or with normal prolactin levels. Other clinical manifestations of hypothyroidism include constipation, cold intolerance, psychomotor retardation, carpal tunnel syndrome, and decreased exercise tolerance. However, patients often appear asymptomatic. Close evaluation can reveal mental slowness, decreased energy, fatigue, poor memory, somnolence, slow speech, a low pitched voice, water retention, periorbital edema, delayed reflexes, or a low body temperature and bradycardia. Hypothyroidism can cause hypertension, cognitive abnormalities, pericardial effusion, asymmetric septal myocardial hypertrophy, myopathy, neuropathy, ataxia, anemia, elevated cholesterol and LDL-cholesterol, or hyponatremia. The increase in cholesterol is due to impaired LDL-cholesterol clearance secondary to a decrease in cell membrane LDL receptors. The mechanism for this LDL effect is attributed to a thyroid response element in the LDL receptor gene.[6]

Serum enzymes may be elevated because of decreased clearance (including creatine phosphokinase [CPK], aspartate aminotransferase [AST,SGOT], alanine aminotransferase [ALT, SGPT], lactic dehydrogenase [LDH], and alkaline phosphatase), triggering a fruitless search for other organ disease. It is worth screening for hypothyroidism in any women with abnormal menses or with complaints of fatigue and depression. In addition, patients should be screened who have elevated levels of cholesterol and LDL-cholesterol.

Diagnosis of Hypothyroidism

With primary thyroid failure, the circulating thyroid hormone levels fall, stimulating the pituitary to increase TSH output. Elevated TSH and low T_4 confirm the diagnosis. Hypothyroidism can occur due to pituitary failure in which case the TSH will be inappropriately low for the T_4. The most common cause will be autoimmune thyroid disease (elevated titers of antithyroid antibodies) in areas with normal iodine intake. However, making an etiologic diagnosis in women adds little to the clinical management.

Subclinical Hypothyroidism

In early hypothyroidism, with undetectable symptoms or signs, a compensated state can be detected by an elevated TSH and normal T_4 (called subclinical hypothyroidism). Many of these patients (but not all) will eventually become clinically hypothyroid with low T_4 concentrations. A good reason to treat subclinical hypothyroidism is to avoid the appearance of a goiter. Furthermore, some patients in retrospect (after treatment) recognize improved physical and mental well-being. In those patients who are asymptomatic, it is worth measuring antithyroid antibodies. A positive test identifies those who are likely to become clinically hypothyroid. With only very slight elevations of TSH, it is reasonable not to treat and to check thyroid function every year to detect further deterioration. Patients with an abnormal cholesterol-lipoprotein profile may show improvement with thyroxine treatment.

**Treatment of
Hypothyroidism**

Initial therapy is straightforward with synthetic thyroxine, T_4, given daily. Mixtures of T_4 and T_3, such as desiccated thyroid, provide T_3 in excess of normal thyroid secretion. It is better to provide T_4 and allow the peripheral conversion process to provide the T_3.[7] "Natural" thyroid preparations are not better, and in fact are potentially detrimental. Patients taking biological preparations should be switched to synthetic thyroxine. Because of a risk of coronary heart disease in older women, the initial dose should be 25–50 µg per day for about 5 weeks, at which time the dose is adjusted according to the clinical and biochemical assessment. Usually the dose required will be close to 1.5 µg/lb body weight, but it may be less in very old women.[8] The average final dose required in the elderly is approximately 70% of that in younger patients. *Patients who have been on thyroid hormone for a long time may have their medication discontinued. Recovery of the hypothalamic-pituitary axis usually requires 8 weeks at which time the TSH and free T_4 levels can be measured.*

Evaluation of Therapy

When the patient appears clinically euthyroid, evaluation of TSH levels will provide the most accurate assessment of the adequacy of thyroid hormone replacement. A patient being treated with thyroid hormone should be evaluated once every year with the sensitive TSH assay. Thyroid hormone requirements tend to decrease with age. If the sensitive TSH assay is low, then the free T_4 should be measured to help adjust the thyroxine dose.[9] *The full response of TSH to changes in T_4 is relatively slow; a minimum of 8 weeks is necessary between changes in dosage and assessment of TSH.*

Hyperthyroidism

The two primary causes of hyperthyroidism are Graves' disease (toxic diffuse goiter) and Plummer's disease (toxic nodular goiter). Plummer's disease is usually encountered in postmenopausal women who have had a long history of goiter. Twenty percent of hyperthyroid patients are over 60, and 25% of older women with hyperthyroidism present with an apathetic or atypical syndrome.

Graves' disease is characterized by the triad of hyperthyroidism, exophthalmos, and pretibial myxedema and is believed to be caused by autoantibodies that have TSH properties and therefore bind to and activate the TSH receptor. Menstrual changes associated with hyperthyroidism are unpredictable, ranging from amenorrhea to oligomenorrhea to normal cycles (hence, the amenorrhea in a thyrotoxic woman can be due to pregnancy).

The classic symptoms of thyrotoxicosis are nervousness, heat intolerance, weight loss, sweating, palpitations, and diarrhea. These symptoms are associated with typical findings on physical examination: proptosis, lid lag, tachycardia, tremor, warm and moist skin, and goiter. Women in the reproductive years usually present with the classic picture. In postmenopausal women, symptoms are often concentrated in a single organ system, especially the cardiovascular or central nervous system. Goiter is absent in 40%. Sinus tachycardia occurs in less than half, but atrial fibrillation occurs in 40% and is resistant to cardioversion or spontaneous reversion to sinus rhythm. The ventricular response is usually rapid and resistant to slowing with digoxin. In old women, there is often a coexistent disease, such as an infection or coronary heart disease, that dominates the clinical picture.

The triad of weight loss, constipation, and loss of appetite, suggesting gastrointestinal malignancy, occurs in about 15% of older patients with hyperthyroidism. Ophthalmopathy is rare in older patients. Hyperthyroidism in older women is sometimes described as "apathetic hyperthyroidism" because the clinical manifestations are different. The clinician should consider the diagnosis in older patients with "failure to thrive," in patients who are progressively deteriorating for unexplained reasons, and in patients with heart disease, unexplained weight loss, and mental or psychologic changes.

Psychologic changes are not unusual in hyperthyroid women. Women who complain of emotional lability and nervousness should be screened for hyperthyroidism.

Diagnosis of Hyperthyroidism

The diagnosis requires laboratory testing. A suppressed TSH with a high T_4 or a high T_3 confirms the diagnosis. Hyperthyroidism caused by high levels of T_3 is more common in older women. Most patients should have a radioactive iodine thyroid uptake and scan after laboratory confirmation of the diagnosis. If the uptake is suppressed then drug therapy is indicated. The scan will indicate whether the patient has a diffuse toxic goiter, a solitary hot nodule, or a hot nodule in a multinodular gland. Toxic multinodular goiters occur more frequently in the elderly. TSH hypersecretion as a cause of hyperthyroidism is extremely rare; the combination of a normal or elevated TSH and elevated thryoid hormone will be the clue to this possibility.

Treatment of Hyperthyroidism

There are multiple objectives of therapy: control of thyroid hormone effects on peripheral tissues by pharmacologic blockade of beta-adrenergic receptors, inhibition of thyroid gland secretion and release of thyroid hormone, and specific treatment of nonthyroidal systemic illnesses which can exacerbate hyperthyroidism or be adversely affected by hyperthyroidism. Antithyroid drugs are usually administered first to achieve euthyroidism, then definitive therapy is accomplished by radioactive iodine treatment. Of course, it is important to make sure a woman is not pregnant before treatment with radioactive iodine, and pregnancy should be postponed for several months after treatment. Monitoring treatment response requires the full 8-week interval for stabilization of the hypothalamic-pituitary-thyroid system.

Antithyroid Drugs

The drug of choice in most circumstances will be methimazole because it has fewer adverse effects. The drug inhibits organification of iodide and decreases production of T_4 and T_3. The dose is 10–15 mg, every 8 hours, orally. The onset of effect takes 2–4 weeks. Remember that the half-life of thyroxine is about one week, and the gland usually has large stores of T_4. Maximal effect occurs at 4–8 weeks. The dose can be titrated down once the disease is controlled. The major side effects are rash, gastrointestinal symptoms, and granulocytopenia. Propranolol and other beta-blockers are effective in rapidly controlling the effects of thyroid hormone on peripheral tissues. The dose is usually 20–40 mg, every 6 hours, orally, and the dose is titrated to maintain a heart rate of about 100 beats/minute. The drug may cause bronchospasm, worsening congestive heart failure, fatigue, and depression. Rarely inorganic iodine will be needed to block release of hormone from the gland. Lugol's solution, 2 drops in water daily, is sufficient. The onset of effect is 1–2 days, with maximal effect in 3–7 days. There may be an escape from protection in 2–6 weeks, and the drug can cause rash, fever, and parotitis.

After the symptoms are controlled, and the patient is euthyroid, a dose of radioactive iodine can be selected, the thiouracil withheld temporarily, and definitive therapy accomplished. Patients with solitary nodules will be treated in the same fashion. Some patients with hot nodules in multinodular glands will require surgery because of the size of the gland and because the hyperthyroidism tends to recur in new nodules after the ablation of the original hot nodule. This can result in repetitive treatments with substantial doses of radioactive iodine, and surgery may be preferable. All patients definitively treated for hyperthyroidism must be monitored for the onset of hypothyroidism.

Osteoporosis and Hyperthyroidism

Because postmenopausal women are at increased risk for osteoporosis, and frequently develop hyperthyroidism or receive levothyroxine treatment for hypothyroidism, the clinician needs to understand how thyroid hormone affects bones.[10] Thyroid hormone excess alters bone integrity via direct effects on bone and gut absorption and indirectly through the effects of vitamin D, calcitonin, and parathyroid hormone.

Thyroid hormone increases bone mineral resorption. In addition, total and ionized calcium increase in hyperthyroid women, leading to increases in serum phosphorous, alkaline phosphatase, and bone Gla protein (osteocalcin), a marker of bone turnover. Parathyroid hormone decreases in response to the increased serum calcium, and this results in decreased hydroxylation of vitamin D. Intestinal calcium and phosphate absorption decrease, while urinary hydroxyproline and calcium excretion increase. The net effect is increased bone resorption and a subsequent decrease in bone density — osteoporosis.[11]

These effects become more clinically important in prolonged exposure to excessive thyroid hormone.[12] This raised concern that mild chronic excess thyroid hormone replacement, especially in postmenopausal women, might increase the risk of osteoporosis, and indeed this subsequently was documented.[13] Bone density has been found to be reduced (9%) in premenopausal women receiving enough thyroxine to suppress TSH for 10 years or more.[14] In another study with lower bone densities in women being treated with levothyroxine, the hormone levels indicated that many were being over treated for their hypothyroidism.[15] On the other hand, a careful comparison of treated patients to controls matched for age and menopausal status failed to detect a difference in bone density.[16] Perhaps this was because the increases in circulating thyroid hormone were relatively mild. It still makes sense to monitor patients receiving thyroxine with the sensitive TSH assay to ensure that levothyroxine doses are "physiologic." Some patients who require TSH suppressive doses of thyroxine, such as patients with nodules, goiters, and cancer, must be considered at increased risk of osteoporosis. The use of hormone therapy, exercise programs, and possibly biphosphate treatment must be seriously considered for these patients. Thus, hyperthyroidism must be added to the risk factors for osteoporosis.

Thyroid Nodules

The major concern with thyroid nodules is the potential for thyroid cancer.[17] Single nodules are 4 times more common in women, and carcinoma of the thyroid is nearly 3 times more common in women than in men. The incidence rises steadily from the age of 55. Mortality from thyroid cancer occurs predominantly in the middle-aged and the elderly. There are 4 major types of primary thyroid carcinoma: papillary, follicular, anaplastic, and medullary. In solitary nodules that are "cold" (those that do not take up radioactive iodine or pertechnetate on thyroid scan), 12% prove to be malignant. This also means that the majority are benign. Surgical excision of nodules can result in vocal cord paralysis, hypoparathyroidism, and other complications. Therefore, the goal is to select patients for curative surgery who have the greatest likelihood of having cancer in the nodule.

Epidemiologic and Clinical Data

The major risk factors for thyroid cancer are family history of this disease and a history of irradiation to head or neck. In those who have received thyroid irradiation, about one-third will have thyroid abnormalities, and about one-third of those with abnormalities will have thyroid cancer (about 10% overall). The carcinogenic risk has been estimated to be 1% per 100 rads in 20 years. A rapidly growing nodule, a hard nodule, the presence of palpable regional lymph nodes, or vocal cord paralysis greatly increase the probability of thyroid cancer.

Thyroid nodules in multinodular thyroid glands, not previously exposed to thyroid irradiation, have no greater risk of thyroid carcinoma than normal glands. Therefore, predominant thyroid nodules in multinodular glands should be followed and, if a nodule grows, then biopsy or surgery considered.

Diagnostic Strategy

In patients with a thyroid nodule, laboratory assessment of thyroid function is essential. When abnormal thyroid function is present, the nodule is almost always benign. Detection of a thyroid nodule is followed by clinical characterization of the nodule, examination of the lymph nodes, and inquiry regarding rapid growth, family history, and history of thyroid irradiation. In the presence of any of these findings, surgery is recommended for excision of the nodule. If none of these is present, proceed directly to fine needle aspiration biopsy. A radionuclide scan is performed if cytologic diagnosis is indeterminate or if thyrotoxicosis is present. Cold nodules require a surgical diagnosis. However, if the patient prefers, one can treat with suppressive doses of levothyroxine and evaluate over time. Unfortunately, many of these thyroid nodules do not regress with thyroid treatment, but it is very reassuring if they do. Growth or lack of disappearance with thyroid suppression is an indication for fine needle aspiration biopsy. Thyroid ultrasound can be utilized to more accurately establish size for comparison over time.

If the fine needle aspiration biopsy reveals suspicious cells, a subtotal thyroidectomy should be performed for diagnosis and treatment. If the aspiration biopsy is benign some would repeat the biopsy in one year to avoid false negatives. Most would provide euthyroid hormone suppressive therapy and follow for growth of the nodule.[18] Growth or lack of disappearance indicates the need for biopsy or surgery. In some cases, especially in older women, nodules can be followed with no therapy and little risk. One of the reasons many are treated with levothyroxine is because of the known growth promoting effects of TSH in carcinoma of the thyroid and the hope that TSH suppression will inhibit the growth of early carcinoma.

Fine Needle Aspiration

The method for fine needle aspiration biopsy requires no anesthetic. Using sterile technique and a 23-gauge needle on a 10 mL syringe, the nodule is fixed with two fingers of one hand and the nodule entered. Aspiration is performed with the syringe while several passes are made through a vertical distance of about 2 mm in the nodule. Suction is stopped when biopsy material becomes visible in the hub of the needle. The contents of the needle should be expelled onto a slide and fixed for pathology. Gentle pressure is applied over the nodule for 10 minutes. Occasionally, a patient will have some bleeding into the nodule or surrounding tissues, but it is usually self-limiting.

The Thyroid Gland and Pregnancy

In response to the metabolic demands of pregnancy, there is an increase in the basal metabolic rate (which is mainly due to fetal metabolism), iodine uptake, and the size of the thyroid gland caused by hyperplasia and increased vascularity. However, a pregnant woman is euthyroid with normal levels of TSH, free T_4, and free T_3; thyroid nodules and goiter require evaluation. During pregnancy, iodide clearance by the kidney increases. For this reason (plus the iodide losses to the fetus), the prevalence of goiter is increased in areas of iodine deficiency. This is not a problem in the U.S., and any goiter should be regarded as pathologic.

The increase in thyroid activity is attributed to the thyrotropic substances secreted by the placenta: a chorionic thyrotropin and the thyrotropic activity in human chorionic gonadotropin (HCG).[19] The increase in thyroid activity in pregnancy is compensated by a marked increase in the circulating levels of TBG in response to estrogen; therefore, a new equilibrium is reached with an increase in the bound portion of the thyroid hormone.

Maternal Thyroid Hormones

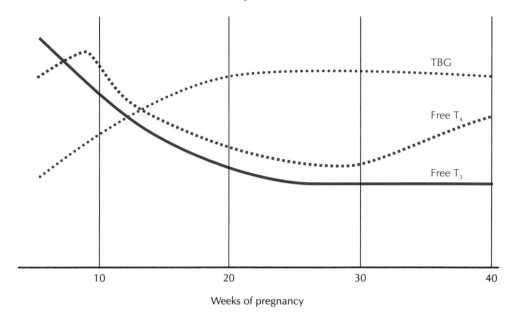

Weeks of pregnancy

The mechanism for the estrogen effect on TBG is an increase in hepatic synthesis and an increase in glycosylation of the TBG molecule that leads to decreased clearance.

TBG levels reach a peak (twice nonpregnant levels) at about 20 weeks, which is maintained throughout the rest of pregnancy.[20] T_4 undergoes a similar change, but T_3 increases more markedly. Because of the increase in TBG, free T_4 and T_3 levels actually decrease, although they remain within the normal range. There is an inverse relationshp between maternal circulation levels of TSH and HCG.[20] TSH reaches a nadir at the same time that HCG reaches a peak at 10 weeks of pregnancy. TSH levels then increase as HCG levels drop to their stable levels throughout the rest of pregnancy. These changes support a role for HCG stimulation of the maternal thyroid gland during early pregnancy.[21,22]

Maternal TSH and HCG

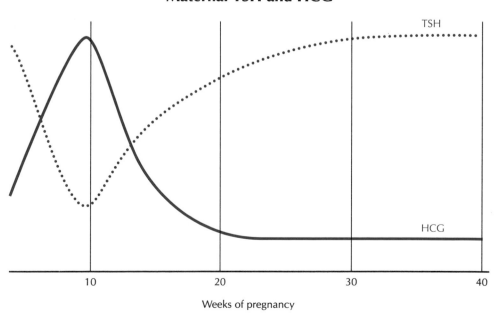

Weeks of pregnancy

In normal pregnancies, placental transfer of TSH, T_4, and T_3 is severely limited in both directions. Indeed, the placenta is essentially impermeable to these substances no matter whether the fetus is euthyroid or hypothyroid. Slight transfer of T_4 and T_3 can occur, however, when maternal levels are very high or when fetal levels are substantially lower than the maternal levels.

The majority of patients with hyperemesis gravidarum have laboratory values consistent with hyperthyroidism, and the severity of the hyperemesis correlates with the degree of hyperthyroidism.[23,24] These patients have higher levels of HCG, and the transient hyperthyroidism and severity of the hyperemesis may be mediated by the thyrotropic and steroidogeneic activity of the HCG.

Thyroid Physiology in the Fetus and the Neonate

The human fetal thyroid gland develops the capacity to concentrate iodine and synthesize hormone between 10 and 12 weeks of gestation, the same time that the pituitary begins to synthesize TSH.[25] Some thyroid development and hormone synthesis are possible in the absence of the pituitary gland, but optimal function requires TSH. By 12–14 weeks, development of the pituitary-thyroid system is complete. Function is minimal, however, until an abrupt increase in fetal TSH occurs at 20 weeks. As with gonadotropin and other pituitary hormone secretion, this thyroid function correlates with the maturation of the hypothalamus and the development of the pituitary portal vascular system, which makes releasing hormone available to the pituitary gland.

Fetal TSH increases and reaches a plateau at 28 weeks and remains at relatively high levels to term. The free T_4 concentration increases progressively. At term, fetal T_4 levels exceed maternal levels. Thus, a state of fetal thyroidal hyperactivity exists near term.

The major thyroid hormone secreted by the fetus is T_4. However, total T_3 and free T_3 levels are low throughout gestation, and levels of RT_3 are elevated, paralleling the rise in T_4. Like T_3, this compound is derived predominantly from conversion of T_4 in peripheral tissues. The increased production of T_4 in fetal life is compensated by rapid conversion to the inactive RT_3, allowing the fetus to conserve its fuel resources.

Fetal Thyroid Hormones

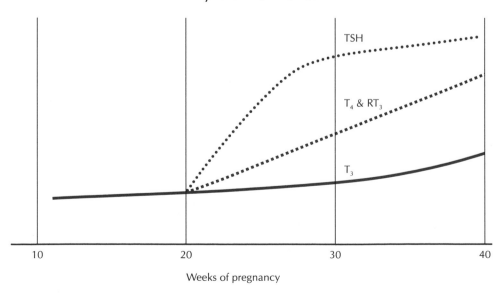

Weeks of pregnancy

Newborn Thyroid Hormones

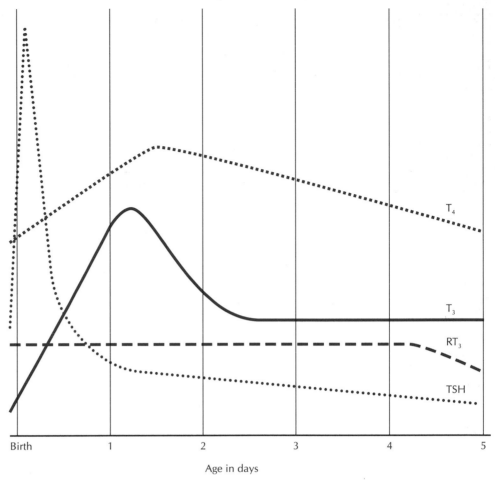

Age in days

With delivery, the newborn moves from a state of relative T_3 deficiency to a state of T_3 thyrotoxicosis. Shortly after birth serum TSH concentrations increase rapidly to a peak at 30 minutes of age. They fall to baseline values by 48–72 hours. In response to this increase in TSH, total T_4 and free T_4 increase to peak values by 24–48 hours of age. T_3 levels increase even more, peaking by 24 hours of age. By 3–4 weeks, the thyroidal hyperactivity has disappeared.

The postnatal surge in TSH is accompanied by a prolactin surge, suggesting that both are increased in response to TRH. The TRH surge is thought to be a response to rapid neonatal cooling. A puzzle is the fact that the early increase in T_3 is independent of TSH and is tied in some way to cutting of the umbilical cord. Delaying cord cutting delays the increase in T_3, but TSH levels still reach their peak at 30 minutes. In some way cord cutting augments peripheral (largely liver) conversion of T_4 to T_3. The later increases in T_3 and T_4 (after 2 hours) are due to increased thyroid gland activity. These thyroid changes after birth probably represent defense mechanisms against the sudden entry into the cold world. The high RT_3 levels during pregnancy continue during the first 3–5 days of life, and then fall gradually to normal levels by 2 weeks.

Summary of Fetal and Newborn Thyroid Changes

1. TSH and T_4 appear in the fetus at 10–13 weeks. Levels are low until an abrupt rise at 20 weeks.

2. T_4 rises rapidly and exceeds maternal values at term.

3. T_3 levels rise, but concentrations are relatively low, similar to hypothyroid adults.

4. RT_3 levels exceed normal adult levels.

5. The fetal pattern of low T_3 and high RT_3 is similar to that seen with calorie malnutrition.

6. After delivery, TSH peaks at 30 minutes of age, followed by a T_3 peak at 24 hours and a T_4 peak at 24–48 hours. The T_3 increase is independent of the TSH change.

7. High RT_3 levels persist for 3–5 days after delivery, then reach normal values by 2 weeks.

Newborn Screening for Hypothyroidism

The incidence of neonatal hypothyroidism is about one in 4,000 live births. The problem is that congenital hypothyroidism is not apparent clinically at birth. Fortunately, infants with congenital hypothyroidism have low T_4 and high TSH concentrations easily detected in blood, and early treatment before 3 months of age is usually associated with normal mental development.[26] Less than normal development can be a consequence of a delay in treatment or extremely low thyroid hormone production in the fetus.

There is a familial tendency for hypothyroidism, and if the diagnosis is made in the antepartum period, intraamniotic injections of thyroxine can raise fetal levels of thyroid hormone.[27] Ultrasonographic examination of patients with polyhydramnios should include a search for a fetal goiter. In addition, the fetus should be monitored for goiter formation in women treated with antithyroid drugs for hyperthyroidism during pregnancy. Amniotic fluid iodothyronines and TSH reflect fetal plasma levels, and abnormal values may allow prenatal diagnosis of fetal hypothyroidism by amniocentesis.[27,28] However, cord blood sampling is advocated for accurate diagnosis.[29] Treatment of fetal hypothyroidism is important because there is a concern that prenatal hypothyroidism can affect some aspects of development, e.g., the full function of physical skills.

Hyperthyroidism in Pregnancy

Untreated thyrotoxicosis in pregnancy is associated with a higher risk of preeclampsia, heart failure, intrauterine growth retardation, and stillbirth.[30] Heart failure is a consequence of the demands of pregnancy superimposed upon the hyperdynamic cardiovascular state induced by the increased thyroid hormone.[31]

The most common cause of thyrotoxicosis in pregnancy is Graves' disease. However, the clinician should always keep in mind that trophoblastic disease can cause hyperthyroidism due to the TSH property inherent in human chorionic gonadotropin. The maternal changes with pregnancy can make diagnosis difficult. Tachycardia upon awakening from sleep and a failure to gain weight should make a clinician suspicious. Hyperemesis gravidarum is a common presentation of hyperthyroidism in pregnancy. Laboratory assessment is unaffected by pregnancy and should follow our algorithm.

The choice of treatment is between surgery and antithyroid drugs. However prior to surgery, the thyroid gland has to be controlled with medical therapy. Most women can be successfully treated with thioamide drugs.[30] Propylthiouracil is preferred for pregnant women because methimazole crosses the placenta more readily.

The aim of treatment should be to maintain mild hyperthyroidism in the mother to avoid thyroid dysfunction in the fetus. Treatment of maternal hyperthyroidism with propylthiouricil, even with moderate doses of 100–200 mg daily, suppresses T_4 and increases TSH levels in newborns.[32] The infants are clinically euthyroid, however, and their laboratory measurements are normal by the 4th to 5th day of life. In addition, follow-up assessment has indicated unimpaired intellectual development in children whose mothers received propylthiouricil during pregnancy.[33] Nevertheless, pregnant women with thyrotoxicosis should be treated with as low a dose of antithyroid drugs as possible. With proper antithyroid drug treatment, very few, if any, deleterious effects are experienced by mother, fetus, or neonate.[34] Although small amounts of antithyroid drugs are transmitted in breast milk, the amount has no impact on neonatal thyroid function, and breastfeeding should be encouraged.

Maternal TSH-like autoantibodies can cross the placenta and cause fetal thyrotoxicosis and demise. Some have advocated fetal cord blood sampling in women with Graves' disease who are euthyroid but who have positive titers of TSH-like antibodies to assess the fetal thyroid status.[35] The fetus can be treated by treating the mother. Neonates have to be observed closely until antithyroid drugs are cleared (a few days) and the true thyroid state can be assessed.

Thyroid Storm
This life-threatening augmentation of thyrotoxicosis is usually precipitated by stress such as labor, cesarean section, or infection. Stress should be limited as much as possible in patients with uncontrolled thyrotoxicosis.

Hypothyroidism in Pregnancy

Serious hypothyroidism is rarely encountered during pregnancy. Patients with this degree of illness probably do not get pregnant. Patients with mild hypothyroidism probably never have a laboratory assessment for thyroid function during pregnancy and go undetected. Preeclampsia and intrauterine growth retardation are more frequent in women with significant hypothyroidism.[36,37] There is also reason to believe that patients with hypothyroidism have an increased rate of spontaneous abortion.[38] The mechanism may be impaired ability of important organs such as the endometrium and the corpus luteum. Women being treated for hypothyroidism require a small increase in thyroxine during pregnancy.[39] TSH should be monitored monthly in the first trimester and again in the postpartum period, and dosage should be adjusted to keep the TSH level in the normal range.

Postpartum Thyroiditis

Autoimmune thyroid disease is suppressed to some degree by the immunologic changes of pregnancy. Thus, there is a relatively high incidence of postpartum thyroiditis (5–10%), usually 3–6 months after delivery, manifested by either hyperthyroidism or hypothyroidism, although commonly transient hyperthyroidism is followed by hypothyroidism.[40] This condition is due to a destructive thyroiditis associated with thyroid microsomal autoantibodies.[41] Women at high risk for postpartum thyroiditis are those with a personal or family history of autoimmune disease, and those with a previous postpartum episode.

Most importantly, the symptoms in these women are often attributed to anxiety or depression, and the obstetrician must have a high index of suspicion for hypothyroidism.

The symptoms usually last 1–3 months and almost all women return to normal thyroid function. Postpartum thyroiditis tends to recur with subsequent pregnancies, and eventually hypothyroidism remains.[42] The symptoms of hyperthyroidism in this condition are not responsive to antithyroid medication, and patients are usually not treated or given beta-adrenergic blocking agents (e.g., propranolol in a dose sufficient to reduce the resting pulse to less than 100 per minute). Because spontaneous remission is common, patients who are treated with hypothyroidism should be reassessed one year after gradual withdrawal of thyroxine. Patients who return to normal should undergo periodic laboratory surveillance of their thyroid status.

References

1. **Medvei VC,** *A History of Endocrinology,* MTP Press Limited, Lancaster, England, 1982.

2. **Melmed S, Hershman J,** The thyroid and aging, in Korenman SG, editor, *Endocrine Aspects of Aging,* Elsevier Science Publishing, New York, 1982, pp 33–53.

3. **Caldwell G, Gow SM, Sweeting VM, Kellett HA, Beckett GJ, Seth J, Toft AD,** A new strategy for thyroid function testing, Lancet 1:1117, 1985.

4. **Robuschi G, Safran M, Braverman LE, Gnudi A, Roti E,** Hypothyroidism in the elderly, Endocrine Rev 8:142, 1987.

5. **Felicetta JV,** Thyroid changes with aging: significance and management, Geriatrics 42:86, 1987.

6. **Wiseman SA, Powell JT, Humphries SE, Press M,** The magnitude of the hypercholesterolemia of hypothyroidism is associated with variation in the low density lipoprotein receptor gene, J Clin Endocrinol Metab 77:108, 1993.

7. **Cooper DS,** Thyroid hormone treatment: new insights into an old therapy, JAMA 261:2694, 1989.

8. **Rosenbaum RL, Barzel US,** Levothyroxine replacement dose for primary hypothyroidism decreases with age, Ann Intern Med 96:53, 1982.

9. **Watts NB,** Use of a sensitive thyrotropin assay for monitoring treatment with levothyroxine, Arch Intern Med 149:309, 1989.

10. **Cooper DS,** Thyroid hormone and the skeleton, JAMA 259:3175, 1988.

11. **Wartofsky L,** Osteoporosis and therapy with thyroid hormone, Endocrinologist 1:57, 1991.

12. **Diamond T, Nery L, Hales I,** A therapeutic dilemma: suppressive doses of thyroxine significantly reduce bone mineral measurements in both premenopausal and postmenopausal women with thyroid carcinoma, J Clin Endocrinol Metab 72:1184, 1991.

13. **Barsony J, Lakatos P, Foldes J, Feher T,** Effect of vitamin D_3 loading and thyroid hormone replacement therapy on the decreased serum 25-hydroxyvitamin D level in patients with hypothyroidism, Acta Endocrinol 113:329, 1986.

14. **Ross DS, Neer RM, Ridgway EC, Daniels GH,** Subclinical hyperthyroidism and reduced bone density as a possible result of prolonged suppression of the pituitary-thyroid axis with L-thyroxine, Am J Med 82:1167, 1987.

15. **Paul TL, Kerrigan J, Kelly AM, Braverman LE, Baran DT,** Long-term L-thyroxine therapy is associated with decreased hip bone density in premenopausal women, JAMA 259:3137, 1988.

16. **Franklyn JA, Betteridge J, Daykin J, Holder R, Oates GD, Parle JV, Lilley J, Heath DA, Sheppard MC,** Long-term thyroxine treatment and bone mineral density, Lancet 340:9, 1992.

17. **Mazzaferri EL,** Management of a solitary thyroid nodule, New Engl J Med 328:553, 1993.

18. **Hamberger B, Gharib H, Melton LJ, Goellner JR, Zinsmeister AR,** Fine-needle aspiration biopsy of thyroid nodules, Am J Med 73:381, 1982.

19. **Kennedy RL, Darne J,** The role of hCG in regulation of the thyroid gland in normal and abnormal pregnancy, Obstet Gynecol 78:298, 1991.

20. **Glinoer D, DeNayer P, Bourdoux P, Lemone M, Robyn C, Van Steirteghem A, Kinthaert J, Lejeune B,** Regulation of maternal thyroid during pregnancy, J Clin Endocrinol Metab 71:276, 1990.

21. **Kimura M, Amino N, Tamaki H, Mitsuda N, Miyai K, Tanizawa O,** Physiologic thyroid activation in normal early pregnancy is induced by circulating hCG, Obstet Gynecol 75:775, 1990.

22. **Ballabio M, Poshyachinda M, Ekins RP,** Pregnancy-induced changes in thyroid function: role of human chorionic gonadotropin as putative regulator of maternal thyroid, J Clin Endocrinol Metab 73:824, 1991.

23. **Goodwin TM, Montoro M, Mestman JH,** Transient hyperthyroidism and hyperemesis gravidarum: clinical aspects, Am J Obstet Gynecol 167:648, 1992.

24. **Goodwin TM, Montoro M, Mestman JH, Pekary AE, Hershman JM,** The role of chorionic gonadotropin in transient hyperthyroidism of hyperemesis gravidarum, J Clin Endocrinol Metab 75:1333, 1992.

25. **Thorpe-Beeston JG, Nicoloaides KH, McGregor AM,** Fetal thyroid function, Thyroid 2:207, 1992.

26. **Fisher DA,** Clinical review 19: management of congenital hypothyroidism, J Clin Endocrinol Metab 72:523, 1991.

27. **Perelman AH, Johnson RL, Clemons RD, Finberg HJ, Clewell WH, Trujillo L,** Intrauterine diagnosis and treatment of fetal goitrous hypothyroidism, J Clin Endocrinol Metab 71:618, 1990.

28. **Klein AH, Murphy BEP, Artal R, Oddie TH, Fisher DA,** Amniotic fluid thyroid hormone concentrations during human gestation, Am J Obstet Gynecol 136:626, 1980.

29. **Davidson KM, Richards DS, Schatz DA, Fisher DA,** Successful in utero treatment of fetal goiter and hypothyroidism, New Engl J Med 324:543, 1991.

30. **Davis LE, Lucas MJ, Hankins GDV, Roark ML, Cunningham FG,** Thyrotoxicosis complicating pregnancy, Am J Obstet Gynecol 160:63, 1989.

31. **Easterling TR, Chmucker BC, Carlson KL, Millard SP, Benedetti TJ,** Maternal hemodynamics in pregnancies complicated by hyperthyroidism, Obstet Gynecol 78:348, 1991.

32. **Cheron RG, Kaplan MM, Larsen PR, Selenkow HA, Crigler JF Jr,** Neonatal thyroid function after propylthiouracil therapy for maternal Graves' disease, New Engl J Med 304:525, 1981.

33. **Burrow GN, Klatskin EH, Genel M,** Intellectual development in children whose mothers received proplythiouracil during pregnancy, Yale J Biol Med 51:151, 1978.

34. **Mitsuda N, Tamaki H, Amino N, Hosono T, Miyai K, Tanizasa O,** Risk factors for developmental disorders in infants born to women with Graves' disease, Obstet Gynecol 80:359, 1992.

35. **Wenstrom KD, Weinger CP, Williamson RA, Grant SS,** Prenatal diagnosis of fetal hyperthyroidism using funipuncture, Obstet Gynecol 76:513, 1990.

36. **Davis LE, Leveno KL, Cunningham FG,** Hypothyroidism complicating pregnancy, Obstet Gynecol 72:108, 1988.

37. **Leung AS, Millar LK, Koonings PP, Montoro M, Mestman JH,** Perinatal outcome in hypothyroid pregnancies, Obstet Gynecol 81:349, 1993.

38. **Maruo T, Katayama K, Matuso H, Anwar M, Mochizuki M,** The role of maternal thyroid hormones in maintaining early pregnancy in threatened abortion, Acta Endocrinol 127:118, 1992.

39. **Mandel SJ, Larsen PR, Seely EW, Brent GA,** Increased need for thyroxine during pregnancy in women with primary hypothyroidism, New Engl J Med 323,91, 1990.

40. **Roti E, Emerson CH,** Clinical review 29: postpartum thyroiditis, J Clin Endocrinol Metab 74:3, 1992.

41. **Vargas MT, Bariones-Urbina R, Gladman D, Papsin FR, Walfish PG,** Antithyroid microsomal autoantibodies and HLA-DR5 are associated with postpartum thyroid dysfunction: evidence supporting an autoimmune pathogenesis, J Clin Endocrinol Metab 67:327, 1988.

42. **Walfish PG, Chan YYC,** Postpartum hyperthyroidism, Clin Endocrinol Metab 14:417, 1985.

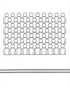

Part III

Contraception

21

Use of Contraception, Sterilization, and Abortion

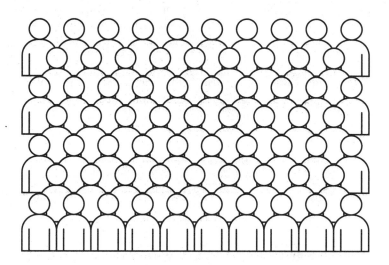

As societies become more affluent, fertility decreases. This decrease is in response to the use of contraception and abortion. During her reproductive lifespan, the average !Kung woman, a member of an African tribe of hunter-gatherers, experienced 15 years of lactational amenorrhea, 4 years of pregnancy, and only 48 menstrual cycles.[1] In contrast, a modern urban woman will experience 420 menstrual cycles. Contemporary women undergo earlier menarche and start having sexual intercourse earlier in their lives than in the past. Even though breastfeeding has increased in recent years, its duration is relatively brief, and its contribution to contraception in the developed world is trivial. Therefore, it is more difficult today to limit the size of a family unless some method of contraception is utilized.

More young women (under age 25) in the United States become pregnant than do their contemporaries in other Western countries.[2] The teenage pregnancy rates in 5 northern European countries and Canada range from 13 to 53% of the U.S. rate. The differences disappear almost completely after age 25. This is largely because American men and women after age 25 utilize surgical sterilization at a great rate.

It is obviously not true that young American women wish to have these higher pregnancy rates. American teenagers abort nearly half of their pregnancies, and this proportion is similar to that seen in other countries. However, from ages 20–34, American women have the highest proportion of pregnancies aborted compared to other countries, indicating an unappreciated, but real, problem of unintended pregnancy existing beyond the teenage years. About half of all pregnancies in the U.S. are estimated to be unplanned, and more than half of these are aborted.[2]

Another possible contribution to the problem of unintended pregnancy is the delay of marriage. Delaying marriage prolongs the period in which women are exposed to the risk of unintended pregnancy. This, however, cannot be documented as a major reason for the large differential between young adults in Europe and the U.S. The evidence available also indicates that a difference in sexual activity is not an important explanation. The major difference between American women and European women is that American women under age 25 are less likely to use any form of contraception.[2,3] Significantly the use of oral contraceptives (the main choice of younger women) is lower in the U.S. than in other countries.

Why are Americans different? The cultures in countries such as Canada and Britain are certainly very similar. A major difference must be attributed to the availability of contraception. In the rest of the world, contraceptive services can be obtained from more accessible resources and relatively inexpensively. In the rest of the world, contraception can be advertised on television. A further problem is the enormous diversity of people as well as the unequal distribution of income in the U.S. These factors influence the ability of our society to effectively provide education regarding sex and contraception and to effectively make contraception services available.

Efficacy of Contraception

A clinician's anecdotal experience is truly insufficient to provide the accurate information necessary for patient counseling. The clinician must be aware of the definitions and measurements used in assessing contraceptive efficacy and must draw upon the talents of appropriate experts in this area to summarize the accurate and comparative failure rates for the various methods of contraception. The publications by Trussell et al. accomplish these purposes and are highly recommended.[4,5]

Definition and Measurement

Contraceptive efficacy is generally assessed by measuring the number of unplanned pregnancies that occur during a specified period of exposure and use of a contraceptive method. The two methods that have been used to measure contraceptive efficacy are the Pearl index and life table analysis.

The Pearl Index

The Pearl index is defined as the number of failures per 100 woman-years of exposure. The denominator is the total months or cycles of exposure from the onset of a method until completion of the study, an unintended pregnancy, or discontinuation of the method. The quotient is multiplied by 1,200 if the denominator consists of months or by 1,300 if the denominator consists of cycles.

With most methods of contraception, failure rates decline with duration of use. The Pearl index is usually based on a lengthy exposure (usually one year) and therefore fails to accurately compare methods at various durations of exposure. This limitation is overcome by using the method of life table analysis.

Life Table Analysis

Life table analysis calculates a failure rate for each month of use. A cumulative failure rate can then compare methods for any specific length of exposure. Women who leave a study for any reason other than unintended pregnancy are removed from the analysis, contributing their exposure until the time of the exit.

Contraceptive failures do occur and for many reasons. Thus, "method effectivness" and "use effectiveness" have been used to designate efficacy with correct and incorrect use of a method. It is less confusing to simply compare the very best performance (the lowest expected failure rate) with the usual experience (typical failure rates) as noted in the table of failure rates during the first year of use. The lowest expected failure rates are determined in clinical trials, where the combination of highly motivated subjects and frequent support from the study personnel yields the best results.

Failure Rates During the First Year of Use, United States[5]

Method	Percent of Women with Pregnancy	
	Lowest Expected	**Typical**
No method	85.0%	85.0%
Combination Pill	0.1	3.0
Progestin only	0.5	3.0
IUDs		3.0
Progesterone IUD	2.0	<2.0
Copper T 380A	0.8	<1.0
Norplant	0.2	0.2
Female sterilization	0.2	0.4
Male sterilization	0.1	0.15
Depo-Provera	0.3	0.3
Spermicides	3.0	21.0
Periodic abstinence		20.0
Calendar	9.0	
Ovulation method	3.0	
Symptothermal	2.0	
Post–ovulation	1.0	
Withdrawal	4.0	18.0
Cervical cap	6.0	18.0
Sponge		
Parous women	9.0	28.0
Nulliparous women	6.0	18.0
Diaphragm and spermicides	6.0	18.0
Condom	2.0	12.0

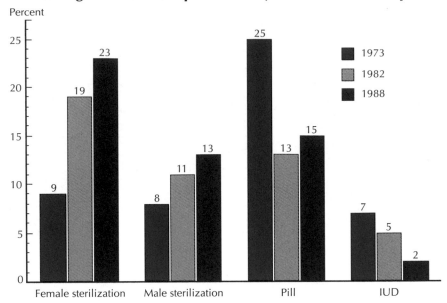

Changes in Contraceptive Use by U.S. Married Couples[6,7]

Contraceptive Use in the United States

The National Survey of Family Growth is conducted every 5–6 years by the National Center for Health Statistics. Data are available from 1972, 1976, 1982, and 1988.[6,7] The sample is very large, and therefore, the estimates are very accurate.

The percent of married couples using sterilization as a method of contraception more than doubled from 1972 to 1988. In contrast, the percent of married couples using oral contraception declined sharply between 1973 and 1982. Recently, however, the use of oral contraception has increased, reaching a new high in 1992. About 10.7 million American women used oral contraceptives in 1988. Among never married women, oral contraception has been the leading method of birth control. Although condom use has not changed significantly among married couples, it did increase among never married women and is the second leading method.

In 1988, 60% of women, 15–44 years of age, were using contraception. Contraceptive sterilization was utilized by 24% of these women (the next leading method was oral contraception, 18.5%) The number of couples using the intrauterine device (IUD) decreased by two-thirds from 1981 to 1988, from 2.2 million to 0.7 million (7.1% to 2%).

The Ortho Pharmaceutical Corporation performs an annual birth control study involving thousands of women.[8] According to this study, the use of oral contraception by U.S. women aged 15–44 has increased from 21% in 1985 to 25% in 1993. The biggest annual increase in oral contraceptive use (9%) in nearly 10 years was recorded in 1991. Women are using oral contraception for longer durations, and more older women are using oral contraception. Oral contraceptive use quadrupled from 1990 to 1993 in women aged 40–45. These changes undoubtedly reflect clinician and patient awareness of the greater safety in low dose formulations. IUD use decreased from 3% in 1985 to 1% in 1991. This percentage has remained stable for the last several years.

A total of 35 million of the 57.9 million women of reproductive age were using some method of contraception in 1988. Of the 40% not using contraception, 7% were at risk of having an unintended pregnancy. Of the other 33%:

•5% — sterilized for medical reasons,
•1% — nonsurgically sterilized,
•5% — pregnant,
•4% — trying to get pregnant,
•18% — not sexually active.

Thus, of those who are at risk of getting pregnant, 90% are using some method of contraception. By ages 35–44, over half of women or their husbands are surgically sterile, either for contraceptive or medical reasons.

U.S. couples have made up for the lack of contraceptive choices by greater reliance on voluntary sterilization. Although the use of sterilization has remained steady for the last several years, approximately one-half of American couples choose sterilization within 15 to 20 years of their last wanted birth. During the years of maximal fertility, oral contraceptives are the most common method peaking at age 20–24. The use of condoms is the second most widely used method of reversible contraception, rising from about 9% in the mid 1980s to approximately 15% of couples in 1991.[8] Most IUD users are concentrated between ages 25 and 40.

The Worldwide Use of Contraception

The world population is expected to stabilize at between 10 and 11 billion by the year 2100.[9] Approximately 95% of the growth will occur in developing countries, so that by 2100, 13% of the population will live in developed countries, a decrease from the current 25%.

World Population
1 billion — achieved in 1800–1850
2 billion — achieved in 1930
3 billion — achieved in 1960
4 billion — achieved in 1976
5 billion — achieved in 1987

Throughout the world, 45% of married women of reproductive age practice contraception. However, there is significant variation from area to area; e.g., 69% in east Asia but only 11% in Africa. Female sterilization and the IUD are most popular in developing countries, while oral contraceptives and condoms are most popular in developed countries. Of the 400 million women of reproductive age, less than 60 million (15%) are using oral contraceptives, and more than half live in the U.S., Brazil, France, and Germany.

The 76% of the world's population living in developing countries account for:

•85% of all births,
•95% of all infant and childhood deaths,
•99% of all maternal deaths.

The problem in the developing world is self-evident. The ability to regulate fertility has a significant impact on infant, child, and maternal mortality and morbidity. A pregnant woman has a 200 times greater chance of dying living in a developing country than in a developed country.[9]

The Impact of Use and Non-use

Inadequate access to contraception is associated with a high abortion rate. Effective contraceptive use largely, although not totally, replaces the resort to abortion.[10] The combination of restrictive abortion laws and the lack of safe abortion services continues to make unsafe abortion a major cause of morbidity and mortality throughout the world. Both safe and unsafe abortions can be minimized by maximizing contraceptive services.

However, the need for safe abortion services will persist. Contraceptive failures account for about half of the 1.6 million annual induced abortions in the U.S.

In the U.S. in the late 1980s, $1 spent on public funding for family planning saved an average of $4.40 spent on medical, welfare, and nutritional services.[11] The investment in family planning leads to short-term reductions in expenditures on maternal and child health services and after 5 years, a reduction in costs for education budgets.

Cutting back on publicly funded family planning services impacts largely on poor women, increasing the number of unintended births and abortions. In California, there is an average of $7.70 saved for every $1 spent to provide contraceptive services.[12] This estimate is higher than the national estimate because the income ceiling for eligibility is higher in California.

There is a gap between the low levels of unintentional pregnancy that can be achieved and the actual levels being obtained, most of which are in couples using reversible contraception. A major thrust, in addition to providing services, must include education and counseling of couples about effective contraception.

STDs and Contraception

The interaction between clinician and patient for the purpose of contraception provides an opportunity to control sexually transmitted diseases (STDs). The modification of unsafe sexual practices reduces the risk of unplanned pregnancy and the risk of infections of the reproductive tract. A patient visit for contraception is an excellent time for STD screening; if an infection is symptomatic, it should be diagnosed and treated during the same visit in which contraception is requested. A positive history for STDs should trigger both screening for asymptomatic infections and counseling for safer sexual practices. Attention should be given to the contraceptive methods that have the greatest influence on the risk of STDs.

The Future

From 1970 to 1986, the number of births in women over 30 quadrupled. As more and more couples defer pregnancy until later in life, the use of sterilization under age 35 will decline, and the need for reversible contraception will increase. In 1988, 75% of pill users were under age 30. Only 5% of women aged 35–44 used oral contraception, compared to 38% under age 25. These numbers will change only if clinicians and patients understand and accept that low dose oral contraception is safe for healthy, nonsmoking older women.

The need for reversible contraception in women over the age of 30 is growing, not diminishing. The highest number of births in the U.S. occurred between 1947 and 1965 — the post World War II baby boom. Women born in this period won't be through reaching their 45th birthday until around 2010. For approximately a 20-year period, therefore, there will be an unprecedented number of women in the later child-bearing years. It is estimated that the number of women aged 35–49 will increase 61% between 1982 and 1995. The proportion of births accounted for by this group of women will increase by about 72%, from 5% in 1982 to 8.6% in 2000.[13] This group of women is not only increasing in number, but it is changing its fertility pattern.

The deferment of marriage is a significant change in our society. In 1960, 28% of women aged 20–24 were single; in 1985, 58.5%. In 1960, 10% of women 25–29 were single; in 1985, 26%. But only 16% of the decline in the total fertility rate is accounted for by the increase in the average age at first marriage. Eighty-three percent of the decline in total fertility rate is accounted for by changes in marital fertility rates. In other words postponement of pregnancy in marriage is the more significant change.[14] This combination of increasing numbers, deferment of marriage, and postponement of pregnancy in marriage is responsible for the fact that we will be seeing more and more older women who will need reversible contraception. In short, there will continue to be longer duration of use in younger women and greater use in older women, the pattern of use which was being observed by 1990.

Change in U.S. Female Demographics 1985–2000 [15]

Age	1985	1990	1995	2000	% Change 1985–2000
15–24	19.5 mill.	17.4 mill.	16.7 mill.	17.7 mill.	-9.2%
25–29	10.9	10.6	9.3	8.6	-21.1
30–34	10.0	11.0	10.8	9.4	-6.0
35–44	16.2	19.1	21.1	21.9	+35.2
Total 15–44	56.6	58.1	57.9	57.6	+1.8

One solution to the problem of a restricted number of choices for American women is to develop new methods. However, experts are pessimistic when it comes to looking forward to new methods. There are many obstacles to the development of new methods, including the attitudes of the American public (besides America's traditionally conservative, religion-oriented views toward sex and family, polarization is produced by responses evoked by specific issues such as sterilization and abortion), the funding available for research, the time and cost required to meet federal regulations, and the problems of product liability.[16]

Fortunately clinicians and patients are beginning to recognize that low dose oral contraception is very safe for healthy, nonsmoking older women. However, as the above statistics indicate, its use is still not sufficient to meet the need. Besides fulfilling a need, this population of women has a series of benefits to be derived from oral contraception that tilt the risk:benefit ratio to the positive side (Chapter 22).

The growing need for reversible contraception would also be served by increased utilization of the IUD. After several years of use, efficacy with the IUD is similar to that of oral contraceptives. The decline in IUD use in the U.S. is in direct contrast to the experience in the rest of the world, a complicated response to publicity and litigation. An increased risk of pelvic infection with contemporary IUDs in use is limited to the act of insertion and the transportation of pathogens to the upper genital tract. This risk is effectively minimized by careful screening with preinsertion cultures and the use of good technique. A return to IUD use by American couples is both warranted and desirable.

If one attempts to sum the impact of the benefits of contraception on public health, as some have done with models focusing on hospital admissions, there is no doubt that the benefits outweigh the risks. The impact can be measured in terms of both morbidity and mortality. But the impact on public health is of little concern during the private clinician-patient interchange in the medical office. Here personal risk is paramount, and compliance with effective contraception requires accurate information.

Contraceptive advice is a component of good preventive health care. The clinician's approach is a key. This is an era of informed choice by the patient. Patients deserve to know the facts and need help in dealing with the state of the art and the uncertainty. But there is no doubt that patients, especially young patients, are influenced in their choice by their clinician's advice and attitude. While the role of a clinician is to provide the education necessary for the patient to make proper choices, one should not lose sight of the powerful influence exerted by the clinician in the choices ultimately made.

In our view, the attitude of the clinician is a crucial influence on the ultimate patient take home message. In the 1970s we approached the patient with great emphasis on risk. In the 1990s the approach should be different, highlighting the benefits and the greater safety of appropriate contraception.

Sterilization

Over the past 20 years, nearly one million Americans each year have undergone a sterilization operation, and recently, more women than men. By 1988, 24% of reproductive aged women relied on contraceptive sterilization: 17% had tubal occlusion, and 7% depended upon their partners' vasectomies.[6,7]

James Blundell proposed in 1823, in lectures at Guy's Hospital in London, that tubectomy ought to be performed at cesarean section to avoid the need for repeat sections.[17] He also proposed a technique for sterilization which he later described so precisely that he must actually have performed the operation, although he never wrote about it. The first report was published in 1881 by Samuel Lungren of Toledo, Ohio, who ligated the tubes at the time of cesarean section, as Blundell had suggested 58 years earlier.[18] The Madlener procedure was devised in Germany in 1910 and reported in 1919. Because of many failures, the Madlener technique was supplanted in the U.S. by the method of Ralph Pomeroy, a prominent physician in Brooklyn, New York. This method, still popular today, was not described to the medical profession by Pomeroy's associates until 1929, 4 years after Pomeroy's death. Frederick Irving of the Harvard Medical School described his technique in 1924, and the Uchida method was not reported until 1946.

Few sterilizations were performed until the 1930s when "family planning" was first suggested as an indication for surgical sterilization by Baird in Aberdeen. He required women to be over 40 and to have had 8 or more children. Mathematical formulas of this kind persisted through the 1960s.

Laparoscopic methods were introduced in the early 1970s. The annual number of vasectomies began to decline, and the number of tubal occlusion operations increased rapidly. By 1973, more sterilization operations were performed for women than for men. This is accurately attributed to dramatic decreases in costs, hospital time, and pain due to the introduction of laparoscopy and minilaparotomy methods. The use of laparoscopy for tubal occlusion increased from only 0.6% of sterilizations in 1970 to more than 35% by 1975.[19] Since 1975, minilaparotomy, a technique popular in the less developed world, has been increasingly performed in the U.S. These methods have allowed women to undergo sterilization operations at times other than immediately after childbirth or during major surgery.

The Pomeroy

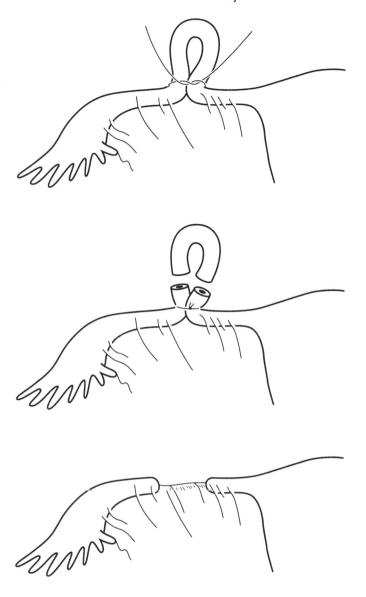

Laparoscopy and minilaparotomy have led to a profound change in the convenience and cost of sterilization operations for women. In 1970, the average woman stayed in the hospital 6.5 days for a tubal sterilization. By 1975, this had declined to 3 days, and today, women rarely remain in the hospital overnight. The shorter length of stay achieved from 1970 to 1975 represented a savings of more than $200 million yearly in health care costs and a tremendous increase in convenience for women eager to return to work and their families.[20] Unlike some advances in technology, laparoscopy and minilaparotomy sterilization are technical innovations that have resulted in large savings in medical care costs.

The Irving

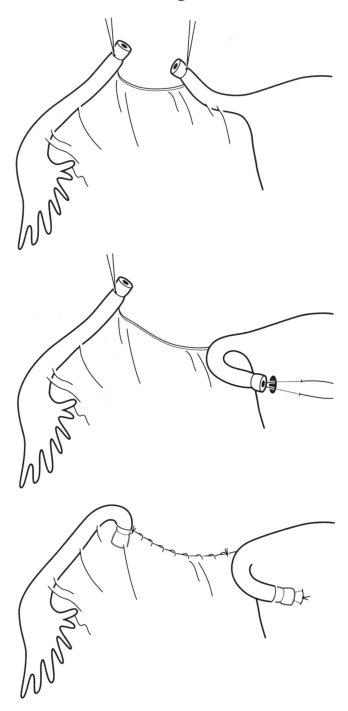

The great majority of sterilization procedures are accomplished in hospitals by physicians in private practice, but a rapidly increasing proportion are performed outside of hospitals in ambulatory surgical settings, including physician's offices. In either hospital or outpatient settings, female sterilization is a very safe operation. Deaths specifically attributed to sterilization now account for a fatality rate of only 1.5 per 100,000 procedures, a mortality rate that is lower than that for childbearing (about 10 per 100,000 births in the U.S.).[21] When the risk of pregnancy from contraceptive method failure is taken into account, sterilization is the safest of all contraceptive methods.

The Uchida

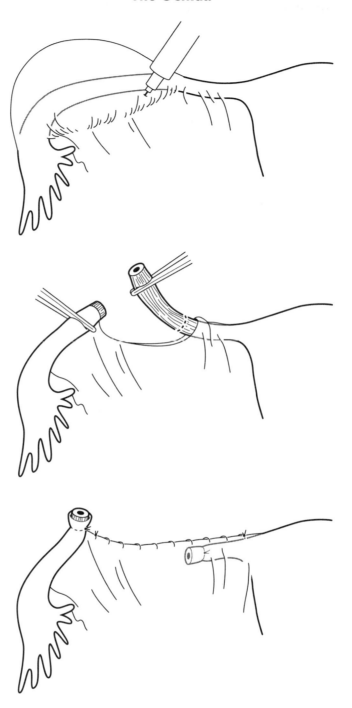

Vasectomy has long been more popular in the U.S. than anywhere else in the world, but why don't more men use it? One explanation is that women have chosen laparoscopic sterilization in increasing numbers. Another is that men have been frightened by reports, often from animal data, of associations with autoimmune diseases, atherosclerosis, and most recently, prostatic cancer. Large epidemiologic studies have failed to confirm any definite adverse consequences.[22] In addition, vasectomy is less expensive than tubal sterilization, morbidity is less, and mortality is essentially zero.

Efficacy of Sterilization

Laparoscopic and minilaparotomy sterilization are not only convenient, they are almost as effective at preventing pregnancy as were the older, more complex operations. Vasectomy is also highly effective once the supply of remaining sperm in the vas deferens is exhausted. After 6 weeks or 15 ejaculations, essentially all men are sterile.

Failure Rates During the First Year, United States[6]

Method	Percent of Women with Pregnancy	
	Lowest Expected	Typical
Female sterilization	0.2%	0.4%
Male sterilization	0.1%	0.15%

Besides the specific operation employed, the skill of the operator and characteristics of the patient make important contributions to the efficacy of female sterilization. Up to 50% of failures are due to technical errors. The methods employing complicated equipment, such as spring-loaded clips and silastic rings, fail for technical reasons more commonly than do simpler procedures such as the Pomeroy tubal ligation.[23] Mini-laparotomy failures, therefore, occur much less frequently from technical errors.

It is hardly surprising that more complicated techniques of tubal occlusion have higher technical failure rates. What is surprising is the finding that characteristics of the patient influence the likelihood of failure even when technical problems are considered. In a careful study of this issue, two patient characteristics, age and lactation, demonstrated a significant impact.[24] Patients younger than 35 years were 1.7 times more likely to become pregnant, and women who were not breastfeeding following sterilization were 5 times more likely to become pregnant. These findings probably reflect the greater fecundity of younger women and the contraceptive contribution of lactation.

Significant numbers of pregnancies after tubal occlusion are present before the procedure. For this reason, some clinicians routinely perform a uterine evacuation or curettage prior to tubal occlusion. It seems more reasonable (and cost effective) to exclude pregnancy by careful history taking, physical examination, and an appropriate pregnancy test prior to the sterilization procedure.[25]

Because method, operator, and patient characteristics all influence sterilization failures, it is difficult to predict which individual will experience a pregnancy after undergoing a tubal occlusion. Therefore, during the course of counseling, all patients should be made aware of the possibility of failure as well as the intent to cause permanent, irreversible sterility. It is important to avoid giving patients the impression that the tubal occlusion procedure is fool proof or guaranteed. Individual clinicians must be cautious judging their own success in accomplishing sterilization because failure is infrequent and many patients who become pregnant after sterilization never reveal the failure to the original surgeon.

Ectopic pregnancies can occur following tubal occlusion, and the incidence is much higher with some types of tubal occlusion. Bipolar tubal coagulation is more likely to result in ectopic pregnancy than is mechanical occlusion.[23,26] The probable explanation is that microscopic fistulae in the coagulated segment connecting to the peritoneal cavity permit sperm to reach the ovum. Ectopic pregnancies following tubal ligation are more likely to occur 2 or more years after sterilization, rather than immediately after. In the first year after sterilization, about 6% of pregnancies will be ectopic, but the majority of pregnancies that occur 2–3 years after occlusion will be ectopic.[27] The rate of intrauterine pregnancies decreases with time, but ectopic rates remain constant. Overall, however, the risk of an ectopic pregnancy in sterilized women is lower than if they had not been sterilized.

Vaginal procedures have higher failure rates than laparoscopy or minilaparotomy, but the principal disadvantage is a higher rate of infection. Intraperitoneal infection is a rare complication of minilap or laparoscopic techniques, but in vaginal procedures, abscess formation approaches 1%.[28] This risk can be reduced by the use of prophylactic antibiotics administered intraoperatively, but open laparoscopy is usually easier and safer than vaginal sterilization even in obese women.

Female Sterilization Techniques

Because laparoscopy permits direct visualization and manipulation of the abdominal and pelvic organs with minimal abdominal disruption, it offers many advantages. Hospitalization is not required; most patients return home within a few hours, and the majority return to full activity within 24 hours. Discomfort is minimal, the incision scars are barely visible, and sexual activity need not be restricted. In addition, the surgeon has an opportunity to inspect the pelvic and abdominal organs for abnormalities. The disadvantages of laparoscopic sterilization include the cost, the expensive, fragile equipment, the special training required, and the risks of inadvertent bowel or vessel injury.

Laparoscopic sterilization can be achieved with any of these methods:

1. Occlusion and partial resection by unipolar electrosurgery.

2. Occlusion and transection by unipolar electrosurgery.

3. Occlusion by bipolar electrocoagulation.

4. Occlusion by mechanical means (clips or silastic rings).

All of these methods can use an operating laparoscope alone, or the diagnostic laparoscope with operating instruments passed through a second trocar, or both the operating laparoscope and secondary puncture equipment. All can be employed using the "open" laparoscopic technique in which the laparoscopic instrument is placed into the abdominal cavity under direct vision to avoid the risk of bowel or blood vessel puncture on blind entry. Patient acceptance and recovery are approximately the same with all methods.

Failure Rates, United States[29]

Pomeroy tubal ligation	4 per 1,000
The Irving tubal ligation	nil
The Uchida tubal ligation	nil
Unipolar electrocoagulation	1 per 1,000
Bipolar electrocoagulation	4 per 1,000
The Hulka-Clemens spring clip	2 per 1,000
The Filshie clip	1 per 1,000
The silastic (Falope or Yoon) ring	4 per 1,000

Tubal Occlusion by Electrosurgical Methods

If electrons from an electrosurgical generator are concentrated in one location, heat within the tissue increases sharply and desiccates the tissue until resistance is so high that no more current can pass. Unipolar methods of sterilization create a dense area of current under the grasping forceps of the unipolar electrode. In order to complete the circuit, however, these electrons must spread through the body and be returned to the generator via a return electrode (the ground plate) that has a broad surface to minimize the density of the current to avoid burns as the electrons leave the body. "Unipolar" refers to the method that requires the patient ground plate.

With the unipolar method, if tissue resistance is high and the electrical pressure (voltage) relatively low, current may cease to flow or may search out alternate pathways with lower resistance. When the voltage is increased, the electrons have more "push" to find another pathway, therefore the surgeon must use the lowest possible voltage necessary to completely coagulate. The return electrode (the ground plate) must be in good contact with the patient.

Unipolar electrosurgery can create a unique electrical "capacitance" problem when an operating laparoscope is used with unipolar forceps. A capacitor is any device that can hold an electric charge, and can exist wherever an insulated material separates two conductors that have different potentials. This property of capacitance explains some of the inadvertent bowel burns that have occurred with laparoscopic sterilization.[30] The operating laparoscope is a hollow metal tube surrounding an active electrode, the forceps used to grasp and coagulate the tubes. When current passes through the active electrode, the laparoscope itself becomes a capacitor. Up to 70% of the current passed through the active electrode can be induced into the laparoscope. Should bowel or other structures touch a laparoscope which is insulated from the abdominal incision (for example, by a fiberglass cannula), the stored electrons will be discharged at high density directly into the vital organ. This potential hazard is eliminated by using a metal trocar sleeve rather than a nonconductive sleeve like fiberglass. Because there is little pressure behind the electrons from a low-voltage generator, not enough heat is generated to burn the skin as the capacitance current leaks out into the patient's body through the sleeve. Even if the active electrode comes in direct contact with the laparoscope, as when a two-incision technique is employed, the current will leak harmlessly through the metal trocar sleeve. The risk of inadvertent coagulation of bowel or other organs cannot be completely eliminated because all body surfaces offer a path back to the ground plate.

The unipolar electrosurgical technique is straightforward. The isthmic portion of the fallopian tube is grasped and elevated away from the surrounding structures, and the electrical energy applied until the tissue blanches, swells, and then collapses. The tube is then grasped, moving toward the uterus, recoagulated, and the steps repeated until 2–3 cm of tube have been coagulated. Some surgeons advise against cornual coagulation for fear it may increase the risk of ectopic pregnancy due to fistula formation.

The coagulation and transection technique is performed in a similar fashion with the same instruments. In order to transect the tube, however, an instrument designed to cut tissue must be utilized. The transection of tissue increases the risk of possible bleeding and does not, by itself, reduce the failure rate over coagulation alone. The specimens obtained by this method are usually coagulated beyond microscopic recognition, and therefore will not provide pathological evidence of successful sterilization.

The bipolar method of sterilization eliminates the ground plate required for unipolar electrosurgery and employs a specially designed forceps. One jaw of the forceps is the active electrode, and the other jaw is the ground electrode. Current density is great at the point of forceps contact with tissue, and the use of a low-voltage, high-frequency current prevents the spread of electrons. By eliminating the return electrode, the chance of an aberrant pathway through bowel or other structures is greatly reduced. There is, however, a disadvantage with this technique. Since electron spread is decreased, more applications of the grasping forceps are necessary to coagulate the same length of tube than with unipolar coagulation. As desiccation occurs at the point of high current density, tissue resistance increases, and the coagulated area eventually provides resistance to flow of the low-voltage current. Should the resistance increase beyond the voltage's capability to push electrons through the tissue, incomplete coagulation of the endosalpinx can result.[31] In addition, the desiccated tissue can adhere to the bipolar forceps, making it difficult to remove from the surface of the tube.

The bipolar method can be used with either a single incision operating laparoscope or with dual incision instruments. The forceps are, however, more delicate than unipolar equipment and must be kept meticulously clean. Damage to the instruments can alter the ability to coagulate, and inadequate or incomplete electrocoagulation is the main cause of failure.

Bipolar cautery is safer than unipolar cautery with regard to burns of abdominal organs, but most studies indicate higher failure rates. Although the bipolar forceps will not burn tissues that are not actually grasped, care must be taken to avoid coagulating structures adherent to the tubes. For example, the ureter can be damaged when the tube is adherent to the pelvic side wall.

Tubal Occlusion with Clips and Rings

Female sterilization by mechanical occlusion eliminates the safety concerns with electrosurgery. However, mechanical devices are subject to flaws in material, defects in manufacturing, and errors in design; all of which can alter efficacy. Three mechanical devices have been widely used and have low failure rates with long-term follow-up: the Hulka-Clemens (spring) clip, the Filshie Clip, and the silastic (Falope or Yoon) ring. Each of the three requires an understanding of its mechanical function, a working knowledge of the intricate applicator necessary to apply the device, meticulous attention to maintenance of the applicators, and skillful tubal placement.

Hulka-Clemens Spring Clip. The spring clip consists of two plastic jaws made of Lexan, hinged by a small metal pin 2 mm from one end. Each jaw has teeth on the opposed surface, and a stainless steel spring is pushed over the jaws to hold them closed over the tube. A special laparoscope for one incision application is most commonly employed, although the spring clip can also be used in a two incision procedure. The spring clip destroys 3 mm of tube and has one-year pregnancy rates of 2 per 1,000 women.[23]

Complications unique to spring clip sterilization result from mechanical difficulties. Should the clip be dislodged or dropped into the abdomen during the procedure, it should be retrieved. Usually it can be removed laparoscopically, but sometimes laparotomy is necessary. Should incomplete occlusion or incorrect alignment of the clip occur, a second clip can be applied without hazard. This clip offers a good chance for reanastomosis, better than electrosurgical methods which destroy more tube.

Filshie Clip. The Filshie clip is made of titanium lined with silicone rubber. The hinged clip is locked over the tube using a special applicator through a second incision or operating laparoscope. The rubber lining of the clip expands on compression to keep the tube blocked. Only 4 mm of the tube is destroyed. Failure rates with the newest model approximate 1 per 1,000 women. Because the Filshie clip is longer, it is reported to occlude dilated tubes more readily than does the spring clip. Both the spring clip and the Filshie clip provide good chances for tubal reanastomosis.

The Hulka-Clemens Spring Clip

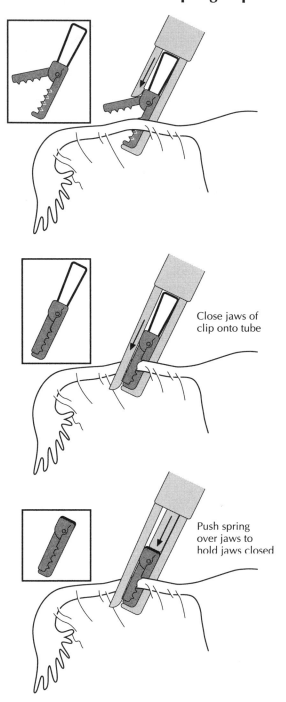

Close jaws of
clip onto tube

Push spring
over jaws to
hold jaws closed

Silastic (Falope or Yoon) Ring. This nonreactive silastic rubber band has an elastic memory of 100% if stretched to no more than 6 mm for a brief time (a few minutes at most). A special applicator, 6 mm in diameter, can be placed through a second cannula or through a standard offset operating laparoscope. The applicator is designed to grasp a knuckle of tube and release the silastic band onto a 2.5 cm loop of tube. The avascular loop of tube can be resected with biopsy forceps to provide a pathology specimen, but this is rarely done (it does not increase efficacy). Ten to 15% of patients experience severe postoperative pelvic cramping from the tight bands (which can be alleviated by the application of a local anesthetic to the tube before or after banding).

The Silastic (Falope-Yoon) Ring

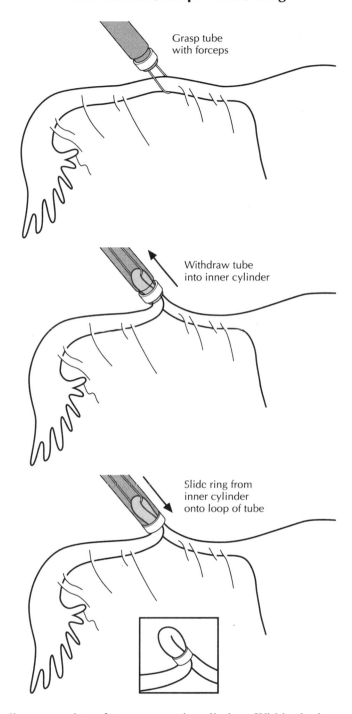

Grasp tube with forceps

Withdraw tube into inner cylinder

Slide ring from inner cylinder onto loop of tube

The ring applicator consists of two concentric cylinders. Within the inner cylinder is a forceps for grasping, elevating, and retracting a segment of the tube. The silastic ring is stretched around the exposed end of the inner cylinder by means of a special ring loader and ring guide. The outer cylinder moves the ring from the inner cylinder on to the tube, a loop of which is held within the inner cylinder by the forceps.

As with application of clips, the ring should be placed at the junction of the proximal and middle third of each fallopian tube. Once the tube is grasped, it is gently withdrawn into the inner cylinder by slowly squeezing the pistol-like handle of the applicator. A final strong pull is needed to slide the ring from the inner applicator cylinder onto the loop of tube. Necrosis occurs promptly and a 2–3 cm segment of the tube is destroyed. Failure rates are about 4 per 1,000 women at one year.[23]

Mesosalpingeal bleeding is the most common complication of silastic ring application. It usually occurs when the forceps grabs not only the tube but also a vascular fold of mesosalpinx. The mesosalpinx can also be torn on the edge of the stainless steel cylinder as the tube is drawn into the applicator. If bleeding is noted, application of the silastic band often controls it. If the placement of additional bands or electrocoagulation fails to stop bleeding, laparotomy may be required.

Silastic rings are occasionally placed on structures other than the tube. If this mistake is recognized, the band can usually be removed from the round ligament or mesosalpingeal folds by grasping the band with the tongs of the applicator and applying gradual, increasing traction. If a gentle attempt fails, removal is not necessary. If rings are inadvertently discharged into the peritoneal cavity, they can safely be left behind.

Patients should be prepared for the use of electrosurgical instruments in case bands or clips cannot be applied (because of adhesions or bleeding).

Minilaparotomy

Tubal ligation accomplished through a small suprapubic incision, "minilaparotomy," is the most frequent method of interval female sterilization around the world. In the U.S. and most of the developed world, laparoscopy is more popular, but minilaparotomy is gaining in favor because of its safety, simplicity, and adaptability to ambulatory surgical settings (particularly when local anesthesia is used).[32]

The fallopian tubes can be occluded through the minilaparotomy incision with bands or clips, but a simple Pomeroy-type tubal ligation is the method most commonly used. Patient characteristics such as obesity, previous pelvic infection, or previous surgery are the principal determinants of complications.[33]

Minilaparotomy is accomplished through an incision that usually measures 3–5 cm in length. Tubal ligation through a suprapubic incision can be accomplished for obese patients, but the incision will necessarily exceed the usual length. Forceful retraction increases the pain associated with the procedure and the time of recovery. For these reasons, we believe that minilaparotomy for ambulatory tubal occlusion should be limited to patients who are not obese (usually less than 150–160 pounds, 70 kg).

Patients who are likely to have adhesions from previous surgery or pelvic infection will probably have a shorter operating and recovery time (and less pain) with open laparoscopic tubal occlusion. In addition, the wide view provided by the laparoscope will make possible a precise description of the pelvic abnormalities that may be useful should the patient develop chronic pelvic pain or recurrent infection.

Tubal occlusion is difficult to accomplish through a minilaparotomy if the uterus is immobile. Laparoscopic tubal occlusion, on the other hand, does not require extreme uterine elevation or rotation and is a better choice for a patient with a uterus fixed in position.

Counseling for Sterilization   All patients undergoing a surgical procedure for permanent contraception should be aware of the nature of the operation, its alternatives, efficacy, safety, and complications. The operation can be described using drawings or pelvic models, as well as films, slides, or video tapes. The description of the operation should emphasize its similarities to and differences from laparoscopy and pelvic surgery, especially hysterectomy or ovariectomy which may be confused with simple tubal ligation. Alternatives, including vasectomy, oral contraception, long-acting hormone methods, barrier methods, and IUDs, should be reviewed. It should be emphasized to the patient that tubal ligation is not intended to be reversible, and that it cannot be guaranteed to prevent intrauterine or ectopic pregnancy. Informed consent is best obtained at a time when a patient is not distracted or distraught, e.g., not immediately before or after a therapeutic abortion.

Sexuality

There is no detrimental effect on sexuality specifically due to sterilization procedures.[34] Indeed, sexual life is usually positively affected. Many couples are less inhibited and more spontaneous in love making when they don't have to worry about an unwanted pregnancy.

Menstrual Function

The effects on menstrual function are less clear and therefore more difficult to explain. The first well-controlled studies of this issue demonstrated no change in menstrual patterns, volume, or pain.[35,36] Subsequently these same authors reported an increase in dysmenorrhea and changes in menstrual bleeding.[37,38] Adding to the confusion, the incidence of hysterectomy for bleeding disorders in women with tubal sterilizations was reported to be increased by some[39] but not by others.[40] On the other hand, in a large cohort of women in a group health plan, hospitalization for menstrual disorders was significantly increased; however, the authors believed this reflected bias by patient and physician preference for surgical treatment.[41] It is possible that extensive electro-coagulation of the fallopian tubes can change ovarian steroid production. Perhaps this is why menstrual changes have been detected with longer (4 years) follow-up, while no changes have been noted with the use of rings or clips.[38,42,43] However, attempts to relate poststerilization menstrual changes with extent of tissue destruction fail to find a correlation.[43] An increase in hospitalization for menstrual disorders after unipolar cautery could not be documented.[41] Still another long-term follow-up study (3–4.5 years) failed to detect any significant changes in menstrual cycles.[44] This inconsistency can reflect differences in sterilization techniques, as well as the fact that a surgical solution is more likely to be chosen if continuing fertility is no longer an issue. More studies with careful attention to the type of tubal occlusion procedure will be necessary. The best answer for now is that some women experience menstrual changes, but most do not. These discordant reports do not make patient counseling about the long-term effects of tubal sterilization an easy task.

Reversibility

An important objective of counseling is to help couples make the right decision about an irreversible decision to become sterile. The active participation of both spouses is a critical factor.[45] Not all couples are pleased following sterilization; in one series, 2% of U.S. women expressed regret one year later and 2.7% after two years.[46] At the two year mark, the main factors associated with regret were age less than 30 and sterilization at the convenient time of a cesarean section. In Europe where tubal sterilization is less common, the most important risk factor for regret was an unstable marriage.[47] A change in marital status is undoubtedly an important reason for a desire to reverse sterilization.[48]

Young women in unstable relationships need special attention in counseling, and both partners should participate in the counseling. Furthermore, for many couples tubal occlusion at the time of cesarean section or immediately after a difficult labor and delivery is not the best time for the procedure. It is important to know that sterilized women have not been observed to develop psychological problems at a greater than expected rate.[49,50]

Microsurgery for tubal reanastomosis is associated with excellent results if only a small segment of the tube has been damaged. Pregnancy rates correlate with the length of remaining tube, a length of 4 cm or more is optimal. Thus, the pregnancy rates are lowest with electrocoagulation, and reach 70–80% with clips, rings, and surgical methods such as the Pomeroy.[51] About 2 per 1,000 sterilized women will eventually undergo tubal reanastomosis.[48]

Male Sterilization: Vasectomy

Vasectomy is safer, easier, and less expensive than female sterilization.[22,52] Hematomas and infection occur rarely and are easily treated with heat, scrotal support, and antibiotics. Most men will develop sperm antibodies following vasectomy, but no long-term sequelae have been observed, including no increased risk of cardiovascular disease.[22] Adverse psychological and sexual effects have not been reported. Since the other constituents of semen are made downstream from the testes, men do not notice a decreased volume or velocity of ejaculate.

Several epidemiologic studies have suggested that vasectomized men subsequently have an increased risk of prostate and testicular cancer, while others have not.[53–56] Because of the rarity of testicular cancer, the studies have been unable to achieve sufficient statistical power. The impressive Nurses' Health Study cohort was able to analyze a cohort of 14,607 vasectomized men.[57,58] There was no relationship apparent between vasectomy and mortality from cancer, and there was no long-term effect on cardiovascular disease. However, an increased risk of nonfatal prostate cancer was observed over time since vasectomy, reaching a relative risk of 1.89 after 20 or more years, in contrast to the negative results of two other cohort studies.[55,56,58] A prospective cohort study of U.S. men again concluded that vasectomy increases the risk of prostate cancer, with an increasing risk over time.[59] An analysis of these studies concluded that these observations are not sufficiently free of bias and confounding factors, and a cause and effect relationship cannot be established.[60] Nevertheless, this controversy is disconcerting and requires review during the informed consent process. Men who have had a vasectomy should follow a preventive program no different than that recommended for all men: annual digital examination and perhaps serial measurement of the prostate antigen level after age 50.

Vasectomy reversal is associated with pregnancy rates greater than 50%. The prospect for pregnancy diminishes with time elapsed from vasectomy, decreasing significantly to 30% after 10 years; the best results are achieved when reversal is performed within 3 years after vasectomy.[61]

Therapeutic Abortion

The number of abortions performed in the United States has remained relatively unchanged since 1980, approximately 1.6 million per year.[62] About 29% of pregnancies not ending in miscarriage or stillbirth are terminated by abortion. American teenagers are especially dependent upon abortion compared to their European counterparts who are better educated about sex and use contraception more often and more effectively. In addition, from ages 20–34, American women have the highest proportion of pregnancies aborted compared to other countries, indicating an unappreciated, but real problem, of unintended pregnancy occurring beyond the teenage years. The lack of perfect contraception and imperfect use of contraception will keep abortion with us.

The proportion of abortions performed in hospitals has steadily declined, reaching 10% in 1988. The proportion handled by specialized abortion clinics increased to 86% by 1988, while the percentage of abortions performed by physicians in their own offices has remained low, about 3–5% of all abortions. More than 50% of abortions are obtained by women younger than 25, with the rate peaking at ages 18–19, and 83% are unmarried.[63]

By 1980, legal abortion became the most common surgical procedure performed in the U.S. Public health authorities have demonstrated that the legalization of abortion reduced maternal morbidity and mortality more than any single development since the advent of antibiotics to treat puerperal infections and blood banking to treat hemorrhage. The number of American women reported as dying from abortion declined from nearly 300 deaths in 1961, to only 6 in 1985 (1 death for every 200,000 legal abortions).[64] For comparison, in 1985, the death rate for childbirth in the U.S. was 10 per 100,000 births and, for ectopic pregnancy, 1 per 2,000 cases.[64]

The most important determinants of abortion mortality are duration of gestation and type of anesthesia: later abortions and general anesthesia are more hazardous.[65] As with mortality, morbidity rates vary primarily with duration of pregnancy, but other factors are important as well, including type of operation, age of patient, type of anesthesia, operator's skill, and method of cervical dilatation.

The possibility that abortion can result in longer-term complications has been examined in over 150 studies.[66] First trimester abortion by vacuum aspiration is not associated with any adverse consequences on the following: subsequent fertility, subsequent pregnancies, or the risk of ectopic pregnancy.[67–71] It is not yet certain if second trimester abortions or multiple first trimester abortions can affect the outcome of later pregnancies.

Preoperative Care of Abortion Patients

The care of the patient who has decided to terminate a pregnancy begins with the diagnosis of intrauterine pregnancy and an accurate estimate of gestational age. Failure to accomplish this is the most common source of abortion complications and subsequent litigation. Tests for pregnancy, including vaginal ultrasound, should be employed when accuracy is difficult.

More than 85% of the abortions performed in the U.S. occur in the first trimester of pregnancy. Morbidity and mortality rates with first trimester abortions are approximately one-tenth those of later abortions. Nearly all women who want to terminate a pregnancy in the first trimester are good candidates for an outpatient procedure under local anesthesia. Possible exceptions include patients with severe cardiorespiratory disease, severe anemias or coagulopathies, mental disorders severe enough to preclude cooperation, and excessive concern about operative pain that is not alleviated by reassurance.

Abortions should not be undertaken for women who have known uterine anomalies or leiomyomata or who have previously had difficult first trimester abortion procedures, unless ultrasonography is immediately available and the surgeon is experienced in its intraoperative use. Previous cesarean section or other pelvic surgery is not a contra-indication to outpatient first trimester abortion.

Counseling Abortion Patients

Counseling has played a critical role in the development of efficient and acceptable abortion services.[72] Whether abortion is accomplished in a clinic, physician's office, or a surgical center, the functions of a counselor must be fulfilled to ensure quality patient care. These include help with decision making, provision of information about the procedure, obtaining informed consent, provision of emotional support for the patient and her family before, during, and after the operation, and providing information about contraception.[73] Referral opportunities should be provided for prenatal care or adoption for women who choose to carry an unplanned pregnancy to term. These responsibilities can be carried out by a physician, nurse, psychologist, social worker, or a trained lay person. An informed consent document should unequivocally state the possibilities of common adverse outcomes such as incomplete abortion, infection, uterine perforation, the need for laparotomy, ectopic pregnancy, and failed abortion. The counselor should document that all preoperative responsibilities have been discharged.

Methods for First Trimester Abortions

The most widely used technique for first trimester abortions is vacuum curettage. The procedure is performed using local anesthesia (a paracervical block). Cervical dilatation is accomplished using tapered dilators (the Pratt dilators). Some surgeons recommend the preoperative insertion of cervical tents. These are osmotic dilators of dried seaweed or synthetic hydrophilic substances left in place from a few hours (synthetic) to overnight (seaweed).[74] RU486, the progesterone antagonist, produces preoperative cervical dilatation equally effectively, and the ease of its single oral dosage makes it a more attractive choice. After the procedure, the patient is observed for 1–2 hours before returning home.

Since September, 1988, RU486 has been available as a medical abortifacient in France and China, and more recently it has become available in other countries. RU486 (the trade name is Mifepristone) is a synthetic relative of the progestational agents in birth control pills. It acts primarily, but not totally, as an antiprogestational agent. RU486 is administered together with a prostaglandin analogue. The combination allows a reduction in dosage of both agents. When administered early in pregnancy, this medical treatment carries with it a success and complication rate similar to that achieved with vacuum curretage.[75] Misoprostol is a stable, orally active synthetic analogue of prostaglandin E_1, available commercially for the treatment of peptic ulcer. By itself it is very ineffective for therapeutic abortion, but combined with RU486 it provides an effective, simple, inexpensive, completely oral method.[76,77]

It is likely that abortion with RU486 is the result of multiple actions. Although RU486 does not induce labor, it does open and soften the cervix (this may be an action secondary to endogenous prostaglandins). Its major action is its blockade of progesterone receptors in the endometrium. This leads to a disruption of the embryo and the production of prostaglandins. The disruption of the embryo and perhaps a direct action on the trophoblast lead to a decrease in human chorionic gonadotropin (HCG) and a withdrawal of support from the corpus luteum. The success rate is dependent upon the length of pregnancy — the more dependent the pregnancy is upon progesterone from the corpus luteum, the more likely the progesterone antagonist, RU486, will result in abortion. The combined RU486-prostaglandin analogue method is usually restricted to pregnancies that are not beyond 9 weeks gestation.

Complications of Abortions

Postoperative complications of elective abortions are classified as either immediate or delayed. Uterine perforation and uterine atony are examples of immediate complications. Delayed complications can occur several hours to several weeks after the operation. These usually present according to the major complaint: bleeding, pain, and continuing symptoms of pregnancy.

Bleeding

By far the most common cause of unusually heavy postabortal bleeding is retained products of conception. Rates in large series vary from 0.2 to 0.6%.[78] Patients with retained products of conception occasionally present several weeks after an abortion, but most report excessive bleeding within one week. Severe pain or pelvic tenderness suggests that infection is also present. Treatment is prompt aspiration of the uterus with the largest cannula that will pass the cervix.

Infection

Infection is sometimes marked by uterine bleeding; although without retained products of conception, the volume of blood loss is usually modest. Fever and uterine tenderness are the most common signs of postabortal endometritis, occurring in about 0.5% of cases.[78] Some studies indicate that prophylactic antibiotics reduce the risk of postabortal infection. Most clinicians agree that women at high risk for pelvic infection (e.g., previous episodes of salpingitis or postabortal endometritis) benefit from the use of prophylactic antibiotics prior to abortion, but some believe that all abortion patients should have prophylactic antibiotics.[79]

Patients who present with uterine tenderness, fever, and bleeding require uterine re-aspiration as well as antibiotic treatment. Patients who have fevers above 38°C (101°F) and signs of peritoneal inflammation, as well as uterine tenderness, require hospitalization and intravenous antibiotics active against anaerobes, gonorrhea, and chlamydia. Outpatient treatment with doxycycline, 100 mg bid for 14 days, should be reserved for patients whose signs and symptoms are confined to the uterus.

Dysfunctional Uterine Bleeding Following Abortion

Women may present with uterine bleeding but without signs or symptoms of retained products of conception or infection. When these two diagnoses have been ruled out by absence of fever, a closed cervix, and a nontender uterus, the bleeding itself can be treated hormonally. Curettage is rarely necessary unless bleeding is excessive.

Ectopic Pregnancy

Failure to diagnose ectopic pregnancy at the time of therapeutic abortion can cause a patient to return with complaints of persistent bleeding with or without pelvic pain. Careful examination of the uterine aspirate for villi at the time of abortion should make a missed ectopic pregnancy an unusual cause of delayed bleeding. If, however, a patient presents with this possibility, quantitative measurement of chorionic gonadotropin and vaginal ultrasonography should be utilized for accurate diagnosis and management.

Cervical Stenosis

Patients who experience amenorrhea or hypomenorrhea and cyclic uterine pain after first trimester abortion may have stenosis of the internal os. This condition occurs in about 0.02% of cases and is more common among women whose abortions are performed in the early first trimester with a minimum of cervical dilatation and a small diameter, flexible plastic cannula. Possibly the tip of this type of cannula abrades the internal os and the minimal dilatation allows the abraded areas to heal in contact. The condition is easily treated with cervical dilatation with Pratt dilators under paracervical block.

Other Late Complications

Amenorrhea, usually without pain, can also be caused by Asherman's syndrome, destruction and scarification of the endometrium. This condition is very rare and usually follows endometrial infection. This problem is best diagnosed and treated at hysteroscopy.

Sensitization of Rh negative women should be prevented. Approximately 4% of these women become sensitized following an induced abortion (the later the abortion the higher the proportion). Subsequent hemolytic disease of the newborn can be prevented by administering 50 μg Rh immune globulin to all Rh negative, Du negative women undergoing early abortion. The standard dose is administered for second trimester abortion.

**Abortion in the
Second Trimester**

Second trimester abortions can be accomplished surgically or medically. The surgical procedure is termed dilatation and evacuation (D and E). Several approaches have been utilized for the medical termination of pregnancy. These include the vaginal, intramuscular, or intramniotic administration of prostaglandins and the intraamniotic injection of hypertonic saline or urea. The D and E procedure is safer and less expensive than the medical methods and is better tolerated (and thus preferred) by patients.[80,81]

The training, experience, and skills of the surgeon are the primary factors which limit the gestational age at which abortion can be safely performed. Advanced gestational age by itself incurs increased risks for all types of complications. These are multiplied when the duration of pregnancy is discovered, after beginning uterine evacuation, to be beyond the experience and skill of the surgeon or capacity of the equipment. Uterine perforation, infection, bleeding, amniotic fluid embolism, and anesthetic reactions are increased as gestational age increases.[80]

When errors in estimating gestational age require the surgeon to use unfamiliar instruments or techniques that are not frequently practiced, the increased duration of the procedure can cause problems. Efforts to sedate or relieve pain by administering additional drugs increase the risk of toxic reactions or overdosage. If a change from local to general anesthesia is undertaken, the patient is at much greater risk of anesthetic complications. Finally, if complications caused by advanced gestational age necessitate transfer of the patient to physicians who are not familiar with uterine evacuation techniques, the patient may undergo unnecessarily extensive surgery, such as hysterectomy, with all the risks inherent in emergency procedures.

Preoperative cervical dilatation with osmotic dilators makes first trimester abortion safer and easier and is essential for second trimester abortion. Local anesthesia instead of general anesthesia also makes abortion safer.[82,83] Some patients are not good candidates for surgical procedures of any kind under local anesthesia, and others may have special reasons to prefer that an abortion be performed under general anesthesia. Patient requests should be seriously considered, but the clinician also has a responsibility to inform the patient of the risks and benefits of local versus general anesthesia.

In the United Kingdom, prostglandin analogues are favored for a noninvasive method of second trimester abortion. A combination of the progesterone antagonist, RU486, (a single oral 200 mg dose of mifepristone administered 36 hours before prostaglandin treatment) and an E prostaglandin analogue (gemeprost) placed vaginally is highly effective, and the combination allows a lesser dose of both agents which results in fewer side effects.[84] In addition this combination does not require the use of cervical laminaria for dilatation.

References

1. **Djerassi C,** *The Politics of Contraception, Vol I. The Present,* Stanford Alumni Association, Stanford, California, 1979.

2. **Westoff CF,** Unintended pregnancy in America and abroad, Fam Plann Perspect 20:254, 1988.

3. **Rimpela A, Rimpela MK, Kosunen EA-L,** Use of oral contraceptives by adolescents and its consequences in Finland 1981-91, Br Med J 305:1053, 1992.

4. **Trussell J, Hatcher RA, Cates W Jr, Stewart FH, Kost K,** A guide to interpreting contraceptive efficacy studies, Obstet Gynecol 76:558, 1990.

5. **Trussell J, Hatcher RA, Cates W Jr, Stewart FH, Kost K,** Contraceptive failure in the United States: an update, Stud Fam Plann 21:51, 1990.

6. **Mosher WD, Pratt WF,** Contraceptive use in the United States, 1973–88, Advance data from vital and health statistics, No. 182, National Center for Health Statistics, Hyattsville, Maryland, 1990.

7. **Mosher WD,** Use of family planning services in the United States: 1982 and 1988, Advance data from vital and health statistics, No. 184, National Center for Health Statistics, Hyattsville, Maryland, 1990.

8. **Ortho Pharmaceutical Corporation,** Annual birth control study, 1993.

9. **Diczfalusy E,** The worldwide use of steroidal contraception, Int J Fertil 34 (Supplement):56, 1989.

10. **Potts M, Rosenfield A,** The fifth freedom revisited: I. Background and existing programs, Lancet 336:1227, 1990.

11. **Forrest JD, Singh S,** Public-sector savings resulting from expenditures for contraceptive services, Fam Plann Perspect 22:6, 1990.

12. **Forrest JD, Singh S,** The impact of public-sector expenditures for contraceptive services in California, Fam Plann Perspect 22:161, 1990.

13. **Spencer G,** Projections of the population of the United States, by age, sex, and race: 1983–2080. Current Population Reports — Population Estimates and Projections, US Department of Commerce, Series P-25, No. 952, Government Printing Office, Washington DC, 1984.

14. **Westoff CF,** Fertility in the United States, Science 234:554, 1986.

15. **Spencer G,** Projections of the population of the United States by age, sex and race: 1988-2080, Current Population Reports 1989, Series P-25, No. 1018, Government Printing Office, Washington, DC, 1989.

16. **Mastroianni L Jr, Donaldson PJ, Kane TT,** editors, *Developing New Contraceptives: Obstacles and Opportunities,* National Academy Press, Washington, DC, 1990.

17. **Speert H,** *Obstetric and Gynecologic Milestones,* The Macmillan Company, New York, 1958, pp 619-629.

18. **Lungren SS,** A case of cesarean section twice successfully performed on the same patient, with remarks on the time, indications, and details of the operation, Am J Obstet 14:78, 1881.

19. **Centers for Disease Control,** Surgical sterilization surveillance: tubal sterilization 1976-1978, 1981.

20. **Layde PM, Ory HW, Peterson HB, Scally MJ, Greenspan JR, Smith JC, Fleming D,** The declining lengths of hospitalization for tubal sterilizations, JAMA 245:714, 1981.

21. **Escobedo LG, Peterson HB, Grubb GS, Franks AL,** Case fatality rates for tubal sterilization in U.S. hospitals, Am J Obstet Gynecol 160:147, 1989.

22. **Peterson HB, Huber DH, Belker AM,** Vasectomy: an appraisal for the obstetrician-gynecologist, Obstet Gynecol 76:568, 1990.

23. **Chi IC, Laufe L, Gardner SD, Tolbert M,** An epidemiologic study of risk factors associated with pregnancy following female sterilizations, Am J Obstet Gynecol 136:768, 1980.

24. **Cheng M, Wong YM, Rochat R, Ratnam SS,** Sterilization failures in Singapore: an examination of ligation techniques and failure rates, Stud Fam Plann 8:109, 1977.

25. **Lichterg E, Laff S, Friedman E,** Value of routine dilatation and curretage at the time of interval sterilization, Obstet Gynecol 67:763, 1986.

26. **McCausland A,** High rate of ectopic pregnancy following laparoscopic tubal coagulation failure, Am J Obstet Gynecol 136:977, 1980.

27. **Chi IC, Laufe LE, Atwed R,** Ectopic pregnancy following female sterilization procedures, Adv Plann Parenthood 16:52, 1981.

28. **Miesfeld R, Gaarontans R, Moyers T,** Vaginal tubal ligation. Is infection a significant risk? Am J Obstet Gynecol 137:183, 1980.

29. **Population Information Program,** Minilaparotomy and laparoscopy: safe, effective, and widely used, Johns Hopkins University, Population Reports, C-9, 1985.

30. **Centers for Disease Control,** Deaths following female sterilization with unipolar electro-coagulating devices, MMWR 30:150, 1981.

31. **Soderstrom RM, Levy BS, Engel T,** Reducing bipolar sterilization failures, Obstet Gynecol 74:60, 1989.

32. **McCann M, Cole L,** Laparoscopy and minilaparotomy: two major advances in female sterilization, Stud Fam Plann 11:119, 1980.

33. **Layde PM, Peterson HB, Dicker RC, DeStefano F, Rubin GL, Ory HW,** Risk factors for complications of interval tubal sterilization by laparotomy, Obstet Gynecol 62:180, 1983.

34. **Kjer J,** Sexual adjustment to tubal sterilization, Eur J Obstet Gynecol 35:211, 1990.

35. **Rulin MC, Turner JH, Dunworth R, Thompson D,** Post tubal sterilization syndrome: a misnomer, Am J Obstet Gynecol 151:13, 1985.

36. **DeStefano F, Huezo CM, Peterson HB, et al,** Menstrual changes after tubal sterilization, Obstet Gynecol 62:673, 1983.

37. **Rulin MC, Davidson AR, Philliber SG, Graves WL, Cushman LF,** Changes in menstrual symptoms among sterilized and comparison women: a prospective study, Obstet Gynecol 79:749, 1989.

38. **DeStefano F, Perlman J, Peterson HB, Diamond E,** Long-term risk of menstrual disturbances after tubal sterilization, Am J Obstet Gynecol 152:835, 1985.

39. **Kjer J, Knudsen L,** Hysterectomy subsequent to laparoscopic sterilization, Eur J Obstet Gynecol 35:63, 1990.

40. **Stergachis A, Shy KK, Gouthaus LC, Wagner EH, Hecht JA, Anderson G, Normand EH, Raboud J,** Tubal sterilization and the long-term risk of hysterectomy, JAMA 264:2893, 1990.

41. **Shy KK, Stergachis A, Grothaus LG, Wagner EH, Hecth J, Anderson G,** Tubal sterilization and risk of subsequent hospital admission for menstrual disorders, Am J Obstet Gynecol 166:1698, 1992.

42. **Thranov I, Hertz JB, Kjer JJ, Andresen A, Micic S, Nielsen J, Hancke S,** Hormonal and menstrual changes after laparoscopic sterilization by Falope-rings or Filshie-clips, Fertil Steril 57:751, 1992.

43. **Wilcox LS, Martinez-Schnell B, Peterson HB, Ware JH, Hughes JM,** Menstrual function after tubal sterilization, Am J Epidemiol 135:1368, 1992.

44. **Rulin MC, Davidson AR, Philliber SG, Graves WL, Cushman LF,** Long-term effect of tubal sterilization on menstrual indices and pelvic pain, Obstet Gynecol 82:118, 1993.

45. **Miller WB, Shain RN, Pasta DJ,** Tubal sterilization or vasectomy: how do married couples make the decision? Fertil Steril 56:278, 1991.

46. **Grubb G, Refoser H, Layde PM, Rubin GL,** Regret after decision to have a tubal sterilization, Fertil Steril 44:248, 1985.

47. **Vemer HM, Colla P, Schoot DC, Willensen WN, Bierkens PB, Rolland R,** Women regretting their sterilization, Fertil Steril 46:724, 1986.

48. **Wilcox LS, Chu SY, Peterson HB,** Characteristics of women who considered or obtained tubal reanastomosis: results from a prospective study of tubal sterilization, Obstet Gynecol 75:661, 1990.

49. **Vessey M, Huggins G, Lawless M, McPherson K, Yeates D,** Tubal sterilization: findings in a large prospective study, Br J Obstet Gynaecol 90:203, 1983.

50. **World Health Organization,** Mental health and female sterilization: report of a WHO collaborative study, J Biosoc Sci 16:1, 1984.

51. **Siegler AM, Hulka J, Peretz A,** Reversibility of female sterilization, Fertil Steril 43:499, 1985.

52. **Smith GL, Taylor GP, Smith KF,** Comparative risks and costs of male and female sterilization, Am J Public Health 75:370, 1985.

53. **Strader CH, Weiss NS, Daling JR,** Vasectomy and the incidence of testicular cancer, Am J Epidemiol 128:56, 1988.

54. **Mettlin G, Natarajan N, Huben R,** Vasectomy and prostate cancer risk, Am J Epidemiol 132:1056, 1990.

55. **Sidney S, Quesenberry CP Jr, Sadler MC, Guess HA, Lydick EG, Cattolica EV,** Vasectomy and the risk of prostate cancer in a cohort of multiphasic health-checkup examinees: second report, Cancer Causes Control 2:113, 1991.

56. **Nienhuis H, Goldacre M, Seagroatt V, Gill L, Vessey M,** Incidence of disease after vasectomy: a record linkage retrospective cohort study, Br Med J 304:743, 1992.

57. **Giovannucci E, Tosteson TD, Speizer FE, Vessey MP, Colditz GA,** A long-term study of mortality in men who have undergone vasectomy, New Engl J Med 326:1392, 1992.

58. **Giovannucci E, Tosteson TD, Speizer FE, Ascherio A, Vessey MP, Colditz GA,** A retrospective cohort study of vasectomy and prostate cancer in US men, JAMA 269:878, 1993.

59. **Giovannucci E, Ascherio A, Rimm EB, Colditz GA, Stampfer MJ, Willett WC,** A prospective cohort study of vasectomy and prostate cancer in US men, JAMA 269:873, 1993.

60. **Howards SS, Peterson HB,** Vasectomy and prostate cancer: chance, bias, or a causal relationship? JAMA 269:913, 1993.

61. **Belker AM, Thomas AJ, Fuchs EF, Konnak JM, Sharlip ID,** Results of 1,469 microsurgical vasectomy reversals by the vasovasostomy group, J Urol 145:505, 1991.

62. **Henshaw SK, Van Vort J,** Abortion services in the United States, 1987 and 1988, Fam Plann Perspect 22:102, 1990.

63. **Henshaw SK,** Induced abortion: a world review, 1990, Fam Plann Perspect22:76, 1990.

64. **Lawson H, Atrash HK, Safflas A, Finch EL,** Ectopic pregnancy surveillance, United States, 1970-1986, Abortion surveillances, 1984–1985. MMWR 38:11, 1989.

65. **Buehler J, Schulz KF, Grimes DA, Hogue C,** The risk of serious complications from induced abortion: do personal characteristics make a difference? Am J Obstet Gynecol 153:14, 1985.

66. **Hogue CJ,** Impact of abortion on subsequent fecundity, Clin Obstet Gynecol 13:95l, 1986.

67. **Stubblefield P, Monson R, Schoenbaum S, et al,** Fertility after induced abortion: A prospective follow-up study, Obstet Gynecol 62:186, 1984.

68. **Daling J, Weiss N, Voigt L, Spadoni L, Soderstrom R, Moore DE, Stadel BV,** Tubal infertility in relation to prior induced abortion, Fertil Steril 43:389, 1985.

69. **Schoenbaum S, Monson R, Stubblefield P, Darney PD, Ryan KJ,** Outcome of the delivery following an induced or spontaneous abortion, Am J Obstet Gynecol 136:19, 1980.

70. **Daling J, Chow W, Weiss N, Metch BJ, Soderstrom R,** Ectopic pregnancy in relation to previous induced abortion, JAMA 253:1005, 1985.

71. **Frank PI, McNamee R, Hannaford PC, Kay RK, Hirsch S,** The effect of induced abortion on subsequent pregnancy outcome, Br J Obstet Gynaecol 98:1015, 1991.

72. **Landy U, Lewit S,** Administrative, counseling, and medical practices in National Abortion Federation facilities, Fam Plann Perspect 14:257, 1982.

73. **Landy U,** Abortion counselling — A new component of medical care, Clin Obstet Gynecol 13:33, 1986.

74. **Darney PD, Atkinson E, Hirabayashi K,** Uterine perforation during second trimester abortion by cervical dilation and instrumental extraction: a review of 15 cases, Obstet Gynecol 75:441, 1990.

75. **Silvestre L, Dubois C, Renault M, Rezvani Y, Baulieu EE, Ulmann A,** Voluntary interruption of pregnancy with Mifepristone (RU 486) and a prostaglandin analogue, New Engl J Med 322:645, 1990.

76. **Thong KJ, Baird DT,** Induction of abortion with mifepristone and misoprostol in early pregnancy, Br J Obstet Gynaecol 99:1004, 1992.

77. **Peyron R, Aubeny E, Targosz V, Silvestre L, Renault M, Elkik F, Leclerc P, Ulmann A, Baulieu EE,** Early termination of pregnancy with mifepristone (RU 486) and the orally active prostaglandin misoprostol, New Engl J Med 328:1509, 1993.

78. **Hakim-Elahi E, Tovell HM, Burnhill MS,** Complications of first trimester abortion: a report of 170,000 cases, Obstet Gynecol 76:929, 1990.

79. **Darj E, Stralin EB, Nilsson S,** The prophylactic effect of doxycycline on postoperative infection rate after first trimester abortion, Obstet Gynecol 70:755, 1987.

80. **Peterson WF, Berry FN, Grace MR, Gulbranson CL,** Second-trimester abortion by dilatation and evacuation: an analysis of 11,747 cases, Obstet Gynecol 62:185, 1983.

81. **Kafrissen M, Schulz K, Grimes D, Cates W Jr,** Midtrimester abortion: intra amniotic instillation of hyperosmolar urea and prostaglandin $F_{2\alpha}$ vs dilatation and evacuation, JAMA 251:916, 1984.

82. **Mackay T, Schulz K, Grimes D,** Safety of local versus general anesthesia for second trimester dilatation and evacuation abortion, Obstet Gynecol 66:661, 1985.

83. **Atrash HK, Check T, Hogue CJ,** Legal abortion and general anesthesia, Am J Obstet Gynecol 158:420, 1988.

84. **Thong KJ, Baird DT,** A study of gemeprost alone, dilapan, or mifepristone in combination with gemeprost for the termination of second trimester pregnancy, Contraception 46:11, 1992.

22 Oral Contraception

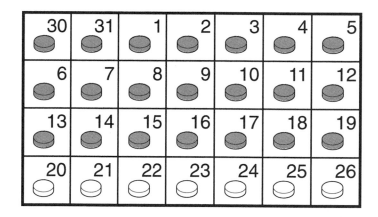

I t wasn't until the early 1900s that inhibition of ovulation was observed to be linked to pregnancy and the corpus luteum. Ludwig Haberlandt, professor of physiology at the University of Innsbruck, Austria, was the first to demonstrate that ovarian extracts given orally could prevent fertility (in mice).[1,2] In the 1920s, Haberlandt and a Viennese gynecologist, Otfried Otto Fellner, were administering steroid extracts to a variety of animals and reporting the inhibition of fertility. By 1931, Haberlandt was proposing the administration of hormones for birth control. An extract was produced, named Infecundin, ready to be used, but Haberlandt's early death in 1932, at age 47, brought an end to this effort. Fellner disappeared after the fall of Austria to Hitler.

The concept was ennunciated by Haberlandt, but steroid chemistry wasn't ready. The extraction and isolation of a few milligrams of the sex steroids required starting points measured in gallons of urine or thousands of pounds of organs. Edward Doisy processed 80,000 sow ovaries to produce 12 mg estradiol.

The supply problem was solved by an eccentric chemist, Russell E. Marker, who completed his thesis, but not his course work, for his Ph.D. After leaving school, Marker worked with the Ethyl Gasoline Corporation, and in 1926, developed the process of octane rating, based on the discovery that knocking in gasoline was due to hydrocarbons with an uneven number of carbons.

From 1927 to 1935, Marker worked at the Rockefeller Institute, publishing a total of 32 papers on configuration and optical rotation as a method of identifying compounds. In 1935, he moved to Pennsylvania State University where he trained himself in steroid chemistry and became interested in solving the problem of producing abundant and cheap amounts of progesterone. At that time it required the ovaries from 2,500 pregnant pigs to produce 1 mg progesterone. In 1939, Marker became convinced that the solution to the problem of obtaining large quantities of steroid hormones was to find plants (in the family that includes the lily, the agave, and the yam) which contained sufficient amounts of sapogenin, a plant steroid which could be used as a starting point for steroid hormone synthesis. This conviction was strengthened with his discovery that a species of *Trillium*, known locally as Beth's root, was collected in North Carolina and used in the preparation of Lydia Pinkham's Compound, popular at the time to relieve menstrual troubles. The active ingredient in Beth's root was diosgenin, a plant steroid.

Marker organized extensive botanical expeditions in the Southwest and Mexico, sending home more than 100,000 pounds of material. In 1942, he collected the roots of the Mexican yam, and back in Pennsylvania, he worked out the degradation of diosgenin to progesterone. United States pharmaceutical companies refused to back Marker, and even the university refused, despite Marker's urging, to patent the process.

In 1943, Marker resigned from Pennsylvania State University and went to Mexico where he collected the roots of *Dioscorea mexicana,* 10 tons worth! In an old pottery shed in Mexico City, he prepared several pounds of progesterone (worth $600,000) in two months. This progesterone gained him entry to Hormone Laboratories in Mexico City. The two partners in Hormone Laboratories and Marker formed a company that they called Syntex. The price of progesterone fell from $200 to $2 a gram.

In 1947, true to his eccentric nature, Marker had a falling out with his partners and sold his share of the company, retiring to Pennsylvania to devote the rest of his life to making replicas of antique works in silver. However, he took his knowhow with him. Fortunately for Syntex, he had published a scientific description of his process, and there still was no patent on his discoveries. Syntex recruited George Rosenkranz, a Hungarian immigrant living in Cuba, to reinstitute the commercial manufacture of progesterone (and testosterone) from Mexican yams, a task that took him 2 years.

In 1949, it was discovered that cortisone relieved arthritis, and the race was on to develop an easy and cheap method to synthesize cortisone. Carl Djerassi joined Syntex to work on this synthesis using the Mexican yam plant steroid diosgenin as the starting point. This was quickly achieved (in 1951), but soon after, an even better method of cortisone production was discovered at Upjohn using microbiologic fermentation. This latter method used progesterone as the starting point, and therefore Syntex found itself as the key supplier to other companies for this important process, at the rate of 10 tons of progesterone per year and a price of 48 cents per gram.

Djerassi and other Syntex chemists then turned their attention to the sex steroids. They discovered that the removal of the 19 carbon from yam-derived progesterone increased the progestational activity of the molecule. Ethisterone had been available for a dozen years, and the Syntex chemists reasoned that removal of the 19 carbon would increase the progestational potency of this orally active compound. In 1951, norethindrone was synthesized; the patent for this drug is the only patent for a drug listed in the National Inventor's Hall of Fame. Two years later, G.D. Searle & Company filed a patent for norethynodrel.

Gregory Pincus of the Worcester Foundation for Experimental Biology in Massachusetts had been studying mammalian fertilization for many years.[3] He attributed his shift of interest to contraception to a visit from Margaret Sanger in 1951. Sanger, president of the International Planned Parenthood Federation, provided a research grant of $2,100 for animal research, and pointed out that Pincus' animal experiments suggested a method of oral contraception for women.

Both the Syntex and Searle compounds (norethindrone and norethynodrel) were tested in animals in 1953–1954 by Gregory Pincus, John Rock, and colleagues, and in the first human trial, in 1956, with the help of Edris Rice-Wray, a pioneer in family planning who was working at the time in Puerto Rico. The initial progestin products were contaminated with about 1% mestranol. In the amounts being used, this added up to 50–500 micrograms mestranol, a sufficient amount of estrogen to inhibit ovulation by itself. When efforts to lower the estrogen content yielded breakthrough bleeding, it was decided to retain the estrogen for cycle control, thus establishing the principle of the combined estrogen-progestin oral contraceptive.

Pincus, a long-time consultant to Searle, picked the Searle compound for extended use. Syntex, a wholesale drug supplier, was without marketing experience or organization. Pincus with great effort convinced Searle that the commercial potential of an oral contraceptive warranted the risk of possible negative public reaction. By the time Syntex had secured arrangements with Ortho for a sales outlet, Searle marketed Enovid in 1960 (150 µg mestranol and 9.85 mg norethynodrel). Ortho-Novum using norethindrone from Syntex appeared in 1962. Wyeth Laboratories introduced norgestrel in 1968, the same year in which the first reliable prospective studies were initiated. It was not until the late 1970s that a dose-response relationship between problems and the amount of steroids in the pill was appreciated. As a result, health care providers and patients, over the years, have been confronted by a bewildering array of different products and formulations. The solution to this clinical dilemma is relatively straightforward: use the lowest doses that provide effective contraception.

The Steroid Components of Oral Contraceptives

The Estrogen Component

Estradiol is the most potent natural estrogen and the major estrogen secreted by the ovaries. The major obstacle to the use of sex steroids for contraception was inactivity of the compounds when given orally. A major breakthrough occurred in 1938 when it was discovered that the addition of an ethinyl group at the 17 position made estradiol orally active. Ethinyl estradiol is a very potent oral estrogen and is one of the two forms of estrogen in every oral contraceptive. The other estrogen is the 3-methyl ether of ethinyl estradiol, mestranol.

Mestranol and ethinyl estradiol are different from natural estradiol and must be regarded as pharmacologic drugs. Animal studies have suggested that mestranol is weaker than ethinyl estradiol, because mestranol must first be converted to ethinyl estradiol in the body. Indeed, mestranol will not bind to the estrogen receptor. Therefore, unconjugated ethinyl estradiol is the active estrogen in the blood for both mestranol and ethinyl estradiol. In the human body, differences in potency between ethinyl estradiol and mestranol do not appear to be significant, certainly not as great as indicated by assays in rodents. This is now a minor point since all of the low dose oral contraceptives contain ethinyl estradiol.

The metabolism of ethinyl estradiol (particularly as reflected in blood levels) varies significantly from individual to individual and from one population to another.[4] There is even a range of variability at different sampling times within the same individual. Therefore, it is not surprising that the same dose can cause side effects in one individual and none in another.

Ethinyl estradiol   Mestranol

The estrogen content (dosage) of the pill is of major clinical importance. Thrombosis is one of the most serious side effects of the pill, playing a key role in the increased risk of death from a variety of circulatory problems. This side effect is related to estrogen, and it is dose related. Therefore, the dose of estrogen is a critical issue in selecting an oral contraceptive.

The Progestin Component

The discovery of ethinyl substitution and oral potency led (at the end of the 1930s) to the preparation of ethisterone, an orally active derivative of testosterone. In 1951, it was demonstrated that removal of the 19 carbon from ethisterone to form norethindrone did not destroy the oral activity, and, most importantly, it changed the major hormonal effect from that of an androgen to that of a progestational agent. Accordingly, the progestational derivatives of testosterone were designated as 19-nortestosterones (denoting the missing 19 carbon). The androgenic properties of these compounds, however, were not totally eliminated, and minimal anabolic and androgenic potential remains within the structure.

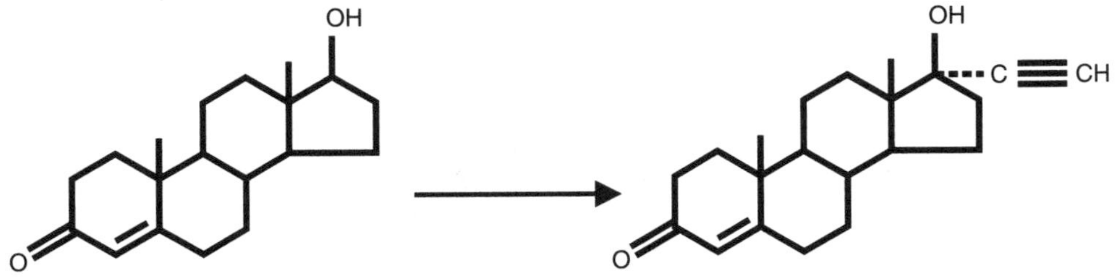

Testosterone → Ethisterone

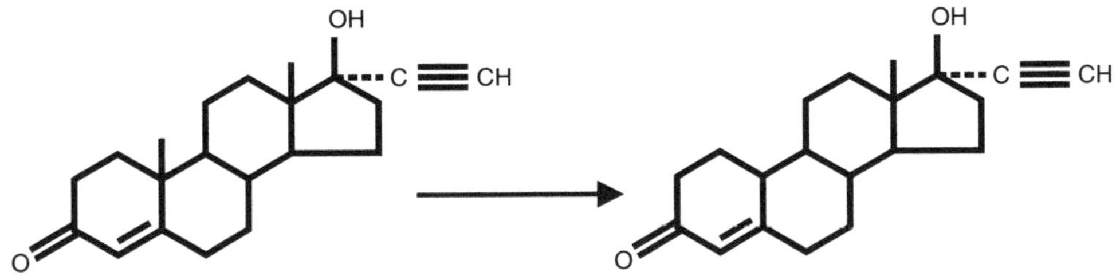

Ethisterone → Norethindrone

The "impurity" of 19-nortestosterones, i.e., androgenic as well as progestational effects, was further complicated in the past by a belief that they were metabolized within the body to estrogenic compounds. This question was restudied, and it was argued that the previous evidence for metabolism to estrogenic compounds was due to an artifact in the laboratory analysis. More recent studies indicate that norethindrone can be converted to ethinyl estradiol. However, the rate of this conversion is so low that insignificant amounts of ethinyl estradiol can be found in the circulation or urine following the administration of the commonly used doses of norethindrone.[5] Any estrogenic activity, therefore, would have to be due to a direct effect activating the estrogen receptor mechanism. In animal and human studies, however, only norethindrone, norethynodrel, and ethynodiol diacetate have estrogen activity, and it is very slight due to weak binding to the estrogen receptor.[6] Clinically, androgenic and estrogenic activities of the progestin component are insignificant because of the low dosage in the current oral contraceptives. As with the estrogen component, serious side effects have been related to the high doses of progestins used in old formulations, not the particular progestin, and routine use of

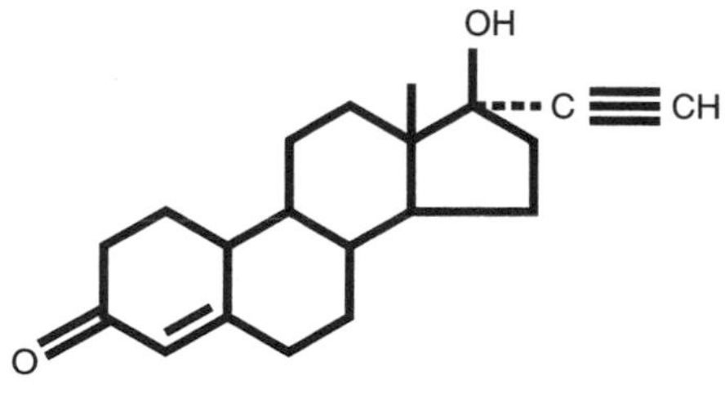

Norethindrone

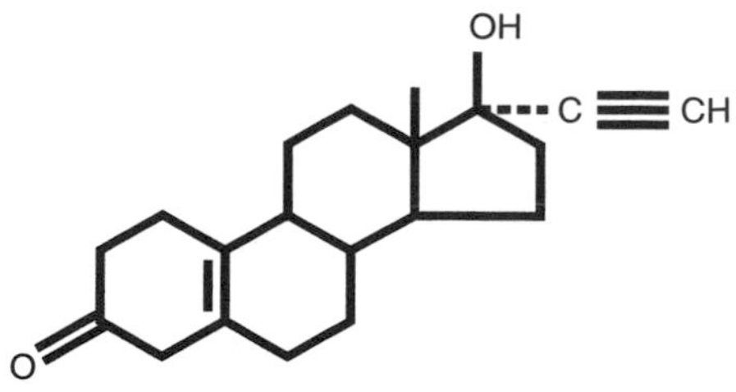

Norethynodrel

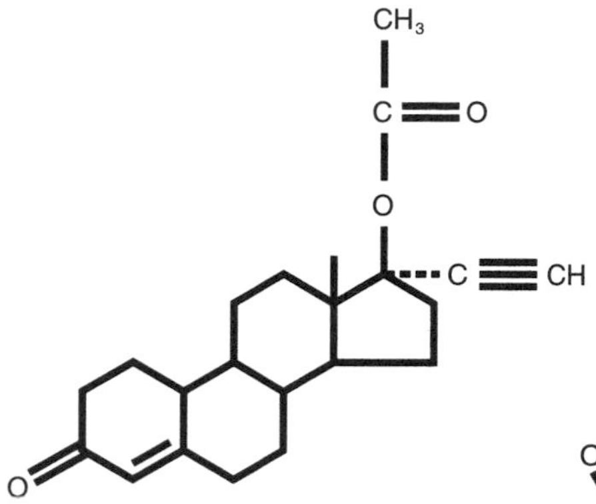

Norethindrone acetate

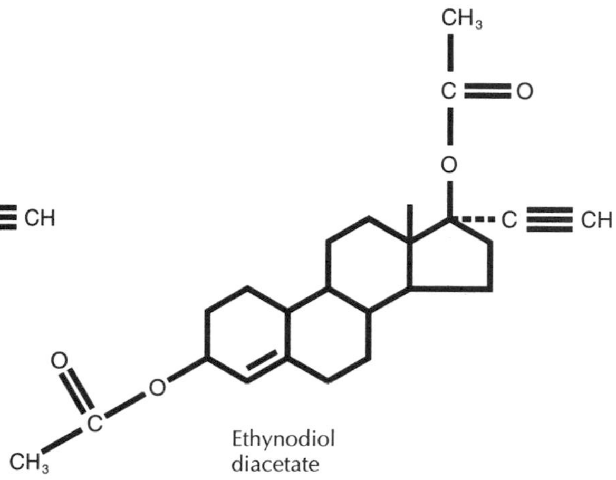

Ethynodiol diacetate

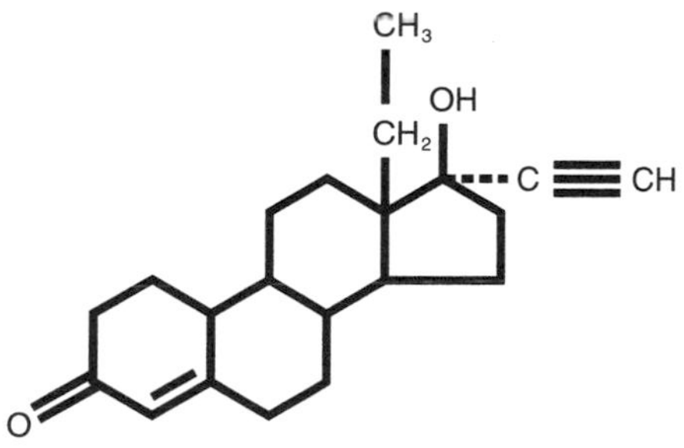

Levonorgestrel

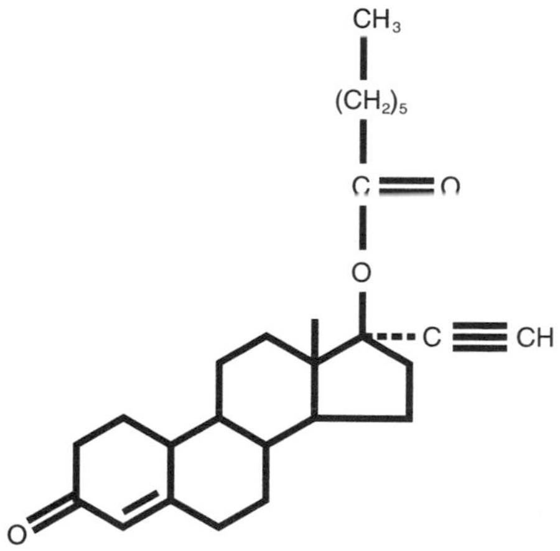

Norethindrone enanthate

oral contraceptives should now be limited to the low dose products.

The norethindrone family contains the following 19-nortestosterone progestins: norethindrone, norethynodrel, norethindrone acetate, ethynodiol diacetate, lynestrenol, norgestrel, norgestimate, desogestrel, and gestodene.

Most of the progestins closely related to norethindrone are converted to the parent compound. Thus the activity of norethynodrel, norethindrone acetate, ethynodiol diacetate, and lynestrenol is due to rapid conversion to norethindrone.

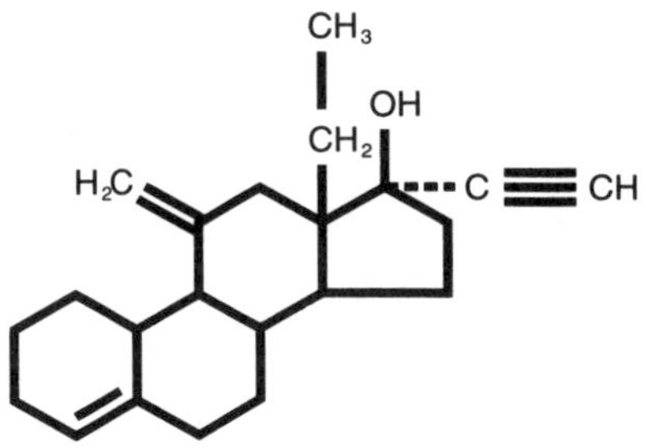

Desogestrel

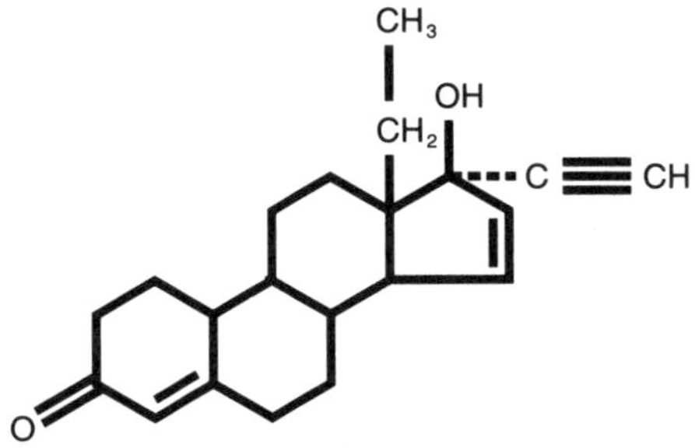

Gestodene

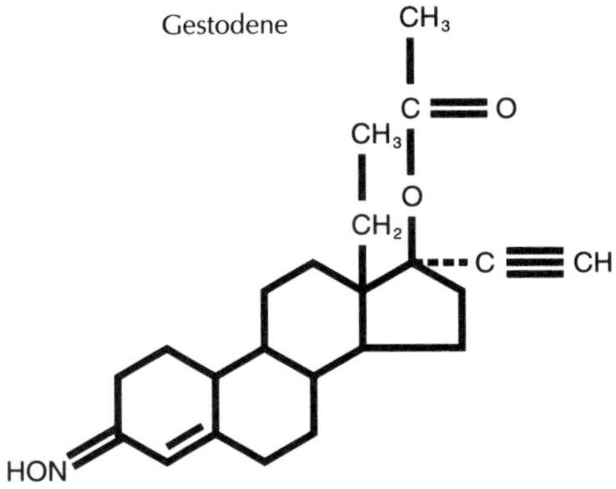

Norgestimate

Norgestrel is a racemic equal mixture of the dextrorotatory enantiomer and the levorotatory enantiomer. These enantiomers are mirror images of each other and rotate the plane of polarized light in opposite directions. The dextrorotatory form is known as *d*-norgestrel, and the levorotatory form is *l*-norgestrel (known as levonorgestrel). Levonorgestrel is the active isomer of norgestrel.

Desogestrel undergoes two metabolic steps before the progestational activity is expressed in its active metabolite, 3-keto-desogestrel. This metabolite differs from levonorgestrel only by a methylene group in the 11 position.

Gestodene differs from levonorgestrel by the presence of a double bond between carbons 15 and 16; thus it is Δ^{15} gestodene. It is metabolized into many derivatives with progestational activity, but not levonorgestrel.

Several metabolites contribute to the activity of norgestimate, including 17-deacetylated norgestimate, 3-keto norgestimate, and levonorgestrel.

A second group of progestins became available for use when it was discovered that acetylation of the 17-hydroxy group of 17-hydroxyprogesterone produced an orally active but weak progestin. An addition at the 6 position is necessary to give sufficient

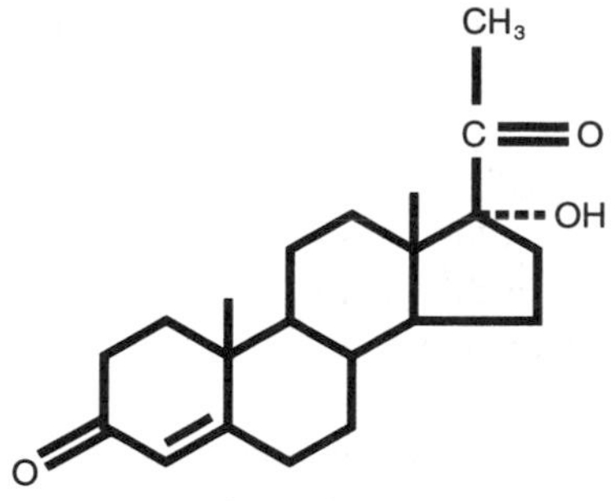

CH$_3$
|
C$=$O
OH

17α-Hydroxyprogesterone

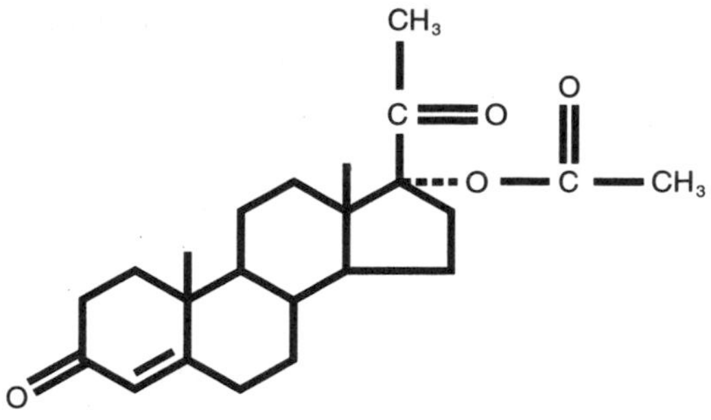

CH$_3$
|
C$=$O   O
‖
O$-$C$-$CH$_3$

17-Acetoxy progesterone

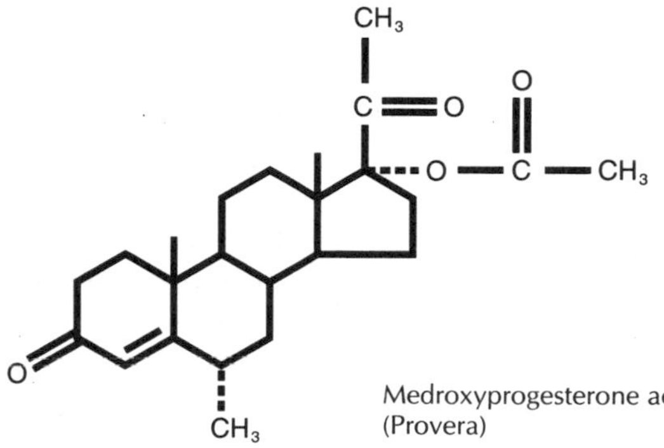

CH$_3$
|
C$=$O   O
‖
O$-$C$-$CH$_3$

Medroxyprogesterone acetate
(Provera)

progestational strength for human use, probably by inhibiting metabolism. Derivatives of progesterone with substituents at the 17 and 6 positions include the widely used medroxyprogesterone acetate.

The New Progestins

Probably the greatest influence on the effort that yielded the new progestins was the belief throughout the 1980s that androgenic metabolic effects were important, especially in terms of cardiovascular disease. Cardiovascular side effects are now known to be due to a dose-related stimulation of thrombosis by estrogen. In the search to find compounds which minimize androgenic effects, however, the pharmaceutical companies succeeded.

The new progestins include desogestrel, gestodene, and norgestimate.[7] With the combined products containing the new progestins, the changes in the coagulation system are very similar to those with the current low dose formulations. A slight prothrombotic effect is characterized by increased levels of fibrinopeptide A that is balanced by antithrombin III and protein C. Thus any coagulation tendency is counteracted. The protime and the activated partial thromboplastin time measure the overall activity of the coagulation pathways — there is no significant increase in these measurements with the new formulations. In a controversial issue, it has been argued that gestodene affects the pharmocokinetics of ethinyl estradiol differently, causing higher circulating levels of the estrogen component. Intense evaluation of this issue, however, has failed to reveal any effects unique to gestodene.[8]

In regard to cycle control (breakthrough bleeding and amenorrhea), the new formulations are comparable to existing low dose products.

All progestins derived from 19-nortestosterone have the potential to decrease glucose tolerance and increase insulin resistance. The impact of the current low dose formulations is very minimal, and the impact of the new progestins is negligible. Most changes are not statistically significant, and when they are, they are so subtle as to be of no

721

clinical significance. For example, there are no changes in hemoglobin A1c.

The decreased androgenicity of the progestins in the new products is reflected in increased sex hormone binding globulin and decreased free testosterone concentrations to a greater degree than the older established oral contraceptives. This difference may be of greater clinical value in the treatment of acne and hirsutism, but whether a better clinical response is possible is yet to be documented in clinical studies.

The new progestins, because of their reduced androgenicity, predictably do not adversely affect the cholesterol-lipoprotein profile. Indeed, the estrogen-progestin balance of combined oral contraceptives containing one of the new progestins may even promote favorable lipid changes. Thus, the new formulations have the potential to offer protection against cardiovascular disease, an important consideration as we enter an era of women using oral contraceptives for longer durations and later in life. But one must be cautious regarding the clinical significance of subtle changes, and it will be a long time before epidemiologic data on this issue are available.

Potency

For many years, clinicians, scientists, medical writers, and even the pharmaceutical industry have attempted to assign potency values to the various progestational components of oral contraceptives. An accurate assessment, however, has been difficult to achieve for many reasons. Progestins act on numerous target organs (e.g., the uterus, the mammary glands, and the liver), and potency varies depending upon the target organ and endpoint being studied. In the past, animal assays, such as the Clauberg test and the rat ventral prostate assay, were used to determine progestin potency. While these were considered acceptable methods at the time, a better understanding of steroid hormone action and metabolism, and a recognition that animal and human responses differ, have led to greater reliance upon data collected from human studies.

Historically, this has been a confusing issue because publications and experts used potency ranking to provide clinical advice. There is absolutely no need for confusion. Oral contraceptive progestin potency is no longer a consideration when it comes to prescribing oral contraception, because the potency of the various progestins has been accounted for by appropriate adjustments of dose. In other words, the biologic effect (in this case the clinical effect) of the various progestational components in current low dose oral contraceptives is approximately the same. The potency of a drug does not determine its efficacy or safety, only the amount of a drug required to achieve an effect.

Clinical advice based on potency ranking is an artificial exercise that has not stood the test of time. There is no clinical evidence that a particular progestin is better or worse in terms of particular side effects or clinical responses. Thus oral contraceptives should be judged by their clinical characteristics: efficacy, side effects, risks, and benefits. Our progress in lowering the doses of the steroids contained in oral contraceptives has yielded products with little serious differences. Potency is no longer an important clinical issue.

Multiphasic Formulations

The multiphasic preparations alter the dosage of both the estrogen and progestin components periodically throughout the pill-taking schedule. The aim of these formulations is to alter steroid levels in an effort to achieve fewer metabolic effects and minimize the occurrence of breakthrough bleeding and amenorrhea, while maintaining efficacy. We are probably at or very near the lowest dose levels which can be achieved without sacrificing efficacy. Metabolic studies with the multiphasic preparations indicate no differences or slight improvements over the metabolic effects of low dose monophasic products. From a clinical point of view, there are no outstanding advantages or disadvantages comparing multiphasic formulations to low dose monophasic products.

Mechanism of Action

The combination oral contraceptive, consisting of the estrogen and progestin components, is given daily for 3 out of every 4 weeks. The combination oral contraceptive prevents ovulation by inhibiting gonadotropin secretion via an effect on both pituitary and hypothalamic centers. The progestational agent primarily suppresses luteinizing hormone (LH) secretion (and thus prevents ovulation), while the estrogenic agent suppresses follicle-stimulating hormone (FSH) secretion (and thus prevents the selection and emergence of a dominant follicle). Therefore, the estrogenic component significantly contributes to the contraceptive efficacy. However, even if follicular growth and development were not sufficiently inhibited, the progestational component would prevent the surge-like release of LH necessary for ovulation.

The estrogen in the oral contraceptive serves two other purposes. It provides stability to the endometrium so that irregular shedding and unwanted breakthrough bleeding can be minimized, and the presence of estrogen is required to potentiate the action of the progestational agents. The latter function of estrogen has allowed reduction of the progestational dose in the oral contraceptive. The mechanism for this action is probably estrogen's effect in increasing the concentration of intracellular progestational receptors. Therefore, a certain pharmacologic level of estrogen is necessary to maintain the potency of the combination oral contraceptive.

Since the effect of a progestational agent will always take precedence over estrogen (unless the dose of estrogen is increased many, many fold), the endometrium, cervical mucus, and perhaps tubal function reflect progestational stimulation. The progestin in the combination pill produces an endometrium which is not receptive to ovum implantation, a decidualized bed with exhausted and atrophied glands. The cervical mucus becomes thick and impervious to sperm transport. It is possible that progestational influences on secretion and peristalsis within the fallopian tubes provide additional contraceptive effects.

Efficacy

With this variety of contraceptive actions, it is hard to understand how the omission of a pill or two can result in a pregnancy. Indeed, careful review of failures suggests that pregnancies usually occur because initiation of the next cycle is delayed allowing escape from ovarian suppression. Strict adherence to 7 pill-free days is critical in order to obtain reliable, effective contraception. For this reason, the 28-day pill package, incorporating 7 pills that do not contain steroids, is a very useful aid to assure adherence to the necessary schedule.

The contraceptive effectiveness of the new progestin and multiphasic formulations are unequivocally comparable to the older low dose (less than 50 µg estrogen) and higher dose monophasic combination birth control pills. While carefully monitored studies with motivated subjects achieve an annual failure rate of 0.1%, typical usage is associated with a 3.0% failure rate during the first year of use.[9] Efficacy decreases significantly when the estrogen component is removed, and only a small dose of the progestin is administered (the progestin-only minipills).

Metabolic Effects of
Oral Contraception

Cardiovascular Disease

In the 1970s, data emerged from two major British prospective cohort studies (the Royal College of General Practitioners [RCGP] study and the Oxford/Family Planning Association [OFPA] study) derived from experience with high dose oral contraceptives (greater than 50 µg estrogen). These reports indicated increased risks for venous thrombosis, myocardial infarction, and stroke. In response to these reports, lower dose formulations (less than 50 µg estrogen) came to dominate the market, and clinicians become more careful in their screening of patients and prescribing of oral contraception. For these reasons, the Walnut Creek study and the Puget Sound study in the United States did not find an increased risk of myocardial infarction with the use of oral contraceptives.[10,11]

It was not until the early 1980s that it became apparent that the major mortality risk was in smokers over the age of 35, and nonsmokers without risk factors for vascular disease could expect the benefits of oral contraception to outweigh the risks. Mortality data using the current low dose pills support this favorable outlook.[11,12]

A review of the massive Medicaid data in the state of Michigan confirms the fact that the risk of venous thrombosis is increased at the 50 µg dose.[13] It is still unknown whether a risk of thrombosis persists at the lower doses. A case-control study of all 794 women in Denmark who suffered a cerebral thromboembolic attack during 1985–1989 concluded that there was an increased relative risk (1.8) associated with oral contraceptives containing 30–40 µg estrogen.[14] Whether the conclusion of this retrospective case-control study (which relied upon questionnaires) is real or not must be verified by the ongoing cohort studies. An analysis of fatal venous thromboembolism in England and Wales between 1986 and 1988 failed to find a statistically significant increase in the relative risk for current users of oral contraceptives.[15]

Studies of the blood coagulation system have concluded that both monophasic and multiphasic low dose oral contraceptives have no significant clinical impact on the coagulation system. Slight increases in thrombin formation are offset by increased fibrinolytic activity.[16,17]

Today, the rare young woman on oral contraception who has a thrombotic episode probably represents someone with an underlying clotting problem, an individual who shows an extreme response to oral contraceptives, or an individual with an unknown lesion of a vessel wall or an unknown local disturbance of circulation. The minimal risk of thrombosis associated with oral contraceptive use does not justify the cost of routine screening for deficiencies in the coagulation system. If a patient develops a thrombotic complication while taking oral contraceptives, an evaluation to search for an underlying abnormality in the coagulation system is warranted (measurement of antithrombin III, protein C, protein S, activated partial thromboplastin time, fibrinogen, and plasminogen).

There is no evidence of an increase in risk of cardiovascular disease among past users of oral contraception.[18–20] Part of the concern for a possible lingering effect of oral contraceptive use was based upon a presumed adverse impact on the atherosclerotic process which would then be added to the effect of aging and thus would be manifested later in life. Instead, the findings are consistent with the contention that cardiovascular disease due to oral contraception is secondary to acute effects, specifically estrogen-induced thrombosis, a dose-related event.

The balance of estrogen and progestin potency in a given oral contraceptive formulation can potentially influence cardiovascular risk by its overall effect on lipoprotein levels. Studies of low dose formulations indicate that the adverse effects of progestins are limited to the fixed dose combination with levonorgestrel, a dose of levonorgestrel that exceeds that in the multiphasic formulation. If certain oral contraceptives had a negative impact on the lipoprotein profile, one would expect to find evidence of atherosclerosis as a cause of an increase in subsequent cardiovascular disease. There is no such evidence. Thus, the mechanism of the cardiovascular complications is undoubtedly a short-term acute mechanism, thrombosis (an estrogen-related effect). Indeed, a case-control study indicated that the risk of myocardial infarction in patients taking levonorgestrel-containing formulations is the same as that experienced with pills containing other progestins.[21]

An important study in monkeys has indicated a protective action of estrogen against atherosclerosis, but by a mechanism independent of the cholesterol-lipoprotein profile. Oral administration of a combination of estrogen and progestin to monkeys fed a high cholesterol, atherogenic diet decreased the extent of coronary atherosclerosis despite a reduction in HDL-cholesterol levels.[22] In considering the impact of progestational agents, lowering of HDL is not necessarily atherogenic if accompanied by other significant estrogen effects. These animal studies help explain why older, higher dose combinations which had an adverse impact on the lipoprotein profile did not increase subsequent cardiovascular disease. The estrogen component provided protection through a direct effect on vessel walls. Perhaps the low dose combinations will even be associated with a favorable impact on the risk of cardiovascular disease.

The first epidemiologic data on this issue derived from low dose oral contraception come from Finland and England. Preliminary analysis of cardiovascular deaths among women under 40 years of age in Finland indicates a statistically significant reduction in low dose oral contraceptive users in the relative risk of myocardial infarction and stroke.[23] In England, studies from the RCGP and OFPA now report no increased risk in *current* users, as previously indicated in studies of higher dose pills.[24] A case-control study of fatal strokes in England and Wales found no statistically significant increase in risk of stroke with low dose oral contraceptives; however, the statistical power was limited because of the relatively small number of stroke cases under the age of 40.[25] The numbers are still small, and the reports still cannot establish whether the reduced risk is due to lower doses or better screening.

These conclusions have significant bearing on the choice of a contraceptive. It certainly is a good pharmacologic principle to utilize a medication with the least impact on normal physiology. However, if this impact is so subtle that it is clinically insignificant, then this issue is of relatively little importance when it comes to selecting an oral contraceptive. Current evidence suggests there is no advantage or disadvantage associated with any of the current low dose formulations in regards to cardiovascular disease. However, it seems prudent to avoid the higher doses of progestins such as 150–250 µg levonorgestrel. The low doses of levonorgestrel (such as in the multiphasic formulations) do not have an adverse impact on the lipid profile.

The new oral contraceptive formulations contain the new progestins: desogestrel, gestodene, and norgestimate. The metabolic effects of these new products are minimal to negligible. It is even possible that the estrogen balance of combined oral contraceptives with the new progestins can promote favorable lipid changes and protect against cardiovascular disease. It will be a long time, however, before epidemiologic data will reveal the clinical impact, if any, of subtle metabolic changes.

Hypertension

Oral contraceptive-induced hypertension was observed in approximately 5% of users of higher dose pills. More recent evidence indicates that small increases in blood pressure can be observed even with 30 μg estrogen, monophasic pills, including those containing the new progestins. However, an increased incidence of clinically significant hypertension has not been reported.[26,27] No significant clinical changes in blood pressure have been noted with any of the multiphasic formulations. It is possible for an occasional patient to experience an idiosyncratic reaction and develop hypertension; therefore, an annual assessment of blood pressure is still an important element of clinical surveillance, even when low dose oral contraceptives are used. Variables such as previous toxemia of pregnancy or previous renal disease do not predict whether a woman will develop hypertension on oral contraception.[28] Likewise, women who have developed hypertension on oral contraception are not more predisposed to develop toxemia of pregnancy.

Carbohydrate Metabolism

With the older high dose oral contraceptives, an impaired glucose tolerance test was present in many women. In these women, plasma levels of insulin as well as the blood sugar were elevated. Generally the effect of oral contraception is to produce an increase in peripheral resistance to insulin action. Most women can meet this challenge by increasing insulin secretion, and there is no change in the glucose tolerance test.

Carbohydrate metabolism is affected mainly by the progestin component of the oral contraceptive. The derangement of carbohydrate metabolism may also be affected by estrogen influences on lipid metabolism, hepatic enzymes, and elevation of unbound cortisol. The glucose intolerance is dose-related, and once again effects are less with the low dose formulations. Insulin and glucose changes with low dose monophasic and multiphasic oral contraceptives are so minimal, that it is now believed that they are of no clinical significance.[29] This includes long-term evaluation with hemoglobin A1c. The one exception is the claim that the levonorgestrel monophasic has an excessively negative impact.

Because long-term, follow-up studies of large populations have failed to detect any increase in the incidence of diabetes mellitus or impaired glucose tolerance (even in past and current users of high dose pills),[30,31] the concern now focuses on the slight impairment as a potential risk for cardiovascular disease. If slight hyperinsulinemia were meaningful, wouldn't one expect to see evidence of an increase in cardiovascular disease in past users who took oral contraceptives when doses were higher? Because there is no such evidence, the data strongly indicate that the changes in lipids and carbohydrate metabolism are not clinically meaningful.

It can be stated definitively that oral contraceptive use does not produce an increase in diabetes mellitus.[30,31] The hyperglycemia associated with oral contraception is not deleterious and is completely reversible. Even women who have risk factors for diabetes in their history do not seem to be affected. In a large study of women with recent gestational diabetes, no significant impact could be demonstrated over 6–13 months comparing a low dose monophasic and a multiphasic to a control group.[32] A high percentage of women with previous gestational diabetes develop overt diabetes and associated vascular complications. Until overt diabetes develops, it is appropriate for these patients to use low dose oral contraception.

In clinical practice, it may, at times, be necessary to prescribe oral contraception for the overt diabetic. The effect on insulin requirement is neither consistent nor predictable, but one would expect little, if any, change with low dose pills. According to the epidemiologic data, the use of oral contraceptives increases the risk of thrombosis in women with insulin-dependent diabetes mellitus; therefore, women with diabetes should be encouraged to use other forms of contraception. However this effect in women under age 35 who are otherwise healthy is probably very minimal with low dose oral contraception, and reliable protection against pregnancy is a benefit for these patients that outweighs the small risk.

Other Effects

In early reports the incidence of gallstones increased after the first 2 years of use, with a return to the level of the control group after 4 years. The latest data, however, have indicated that this apparent increase was due to an acceleration of gallbladder disease in women already susceptible.[33] In other words, the overall risk of gallbladder disease is not increased, but in the first years of use disease is activated or accelerated in women who are vulnerable because of asymptomatic disease or a tendency toward gallbladder disease. The mechanism appears to be induced alterations in the composition of gallbladder bile, specifically a rise in cholesterol saturation that is presumably an estrogen effect. One anticipates a lesser effect in the forthcoming reports describing the impact of low dose oral contraceptives. Keep in mind that while studies have found a statistically significant modest increase in the relative risk of gallbladder disease, because the actual incidence of this problem is low, the effect is of minimal clinical importance.

The only absolute hepatic contraindication to oral contraceptive use is acute or chronic cholestatic liver disease. Cirrhosis and previous hepatitis are not aggravated. Once recovered from the acute phase of liver disease, a woman can use oral contraception.

Nausea, breast discomfort, and weight gain continue to be disturbing effects, but their incidence is significantly less with low dose oral contraception. Fortunately, these effects are most intense in the first few months of use and, in most cases, gradually disappear. Weight gain usually responds to dietary restriction, but for some patients, the weight gain is an anabolic response to the sex steroids, and discontinuation of oral contraception is the only way that weight loss can be achieved. This must be rare with low dose oral contraception because the data in published studies fail to indicate a difference in body weight between users and nonusers. There is no association between oral contraception and peptic ulcer disease or inflammatory bowel disease.[34,35] Oral contraception is not recommended for patients with problems of gastrointestinal malabsorption because of the possibility of contraceptive failure.

Chloasma, a patchy increase in facial pigment, was, at one time, found to occur in approximately 5% of oral contraceptive users. It is now a rare problem due to the decrease in estrogen dose. Unfortunately, once chloasma appears, it fades only gradually following discontinuation of the pill and may never disappear completely. Skin blanching medications may be useful.

Hematologic effects include an increased sedimentation rate due to increased levels of fibrinogen, increased total iron binding capacity due to the increase in globulins, and a decrease in prothrombin time. The continuous use of oral contraceptives may prevent the appearance of symptoms in porphyria precipitated by menses. Changes in vitamin metabolism have been noted: a small nonharmful increase in vitamin A and decreases in blood levels of pyridoxine (B_6) and the other B vitamins, folic acid, and ascorbic acid. Despite these changes, routine vitamin supplements have not been shown to be of benefit for women eating adequate, normal diets.

Mental depression is very rarely associated with oral contraceptives. In studies with higher dose oral contraceptives, the effect was due to estrogen interference with the synthesis of tryptophan that could be reversed with pyridoxine treatment. It seems wiser, however, to discontinue oral contraception if depression is encountered. Though infrequent, a reduction in libido is occasionally a problem and may be a cause for seeking an alternative method of contraception.

Because estrogen is known to stimulate prolactin secretion and to cause hypertrophy of the pituitary lactotrophs, it was appropriate to be concerned over a possible relationship between oral contraception and prolactin-secreting pituitary adenomas. Several case-control studies have uniformly concluded that no such relationship exists. Previous use of oral contraceptives is not related to the size of prolactinomas at presentation and diagnosis.[36] Oral contraception can be prescribed to patients with pituitary micro-adenomas without fear of subsequent tumor growth.[37]

Oral Contraception and Cancer

Cancer of the Endometrium

The use of oral contraception protects against endometrial cancer. Use for at least 12 months reduces the risk of developing endometrial cancer by *50%*, with the greatest protective effect gained by use for more than 3 years.[38,39] This protection persists for 15 or more years after discontinuation (the actual length of duration of protection is unknown) and is greatest in women at highest risk: nulliparous and low parity women. This protection is equally protective for all 3 major histologic subtypes of endometrial cancer: adenocarcinoma, adenoacanthoma, and adenosquamous cancers. Finally, protection is seen with all monophasic formulations of oral contraceptives, including pills with less than 50 μg estrogen. There are no data as yet with multiphasic preparations or the new progestin formulations, but since these products are still dominated by their progestational component, there is every reason to believe that they will be protective.

Cancer of the Ovary

Protection against ovarian cancer, the most lethal of female reproductive tract cancers, is one of the most important benefits of oral contraception. Because this cancer is detected late and prognosis is poor, the impact of this protection is very significant. The risk of developing epithelial ovarian cancer in users of oral contraception is reduced by *40%* compared to that of nonusers.[40,41] This protective effect increases with duration of use (taking 5–10 years to become apparent) and continues for at least 10–15 years after stopping the medication. This protection is seen in women who use oral contraception for as little as 3 to 6 months, reaches an 80% reduction in risk with more than 10 years of use, and is a benefit associated with all monophasic formulations, including the low dose formulations. Again, the multiphasic and new progestin products have not been in use long enough to yield any data on this issue, but because ovulation is effectively inhibited by these formulations, protection against ovarian cancer should be exerted.

Cancer of the Cervix

Studies have indicated that the risk for dysplasia and carcinoma-in-situ of the uterine cervix increases with the use of oral contraception for more than one year.[42–44] Invasive cervical cancer may be increased after 5 years of use, reaching a two-fold increase after 10 years. It is well recognized, however, that the number of partners a woman has had and age at first coitus are the most important risk factors for cervical neoplasia. Other confounding factors include exposure to human papillomavirus, the use of barrier contraception (protective), and smoking. These are difficult factors to control, and therefore, the conclusions regarding cervical cancer are not definitive. An excellent study from the Centers for Disease Control and Prevention (CDC) concluded there is no increased risk of invasive cervical cancer in uses of oral contraception, and an apparent increased risk of carcinoma-in-situ is due to enhanced detection of disease (because oral contraceptive users have more frequent Pap smears).[45] On the other hand, an excellent case-control study of patients in Panama, Costa Rica, Colombia, and Mexico concluded that there is a minimal risk for invasive squamous cell carcinoma, but there is a significantly increased risk for invasive adenocarcinoma.[46]

This concern obviously is an important reason for annual Pap smear surveillance. Fortunately, steroid contraception does not mask abnormal cervical changes, and the necessity for prescription renewals offers the opportunity for improved screening for cervical disease. It is reasonable to perform Pap smears every 6 months in women using oral contraception for 5 or more years who are also at higher risk because of their sexual behavior (multiple partners, history of sexually transmitted diseases).

Tumors of the Liver

Hepatocellular adenomas can be produced by steroids of both the estrogen and androgen families. Actually, there are two different lesions, peliosis and adenomas. Peliosis is characterized by dilated vascular spaces without endothelial lining and may occur in the absence of adenomatous changes. The adenomas are not malignant; their significance lies in the potential for hemorrhage. The most common presentation is acute right upper quadrant or epigastric pain. The tumors may be asymptomatic, or they may present suddenly with hematoperitoneum. There is some evidence that the tumors regress when oral contraception is stopped. Epidemiologic data have not supported the contention that mestranol increased the risk more than ethinyl estradiol.

The risk appears to be related to duration of oral contraceptive use and to the steroid dose in the pills. This is reinforced by the rarity of the condition ever since low dose oral contraception became available. The ongoing prospective studies have accumulated many woman-years of use and have not identified a single case of such a tumor.

No reliable screening test or procedure is currently available. Routine liver function tests are normal. Computed tomography (CT) scanning may be the best means of diagnosis; angiography and ultrasonography are not reliable. Palpation of the liver should be part of the periodic evaluation in oral contraceptive users. If an enlarged liver is found, oral contraception should be stopped, and regression should be evaluated and followed by CT scan.

Oral contraception has been linked to the development of hepatocellular carcinoma. However, the very small number of cases, and thus the limited statistical power, requires great caution in interpretation. The largest study on this question, the World Health Organization Collaborative Study of Neoplasia and Steroid Contraceptives, found no association between oral contraception and liver cancer.[47] In the United States, the death rates from liver cancer have not changed over the last 3 decades despite introduction and widespread use of oral contraception.

Cancer of the Breast

Because of its prevalence and its long latent phase, concern over the relationship between oral contraception and breast cancer continues to be an issue in the minds of both patients and clinicians. Unfortunately, the issue is not resolved and probably will not be until another decade passes, until data emerge from the modern era of lower dose oral contraception.

Worth emphasizing is the protective effect of higher dose oral contraception on benign breast disease, an effect that becomes apparent after 2 years of use.[48] After 2 years there is a progressive reduction (about 40%) in the incidence of fibrocystic disease of the breast. Women who used oral contraception were one-fourth as likely to develop benign breast disease as nonusers, but this protection was limited to current and recent users. It is still unkown whether this same protection is provided by the lower dose products.

The RCGP,[49] OFPA,[50] and Walnut Creek[10] cohort studies (and more recently, the Nurses' Health Study[51]) indicated no significant differences in breast cancer rates between users and nonusers. However, patients were enrolled in these studies at a time when oral contraception was used primarily by married couples spacing out their children. By the 1980s, oral contraception was primarily being used by women early in life, for longer durations, and to delay an initial pregnancy (remember, a full-term pregnancy early in life protects against breast cancer).

Over the last decade, case-control studies have focused on the use of oral contraception early in life, for long duration, and to delay a first, full-term pregnancy. Because the cohort of women who have used oral contraception in this fashion is just now beginning to reach the ages of postmenopausal breast cancer, the studies had to examine the risk of breast cancer diagnosed before age 45 (only 13% of all breast cancer). The results of these studies have not been clear-cut. The most impressive finding indicates a link in most studies[52-58] but not all,[59,60] of early breast cancer before age 40 in women who used oral contraception for long durations of time.

The Centers for Disease Control study is the largest case-control study on the subject.[61-63] No overall increased risk of breast cancer was found in women using oral contraceptives before the age of 20 with a duration of use greater than 4 years, before the age of 25 with a duration of use greater than 6 years, or with greater than 4 years use before a first pregnancy. In addition, no overall increased risk of breast cancer was found among any subgroups of users including women with benign breast disease or a family history of breast cancer.

In further analysis of the CDC study, there was no increased risk associated with any specific type of oral contraceptive, progestin only pills, or the use of 2 or more types. In addition, there was no increased risk associated with any specific progestin or estrogen component, and, most importantly, it was demonstrated that long-term use (15 or more years) was not associated with an increased risk of breast cancer. The reliability of the CDC study is reinforced by the fact that the data confirmed the previously identified risk factors, such as nulliparity, late age at first birth, history of benign breast disease, and a family history of breast cancer. Thus far, the CDC study has found no evidence for a latent effect (increased risk many years later) on breast cancer risk through age 54.[64]

In view of the confusing and contradictory findings among the many case-control studies, the CDC reexamined their data to determine whether oral contraceptive use had different effects on the risk of breast cancer diagnosed at different ages.[65] The data indicated that oral contraceptive use increased slightly the risk of breast cancer diagnosed under the age of 35, and had no effect on women diagnosed from age 35 to 44, and in women diagnosed from age 45 to 54, oral contraceptive use appeared to decrease the risk of breast cancer. However, these estimates were of borderline statistical significance. Nevertheless, the protection that oral contraceptive use appears to provide to older women is a more convincing argument because it was supported by several dose-response relationships (age with first use and time since first and last use). The elevated risk among the women with early breast cancer is a more tenuous conclusion, not strengthened by supporting dose-response patterns.

The crucial question is this: as studies gain more statistical power, will they confirm a slightly increased risk for premenopausal breast cancer or will the present suggestion of an increased risk disappear? For some time to come, probably a decade or more, clinical advice will have to be based on the current conflicting findings. With considerable confidence, it can be stated that long-term use of oral contraception during the reproductive years is **NOT** associated with a significant increase in the risk of breast cancer after age 45. There is the possibility that a subgroup of young women who use contraception early and for a long time (greater than 4 years) has a slightly increased risk of breast cancer before the age of 45, a relative risk of less than 1.5.[66] It is not cost-effective to promote mammographic surveillance of this group of patients, but it should not be denied to any woman of this group who makes the request. There is also the possibility that previous users of oral contraception are provided some protection against postmenopausal breast cancer. Keep in mind that these conclusions depend upon data derived from use of higher dose oral contraception. It is important to be aware that there has been consistent failure to demonstrate an increased risk with oral contraceptive use in women with positive family histories of breast cancer or in women with proven benign breast disease.[62,67]

Other Cancers

The Walnut Creek study suggested that melanoma was linked to oral contraception; however, the major risk factor for melanoma is exposure to sunlight. More recent and accurate evaluation utilizing both of the RCGP and OFPA prospective cohorts and accounting for exposure to sunlight has not indicated a significant difference in the risk of melanoma comparing users to nonusers.[68,69] There is no evidence linking oral contraceptive use to kidney cancer, colon cancer, gallbladder cancer, or pituitary tumors.[70]

Endocrine Effects

Adrenal Gland

For some time it has been known that estrogen increases the cortisol-binding globulin, transcortin. It had been thought that the increase in plasma cortisol while on oral contraception was due to increased binding by this globulin and not an increase in free active cortisol. Now it is apparent that free and active cortisol levels are also elevated. Estrogen decreases the ability of the liver to metabolize cortisol, and in addition, progesterone and related compounds can displace cortisol from transcortin and thus contribute to the elevation of unbound cortisol. The effects of these elevated levels over prolonged periods of time are unknown. To put this into perspective, the increase is not as great as that which occurs in pregnancy, and, in fact it is within the normal range for nonpregnant women.

The adrenal gland responds to adrenocorticotropic hormone (ACTH) normally in women on oral contraceptives; therefore there is no suppression of the adrenal gland itself. Initial studies showed that the response to metyrapone (a 11-hydroxylase blocker) was abnormal, suggesting that the pituitary was suppressed. However estrogen accelerates the conjugation of metyrapone by the liver, and therefore the drug has less effect, thus explaining the subnormal responses. The pituitary-adrenal reaction to stress is normal in women on oral contraceptive pills.

Thyroid

As with transcortin, estrogen increases thyroxine-binding globulin. Prior to the introduction of new methods for measuring free thyroxine levels, evaluation of thyroid function was a problem. Measurement of TSH (thyroid-stimulating hormone) and the free thyroxine level in a woman on oral contraception provides an accurate assessment of a patient's thyroid state. Oral contraception affects the total thyroxine level in the blood as well as the amount of binding globulin, but the free thyroxine level is unchanged.

Oral Contraception and Reproduction

Inadvertent Use While Pregnant

One of the reasons, if not the major reason, why a lack of withdrawal bleeding while using oral contraceptives is such a problem is the anxiety produced in both patient and clinician. The patient is anxious because of the uncertainty regarding pregnancy, and the clinician is anxious because of the concerns stemming from early retrospective studies which indicated an increased risk of congenital malformations among the offspring of women who were pregnant and using oral contraception.

The initial positive reports linking the use of contraceptive steroids to congenital malformations have not been substantiated. Many suspect a strong component of recall bias in the few positive studies due to a tendency of patients with malformed infants to recall details better than those with normal children. Other confounding problems have included a failure to consider the reasons for the administration of hormones (e.g., bleeding in an already abnormal pregnancy), and a failure to delineate the exact timing of the treatment (e.g., treatment was sometimes confined to a period of time during which the heart could not have been affected).

An association with cardiac anomalies was first claimed in the 1970s. Subsequently, analysis of these data uncovered several methodologic shortcomings. Simpson, in a very thorough and critical review in 1990, concluded that there is no reliable evidence implicating sex steroids as cardiac teratogens.[71] In fact, Simpson found no relationship between oral contraception and the following problems: hypospadias, limb reduction anomalies, neural tube defects, and mutagenic effects which would be responsible for chromosomally abnormal fetuses. Even virilization is not a practical consideration because the doses required (e.g., 20–40 mg norethindrone per day) are in excess of anything currently used. These conclusions reflect use of combined oral contraceptives as well as progestins alone.

In the past there was a concern regarding the VACTERL complex. VACTERL refers to a complex of vertebral, anal, cardiac, tracheoesophageal, renal, and limb anomalies. While case-control studies indicated a relationship with oral contraception, prospective studies have failed to observe any connection between sex steroids and the VACTERL complex. A meta-analysis of 26 prospective studies of the risk of birth defects with oral contraceptive ingestion during pregnancy concluded that there was no increase in risk for major malformations, congenital heart defects, or limb reduction defects.[72]

Women who become pregnant while taking oral contraceptives or women who inadvertently take birth control pills early in pregnancy should be advised that the risk of a significant congenital anomaly is no greater than the general rate of 2–3%. This recommendation can be extended to those pregnant woman who have been exposed to a progestational agent such as medroxyprogesterone acetate or 17-hydroxyprogesterone caproate.[73]

Subsequent Fertility

The early reports from the English prospective studies indicated that former users of oral contraception had a delay in achieving pregnancy. In the OFPA study, former use had an effect on fertility for up to 42 months in nulligravida women and for up to 30 months in multigravida women.[74] Presumably the delay is due to lingering suppression of the hypothalamic-pituitary reproductive system.

A later analysis of the Oxford data indicated that the delay is concentrated in women age 30–34 who have never given birth.[75] At 48 months 82% of these women had given birth compared to 89% of users of other contraceptive methods, not a large difference. No effect was observed in women younger than 30 or in women who had previously given birth. Childless women age 25–29 experienced some delay in return to fertility, but by 48 months, 91% had given birth compared to 92% in users of other methods. It should be noted that after 72 months the proportions of women who remained undelivered were the same in both groups of women.

This delay has been observed in the United States as well. In the Boston area, the interval from cessation of contraception to conception was 13 months or greater for 24.8% of prior oral contraceptive users compared to 10.6% for former users of all other methods (12.4% for intrauterine device users, 8.5% for diaphragm users, and 11.9% for other methods).[76] Oral contraceptive users had a lower monthly percentage of conceptions for the first 3 months, and somewhat lower percentage from 4 to 10 months. It took 24 months for 90% of previous oral contraceptive users to become pregnant, 14 months for intrauterine device users, and 10 months for diaphragm users. Similar findings in Connecticut indicate that this delay lasts at least one year, and the effect is greater with higher dose preparations.[77] Despite this delay, there is no evidence that infertility is increased by the use of oral contraception.

Spontaneous Abortion

There is no increase in the incidence of spontaneous abortion in pregnancies after the cessation of oral contraception.[78] Indeed, the rate of spontaneous abortion and stillbirths is slightly less in former oral contraceptive users, about 1% and 0.3%, respectively.

Pregnancy Outcome

There is no evidence that oral contraceptives cause changes in individual germ cells that would yield an abnormal child at a later time.[71] There is no increase in the number of abnormal children born to former oral contraceptive users, and there is no change in the sex ratio (a sign of sex-linked recessive mutations).[79] These observations are not altered when analyzed for duration of use. Initial observations that women who had previously used oral contraception had an increase in chromosomally abnormal fetuses have not been confirmed. Furthermore, as noted above, there is no increase in the abortion rate after discontinuation, something one would expect if oral contraceptives induce chromosomal abnormalities since these are the principal cause of spontaneous abortion.

In a 3-year follow-up of children whose mothers used oral contraceptives prior to conception, no differences could be detected in weight, anemia, intelligence, or development.[80] Former oral contraceptive users have no increased risks for the following: perinatal morbidity or mortality, prematurity, and low birth weight.[81] Dizygous twinning has been observed to be nearly two-fold (1.6% vs 1.0%) increased in women who conceive soon after cessation of oral contraception.[78] This effect was greater with greater duration of use.

The only reason (and it is a good one) to recommend that women defer attempts to conceive for a month or two after stopping the oral contraceptive is to improve the accuracy of gestational dating by allowing accurate identification of the last menstrual period.

Oral Contraception and Breastfeeding

Oral contraception has been demonstrated to diminish the quantity and quality of lactation in postpartum women. Also of concern is the potential hazard of transfer of contraceptive steroids to the infant (a significant amount of the progestational component is transferred into breast milk).[82] However no adverse effects have thus far been identified. Women who use oral contraception have a lower incidence of breastfeeding after the 6th postpartum month, regardless of whether oral contraception is started at the first, second, or third postpartum month.[83,84]

In adequately nourished women, no impairment of infant growth can be detected; presumably compensation is achieved either through supplementary feedings or increased suckling.[85] In an 8 year follow-up study of children breastfed by mothers using oral contraceptives, no effect could be detected on diseases, intelligence, or psychological behavior.[86] This study also found that mothers on birth control pills lactated a significantly shorter period of time than controls, a mean of 3.7 months vs 4.6 months in controls.

Because the above considerations indicate that oral contraception shortens the duration of breastfeeding, it is worthwhile to consider the contraceptive effectiveness of lactation. In Scotland, no ovulation could be detected in women during exclusive breastfeeding.[87] However, in Chile, 14% of women ovulated during full breastfeeding, although full breastfeeding provided effective contraception up to 3 months postpartum.[88,89] It has been argued that the threshold for suppression of ovulation is at least 5 feedings for a total of at least 65 minutes per day of suckling duration.[90] However, in the studies from Chile, the frequency of nursing was the same in breastfeeders who ovulated and those who did not.

In Mexico, a study of 29 breastfeeding mothers and 10 nonbreastfeeders observed that in the absence of bleeding and supplementary feedings, 100% of the breastfeeders remained anovulatory for 3 months postpartum and 96% up to 6 months.[91] The median time from delivery to first ovulation was 259 days for breastfeeders compared to 119 days for nonbreastfeeders. However, by the third postpartum month, 18% of the breastfeeders had ovulated. *Only amenorrheic women who exclusively breastfeed at regular intervals, including nighttime, during the first 6 months have the contraceptive protection equivalent to that provided by oral contraception; with menstruation or after 6 months, the risk of ovulation increases.*[92] Supplemental feeding increases the risk of ovulation (and pregnancy) even in amenorrheic women.[93] Total protection against pregnancy is achieved by the exclusively breastfeeding woman for a duration of only 10 weeks.

Lactation provides a contraceptive effect, but it is variable and not reliable for every woman. Furthermore, because frequent suckling is required to maintain full milk production, women who use oral contraception and also breastfeed less frequently (e.g., because they work outside their home) have two reasons for decreased milk volume. This combination can make it especially difficult to continue nursing.

Because of the concerns regarding the impact of oral contraceptives on breastfeeding, a useful alternative is to combine the contraceptive effect of lactation with the progestin-only minipill. This low dose of progestin has no negative impact on breast milk, and some studies document an increase in milk quantity and nutritional quality. Highly effective (near total) protection can be achieved with the combination of lactation and the minipill.

Initiation of Oral Contraception in the Postpartum Period

The individual woman is in need of contraception early in the postpartum period. In a careful study of 22 postpartum, nonbreastfeeding women, the mean time from delivery to the first menses was 45 ± 10.1 days, and no woman ovulated before 25 days after delivery.[94] A high proportion of the first cycles (81.8%) and the subsequent cycles (37%) were not normal; however, this is certainly not predictable in individual women. Others have documented a mean delay of 7 weeks before resumption of ovulation, but half of the women studied ovulated before the 6th week, the time of the traditional postpartum visit. The obstetrical tradition of scheduling the postpartum visit at 6 weeks should be changed. A 3-week visit would be more effective for avoiding postpartum surprises.

Rule of 3's for Postpartum Initiation of Contraception
Full breastfeeding: **Begin in *3rd postpartum month.***
Partial or no breastfeeding: **Begin in *3rd postpartum week.***

After the termination of a pregnancy of less than 12 weeks, oral contraception can be started immediately. After a pregnancy of 12 or more weeks, oral contraception has traditionally been started 2 weeks after delivery to avoid an increased risk of thrombosis during the initial postpartum period. This practice has been based on a theoretical concern that is probably no longer an issue with low dose oral contraception. Oral contraception can be started immediately after a second trimester abortion or premature delivery.

Postpill Amenorrhea

The approximate incidence of "postpill amenorrhea" is 0.7–0.8%, which is equal to the incidence of spontaneous secondary amenorrhea,[81,95] and there is no evidence to support the idea that oral contraception causes secondary amenorrhea. If a cause and effect relationship exists between oral contraception and subsequent amenorrhea, one would expect the incidence of infertility to be increased after a given population discontinues use of oral contraception. In those women who discontinue oral contraception in order to get pregnant, 50% conceive by 3 months, and after 2 years, a maximum of 15% of nulliparous women and 7% of parous women fail to conceive,[81] figures comparable to those quoted for the prevalence of spontaneous infertility. While patients with this problem come more quickly to our attention because of previous oral contraceptive use and follow-up, there is no cause and effect relationship. Women who have not resumed menstrual function within 12 months should be evaluated as any other patient with secondary amenorrhea.

Use During Puberty

Should oral contraception be advised for a young woman with irregular menses and oligoovulation or anovulation? The fear of subsequent infertility should not be a deterrent to providing appropriate contraception. Women who have irregular menstrual periods are more likely to develop secondary amenorrhea whether they use oral contraception or not. The possibility of subsequent secondary amenorrhea is less of a risk and a less urgent problem for a young woman than leaving her unprotected. The need for contraception takes precedence.

There is no evidence that the use of oral contraceptives in the pubertal, sexually active girl impairs growth and development of the reproductive system. Again, the most important concern is and should be the prevention of an unwanted pregnancy. For most teenagers oral contraception, dispensed in the 28-day package for better compliance, is the contraceptive method of choice.

Oral Contraception and Infections

Bacterial STDs

Sexually transmitted diseases (STDs) are one of the most common public health problems in the United States. Pelvic inflammatory disease (PID) is usually a consequence of STDs. The best estimate of subsequent tubal infertility is approximately 12% after one episode of PID, 23% after 2 episodes, and 54% after 3 episodes.[96] Because pelvic infection is the single greatest threat to the reproductive future of a young woman, the now recognized protection offered by oral contraception against pelvic inflammatory disease is very important.[97] The risk of hospitalization for PID is reduced by approximately 50%–60%, but at least 12 months of use is necessary, and the protection is limited to current users.[98] If a woman does get a pelvic infection, the severity of the salpingitis found at laparoscopy is decreased.[99] The mechanism of this protection remains unknown. Speculation includes thickening of the cervical mucus to prevent movement of pathogens and bacteria-laden sperm into the uterus and tubes, and decreased menstrual bleeding which reduces movement of pathogens into the tubes as well as a reduction in "culture medium."

The argument has been made that this protection is limited to gonococcal disease, and chlamydia infections may even be enhanced. Fifteen of 17 published studies by 1985 reported a positive association of oral contraceptives with lower genital tract chlamydia cervicitis.[100] Because lower genital tract infections caused by chlamydia are on the rise (now the most prevalent bacterial STD in the U.S.) and the rate of hospitalization for PID is also increased, it is worthwhile for both patients and clinicians to be alert for symptoms of cervicitis or salpingitis in women on oral contraception who are at high risk of sexually transmitted disease (multiple sexual partners, a history of STD, or cervical discharge).

Despite this potential relationship between oral contraception and chlamydia infections, it should be emphasized that there is no evidence that oral contraceptives increase the incidence of tubal infertility.[101] In fact, a case-control study indicates that oral contraceptive users with chlamydia infection are protected against symptomatic PID.[102] Thus, the influence of oral contraception on the upper reproductive tract may be different than on the lower tract. These observations on fertility are derived mostly, if not totally, from women using oral contraceptives containing 50 μg estrogen. The continued progestin dominance of the lower dose formulations should produce the same protective impact, and evidence is appearing that this is so.[98]

Viral STDs

The viral STDs include human immunodeficiency virus (HIV), human papillomavirus (HPV), herpes simplex virus (HSV), and hepatitis B (HBV). At the present time, no proven associations exist between oral contraception and the viral STDs.[103] Of course, significant prevention includes barrier methods of contraception. Thus far, most studies have found no association beween oral contraceptive use and HIV seropositivity. For women not in a stable, monogamous relationship, a dual approach is recommended, combining the contraceptive efficacy and protection against PID offered by oral contraception with the use of a barrier method (and spermicide) for prevention of viral STDs.

Other Infections

In the British prospective studies, urinary tract infections were increased by 20% in users of oral contraception, and a correlation was noted with estrogen dose. An increased incidence of cervicitis was also reported, an effect related to the progestin dose. The incidence of cervicitis increased with the length of time the pill was used, from no higher after 6 months to 3 times higher by the 6th year of use. A significant increase in a variety of viral diseases, e.g., chickenpox, was observed, suggesting steroid effects on the immune system. The prevalence of these effects with low dose oral contraception is yet unknown.

Oral contraception is not linked to bacterial vaginosis and appears to protect against infections with *Trichomonas*.[104] Evidence is lacking to convincingly implicate oral contraception with vaginal infections with *Candida* species.[104] However, clinical experience is sometimes impressive when recurrence and cure repeatedly follow use and discontinuation of oral contraception.

Patient Management

Absolute Contraindications to the Use of Oral Contraception

1. Thrombophlebitis, thromboembolic disorders, cerebral vascular disease, coronary occlusion, a past history of these conditions, or conditions predisposing to these problems.

2. Markedly impaired liver function. Steroid hormones are contraindicated in patients with hepatitis until liver function tests return to normal.

3. Known or suspected breast cancer.

4. Undiagnosed abnormal vaginal bleeding.

5. Known or suspected pregnancy.

6. Smokers over the age of 35.

Relative Contraindications Requiring Clinical Judgment and Informed Consent

1. Migraine headaches. In retrospective studies of high dose pills, migraine headaches have been associated with an increased risk of stroke; however, some women report an improvement in their headaches.

2. Hypertension. A woman under 35 who is otherwise healthy and whose blood pressure is controlled by medication can elect to use oral contraception.

3. Uterine leiomyoma. This is not a contraindication with the low dose formulations. There is evidence that the risk of leiomyomas is decreased by 31% in women who used higher dose oral contraception for 10 years.[105] However, a case-control study found neither a decrease nor an increase in risk.[106]

4. Gestational diabetes. Low dose formulations do not produce a diabetic glucose tolerance response in women with previous gestational diabetes, and there is no evidence that oral contraception increases the incidence of overt diabetes mellitus. We believe that women with previous gestational diabetes can use oral contraception with annual assessment of the fasting glucose level.

5. Diabetes mellitus. Effective prevention of pregnancy outweighs the small risk in diabetic women who are under age 35 and otherwise healthy.

6. Elective surgery. The recommendation that oral contraception should be discontinued 4 weeks before elective surgery to avoid an increased risk of postoperative thrombosis is based upon data derived from high dose pills. It is safer to follow this recommendation if possible, but it is probably less critical with low dose oral contraceptives. It is prudent to maintain contraception right up to the performance of a sterilization procedure, and this short, outpatient operation probably carries very minimal risk.

7. Epilepsy. Oral contraceptives do not exacerbate epilepsy, and in some women, improvement in seizure control has occurred.[107] Antiepileptic drugs, however, may decrease the effectiveness of oral contraception.

8. Obstructive jaundice in pregnancy. Not all patients with this history will develop jaundice on oral contraception, especially with the low dose formulations.

9. Sickle cell disease or sickle C disease. Patients with sickle cell trait can use oral contraception. The risk of thrombosis in women with sickle cell disease or sickle C diseases is theoretical and it has medical-legal implications. We believe effective protection against pregnancy in these patients warrants the use of low dose oral contraception.

10. Gallbladder disease.

Surveillance of Patients on Oral Contraception

In view of the increased safety of low dose preparations for healthy young women with no risk factors, patients need be seen only every 12 months for exclusion of problems by history, measurement of the blood pressure, urinalysis, breast examination, palpation of the liver, and pelvic examination with Pap smear. Women with risk factors should be seen every 6 months by appropriately trained personnel for screening of problems by history and blood pressure measurement. Breast and pelvic examinations are necessary only yearly. It is worth emphasizing that better compliance is achieved by reassessing new users within 3 months. It is at this time that subtle fears and unvoiced concerns need to be confronted and resolved.

Oral contraception is safer than we thought it was, and the low dose preparations are extremely safe. Health care providers should make a significant effort to get this message to patients and our colleagues. We must make sure our patients receive adequate counseling, either from ourselves or our professional staff. The major reason why patients discontinue oral contraception is fear of side effects. Let's take time to put the risks into proper perspective and to emphasize the benefits as well as the risks.

Laboratory surveillance should be used only when indicated. Routine biochemical measurements fail to yield sufficient information to warrant the expense. Assessing the cholesterol-lipoprotein profile and carbohydrate metabolism should follow the same guidelines applied to all patients, users and nonusers of contraception. The following is a useful guide for who should be screened prior to treatment with blood tests for glucose, lipids, and lipoproteins:

Women 35 years or older.
Women with a strong family history of heart disease, diabetes mellitus, or hypertension.
Women with gestational diabetes mellitus.
Women with xanthomatosis.
Obese women.
Diabetic women.

Choice of Pill

The therapeutic principle remains: utilize the formulations that give effective contraception and the greatest margin of safety. The multiphasic preparations do have a reduced progestin dosage compared to some of the existing monophasic products; however, based on currently available information there is little difference between the low dose monophasics and the multiphasics. It remains to be seen whether formulations with the new progestins will provide protection against cardiovascular disease. Nevertheless, the new progestin combinations offer minimal metabolic impact, although it is by no means certain yet that this provides an advantage over the available low dose formulations. The one exception is monophasic preparations containing relatively high doses of levonorgestrel (150–250 μg); these should be avoided in favor of low dose formulations.

Patients should be urged to choose a low dose preparation containing less than 50 μg estrogen, combined with low doses of new or old progestins, avoiding the high doses of levonorgestrel. Patients on higher dose oral contraception should be changed to the low dose preparations. Stepping down to a lower dose can be accomplished immediately with no adverse reactions such as increased bleeding or failure of contraception.

The pharmacologic effects in animals of various formulations have been used as a basis for therapeutic recommendations in selecting the optimal oral contraceptive pill. ***These recommendations (tailor-making the pill to the patient) have not been supported by appropriately controlled clinical trials. All too often this leads to the prescribing of a pill of excessive dosage with its attendant increased risk of serious side effects.*** It is worth repeating our earlier comments on potency. Oral contraceptive potency (specifically progestin potency) is no longer a consideration when it comes to prescribing birth control pills. The potency of the various progestins has been accounted for by appropriate adjustments of dose. Progress in lowering the doses of the steroids contained in oral contraceptives has yielded products with little serious differences.

Proper Pill Taking

Effective contraception is present during the first cycle of pill use, provided the pills are started no later than the 5th day of the cycle, and no pills are missed. Thus, starting oral contraception on the first day of menses assures immediate protection. In the United States, most clinicians and patients prefer the Sunday start packages, beginning on the first Sunday following menstruation. This is easy to remember, and it usually avoids menstrual bleeding on weekends. It is probable, but not totally certain, that even if a dominant follicle should emerge after a Sunday start, an LH surge and ovulation will still be prevented.[108,109] Some clinicians prefer to advise patients to use added protection in the first week of use.

Occasionally patients would like to postpone a menstrual period, e.g., for a wedding, holiday, or vacation. This can be easily achieved by omitting the 7-day hormone-free interval. Simply start a new package of pills the next day after finishing the series of 21 pills in the previous package. Remember, when using a 28 pill package, the patient would start a new package after using the 21 *active* pills.

There is no rationale for recommending a pill-free interval "to rest." Side effects are not eliminated by pill-free intervals. This practice all too often results in unwanted pregnancies.

What to do when pills are missed. *If a woman misses 1 pill,* she should take that pill as soon as she remembers and take the next pill as usual. No back-up is needed.

If a woman misses 2 pills in the first two weeks, she should take two pills on each of the next two days; it is unlikely that a back-up method is needed, but the official consensus is to recommend back-up for the next 7 days.

If 2 pills are missed in the third week, or if more than 2 pills are missed at any time, another form of contraception should be used as back-up immediately and for 7 days; if a Sunday starter, the patient should keep taking a pill every day until Sunday, on Sunday she should start a new package; if a non Sunday starter, start a new package the same day.

Recent studies have questioned whether missing pills has an impact on contraception. One study demonstrated that skipping 4 consecutive pills at varying times in the cycle did not result in ovulation.[108] Studies in which women deliberately lengthen their pill-fee interval up to 11 days have failed to show signs of ovulation.[109] So far there is no evidence that moving to lower doses has had an impact on the margin of error. However, the studies have involved small numbers of women and given the large individual variation, it still is possible that some women might be at risk with a small increase in the pill-free interval. The current recommendations may well be proven to be too conservative, and a woman's chance of getting pregnant with missing pills is nearly zero. Nevertheless, the above conservative advice is the safest message to convey.

Clinical Problems

Breakthrough Bleeding

A problem that impacts in a major way on compliance is breakthrough bleeding. Breakthrough bleeding gives rise to fears and concerns; it is aggravating and even embarrassing. Therefore, upon starting oral contraception, patients need to be fully informed regarding breakthrough bleeding. There is no evidence that indicates that the onset of bleeding is associated with decreased efficacy, no matter what oral contraceptive formulation is used, even the lowest dose products. Indeed, in a careful study, breakthrough bleeding did not correlate with changes in the blood levels of the contraceptive steroids.[110]

The most frequently encountered breakthrough bleeding occurs in the first few months of use. The incidence is greatest in the first 3 months, ranging from 10–30% in the first month to 1–10% in the third. It is best managed by encouragement and reassurance. This bleeding usually disappears by the third cycle in the majority of women. If necessary, even this early pattern of breakthrough bleeding can be treated as outlined below. It is helpful to explain to the patient that this bleeding represents tissue breakdown as the endometrium adjusts from its usual thick state to the relatively thin state allowed by the hormones in oral contraceptives.

Breakthrough bleeding that occurs after many months of oral contraceptive use is a consequence of the progestin-induced decidualization. This endometrium is shallow and tends to be fragile and prone to breakdown and asynchronous bleeding.

If bleeding occurs just before the end of the pill cycle, it can be managed by having the patient stop the pills, wait 7 days and start a new cycle. If breakthrough bleeding is prolonged or if it is aggravating for the patient, regardless of the point in the pill cycle, control of the bleeding can be achieved with a short course of exogenous estrogen. Conjugated estrogens, 1.25 mg, or estradiol, 2 mg, is administered daily for 7 days when the bleeding is present, no matter where the patient is in her pill cycle. The patient continues to adhere to the schedule of pill taking. Usually one course of estrogen solves the problem, and recurrence of bleeding is unusual (but if it does recur, another 7-day course of estrogen is effective).

Responding to irregular bleeding by having the patient take 2 or 3 pills is not effective. The progestin component of the pill will always dominate, hence doubling the number of pills will also double the progestational impact and its decidualizing, atrophic effect on the endometrium. The addition of extra estrogen while keeping the progestin dose unchanged is logical and effective. This allows the patient to remain on the low dose formulation with its advantage of greater safety. Breakthrough bleeding is not sufficient reason to expose patients to the increased risks associated with higher dose oral contraceptives. Any bleeding that is not handled by this routine requires investigation for the presence of pathology.

There is no evidence that any specific formulation is significantly superior to any other in terms of the rate of breakthrough bleeding. Clinicians often become impressed that switching to another specific product effectively stops the breakthrough bleeding. It is more likely that the passage of time is the responsible factor, and bleeding would have stopped regardless of switching and regardless of product.

Amenorrhea

With low dose pills, the estrogen content is insufficient to stimulate endometrial growth in some women. The progestational effect dominates to such a degree that a shallow atrophic endometrium is produced, lacking sufficient tissue to yield withdrawal bleeding. It should be emphasized that permanent atrophy of the endometrium does not occur, and resumption of normal ovarian function will restore endometrial growth and development. Indeed, there is no harmful, permanent consequence of developing amenorrhea while on oral contraception.

The major problem with amenorrhea while on oral contraception is the anxiety produced in both patient and clinician because the lack of bleeding may be a sign of pregnancy. The patient is anxious because of the uncertainty regarding pregnancy, and the clinician is anxious because of the medical-legal concerns stemming from the old studies that indicated an increased risk of congenital abnormalities among the offspring of women who inadvertently used oral contraception in early pregnancy. However, there is no association between oral contraception and an increased risk of congenital malformations.

The incidence of amenorrhea in the first year of use with low dose oral contraception is approximately 1%. This incidence increases with duration, reaching perhaps 5% after several years of use. It is important to alert patients upon starting oral contraception that diminished bleeding and possibly no bleeding may ensue.

Amenorrhea is a difficult management problem. A pregnancy test will allow reliable assessment for the presence of pregnancy even at this early stage. However, routine, repeated use of such testing is expensive and annoying, and may lead to discontinuation of oral contraception. *A simple test for pregnancy is to assess the basal body temperature during the END of the pill-free week; a basal body temperature of less than 98 °F (36.8 °C) is inconsistent with pregnancy, and oral contraception can be continued.*

Many women are reassured with an understanding of why there is no bleeding and are able to continue on the pill despite the amenorrhea. Some women cannot reconcile themselves to a lack of bleeding, and this is an indication for trying other formulations (a practice unsupported by any clinical trials, and therefore, the expectations are uncertain). But again, this problem does not warrant exposing patients to the greater risks of major side effects associated with higher dose products.

Weight Gain

The complaint of weight gain is frequently cited as a major problem with compliance. Yet studies of the low dose preparations fail to demonstrate a significant weight gain with oral contraception, and no major differences among the various products. This is obviously a problem of perception. The clinician has to carefully reinforce the lack of association between low dose oral contraceptives and weight gain and focus the patient on the real culprits: diet and level of exercise.

Acne

Low dose oral contraceptives improve acne regardless of which product is used. The low progestin doses (including levonorgestrel formulations) currently used are insufficient to stimulate an androgenic response.

741

Ovarian Cysts

Anecdotal reports suggested that ovarian cysts are encountered more frequently and suppress less easily with multiphasic formulations. This observation failed to withstand careful scrutiny.[111] Functional ovarian cysts occurred less frequently in women on higher dose oral contraception.[112] This protection appears to be reduced with the current lower dose products. Thus, the risk of such cysts is not eliminated, and therefore, clinicians can encounter such cysts in patients taking any of the oral contraceptive formulations.

Drugs That Affect Efficacy

There are many anecdotal reports of patients who conceived on oral contraceptives while taking antibiotics. There is little evidence, however, that antibiotics such as ampicillin, metronidazole, quinolone, doxycycline and tetracycline, which reduce the bacterial flora of the gastrointestinal tract, affect oral contraceptive efficacy. Studies indicate that while antibiotics can alter the excretion of contraceptive steroids, plasma levels are unchanged, and there is no evidence of ovulation.[113,114]

There is good reason to believe that drugs which stimulate the liver's metabolic capacity can affect oral contraceptive efficacy. On the other hand, a search of a large database failed to discover any evidence that lower dose oral contraceptives are more likely to fail or to have more drug interaction problems when other drugs are used.[115]

To be cautious, patients on medications that affect liver metabolism should choose an alternative contraceptive. These drugs are as follows:

> Rifampin
> Phenobarbital
> Phenytoin (Dilantin)
> Primidone (Mysoline)
> Carbamazepine (Tegretol)
> Possibly primidone, ethosuximide, and griseofulvin

Other Drug Interactions

Although not extensively documented, there is reason to believe that oral contraceptives potentiate the action of diazepam (Valium), chlordiazepoxide (Librium), tricyclic antidepressants, and theophylline. Thus, lower doses of these agents may be effective in oral contraceptive users. Because of an influence on clearance rates, oral contraceptive users may require larger doses of acetaminophen and aspirin.

Migraine Headaches

True migraine headaches are more common in women, while tension headaches occur equally in men and women. There have been no well-done studies to determine the impact of oral contraception on migraine headaches. Patients may report that their headaches are worse or better.

Studies with high dose pills indicated that migraine headaches were linked to a risk of stroke. There is reason to believe that the combination of good patient screening and the use of low dose oral contraception has virtually eliminated the risk of stroke. Nevertheless, because of the seriousness of this potential complication, the onset of visual symptoms or severe headaches requires a serious response. Certainly if the patient is at a higher dose, a move to a low dose formulation often relieves the symptom. Switching to a different brand is worthwhile, if only to evoke a placebo response. True vascular headaches are an indication to discontinue oral contraception.

Clues to severe vascular headaches:
- Headaches that last a long time.
- Dizziness, nausea, or vomiting with headaches.
- Scotomata or blurred vision.
- Episodes of blindness.
- Unilateral, unremitting headaches.
- Headaches that continue despite medication.

In some women, a relationship exists between their fluctuating hormone levels during a menstrual cycle and migraine headaches, with the onset of headaches characteristically coinciding with menses. We have had personal success (anecdotal to be sure) alleviating headaches by eliminating the menstrual cycle, either with the use of *daily* oral contraceptives or the daily administration of a progestational agent (such as 10 mg medroxyprogesterone acetate). Some women with migraine headaches have extremely gratifying responses.

Summary: Oral Contraceptive Use and Medical Problems

Gestational Diabetes
There is no contraindication to oral contraceptive use following gestational diabetes.

Diabetes Mellitus
Oral contraception can be used by diabetic women less than 35 years old who do not smoke and are otherwise healthy (especially an absence of diabetic vascular complications).

Hypertension
Low dose oral contraception can be used in women less than age 35 years old with hypertension controlled by medication, and who are otherwise healthy and do not smoke.

Pregnancy-Induced Hypertension
Women with pregnancy-induced hypertension can use oral contraception as soon as the blood pressure is normal in the postpartum period.

Gallbladder Disease
Oral contraception use may precipitate a symptomatic attack in women known to have stones or a positive history for gallbladder disease and, therefore, should either be used very cautiously or not at all.

Obesity
An obese woman who is otherwise healthy can use low dose oral contraception.

Hepatic Disease
Oral contraception can be utilized when liver function tests return to normal. Follow-up liver function tests should be obtained after 2–3 months of use.

Seizure Disorders
There is no impact of oral contraceptives on pattern or frequency of seizures. The concern is that anticonvulsant-induced hepatic enzyme activity can increase the risk of contraceptive failure. Some clinicians advocate the use of higher dose (50 µg estrogen) products; however, no studies have been performed to demonstrate that this higher dose is necessary.

Mitral Valve Prolapse
Oral contraception use is limited to nonsmoking patients who have only the echocardiographic diagnosis and are free of the clinical findings of mitral regurgitation.

Systemic Lupus Erythematosus

Oral contraceptive use can excacerbate systemic lupus erythematous, and the vascular disease associated with lupus represents a contraindication to estrogen-containing oral contraceptives.[116] The progestin-only methods can be considered.

Migraine Headaches

Low dose oral contraception can be tried with careful surveillance in women with common migraine headaches. Daily administration can prevent menstrual migraine headaches. Oral contraception is best avoided in women with classic migraine headaches associated with neurologic symptoms.

Sickle Cell Disease

Patients with sickle cell trait can use oral contraception. The risk of thrombosis in women with sickle cell disease or sickle C diseases is theoretical (and medical-legal). We believe effective protection against pregnancy in these patients warrants the use of low dose oral contraception.

Benign Breast Disease

Benign breast disease is not a contraindication for oral contraception; with 2 years of use, the condition can improve.

Congenital Heart Disease or Valvular Heart Disease

Oral contraception is contraindicated only if there is marginal cardiac reserve or a condition that predisposes to thrombosis.

Hyperlipidemia

Because low dose oral contraceptives have negligible impact on the lipoprotein profile, hyperlipidemia is not an absolute contraindication, with the exception of very high levels of triglycerides (which can be made worse by oral contraception). If vascular disease is already present, oral contraception should be avoided. If other risk factors are present, especially smoking, oral contraception is not recommended. Dyslipidemic patients who begin oral contraception should have their lipoprotein profiles monitored monthly for a few visits to ensure no adverse impact. If the lipid abnormality cannot be held in control, an alternative method of contraception should be used.[117]

Depression

Low dose oral contraceptives have minimal, if any, impact on mood.

Smoking

Oral contraception is absolutely contraindicated in smokers over the age of 35. In patients 35 years old and younger, heavy smoking (15 or more cigarettes per day) is a relative contraindication. The data indicate no increased risk of dying of a cardiovascular event in smokers under the age of 30. An exsmoker should be regarded as a nonsmoker. Risk is only linked to active smoking. Is there room for judgment? Given the right circumstances, low dose oral contraceptives might be appropriate for a light smoker or the user of a nicotine patch.

Pituitary Prolalctin-Secreting Adenomas

Low dose oral contraception can be used in the presence of microadenomas.

Infectious Mononucleosis

Oral contraception can be used as long as liver function tests are normal.

Ulcerative Colitis

There is no association between oral contraception and ulcerative colitis. Women with this problem can use oral contraceptives.[118] Oral contraceptives are absorbed mainly in the small bowel.

An Alternate Route of Administration

Occasionally a situation may be encountered when an alternative to oral administration of contraceptive pills is required. For example, patients receiving chemotherapy can either have significant nausea and vomiting, or mucocitis, both of which would prevent oral drug administration. The low dose oral contraceptives can be administered vaginally. Initially it was claimed that two pills must be placed high in the vagina daily in order to produce contraceptive steroid blood levels comparable to the oral administration of one pill.[119,120] However, a large clinical trial has demonstrated typical contraceptive efficacy with one pill per day.[121]

The Noncontraceptive Benefits of Oral Contraception

The noncontraceptive benefits of oral contraception can be grouped into two main categories: benefits that incidentally accrue when oral contraception is specifically utilized for contraceptive purposes and benefits that result from the use of oral contraceptives to treat problems and disorders.

The noncontraceptive incidental benefits can be listed as follows:

Effective Contraception.
   —less need for therapeutic abortion.
   —less need for surgical sterilization.
Less Endometrial Cancer.
Less Ovarian Cancer.
Less Benign Breast Disease.
Fewer Ectopic Pregnancies.
More Regular Menses.
   —less flow.
   —less dysmenorrhea.
   —less anemia.
Less Salpingitis.
Less Rheumatoid Arthritis.
Increased Bone Density.
Probably Less Endometriosis.
Possibly Protection against Atherosclerosis.
Possibly Fewer Fibroids.
Possibly Fewer Ovarian Cysts.

Protection against pelvic inflammatory disease is especially noteworthy and a major contribution to not only preservation of fertility but to lower health care costs. Also important is the prevention of ectopic pregnancies. Ectopic pregnancies have increased in incidence (partly due to an increase in STDs) and represent a major cost for our society and a threat to both fertility and life for individual patients.

Of course, prevention of benign and malignant neoplasia is an outstanding feature of oral contraception. Oral contraceptive use decreases the incidence of benign breast disease diagnosed clinically as well as fibrocystic disease and fibroadenomas diagnosed by biopsy. A 40% reduction in ovarian cancer and a 50% reduction in endometrial cancer represent substantial protection. Studies with higher dose formulations have documented in long-term users a 31% reduction in uterine leiomyomata and in current users a 78% reduction in corpus luteum cysts and a 49% reduction in functional ovarian cysts.[105,112] The impact of low dose preparations on these problems remains to be accurately measured and may be less. A case-control study with low dose oral contraceptives found no impact on the risk of uterine fibroids, neither increased nor decreased.[106] Two epidemiologic studies have indicated that a progressive decline in the incidence of ovarian cysts is proprotional to the steroid doses in oral contraceptives.[122,123] In one of these studies, current low dose monophasic and multiphasic formulations provided no protection against functional ovarian cysts.[123] This apparent weaker protection afforded by the current low dose formulations makes it very likely that clinicians will encounter such cysts in their patients on oral contraceptives.

The low dose contraceptives are as effective as higher dose preparations in reducing menstrual flow and the prevalence and severity of dysmenorrhea.[124,125] Previous use of oral contraception is associated with a lower incidence of endometriosis.[126] An Austrian study concluded that osteoporosis occurs later and is less frequent in women who have used long-term oral contraception.[127] Cross-sectional studies of postmenopausal women indicate that prior use of oral contraception is associated with higher levels of bone density and that the degree of protection is related to duration of exposure.[128,129] Because women who have had the opportunity to use oral contraception are just now entering the postmenopausal years, it will be several years before we know if previous oral contraceptive users have fewer fractures.

The literature on rheumatoid arthritis has been controversial, with studies in Europe finding evidence of protection and studies in North America failing to demonstrate such an effect. An excellent Danish case-control study was designed to answer criticisms of shortcomings in the previous literature.[130] Ever-use of oral contraception reduced the relative risk of rheumatoid arthritis by 60%, and the strongest protection was present in women with a positive family history. A meta-analysis concluded that the evidence consistently indicated a protective effect, but that rather than preventing the development of rheumatoid arthritis, oral contraception may modify the course of disease, inhibiting the progression from mild to severe disease.[131]

Oral contraceptives are frequently utilized to manage the following problems and disorders:

Definitely Beneficial:
—**dysfunctional uterine bleeding.**
—**dysmenorrhea.**
—**mittelschmerz.**
—**endometriosis prophylaxis.**
—**acne and hirsutism.**
—**hormone replacement for hypothalamic amenorrhea.**
—**prevention of menstrual porphyria.**

Probably Beneficial:
—**functional ovarian cysts.**
—**premenstrual syndrome.**
—**control of bleeding (dyscrasias, anovulation).**

Oral contraceptives have been a cornerstone for the treatment of anovulatory, dysfunctional uterine bleeding. For patients who need effective contraception, oral contraceptives are a good choice to provide hormone therapy to amenorrheic patients, as well as to treat dysmenorrhea. Oral contraceptives are also a good choice to provide prophylaxis against the recurrence of endometriosis in a woman who has already undergone more vigorous treatment with surgery or the GnRH analogues. To protect against endometriosis, oral contraceptives should be taken daily, with no break and no withdrawal bleeding.

The low dose oral contraceptives are effective in treating acne and hirsutism. Suppression of free testosterone levels is comparable to that achieved with higher dosage.[132] The beneficial clinical effect is the same with low dose preparations containing levonorgestrel, previously recognized to cause acne at high dosage.[133] Formulations with desogestrel, gestodene, and norgestimate are associated with greater increases in sex hormone binding globulin and decreases in free testosterone levels. Theoretically these products would be more effective in the treatment of acne and hirsutism; however, this is yet to be documented by clinical studies.

Oral contraceptives have long been used to speed the resolution of ovarian cysts, but the efficacy of this treatment has not been established. In a small study, 24 patients who had persistent cysts after exogenous gonadotropin treatment were randomized to receive an oral contraceptive or expectant management.[134] No advantage for the contraceptive treatment could be demonstrated. The cysts resolved completely and equally fast in both groups. Of course, these were functional cysts secondary to ovulation induction, and this experience may not apply to spontaneously appearing cysts. Oral contraception does provide protection in women who repetitively form ovarian cysts.

Oral contraceptives are associated with a collection of effects which yield an overall improvement in individual health. From a public health point of view, the combined impact leads to a decrease in the cost of health care. For both the individual and the public health, these impacts are especially significant in older women. These considerations allow the clinician to present oral contraception with a very positive attitude, an approach which makes an important contribution to a patient's ability to make appropriate health choices.

Maintaining Good Compliance with Oral Contraception

Despite the fact that oral contraception is highly effective, hundreds of thousands of unintended pregnancies occur each year in the United States because of the failure of oral contraception. Worldwide, literally millions of unintended pregnancies result from poor compliance. In general, young, unmarried, poor, and minority women are more likely to have failures, reaching rates of 10–20%.[135] Overall, the failure rate with actual use ranges from 3 to 6%. This difference between the theoretical efficacy and actual use reflects compliance and noncompliance. Noncompliance includes a wide variety of behavior: failure to fill the initial prescription, failure to continue on the medication, and incorrect ingestion of oral contraception. Compliance is an area in which personal behavior, biology, and pharmacology come together. Oral contraceptive compliance reflects the interaction of these influences.

There are 3 major factors that affect compliance:

1. Fears and concerns regarding cancer, cardiovascular disease, and the impact of oral contraception on future fertility.

2. The experience of side effects such as breakthrough bleeding and amenorrhea and perceived experience of "minor" problems such as headaches, nausea, and weight gain.

3. Nonmedical issues such as inadequate instructions on pill-taking, complicated pill packaging, and difficulties arising from the patient package insert.

The information in this chapter is the foundation for good compliance, but the clinician must go beyond the presentation of information and develop an effective means of communicating that information. We recommend the following approach to the clinician-patient encounter as one way to improve compliance with oral contraception.

1. Explain how oral contraception works.

2. Review briefly the risks and benefits of oral contraception, but be careful to put the risks in proper perspective, and to emphasize the safety and noncontraceptive benefits of low dose oral contraceptives.

3. Show and demonstrate to the patient the package of pills she will use.

4. Explain how to take the pills:
    —When to start.
    —How to develop a daily routine to avoid missing pills.
    —What to do if pills are missed.

5. Review the side effects that can affect compliance: amenorrhea, break-through bleeding, headaches, weight gain, nausea, etc., and what to do if one or more occurs.

6. Explain the warning signs of potential problems: abdominal or chest pain, trouble breathing, severe headaches, visual problems, leg pain or swelling.

7. Ask the patient to be sure to call if another clinician prescribes other medications.

8. Ask the patient to repeat critical information to make sure she understands what has been said. Ask if the patient has any questions.

9. Schedule a return appointment in 2–3 months to review understanding and address fears and concerns.

10. Make sure a line of communication is open to a clinician or office personnel. Ask the patient to call for any problem or concern before she stops taking the oral contraceptives.

The Progestin-Only Minipill

The minipill contains a small dose of a progestational agent and must be taken daily, in a continuous fashion.[136] There is no evidence for any difference in clinical behavior with any of the products.

Minipills available worldwide:

1. Micronor, NOR-QD, Noriday, Norod   0.350 mg norethindrone.

2. Microval, Noregeston, Microlut   0.030 mg levonorgestrel.

3. Ovrette, Neogest   0.075 mg norgestrel.

4. Exluton   0.500 mg lynestrenol.

5. Femulen   0.500 mg ethynodial diacetate.

Mechanism of Action

The small amount of progestin in the circulation will have a significant impact only on those tissues very sensitive to the female sex steroids, estrogen and progesterone. The contraceptive effect is more dependent upon endometrial and cervical mucus effects, since gonadotropins are not consistently suppressed. The endometrium involutes and becomes hostile to implantation, and the cervical mucus becomes thick and impermeable. Approximately 40% of patients will ovulate normally. Tubal physiology may also be affected, but this is speculative.

Because of the low dose, the minipill must be taken daily at the same time of day. The change in the cervical mucus requires 2–4 hours to take effect, and, most importantly, the impermeability diminishes 22 hours after administration.

Ectopic pregnancy is not prevented as effectively as intrauterine pregnancy. Although the overall incidence of ectopic pregnancy is not increased, when pregnancy occurs, the clinician must suspect that it is more likely to be ectopic.

There are no significant metabolic effects,[137] and there is an immediate return to fertility upon discontinuation (unlike the delay seen with the combination oral contraceptive).

Efficacy

Failure rates have been documented to range from 1.1 to 9.6 per 100 women in the first year of use.[9] The failure rate is higher in younger women (3.1 per 100 woman-years) compared to women over age 40 (0.3 per 100 woman-years).[138] In motivated women, the failure rate is comparable to the actual use rate with combination oral contraception.[139,140]

Pill Taking

The minipill should be started on the first day of menses, and a back-up method must be used for the first 7 days. The pill should be keyed to a daily event to ensure regular administration at the same time of the day. If pills are forgotten or gastrointestinal illness impairs absorption, the minipill should be resumed as soon as possible, and a back-up method should be used immediately and until the pills have been resumed for at least 2 days. If 2 or more pills are missed in a row and there is no menstrual bleeding in 4–6 weeks, a pregnancy test should be obtained. *If more than 3 hours late in taking a pill, a back-up method should be used for 48 hours.*

Problems

In view of the unpredictable effect on ovulation, it is not surprising that irregular menstrual bleeding is the major clinical problem. The daily progestational impact on the endometrium also contributes to this problem. Patients can expect to have normal, ovulatory cycles (40%), short, irregular cycles (40%), or a total lack of cycles ranging from irregular bleeding to spotting and amenorrhea (20%). This is the major reason why women discontinue the minipill method of contraception.[139]

Women on progestin-only contraception develop more functional, ovarian follicular cysts.[141] Nearly all, if not all, regress. This is not a clinical problem of any significance.

The levonorgestrel minipill may be associated with acne. The mechanism is similar to that seen with Norplant. The androgenic activity of levonorgestrel decreases the circulating levels of sex hormone binding globulin (SHBG). Therefore free steroid levels (levonorgestrel and testosterone) will be increased. This is in contrast to the action of combined oral contraception where the effect of the progestin is countered by the estrogen-induced increase in SHBG.

The incidence of the minor side effects is very low, probably at the same rate that would be encountered with a placebo.

Clinical Decisions

There are two situations where excellent efficacy, probably near total effectiveness, is achieved: lactating women and women over age 40. In lactating women, the contribution of the minipill is combined with prolactin-induced suppression of ovulation, adding up to very effective protection.[142] In women over age 40, reduced fecundity adds to the minipill's effects.

There is another reason why the minipill is a good choice for the breastfeeding woman. There is no evidence for any adverse effect on breastfeeding as measured by milk volume and infant growth.[143] In fact, there is a modest positive impact; women using the minipill breastfeed longer and add supplementary feeding at a later time.[144] Because of the slight positive impact on lactation, the minipill can be started immediately after delivery.

The minipill is a good choice in situations where estrogen is contraindicated, such as patients with serious medical conditions (diabetes with vascular disease, severe systemic lupus erythematosus, cardiovascular disease). It should be noted that the freedom from estrogen effects, although likely, is presumptive. Substantial data, e.g., on associations with vascular disease, blood pressure, and cancer, are not available because relatively small numbers have chosen to use this method of contraception. On the other hand, it is very logical to conclude that any of the progestin effects associated with the combination oral contraceptives can be related to the minipill according to a dose-response curve; all effects should be reduced.

No impact can be measured on the coagulation system.[145] The minipill can probably be used in women with previous episodes of thrombosis, but the package insert in the United States carries the same precautions and warnings that combined oral contraceptives carry. This is not appropriate in view of the absence of estrogen and the lower dose of progestin. Theoretically, minipills should be free of serious complications. Unfortunately, the package insert injects an element of medical-legal risk for the clinician.

The minipill is a good alternative for the occasional woman who reports diminished libido on combination oral contraceptives, presumably due to decreased androgen levels. The minipill should also be considered for the few patients who report minor side effects (gastrointestinal upset, breast tenderness, headaches) of such a degree that the combination oral contraceptive is not acceptable.

Do the noncontraceptive benefits associated with combination oral contraception apply to the minipill? Studies are unable to help us with this issue, again because of relatively small numbers of users. However, the progestin impact on cervical mucus, endometrium, and ovulation leads one to think the benefits will be present, but probably at a reduced level.

Good efficacy with the minipill requires regularity, taking the pill at the same time each day. There is less room for forgetting, and therefore the minipill is probably not a good choice for the noncompulsive, disorganized woman or for the average adolescent.

Emergency Postcoital Contraception

The use of large doses of estrogen to prevent implantation was pioneered by Morris and van Wagenen at Yale in the 1960s. The initial work in monkeys led to the use of high doses of diethylstilbestrol (25–50 mg/day) and ethinyl estradiol in women.[146] It was quickly appreciated that these extremely large doses of estrogen were associated with a high rate of gastrointestinal side effects. Yuzpe developed a method utilizing a combination oral contraceptive, resulting in an important reduction in dosage.[147] The following treatment regimens have been documented to be effective:

Conjugated Estrogens, 15 mg bid for 5 days or 50 mg iv on each of 2 consecutive days.

Ethinyl Estradiol, 2.5 mg bid for 5 days.

Ovral, 4 tablets (2 given 12 hours apart).

LoOvral or Levelen, 8 tablets (4 given 12 hours apart).

This method has been more commonly called postcoital contraception or the "morning after" treatment. Emergency contraception is a more accurate and appropriate name, indicating the intention to be one-time protection. It is an important option for patients and should be considered when condoms break, sexual assault occurs, or diaphragms or cervical caps dislodge or with the lapsed use of any method. In a study at an abortion service, fully half of the patients would have been suitable for emergency contraception.[148] Emergency contraception is another component of contraception that cries for public education and media publicity.

Mechanism and Efficacy

The mechanism of action is not known with certainty, but it is believed with justification that this treatment interferes with implantation. The efficacy has been confirmed in large clinical trials and summarized in a complete review of the literature.[149] Treatment with high doses of estrogen yields a failure rate of approximately 1%, with the combination oral contraceptive, about 2%. The failure rate is lowest with high doses of ethinyl estradiol given within 72 hours (0.1%), but the side effects make the combination oral contraceptive a better choice.

Treatment Method

Treatment should be initiated as soon after exposure as possible but no later than 72 hours. Because of possible, but unlikely, harmful effects of these high doses to a fetus, an already existing pregnancy should be ruled out prior to use of postcoital hormones. Furthermore, the patient should be offered therapeutic abortion if the method fails. This patient encounter also provides an important opportunity to screen for STDs.

The combination oral contraceptive method delivers significantly less steroid hormone, and this reduction in the total dose and the number of doses reduces the side effects and limits them to a shorter time period. It is worth adding an antiemetic, oral or suppository, to the treatment. Side effects reflect the high doses used: nausea, vomiting, breast tenderness, headache, and dizziness. The usual contraindications for oral contraception apply to this use.

A 3-week follow-up visit should be scheduled to assess the result and to counsel for regular contraception.

Could other combination oral contraceptive products be used? Since other doses and other formulations have never been tested, the efficacy is unknown. It would not be appropriate to expose patients to an unknown failure rate. Levonorgestrel in a dose of 0.75 mg given twice, 12 hours apart, is as successful as the combination oral contraceptive method, but this dose is equivalent to 25 pills of the levonorgestrel progestin-only minipill.[150] The use of danazol for this purpose is relatively untested, but RU486, the progesterone antagonist, has been without failures and with lower side effects in preliminary trials.

The two major problems with the available methods of emergency contraception are the high rate of side effects and the small, but important, failure rate. Mifepristone (RU486) in a single oral dose of 600 mg is associated with markedly less nausea and vomiting and. in nearly 1,000 women, a pregnancy rate of zero.[151,152] Because the next menstrual cycle is delayed after mifepristone, contraception should be initiated immediately after treatment. Ironically, RU486, around which swirls the abortion controversy, can make an effective contribution to preventing unwanted pregnancies and therapeutic abortions.

Another method of emergency contraception is the insertion of a copper IUD, up to 5 days after unprotected intercourse. The failure rate (in a small number of studies) is very low, 0.1%.[149] This method definitely prevents implantation, but it is not suitable for women at risk for infection (multiple sexual partners, rape victim).

Oral Contraception for Older Women

The years from age 35 to menopause can be referred to as the transition years. During this period of time, there are several medical needs that must be addressed: the need for contraception, the management of persistent anovulation, and finally, menopausal and postmenopausal hormone therapy.

At approximately 40 years of age, the frequency of ovulation decreases. This initiates a period of waning ovarian function called the climacteric that will last several years, carrying a woman through decreased fertility and menopause to the postmenopausal years. Prior to menopause, the remaining follicles perform less well. As cycles become irregular, vaginal bleeding occurs at the end of an indequate luteal phase or after a peak of estradiol without subsequent ovulation and corpus luteum formation. Eventually, many women will live through a period of anovulation. Occasionally corpus luteum formation and function occur, and therefore the older woman is not totally safe from the threat of an unplanned and unexpected pregnancy.

Fortunately clinicians and patients have recognized that low dose oral contraception is very safe for healthy, nonsmoking older women. However, its use is still not sufficient to meet the need. Among women using contraception in 1988, only 5% of women aged 35–44 used oral contraception and only 3% aged 40–44, compared to 68% aged 20–24.[153] Besides fulfilling a need, we would argue that this population of women has a series of benefits to be derived from oral contraception that tilts the risk:benefit ratio to the positive side.

The most up-to-date conclusion now indicates that the risk of dying from circulatory diseases is confined to smokers over the age of 35 who use oral contraception, and that conclusion is based upon data from women using higher dose pills. Nonsmoking, healthy women over 35 can expect no adverse impact from low dose oral contraception.

Presently there is no reason why low dose oral contraception cannot be utilized by appropriate patients until menopause. Menopause occurs in American women between the ages of 48 and 55, with the median age being approximately 50. Because the age of menopause occurs over such a relatively large age range, it is difficult to know when it is safe to change from oral contraception to a postmenopausal hormone program. And it should be emphasized that this change is important because the estrogen dose in even the lowest contraceptive formulations available is at least four times greater than what is needed for postmenopausal treatment. However, even this dose of estrogen has an insignificant impact on the coagulation system.[154,155]

The therapeutic principle remains to utilize the formulation that gives effective contraception and the greatest margin of safety. Because we now appreciate the dose-response relationship between the steroid components and side effects, it makes sense to use the lowest doses that are still effective. For this reason products with less than 30 μg of estrogen might be especially useful for older women.

Over the years, the debate over the cause of circulatory complications attributed to oral contraception turned from thrombosis to atherosclerosis. Today, belief is firmly back in the camp of thrombosis. A significant reason is the failure to detect any lingering risk of cardiovascular disease in former pill users. Most noteworthy is the Nurses' Health Study.[18] Now that the nurses initially enrolled in this follow-up study have aged sufficiently, we have statistically and clinically significant data from women who have reached the age of major risk for cardiovascular disease. Even the use of higher-dose oral contraceptives is not associated with a subsequent increased risk of coronary heart disease and stroke. The fact that an increased risk of cardiovascular disease is limited to current use (of higher dose pills) is a very strong indicator that the mechanism is a short-term acute mechanism, specifically thrombosis, an estrogen-related effect. Therefore, our return to the belief that cardiovascular disease is linked to thrombosis makes the role, and the dose, of estrogen very important.

A product containing 20 μg ethinyl estradiol and 150 μg desogestrel has been demonstrated in multicenter studies of women over age 30 to have the same efficacy and side effects as pills containing 30 and 35 μg of estrogen.[156,157] In a randomized study, this formulation was associated with the virtual elimination of any effects on coagulation factors.[155]

It seems to us that the time is right for the lowest estrogen dose products for older women. While it is true that the implied safety of the lowest estrogen dose remains to be documented by epidemiologic studies, it seems clinically prudent to maximize the safety margin in this older age group of women. With avoidance of risk factors and use of lowest dose pills, health risks are probably negligible for healthy, nonsmoking women. For healthy nonsmoking women, no specific laboratory screening is necessary beyond that which is usually incorporated in a program of preventive health care.

We should also mention the progestin-only minipill. Because of reduced fecundity, the minipill achieves near total efficacy in women over age 40. Therefore, the progestin-only minipill is a good choice for older women, and especially for those women in whom estrogen is contraindicated. Older women are more accepting of irregular menstrual bleeding when they understand its mechanism and thus are more accepting of the progestin-only minipill.

When to Change from Oral Contraception to Postmenopausal Hormone Therapy
One approach to establish the onset of the postmenopausal years is to measure the FSH level, beginning at age 50, on an annual basis, being careful to obtain the blood sample on day 5–7 of the pill-free week. By then, the steroid levels will have declined sufficiently to allow FSH to rise. When FSH is greater than 30 IU/L, it is time to change to a postmenopausal hormone program. Some clinicians are comfortable allowing patients to enter their mid-fifties on low dose oral contraception, and then empirically switching to a postmenopausal hormone regimen.

Anovulation and Bleeding

Throughout the transitional period of life there is a significant incidence of dysfunctional uterine bleeding due to anovulation. While the clinician is usually alerted to this problem because of irregular bleeding, clinician and patient often fail to diagnose anovulation when bleeding is not abnormal in schedule, flow, or duration. As a woman approaches menopause, a more aggressive attempt to document ovulation is warranted. A serum progesterone level measured approximately one week before menses is simple enough to obtain and worth the cost. The prompt diagnosis of anovulation (serum progesterone less than 300 ng/dL) will lead to appropriate therapeutic management which will have a significant impact on the risk of endometrial cancer.

In an anovulatory woman with proliferative or hyperplastic endometrium (unaccompanied by atypia), periodic oral progestin therapy is mandatory, such as 10 mg medroxyprogesterone acetate given daily the first 10 days of each month. If hyperplasia is already present, follow-up aspiration office curettage after 3–4 months is required. If progestin treatment is ineffective and histological regression is not observed, more aggressive treatment is warranted.

Monthly progestin treatment should be continued until withdrawal bleeding ceases or menopausal symptoms are experienced. These are reliable signs (in effect, a bioassay) indicating the onset of estrogen deprivation and the need for the addition of estrogen in a postmenopausal hormone program.

If contraception is desired, the clinician and patient should seriously consider the use of oral contraception. The anovulatory woman cannot be guaranteed that spontaneous ovulation and pregnancy will not occur. The use of a low dose oral contraceptive will at the same time provide contraception and prophylaxis against irregular, heavy anovulatory bleeding and the risk of endometrial hyperplasia and neoplasia.

Clinicians have been made so wary of providing oral contraceptives to older women that a traditional postmenopausal hormone regimen is often utilized to treat a woman with the kind of irregular cycles usually experienced in the transitional years. This addition of exogenous estrogen when a woman is not amenorrheic or experiencing menopausal symptoms is inappropriate and even risky (exposing the endometrium to excessively high levels of estrogen). The appropriate response is to regulate anovulatory cycles with monthly progestational treatment or to utilize low dose oral contraception.

Preventive Health Care for Older Women

Preventive health care for women is especially important during the transition years. The issues of preventive health care are familiar ones. They include contraception, cessation of smoking, prevention of heart disease and osteoporosis, maintenance of mental well-being (including sexuality), and cancer screening. Management of the transition years should be significantly oriented to preventive health care, and the use of low dose oral contraception can now legitimately be viewed as a component of preventive health care. A discussion of the noncontraceptive health benefits of low dose oral contraception is especially important with patients in their transition years. This group of women appreciates and understands decisions made with the risk:benefit ratio in mind.

References

1. **Goldzieher JW,** Hormonal contraception - whence, how, and whither? in Givens J, editor, *Clinical Uses of Steroids,* Yearbook, Chicago, 1980, pp 31-43.

2. **Medvei VC,** *A History of Endocrinology,* MTB Press, Hingham, Massachusetts, 1982.

3. **Pincus, G,** *The Control of Fertility,* Academic Press, New York, 1965.

4. **Goldzieher JW,** Selected aspects of the pharmacokinetics and metabolism of ethinyl estrogens and their clinical implications, Am J Obstet Gynecol 163:318, 1990.

5. **Stanczyk FZ, Roy S,** Metabolism of levonorgestrel, norethindrone, and structurally related contraceptive steroids, Contraception 42:67, 1990.

6. **Edgren RA,** Progestagens, in Givens J, editor, *Clinical Uses of Steroids,* Yearbook, Chicago, 1980, pp 1-29.

7. **Speroff L, DeCherney A,** Evaluation of a new generation of oral contraceptives, Obstet Gynecol 81:1034, 1993.

8. **Hammerstein J, Daume E, Simon A, Winkler UH, Schindler AE, Back DJ, Ward S, Neiss A,** Influence of gestodene and desogestrel as components of low-dose oral contraceptives on the pharmacokinetics of ethinyl estradiol (EE), on serum CBG and on urinary cortisol and 6β-hydroxycortisol, Contraception 47:263, 1993.

9. **Trussell J, Hatcher RA, Cates W Jr, Stewart FH, Kost K,** Contraceptive failure in the United States: an update, Stud Fam Plann 21:51, 1990.

10. **Ramcharan S, Pellegrin FA, Ray RM, Hsu J-P,** The Walnut Creek Contraceptive Drug Study. A prospective study of the side effects of oral contraceptives, J Reprod Med 25:366,360, 1980.

11. **Porter JB, Hershel J, Walker AM,** Mortality among oral contraceptive users, Obstet Gynecol 70:29, 1987.

12. **Vessey MP, Villard-Mackintosh I, McPherson K, Yeates D,** Mortality among oral contraceptive users: 20 year follow up of women in a cohort study, Br Med J 299:1487, 1989.

13. **Gerstman BB, Piper JM, Tomita DK, Ferguson WJ, Stadel BV, Lundin FE,** Oral contraceptive estrogen dose and the risk of deep venous thromboembolic disease, Am J Epidemiol 133:32, 1991.

14. **Lidegaard O,** Oral contraception and risk of a cerebral thromboembolic attack: results of a case-control study, Br Med J 306:956, 1993.

15. **Thorogood M, Mann J, Murphy M, Vessey M,** Risk factors for fatal venous thromboembolism in young women: a case-control study, Int J Epidemiol 21:48, 1992.

16. **Jespersen J, Petersen KR, Skouby SO,** Effects of newer oral contraceptives on the inhibition of coagulation and fibrinolysis in relation to dosage and type of steroid, Am J Obstet Gynecol 163:396, 1990.

17. **Notelovitz M, Kitchens CS, Khan FY,** Changes in coagulation and anticoagulation in women taking low-dose triphasic oral contraceptives: a controlled comparative 12-month clinical trial, Am J Obstet Gynecol 167:1255, 1992.

18. **Stampfer MJ, Willett WC, Colditz GA, Speizer FE, Hennekens CH,** Past use of oral contraceptives and cardiovascular disease: a meta-analysis in the context of the Nurses' Health Study, Am J Obstet Gynecol 163:285, 1990.

19. **Rosenberg L, Palmer JR, Lesko SM, Shapiro S,** Oral contraceptive use and the risk of myocardial infarction, Am J Epidemiol 131:1009, 1990.

20. **Croft P, Hannaford PC,** Risk factors for acute myocardial infarction in women: evidence from the Royal College of General Practitioners' oral contraception study, Br Med J 298:165, 1989.

21. **Croft P, Hannaford PC,** Risk factors for acute myocardial infarction in women, Br Med J 298:674, 1989.

22. **Clarkson TB, Shively CA, Morgan TM, Koritnik DR, Adams MR, Kaplan JR,** Oral contraceptives and coronary artery atherosclerosis of cynomolgus monkeys, Obstet Gynecol 75:217. 1990.

23. **Hirvonen E, Heikkila-Idanpaan J,** Cardiovascular death among women under 40 years of age using low-estrogen oral contraceptives and intrauterine devices in Finland from 1975 to 1984, Am J Obstet Gynecol 163:281, 1990.

24. **Mant D, Villard-Mackintosh L, Vessey MP, Yeates D,** Myocardial infarction and angina pectoris in young women, J Epidemiol Community Health 41:215, 1987.

25. **Thorogood M, Mann J, Murphy M, Vessey M,** Fatal stroke and use of oral contraceptives: findings from a case-control study, Am J Epidemiol 136:35, 1992.

26. **Kovacs L, Bartfai G, Apro G, Annus J, Bulpitt C, Belsey E, Pinol A,** The effect of the contraceptive pill on blood pressure: a randomized controlled trial of three progestogen-oestrogen combinations in Szeged, Hungary, Contraception 33:69, 1986.

27. **Nichols M, Robinson G, Bounds W, Newman B, Guillebaud J,** Effect of four combined oral contraceptives on blood pressure in the pill-free interval, Contraception 47:367, 1993.

28. **Pritchard JA, Pritchard SA,** Blood pressure response to estrogen-progestin oral contraceptives after pregnancy-induced hypertension, Am J Obstet Gynecol 129:733, 1977.

29. **van der Vange N, Kloosterboer HJ, Haspels AA,** Effect of seven low-dose combined oral contraceptive preparations on carbohydrate metabolism, Am J Obstet Gynecol 156:918, 1987.

30. **Duffy TJ, Ray R,** Oral contraceptive use: prospective follow-up of women with suspected glucose intolerance, Contraception 30:197, 1984.

31. **Hannaford PC, Kay CR,** Oral contraceptives and diabetes mellitus, Br Med J 299:315, 1989.

32. **Kjos SL, Shoupe D, Douyan S, Friedman RL, Bernstein GS, Mestman JH, Mishell DR Jr,** Effect of low-dose oral contraceptives on carbohydrate and lipid metabolism in women with recent gestational diabetes: results of a controlled, randomized, prospective study, Am J Obstet Gynecol 163:1822, 1990.

33. **Royal College of General Practitioners' Oral Contraception Study,** Oral contraceptives and gallbladder disease, Lancet 2:957, 1982.

34. **Vessey MP, Villard-Mackintosh L, Painter R,** Oral contraceptives and pregnancy in relation to peptic ulcer, Contraception 46:349, 1992.

35. **Lashner BA, Kane SV, Hanauer SB,** Lack of association between oral contraceptive use and ulcerative colitis, Gastroenterology 99:1032, 1990.

36. **Hulting A-L, Werner S, Hagenfeldt K,** Oral contraceptives do not promote the development or growth of prolactinomas, Contraception 27:69, 1983.

37. **Corenblum B, Donovan L,** The safety of physiological estrogen plus progestin replacement therapy and with oral contraceptive therapy in women with pathological hyperprolactinemia, Fertil Steril 59:671, 1993.

38. **The Cancer and Steroid Hormone Study of the CDC and NICHD,** Combination oral contraceptive use and the risk of endometrial cancer, JAMA 257:796, 1987.

39. **Schlesselman JJ,** Oral contraceptives and neoplasia of the uterine corpus, Contraception 43:557, 1991.

40. **The Cancer and Steroid Hormone Study of the CDC and NICHD,** The reduction in risk of ovarian cancer associated with oral-contraceptive use, New Engl J Med 316:650, 1987.

41. **Hankinson SE, Colditz GA, Hunter DJ, Spencer TL, Rosner B, Stampfer MJ,** A quantitative assessment of oral contraceptive use and risk of ovarian cancer, Obstet Gynecol 80:708, 1992.

42. **Brinton LA,** Oral contraceptives and cervical neoplasia, Contraception 43:581, 1991.

43. **Delgado-Rodriguez M, Sillero-Arenas M, Martin-Moreno JM, Galvez-Vargas R,** Oral contraceptives and cancer of the cervix uteri. A meta-analysis, Acta Obstet Gynecol Scand 71:368, 1992.

44. **Gram IT, Macaluso M, Stalsberg H,** Oral contraceptive use and the incidence of cervical intraepithelial neoplasia, Am J Obstet Gynecol 167:40, 1992.

45. **Irwin KL, Rosero-Bixby L, Oberle MW, Lee NC, Whatley AS, Fortney JA, Bonhomme MG,** Oral contraceptives and cervical cancer risk in Costa Rica: detection bias or causal association? JAMA 259:59, 1988.

46. **Brinton LA, Reeves WC, Brenes MM, et al,** Oral contraceptive use and risk of invasive cervical cancer, Int J Epidemiol 19:4, 1990.

47. **WHO Collaborative Study of Neoplasia and Steroid Contraceptives,** Combined oral contraceptives and liver cancer, Int J Cancer 43:254, 1989.

48. **Brinton LA, Vessey MP, Flavel R, Yeates D,** Risk factors for benign breast disease, Am J Epidemiol 113:203, 1981.

49. **Royal College of General Practitioners Oral Contraceptive Study,** Further analyses of mortality in oral contraceptive users, Lancet 1:541, 1981.

50. **Vessey M, McPherson K, Villard-Mackintosh L, Yeates D,** Oral contraceptives and breast cancer: latest findings in a large cohort study, Br J Cancer 59:613, 1989.

51. **Romieu I, Willett WC, Colditz GA, Stampfer MJ, Rosner B, Hennekens, CH, Speizer FE,** Prospective study of oral contraceptive use and risk of breast cancer in women, J Natl Cancer Inst 81:1313, 1989.

52. **Meirik O, Dami H, Christoffersen T, Lund E, Bergstrom R, Bergsjo P,** Oral contraceptive use and breast cancer in young women, Lancet 2:650, 1986.

53. **Miller DR, Rosenberg L, Kaufman DW, Stolley P, Warshauer ME, Shapiro S,** Breast cancer before age 45 and oral contraceptive use: new findings, Am J Epidemiol 129:269, 1989.

54. **UK National Case-Control Study Group,** Oral contraceptive use and breast cancer risk in young women, Lancet 1:973, 1989.

55. **McPherson K, Vessey MP, Neil A, Doll R, Jones L, Roberts M,** Early oral contraceptive use and breast cancer: results of another case-control study, Br J Cancer 56:653, 1987.

56. **Stadel BV, Lai SL,** Oral contraceptives and premenopausal breast cancer in nulliparous women, Contraception 38:287, 1988.

57. **Pike MC, Krailo MD, Henderson BE, Duke A, Roy S,** Breast cancer in young women and use of oral contraceptives: possible modifying effect of formulation and age at use, Lancet 2:926, 1983.

58. **Ursin G, Aragaki CC, Paganini-Hill A, Siemiatycki J, Thompson WD, Haile RW,** Oral contraceptives and premenopausal bilateral breast cancer: a case-control study, Epidemiology 3:414, 1992.

59. **Stanford JL, Brinton LA, Hoover RN,** Oral contraceptives and breast cancer: results from an expanded case-control study, Br J Cancer 60:375, 1989.

60. **Schildkraut JM, Hulka BS, Wilkinson WE,** Oral contraceptives and breast cancer: a case-control study with hospital and community controls, Obstet Gynecol 76:395, 1990.

61. **Cancer and Steroid Hormone Study, CDC and NICHD,** Oral contraceptive use and the risk of breast cancer, New Engl J Med 315:405, 1986.

62. **Murray P, Schlesselman JJ, Stadel BV, Shenghan L,** Oral contraceptives and breast cancer risk in women with a family history of breast cancer, Am J Obstet Gynecol 73:977, 1989.

63. **Schlesselman JJ, Stadel BV, Murray P, Shenghan L,** Breast cancer risk in relation to type of estrogen contained in oral contraceptives, Contraception 36:595, 1987.

64. **Schlesselman JJ, Stadel BV, Murray P, Lai S,** Breast cancer in relation to early use of oral contracpetives. No evidence of a latent effect, JAMA 259:1828, 1988.

65. **Wingo PA, Lee NC, Ory HW, Beral V, Peterson HB, Rhodes P,** Age-specific differences in the relationship between oral contraceptive use and breast cancer, Obstet Gynecol 78:161. 1991.

66. **Rushton L, Jones DR,** Oral contraceptive use and breast cancer risk: a meta-analysis of variations with age at diagnosis, parity and total duration of oral contraceptive use, Br J Obstet Gynaecol 99:239, 1992.

67. **Stadel BV, Schlesselman JJ,** Oral contraceptive use and the risk of breast cancer in women with a "prior" history of benign breast disease, Am J Epidemiol 123:373, 1986.

68. **Green A,** Oral contraceptives and skin neoplasia, Contraception 43:653, 1991.

69. **Hannaford PC, Villard-Mackintosh L, Vessey MP, Kay CR,** Oral contraceptives and malignant melanoma, Br J Cancer 63:430, 1991.

70. **Milne R, Vessey M,** The association of oral contraception with kidney cancer, colon cancer, gallbladder cancer (including extrahepatic bile duct cancer) and pituitary tumors, Contraception 43:667, 1991.

71. **Simpson JL, Phillips OP,** Spermicides, hormonal contraception and congenital malformations, Adv Contracept 6:141, 1990.

72. **Bracken MB,** Oral contraception and congenital malformations in offspring: a review and meta-analysis of the prospective studies, Obstet Gynecol 76:552, 1990.

73. **Katz Z, Lancet M, Skornik J, Chemke J, Mogilemer B, Klinberg M,** Teratogenicity of progestogens given during the first trimester of pregnancy, Obstet Gynecol 65:775, 1985.

74. **Vessey MP, Wright NH, McPherson K, Wiggins P,** Fertility after stopping different methods of contraception, Br Med J 1:265, 1978.

75. **Vessey MP, Smith MA, Yates D,** Return of fertility after discontinuation of oral contraceptives: influence of age and parity, Br J Fam Plann 11:120, 1986.

76. **Linn S, Schoenbaum SC, Monson RR, Rosner B, Ryan KJ,** Delay in conception for former 'pill' users, JAMA 247:629, 1982.

77. **Bracken MB, Hellenbrand KG, Holford TR,** Conception delay after oral contraceptive use: the effect of estrogen dose, Fertil Steril 53:21, 1990.

78. **Rothman KJ,** Fetal loss, twinning, and birth weight after oral-contraceptive use, New Engl J Med 297:468, 1977.

79. **Rothman KJ, Liess J,** Gender of offspring after oral-contraceptive use, New Engl J Med 295:859, 1976.

80. **Magidor S, Poalti H, Harlap S, Baras M,** Long-term follow-up of children whose mothers used oral contraceptives prior to contraception, Contraception 29:203, 1984.

81. **Royal College of General Practitioners,** The outcome of pregnancy in former oral contraceptive users, Br J Obstet Gynaecol 83:608, 1976.

82. **Betrabet SS, Shikary ZK, Toddywalla VS, Toddywalla SP, Patel D, Saxena BN,** Transfer of norethisterone (NET) and levonorgestrel (LNG) from a single tablet into the infant's circulation through the mother's milk, Contraception 35:517, 1987.

83. **Croxatto HB, Diaz S, Peralta O, Juez G, Herreros C, Casado ME, Salvatierra AM, Miranda P, Durn E,** Fertility regulation in nursing women: IV. Long-term influence of a low-dose combined oral contraceptive initiated at day 30 postpartum upon lactation and child growth, Contraception 27:13, 1983.

84. **Peralta O, Diaz S, Juez G, Herreros C, Casado ME, Salvatierra AM, Miranda P, Durn E, Croxatto HB,** Fertility regulation in nursing women. V. Long-term influence of a low-dose combined oral contraceptive initiated at day 90 postpartum upon lactation and infant growth, Contraception 27:27, 1983.

759

85. **WHO Task Force on Oral Contraceptives,** Effects of hormonal contraceptives on milk volume and infant growth, Contraception 30:505, 1984.

86. **Nilsson S, Mellbin T, Hofvander Y, Sundelin C, Valentin J, Nygren KG,** Long-term follow-up of children breast-fed by mothers using oral contraceptives, Contraception 34:443, 1986.

87. **Howie PW, McNeilly AS, Houston MJ, Cook A, Boyle H,** Effect of supplementary food on suckling patterns and ovarian activity during lactation, Br Med J 283:757, 1981.

88. **Perez A, Vela P, Masnick GS, Potter RG,** First ovulation after childbirth: the effect of breastfeeding, Am J Obstet Gynecol 114:1041, 1972.

89. **Diaz S, Peralta O, Juez G, Salvatierra AM, Casado ME, Duran E, Croxatto HB,** Fertility regulation in nursing women. I. The probablity of conception in full nursing women living in an urban setting, J Biosoc Sci 14:329, 1982.

90. **McNeilly AS, Glasier A, Howie PW,** Endocrine control of lactational infertility, in Dobbing J, editor, *Maternal Nutrition and Lactational Infertility,* Nevey/Raven Press, New York, 1985, p 177.

91. **Rivera R, Kennedy KI, Ortiz E, Barrera M, Bhiwandiwala PP,** Breast-feeding and the return to ovulation in Durango, Mexico, Fertil Steril 49:780, 1988.

92. **Gray RH, Campbell OM, Apelo R, Eslami SS, Zacur H, Ramos RM, Gehret JC, Labbok MH,** Risk of ovulation during lactation, Lancet 335:25, 1990.

93. **Diaz S, Aravena R, Cardenas H, Casado ME, Miranda P, Schiappacasse V, Croxatto HB,** Contraceptive efficacy of lactational amenorrhea in urban Chilean women, Contraception 43:335, 1991.

94. **Campbell OM, Gray RH,** Characteristics and determinants of postpartum ovarian function in women in the United States, Am J Obstet Gynecol 169:55, 1993.

95. **Furuhjelm M, Carlstrom K,** Amenorrhea following use of combined oral contraceptives, Acta Obstet Gynecol Scand 52:373, 1973.

96. **Westrom L,** Incidence, prevalence, and trends of acute pelvic inflammatory disease and its consequences in industrialized countries, Am J Obstet Gynecol 138:880, 1980.

97. **Rubin GL, Ory WH, Layde PM,** Oral contraceptives and pelvic inflammatory disease, Am J Obstet Gynecol 140:630, 1980.

98. **Panser LA, Phipps WR,** Type of oral contraceptive in relation to acute, initial episodes of pelvic inflammatory disease, Contraception 43:91, 1991.

99. **Svensson L, Westrom L, Mardh P,** Contraceptives and acute salpingitis, JAMA 251:2553, 1984.

100. **Cates W Jr, Washington AE, Rubin GL, Peterson HB,** The pill, chlamydia and PID, Fam Plann Perspect 17:175, 1985.

101. **Cramer DW, Goldman MB, Schiff I, Belisla S, Albrecht B, Stadel B, Gibson M, Wilson E, Stillman R, Thompson I,** The relationship of tubal infertility to barrier method and oral contraceptive use, JAMA 257:2446, 1987.

102. **Wolner-Hanssen P, Eschenbach DA, Paavonen J, Kiviat N, Stevens CE, Critchlow C, DeRouen T, Holmes KK,** Decreased risk of symptomatic chlamydial pelvic inflammatory disease associated with oral contraceptive use, JAMA 263:54, 1990.

103. **Hunter DJ, Mati JK,** Contraception, family planning, and HIV, presented at the Conference on AIDS and Reproductive Health, Bellagio, Italy, 1990.

104. **Barbone F, Austin H, Louv WC, Alexander WJ,** A follow-up study of methods of contraception, sexual activity, and rates of trichomoniasis, candidiasis, and bacterial vaginosis, Am J Obstet Gynecol 163:510, 1990.

105. **Ross RK, Pike MC, Vessey MP, Bull D, Yeates D, Casagrande JT,** Risk factors for uterine fibroids: reduced risk associated with oral contraceptives, Br J Med 293:359, 1986.

106. **Parazzini F, Negri E, Lavecchia C, Fedele L, Rabaiotti M, Luchini L,** Oral contraceptive use and risk of uterine fibroids, Obstet Gynecol 79:430, 1992.

107. **Mattson RH, Cramer JA, Darney PD, Naftolin F,** Use of oral contraceptives by women with epilepsy, JAMA 256:238, 1986

108. **Letterie GS, Chow GE,** Effect of "missed" pills on oral contraceptive effectiveness, Obstet Gynecol 79:979, 1992.

109. **Killick SR, Bancroft K, Oelbaum S, Morris J, Elstein M,** Extending the duration of the pill-free interval during combined oral contraception, Adv Contraception 6:33, 1990.

110. **Jung-Hoffman C, Kuhl H,** Intra- and interindividual variations in contraceptive steroid levels during 12 treatment cycles: no relation to irregular bleedings, Contraception 42:423, 1990.

111. **Grimes DA, Hughes JM,** Use of multiphasic oral contraceptives and hospitalizations of women with functional ovarian cysts in the United States, Obstet Gynecol 73:1037, 1989.

112. **Vessey M, Metcalfe A, Wells C, McPherson K, Westhoff C, Yeates D,** Ovarian neoplasms, functional ovarian cysts, and oral contraceptives, Br Med J 294:1518, 1987.

113. **Neely JL, Abate M, Swinker M, D'Angio R,** The effect of doxycycline on serum levels of ethinyl estradiol, norethindrone, and endogenous progesterone, Obstet Gynecol 77:416, 1991.

114. **Murphy AA, Zacur HA, Charache P, Burkman RT,** The effect of tetracycline on levels of oral contraceptives, Am J Obstet Gynecol 164:28, 1991.

115. **Szoka PR, Edgren RA,** Drug interactions with oral contraceptives: compilation and analysis of an adverse experience report database, Fertil Steril 49(Suppl):31S, 1988.

116. **Jungers P, Dougados M, Pelissier L, Kuttenn F, Tron F, Lesavre P, Bach JF,** Influence of oral contraceptive therapy on the activity of systemic lupus erythematosus, Arthritis Rheum 25:618, 1982.

117. **Knopp RH, LaRosa JC, Burkman RT Jr,** Contraception and dyslipidemia, Am J Obstet Gynecol 168:1994, 1993.

118. **Lashner BA, Kane SV, Hanauer SB,** Lack of association between OC use and ulcerative colitis, Gastroenterology 99:1032, 1990.

119. **Coutinho EM, da Silva AR, Carreira C, Rodrigues V, Goncalves MT,** Conception control by vaginal administration of pills containing ethinyl estradiol and dl-norgestrel, Fertil Steril 42:478, 1984.

120. **Sullivan-Nelson M, Kuller JA, Zacur HA,** Clinical use of oral contraceptives administered vaginally: a case report, Fertil Steril 52:864, 1989.

121. **Coutinho EM, de Souza JC, da Silva AR, de Acosta OM, et al,** Comparative study on the efficacy and acceptability of two contraceptive pills administered by the vaginal route: an international multicenter clinical trial, Clin Pharmacol Ther 53:65, 1993.

122. **Lanes SF, Birmann B, Walker AM, Singer S,** Oral Contraceptive type and functional ovarian cysts, Am J Obstet Gynecol 166:956, 1992.

123. **Holt VL, Daling JR, McKnight B, Moore D, Stergachis A, Weiss NS,** Functional ovarian cysts in relation to the use of monophasic and triphasic oral contraceptives, Obstet Gynecol 79:529, 1992.

124. **Milsom E, Sundell G, Andersch B,** The influence of different combined oral contraceptives on the prevalence and severity of dysmenorrhea, Contraception 42:497, 1990.

125. **Larsson G, Milsom I, Lindstedt G, Rybo G,** The influence of a low-dose combined oral contraceptive on menstrual blood loss and iron status, Contraception 46:327, 1992.

126. **Kirshon B, Poindexter AN III,** Contraception: a risk factor for endometriosis, Obstet Gynecol 71:829, 1988.

127. **Enzelsberger H, Metka M, Heytmanek G, Schurz B, Kurz C, Kusztrich M,** Influence of oral contraceptive use on bone density in climacteric women, Maturitas 9:375, 1988.

128. **Kleerekoper M, Brienza RS, Schultz LR, Johnson CC,** Oral contraceptive use may protect against low bone mass, Arch Intern Med 151:1971, 1991.

129. **Kritz-Silverstein D, Barrett-Connor E,** Bone mineral density in postmenopausal women as determined by prior oral contraceptive use, Am J Public Health 83:100, 1993.

130. **Hazes JMW, Dijkmans BAC, Vandenbroucke JP, De Vries RRP, Cats A,** Reduction of the risk of rheumatoid arthritis among women who take oral contraceptives, Arthritis Rheum 33:173, 1990.

131. **Spector TD, Hochberg MC,** The protective effect of the oral contraceptive pill on rheumatoid arthritis: an overview of the analytical epidemiological studies using meta-analysis, J Clin Epidemiol 43:1221, 1990.

132. **van der Vange N, Blankenstein MA, Kloosterboer HJ, Haspels AA, Thijssen JHH,** Effects of seven low-dose combined oral contraceptives on sex hormone binding globulin, corticosteroid binding globulin, total and free testsosterone, Contraception 41:345, 1990.

133. **Lemay A, Dewailly SD, Grenier R, Huard J,** Attenuation of mild hyperandrogenic activity in postpubertal acne by a triphasic oral contraceptive containing low doses of ethynyl estradiol and d,l-norgestrel, J Clin Endocrinol Metab 71:8, 1990.

134. **Steinkampf MP, Hammond KR, Blackwell RE,** Hormonal treatment of functional ovarian cysts: a randomized, prospective study, Fertil Steril 54:775, 1990.

135. **Jones EF, Forrest JD,** Contraceptive failure in the United States: revised estimates from the 1982 National Survey of Family Growth, Fam Plann Perspect 21:103, 1989.

136. **Chi I,** The safety and efficacy issues of progestin-only oral contraceptives — an epidemiologic perspective, Contraception 47:1, 1993.

137. **Ball MJ, Gillmer AE,** Progestagen-only oral contraceptives: comparison of the metabolic effects of levonorgestrel and norethisterone, Contraception 44:223, 1991.

138. **Vessey MP, Lawless M, Yeates D, McPherson K,** Progestogen-only contraception: findings in a large prospective study with special reference to effectiveness, Br J Fam Plann 10:117, 1985.

139. **Broome M, Fotherby K,** Clinical experience with the progestogen-only pill, Contraception 42:489, 1990.

140. **Sheth A, Jain U, Sharma S, Adatia A, Patankar S, Andolsek L, Pretnar-Darovec A, Belsey MA, Hall PE, Parker RA, Ayeni S, Pinol A, Li Hoi Foo C,** A randomized, double-blind study of two combined and two progestogen-only oral contraceptives, Contraception 25:243, 1982.

141. **Tayob Y, Adams J, Jacobs HS, Guillebaud J,** Ultrasound demonstration of increased frequency of functional ovarian cysts in women using progestogen-only oral contraception, Br J Obstet Gynaecol 92:1003, 1985.

142. **Dunson TR, McLaurin VL, Grubb GS, Rosman AW,** A multicenter clinical trial of a progestin-only oral contraceptive in lactating women, Contraception 47:23, 1993.

143. **WHO Special Programme of Research, Development, and Research Training in Human Reproduction, Task Force on Oral Contraceptives,** Effects of hormonal contraceptives on milk volume and infant growth, Contraception 30:505, 1984.

144. **McCann MF, Moggia AV, Hibbins JE, Potts M, Becker C,** The effects of a progestin-only oral contraceptive (levonorgestrel 0.03 mg) on breast-feeding, Contraception 40:635, 1989.

145. **Fotherby K,** The progestogen-only pill and thrombosis, Br J Fam Plann 15:83, 1989.

146. **Morris J McL, van Wagenen G,** Compounds interfering with ovum implantation and development. III. The role of estrogens, Am J Obstet Gynecol 96:804, 1966.

147. **Yuzpe AA, Smith RP, Rademaker AW,** A multicenter clinical investigation employing ethinyl estradiol combined with dl-norgestrel as a postcoital contraceptive agent, Fertil Steril 37:508, 1982.

148. **Burton R, Savage W, Reader F,** The "morning after pill." Is this the wrong name for it? Br J Fam Plann 15:119, 1990.

149. **Fasoli M, Parazzini F, Cecchetti G, La Vecchia C,** Post-coital contraception: an overview of published studies, Contraception 39:459, 1989.

150. **Ho PC, Kwan MSW,** A prospective randomized comparison of levonorgestrel with the Yuzpe regimen in post-coital contraception, Hum Reprod 8:389, 1993.

151. **Webb AMC, Russell J, Elstein M,** Comparison of Yuzpe regimen, danazol, and mifepristone (RU486) in oral postcoital contraception, Br Med J 305:927, 1992.

152. **Glasier A, Thong KJ, Dewar M, Mackie M, Baird DT,** Mifepristone (RU 486) compared with high-dose estrogen and progestogen for emergency postcoital contraception, New Engl J Med 327:1041, 1992.

153. **Mosher WD,** Contraceptive practice in the United States, 1982–1988, Fam Plann Perspect 22:198, 1990.

154. **Gordon MG, Williams SR, Frenchek B, Maxur CH, Speroff L,** Dose-dependent effects of postmenopausal estrogen/progestin on antithrombin III and factor XII, J Lab Clin Med 111:52, 1988.

155. **Mellis GB, Fruzzetti F, Nicoletti I, Ricci C, Lammers P, Atsma WJ, Fioretti P,** A comparative study on the effects of a monophasic pill containing desogestrel plus 20 μg ethinylestradiol, a triphasic combination containing levonorgestel and a monophasic combination containing gestodene on coagulatory factors, Contraception 43:23, 1991.

156. **Volpe A, Silferi M, Genazzani AD, Genazzani AR,** Contraception in older women, Contraception 47:229, 1993.

157. **Kirkman RJE, Pedersen JH, Fioretti P, Roberts HE,** Clinical comparison of two low-dose oral contraceptives, Minulet and Mercilon, in women over 30 years of age, Contraception 49:33, 1994.

23 Long-Acting Methods of Contraception

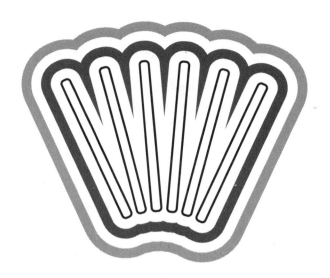

The high rate of unintended pregnancies and the relatively high failure rates with the typical use of reversible methods of contraception are strong indications of a need for long-acting contraceptive methods that simplify compliance. Two effective and popular methods are available, the Norplant system and depot-medroxy-progesterone acetate (Depo-Provera). Other products are in development.

Norplant employs silastic tubing permeable to steroid molecules to provide stable circulating levels of synthetic progestins over months and years. The progestins, circulating at levels one-fourth to one-tenth of those obtained with combined oral contraceptives, prevent conception by suppressing ovulation and thickening cervical mucus to inhibit sperm penetration so that fertilization rarely occurs.[1]

Injectable medroxyprogesterone acetate is a long-acting (3–6 months) agent which has been part of the contraceptive programs of many countries for more than 20 years. This experience has demonstrated it to be safe, effective, and acceptable. It is not a "sustained release" system, but its action is the same.

Because serum levels of progestin remain low and because no estrogen is administered, these long-acting contraceptive methods have not caused any serious health effects.[2] These methods do, however, cause many of the same minor, but bothersome, side effects associated with the progestin component of combined oral contraceptives. The continuous presence of low levels of progestin leads to irregular endometrial sloughing, a problem common to all of these methods, and one that is highly variable from one woman to another.

The Norplant System

The Norplant system consists of 6 capsules, each measuring 34 mm in length with a 2.4 mm outer diameter and containing levonorgestrel. The capsule is made of flexible, medical grade silastic (polydimethylsiloxane) tubing which is sealed shut with silastic medical adhesive, silicone type A. The cavity of the capsule has an inner diameter of 1.57 mm, with an inner length of 30 mm. Each capsule contains 36 mg dry crystalline levonorgestrel for a total of 216 mg in the 6 capsules. The levonorgestrel is very stable and has remained unchanged in capsules examined after more than 7 years of use. Norplant II, which consists of two implants, is a system nearing completion of clinical trials.

The release rate of the capsule is determined by its total surface area and the thickness of the capsule wall. The levonorgestrel diffuses through the wall of the tubing into the surrounding tissues where it is absorbed by the circulatory system and distributed systemically, avoiding an initial high level in the hepatic circulation. Within 24 hours after insertion, plasma concentrations of levonorgestrel range from 0.4 to 0.5 ng/mL, high enough to prevent conception.[3] This level corresponds to the level reached 12 hours after taking the levonorgestrel progestin-only oral minipill. The capsules release approximately 80 μg levonorgestrel per 24 hours during the first 6–12 months of use. This rate declines gradually to 30–35 μg per day for the remaining duration of use. After 5 years, the implants release about 25 μg per day. The 80 μg per day of hormone released by the implants during the first 2–6 months of use is about the same as the daily dose of levonorgestrel delivered by the progestin-only, minipill oral contraceptive, and 25–50% of the dose delivered by low dose combined oral contraceptives. Mean plasma concentrations below 0.20 ng/mL are associated with increased pregnancy rates. After 6 months of use, daily levonorgestrel concentrations are about 0.35 ng/mL; at 2.5 years, the levels decrease to 0.25–0.35 ng/mL. Until the 5 year mark, mean levels remain above 0.25 ng/mL.[4]

Mechanism of Action

The mechanism by which Norplant prevents conception is only partially explained. There are three probable modes of action, which are similar to those attributed to the contraceptive effect of the progestin-only minipills:

1. The levonorgestrel suppresses, at both the hypothalamus and the pituitary, the luteinizing hormone (LH) surge necessary for ovulation. As determined by progesterone levels in many users over several years, about one-third of all cycles are ovulatory.[4,5]

2. The levonorgestrel has a marked effect on the cervical mucus. The mucus thickens and decreases in amount, forming a barrier to sperm penetration.[3,6]

3. The constant level of levonorgestrel suppresses the estradiol-induced cyclic maturation of the endometrium and eventually causes atrophy. These changes could prevent implantation should fertilization occur; however, no evidence of fertilization can be detected in Norplant users.[1]

The Advantages of Norplant

Norplant is a safe, highly effective, continuous method of contraception that requires little user compliance or motivation and is rapidly reversible. Because this is a progestin-only method, it may be utilized by women who have contraindications for the use of estrogen-containing oral contraceptives. The sustained release of low doses of progestin avoids the high initial dose delivered by injectables and the daily hormone surge associated with oral contraceptives. Norplant is not a coitus-related contraceptive method. The use-effectiveness closely approximates the theoretical effectiveness.[7] Norplant is an excellent choice for a breastfeeding woman (there is no effect on breastfeeding) and can be inserted immediately postpartum.

The Disadvantages of Norplant	There are some disadvantages associated with the use of the Norplant system. Norplant frequently causes disruption of bleeding patterns in up to 80% of users, especially during the first year of use, and some women or their partners find these changes unacceptable.[8] Endogenous estrogen is variably suppressed, and unlike the combined oral contraceptives, no exogenous estrogen is provided to maintain a stable endometrium. The absence of cyclic administration does not allow for regular withdrawal bleeding. Consequently, the relatively unstable endometrium sheds at unpredictable intervals. The implants must be inserted and removed in a surgical procedure performed by trained personnel. Women cannot initiate or discontinue the method without the assistance of a clinician. Because the insertion and removal of Norplant requires a minor surgical procedure, initiation and discontinuation costs will be higher than with oral contraceptives or barrier methods. The implants can be visible under the skin. This sign of the use of contraception may be unacceptable for some women, and for some partners.[8] Norplant is not known to provide protection against sexually transmitted diseases (STDs) such as herpes, human papillomavirus, human immunodeficiency virus (HIV), gonorrhea, or chlamydia. Users at risk for STDs must consider adding a barrier method to prevent infection.

Absolute Contraindications for Norplant Use	Norplant use is contraindicated in women who have:

1. Active thrombophlebitis or thromboembolic disease.

2. Undiagnosed genital bleeding.

3. Acute liver disease.

4. Benign or malignant liver tumors.

5. Known or suspected breast cancer.

Relative Contraindications for Norplant Use	Based on clinical judgment and appropriate medical management, Norplant may be used by women with a history of or current diagnosis of the following conditions:

1. Heavy cigarette smoking (15 or more daily) in women older than 35 years.

2. History of ectopic pregnancy.

3. Diabetes mellitus. Because multiple studies have failed to observe a significant impact on carbohydrate metabolism, Norplant is particularly well-suited for diabetic women.

4. Hypercholesterolemia.

5. Severe acne.

6. Hypertension.

7. History of cardiovascular disease, including myocardial infarction, cerebral vascular accident, coronary artery disease, or angina. Patients with artificial heart valves.

8. Gallbladder disease.

9. Severe vascular or migraine headaches.

10. Severe depression.

11. Chronic disease, such as immunocompromised patients.

12. Concomitant use of medications that induce microsomal liver enzymes (phenytoin, phenobarbital, carbamazepine, rifampin). Norplant is not recommended because of a likely increased risk of pregnancy due to lower blood levels of levonorgestrel.

The Efficacy of Norplant

Norplant is a more effective method of birth control than any of the other reversible methods. In studies conducted in 11 countries, totaling 12,133 woman-years of use, the pregnancy rate was 0.2 pregnancies per 100 woman-years of use.[9] All but one of the pregnancies that occurred during this evaluation were present at the time of implant insertion. If these luteal phase insertions are excluded from analysis, the first year pregnancy rate was 0.01 per 100 woman-years.

Pregnancy Rates According to Years of Use[2]

First Year	Second Year	Third Year	Fourth Year	Fifth Year
0.2%	0.2%	0.9%	0.5%	1.1%

The overall pregnancy rate after 2 years of use in 9 countries was 0.2 per 100 woman-years of use.[2] The pregnancy rate achieved in the U.S. trials during the second year of use was higher (2.1 per 100 woman-years). Two factors may account for this difference. First, users in the U.S. weighed, on the average, more than study participants in other countries. Clinical trials have demonstrated a direct correlation between weight greater than 70 kg (154 pounds) and an increased risk of pregnancy, but even for heavy women, pregnancy rates are lower than with oral contraception. Second, two different types of silastic tubing were used in the manufacture of Norplant capsules.[8] The first type contained a larger proportion of inert filler and was more dense, while the second type contained less filler and was less dense. Higher pregnancy rates have been observed among women using the more dense capsules, and in the U.S. trials, capsules were more often of the more dense variety. The less dense tubing is now the only one used in the manufacture of Norplant and has a 15% higher release rate than denser tubing.

Using the less dense tubing, there now are no weight restrictions for Norplant users, but heavier women (more than 70 kg) may experience slightly higher pregnancy rates in the fourth and fifth years of use compared to lighter women. Even in the later years, however, pregnancy rates for heavier women using Norplant are lower than with oral contraception. The differences in pregnancy rates by weight are probably due to the dilutional effect of larger body size on the low, sustained serum levels of levonorgestrel. Heavier women should not rely on Norplant beyond the 5-year limit. For slender women the duration of Norplant's efficacy may extend well into the fifth year of use.

The ectopic pregnancy rate during Norplant use has been 0.28 per 1,000 woman-years.[2] This compares to the rate of 1.5 per 1,000 among U.S. women aged 15–44. Although the risk of developing an ectopic pregnancy during use of Norplant is low, when pregnancy does occur, ectopic pregnancy should be suspected, especially if the patient has additional risk factors.

Ectopic Pregnancy Rates per 1,000 Woman-Years [2]

All U.S. women	1.50
Non-contraceptive users	3.00
Copper T-380 IUD	0.20
Norplant	0.28

The return of fertility after Norplant removal is prompt and pregnancy outcomes are within normal limits.[9] The rate and outcome of subsequent pregnancies are not influenced by duration of use.

Side Effects with Norplant

Menstrual bleeding patterns are highly variable among users of Norplant. Some alteration of menstrual patterns will occur during the first year of use in approximately 60% of users. The changes include alterations in the interval between bleeding, the duration and volume of menstrual flow, and spotting. Oligomenorrhea and amenorrhea also occur but are less common. Irregular and prolonged bleeding usually occurs during the first year. Although bleeding problems occur much less frequently after the second year, they can occur at any time.[10] Despite an increase in the number of spotting and bleeding days over preinsertion menstrual patterns, hemoglobin concentrations rise in Norplant users because of a decrease in the average amount of menstrual blood loss.

Patients who can no longer tolerate the presence of prolonged bleeding will benefit from a short course of oral estrogen: conjugated estrogens, 1.25 mg, or estradiol, 2 mg, administered daily for 7 days. A therapeutic dose of one of the prostaglandin inhibitors given during the bleeding will help to diminish flow, but estrogen is more effective.[11]

Although the Norplant system is very effective, pregnancy must be considered in women reporting amenorrhea who have been ovulating previously, as evidenced by regular menses prior to an episode of amenorrhea. A sensitive urine pregnancy test should be obtained. Women who remain amenorrheic throughout their use of Norplant are unlikely to become pregnant.[10] It is important to explain to patients the mechanism of the amenorrhea: the local progestational effect causing decidualization and atrophy.

Exposure to the sustained, low dose of levonorgestrel delivered by the implants is not associated with significant metabolic changes.[12–16] Studies of carbohydrate metabolism, liver function, blood coagulation, immunoglobulin levels, serum cortisol levels, and blood chemistries have failed to detect changes outside of normal ranges.

No major impact on the lipoprotein profile can be demonstrated. Minor changes are transient, and with prolonged duration of use, lipoproteins return to preinsertion levels. Long-term exposure to the low dose of levonorgestrel released by Norplant is unlikely to affect user's risk of atherosclerosis, just as prolonged exposure to combined oral contraception has not.

Circulating levels of levonorgestrel become too low to measure within 48 hours after removal of Norplant. Most women resume normal ovulatory cycles during the first month after removal. The pregnancy rates during the first year after removal are comparable to those of women not using contraceptive methods and trying to become pregnant. There are no long-term effects on future fertility, nor are there any effects on sex ratios, rates of ectopic pregnancy, spontaneous abortion, stillbirth, or congenital malformations.[9]

In addition to the menstrual changes, the following side effects have been reported: headache, acne, weight change, mastalgia, hyperpigmentation over the implants, hirsutism, depression, mood changes, anxiety, nervousness, ovarian cyst formation, and galactorrhea.[2,8] It is difficult, of course, to be certain which of these effects were actually caused by the levonorgestrel. Although these side effects are minor in nature, they can cause patients to discontinue the method. Patients often find common side effects tolerable after assurance that they do not represent a health hazard.[8] Many complaints respond to reassurance; others can be treated with simple therapies. The most common side effect experienced by users is headache; about 20% of women who discontinue use do so because of headache.

Women using Norplant more frequently complain of weight gain than of weight loss, but findings are variable. Assessment of weight change in Norplant users is confounded by changes in exercise, diet, and aging. Although an increase in appetite can be attributed to the androgenic activity of levonorgestrel, it is unlikely that the low levels with Norplant have any clinical impact. Counseling for weight changes should include dietary review and focus on dietary changes.

Bilateral mastalgia, often occurring premenstrually, is usually associated with complaints of fluid retention. After pregnancy has been ruled out, reassurance and therapy aimed at symptomatic relief are indicated. This symptom decreases with increasing duration of Norplant use. Most Norplant users respond to treatment and do not elect to remove the implants. Careful assessments of the relationship between methylxanthines and mastalgia have failed to demonstrate a link. The most effective treatments are the following: danazol (200 mg/day), vitamin E (600 units/day), bromocriptine (2.5 mg/day), or tamoxifen (20 mg/day).

Galactorrhea is more common among women who have had insertion of the implants upon discontinuation of lactation. Pregnancy and other possible causes should be ruled out by performing a pregnancy test and a thorough breast examination. Patients should be reassured that this is a common occurrence among implant and oral contraceptive users. Decreasing the amount of breast and nipple stimulation during sexual relations can alleviate the symptom, but if amenorrhea accompanies persistent galactorrhea, a prolactin level should be obtained.

Acne, with or without an increase in oil production, is the most common skin complaint among Norplant users. The acne is caused by the androgenic activity of the levonorgestrel that produces a direct impact and also causes a decrease in sex hormone binding globulin (SHBG) levels leading to an increase in free steroid levels (both levonorgestrel and testosterone). This is in contrast to combined oral contraceptives that contain levonorgestrel, where the estrogen effect on SHBG (an increase) produces a decrease in unbound, free androgens. Common therapies for complaints of acne include dietary change, practice of good skin hygiene with the use of soaps or skin cleansers, and application of topical antibiotics (e.g., 1% clindamycin solution or gel, or topical erythromycin). Use of local antibiotics helps most users to continue Norplant.

Unlike oral contraception, the low serum progestin levels maintained by Norplant do not suppress follicle-stimulating hormone (FSH) which continues to stimulate ovarian follicle growth in some users. The luteinizing hormone (LH) peak, on the other hand, is usually abolished so that these follicles do not ovulate. However, some continue to grow and cause pain or are palpated at the time of pelvic examination. Adnexal masses are approximately 8 times more frequent in Norplant users compared to normally cycling women. Because these are simple cysts (and most regress spontaneously within one month of detection), they need not be sonographically or laparoscopically evaluated. Further evaluation is indicated if they became large and painful or fail to regress. Regular ovulators are less likely to form cysts.

Some users have complained of outbreaks of genital herpes simplex lesions occurring more frequently than prior to insertion. Most commonly, the lesions develop during periods of prolonged spotting or bleeding with the wearing of sanitary napkins. Use of vaginal tampons for bleeding and suppression of the virus with oral acyclovir (200 mg tid for up to 6 months) have been successful in dealing with this problem.

Depo-Provera (Medroxyprogesterone Acetate)

Medroxyprogesterone acetate (Depo-Provera) for contraception is administered as microcrystals, suspended in an aqueous solution, which dissolve very slowly. The dose of medroxyprogesterone acetate for contraceptive purposes is 150 mg intramuscularly every 3 months. The injection should be given within the first 5 days of the current menstrual cycle, otherwise a back-up method is necessary for 2 weeks. The effective contraceptive level is maintained for 4 months, providing a safety margin for reliable contraception. The efficacy of this method is equal to that of sterilization.[17] The mechanism of action is the same as with all progestin-only methods, except the circulating level of the progestin is high enough to effectively block the LH surge, and therefore it is unlikely that any patient will ovulate with this method. Depo-Provera also affects the endometrium and cervical mucus, producing barriers to implantation and sperm penetration, as with Norplant. Suppression of FSH is not as intense as with the combination oral contraceptive, therefore follicular growth is maintained sufficiently to produce estrogen levels comparable to those in the early folllicular phase of a normal menstrual cycle. Symptoms of estrogen deficiency, such as vaginal atrophy or a decrease in breast size, do not occur.

Problems with Depo-Provera

Major problems with Depo-Provera are irregular menstrual bleeding, breast tenderness, weight gain, and depression.[17] The incidence of irregular bleeding is 30% in the first year, and 10% thereafter. After several injections, the majority of women become totally amenorrheic. If necessary, the bleeding can be treated with exogenous estrogen, 1.25 mg conjugated estrogens, or 2 mg estradiol, given daily for 7 days. Serious weight gain and depression (less than 5% incidence) are not relieved until the drug clears the body 6–8 months after the last injection.

This progestin, in large continuous doses, produced breast tumors in beagle dogs. This is an effect unique to the beagle dog, and has not appeared in other animals or in women after years of use. A very large, hospital-based case-control WHO study conducted over 9 years in 3 developing countries indicated that exposure to Depo-Provera is associated with a very slightly increased risk in breast cancer in the first 4 years of use, but there was no evidence for an increase in risk with increased duration of use.[18] The results were interpreted to suggest that growth of already existing tumors is enhanced. The number of cases was not large, and the confidence intervals reflected this. Two earlier population-based case-control studies indicated a possible association beween breast cancer and Depo-Provera. One, from Costa Rica, was subject to several biases.[19] The other, from New Zealand, did not find an increased relative risk in ever-users but did find an indication of increased risk shortly after initiating use at an early age.[20] These studies have been all limited by very small numbers and thus have been inconclusive. Certainly the risk, if real, is very slight, and it is equally possible that the suggestions of increased risk have not been free of confounding variables. It is more appropriate to emphasize that these studies did not find evidence for an increased risk of breast cancer with long durations of use.

The impact of Depo-Provera on the lipoprotein profile is uncertain. While some fail to detect an adverse impact, and claim that this is due to the avoidance of a first pass through effect in the liver,[21] others have demonstrated a decrease in HDL-cholesterol and increases in total cholesterol and LDL-cholesterol.[22,23] In a multicenter clinical trial by the World Health Organization, a transient adverse impact was present only in the few weeks after injection when blood levels were high.[24] The clinical impact of these changes, if any, have yet to be reported. It seems prudent to monitor the lipid profile annually in women using Depo-Provera for long durations. The emergence of significant adverse changes in LDL-cholesterol and HDL-cholesterol warrant reconsideration of contraceptive choice. There are no clinically significant changes in carbohydrate metabolism or in coagulation factors.[22,25]

There is some concern that the blood levels of estrogen with this method of contraception are relatively lower over a period of time compared to a normal menstrual cycle, and therefore patients can lose bone to some degree.[26] Another possible mechanism is displacement of cortisol by the progestin from its binding globulin in the circulation, resulting in elevated levels of free cortisol. It is unlikely that this bone loss is sufficient to raise the risk of osteoporosis later in life. Furthermore, it is probable that any loss is regained with discontinuation of the method. This concern will require on-going surveillance, especially of past users, but at the present time, this should not be a reason to avoid this method of contraception.

The concern that infertility with suppressed menstrual function may be caused by Depo-Provera has not been supported by epidemiologic data. The pregnancy rate in women discontinuing the injections because of a desire to become pregnant is normal.[27] The delay to conception is about 9 months after the last injection, and the delay does not increase with increasing duration of use. Suppressed menstrual function persisting beyond 12 months after the last injection is not due to the drug and deserves evaluation.

Accidental pregnancies occurring at the time of the initial injection of Depo-Provera have been reported to be associated with higher neonatal and infant mortality rates, probably due to an increased risk of intrauterine growth retardation.[28,29] The timing of the first injection is, therefore, very important. To ensure effective contraception, the first injection should be administered within the first 5 days of the menstrual cycle (before a dominant follicle emerges), or a back-up method is necessary for 2 weeks.

The Advantages of Depo-Provera

Like other sustained release forms of contraception, this method is not associated with compliance problems and is not related to the coital event. The freedom from the side effects of estrogen allows Depo-Provera to be considered for patients with congenital heart disease, sickle cell anemia, patients with a previous history of thromboembolism, and women over 30 who smoke or have other risk factors. The absolute safety in regard to thrombosis is mainly theoretical; it has not been proven in a controlled study. However, an increased rate of thrombosis has not been observed in epidemiologic evaluation of Depo-Provera users.

A further advantage in patients with sickle-cell disease is evidence indicating an inhibition of in vivo sickling with hematologic improvement during treatment.[30] Depo-

Provera is useful for cases where compliance is a problem, e.g., mentally retarded young women. Another advantage is the finding that Depo-Provera increases the quantity of milk in nursing mothers, a direct contrast to the effect seen with combination oral contraception. The concentration of the drug in the breast milk is very small, and no effects of the drug on infant growth and development have been observed.[31,32] Depo-Provera should be considered in patients with seizure disorders; an improvement in seizure control can be achieved probably because of the sedative properties of progestins.[33]

Other benefits associated with Depo-Provera use include a decreased risk of endometrial cancer[34,35] and probably the same benefits associated with the progestin impact of oral contraceptives: reduced menstrual flow and anemia, less pelvic inflammatory disease, less endometriosis, and fewer ectopic pregnancies. A failure to document a reduced risk of ovarian cancer by the World Health Organization probably reflects the study's low statistical power and the high parity in the Depo-Provera users.[36] A large case-control study could detect no increase in risk of invasive cervical cancer even after over 12 years since exposure.[37] However, women at higher risk because of their sexual behavior (multiple partners, history of STDs) should have Pap smears every 6 months.

Norethindrone Enanthate

Norethindrone enanthate is available in many countries throughout the world. It is administered as an injection of 200 mg every 2 months.[34] The efficacy and side effects are comparable to Depo-Provera, but the incidence of amenorrhea is less, and a greater adverse impact on the cholesterol lipoprotein profile is associated with norethindrone enanthate.[23]

Long-Acting Methods for Older Women

The long-acting methods of hormonal contraception (Norplant and Depo-Provera) deserve consideration in those situations where combination estrogen-progestin is unacceptable because of health problems (where estrogen is contraindicated), or where oral contraception has already proved to be unsuccessful. Older women, as they approach the menopause, may be more comfortable with the irregular bleeding or amenorrhea associated with these methods. However, the irregular bleeding patterns associated with these methods can cause more concern in some women regarding possible pathology. Hormone treatment can be initiated if menopausal symptoms develop or when annual measurement of the FSH level (beginning at age 50) indicates a rise above 30 IU/L.

References

1. **Segal SJ, Alvarez-Sanchez F, Brache V, Faundes A, Vilja P, Tuohimaa P,** Norplant implants: the mechanism of contraceptive action, Fertil Steril 56:273, 1991.

2. **Sivin I,** International experience with Norplant and Norplant-2 contraceptives, Stud Fam Plann 19:81, 1988.

3. **Brache V, Faundes A, Johansson E, Alvarez F,** Anovulation, inadequate luteal phase, and poor sperm penetration in cervical mucus during prolonged use of Norplant implants, Contraception 31:261, 1985.

4. **Brache V, Alvarez-Sanchez F, Faundes A, Tejada AS, Cochon L,** Ovarian endocrine function through five years of continuous treatment with Norplant subdermal contraceptive implants, Contraception 41:169, 1990.

5. **Alvarez F, Brache V, Tejada AS, Faundes A,** Abnormal endocrine profile among women with confirmed or presumed ovulation during long-term Norplant use, Contraception 33:111, 1986.

6. **Croxatto HB, Diaz S, Salvatierra AM, Morales P, Ebensperger C, Brandeis A,** Treatment with Norplant subdermal implants inhibits sperm penetration through cervical mucus in vitro, Contraception 36:193, 1987.

7. **Trussell J, Hatcher RA, Cates W Jr, Stewart FH, Kost K,** Contraceptive failure in the United States: an update, Stud Fam Plann 21:51, 1990.

8. **Darney PD, Klaisle CM, Tanner ST, Alvarado AM,** Sustained release contraceptives, Curr Prob Obstet Gynecol Fertil 13:87, 1990.

9. **Sivin I, Stern J, Diaz S, Pavez M, Alvarez F, Brache V, Mishell DR Jr, Lacarra M, McCarthy T, Holma P, Darney P, Klaisle C, Olsson S-E, Odlind V,** Rates and outcomes of planned pregnancy after use of Norplant capsules, Norplant II rods, or levonorgestrel-releasing or copper TCu 380Ag intrauterine contraceptive devices, Am J Obstet Gynecol 166:1208, 1992.

10. **Shoupe D, Mishell DR Jr, Bopp B, Fiedling M,** The significance of bleeding patterns in Norplant implant users, Obstet Gynecol 77:256, 1991.

11. **Diaz S, Croxatto HB, Pavez M, Belhadj H, Stern J, Sivin I,** Clinical assessment of treatments for prolonged bleeding in users of Norplant implants, Contraception 42:97, 1990.

12. **Konje JC, Otolorin EO, Ladipo OA,** Changes in carbohydrate metabolism during 30 months on Norplant, Contraception 44:163, 1991.

13. **Singh K, Viegas OAC, Liew D, Singh P, Ratnam SS,** Two-year follow-up of changes in clinical chemistry in Singaporean Norplant acceptors: metabolic changes, Contraception 39:129, 1989.

14. **Singh K, Viegas OAC, Loke DFM, Ratnam SS,** Effect of Norplant implants on liver, lipid and carbohydrate metabolism, Contraception 45:141, 1992.

15. **Otubu JAM, Towobola OA, Aisien AO, Ogunkeye OO,** Effects of Norplant contraceptive subdermal implants on serum lipids and lipoproteins, Contraception 47:149, 1993.

16. **Singh K, Viegas OAC, Koh SCL, Ratnam SS,** Effect of long-term use of Norplant implants on haemostatic function, Contraception 45:203, 1992.

17. **WHO,** A multicentered phase III comparative clinical trial of depot-medroxyprogesterone acetate given three-monthly at doses of 100 mg or 150 mg: I. Contraceptive efficacy and side effects, Contraception 34:223, 1986.

18. **WHO Collaborative Study of Neoplasia and Steroid Contraceptives,** Breast cancer and depot-medroxyprogesterone acetate: a multinational study, Lancet 338:833, 1991.

19. **Lee NC, Rosero-Bixby L, Oberle MW, Grimaldo C, Whatley AS, Rovira EZ,** A case-control study of breast cancer and hormonal contraception in Costa Rica, J Natl Cancer Inst 79:1247, 1987.

20. **Paul C, Skegg DCG, Spears GFS,** Depot medroxyprogesterone (Depo-Provera) and risk of breast cancer, Br Med J 299:759, 1989.

21. **Garza-Flores J, De la Cruz DL, Valles de Bourges V, Sanchez-Nuncio R, Martinez M, Fuziwara JL, Perez-Palacios G,** Long-term effects of depot-medroxyprogesterone acetate on lipoprotein metabolism, Contraception 44:61, 1991.

22. **Fahmy K, Khairy M, Allam G, Gobran F, Allush M,** Effect of depo-medroxyprogesterone acetate on coagulation factors and serum lipids in Egyptian women, Contraception 44:431, 1991.

23. **Enk L, Landgren BM, Lindberg U-B, Silverstolpe G, Crona N,** A prospective, one-year study on the effects of two long acting injectable contraceptives (depot-medroxyprogesterone acetate and norethisterone oenanthate) on serum and lipoprotein lipids, Horm Metab Res 24:85, 1992.

24. **WHO,** A multicentre comparative study of serum lipids and apolipoproteins in long-term users of DMPA and a control group of IUD users, Contraception 47:177, 1993.

25. **Fahmy K, Abdel-Razik M, Shaaraway M, Al-Kholy G, Saad S, Wagdi A, Al-Azzony M,** Effect of long-acting progestagen-only injectable contraceptives on carbohydrate metabolism and its hormonal profile, Contraception 44:419, 1991.

26. **Cundy T, Evans M, Roberts H, Wattie D, Ames R, Reid IR,** Bone density in women receiving depot medroxyprogesterone acetate for contraception, Br Med J 303:13, 1991.

27. **Pardthaisong T,** Return of fertility after use of the injectable contraceptive Depo Provera: updated analysis, J Biosoc Sci 16:23, 1984.

28. **Pardthaisong T, Gray RH,** In utero exposure to steroid contraceptives and outcome of pregnancy, Am J Epidemiol 134:795, 1991.

29. **Gray RH, Pardthaisong T,** In utero exposure to steroid contraceptives and survival during infancy, Am J Epidemiol 134:804, 1991.

30. **DeCeular K, Gruber C, Hayes R, Serjeant GR,** Medroxyprogesterone acetate and homozygous sickle-cell disease, Lancet 2:229, 1982.

31. **Jimenez J, Ochoa M, Soler MP, Portales P,** Long-term follow-up of children breast-fed by mothers receiving depot-medroxyprogesterone acetate, Contraception 30:5232, 1984.

32. **Pardthaisong T, Yenchit C, Gray R,** The long-term growth and development of children exposed to Depo-Provera during pregnancy or lactation, Contraception 45:313, 1992.

33. **Mattson RH, Cramer JA, Caldwell BV, Siconolfi BC,** Treatment of seizures with medroxyprogesterone acetate: preliminary report, Neurology 34:1255, 1984.

34. **WHO,** Multinational comparative clinical evaluation of two long-acting injectable contraceptive steroids: norethisterone enanthate and medroxyprogesterone acetate. Final report, Contraception 28:1, 1983.

35. **WHO, Collaborative Study of Neoplasia and Steroid Contraceptives,** Depot-medroxyprogesterone acetate (DMPA) and risk of endometrial cancer, Int J Cancer 49:186, 1991.

36. **WHO, Collaborative Study of Neoplasia and Steroid Contraceptives,** Depot-medroxyprogesterone acetate (DMPA) and risk of epithelial ovarian cancer, Int J Cancer 49:191, 1991.

37. **WHO Collaborative Study of Neoplasia and Steroid Contraceptives,** Depot-medroxyprogesterone acetate (DMPA) and risk of invasive squamous cell cervical cancer, Contraception 45:299, 1992.

24   The Intrauterine Device (IUD)

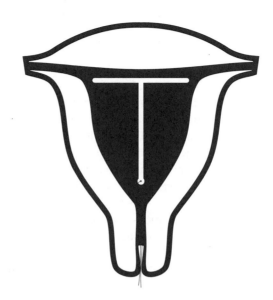

A frequently told, but not well-documented, story assigns the first use of intrauterine devices (IUDs) to caravan drivers who allegedly used intrauterine stones to prevent pregnancies in their camels during long journeys. The forerunners of the modern IUD were small stem pessaries used in the 1800s, small button-like structures that covered the opening of the cervix and that were attached to stems extending into the cervical canal.[1] It is not certain these pessaries were used for contraception, but this seems to have been intended. In 1902, a pessary which extended into the uterus was developed by Hollweg in Germany and used for contraception. This pessary was sold for self-insertion, but the hazard of infection was great, earning the condemnation of the medical community.

In 1909, Richter, in Germany, reported success with a silkworm catgut ring having a nickle and bronze wire protruding through the cervix.[2] Shortly after, Pust combined Richter's ring with the old button-type pessary, and replaced the wire with a catgut thread.[3] This IUD was used during World War I in Germany, although the German literature was quick to report infections with its insertion and use. In the 1920s, Gräfenberg removed the tail and pessary because he believed this was the cause of infection. He reported his experience in 1930, using rings made of coiled silver and gold, then steel.[4]

The Gräfenberg ring was short-lived, falling victim to Nazi political philosophy that was bitterly opposed to contraception. The nonAryan Gräfenberg was finally sent to jail, but he managed to flee Germany, dying in New York City in 1955. He never received the recognition which was his just due.

The Gräfenberg ring was associated with a high rate of expulsion. This was solved by Ota in Japan who added a supportive structure to the center of his gold or silver plated ring in 1934.[5] Ota also fell victim to World War II politics, being sent into exile, but his ring continued to be used.

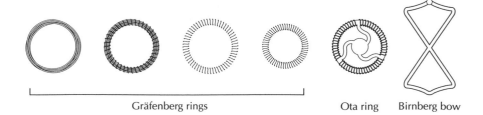

Gräfenberg rings   Ota ring   Birnberg bow

The Gräfenberg and Ota rings were essentially forgotten by the rest of the world throughout the World War II period. An awareness of the explosion in population and its impact began to grow in the first two decades after World War II. In 1959, reports from Japan and Israel by Ishihama and Oppenheimer once again stirred interest in the rings.[6,7] The Oppenheimer report was in the *American Journal of Obstetrics and Gynecology,* and several American gynecologists were stimulated to use rings of silver or silk, and others to develop their own devices.

In the 1960s and 1970s, the IUD thrived. Techniques were modified and a plethora of types introduced. The various devices developed in the 1960s were made of plastic (polyethylene) impregnated with barium sulfate so that they would be visible on an x-ray. The Margulies Coil, developed by Lazer Margulies in 1960 at Mt. Sinai Hospital in New York City, was the first plastic device with a memory, allowing the use of an inserter and reconfiguration of the shape when it was expelled into the uterus. The Coil was a large device (sure to cause cramping and bleeding), and its hard plastic tail proved risky for the male partner.

In 1962, the Population Council, at the suggestion of Alan Guttmacher who that year became president of the Planned Parenthood Federation of America, organized the first international conference on IUDs in New York City. It was at this conference that Jack Lippes of Buffalo presented experience with his device, which fortunately as we will see, had a single filament thread as a tail. The Margulies Coil was rapidly replaced by the Lippes Loop, which quickly became the most widely prescribed IUD in the United States in the 1970s.

The 1962 conference also led to the organization of a program established by the Population Council, under the direction of Christopher Tietze, to evaluate IUDs, the Cooperative Statistical Program. The Ninth Progress Report in 1970 was a landmark comparison of efficacy and problems with the various IUDs being used.[8]

Many other devices came along, but with the exception of the four sizes of Lippes Loops and the two Saf-T-Coils, they had limited use. Stainless steel devices incorporating springs were designed to compress for easy insertion, but the movement of these devices allowed them to embed in the uterus, making them too difficult to remove. The Majzlin Spring is a memorable example.

The Dalkon Shield was introduced in 1970. Within 3 years, a high incidence of pelvic infection was recognized. There is no doubt that the problems with the Dalkon Shield were due to defective construction, pointed out as early as 1975 by Tatum.[9] The multifilamented tail (hundreds of fibers enclosed in a sheath) of the Dalkon Shield provided a pathway for bacteria to ascend protected from the barrier of cervical mucus.

Although sales were discontinued in 1975, a call for removal of all Dalkon Shields was not issued until the early 1980s. The large number of women with pelvic infections led to many lawsuits against the pharmaceutical company, ultimately causing its bank-

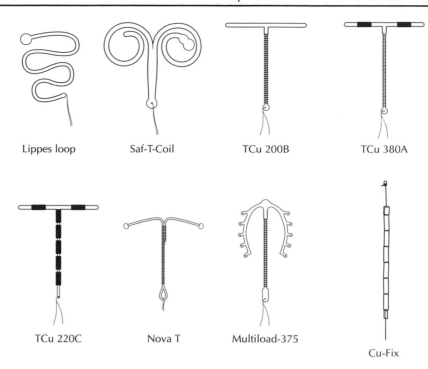

| Lippes loop | Saf-T-Coil | TCu 200B | TCu 380A |

| TCu 220C | Nova T | Multiload-375 | Cu-Fix |

ruptcy. Unfortunately, the Dalkon Shield problem tainted all IUDs, and ever since, media and the public have inappropriately regarded all IUDs in a single, generic fashion.

About the time of the introduction of the Dalkon Shield, the U.S. Senate conducted hearings on the safety of oral contraception. Young women who were discouraged from using oral contraceptives following these hearings turned to IUDs, principally the Dalkon Shield which was promoted as suitable for nulliparous women. Changes in sexual behavior in the 1960s and 1970s, and failure to use protective contraception (condoms and oral contraceptives), led to an epidemic of sexually transmitted diseases (STDs) and pelvic inflammatory disease (PID) for which IUDs were held partially responsible.[10]

The first epidemiologic studies of the relationship between IUDs and PID used as controls women who depended on oral contraception or barrier methods and who were, therefore, at reduced risk of PID compared to noncontraceptors and IUD users.[11,12] In addition, these first studies failed to control for the characteristics of sexual behavior that are now accepted as risk factors for PID (multiple partners, early age at first intercourse, and increased frequency of intercourse).[13] The Dalkon Shield magnified the risk attributed to IUDs because its high failure rate in young women who were already at risk of STDs led to septic spontaneous abortions and, in some cases, death.[14] Reports of these events led the American public to regard all IUDs as dangerous, including those that, unlike the Dalkon Shield, had undergone extensive clinical trials and post-marketing surveillance.

The 1980s saw the decline of IUD use in the United States as manufacturers discontinued marketing in response to the burden of litigation. Despite the fact that most of the lawsuits against the copper devices were won by the manufacturer, the cost of the defense combined with declining use affected the financial return. It should be emphasized that this action was the result of corporate business decisions related to concerns for profit and liability, not for medical or scientific reasons. The number of women using the IUD in the U.S. decreased by two-thirds from 1981 to 1988, from 2.2 million to 0.7 million (7.1% to 2% of married couples).[15]

The reason for the decline in the U.S. is the consumer fear of IUD-related pelvic infection. The final blow to the IUD in the U.S. came in 1985 with the publication of two reports indicating that the use of IUDs was associated with tubal infertility.[16,17] Later, better controlled studies identified the Dalkon Shield as a high risk device, and failed to demonstrate an association between PID and other IUDs, except during the period shortly after insertion. Efforts to point out that the situation was different for the copper IUDs, and that in fact, pelvic inflammatory disease was not increased in women with a single sexual partner,[18] failed to prevent the withdrawal of IUDs from the American market and the negative reaction to IUDs by the American public.

Worldwide, the IUD is the most popular method of reversible contraception. Ironically, the IUD declined in the country that developed the modern IUD.

The Modern IUD

The addition of copper to the IUD was suggested by Jaime Zipper of Chile, whose experiments with metals indicated that copper acted locally on the endometrium.[19] Howard Tatum combined Zipper's suggestion with the development of the T-shape to diminish the uterine reaction to the structural frame, and produced the copper-T. The first copper IUD had copper wire wound around the straight shaft of the T, the TCu-200 (200 mm^2 of exposed copper wire), also known as the Tatum-T.[20] Tatum's reasoning was that the T-shape would conform to the shape of the uterus in contrast to the other IUDs which required the uterus to conform to their shape. Furthermore, the copper IUDs could be much smaller than those of simple, inert plastic devices and still provide effective contraception. Recent studies indicate that copper exerts its effect before implantation of a fertilized ovum; it may be spermicidal, or it may diminish sperm motility or fertilizing capacity. The addition of copper to the IUD and reduction in the size and structure of the frame improved tolerance, resulting in fewer removals for pain and bleeding.

The Cu-7 with a copper wound stem was developed in 1971, and quickly became the most popular device in the U.S. Both the Cu-7 and the Tatum-T were withdrawn from the U.S. market in 1986 by G. D. Searle and Company.

IUD development continued, however. More copper was added by Population Council investigators, leading to the TCu-380A (380 mm^2 exposed copper surface area — copper wound around the stem plus a copper sleeve on each horizontal arm).[21] It has been in use in more than 30 countries since 1982, and in 1988, it was marketed in the U.S. by the GynoPharma Corporation as the "ParaGard."

The Progestasert was developed by the Alza Corporation at the same time that the copper IUDs were developed. This T-shaped device releases 65 µg progesterone per day for at least one year. The progesterone diminishes the amount of cramping and the amount of blood loss; thus, it is especially useful for women who have heavy periods and cramping. The short lifespan can be and has been solved by using a more potent progestin, such as levonorgestrel.

Efforts continue to develop IUDs that address the main problems of bleeding and cramping. The IUDs of the future will probably be medicated with alterations in the frame (size and flexibility).

Types of IUDs

Unmedicated IUDs

The Lippes Loop, made of plastic (polyethylene) impregnated with barium sulfate, is still used throughout the world (except in the U.S.). Flexible stainless steel rings are widely used in China, but not elsewhere.[22]

Copper IUDs

The first copper IUDs were wound with 200 to 250 mm² of wire, and two of these are still available (except in the U.S.), the TCu-200 and the Multiload-250. The more modern copper IUDs contain more copper, and part of the copper is in the form of solid tubular sleeves, rather than wire, increasing efficacy and extending lifespan. This group of IUDs is represented in the U.S. by the TCu-380A (the ParaGard), and in the rest of the world by the TCu-220C, the Nova T, and the Multiload-375. Theoretically, the copper content will provide effective contraception longer than that demonstrated thus far in clinical trials, probably up to 10 years.

The TCu-380A is a T-shaped device with a polyethylene frame holding 380 mm² of exposed surface area of copper. The pure electrolytic copper wire wound around the stem weighs 176 mg, and copper sleeves on the horizontal arms weigh 66.5 mg. A polyethylene monofiliment is tied through the ball on the stem, providing two white threads for detection and removal. The ball at the bottom of the stem helps reduce the risk of cervical perforation. The IUD frame contains barium sulfate, making it radiopaque. The TCu-380Ag is identical to the TCu-380A, but the copper wire on the stem has a silver core (to extend the lifespan of the copper). Its performance is equal to that of the TCu-380A.[23]

The Multiload-375 has 375 mm² of copper wire wound around its stem. The flexible arms were designed to minimize expulsions. This is a popular device in many parts of the world. The Multiload-375 and the TCu-380A are similar in their efficacy and performance.[24]

The Nova T is similar to the TCu-200, containing 200 mm² of copper; however, the Nova T has a silver core to the copper wire, flexible arms, and a large, flexible loop at the bottom to avoid injury to cervical tissue. There is some concern that the Nova-T loses efficacy after 3 years.[24]

Hormone-Releasing IUDs

The only hormone-releasing device marketed in the U.S. (since 1976) is the Progestasert. The Progestasert is a T-shaped IUD made of ethylene/vinyl acetate copolymer containing titanium dioxide. The vertical stem contains a reservoir of 38 mg progesterone together with barium sulfate dispersed in silicone fluid. The horizontal arms are solid and made of the same copolymer. Two blue-black, monofiliment strings are attached at a hole in the base of the stem. Progesterone is released at a rate of 65 µg per day.

The LNG-20, developed by the Population Council, releases 20 µg levonorgestrel per day. It has been marketed in Europe.[25] This T-shaped device (similar to the Nova-T) has a polydimethylsiloxane collar attached to the vertical arm, which contains 46 mg levonorgestrel, released at a rate of 20 µg per day. It has been demonstrated to be effective for 7 years.[23]

Future IUDs	Modifications of the copper IUD are being studied throughout the world. The Ombrelle-250 has been marketed in France; it is designed to be more flexible in order to reduce expulsion and side effects. A frameless IUD, the FlexiGard (also known as the Cu-Fix), is undergoing worldwide testing.[26] It consists of 6 copper sleeves (330 mm² copper) strung on a surgical nylon (polypropylene) thread that is knotted at one end. The knot is pushed into the myometrium during insertion with a notched needle which works like a miniature harpoon. Because it is frameless, it is expected to have low rates of expulsion and removal for bleeding or pain. The TCu-380 Slimline has copper sleeves set at the end of the crossbar that do not rise above the plastic surface of the crossbar, thus facilitating loading of the inserter tube and insertion itself.[27]

Mechanism of Action	The contraceptive action of all IUDs is mainly in the uterine cavity. Ovulation is not affected, nor is the IUD an abortifacient.[28,29] It is currently believed that the major mechanism of action for IUDs is the production of an intrauterine environment that is spermicidal. The protection provided by IUDs against ectopic pregnancy (see below) argues that there exists an extrauterine action as well, perhaps a cytotoxic effect on ova or a disruption of tubal function.

Nonmedicated IUDs depend for contraception upon the general reaction of the uterus to a foreign body. It is believed that this reaction, a sterile inflammatory response, produces tissue injury of a minor degree, but sufficient enough to be spermicidal. Very few, if any, sperm reach the ovum in the fallopian tube. Normally cleaving, fertilized ova cannot be obtained by tubal flushing in women with IUDs in contrast to noncontraceptors, indicating the failure of sperm to reach the ovum, and thus fertilization does not occur.[30] If this action should fail, the inflammatory response would also prevent implantation. In women using copper IUDs, sensitive assays for human chorionic gonadotropin (HCG) find evidence of fertilization in less than 1% of menstrual cycles.[31,32]

The copper IUD releases free copper and copper salts which have both a biochemical and morphological impact on the endometrium. There is no measurable increase in the serum copper level. Copper has many specific actions, including the enhancement of prostaglandin production and the inhibition of various endometrial enzymes. Perhaps the overall inflammatory response is intensified.

The progestin-releasing IUDs add the endometrial action of the progestin to the foreign body reaction. The endometrium becomes decidualized with atrophy of the glands. The progesterone IUD probably has two mechanisms of action: inhibition of implantation and inhibition of sperm capacitation and survival. The levonorgestrel IUD also partially inhibits ovarian follicular development and ovulation. Finally, the progestin IUDs thicken the cervical mucus, creating a barrier to sperm penetration.

With the exception of the progestin-releasing IUDs, no major noncontraceptive benefits are associated with IUD use. The progestin IUDs decrease menstrual blood loss (about 40–50%) and dysmenorrhea. Average hemoglobin and iron levels increase over time compared to preinsertion values.

Following removal of IUDs, the normal intrauterine environment is rapidly restored. In large studies, there is no delay in achieving pregnancy, which belies the assertion that IUD use is associated with infection leading to infertility.[33,34]

Efficacy of IUDs

Intrauterine Pregnancy

The TCu-380A is approved for use in the United States for 8 years; however, it has a theoretical lifespan of 10 years.[35] The Multiload-375 should also be effective for 10 years. Pending future studies, leaving the modern copper IUD in for longer than 8 years (up to 10 years) means that clinician and patient would have to accept the possibility of a small loss of contraceptive efficacy, although we hasten to add this has not yet been documented. The Nova-T is approved for 5 years.

The progesterone-releasing IUD must be replaced every year because the reservoir of progesterone is depleted in 12–18 months. The levonorgestrel IUD can be used for at least 7 years, and probably 10.[23] The progesterone IUD has a slightly higher failure rate, but the levonorgestrel device that releases 20 µg levonorgestrel per day is as effective as the new copper IUDs.[23,36]

The nonmedicated IUDs never have to be replaced. The deposition of calcium salts on the IUD can produce a structure that is irritating to the endometrium. If bleeding increases after a nonmedicated IUD has been in place for some time, it is worth replacing.

The actual use failure rate in the first year of use for all IUDs is approximately 3%, with a 10% expulsion rate and a 15% rate of removal, mainly for bleeding and pain. With increasing duration of use and increasing age, the failure rate decreases, as do removals for pain and bleeding.

First Year Clinical Trial Experience in Parous Women[22, 37]

Device	Pregnancy Rate	Expulsion Rate	Removal Rate
Lippes Loop	3%	12–20%	12–15%
Cu–7	2–3	6	11
TCu–200	3	8	11
TCu–380A	0.5–0.8	5	14
Progesterone IUD	1.3–1.6	2.7	9.3
Levonorgestrel IUD	0.2	6	17

In careful studies, with attention to technique and participation by motivated patients, the failure rate with the TCu-380A and the other newer copper IUDs is less than one per 100 women per year.[22,37] The cumulative net pregnancy rate after 7 years of use is 1.5 per 100 woman-years.[38] In developing countries, the failure rate with IUDs is less than that with oral contraception. Failure rates are slightly higher in younger (less than age 25), more fertile women.

Women use IUDs longer than other reversible methods of contraception. The IUD continuation rate is higher than that with oral contraception, condoms, or diaphragms. This may reflect the circumstances surrounding the choice of an IUD (older, parous women).

Ectopic Pregnancy

IUDs do not increase the risk of ectopic pregnancy, and they offer some protection.[39-41] The largest study, a World Health Organization multicenter study, concluded that IUD users were 50% less likely to have an ectopic pregnancy when compared to women using no contraception.[42] This protection is not as great as that achieved by inhibition of ovulation with oral contraception. Therefore, when an IUD user becomes pregnant, the pregnancy is more likely to be ectopic. About 3–4% of IUD pregnancies have been ectopic, making the actual occurrence a rare event.

Ectopic Pregnancy Rates per 1,000 Woman-Years [43, 46]

All U.S. women	1.50
Non-contraceptive users	3.00
Copper T-380A IUD	0.20
Copper T-200 IUD	0.60
Progesterone IUD	6.80
Levonorgestrel IUD	0.20

The lowest ectopic pregnancy rates are seen with the most effective IUDs, the newer copper devices (90% less likely compared to noncontraceptors).[43] The rate is about one-tenth the ectopic pregnancy rate associated with the Lippes Loop or TCu-200.[43] The progesterone-releasing IUD has a higher rate that, in fact, is about 50–80% greater than noncontraceptors.[43] Very few ectopic pregnancies have been reported with the levonorgestrel IUD, presumably because it is associated with a partial suppression of gonadotropins with subsequent disruption of normal follicular growth and development and, in a significant number of cycles (20–30%), inhibition of ovulation.[23,44,45]

The protection against ectopic pregnancy provided by the TCu-380A and the levonorgestrel IUD makes these IUDs acceptable choices for contraception in women with previous ectopic pregnancies.

Side Effects of IUDs

With effective patient screening and good insertion technique, the copper and medicated IUDs are not associated with an increased risk of infertility after their removal. Even if IUDs are removed for problems, subsequent fertility rates are normal.[47]

The symptoms most often responsible for IUD discontinuation are increased uterine bleeding and increased menstrual pain. Within one year, 5–15% of women discontinue IUD use because of these problems. Smaller copper and progestin IUDs have reduced the incidence of pain and bleeding considerably, but a careful menstrual history is still important in helping a woman consider an IUD. Women with prolonged, heavy menstrual bleeding or significant dysmenorrhea may not be able to tolerate copper IUDs but may benefit from a progestin IUD.[48] Because bleeding and cramping are most severe in the first few months after IUD insertion, treatment with a nonsteroidal anti-inflammatory (NSAID) agent (an inhibitor of prostaglandin synthesis) during the first several menstrual periods can reduce bleeding and cramping and help a patient through this difficult time. IUDs rarely cause intermenstrual bleeding, and such bleeding deserves the usual evaluation for cervical or endometrial pathology.

Because of a decidualizing, atrophic impact on the endometrium, amenorrhea can develop over time with the progestin-containing IUDs. For some women, the lack of periods is so disconcerting that they request removal. Sufficient progestin reaches the systemic circulation from the levonorgestrel-containing IUD so that androgenic side effects can occur such as acne and hirsutism. More extensive clinical studies are needed to assess the impact of this IUD on the lipoprotein profile; however, it is unlikely that the low dose of levonorgestrel has an important effect on cardiovascular risk.

Some women report an increased vaginal discharge while wearing an IUD. This complaint deserves examination for the presence of vaginal or cervical infection. Treatment can be provided with the IUD remaining in place.

Infections

IUD-related infection is now believed to be due to contamination of the endometrial cavity at the time of insertion. Infections that occur 3–4 months after insertion are believed to be due to acquired STDs, not the direct result of the IUD. The early, insertion-related infections, therefore, are polymicrobial, derived from the endogenous cervicovaginal flora, with a predominance of anaerobes.

A review of the World Health Organization data base derived from all of the WHO IUD clinical trials concluded that the risk of pelvic inflammatory disease was 6 times higher during the 20 days after the insertion compared to later times during follow-up, but, most importantly, PID was extremely rare beyond the first 20 days after insertion.[49] In nearly 23,000 insertions, however, only 81 cases of PID were diagnosed, and a scarcity of PID was observed in those situations where STDs are rare. There was no statistically significant difference comparing the copper IUD to the inert Lippes Loop or progestin-containing IUDs. These data confirm that the risk of infection is highest immediately after insertion and that PID risk does not increase with long-term use. The problem of infection can be minimized with careful screening and the use of aseptic technique.

Compared with oral contraception, barrier methods, and hormonal IUDs, there is no reason to think that nonmedicated or copper IUDs can confer protection against STDs.[50] However, the levonorgestrel-releasing IUD has been reported to be associated with a protective effect against pelvic infection.[51] Even though the association between IUD use and pelvic infection (and infertility) is now seriously questioned,[10,52] women who use IUDs should be those at low risk for STDs by virtue of a mutually monogamous sexual relationship, or users must be counseled to employ condoms along with the IUD whenever they have intercourse with a partner who could be an STD carrier. Because sexual behavior is the most important modifier of the risk of infection, clinicians should ask prospective IUD users about numbers of partners, their partner's sexual practices, the frequency and age of onset of intercourse, and history of STDs.[53] Women at low risk are unlikely to have pelvic infections while using IUDs.[18]

The IUD is not recommended for women who are at increased risk of bacterial endocarditis (previous endocarditis, rheumatic heart disease, or the presence of prosthetic heart valves). *Women with mitral valve prolapse can use an IUD, but antibiotic prophylaxis (amoxicillin 2 g) should be provided one hour before insertion.*

Asymptomatic IUD users whose cervical cultures show gonorrheal or chlamydia infection should be treated with the recommended drugs without removal of the IUD. If, however, there is evidence that an infection has ascended to the endometrium or fallopian tubes, treatment must be instituted and the IUD removed promptly. Bacterial vaginosis should be treated (metronidazole, 500 mg bid for 7 days), but the IUD need not be removed unless pelvic inflammation is present.

For simple endometritis, in which uterine tenderness is the only physical finding, doxycycline (100 mg bid for 14 days) is adequate. If tubal infection is present, as evidenced by cervical motion tenderness, abdominal rebound tenderness, adnexal tenderness or masses, or elevated white blood count and sedimentation rate, parenteral treatment is indicated with removal of the IUD as soon as antibiotic serum levels are adequate. The previous presence of an IUD does not alter the treatment of PID.

Appropriate outpatient management of less severe infections:
   Cefoxitin (2 g im) plus probenecid (1 g orally), or
   Ceftriaxone (250 mg im) plus doxycycline (100 mg bid orally)for 14 days.

Severe infections require hospitalization and treatment with:
   Cefoxitin (2 g iv q 6 h), or
   Cefotetan (2 g iv q 12 h)
   Plus doxycycline (100 mg bid orally or iv)

   Followed by 14 days of an oral regimen of antibiotics.

The following is an alternative regimen:
   Clindamycin (900 mg iv q 8 h), plus
   Gentamicin (2 mg/kg iv or im followed by 1.5 mg/kg q 8 h).

Actinomyces

The significance of actinomycosis infection in IUD users is unclear. There are several reports of IUD users with unilateral pelvic abscesses containing *actinomyces*.[54,55] However, *actinomyces* are found in Pap smears of up to 30% of plastic IUD wearers when cytologists take special care to look for the organisms. The rate is much lower (less than 1%) with copper devices and varies with duration of use.[54–57] The clinician must decide whether to remove the IUD and treat the patient, treat with the IUD in place, or simply remove the IUD. These patients are almost always asymptomatic and without clinical signs of infection. If uterine tenderness or a pelvic mass is present, the IUD should always be removed after the initiation of treatment with oral penicllin G, 500 mg qid for one month. If *actinomyces* are present on the Pap smear of a well woman, the IUD should be removed and replaced with a copper-containing device when a repeat Pap smear is negative.

Pregnancy with an IUD in Situ

Spontaneous abortion occurs more frequently among women who become pregnant with IUDs in place, a rate of approximately 50%. Because of this high rate of spontaneous abortion and the hazard of septic abortion, IUDs should always be removed if pregnancy is diagnosed and the string is visible. Use of instruments inside the uterus should be avoided if the pregnancy is desired, unless sonographic guidance can help avoid rupture of the membranes.[58] After removal of an IUD with visible strings, the spontaneous abortion rate is approximately 30%. Combining ultrasonography guidance with carbon dioxide hysteroscopy, an IUD with a missing tail can be identified and removed during early pregnancy.[59] If the IUD cannot be easily removed, the patient should be offered therapeutic abortion because the risk of life-threatening septic, spontaneous abortion in the second trimester is increased 20-fold if the pregnancy continues with the IUD in utero. Even if a patient plans to terminate a pregnancy that has occurred with an IUD in place, the IUD should be removed immediately rather than waiting until the time of the abortion, because septic abortion could ensue in the interval. If there is no evidence of infection, the IUD can safely be removed in a clinic or office.

If an IUD is in an infected, pregnant uterus, removal of the device should be undertaken only after antibiotic therapy has been initiated, and equipment for cardiovascular support and resuscitation is immediately available. These precautions are necessary because removal of an IUD from an infected, pregnant uterus can lead to septic shock.

IUD Insertion

Patient Selection

Patient selection for successful IUD use requires attention to menstrual history and the risk for STDs. Age and parity are not the critical factors in selection; the risk factors for STDs are the most important consideration. In addition, there are other conditions that can compromise success. Women who have abnormalities of uterine anatomy (bicornuate uterus, submucous myoma, cervical stenosis) may not accommodate an IUD. The few individuals who have allergies to copper or have Wilson's disease (a prevalence of about 1 in 200,000) should not use copper IUDs. Immunosuppressed patients and patients at risk for endocarditis should not use IUDs. The IUD can be used by women with mitral valve prolapse, but prophylactic antibiotics are recommended at the time of insertion if mitral regurgitation is present. The IUD is a good choice for women with diabetes mellitus.

Preferably, the absence of cervical infection should be established before insertion. If this is not feasible, insertion should definitely be delayed if a mucopurulent discharge is present.

A careful speculum and bimanual examination is essential prior to IUD insertion. It is important to know the position of the uterus; undetected extreme posterior uterine position is the most common reason for perforation at the time of IUD insertion. A very small or large uterus, determined by examination and sounding, can preclude insertion. For successful IUD use, the uterus should not sound less than 6 cm or more than 10 cm.

Timing

An IUD can be safely inserted at any time after delivery, abortion, or during the menstrual cycle. Expulsion rates were higher when the older, large plastic IUDs were inserted sooner than 8 weeks postpartum; however, studies indicate that the copper IUDs can be inserted between 4 and 8 weeks postpartum without an increase in pregnancy rates, expulsion, or removals for bleeding and/or pain.[60] Postpartum insertions immediately after expulsion of the placenta or during the first postpartum week can be safely accomplished; however, an expulsion rate of 7–15 per 100 users can be expected in the first 6 months.[61] Expulsion rates are lower after placement at cesarean section. High fundal placement is a key to minimizing expulsion rates. Insertion is easier and tolerance is better with the TCu-380A in breastfeeding women.[62]

Insertions can be more difficult if the cervix is closed between menses. The advantages of insertion during or shortly after a menstrual period include a more open cervical canal, the masking of insertion-related bleeding, and the knowledge that the patient is not pregnant. These relative advantages may be outweighed by the risk of unintended pregnancy if insertion is delayed to await menstrual bleeding.

Prophylactic Antibiotics

Doxycycline (200 mg) administered orally one hour prior to insertion will provide protection against insertion-associated pelvic infection, but it is probably of little benefit to women at low risk for STDs.[63]

IUD Removal

Removal of an IUD can usually be accomplished by grasping the string with a ring forceps or uterine dressing forceps and exerting firm traction. If strings cannot be seen, they can often be extracted from the cervical canal by rotating two cotton-tipped applicators or a Pap smear cytobrush in the endocervical canal. If further maneuvers are required, a paracervical block should be administered. Oral administration of a prostaglandin inhibitor beforehand will reduce uterine cramping.

If IUD strings cannot be identified or extracted from the endocervical canal, a light plastic uterine sound should be passed into the endometrial cavity after administration of a paracervical block. A standard metal sound is too heavy and insensitive for this purpose. The IUD can frequently be felt with the sound and localized against the anterior or posterior wall of the uterus. The device can then be removed using a Facit ureteral stone or alligator type forceps directed to where the device was felt, taking care to open the forceps widely immediately on passing it through the internal cervical os so that the IUD can be caught between the jaws. If removal is not easily accomplished using this forceps, direct visualization of the IUD with sonography or hysteroscopy can facilitate removal. Sonography is less painful and more convenient and should be tried first.

Fertility returns promptly and pregnancies after removal of an IUD occur sooner than after oral contraception, but later than after using the diaphragm. Pregnancy outcomes are within normal limits, and duration of use does not affect the return of fertility.[64] If a patient wishes to continue use of an IUD, a new device can be placed immediately after removal of the old one. In this case, antibiotic prophylaxis is advised.

Finding a Displaced IUD

When an IUD cannot be found, one has to consider, besides expulsion, perforation of the uterus into the abdominal cavity (a very rare event) or embedment into the myometrium. All IUDs are radiopaque, but localizing them radiographically requires 2–3 views, is time-consuming and expensive, and does not allow intrauterine direction of instruments. A quick, real-time sonographic scan in the office is the best method to locate a lost IUD, whether or not removal is desired.

If the IUD is identified perforating the myometrium or in the abdominal cavity, it should be removed using operative laparoscopy, usually under general anesthesia. If the IUD is in the uterine cavity, but cannot be grasped with a forceps under sonographic guidance, hysteroscopy is the best approach. Both routes may be helpful if an IUD is partially perforated.

Copper in the abdominal cavity can lead to adhesion formation, making laparoscopic removal difficult.[65] Although inert perforated devices without closed loops were previously allowed to remain in the abdominal cavity, current practice is to remove any perforated IUD. Because IUD perforations usually occur at the time of insertion, it is important to check for correct position by identifying the string within a few weeks after insertion. Uterine perforation itself is unlikely to cause more than transient pain and bleeding, and can go undetected at the time of IUD insertion. If you believe perforation has occurred, prompt sonography is indicated so that the device can be removed before adhesion formation can occur.

This problem should be put into perspective. With the new generation of IUDs (copper and medicated), adhesion formation appears to be an immediate reaction which does not progress and rarely leads to serious complications.[66] In appropriate situations (where the risk of surgery is considerable), clinician and patient may elect not to remove the translocated IUD. However, a case has been reported of sigmoid perforation occurring

5 years after insertion, and the general consensus continues to favor removal of a perforated IUD immediately upon diagnosis.[67]

The IUD for Older Women

The IUD is a good reversible contraceptive choice for older women. An older woman is more likely to be mutually monogamous and less likely to develop PID, and for those women who have already had their children, concern with fertility and problems with cramping and bleeding are both lesser issues. If protection from STDs is not a concern, insertion of a copper IUD can provide very effective contraception until the menopause without the need to do anything other than check the string occasionally. On the other hand, because alterations of bleeding patterns become more common in this age group, it may be necessary to remove an IUD.

References

1. **Huber SC, Piotrow PT, Orlans B, Dommer G,** Intrauterine devices, Popul Reports, Series B, No.2, 1975.

2. **Richter R,** Ein mittel zur verhutung der konzeption, Deutsche Med Wochenschr 35:1525, 1909.

3. **Pust K,** Ein brauchbarer frauenschutz, Dtsch Med Wochenschrift 49:952, 1923.

4. **Gräfenberg E,** An intrauterine contraceptive method, in Sanger M, Stone HM, editors, *The Practice of Contraception: Proceedings of the 7th International Birth Control Conference, Zurich, Switzerland,* Williams & Wilkins, Baltimore, Maryland, 1930, pp 33-47.

5. **Ota T,** A study on birth control with an intra-uterine instrument, Jpn J Obstet Gynecol 17:210, 1934.

6. **Ishihama A,** Clinical studies on intrauterine rings, especially the present state of contraception in Japan and the experiences in the use of intra-uterine rings, Yokohama Med Bull 10:89, 1959.

7. **Oppenheimer W,** Prevention of pregnancy by the Graefenberg ring method: a re-evaluation after 28 years' experience, Am J Obstet Gynecol 78:446, 1959.

8. **Tietze C,** Evaluation of intrauterine devices. Ninth progress report of the cooperative statistical program, Stud Fam Plann 1:1, 1970.

9. **Tatum HJ, Schmidt FH, Phillips DM, McCarty M, O'Leary WM,** The Dalkon shield controversy, structural and bacteriologic studies of IUD tails, JAMA 231:711, 1975.

10. **Kessel E,** Pelvic inflammatory disease with intrauterine device use: a reassessment, Fertil Steril 51:1, 1989.

11. **Eschenbach DA, Harnisch JP, Holmes KK,** Pathogenesis of acute pelvic inflammatory disease: role of contraception and other risk factors, Am J Obstet Gynecol 128:838, 1977.

12. **Kaufman DW, Shapiro S, Rosenberg L, Monson RR, Mietinen OS, Stolley PD, Slone D,** Intrauterine contraceptive device use and pelvic inflammatory disease, Am J Obstet Gynecol 136:159, 1980.

13. **Kaufman DW, Watson J, Rosenberg L, Helmrich SP, Miller DR, Miettinen DS, Stolley PD, Shapiro S,** The effect of different types of intrauterine devices on the risk of pelvic inflammatory disease, JAMA 250:759, 1983.

14. **Lee NC, Rubin GL, Ory HW, Burkman RT,** Type of intrauterine device and the risk of pelvic inflammatory disease, Obstet Gynecol 62:1, 1983.

15. **Mosher WD, Pratt WF,** Contraceptive use in the United States, 1973-1988, Advance data from vital and health statistics; No. 182, National Center for Health Statistics, Hyattsville, Maryland, 1990.

16. **Daling JR, Weiss NS, Metch BJ, Chow WH, Soderstrom RM, Moore DE, Spadoni LR, Stadel BV,** Primary tubal infertility in relation to the use of an intrauterine device, New Engl J Med 312:937, 1985.

17. **Cramer DW, Schiff I, Schoenbaum SC, Gibson M, Belisle S, Albrecht B, Stillman RJ, Berger MJ, Wilson E, Stadel BV, Seible M,** Tubal infertility and the intrauterine device, New Engl J Med 312:941, 1985.

18. **Lee NC, Rubin GL, Borucki R,** The intrauterine device and pelvic inflammatory disease revisited: new results from the Women' Health Study, Obstet Gynecol 72:1, 1988.

19. **Zipper JA, Medel M, Prager R,** Suppression of fertility by intrauterine copper and zinc in rabbits: a new approach to intrauterine contraception, Am J Obstet Gynecol 105:529, 1969.

20. **Tatum HJ,** Milestones in intrauterine device development, Fertil Steril 39:141, 1983.

21. **Sivin I, Tatum HJ,** Four years of experience with the TCu 380A intrauterine contraceptive device, Fertil Steril 36:159, 1981.

22. **Treiman K, Liskin L,** Intrauterine devices, Pop Reports, Series B, No. 5, Population Information Program, Johns Hopkins University, Baltimore, 1988.

23. **Sivin I, Stern J, International Committee for Contraception Research,** Health during prolonged use of levonorgestrel 20 µg/d and the copper TCu 380 Ag intrauterine contraceptive devices: a multicenter study, Fertil Steril 61:70, 1994.

24. **Chi I,** The TCu-380A (AG), MLCu375, and Nova-T IUDs and the IUD daily releasing 20 µg levonorgestrel-four pillars of IUD contraception for the nineties and beyond? Contraception 47:325, 1993.

25. **Luukkainen T, Allonen H, Haukkamaa M, Lahteenmake P, Nilsson CG, Toivonen J,** Five years' experience with levonorgestrel-releasing IUDs, Contraception 33:139, 1986.

26. **Wildemeersch D, Van Der Pas H, Thiery M, Van Kets H, Parewijck W, Delbarge W,** The copper-fix (Cu-Fix): a new concept in IUD technology, Adv Contracept 4:197, 1988.

27. **Sivin I, Diaz S, Pavez M, Alvarez F, Brasche V, Diaz J, Odlind V, Olsson S-E, Stern J,** Two-year comparative trial of the gyne T 380 slimline and gyne T 380 intrauterine copper devices, Contraception 44:481, 1991.

28. **Sivin I,** IUDs are contraceptives, not abortifacients: a comment on research and belief, Stud Fam Plann 20:355, 1989.

29. **Ortiz ME, Croxatto HB,** The mode of action of IUDs, Contraception 36:37, 1987.

30. **Alvarez F, Guiloff E, Brache V, Hess R, Fernandez E, Salvatierra AM, Guerrero B, Zacharias S,** New insights on the mode of action of intrauterine contraceptive devices in women, Fertil Steril 49:768, 1988.

31. **Segal SJ, Alvarez-Sanchez F, Adejuwon CA, Brache De Mejla V, Leon P, Faundes A,** Absence of chorionic gonadotropin in sera of women who use intrauterine devices, Fertil Steril 44:214, 1985.

32. **Wilcox AJ, Weinberg CR, Armstrong EG, Canfield RE,** Urinary human chorionic gonadotropin among intrauterine device users: detection with a highly specific and sensitive assay, Fertil Steril 47:265, 1987.

33. **Vessey M, Meisler L, Flavel R, Yeates D,** Outcome of pregnancy in women using different methods of contraception, Br J Obstet Gynaecol 86:548, 1979.

34. **Belhadj H, Sivin I, Diaz S, Pavez M, Tejada A-S, Brache V, Alvarez F, Shoupe D, Breaux H, Mishell DR Jr, McCarthy T, Yo V,** Recovery of fertility after use of the levonorgestrel 20 mcg/day or copper T 380Ag intrauterine device, Contraception 34:261, 1986.

35. **Newton J, Tacchi D,** Long-term use of copper intrauterine devices, Lancet 335:1322, 1990.

36. **Sivin I, Stern J, Diaz J, Diaz MM, Faundes A, Mahgoub SE, Diaz S, Pavez M, Coutinho E, Mattos CER, McCarthy T, Mishell DR Jr, Shoupe D, Alvarez F, Brache V, Jimenez E,** Two years of intrauterine contraception with levonorgestrel and with copper: A randomized comparison of the TCu 380Ag and levonorgestrel 20 mcg/day devices, Contraception 35:245, 1987.

37. **Sivin I, Schmidt F,** Effectiveness of IUDs: a review, Contraception 36:55, 1987.

38. **WHO Special Programme of Research, Development and Research Training in Human Reproduction. Task Force on the Safety and Efficacy of Fertility Regulating Methods,** The TCu 380A, TCu 220C, Multiload 250, and Nova T IUDs at 3, 5, and 7 years of use, Contraception 42:141, 1990.

39. **Ory HW,** Ectopic pregnancy and intrauterine contraceptive devices: new perspectives, Obstet Gynecol 57:2, 1981.

40. **Makinen JI, Erkkola RU, Laippala PJ,** Causes of the increase in incidence of ectopic pregnancy — a study on 1017 patients from 1966 to 1985 in Turku, Finland, Am J Obstet Gynecol 160:642, 1989.

41. **Edelman DA, Porter CW,** The intrauterine device and ectopic pregnancy, Contraception 36:85, 1987.

42. **WHO Special Programme of Research, Development and Research Training in Human Reproduction. Task Force on Intrauterine Devices for Fertility Regulation,** A multinational case-control study of ectopic pregnancy, Clin Reprod Fertil 3:131, 1985.

43. **Sivin I,** Dose- and age-dependent ectopic pregnancy risks with intrauterine contraception, Obstet Gynecol 78:291, 1991.

44. **Barbosa I, Bakos O, Olsson S-E, Odlind V, Johansson EDB,** Ovarian function during use of a levonorgestrel-releasing IUD, Contraception 42:51, 1990.

45. **Bilian X, Liying Z, Xuling Z, Mengchun J, Luukkainen T, Allonen H,** Pharmacokinetic and pharmacodynamic studies of levonorgestrel-releasing intrauterine device, Contraception 41:353, 1990.

46. **Franks AL, Beral V, Cates W Jr, Hogue CJ,** Contraception and ectopic pregnancy risk, Am J Obstet Gynecol 163:1120, 1990.

47. **Wilson JC,** A prospective New Zealand study of fertility after removal of copper intrauterine devices for conception and because of complications: a four-year study, Am J Obstet Gynecol 160:391, 1989.

48. **Andersson J, Rybo G,** Levonorgestrel-releasing intrauterine device in the treatment of menorrhagia, Br J Obstet Gynaecol 97:697, 1990.

49. **Farley MM, Rosenberg MJ, Rowe PJ, Chen J-H, Meirik O,** Intrauterine devices and pelvic inflammatory disease: an international perspective, Lancet 339:785, 1992.

50. **Buchan H, Villard-Mackintosh L, Vessey M, Yeates D, McPherson K,** Epidemiology of pelvic inflammatory disease in parous women with special reference to intrauterine device use, Br J Obstet Gynaecol 97:780, 1990.

51. **Toivonen J, Luukkainen T, Alloven H,** Protective effect of intrauterine release of levonorgestrel on pelvic infection: three years' comparative experience of levonorgestrel and copper-releasing intrauterine devices, Obstet Gynecol 77:261, 1991.

52. **Kronmal RA, Whitney CW, Mumford SD,** The intrauterine device and pelvic inflammatory disease; the Women's Health Study reanalyzed, J Clin Epidemiol 44:109, 1991.

53. **Lee NC, Rubin GL, Grimes DA,** Measures of sexual behavior and the risk of pelvic inflammatory disease, Obstet Gynecol 77:425, 1991.

54. **Chapin DS, Sullinger JC,** A 43-year old woman with left buttock pain and a presacral mass, New Engl J Med 323:183, 1990.

55. **Keebler C, Chatwani A, Schwartz R,** Actinomycosis infection associated with intrauterine contraceptive devices, Am J Obstet Gynecol 145:596, 1983.

56. **Duguid HLD,** Actinomycosis and IUDs, Int Plann Parenthood Fed Med Bull 17:3, 1983.

57. **Petitti DB, Yamamoto D, Morgenstern N,** Factors associated with actinomyces-like organisms on Papanicolau smear in users of IUDs, Am J Obstet Gynecol 145:338, 1983.

58. **Stubblefield P, Fuller A, Foster S,** Ultrasound-guided intrauterine removal of intrauterine contraceptive devices in pregnancy, Obstet Gynecol 72:961, 1988.

59. **Assaf A, Gohar M, Saad S, El-Nashar A, Abdel Aziz A,** Removal of intrauterine devices with missing tails during early pregnancy, Contraception 45:541, 1992.

60. **Mishell DR Jr, Roy S,** Copper intrauterine contraceptive device event rates following insertion 4 to 8 weeks post partum, Am J Obstet Gynecol 143:29, 1982.

61. **O'Hanley K, Huber DH,** Postpartum IUDs: keys for success, Contraception 45:351, 1992.

62. **Farr G, Rivera R,** Interaction between IUD use and breast-feeding status at time of IUD insertion: analysis of TCu-380A acceptors in developing countries, Am J Obstet Gynecol 167:144, 1992.

63. **Sinei SKA, Schulz KF, Laptey PR, Grimes D, Arnsi J, Rosenthal S, Rosenberg M, Rivon G, Njage P, Bhullar V, Ogendo H,** Preventing IUCD-related pelvic infection: the efficacy of prophylactic doxycycline at insertion, Br J Obstet Gynaecol 97:412, 1990.

64. **Sivin I, Stern J, Diaz S, Pavez M, Alvarez F, Brache V, Mishell DR Jr, Lacarra M, McCarthy T, Holma P, Darney P, Klaisle C, Olsson S-E, Odlind V,** Rates and outcomes of planned pregnancy after use of Norplant capsules, Norplant II rods, or levonorgestrel-releasing or copper TCu 380Ag intrauterine contraceptive devices, Am J Obstet Gynecol 166:1208, 1992.

65. **Gorsline J, Osborne N,** Management of the missing intrauterine contraceptive device: report of a case, Am J Obstet Gynecol 153:228, 1985.

66. **Adoni A, Chetrit AB,** The management of intrauterine devices following uterine perforation, Contraception 43:77, 1991.

67. **Gronlund B, Blaabjerg J,** Serious intestinal complication five years after insertion of a Nova-T, Contraception 44:517, 1991.

25 Barrier Methods of Contraception

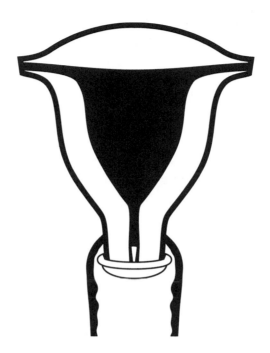

The use of vaginal contraceptives is as ancient as civilization. References to sponges and plugs appear in the earliest of writings. Substances with either barrier or spermicidal properties (or both) have included honey, alum, spices, oils, tannic acids, lemon juice, and even crocodile dung. However, the diaphragm and the cervical cap were not invented until the late 1800s, the same time period that saw the beginning of investigations with spermicidal agents.

Intravaginal contraception was widespread in isolated cultures throughout the world. The Japanese used balls of bamboo paper; Islamic women used willow leaves, and the women in the Pacific Islands used seaweed. References can be found throughout ancient writings to sticky plugs, made of gumlike substances, to be placed in the vagina prior to intercourse. In preliterate societies, an effective method had to have been the result of trial and error, with some good luck thrown in.

How was contraceptive knowledge spread? Certainly, until modern times, individuals did not consult physicians for contraception. Contraceptive knowledge was folk knowledge, undoubtedly perpetuated by the oral tradition. The social and technical circumstances of ancient times conspired to make communication of knowledge very difficult. But even when knowledge was lacking, the desire to prevent conception was not. Hence, the widespread use of potions, body movements, and amulets — all of which can be best described as magic.

Egyptian papyri dating from 1850 B.C. refer to plugs of honey, gum, acacia, and crocodile dung. The descriptions of contraceptive techniques by Soranus are viewed as the best in history until modern times.[1] Soranus gave explicit directions how to make concoctions that probably combined a barrier with spermicidal action. He favored making pulps from nuts and fruits (probably very acidic and spermicidal) and advocated the use of soft wool placed at the cervical os. He actually described up to 40 different combinations.

The earliest penis protectors were just that, intended to provide prophylaxis against infection. Gabriello Fallopius, one of the early authorities on syphilis, described, in 1564, a linen condom that covered the glans penis. The linen condom of Fallopius was followed by full covering with animal skins and intestines, but use for contraception cannot be dated to earlier than the 1700s.

There are many versions accounting for the origin of the word condom. Most attribute the word to a Dr. Condom, a physician in England in the 1600s. The most famous story declares that Dr. Condom invented the sheath in response to the annoyance displayed by Charles II at the number of his illegitimate children. All attempts to trace this physician have failed. This origin of the word can neither be proved nor disproved. By 1800, condoms were available at brothels throughout Europe, but nobody wanted to claim responsibility. The French called the condom the English cape; the English called condoms French letters.

Vulcanization of rubber dates to 1844, and by 1850 rubber condoms were available in the U.S. The vulcanization of rubber revolutionized transportation and contraception. The introduction of liquid latex and automatic machinery ultimately made reliable condoms both plentiful and affordable. Diaphragms first appeared in publication in Germany in the 1880s. A practicing German gynecologist, C. Haase, wrote extensively about his diaphragm, using a pseudonym of Wilhelm P.J. Mensinga. The Mensinga diaphragm retained its original design with little change until modern times.

The cervical cap was available for use before the diaphragm. A New York gynecologist, E.B. Foote, wrote a pamphlet describing its use around 1860. By the 1930s, the cervical cap was the most widely prescribed method of contraception in Europe. Why was the cervical cap not accepted in the U.S.? The answer is not clear. Some blame the more prudish attitude toward sexuality as an explanation for why American women had difficulty learning self-insertion techniques.

Scientific experimentation with chemical inhibitors of sperm began in the 1800s. By the 1950s, more than 90 different spermicidal products were being marketed.[2] With the availability of the intrauterine device and the development of oral contraception, interest in spermicidal agents waned, and the number of products declined.

In the last decades of the 1800s, condoms, diaphragms, pessaries, and douching syringes were widely advertised; however, they were not widely utilized. It is only since 1900 that the knowledge and application of contraception have been democratized, encouraged, and promoted.

Risks and Benefits Common to All Barrier Methods

Barrier and spermicide methods provide protection (about a 50% reduction) against sexually transmitted diseases and pelvic inflammatory disease.[4–6] This includes chlamydia, gonorrhea, herpes simplex, cytomegalovirus, human papillomavirus, and human immunodeficiency virus (HIV). This protection has a beneficial impact on the risk of tubal infertility and ectopic pregnancy.[7] In addition, women who have never used barrier methods of contraception are almost twice as likely to develop cancer of the cervix.[7,8] The risk of toxic shock syndrome is increased with barrier methods, but the actual incidence is so rare that this is not a significant clinical consideration.[9] Patients who have had toxic shock syndrome, however, should be advised to avoid barrier methods.

Failure Rates During the First Year of Use, United States[3]

Method	Percent of Women with Pregnancy Lowest Expected	Typical
No method	85.0%	85.0%
Diaphragm and spermicides	6.0	18.0
Cervical cap	6.0	18.0
Sponge		
Parous women	9.0	28.0
Nulliparous women	6.0	18.0
Spermicides	3.0	21.0
Condom	2.0	12.0

Barrier Methods and Preeclampsia

An initial case-control study indicated that methods of contraception that prevented exposure to sperm were associated with an increased risk of preeclampsia.[10] This was not confirmed in a careful analysis of two large cohort prospective pregnancy studies.[11] This latter conclusion was more compelling in that it was derived from a large prospective cohort data base.

The Diaphragm

The first effective contraceptive method under a woman's control was the vaginal diaphragm. Distribution of diaphragms led to Margaret Sanger's arrest in New York City in 1918. This was still a contentious issue in 1965 when the Supreme Court's decision in Griswold v. Connecticut ended the ban on contraception in that state. By 1940, one-third of contracepting American couples were using the diaphragm. This decreased to 10% by 1965 after the introduction of oral contraceptives and intrauterine devices, and fell to about 3% by 1988.

Efficacy

Failure rates for diaphragm users vary from as low as 2% per year of use to a high of 23%. The typical use failure rate after one year of use is 18%.[3] Older, married women with longer use achieve the highest efficacy, but young women can use diaphragms very successfully if they are properly encouraged and counseled. There have been no adequate studies to determine whether efficacy is different with and without spermicides.[12]

Side Effects

The diaphragm is a safe method of contraception that rarely causes even minor side effects. Occasionally women report vaginal irritation due to the latex rubber or the spermicidal jelly or cream used with the diaphragm. Less than 1% discontinue diaphragm use for these reasons. Urinary tract infections are approximately twice as common among diaphragm users as among women using oral contraception.[13] Possibly the rim of the diaphragm presses against the urethra and causes irritation which is perceived as infectious in origin, or true infection may result from touching the perineal area or incomplete emptying of the bladder. Studies also indicate that spermicide use can increase the risk of bacteriuria with *E coli*, perhaps due to an alteration in the normal vaginal flora.[14] Clinical experience suggests that voiding after sexual intercourse is helpful, and if necessary, a single postcoital dose of a prophylactic antibiotic can be recommended.

Improper fitting or prolonged retention (beyond 24 hours) can cause vaginal irritation or mucosal irritation. There is no link between the normal use of diaphragms and the toxic shock syndrome.[15] It makes sense, however, to minimize the risk of toxic shock by removing the diaphragm after 24 hours and during menses.

Benefits

Diaphragm use reduces the incidence of cervical gonorrhea,[16] pelvic inflammatory disease,[17] and tubal infertility.[4,7] This protection may be due in part to the simultaneous use of a spermicide. There are no data, as of yet, regarding the effect of diaphragm use on the transmission of the AIDS virus (HIV). An important advantage of the diaphragm is low cost. Diaphragms are durable and, with proper care, can last for several years.

Choice and Use of the Diaphragm

There are three types of diaphragms, and most manufacturers produce them in sizes ranging from 50 to 105 mm diameter, in increments of 2.5 to 5 mm. Most women use sizes between 65 and 80 mm.

The diaphragm made with a *flat metal spring* or a *coil spring* remains in a straight line when pinched at the edges. This type is suitable for women with good vaginal muscle tone and an adequate recess behind the pubic arch. However, many women find it difficult to place the posterior edge of these flat diaphragms into the posterior cul-de-sac and over the cervix.

Arcing diaphragms are easier to use for most women. They come in two types. The All-Flex type bends into an arc when the edges are pinched together. The hinged type must be pinched between the hinges in order to form a symmetrical arc. The hinged type forms a narrower shape when pinched together. These diaphragms allow the posterior edge of the diaphragm to slip more easily past the cervix and into the posterior cul-de-sac. Arcing diaphragms are used more successfully by women with poor vaginal muscle tone, cystocele, rectocele, a long cervix, or an anterior cervix with a retroverted uterus.

Fitting

Successful use of a diaphragm depends upon proper fitting. The clinician must have available aseptic fitting rings or diaphragms themselves in all diameters. These devices should be scrupulously disinfected. At the time of the pelvic examination, the middle finger is placed against the vaginal wall and the posterior cul-de-sac, while the hand is lifted anteriorly until the pubic symphysis abuts the index finger. This point is marked with the examiner's thumb to approximate the diameter of the diaphragm. The corresponding fitting ring or diaphragm is inserted, the fit to be assessed by both clinician and patient.

If the diaphragm is too tightly pressed against the pubic symphysis, a smaller size is selected. If the diaphragm is too loose (comes out with a cough or bearing down), the next larger size is selected. After a good fit is obtained, the diaphragm is removed by hooking the index finger under the rim and pulling. It is useful to instruct the patient in these procedures as they are experienced. The patient should then insert the diaphragm, practicing checking for proper placement as well as removal.

Timing

Diaphragm users need additional instruction about the timing of diaphragm use in relation to sexual intercourse and the use of spermicide. None of this advice has been rigorously assessed in clinical studies; therefore these recommendations represent the consensus of clinical experience.

The diaphragm should be inserted no longer than 6 hours prior to sexual intercourse. About a teaspoonful of spermicidal cream or jelly, designated for use in conjunction with a diaphragm, should be placed in the dome of the diaphragm prior to insertion. Some of the spermicide should be spread around the rim with a finger. The diaphragm should be left in place for approximately 6 hours (but no more than 24 hours) after coitus. Additional spermicide (an applicatorful) should be placed in the vagina before each additional episode of sexual intercourse while the diaphragm is in place.

Reassessment

Weight loss, weight gain, vaginal delivery, and even sexual intercourse can change vaginal caliber. The fit of a diaphragm should be assessed every year at the time of the regular examination.

Care of the Diaphragm

After removal, the diaphragm should be washed with soap and water, rinsed, and dried. Powders of any sort need not and should not be applied to diaphragm. It is wise to use water to periodically check for leaks. Diaphragms should be stored in a cool and dark location.

The Cervical Cap

The cervical cap was popular in Europe long before its recent reintroduction into the United States. There are several types of cervical caps, but only the cavity rim (Prentif) cap is approved in the U.S. U.S. trials have demonstrated the cervical cap to be about as effective as the diaphragm but somewhat harder to fit (it comes in only four sizes) and more difficult to insert (it must be placed precisely over the cervix).[18]

The cervical cap has several advantages over the diaphragm. It can be left in place for a longer time (up to 36 hours), and it need not be used with a spermicide. However, spermicide filling one-third of the dome before application is reported to prolong wearing time by decreasing the incidence of foul-smelling discharge (a common complaint after 24 hours). The cap should be inserted at least 20 minutes and not more than 4 hours before intercourse.

The size of the cervix varies considerably from woman to woman, and the cervix changes in individual women in response to pregnancy or surgery. Proper fitting, therefore, can be accomplished in only 50% of women. Women with a cervix that is too long or too short, or with a cervix that is far forward in the vagina, may not be suited for cap use. However, women with vaginal wall or pelvic relaxation may be able to use the cap. The cap should completely cover the cervix and the rim should extend back to the vaginal fornices.

Those women who can be fitted with one of the 4 sizes must first learn how to identify the cervix and then how to slide the cap into the vagina, up the posterior vaginal wall, and onto the cervix. After insertion, and after each act of sexual intercourse, the cervix should be checked to make sure it is covered. The best position for insertion and removal is squatting.

To remove the cap (at least 6 hours after coitus), pressure must be exerted with a finger tip to break the seal. The finger is hooked over the cap rim to pull it out of the vagina. Bearing down can help to bring the cervix within reach of the finger.

The cervical cap can be left in place for several days, but most women experience a foul-smelling discharge by 3 days. Like the diaphragm, it must be left in place for at least 6 hours after sexual intercourse in order to ensure that no motile sperm are left in the vagina.

The most common cause of failure is dislodgment of the cap from the cervix during sexual intercourse. There is no evidence that cervical caps cause toxic shock syndrome or dysplastic changes in the cervical mucosa.[19] It seems likely (although not yet documented) that cervical caps would provide the same protection from sexually transmitted diseases as the diaphragm.

The Contraceptive Sponge

The vaginal contraceptive sponge is a sustained release system for the spermicide, Nonoxynol-9. The sponge also absorbs semen and blocks the entrance to the cervical canal. The "Today" sponge is a dimpled polyurethaned disc impregnated with one g of Nonoxynol-9. About 20% of the Nonoxynol-9 is released over the 24 hours the sponge is left in the vagina.

The sponge must be throughly moistened with water to activate the spermicide. The sponge can be inserted immediately before sexual intercourse or up to 14 hours beforehand. There should always be a lapse of at least 6 hours after sexual intercourse before removal, even if the sponge has been in place for 24 hours before intercourse (maximal wear time, therefore, is 30 hours).

Obviously, the sponge is not a good choice for women with anatomical changes that make proper insertion and placement difficult. In most studies, the effectiveness of the sponge exceeds that of foam, jellies, and tablets, but it is lower than that associated with diaphragm or condom use.[3,20] Some studies indicated higher failure rates (twice as high) in parous women, suggesting that one size may not fit all users.[21]

Discontinuation rates are generally higher among sponge users, compared to diaphragm and spermicide use. For some women, however, the sponge is preferred because it provides continuous protection for 24 hours regardless of the frequency of coitus. In addition, it is easier to use and less messy.

Side effects associated with the sponge include allergic reactions in about 4% of users. Another 8% complain of vaginal dryness, soreness, or itching. There is no risk of toxic shock syndrome, and in fact the Nonoxynol-9 retards staphylococcal replication and toxin production.

Spermicides

Jellies, creams, foams, melting suppositories, foaming tablets, foaming suppositories, and soluble films are used as vehicles for chemical agents that inactivate sperm in the vagina before they can move into the upper genital tract. Some are used together with diaphragms, caps, and condoms, but even used alone, they can provide protection against pregnancy.

Various chemicals and a wide array of vehicles have been used vaginally as contraceptives for centuries. The first commercially available spermicidal pessaries were made in England in 1885 of cocoa butter and quinine sulfite. These or similar materials were used until the 1920s when effervescent tablets that released carbon dioxide and phenyl mercuric acetate were marketed. Modern spermicides, introduced in the 1950s, contain surface active agents that damage the sperm cell membranes (this same action occurs with bacteria and viruses, explaining the protection against STDs). The agents currently used are Nonoxynol-9, Octoxynol-9, and Menfegol. Most preparations contain 60–100 mg of these agents in each vaginal application.

Representative Products:

Vaginal Contraceptive Film — VCF.

Foams — Delfen, Emko, Koromex.

Jellies and Creams — Conceptrol, Koromex Jel, Gyneol, Ortho Gynol, Ramses, Koromex Cream.

Suppositories — Encare, Intercept, Prevent, Semicid, Conceptrol Inserts, Koromex Inserts.

Efficacy of Spermicides

Only periodic abstinence demonstrates as wide a range of efficacy in different studies as do the studies of spermicides. Efficacy seems to depend more on the population studied than the agent used. Efficacy ranges from less than 1% to nearly one-third in the first year of use.[22] Failure rates of approximately 20% during a year's use are most typical.[3] There are no comparative studies to indicate which preparations, if any, are better or worse.

Spermicides require application 10–30 minutes prior to sexual intercourse. Jellies, creams, and foams remain effective for as long as 8 hours, but tablets and suppositories are good for less than one hour. If ejaculation does not occur within the period of effectiveness, the spermicide should be reapplied. Reapplication should definitely take place for each coital episode.

Vaginal douches are ineffective contraceptives even if they contain spermicidal agents. Postcoital douching is too late to prevent the rapid ascent of sperm (within seconds) to the fallopian tubes.

Advantages of Spermicides

Spermicides are relatively inexpensive and widely available in many retail outlets without prescription. This makes spermicides popular among adolescents and others who have infrequent or unpredictable sexual intercourse. In addition, spermicides are simple to use.

Spermicides provide protection against sexually transmitted diseases. In vitro studies have demonstrated that contraceptive spermicides kill or inactivate most STD pathogens, including HIV. However, there is no evidence as of yet that spermicides can prevent HIV infection.[23,24] Clinical studies indicate reductions in the risk of gonorrhea,[25–27] pelvic infections,[28] and chlamydial infection.[25,27] There is little difference in the incidence of trichomoniasis, candidiasis, or bacterial vaginosis among spermicide users.[29] Spermicidal agents used in combination with condoms confer added protection against STDs.

Side Effects of Spermicides

No serious side effects or safety problems have arisen in all the years that spermicides have been used. The only serious question raised is that of a possible association between spermicide use and congenital abnormalities or spontaneous abortions. Epidemiologic analysis, including a meta-analysis, concludes that there is insufficient evidence to support these associations.[30–32] Spermicides are not absorbed through the vaginal mucosa in concentrations high enough to have systemic effects.[33]

The principal minor problem is allergy, which occurs in 1–5% of users, related to either the vehicle or the spermicidal agent. Utilizing a different product often solves the problem.

Condoms

Six billion condoms were used world-wide in 1990. However, if condoms had been used in every sex act where they were needed, more than 12 billion would have been used. Although awareness of condoms as an effective contraceptive method as well as protectors against STDs has increased tremendously in recent years, a great deal remains to be accomplished in order to reach the appropriate level of condom use.[34] Contraceptive efficacy and STD prevention must be linked together and publicly promoted.

There are three specific goals: correct use, consistent use, and affordable, easy availability. If these goals are met, the year 2000 will see the annual manufacture of 20 billion condoms.

Two types of condoms are available. Most are made of latex. "Natural skin" (lamb's intestine) condoms are still obtainable (about 1% of sales). Latex condoms are 0.3–0.8 mm thick. Sperm which are 0.003 mm in diameter cannot penetrate condoms. The organisms that cause STDs and AIDS also do not penetrate latex condoms, but they can penetrate condoms made from intestine.[35,36] Condom use (latex) also probably prevents transmission of human papillomavirus (HPV), the cause of condylomata acuminata. Because spermicides also provide significant protection against STDs, condoms and spermicides used together offer more protection than either method used alone.

Condoms can be straight or tapered, smooth or ribbed, colored or clear, lubricated or nonlubricated. These are all marketing ventures aimed at attracting individual notions of pleasure and enjoyment.[37] Condoms that incorporate a spermicidal agent coating the inner and outer surfaces logically promise greater efficacy and may reduce STD transmission, but these remain to be determined.

Allergic reactions can occur, either to the latex or to chemicals in the latex.[38] The typical symptoms of an allergic reaction can occur immediately, or they can be delayed. Switching condom brands is worth trying because the only other alternative is the wearing of two condoms, one latex and one lamb's intestine.

An often repeated concern is the alleged reduction in penile glans sensitivity that accompanies condom use.[37] This has never been objectively studied, and it is likely that this complaint is perception (or excuse) not based on reality. A clinician can overcome this obstruction by advocating the use of thinner (and more esoteric) condoms, knowing that any difference is also more of perception than reality.

As is true for most contraceptive methods, older, married couples experienced in using condoms and strongly motivated to avoid another pregnancy are much more effective users than young, unmarried couples with little contraceptive experience. This does not mean that condoms are not useful contraceptives for adolescents, who are likely to have sex unexpectedly or infrequently.

Prospective users need instructions if they are to avoid pregnancy and STDs. A condom must be placed on the penis before it touches a partner. Uncircumcised men must pull the foreskin back. Prior to unrolling the condom to the base of the penis, air should be squeezed out of the reservoir tip with a thumb and forefinger. The tip of the condom should extend beyond the end of the penis to provide a reservoir to collect the ejaculate (a half inch of pinched tip). If lubricants are used, they must be water based. Oil based lubricants (such as Vaseline) will weaken the latex. Couples should understand that any vaginal medication can compromise condom integrity. After intercourse, the condom should be held at the base as the still erect penis is withdrawn. Semen must not be allowed to spill or leak. The condom should be handled gently as finger nails and rings can penetrate the latex and cause leakage. If there is evidence of spill or leakage, a spermicidal agent should be quickly inserted into the vagina.

These instructions should be provided to new users of condoms who are likely to be reluctant to ask questions. Most condoms are acquired without medical supervision, and therefore clinicians should use every opportunity to inform patients about their proper use.

Inconsistent use explains most condom failures. Incorrect use accounts for additional failures, and also, condoms sometimes break. Breakage rates range from 1–12 per 100 episodes of vaginal intercourse (and somewhat higher for anal intercourse). In a U.S. survey, one pregnancy resulted for every 3 condom breakages. Concomitant use of spermicides lowers failure rates in case of breakage.[39]

Breakage is a greater problem for couples at risk for STDs. An infected man transmits gonorrhea to a susceptible woman about two-thirds of the time.[40] If the woman is infected, transmission to the man occurs one-third of the time.[41] The chance of HIV infection after a single sexual exposure ranges from one in 1,000 to one in 10.[42,43]

Condom breakage rates depend upon sexual behavior and practices, experience with condom use, the condition of the condoms, and manufacturing quality. Condoms remain in good condition for up to 5 years unless exposed to ultraviolet light, excessive heat or humidity, ozone, or oils. Condom manufacturers regularly check samples of their products to make sure they meet national standards. These procedures limit the proportion of defects to less than 0.1% of all condoms used.[44] Contraceptive failure is more likely to be due to nonuse or incorrect use.

For the immediate future, prevention of STDs and control of the AIDS epidemic will require a great increase in the use of condoms. We must all be involved in the effort to promote condom use. Condom use must be portrayed in the positive light of STD prevention. An important area of concentration is the teaching of the social skills required to ensure use by a reluctant partner.

Using scare tactics about STDs in order to encourage condom use is not sufficient. A more positive approach can yield better compliance. It is useful to emphasize that prevention of STDs will preserve future fertility. We would suggest that clinicians consider making free condoms available within their office setting. Manufacturers will sell condoms at a bulk rate, from $50–$100 per 1,000, depending upon style and lubrication.

Female Condoms

Female condoms are pouches made of polyurethane or latex, which line the vagina.[45] The female condom should be an effective barrier to STD infection; however, high cost and acceptability are major problems. The devices are more cumbersome than condoms. Women who have successfully used barrier methods and who are strongly motivated to avoid STDs are more likely to choose the female condom.

Barrier Methods for Older Couples

Some women use barrier methods throughout their reproductive years, but most change to easier, more effective methods as their sexual lives become more stable, their risk of STDs decreases accordingly, and they need contraception for avoiding rather than spacing pregnancies. Some women begin new relationships as they age and may require reminding about the risks of STDs and the need to use condoms with new partners whose sexual and drug use histories are unknown. Perimenopausal women whose earlier use of contraception was not directed at avoiding HIV infection may need to learn how and with whom to use condoms.

References

1. **Himes NE,** *Medical History of Contraception,* Williams & Wilkins, Baltimore, 1936.

2. **Gamble CJ,** Spermicidal times as aids to the clinician's choice of contraceptive materials, Fertil Steril 8:174, 1957.

3. **Trussell J, Hatcher RA, Cates W Jr, Stewart FH, Kost K,** Contraceptive failure in the United States: an update, Stud Fam Plann 21:51, 1990.

4. **Cramer DW, Goldman MB, Schiff I, Belisla S, Albrecht B, Stadel B, Gibson M, Wilson E, Stillman R, Thompson I,** The relationship of tubal infertility to barrier method and oral contraceptive use, JAMA 257:2446, 1987.

5. **Cates W, Stone K,** Family planning, sexually transmitted diseases and contraceptive choice: a literature update: part I, Fam Plann Perspect 24:75, 1992.

6. **Rosenberg MJ, Davidson AJ, Chen J-H, Judson FN, Douglas JM,** Barrier contraceptives and sexually transmitted diseases in women: a comparison of female-dependent methods and condoms, Am J Public Health 82:669, 1992.

7. **Kost K, Forrest JD, Harlap S,** Comparing the health risks and benefits of contraceptive choices, Fam Plann Persp 23:54, 1991.

8. **Coker AL, Hulka BS, McCann MF, Walton LA,** Barrier methods of contraception and cervical intraepithelial neoplasia, Contraception 45:1, 1992.

9. **Schwartz B, Gaventa S, Broome CV, Reingold AL, Hightower AW, Perlman JA, Wolf PH,** Nonmenstrual toxic shock syndrome associated with barrier contraceptives: report of a case-control study, Rev Infect Dis 11(Suppl 1):S43, 1989.

10. **Klonoff-Cohen HS, Savitz DA, Cefalo RC, McCann MF,** An epidemiologic study of contraception and preeclampsia, JAMA 62:3143, 1989.

11. **Mills JL, Klebanoff MA, Graubard BI, Carey JC, Berendes HW,** Barrier contraceptive methods and preeclampsia, JAMA 265:70, 1991.

12. **Craig S, Hepburn S,** The effectiveness of barrier methods of contraception with and without spermicide, Contraception 26:347, 1982.

13. **Fihn SD, Latham RH, Roberts P, Running K, Stamm WE,** Association between diaphragm use and urinary tract infection, JAMA 254:240, 1985.

14. **Hooton TM, Hillier S, Johnson C, Roberts P, Stamm WE,** *Escherichia coli* bacteriuria and contraceptive method, JAMA 265:64, 1991.

15. **Centers for Disease Control,** Toxic shock syndrome, United States, 1970–1982, MMWR 31:201, 1982.

16. **Keith L, Berger G, Moss W,** Prevalence of gonorrhea among women using various methods of contraception, Br J Venereal Dis 51:307, 1975.

17. **Kelaghan J, Rubin GL, Ory HW, Layde PM,** Barrier method contraceptives and pelvic inflammatory disease, JAMA 248:184, 1982.

18. **Bernstein G, Kilzer LH, Coulson AH, Nakamara RM, Smith GC, Bernstein R, Frezieres R, Clark VA, Coan C,** Studies of cervical caps, Contraception 26:443, 1982.

19. **Gollub EL, Sivin I,** The Prentif cervical cap and pap smear results: a critical appraisal, Contraception 40:343, 1989.

20. **Edelman DA, McIntyre SL, Harper J,** A comparative trial of the Today contraceptive sponge and diaphragm: a preliminary report, Am J Obstet Gynecol 150:869, 1984.

21. **McIntyre SL, Higgins JE,** Parity and use-effectiveness with the contraceptive sponge, Am J Obstet Gynecol 155:796, 1986.

22. **Ryder NB,** Contraceptive failure in the United States, Fam Plann Perspect 5:133, 1973.

23. **Hicks DR, Martin LS, Getchell JP, Heath JL, Francis DP, McDougal JS, Curran JW, Voeller B,** Inactivation of HTLV-III/LAV-infected cultures of normal human lymphocytes by nonoxynol-9 in vitro, Lancet 2:1422, 1985.

24. **Kreiss J, Ngugi E, Holmes K, Ndinya-Achola J, Waiyaki P, Roberts PL, Ruminjo I, Sajabi R, Kimata J, Fleming TR, Anzala A, Holton D, Plummer F,** Efficacy of nonoxynol-9 contraceptive sponge use in preventing heterosexual acquisition of HIV in Nairobi prostitutes, JAMA 268:477, 1992.

25. **Louv WC, Austin H, Alexander WJ, Stagno S, Cheeks J,** A clinical trial of nonoxynol-9 as a prophylaxis for cervical Neisseria gonorrhoeae and Chlamydia trachomatis infections, J Infect Dis 158:518, 1988.

26. **Austin H, Louv WC, Alexander WJ,** A case-control study of spermicides and gonorrhea, JAMA 251:2822, 1984.

27. **Niruthisard S, Roddy RE, Chutivongse S,** Use of nonoxynol-9 and reduction in rate of gonococcal and chlamydial cervical infections, Lancet 339:1371, 1992.

28. **Kelaghan J, Rubin GL, Ory HW, Layde PM,** Barrier-method contraceptives and pelvic inflammatory disease, JAMA 248:184, 1982.

29. **Barbone F, Austin H, Louv WC, Alexander WJ,** A follow-up study of methods of contraception, sexual activity, and rates of trichomoniasis, candidiasis, and bacterial vaginosis, Am J Obstet Gynecol 163:510, 1990.

30. **Louik C, Mitchell AA, Werler MM, Hanson JW, Shapiro S,** Maternal exposure to spermicides in relation to certain birth defects, New Engl J Med 317:474, 1987.

31. **Bracken MB, Vita K,** Frequency of non-hormonal contraception around conception and association with congenital malformations in offspring, Am J Epidemiol 117:281, 1983.

32. **Einarson TR, Koren G, Mattice D, Schechter-Tsafriri O,** Maternal spermicide use and adverse reproductive outcome: a meta-analysis, Am J Obstet Gynecol 162:655, 1990.

33. **Malyk B,** Preliminary results: serum chemistry values before and after the intravaginal administration of 5% nonoxynol-9 cream, Fertil Steril 35:647, 1981.

34. **Tanfer K, Grady WR, Klepinger DH, Billy JOG,** Condom use among U.S. men, 1991, Fam Plann Perspect 25:61, 1993.

35. **Stone KM, Grimes DA, Magder LS,** Primary prevention of sexually transmitted diseases. A primer for clinicians, JAMA 255:1763, 1986.

36. **Van de Perre P, Jacobs D, Sprecher-Goldberger S,** The latex condom, an efficient barrier against sexual transmission of AIDS-related viruses, AIDS 1:49, 1987.

37. **Grady WR, Klepinger DH, Billy JOG, Tanfer K,** Condom characteristics: the perceptions and preferences of men in the United States, Fam Plann Perspect 25:67, 1993.

38. **Turjanmaa K, Reunala T,** Condoms as a source of latex allergen and cause of contact urticaria, Contact Dermatitits 20:360, 1989.

39. **Population Information Program,** Condoms, now more than ever, Population Reports, H-8l, The Johns Hopkins University, Baltimore, 1990, p 11.

40. **Platt R, Rice PA, McCormack WM,** Risk of acquiring gonorrhea and prevalence of abnormal adnexal findings among women recently exposed to gonorrhea, JAMA 250:3205, 1983.

41. **Hooper RR, Reynolds GM, Jones OG, Zaidi A, Wiesner RJ, Latimer KP, Lester A, Campbell AF, Harrison WO, Karney WW, Holmes KK,** Cohort study of venereal disease. I. The risk of gonorrhea transmission from infected women to men, Am J Epidemiol 108:136, 1978.

42. **Anderson RM, Medley GF,** Epidemiology of HIV infection and AIDS: incubation and infectious periods, survival and vertical transmissions, AIDS 2 (Suppl 1):557, 1988.

43. **Cameron DW, Simonsen JN, D'Costa LJ, et al,** Female to male transmission of human immunodeficiency virus type 1: Risk factors for seroconverison in men, Lancet 2:403, 1989.

44. **Free MJ, Skiens EW, Morrow MM,** Relationship between condom strength and failure during use, Contraception 22:31, 1980.

45. **Soper DE, Brockwell NJ, Dalton JP,** Evaluation of the effects of a female condom on the female lower genital tract, Contraception 44:21, 1991.

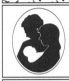

Part IV

Infertility

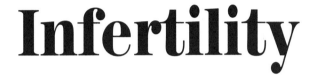

26   Female Infertility

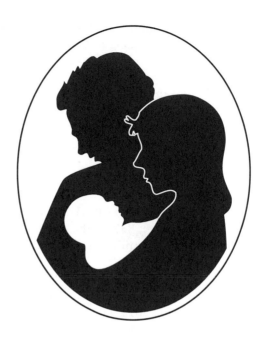

Infertility is defined as one year of unprotected coitus without conception. It affects approximately 10–15% of couples in the reproductive age group which makes it an important component of the practices of many physicians.[1] *Fecundability* is the probability of *achieving a pregnancy* within one menstrual cycle (about 25% in normal couples); *fecundity* is the ability to *achieve a live birth* within one menstrual cycle.

There have been 3 striking changes in infertility practice during the past 2 decades. First was the introduction of in vitro fertilization and other assisted reproductive technologies (ART) which have enlarged the possibilities for successful treatment and provided an opportunity to study basic reproductive processes. ART refers to all techniques involving direct retrieval of oocytes from the ovary (Chapter 31). Second, and partially because of the media attention focused on ART, the public has become more aware of potential treatments, and this has generated a marked increase in patient visits for infertility. There has been no recent dramatic change in the proportion of couples considered infertile; however, there is an increasing number of infertile couples, due, in part, to the aging of the large post World War II population boom generation. The third change is the increase in the proportion of women over 35 seeking medical attention for infertility. One of every five women in the United States is having a first child after 35, a marked increase over earlier figures. This reflects both a later age for marriage and postponement of pregnancy in marriage as women, by choice or by circumstances, commit to the work place.

The Epidemiology of Infertility

The first United States census was in 1790. At that time, the birth rate was 55 per 1,000 population; 200 years later, it is 15.5 per 1,000 population, a decrease from 8 births per woman to 1.8.[2] There are some obvious and some speculative explanations for the decline in U.S. fertility.

Popular Explantations for the Decline in U.S. Fertility
- Changing roles and aspirations for women.
- Postponement of marriage.
- Delayed age of childbearing.
- Increasing use of contraception.
- Liberalized abortion.
- Concern over the environment.
- Unfavorable economic conditions.

The deferment of marriage and postponement of pregnancy in marriage are the most significant changes in modern society. However, only 16% of the decline in the total fertility rate in the U.S. is accounted for by the increase in the average age at first marriage; 83% of the decline in the total fertility rate is accounted for by a change in marital fertility rates (avoiding pregnancy in the first years of marriage).[1,2]

After World War II, the U.S. total fertility rate reached a modern high of 3.8 births per woman. The last women born in this period won't be reaching their 45th birthday until around 2010. For approximately a 20-year period, therefore, there will be an unprecedented number of women in the later childbearing years. The aging of the World War II population boom is giving current times a greater number of women who are delaying marriage and childbirth. This demographic change has 3 specific impacts on couples.

1. A need for effective contraception.

2. The problem of achieving pregnancy later in life.

3. The problem of being pregnant later in life.

The proportion of births accounted for by this older group of women will increase by about 72% from 1982 to 2000.[3] These couples, pressed for time, have a desire to get pregnancies accomplished in a shorter time period.

Concern with Infertility

During 1982, nearly one in 5 ever-married women of reproductive age reported that they had sought professional help during their lifetimes because of infertility.[1] A sharp escalation of demand for infertility services began in 1981. From approximately 600,000 visits in 1968, the total increased to nearly 1 million in the early 1970s, then in the early 1980s, the total went over 2 million. From 1982 to 1988, the number of women who used infertility services increased by 25%, from 1.1 million to 1.35 million.[4]

There have been no significant changes in the proportion of infertile couples in the 1980s.[4] In 1988, 7.9% of all currently married couples in the United States with a wife in childbearing age were considered infertile. Eliminating those who were surgically sterile, the percentage was 13.9%. Of all U.S. women aged 15–44, 8.4% reported impaired fecundity in 1988 (4.9 million women).[4] Approximately 25% of women will experience an episode of infertility during their reproductive life.[5]

Why then is there this increasing concern for infertility? First, although the proportion of married couples considered infertile has demonstrated no recent change, there is an increasing number of infertile couples. As noted, the aging of the post World War II generation is yielding a greater number of women who are delaying marriage and childbirth. From 1982 to 1988, the number of childless women aged 35–44 years increased by over 1 million, from 1.8 million in 1982 to 2.9 million in 1988.[4] About 4% of women aged 15–24 have impaired fecundity, compared to 13% at age 25–34, and 30% at age 35–44. In addition, there is a greater awareness of modern treatments and a greater ability to afford health care. The impact of widespread publicity is significant. Furthermore, the current effectiveness of the control of fertility allows more attention to be given to infertility. Also to be considered is the decreased supply of infants for adoption. There is an increased availability of services, and there is a greater knowledge of the diagnosis and management of infertility among clinicians. Finally, infertility is now more socially acceptable as a problem.

The post World War II generation has faced an unique evolutionary change. They were the first to be able to exercise control over their fertility, and then as they aged and deferred pregnancy, they had to deal with the problem of unintended infertility. Because many couples defer pregnancy and then desire their families within a condensed interval of time, there is a growing demand for infertility services. These factors have combined to substantially increase the number of couples seeking and using infertility services. Nevertheless, in the 1988 U.S. National Survey of Family Growth, the majority of women with impaired fecundity had not obtained professional services.[6] Of U.S. women with impaired fecundity, 43% had obtained some form of infertility service; 24% had specialized infertility treatment, and only 2% had received in vitro fertilization.

Age alone impacts on fertility. Certainly, aging of the reproductive system plays a role and spontaneous abortion provides another factor. The majority of early abortions after age 35 are due to autosomal trisomies, the incidence of which increases with maternal age. The risk of clinically recognized spontaneous abortion increases from about 10% until age 30, to 18% in the late 30s, and 34% in the early 40s.[7] In addition, as women enter their 30s, there is a greater likelihood of being affected by a number of diseases, for example endometriosis, that can interfere with fertility. Cumulative exposures to occupational or environmental hazards also could lessen fertility as a woman ages. An additional factor that has contributed to infertility at all ages is the spread of sexually transmitted diseases with their damaging effect on the fallopian tubes.

Aging and Fertility

What is the impact of age on fertility? The classic study is that of the Hutterites who live in the Dakotas, Montana, and the adjacent parts of Canada. The sect originated in Switzerland in 1528, and practically all of the living Hutterites came to South Dakota in the 1870s. Four colonies of 443 Hutterites grew by 1950 to 93 colonies containing 8,542 Hutterites. Contraception is condemned, and because of the communal arrangement of their society, there is no incentive to limit the size of families. All families are provided for equally.

In the 1950s, Joseph Eaton of Western Reserve University studied the Hutterites, focusing on the incidence of mental disorders. He provided his demographic data to Tietze who analyzed the fertility rates.[8] Only 5 of 209 women had no children for an infertility rate of 2.4%. The average age of the women at the last pregnancy was 40.9 years, and there was a definite decrease in fertility with age. Eleven percent of the women bore no children after age 34; 33% of the women were infertile by age 40, and 87% were infertile at age 45.

The fertility of the Hutterites has become legendary. Their fertility rate is an example of how high fertility can be when a population is healthy, stable, and not using contraception. Based on the Hutterite data, it can be concluded that a population which marries relatively late (age 22), has some lactational amenorrhea, and some age-related and parity-related decline in coital frequency, can produce 11 live births per married woman. Hypothetically, if marriage were earlier, there were no lactational amenorrhea, and no sterilization or decline in coitus, the total fertility rate would be about 15 live births per woman.[9]

The French studied the pregnancy rate in a donor insemination program, including only women with azoospermic husbands.[10] These women are less likely to have infertility factors than those women married to oligospermic males. A decrease in conception rate with age was noted. Below the age of 31 the pregnancy rate over one year was 74%. This decreased to 62% at ages 31 to 35 and to 54% when the women were older than 35. An American study with therapeutic insemination has demonstrated a similar relationship with age.[11] Of note was the requirement for more treatment cycles to achieve pregnancy in older women, 9–10 cycles rather than the usual 6. In a donor insemination program in the Netherlands, the probability of having a healthy baby decreased 3.5% per year after age 30.[12] A woman age 35 had 50% the chance of having a healthy baby compared to a woman age 25.

The decline of fertility among married couples with advancing age has been repeatedly documented. It is safe to say that about one-third of women who defer pregnancy until the mid to late 30s will have an infertility problem, and at least half of women over age 40. In programs of assisted reproductive technologies, delivery rates in women over age 40 are one-third to one-half of those in younger women, and many programs have only rare successful pregnancies in women over age 40.[13,14]

The oldest spontaneous pregnancy in modern times (according to The Guinness Book of World Records) occurred in a woman from Portland, Oregon, who delivered when she was 57 years and 120 days old. In older times, a Scottish woman was reputed to have delivered 6 children after the age of 47, the last at age 62![15]

Keep in mind that a major contributor to the decline in delivery rates associated with increasing age is the risk of spontaneous abortion. Indeed, once pregnancy is achieved, the greatest obstacle to successful delivery is the risk of spontaneous loss. The frequency of both euploid (normal) and aneuploid (abnormal) abortuses increases with maternal age. Clinically recognized abortion occurs in only 12% of women younger than age 20, but the incidence increases to 26% in women older than age 40.[16,17] The overall abortion risk (recognized and unrecognized) in women over age 40 is approximately 75%!

It has been assumed that male fertility is immortal because so many very old men have been able to produce pregnancies. A short report in 1935 told of a North Carolina farmer born in 1840.[18] Over a period of 30 years, his first wife had 16 children. At age 93, he remarried to a 27-year-old widow; one year later, a child was born. Reading the detailed physical examination provided in this report, it is obvious that this 94-year-old man was very unattractive, with leathery, wrinkled skin and no teeth. It is by no means certain that he was the father of the child.

The changes in the male with aging are modest, but significant. There are at least two reasons to believe that the quality of sperm decreases with aging. New autosomal disease can be attributed to an increase in the frequency of male gene mutations, and paternal age is related to the risk of trisomies, indicating an increase in nondisjunction in the male.[19] It is possible, however, that the decrease in sperm in older men is not correlated with fecundability. To perform the appropriate study is probably impossible; the arrangements are forbidding (such as old sperm into young recipients).

Pregnancy Outcome with Increasing Age

Traditional teaching has emphasized an increased risk of obstetrical complications with increasing age. Indeed, statistics indicate that older women have had a higher mortality rate with pregnancy.[20] In Swedish data, delayed childbearing has been associated with an increase in poor outcome measures even after adjusting for maternal complications and other risk factors.[21]

There is reason to believe, however, that the obstetrical risks associated with advancing age can be minimized by good screening and modern obstetrical care. Experience in the United States indicates that good pregnancy outcome with no increase in maternal mortality is possible with exemplary care.[22,23]

Endocrine Changes with Aging

The early fetal mitotic multiplication of germ cells produces a total of 6–7 million oogonia by 16–20 weeks of pregnancy. From this point in time, the germ cell content will irretrievably decrease. At the onset of puberty, the germ cell mass has already been reduced to approximately 300,000 units. During the next 35–40 years of reproductive life, these units will be depleted further to a point at menopause when only a few hundred remain.

In the last 10–15 years before menopause, there is an acceleration of follicular loss. This accelerated loss begins when the total number of follicles reaches approximately 25,000, a number reached in normal women at age 37–38.[24] This loss correlates with a subtle but real increase in follicle-stimulating hormone (FSH) and decrease in inhibin. These changes, including the increase in FSH, reflect the reduced quality and capability of aging follicles. These subtle changes (which influence fertility) are not associated with any noteworthy and observable changes, such as a major alteration in menstrual cycle characteristics.

Prior to the menopause, there is a period with shorter follicular phases, with increased FSH levels, but normal luteinizing hormone (LH) levels and luteal phases.[25] The menstrual periods for 10–15 years before the menopause are regular, but there is a steady decrease in cycle length due to the shortened follicular phase. Cycle lengths are the shortest (with the least variability) in the late 30s, a time when subtle but real increases in FSH and decreases in inhibin are occurring.[26–29] For a period of several years (as much as 10 years in some women) prior to menopause, the cycles lengthen again.

Women who present with "incipient" ovarian failure have elevated FSH levels and decreased levels of inhibin, but normal levels of estradiol.[30] The rise in FSH during the later years is in response to declining inhibin production by the less competent ovarian follicles.[31,32] Inhibin levels are lower in the follicular phase in women 45–49 years old compared to younger women. This decline begins early, but accelerates after 40 years of age. The rise in FSH is not apparent until age 40, and there is no change in LH levels until menopause. The changes in the later reproductive years reflect lesser follicular competence as the better primordial follicles respond early in life, leaving the lesser follicles for later. This is correlated with the decrease in fecundability that occurs with aging.

Elevated FSH levels on cycle day 3 (greater than 15 IU/L, but especially greater than 20 IU/L) are associated with poor performance with in vitro fertilization.[33] A cycle day 3 FSH level that is 25 IU/L or more, or an age of 44 years or more, both independently are associated with a chance of pregnancy close to zero during ovulation induction or with assisted reproductive technology.[34] Women with one ovary have higher day 3 FSH levels that correlate with reduced outcomes in in vitro fertilization.[35] It is not certain whether this reflects the loss of the other ovary or the factors which were responsible for the unilateral oophorectomy.

Keep in mind that there is no abrupt change at age 40, and therefore, these changes can apply to younger women. The age of change is determined by the rate of oocyte loss, a rate that is genetically programmed in most women.

Is the Decline in Fecundity with Aging Due to the Uterus or the Oocytes?

Experience has repeatedly demonstrated a reduction in in vitro fertilization pregnancy rates when the oocytes are of advanced age. When embryos from the same cohort of young donated oocytes were simultaneously transferred to young and older recipients, pregnancy rates were similar.[36] The high rate of implantation and pregnancy in older women receiving donated younger oocytes has argued that uterine factors are not involved with the decline in fecundity with aging. However, it is possible that the stimulation protocols overcome any contribution from a uterine factor.

In 100 consecutive patients in an oocyte donor program, there was no decline in success over the age range from 40 to 50.[37] Furthermore, excellent outcomes have been achieved in women aged 50–59.[38] The good obstetrical outcomes in these patients must reflect to a significant degree the youthful good health of this older group of women, as determined by extensive medical and psychological assessment. Of importance is the fact that the stimulation protocol utilized a 100 mg dose of progesterone.

Meldrum reported a lesser percentage of delivered pregnancies in women over 40 compared to women under 40 going through an identical donor oocyte-in vitro fertilization program.[13] However, he then achieved pregnancy rates in women over 40 similar to those in women under 40 by increasing the progesterone dose in the stimulation protocol from 50 mg to 100 mg per day. The uterine contribution to the decline in fecundity with aging can thus be overcome by the hormone stimulation provided in the stimulation protocols. The experience with donor oocyte programs argues, therefore, that the age-related decline in fecundity is primarily due to aging oocytes.

A pregnancy rate in older women of approximately 30% per cycle can be achieved in a donor oocyte program. In a large series, the rate of spontaneous abortion in recipients correlated with the age of the donors. The abortion rate increased from 14% in recipients who received oocytes from donors aged 20–24 years to 44.5% when the recipient received oocytes from donors older than age 35.[39] These results further point out that the increased risks of spontaneous abortion and chromosomal anomalies associated with older age are also due primarily to aging oocytes. Pregnancy wastage directly correlates with the age of the woman who produces the oocytes.

Clinicians can appropriately advise older women that there is no time to waste, and serious consideration should be given to an early resort to hormonal stimulation for both oocyte response and support of the endometrium. Older couples should be provided the option of oocyte donation from young donors instead of standard assisted reproductive technologies.

The Role of the Physician

When is a medical success really a success? There is an incidence of spontaneous pregnancy among infertile couples. About one-half of couples presenting after one year of infertility can be expected to become pregnant spontaneously in the following year. In an English study, only 20% of women who had failed to have a birth within the first two years of marriage never had a child.[40] In a life-table analysis of 58 untreated apparently normal infertile couples, 74% were pregnant by two years; however, normal couples achieve this rate in 9 months.[41] Overall, approximately 40% of couples become pregnant after discontinuation of treatment, and 35% of couples never treated can expect to become pregnant.[42]

One of the important missions for the infertility physician is not necessarily to take credit for achieving a pregnancy, but to speed up the period of time required for that achievement. For couples in their 30s, the recommendation to seek help promptly is valid — the sooner a problem is detected, the better.

In response to the needs of infertile individuals, physicians should have four goals in mind:

1. The first goal is to seek out and to correct the causes of infertility. With proper evaluation and therapy, the majority of women will become pregnant.

2. The second goal is to provide accurate information and to dispel the misinformation commonly gained from friends and mass media.

3. The third goal is to provide emotional support for the couple during a trying period. The inability to conceive generates a feeling in many couples that they have lost control over a very significant segment of their lives. The burden is aggravated by the manipulations that couples have to undergo during the infertility investigation, including the need to have intercourse on schedule. Couples need to have an opportunity to ventilate their concerns and dispel some of their fears. A valuable adjunct to the efforts of the physician are support groups for infertile couples such as those organized by RESOLVE.

   Meetings in groups allows individuals to realize that their problem is not unique, and it enables them to obtain information on how others cope with infertility. It must be emphasized that, while severe anxieties can interfere with ovulation and frequency of intercourse, there is no evidence that infertility is caused by the usual anxieties besetting a couple trying to conceive.

4. An often neglected goal is that of counseling a couple concerning the proper time to discontinue investigation and treatment. This is especially important in the 10–15% of couples with no known cause for their infertility. Despite the absence of pathology, couples with 3 years or more of infertility have a poor prognosis. Counseling must include consideration of assisted reproductive technologies.

   Counseling also should be an ongoing process during the infertility investigation and treatment. At least every 3 months the physician and couple should review the status of their care and outline the anticipated management. Thereby, changes in plans due to medical, emotional or financial reasons can be instituted in a timely fashion.

Causes of Infertility

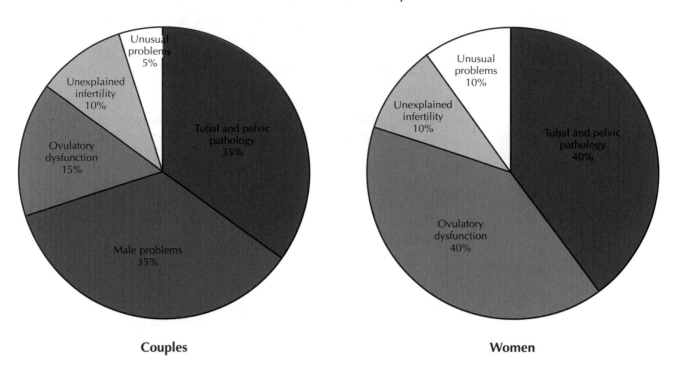

Couples   Women

The Female Infertility Investigation

We find it very helpful to mail a detailed questionnaire to our patients prior to their initial visit. The questionnaire is very complete, providing information that ranges from previous medical events and sexuality to recreational, social, and vocational activities. Patients often write comments regarding their past history and their feelings that are difficult to express during an office interview.

There are advantages to having the male present during the initial interview. He may contribute valuable historical information. It also gives the physician the opportunity to emphasize that both partners are involved in the infertility investigation. A male who has been acquainted at its inception with the physician's treatment of the infertility problem will be less reluctant, as time progresses, to ask for clarification of any aspect of the testing. This can prevent misunderstandings engendered when the male partner's only source of information is the woman. Early in the physician-couple interaction, frequency of coitus, and possible sexual problems should be ascertained.

Failure to ovulate is the major problem in approximately 40% of female infertility, another 40% is due to tubal pathology, and less than 10% is due to problems such as anatomic abnormalities or thyroid disease. It should be noted that induced abortions do not influence subsequent pregnancy rates.[43] Fetal wastage is definitely higher in diethylstilbestrol-exposed women, and while there is still some uncertainty, evidence suggests that primary infertility is also more common.[44] Besides the well-known impact of smoking on pregnancy, there is a growing story that fecundity is reduced in men and women who smoke, and the risk is greater with smoking at an early age.[45,46] Marijuana inhibits the secretion of GnRH and can suppress reproductive function in both men and women, and cocaine use is known to reduce spermatogenesis.[47,48] Studies have failed to confirm an adverse impact of caffeine.[49]

Couples need to be aware that there is a normal time requirement to achieve pregnancy. In each ovulatory cycle normal couples have only about a 25% chance of becoming pregnant. Guttmacher's classic table has been a standard since 1956.[50]

Time Required for Conception in Couples Who Will Attain Pregnancy

Months of Exposure	% Pregnant
3 months	57%
6 months	72%
1 year	85%
2 years	93%

Because the male factor accounts for approximately 35% of infertility, examination of the semen should be an early diagnostic step in the investigation. If abnormal, further diagnostic procedures in the woman should be deferred until decisions are reached regarding the man (see Chapter 29). If normal, attention is directed to the woman.

Laboratory testing should be directed by clinical judgment. However, there are a few specific recommendations. Women with a negative rubella titer should be immunized before becoming pregnant. Testing for the human immunodeficiency virus is essential in high risk couples, but especially necessary for couples participating in one of the techniques of assisted reproduction.

The Postcoital Test

The postcoital test provides information regarding both the receptivity of cervical mucus and the ability of sperm to reach and survive in the mucus. Estrogen levels peak just prior to ovulation, and this provides maximal stimulation of the cervical glands. An outpouring of clear, watery mucus is fostered which may be of sufficient quantity to be noted by the woman. Earlier in the cycle, when estrogen output is lower, and starting 2 to 3 days after ovulation when progesterone levels increase and counteract the estrogen, the mucus is thick, viscid, and opaque.

The postcoital test is performed around the time of the expected luteinizing hormone (LH) surge as determined by a previous basal body temperature chart or by the length of prior cycles. Timing also can be obtained with ultrasonography and LH monitoring, but this usually is not necessary. Between 2 and 8 hours after coitus, cervical mucus is removed with a nasal polyp forceps or tuberculin syringe and examined for macroscopic and microscopic characteristics. Attempts to refine the postcoital test by studying individual fractions from different levels in the cervical canal, with emphasis on the sample from the internal os, have not produced convincing evidence of value. Sperm distribution is uniform throughout the cervical canal, and selective sampling at the level of the internal os is not necessary.[51] A less than 2-hour interval between coitus and examination has been recommended as giving maximal information, but this early evaluation may be deceptive because complement dependent reactions in mucus which can immobilize sperm may not be apparent for a few hours. Others have suggested that a 16- to 24-hour interval provides a better assessment of sperm longevity, and a study has indicated that there is no drop in the number of sperm at any time during the first 24 hours.[52] There are other indications, however, that the number of sperm does decrease after 8 hours, and this is more in keeping with our experience. Therefore, we suggest that the couple have coitus in the morning or late at night, and that the test be performed 2 to 8 hours later. It is also suggested that the couple abstain from intercourse for 48 hours prior to the postcoital test.

The stretchability *(spinnbarkeit)* of the mucus at midcycle should be 8–10 cm or more. This characteristic can be assessed as the mucus is pulled from the cervix, or alternatively, by placing the mucus on a slide, covering it with a coverslip and then lifting the coverslip. At midcycle the mucus contains 95–98% water and should be watery, thin, clear, acellular, and abundant. When dried on a slide, it should form a distinct fern pattern.

Fern pattern

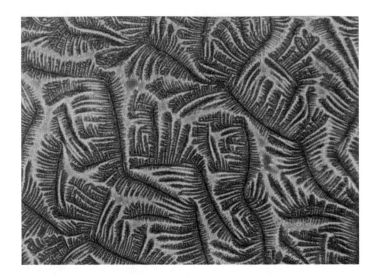

Lack of fern

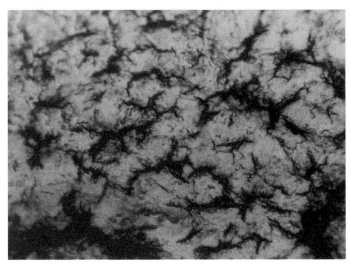

If the mucus is thick rather than thin, opaque instead of clear, the proximity of the test to ovulation should be determined by the onset of the next period (or by the temperature chart if one is being taken during that cycle). If poor mucus quality is related to inaccurate timing, the test should be repeated in a subsequent cycle with scheduling based on self-monitoring of urinary LH. Poor mucus at midcycle is a physical barrier that decreases sperm penetration and requires alteration to enhance fertility. In one study 54% of women with good mucus became pregnant, compared to 37% with poor mucus, a statistically significant difference.[53] In all likelihood some of these poor tests were reflections of inaccurate timing, and pregnancies do occur even with poor mucus at ovulation time.[54] It remains our impression, however, that poor mucus is associated with a decreased chance for fertility.

Treatment of poor mucus has been attempted by giving 0.625 mg of conjugated estrogens daily for the 8 or 9 days preceding the expected time of ovulation. In a 28-day cycle that would be between days 5 and 13. There is no advantage to continuing the hormone treatment through the luteal phase of the cycle. If the initial treatment with estrogen fails to produce a change in the mucus, the dose is increased to 1.25 mg/day. In refractory cases, 5 mg of conjugated estrogens can be given starting a few days prior to expected ovulation. However, evidence for the value of estrogen therapy is lacking, and it has no demonstrable benefit for the poor mucus which is, on occasion, associated with use of clomiphene citrate.[55] Guaifenesin, a mucolytic agent found in some over the counter cough syrups has been used to treat thick mucus, but its efficacy is questionable. If there is evidence of chronic cervicitis with thick yellowish mucus, culture for chlamydia is important, and, where appropriate, systemic antibiotics should be used. On rare occasions, the cervix is treated with electrocautery or cryosurgery.

An alternate treatment for poor mucus utilizes stimulation with human menopausal gonadotropins to enhance estrogen production, and, as a result, increased mucus formation occurs. This treatment is seldom warranted, because it is expensive and entails the risks of multiple births and ovarian hyperstimulation. The most logical approach to overcome the barrier of thick cervical mucus is the method we prefer, the use of intrauterine insemination (IUI) of washed sperm (see Chapter 29). If poor mucus is the sole problem, IUI for 3–4 cycles is associated with a cumulative pregnancy rate of 35%.

In addition to providing an evaluation of mucus the postcoital test also gives information concerning the male. Absence of sperm requires a review of the couple's coital technique. Repeated cancellations of appointments for the postcoital test may be a clue that there are sexual problems that have not been uncovered by the interview. More importantly, absence of sperm necessitates a detailed review of the semen specimen.

One of the most difficult problems in infertility is the postcoital test which repeatedly shows no sperm or only dead sperm despite good mucus. The patient should be cautioned that lubricants such as K-Y Jelly and Surgilube have a spermicidal effect in vitro and should not be used by infertile couples. If lubrication is necessary, vegetable oil can be used without interfering with sperm movement. As noted earlier, re-examination of the semen to check sperm count and motility is a necessity if the postcoital test is poor.

If the semen is normal, the pH of the cervical mucus at midcycle should be determined. Good results have been reported using a precoital douche of 1 tablespoon of sodium bicarbonate in 1 quart of water when a poor postcoital test was associated with a pH below 7.[56] Cervical cultures should be obtained for chlamydia if the mucus is yellowish, and sperm antibody testing should be performed in cases where there are no sperm or mostly nonmotile sperm. In addition, sperm antibody testing (Chapter 29) is mandatory when, in a postcoital test with good mucus, the sperm are found shaking in place but not moving progressively. This shaking movement is a common finding in immunologic infertility.

In vitro cross testing, utilizing donor or bovine mucus and donor sperm, can help to determine whether the poor postcoital test is due to factors in the mucus or to defects in the sperm. A drop of the consort's sperm and a drop of donor sperm separately are placed in contact with the patient's mucus on a slide. Penetration of the mucus by the two specimens is compared under a microscope. A similar test can be performed with donor mucus. A commercially available test, consisting of bovine cervical mucus in capillary tubes, can be substituted for donor mucus. In this test the sperm are allowed to swim into the capillary tube and the depth of penetration measured.

A postcoital test cannot be considered a substitute for a semen analysis. While 21 or more sperm/HPF is almost always associated with a sperm count above 20 million/mL, the postcoital test gives little information concerning the morphology of sperm in the ejaculate. There are considerably fewer abnormal forms in the cervical mucus compared to the ejaculate. This may represent a filtering effect of the cervical mucus or may indicate that abnormal forms do not have the motility to penetrate the cervical mucus.

The postcoital test has had a role in the infertility investigation for over 100 years.[57] The postcoital examination first received prominence in the late 1800s in the writings of J. Marion Sims who was primarily interested in how long sperm survived in the mucus. Sim's son, Harry, reported to the American Gynecological Society in 1888 the details and purpose of the postcoital test, essentially as still performed today. The major impetus to general clinical use can be attributed to a book published in 1913 by Max Hühner, entitled *Sterility in the Male and Female*. Hühner, born in Berlin and a graduate of the College of Physicians and Surgeons of Columbia University, was a urologist in New York City. His second book, *A Practical Treatise on Disorders of the Sexual Function in the Male and Female*, was published in 1916 and went through 3 editions and a Spanish translation; this was followed by a third book in 1937. Thus, the postcoital test is also known as the Sims-Hühner test.

The place of the postcoital test in the infertility investigation has recently been called into question. There has always been an undercurrent of discontent concerning standardization of the test, its interpretation, and most importantly, its prognostic significance. Griffith and Grimes reviewed the literature pertaining to the postcoital test and concluded that the sensitivity (the ability of the test to detect infertility) ranged from 0.09 to 0.71 (a value of 1.00 would represent the ability to detect all cases).[58] The specificity (ability to identify fertility) ranged from 0.62 to 1.00 indicating that the test identified anywhere from 62% to 100% of fertile couples. They emphasized that the postcoital test suffers from poor validity, a lack of standard methodology, and confusion over the definition of normality. Others could find no difference in the subsequent pregnancy rates among groups having no sperm, no motile sperm, 1–5 motile sperm, 6–10 motile sperm, and 11 or more motile sperm.[54] Another study indicated that there was a statistically significant increase in the percentage of pregnancies only when there were more than 20 sperm/HPF.[53] Moreover, in a study of postcoital tests in *fertile* couples, 20% had either no sperm or less than one sperm/HPF.[59] Asch aspirated the cul-de-sac 8–36 hours after intercourse and found that of 8 women with a negative postcoital test, 6 had sperm in the peritoneal fluid.[60] Thus, the postcoital test would have led to the erroneous conclusion that sperm had not entered the female reproductive tract.

A newer argument raised against use of the postcoital test is that widespread use of intrauterine inseminations (IUI) combined with superovulation has made the assessment of sperm-cervical mucus interactions merely an academic exercise. In this view, whether the postcoital test is normal or abnormal, the treatment is the same. An important underlying assumption is that combined IUI and superovulation is, in fact, effective therapy (see Chapters 29 and 30). Support for this as yet unproven premise may be forthcoming from the results of a prospective controlled trial now in progress.

Given the array of negative assessments of the postcoital test, what can be said in its defense beyond that it provides an opportunity to observe interactions of sperm and a product of the female reproductive tract. If the mucus is clear and abundant with good spinnbarkeit, the patient has a better chance for pregnancy than if it is thick and sparse. If sperm are found in the mucus, it is reasonable assurance that coital technique is adequate. Additional reassurance is provided by the finding of motile sperm in the postcoital test. If live sperm are found in the cervical mucus, the pH is not hostile and the pregnancy rate is higher than if the sperm are all immotile. If there are more than 20 sperm/HPF, the male, in all likelihood, has a sperm count above 20 million/mL, and the couple has a significantly better chance for pregnancy than if the postcoital test contains fewer than 20 sperm/HPF. A poor result in the postcoital test can raise a suspicion of an immunologic problem. A poor result also can suggest the need for intrauterine inseminations. Individuals with progressively motile sperm in the postcoital test have significantly higher pregnancy rates.[61] In addition, sperm numbers in the postcoital test correlate with the length of time it takes to become pregnant. A postcoital test can guide treatment. *We believe that appropriate therapy for a poor postcoital test is IUI without the need for ancillary superovulation.* This decreases the risk of multiple births and hyperstimulation, and at a significantly lower expense.

What constitutes a poor postcoital test in terms of sperm numbers is controversial. Intrauterine insemination has been reported to enhance the chances for pregnancy when there were 3 or fewer sperm/HPF in the postcoital test but not when there were 5 or more sperm/HPF.[62] We continue to support a minimum level of one motile progressive sperm/HPF as compatible with normality. The finding of no sperm, all dead sperm or a large proportion of shaking sperm suggests a possible immunologic factor. These findings, specifically immotile or absent sperm, also should prompt inquiry concerning use of vaginal lubricants. Both Surgilube and KY Jelly can immobilize sperm and they should be avoided. If there are no motile sperm in the postcoital test, the pH of the mucus should be determined. Thus, whereas the usefulness of the postcoital test may be limited, it still has a place in the investigation of infertility.

The need for scheduling the postcoital test at precise times in the cycle may produce problems for the couple who cannot have sex on demand. This may further burden a couple already troubled by the need to cope with their infertility and the loss of control involved in the infertility investigation. A physician must be sympathetic to this problem, and on occasion, precise timing must be sacrificed and the woman told to come to the office following unscheduled intercourse.

Hysterosalpingography

A history of pelvic inflammatory disease, septic abortion, ruptured appendix, tubal surgery, or ectopic pregnancy alerts the physician to the possibility of tubal damage. Pelvic inflammatory disease is unquestionably the major contributor to tubal infertility and ectopic pregnancies. Westrom's classic studies with laparoscopically confirmed pelvic inflammatory disease indicated that the incidence of subsequent tubal infertility is approximately 12% after one episode of pelvic infection, 23% after two episodes, and 54% after three episodes.[63] The risk of ectopic pregnancy is increased 6–7-fold after pelvic infection. Almost one-half of patients who are eventually found to have tubal damage and/or pelvic adhesions, however, have no history of antecedent disease. Many of these women will have elevated anti-chlamydia antibodies, suggestive of prior infection. There have been a few reports of damaged tubes showing histologic evidence of viral infection which could explain the absence of traditional causes of tubal damage.

Tubal disease is diagnosed by the hysterosalpingogram (HSG) and by laparoscopy. The HSG is performed 2 to 5 days after cessation of a menstrual flow. If there is a history suggestive of pelvic inflammatory disease, a sedimentation rate is obtained prior to the HSG and, if elevated, antibiotic therapy is given. The procedure is than postponed for a month when a repeat sedimentation rate is obtained. Only if this is normal is the HSG scheduled. If masses or tenderness are revealed by the pelvic examination at any time, the HSG should be bypassed and the pelvis evaluated by laparoscopy. If there is a documented history of pelvic inflammatory disease, the risk of a serious reinfection following HSG is too high, and it should be replaced by laparoscopy. If an HSG is performed in a patient who is at questionable risk for infection, a water-soluble rather than an oil dye should be used because of the faster absorption. The overall risk of infection with HSG is probably less than 1%, although in a high-risk population serious infection can occur in approximately 3% of cases.[64] Clinically apparent infections were not present in 398 women who had nondilated tubes on HSG; however, 11% of those with dilated tubes developed pelvic inflammatory disease.[65] Doxycycline, 200 mg after the procedure, can be administered if the tubes are dilated, followed by 100 mg bid for 5 days. Many clinicians routinely administer prophylactic antibiotics (doxycycline, 100 mg bid for 5 days, beginning 2 days before the procedure).

HSG should be performed under image intensification fluoroscopy, and a minimal number of films taken. Too often, multiple oblique views are taken to delineate small filling defects in the uterus which are of no clinical significance. In our experience the oblique films are of little help even in diagnosing tubal patency. Only 3 films are usually required — a preliminary before dye is injected, a film showing spill of dye from one or both tubes, and a delayed film to show spread of dye through the peritoneal cavity. It is advantageous if the gynecologist does the actual injection of the dye, but in most instances this is now done by the radiologist. The dye can be injected either using a classic Jarcho cannula with a single-tooth tenaculum, or a suction apparatus appended to the cervix with dye injected through a contained cannula. A third technique involves threading a pediatric Foley catheter through the cervix into the uterus. This is a relatively atraumatic method. The balloon on the catheter does, however, obscure portions of the uterine cavity and both myomas and polyps can be missed. Use of a prostaglandin synthesis inhibitor which can be purchased over the counter and taken 30 minutes prior to the procedure can decrease the pain which many women experience with HSG.

The dye should be injected slowly so that abnormalities of the uterine cavity are not missed. This is of special importance in diethylstilbestrol-exposed daughters, many of whom have abnormalities of uterine contour. Usually no more than 3 to 6 mL of dye are required to fill the uterus and tubes. If the patient complains of cramping, the injection of dye should be stopped for a few minutes and fluoroscopy temporarily discontinued. Spasm is rare with Ethiodol, an oil dye which is our preferred medium; if it does occur, slow injection with pauses is helpful. If the tubes fill but dye droplets do not spill from the ends of the tubes, the uterus should be pushed up in the abdomen by means of the tenaculum or suction cup. This puts the tubes on stretch and may help to release dye from the fimbriated ends. The droplets seen coming from the tube are the result of mixing of the oil dye and peritoneal fluid On occasion, injection of dye into a hydrosalpinx will produce a similar pattern, and a delayed film to show loculation of dye is crucial in differentiating this condition from normal spill where the dye is distributed throughout the pelvis. If dye does not pass into the tubes, changing the woman to a prone position will sometimes facilitate passage of dye.[66]

If dye goes through one tube rapidly and fails to enter the other tube, it usually means that the dye-containing tube presents the path of least resistance. In this situation, the nonfilling tube is usually normal. In our own series, when both tubes were patent on x-ray, the pregnancy rate was only slightly higher (58%) than when there was unilateral patency and nonfilling of the other tube (50%).[67]

While the diagnostic usefulness of the HSG is established, its value as a therapeutic procedure in infertility is a subject of some controversy. Does an HSG enhance fertility, and, if so, is the effect seen with both oil and water-soluble dyes? A conception rate of 41.3% within 1 year of an HSG with oil media has been reported, whereas the rate was only 27.3% when water-soluble agents were employed.[68] This is in accord with other reports where the great majority of pregnancies that followed HSG occurred within 7 months of the procedure. A review of the question of oil versus aqueous dye noted that in every retrospective study in which increased pregnancy rates were noted after HSG, an oil dye was used.[69]

In a randomized, prospective study of close to 400 women, the pregnancy and live birth rates were increased in women who had their HSG performed with oil dye. Within 9 ovulation cycles following an HSG, the pregnancy rate was 33% in the oil dye group and 17% in the water dye group.[70] Thus, HSG with Ethiodol is a very useful therapeutic as well as diagnostic tool in women with infertility.

How does the oil dye increase fertility?

1. It may effect a mechanical lavage of the tubes, dislodging mucus plugs.

2. It may straighten the tubes and thus break down peritoneal adhesions.

3. It may provide a stimulatory effect for the cilia of the tube.

4. It may improve the cervical mucus.

5. The iodine may exert a bacteriostatic effect on the mucous membranes.

6. Ethiodol decreases in vitro phagocytosis by peritoneal macrophages. If the same effect occurs in vivo it could decrease macrophage activity and thus aid fertility by inhibiting the release of cytokines and decreasing phagocytosis of sperm.[71,72]

The use of an oil medium has been criticized on grounds that it is only slowly absorbed and may cause granuloma formation. Granulomas are found very infrequently, and they also may follow the use of water dyes. An additional fear with oil dye is embolization. However, only 13 cases of dye intravasation were encountered in 533 HSGs performed with Ethiodol.[73] Six of these women had embolization of the dye but there were no symptoms and no morbidity was noted. When fluoroscopy is used, venous or lymphatic intravasation can be detected immediately and injection of dye halted.

Hysteroscopy

Hysteroscopy is a technique which complements hysterosalpingography. The hysteroscope is good for differentiating between endometrial polyps and submucous leiomyomas, establishing the definitive diagnosis and treatment of intrauterine adhesions, and for the diagnosis and treatment of intrauterine congenital anomalies. One can argue from a cost-effective point of view that hysterosalpingography is the more useful screening procedure, and the hysteroscope should be reserved to pursue abnormalities identified on the hysterogram.

Falloposcopy

Because of its narrow and tortuous character, it has been difficult to pass probes via the uterine cavity into the fallopian tube. This problem has been overcome by the development of self-seeking guidewires and the adaptation of techniques used for coronary angioplasty. Hysteroscopic directed falloposcopy can be utilized to transvaginally examine the entire length of the tubal lumen.[74] This technique requires considerable expertise, but it has already verifed that the tubal ostium can undergo spasm, and intraluminal debris is present that can be a cause of tubal obstruction (and treated by cannulation or balloon tuboplasty, or even be cleared by hysterosalpingography). This is a technique that can more precisely select patients who are good candidates for tubal surgery.

Outpatient Canalization of the Tube

Proximal tubal obstruction can be treated by outpatient tubal cannulation or balloon tuboplasty. Transcervical tuboplasty can be performed by either a fluoroscopic or hysteroscopic approach, although most of the experience thus far is with the fluoroscopic technique.[75-77] The level of discomfort is similar to that with hysterosalpingography; intravenous sedation and a paracervical block are usually sufficient. Cannulation and balloon tuboplasty success is achieved in at least one tube in 80–90% of attempts, Approximately 30% of patients will become pregnant in the 3–6 months following the procedure. Further technical developments may eventually allow canalization of the tube to be performed in the office, e.g., with ultrasonography. The advantage of these accomplishments is the avoidance of general anesthesia, surgery, and expensive hospitalization. Eventually, treatment of proximal tubal obstruction will immediately follow diagnosis.

Disorders of Ovulation

Disorders of ovulation account for approximately 15% of all infertility problems in couples. These may be anovulation or severe oligoovulation. In the latter cases, even though ovulation does occur, its relative infrequency decreases the woman's chances for pregnancy. If periods occur only every 3 or 4 months, for practical purposes it matters little whether these are ovulatory or anovulatory. Anovulatory or oligoovulatory women should be promptly treated with clomiphene citrate to increase the frequency of, or to initiate, ovulation (see Chapter 30), and the drug can be started immediately, even before other areas have been investigated. If anovulation is the only infertility factor, most couples will become pregnant within 3 months of ovulation induction. Women with amenorrhea or hyperandrogenic anovulation should be evaluated and managed according to the clinical approaches detailed in Chapters 12, 13, and 14.

Basal Body Temperature

Women who have menstrual periods at monthly intervals marked by premenstrual symptoms and dysmenorrhea are almost always ovulatory, but not always; 5% are anovulatory. Indirect confirmatory evidence of ovulation should be obtained by use of basal body temperature (BBT) charts. The temperature can be taken orally with a regular thermometer or with special instruments (unnecessarily expensive however) that show a range of only a few degrees and thus are easier to read. It is worth emphasizing that the temperature is best taken immediately upon awakening and before any activity. The woman may be surprised to find that the basal temperatures are substantially lower than the usual 98.6° F (37° C). Days when intercourse takes place should be noted on the chart, and this may give the physician an indication that coital frequency is a problem.

Use of the BBT chart has been criticized because a small percentage of women who ovulate have monophasic graphs, and there is often disagreement among physicians concerning interpretation of individual charts. Moreover, the time of ovulation predicted by the BBT does not always correlate well with measurements of the LH surge or with perceptions of maximal cervical mucus production. There is a relationship between a nadir in the BBT and the LH surge, but the BBT is reliable in predicting the day of the LH surge only within 2–3 days.[78] Although the nadir is believed to represent the beginning of the LH surge, the occurrence of a nadir is variable and often is not detected. To be used prospectively to predict ovulation, nearly absolute cycle regularity is required.

Nevertheless, we still find the BBT helpful as a preliminary indicator of ovulation and as a tool for examining with patients the timing of intercourse. Patients should not become fixated on taking their temperatures, and usually one or two months of charts are sufficient.

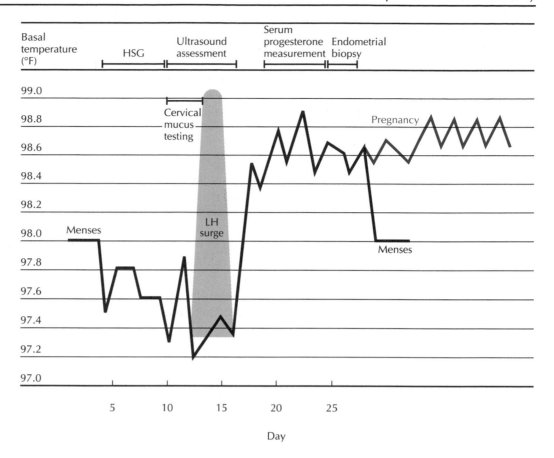

A significant increase in temperature is not noted until 2 days after the LH peak, coinciding with a rise in peripheral levels of progesterone to greater than 4 ng/mL.[79] Physical release of the ovum probably occurs on the day prior to the time of the first temperature elevation. The temperature rise should be sustained for 11 to 16 days, and it will then drop at the time of the subsequent menstrual period.

If an approximate time of ovulation can be determined by temperature charts, a sensible schedule for coitus is every 36 to 48 hours in a period encompassed by 3 to 4 days prior to and 2 days after expected ovulation. It is unwise, however, to demand rigid adherence to a schedule. This may produce psychologic stress sufficient to inhibit sexual relations. In discussing coital timing, the patient will usually want to know the fertilizable life of the sperm and the egg. The information on human gametes is speculative. Cases have been reported in which isolated coitus even up to 7 days prior to the rise in basal body temperature has resulted in pregnancy, but this probably represents the limits of biologic variation. It is estimated that sperm retain their ability to fertilize for 24 to 48 hours and that the human egg is fertilizable for 12 to 24 hours. However, immature human eggs aspirated from follicles for in vitro fertilization can be fertilized after incubation in vitro for even as long as 36 hours.

Home urinary LH testing is commonly used to assist diagnostic and therapeutic timing. The postcoital test should be performed within 12 hours of a positive urinary LH test.[80] However, appropriate use of the basal body temperature chart yields results equivalent to those obtained with the more expensive methods of urinary LH assays.[81]

Endometrial Biopsy

A reliable assessment of ovulation can be obtained by endometrial biopsy. Endometrial biopsy is performed 2 to 3 days prior to the expected period (although some feel that biopsy done in the midluteal phase is superior for diagnosing luteal phase defects), and the histology is read by the criteria outlined by Noyes, Hertig, and Rock.[82] Although premenstrual biopsy could interrupt a pregnancy if performed in a conception cycle, the danger is not great.[83] An alternative, taking the biopsy on the first day of menses, has three disadvantages:

1. Inconvenient time for patient and physician.

2. The tissue is disrupted and often more difficult to interpret.

3. A slight amount of bleeding can occur at the time of the expected period even if the patient is pregnant.

We recommend the use of the plastic endometrial suction curette. It is easy to use, requires no cervical dilation (3 mm diameter), and is usually painless.

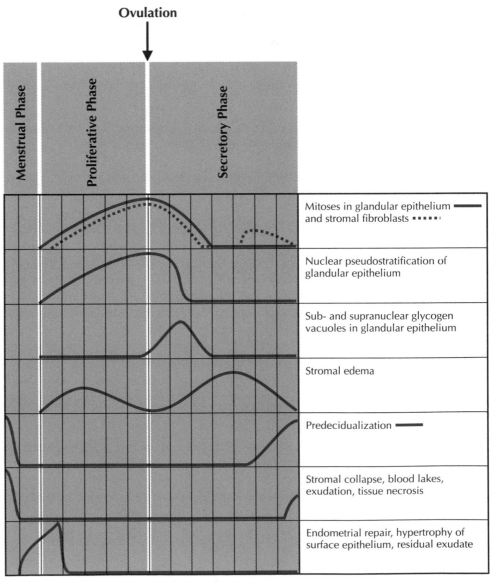

After Noyes, et al [82]

Progesterone Measurements

A serum progesterone level of less than 3 ng/mL (10 nmol/L) is consistent with follicular phase levels.[84] To confirm ovulation, values at the midluteal phase, just at the midpoint between ovulation and the onset of the subsequent menstrual period, should be at least 6.5 ng/mL (21 nmol/L) and preferably 10 ng/mL (32 nmol/L) or more. The consensus of opinion is that a single midluteal phase progesterone level is *insufficient* evidence upon which to judge the adequacy of the luteal phase.[85–90] The progesterone level is subject to the variation associated with pulsatile secretion, but more importantly, there is often poor correlation with the histologic state of the endometrium.

Luteal Phase Defect (Inadequate Luteal Phase)

A luteal phase defect, defined as a lag of more than two days in histologic development of the endometrium compared to day of the cycle (presumably due to inadequate progesterone secretion or action), can be found in up to 30% of isolated cycles of normal women, and only if the defect is found in 2 cycles is it thought to be a possible factor in infertility. Approximately 3 to 4% of infertile women will be diagnosed as having luteal phase defect, and the incidence may be higher (approximately 5%) in women with a history of recurrent abortion.[91]

Although luteal phase defect is often a direct result of decreased hormone production by the corpus luteum, the underlying causes of this dysfunction can be multiple. Decreased levels of FSH in the follicular phase of the cycle, abnormal patterns of LH secretion, decreased levels of LH and FSH at the time of the ovulatory surge, or decreased response of the endometrium to progesterone have been implicated.[89] Elevated prolactin levels also may be associated with luteal phase defect. The preponderance of evidence supports a preovulatory cause. Nuclear progesterone receptor concentrations are normal in luteal phase endometrial samples from women with luteal phase defect, but the concentration is reduced during the proliferative phase (suggesting an alteration, such as lesser estrogen stimulation, during the proliferative phase).[92]

The diagnosis should be considered in women with normal cycles and unexplained infertility, women with short luteal phases demonstrated by basal body temperature charts, and women with a history of recurrent spontaneous abortion. Women taking clomiphene citrate for ovulation induction also are at risk.

In the past, the controversies surrounding the concept of luteal phase defect have revolved around issues of diagnosis, endometrial biopsy versus progesterone levels, and treatment, progesterone versus clomiphene citrate. While space in journals and much time in postgraduate courses are devoted to these questions, a fundamental concern must be addressed. Is there really such an entity as luteal phase defect, and even if there is, does it play any role in infertility?

As noted above, although measuring progesterone levels has been advocated as a means of diagnosing luteal phase defect, the majority of clinical studies on this subject have used endometrial biopsy as the gold standard. The endometrium must lag behind the day of the cycle by greater than two days, and the lag must occur in more than one cycle. Whereas it has been common to date the cycle day from the onset of the subsequent menstrual period, there is evidence that better dating can be achieved by counting forward from the LH surge.[93,94]

An important issue is how well can the physician, usually a pathologist, date the endometrium. When the same observer viewed 63 endometrial biopsies on two separate occasions, there was exact agreement in only 15 (24%).[95] Disagreement of more than two days in the dating of the endometrium occurred in six instances (10%). A further problem in establishing luteal phase defect as a clinical entity is the finding in most studies of an out-of-phase biopsy in approximately 20% to 30% of normal cycles and repetitive lags in more than one normal cycle of approximately 5%.[94,96] These figures suggest that luteal phase defect occurs by chance alone.

The frequency of luteal phase defect in women with infertility, when strictly defined, is no greater than that found by chance in normal cycles.[96] In a series of 1,492 biopsies in 1,055 women reported by Balasch, there were 26 biopsies in conception cycles.[97] With an in-phase biopsy, 15 of 20 pregnancies went to term but 4 out of 6 pregnancies with out-of-phase biopsies also went to term. Similarly, the term pregnancy rates were almost identical in women treated and untreated for luteal phase defect. There is a window of endometrial development during which successful embryo transfer in in vitro fertilization can occur.[98] The window extends over a 6-day period, and this indicates that precise synchronization of the endometrium and the embryo may not be needed for successful implantation.

Given the uncertainties surrounding the diagnosis of luteal phase defect in unexplained infertility, it becomes difficult to justify putting women through the expense and possible pain of endometrial biopsy. However, Downs and Gibson made the interesting observation that there may be degrees of luteal phase defect.[99] In a group with a lag on biopsy of 5 days or more, treatment with clomiphene citrate yielded a conception rate of 79%. In contrast, in those with a less severe defect, clomiphene citrate therapy was associated with a rate of only 8.9%. Thus, with a redefinition of what constitutes luteal phase defect, it may prove useful to make the diagnosis.

In common practice, again because of the discomfort and expense associated with endometrial biopsy, attention has turned to measurements of serum progesterone levels as a means of diagnosing, if not luteal phase defect, then at least a "hormone deficiency." Whereas exact normal values for progesterone are in some dispute, many physicians believe that a level of less than 10 to 12 ng/mL one week prior to the onset of menstruation is a good indication of a luteal phase defect. Frequently a diagnosis of "hormone deficiency" is made based on an isolated and not always well-timed progesterone level of less than 10 ng/mL (32 nmol/L). It is also common practice to utilize such a finding as a rationale for treating as if a luteal phase defect were present. Daily progesterone measurements taken throughout the luteal phase could provide strong evidence for luteal phase defect if the values are low, but such frequent sampling is impractical. Most important, however, is the impressive evidence documenting a lack of correlation between progesterone measurements and endometrial histology.[85–90]

Treatment of Luteal Phase Defect

Based on findings that low FSH values prior to ovulation can be associated with luteal phase defect, it would seem reasonable, in selected cases, to use human menopausal gonadotropins or clomiphene citrate. Gonadotroopin treatment has the potential for causing hyperstimulation of the ovaries, and it creates an increased risk of multiple births. Because of these effects, gonadotropin treatment is seldom used for this indication. Clomiphene citrate is the first choice of many physicians for the treatment of luteal phase defect. The only significant risk is a 5% (twice normal) chance of multiple births, essentially all twins. The initial dose is 50 mg a day for 5 days starting on day 3, 4, or 5 of the cycle (Chapter 30).

Because there is a suspected deficiency of progesterone in luteal phase defect exogenous progesterone has been utilized. A vaginal suppository containing 25 mg of progesterone is inserted twice a day starting approximately 3 days after ovulation. Treatment is maintained until menstruation occurs or until a pregnancy is diagnosed. If the latter, a switch is made to weekly injections of 17-hydroxyprogesterone caproate (250 mg) through the 10th week of pregnancy. Using this therapy, success rates of approximately 50% have been achieved, but good control studies are lacking.

There is no difference in pregnancy rates in studies comparing clomiphene and progesterone treatment.[100,101] In our view, this is an argument in favor of clomiphene because of a significant disadvantage associated with progesterone therapy. Progesterone supplementation prolongs the luteal phase and can delay the onset of menses. This is not a problem for the physician, but for the couple the disappointment at the time of delayed menses or a negative pregnancy test is even more profound.

Dopamine agonist treatment has been reported to correct luteal phase defect associated with hyperprolactinemia, but its value in women with normal prolactin levels has not been demonstrated. In a subgroup of patients with unexplained infertility, high normal prolactin levels, and expressible galactorrhea, treatment with bromocriptine enhanced fertility compared to similar women treated with pyridoxine.[102] If galactorrhea is present, even if the prolactin is normal, ovulatory dysfunction responds well to dopamine agonist therapy.[103] In the absence of galactorrhea, a prolactin elevation may be subtle (such as an increase in nocturnal peaks), and this could explain occasional good responses to dopamine agonist treatment. In evaluating any therapy it is important to keep in mind that pregnancies can occur without treatment in women who are diagnosed as having luteal phase defect.

Many physicians short circuit the diagnostic evaluation of hormone adequacy and automatically proceed to treatment of unexplained infertility with clomiphene citrate. They argue that there may be subtle hormonal abnormalities that cannot be diagnosed with current technology but which can be successfully treated by stimulating the ovaries. Moreover, there is a theoretical advantage in having more than one oocyte in the fallopian tube at the time of fertilization. Randomized placebo-controlled studies seem to support the efficacy of this approach (reviewed with references in Chapter 30). By contrast, some have not found a benefit for the use of clomiphene citrate in unexplained infertility.[104]

The attraction of clomiphene citrate for patients is most often based on three factors:

1. The anecdotal experience of friends.

2. The desire to have some treatment, especially since clomiphene citrate is known as the fertility pill.

3. The hypothetical advantages of ovulating more than one oocyte and increasing luteal phase progesterone levels.

The drawbacks to clomiphene citrate use are the risk of multiple births, occasional hot flushes, and sometimes severe mood changes that some women experience. The most concerning side effects are visual changes which occur only rarely (and are always reversible) and usually with doses of 150 mg or higher. We do not object to the use of clomiphene, provided there is a clear understanding of the potential side effects and the uncertain efficacy of the medication.

Mycoplasma

Mycoplasma, a pleuropneumonia-like organism, has been implicated as a possible cause of recurrent abortion and salpingitis. A markedly higher prevalence of T mycoplasma (now called *ureaplasma urealyticum*) has been detected in cervical mucus and semen of infertile couples compared with a group of fertile women and men.[105] Treatment with doxycycline decreased the number of couples with mycoplasma and also was associated with pregnancy in 15 of 52 couples (29%), all of whom had had primary infertility of at least 5 years duration. However, a series of reports from England agreed with these findings in only one respect.[106,107] They confirmed that treatment with doxycycline could eliminate mycoplasma from the genital tract of the majority of individuals. There was no difference, however, in the frequency of either T strain or *Mycoplasma hominis* between infertile and fertile couples. In a double-blind study, treatment with doxycycline for 28 days had no effect on the rate of conception, and the English group suggested that culturing for mycoplasma in the routine investigation of infertility was unrewarding.

Since those early publications, a number of studies have established the widespread distribution of *ureaplasma urealyticum* in both fertile and infertile populations. Some have found higher colonization in infertile couples, whereas others have found no relationship between the organisms and infertility. In a study that received a great deal of media attention, it was reported that 60% of males who were culture positive for *ureaplasma urealyticum* and were cleared of infection by antibiotic treatment achieved a pregnancy.[108] Failure to clear the infection resulted in a 5% pregnant rate. This study suffers from lack of clarity on the criteria for entry into treatment and from any mention of individuals lost to follow-up. The incidence of ureaplasma infection is only significantly higher in those women whose male partners have semen abnormalities.[109]

It can be concluded that culturing for ureaplasma may be reasonable with male infertility but is not worthwhile in cases of unexplained infertility, and indiscriminate treatment with antibiotics is not warranted.

Endoscopy

Laparoscopy is the final diagnostic procedure of any infertility investigation. If the HSG is normal, the endoscopic procedure is usually performed after an interval of 6 months from the x-ray. This allows time for the fertility enhancing effect of the x-ray procedure. Because of the possible benefit from the HSG, we disagree with physicians who bypass it and go directly to laparoscopy. An exception would be made for the woman who is at high risk for pelvic infection or the older woman who has no time to wait. Obviously, if the HSG shows tubal occlusion or other major abnormalities, we do not hold to the 6 month delay. The findings at laparoscopy agree with those of HSG in approximately two-thirds of the cases. The major area of disagreement is the failure of the HSG to detect pelvic adhesions or endometriosis. Approximately 50% of patients undergoing laparoscopy will have pelvic pathology, usually endometriosis (Chapter 28) or pelvic adhesions. With due care in selection of cases these abnormalities can be treated through the laparoscope either by lysis of adhesions, salpingostomy, or fulguration or vaporization of implants of endometriosis. Patients with significant tubal disease are best advised to proceed to in vitro fertilization.

When findings at laparoscopy are combined with those of other test procedures, the majority of couples will have a discoverable cause for their inability to conceive. Still there will be a significant number of couples in whom no abnormality is found.

Laparoscopic Treatment of Distal Tubal Pathology[110]

Lysis of adhesions	50% pregnancy rate
Distal tubal obstruction:	
Mild disease	80% pregnancy rate
Moderate disease	30% pregnancy rate
Severe disease	15% pregnancy rate

Unexplained Infertility

An infertile couple has what is called unexplained infertility when all standard clinical investigations (semen analysis, the postcoital test, assessment of ovulation, demonstration of tubal patency) yield normal results. It is estimated that from 10% to 15% of infertile couples will ultimately reach this clinical diagnosis, and, using normal findings on laparoscopy as a criterion, the prevalence may be less than 10%.[111] Important variables are age of the woman and duration of the infertility.[42]

The average monthly fecundity in normal couples is 25%; the monthly pregnancy rate in couples with unexplained infertility is 1.5–3%. After 3 years of infertility, the prospect of pregnancy decreases by 24% each year.[111] Approximately 60% of couples with unexplained infertility of less than 3 years duration will become pregnant with 3 years of *expectant* management.[112,113] Because the incidence of spontaneous pregnancy is significant until 3 years have passed, it is appropriate to require 3 years of infertility in women less than 35 years old before making this diagnosis. Further evaluation and therapy should not be deferred in older women.

A meticulous review of available results is essential to avoid overlooking a treatable factor. The use of sperm function tests can be helpful. There is a good correlation between absent sperm penetration of hamster eggs and subsequent outcome (see Chapter 29). If these tests are not available, keep in mind that a definite diagnosis of unexplained infertility requires successful fertilization in vitro. Thus, a human egg test (in vitro fertilization) is worth doing.

Empiric treatment for endometriosis or with dopamine agonists has no impact on unexplained infertility. However, the methods of assisted reproductive technology and superovulation with intrauterine insemination do increase the prospect of pregnancy (superovulation is probably the key factor and not intrauterine insemination[114]). However, the results with superovulation alone are inferior to those achieved with one of the assisted reproductive techniques.[115] The lower fertilization rate using in vitro fertilization, but a normal conception rate following embryo transfer, indicates that at least one subgroup of women with unexplained infertility has impaired oocytes.[116]

A cumulative pregnancy rate of 40% can be achieved after 6 cycles of superovulation or 3 cycles of in vitro fertilization.[117] In randomized, controlled clinical trials, the monthly pregnancy rates in couples with unexplained infertility is increased 3-fold (a monthly fecundity rate of 9%) with clomiphene treatment, and with human menopausal gonadotropins, the monthly fecundity rate is approximately 10–15%.[118–120] *Therefore couples with unexplained infertility should be offered superovulation or one of the assisted reproductive technologies.*

Luteinized Unruptured Follicle

On occasion, a corpus luteum will form despite the failure of release of the oocyte. Initially it was thought that this problem could be identified at laparoscopy by noting an absence of the ovulatory stigma, but now it is apparent that the stigma can be epithelialized rapidly and thus obscured from view.[121] Currently, clinical diagnosis of a luteinized unruptured follicle (LUF) is made on the basis of ultrasound monitoring. The preovulatory growth of the follicle usually is normal but the follicle does not collapse following the LH surge, and there may be increased growth in the luteal phase. The interior of the follicle lacks the echoes often seen in corpora lutea. Whereas these criteria seem straightforward, establishing the diagnosis of LUF is often difficult. Even if ultrasonography is performed daily, the collapse of the follicle can be missed, and a corpus luteum refilled with blood can be mistaken for a persistent follicle. Therefore, routine ultrasound screening of women with unexplained infertility is of questionable value. It is doubtful that LUF is a significant cause of infertility, and furthermore, the only treatment worth considering is superovulation or one of the assisted reproductive technologies, treatment choices that will be empirically offered anyway. Because inhibition of prostaglandin synthesis can cause a luteinized unruptured follicle, patients should be cautioned to avoid the use of nonsteroidal anti-inflammatory agents.

When Should Adoption Be Advised?

With proper evaluation and therapy, the majority of couples attending an infertility clinic will become pregnant. Of those who do not achieve a pregnancy, the individuals most in need of counseling are those with unexplained infertility. Despite the absence of pathology, couples with 3 or more years of infertility have a poor prognosis and for these patients, as well as those who have exhausted their treatment options, the physician should encourage consideration of either assisted reproductive technology or adoption.

People who turn to the social agencies involved with adoption may be accorded a bleak picture of their prospects for adoption. This can compound the depression that the individuals may already feel from their inability to conceive. An alternative is private adoption, which can provide babies more rapidly, at reasonable cost, and without resort to foreign countries. In private adoption a fee should not be paid to the biologic mother for giving up the baby. In most cases the biologic mother will know who adopted the child and this lack of anonymity may direct some couples away from private adoption. In addition, there is a short time period during which the biologic mother can reclaim the baby. In our experience this devastating event occurs in approximately 5% of private adoptions.

Patients should be encouraged to "spread the word" that they are interested in adoption. In addition, letters can be directed to obstetricians throughout the country describing the couple and their desires for adoption. Consultation with a lawyer is necessary to obtain information concerning the adoption laws in the individual states because a number of states do not allow private adoption. An excellent review of private adoption, including the legal aspects, can be found in Friedman and Gradstein's book, *Surviving Pregnancy Loss,* and another superb resource is the book, *Beating the Adoption Game,* by Martin.[122,123]

Myths and Appropriate Goals

It is important for physicians and other health care professionals to dispel the myths that are associated with infertility. Women should not be told that they are infertile because they are too nervous. Unless anxiety interferes with ovulation or coital frequency, there is no present evidence that infertility is caused by the usual anxieties besetting a couple attempting to conceive. Despite many anecdotes to the contrary, adoption does not increase a couple's fertility.[124] The treatment of euthyroid infertile women with thyroid has been shown repeatedly to be worthless. A dilatation and curettage (D and C) is not a legitimate part of a routine infertility investigation. It provides minimal information beyond that obtained by endometrial biopsy and is both expensive and potentially hazardous because it subjects the woman to the risk of general anesthesia. There is also no evidence to support the old belief that a woman becomes more fertile following D and C. Quite the contrary, one study indicates a decreased fertility potential for those women undergoing D and C.[125]

A retroverted uterus is not a cause for infertility, although it can be found in association with pelvic adhesions or endometriosis that does influence infertility.

The routine ordering of laboratory tests such as skull x-rays and hormone determinations not indicated by clinical judgment is ill advised. These may be of value in selected cases but certainly not in every case.

Be aware that a substantial number of pregnancies occur in infertile couples without treatment, irrespective of the diagnosis.[42] Thus, the physician should not feel obligated to render a treatment just to do something. The goals of the practitioner should be to accomplish a thorough investigation, to treat any abnormalities that are uncovered, to educate the couple in the workings of the reproductive system, to give the couple some estimate of their fertility potential, to counsel for adoption where appropriate, and to provide emotional support. If these goals are achieved by a sympathetic, understanding physician, they will satisfy most couples who suffer from infertility.

References

1. **Mosher WD, Pratt WF,** Fecundity and infertility in the United States: incidence and trends, Fertil Steril 56:192, 1991.

2. **Westoff CF,** Fertility in the United States, Science, 234:554, 1986.

3. **Spencer G,** Projections of the population of the United States by age, sex, and race: 1983–2080, Current population reports — Population estimates and projections, U.S. Department of Commerce, May, 1984, Series P-25, No. 952.

4. **Mosher WD, Pratt WF,** The demography of infertility in the United States, in Asch RH, Studd JW, editors, *Annual Progress in Reproductive Medicine,* Parthenon Publishing Group, Pearl River, New York, 1993, pp 37–43.

5. **Greenhill E, Vessey M,** The prevalence of subfertility: a review of the current confusion and a report of two new studies, Fertil Steril 54:978, 1990.

6. **Wilcox LS, Mosher WD,** Use of infertility services in the United States, Obstet Gynecol 82:122, 1993.

7. **Warburton D, Kline J, Stein Z, Strobino B**, Cytogenetic abnormalities in spontaneous abortions of recognized conceptions, in Porter IH, editor, *Perinatal Genetics: Diagnosis and Treatment*, Academic Press, New York, 1986, p 133.

8. **Tietze C**, Reproductive span and rate of reproduction among Hutterite women, Fertil Steril 8:89, 1957.

9. **Robinson WC**, Another look at the Hutterites and natural fertility, Soc Biol 33:65, 1986.

10. **Federation CECOS, Schwartz D, Mayaux JM,** Female fecundity as a function of age: results of artificial insemination in 2193 nulliparous women with azoospermic husbands, New Engl J Med 306:404, 1982.

11. **Virro MS, Shewchuk AB,** Pregnancy outcome in 242 conceptions after artificial insemination with donor sperm and effects of maternal age on the prognosis for successful pregnancy, Am J Obstet Gynecol 148:518, 1984.

12. **van Noord-Zaadstra BM, Looman CW, Alsbach H, Habbena JDF, te Velde ER, Karbaat J,** Delaying child-bearing: effect of age on fecundity and outcome of pregnancy, Br Med J 302:1361, 1991.

13. **Meldrum DR,** Female reproductive aging — ovarian and uterine factors, Fertil Steril 59:1, 1993.

14. **Wood C, Calderon I, Crombie A,** Age and fertility: results of assisted reproductive technology in women over 40 years, J Assist Reprod Genetics 9:482, 1992.

15. **Kennedy WJ,** Edinburgh Med J, 27:1086, 1882.

16. **Warburton D,** Reproductive loss: how much is preventable? New Engl J Med 316:158, 1987.

17. **Wilcox AJ, Weibereg CR, O'Connor JF, Baird DD, Schlatterer JP, Canfield RE, Armstrong EG, Nisula BC,** Incidence of early loss of pregnancy, New Engl J Med 319:189, 1988.

18. **Seymour FI, Duffy C, Koerner A,** A case of authenticated fertility in a man of 94, JAMA 105:423, 1935.

19. **Stene J, Fischer G, Stene B, Mikhelson M, Petersen E,** Paternal age effect in Down's syndrome, Ann Hum Genet 40:299, 1977.

20. **Buehler JW, Kaunitz AM, Hogue CJR, Hughes JM, Smith JC, Rochate RW,** Maternal mortality in women aged 35 years and older: United States, JAMA 255:53, 1986.

21. **Cnattingius S, Forman MR, Berendes HW, Isotalo L,** Delayed childbearing and risk of adverse perinatal outcome, JAMA 268:886, 1992.

22. **Spellacy WN, Miller SL, Winegar A,** Pregnancy after 40 years of age, Obstet Gynecol 68:452, 1986.

23. **Berkowitz GS, Skovron MD, Lapinsmki RH, Berkowitz RL,** Delayed childbearing and the outcome of pregnancy, New Engl J Med 322:659, 1990.

24. **Faddy MJ, Gosden RG, Gougeon A, Richardson SJ, Nelson JF,** Accelerated disappearance of ovarian follicles in mid-life: implications for forecasting menopause, Hum Reprod 7:1342, 1992.

25. **Metcalf M, Livesey J,** Gonadotropin excretion in fertile women: effect of age and the onset of the menopausal transition, J Endocrinol 105:357, 1985.

26. **Lenton EA, Landgren B, Sexton L, Harper R,** Normal variation in the length of the follicular phase of the menstrual cycle: effect of chronological age, Br J Obstet Gynaecol 91:681, 1984.

27. **Lee SJ, Lenton EA, Sexton L, Cooke ID,** The effect of age on the cyclical patterns of plasma LH, FSH, oestradiol and progesterone in women with regular menstrual cycles, Hum Reprod 3:851, 1988.

28. **Musey VC, Collins DC, Musey PI, Saltzman-Martino D, Preedy JRK,** Age-related changes in the female hormonal environment during reproductive life, Am J Obstet Gynecol 157:312, 1987.

29. **Hughes EG, Robertson DM, Handelsman DJ, Hayward S, Healey DL, de Kretser DM,** Inhibin and estradiol responses to ovarian hyperstimulation: effects of age and predictive value for in vitro fertilization outcome, J Clin Endocrinol Metab 70:358, 1990.

30. **Buckler HM, Evans A, Mamlora H, Burger HG, Anderson DC,** Gonadotropin, steroid and inhibin levels in women with incipient ovarian failure during anovulatory and ovulatory 'rebound' cycles, J Clin Endocrinol Metab 72:116, 1991.

31. **Lenton EA, de Kretser DM, Woodward AJ, Robertson DM,** Inhibin concentrations throughout the menstrual cycles of normal, infertile, and older women compared with those during spontaneous conception cycles, J Clin Endocrinol Metab 73:1180, 1991.

32. **McNaughton J, Banah M, McCloud P, Hee J, Burger H,** Age related changes in follicle stimulating hormone, luteinizing hormone, oestradiol and immunoreactive inhibin in women of reproductive age, Clin Endocrinol 36:339, 1992.

33. **Toner JP, Philput CB, Jones GS, Muasher SJ,** Basal follicle-stimulating hormone level is a better predictor of in vitro fertilization performance than age, Fertil Steril 55:784, 1991.

34. **Pearlstone AC, Fournet N, Gambone JC, Pang SC, Buyalos RP,** Ovulation induction in women age 40 and older: the importance of basal follicle-stimulating hormone level and chronological age, Fertil Steril 58:674, 1992.

35. **Khalifa E, Toner JP, Muasher SJ, Acosta AA,** Significance of basal follicle-stimulating hormone levels in women with one ovary in a program of in vitro fertilization, Fertil Steril 57:835, 1992.

36. **Navot D, Drews MR, Bergh PA, Guzman I, Karstaedt A, Scott RT Jr, Garrisi GJ, Hofmann GE,** Age-related decline in female fertility is not due to diminished capacity of the uterus to sustain embryo implantation, Fertil Steril 61:97, 1994.

37. **Sauer MV, Paulson RJ, Lobo RA,** Reversing the natural decline in human fertility: an extended clinical trial of ooctye donation to women of advanced reproductive age, JAMA 268:1275, 1992.

38. **Sauer MV, Paulson RJ, Lobo RA,** Pregnancy after age 50: application of oocyte donation to women after natural menopause, Lancet 341:321, 1993.

39. **Abdalla HI, Burton G, Kirkland A, Johnson MR, Leonard T, Brooks AA, Studd JW,** Age, pregnancy and miscarriage: uterine versus ovarian factors, Hum Reprod 8:1512, 1993.

40. **Menken J, Trussell J, Larsen U,** Age and infertility, Science 233:1389, 1986.

41. **Barnea ER, Holford TR, McInnes DRA,** Long-term prognosis of infertile couples with normal basic investigations: a life-table analysis, Obstet Gynecol 66:24, 1985.

42. **Collins JA, Wrixon W, Janes LB, Wilson EH,** Treatment-independent pregnancy among infertile couples, New Engl J Med 309:1201, 1983.

43. **Stubblefield PG, Monson RR, Schoenbaum SC, Wolfson CE, Cookson DJ, Ryan KJ,** Fertility after induced abortion: a prospective follow-up study, Obstet Gynecol 63:186, 1984.

835

44. **Senekjian EK, Potkul RK, Frey K, Herbst A**, Infertility among daughters either exposed or not exposed to diethylstilbestrol, Am J Obstet Gynecol 184:493, 1988.

45. **Stillman RJ, Rosenberg MJ, Sachs BP**, Smoking and reproduction, Fertil Steril 46:545, 1986.

46. **Laurent SL, Thompson SJ, Addy C, Garrison CZ, Moore EE,** An epidemiologic study of smoking and primary infertility in women, Fertil Steril 57:565, 1992.

47. **Smith CG, Asch RH**, Drug abuse and reproduction, Fertil Steril 48:355, 1987.

48. **Bracken MB, Eskenazi B, Sachse K, McSharry J-E, Hellenbrand K, Leon-Summers L,** Association of cocaine use with sperm concentration, motility, and morphology, Fertil Steril 53:315, 1990.

49. **Joesoef MR, Beral V, Rolfs RT, Aral SO, Cramer DW,** Are caffeinated beverages risk factors for delayed conception? Lancet 335:136, 1990.

50. **Guttmacher AF**, Factors affecting normal expectancy of conception, JAMA 161:855, 1956.

51. **Drake TS, Tredway DR, Buchanan GC**, A reassessment of the fractional postcoital test, Am J Obstet Gynecol 133:382, 1979.

52. **Gibor Y, Garcia CJ, Cohen MR, Scommegna A**, The cyclical changes in the physical properties of the cervical mucus and the results of the postcoital test, Fertil Steril 21:20, 1970.

53. **Jette NT, Glass RH**, Prognostic value of the postcoital test, Fertil Steril 23:29, 1972.

54. **Collins JA, So Y, Wilson EH, Wrixon W, Casper RF**, The postcoital test as a predictor of pregnancy among 355 infertile couples, Fertil Steril 41:703, 1984.

55. **Bateman BG, Nunley WCJr, Kolp LA**, Exogenous estrogen therapy for the treatment of clomiphene citrate-induced cervical mucus abnormalities: is it effective? Fertil Steril 54:577, 1990.

56. **Ansari AH, Gould KG, Ansari VM**, Sodium bicarbonate douching for improvement of the postcoital test, Fertil Steril 33:608, 1980.

57. **Speert H,** *Obstetric and Gynecologic Milestones,* The Macmillan Company, New York, 1958, pp 271–276.

58. **Griffith CS, Grimes DA**, The validity of the postcoital test, Am J Obstet Gynecol 162:615, 1990.

59. **Kovacs GT, Newman GB, Henson GL**, The postcoital test: What is normal?, Br Med J 1:818, 1978.

60. **Asch RH**, Laparoscopic recovery of sperm from peritoneal fluid in patients with negative or poor Sims-Hühner test, Fertil Steril 27:1111, 1976.

61. **Hull MGR, Savage PE, Bromham DR**, Prognostic value of the postcoital test: prospective study based on time-specific conception rates, Br J Obstet Gynaecol 89:299, 1982.

62. **Quagliarello J, Arny M**, Intracervical versus intrauterine insemination: correlation of outcome with antecedent postcoital testing, Fertil Steril 46:870, 1986.

63. **Westrom L,** Incidence, prevalence, and trends of acute pelvic inflammatory disease and its consequences in industrialized countries, Am J Obstet Gynecol 138:880, 1980.

64. **Stumpf PG, March CM**, Febrile morbidity following hysterosalpingography: identification of risk factors and recommendations for prophylaxis, Fertil Steril 33:487, 1980.

65. **Pittaway DE, Winfield AC, Maxson W, Daniell J, Herbert C, Wentz AC**, Prevention of acute pelvic inflammatory disease after hysterosalpingography: efficacy of doxycycline prophylaxis, Am J Obstet Gynecol 147:623, 1983.

66. **Spring D**, Prone hysterosalpingography, Radiology 136:235, 1980.

67. **Mackey RA, Glass RH, Olson LE, Vaidya RA**, Pregnancy following hysterosalpingography with oil and water soluble dye, Fertil Steril 22:504, 1971.

68. **Gillespie HW**, The therapeutic aspect of hysterosalpingography, Br J Radiol 38:301, 1965.

69. **Soules MR, Spadoni LR**, Oil versus aqueous media for hysterosalpingography: a continuing debate based on many opinions and few facts, Fertil Steril 38:1, 1982.

70. **Rasmussen F, Lindequist S, Larsen C, Justesen P**, Therapeutic effect of hysterosalpingography: oil versus water soluble contrast media — a randomized prospective study, Radiology 179:75, 1991.

71. **Boyer P, Territo MC, de Ziegler D, Meldrum DR**, Ethiodol inhibits phagocytosis by pelvic peritoneal macrophages, Fertil Steril 46:715, 1986.

72. **Johnson JV, Montoya IA, Olive DL**, Ethiodol oil contrast medium inhibits macrophage phagocytosis and adherence by altering membrane electronegativity and microviscosity, Fertil Steril 58:511, 1992.

73. **Bateman BG, Nunley WC Jr, Kitchin JD**, Intravasation during hysterosalpingography using oilbase contrast media, Fertil Steril 34:439, 1980.

74. **Kerin JF, Williams DB, San Roman GA, Pearlstone AC, Grundfest WS, Surrey ES**, Falloposcopic classification and treatment of fallopian tube lumen disease, Fertil Steril 57:731, 1992.

75. **Novy MJ, Thurmond AS, Patton P, Uchida BT, Rosch J**, Diagnosis of cornual obstruction by transcervical fallopian tube cannulation, Fertil Steril 50:434, 1988.

76. **Thurmond AS, Rosch J**, Nonsurgical fallopian tube recanalization for treatment of infertility, Radiology 174:371, 1990.

77. **Confino E, Tur-Kaspa I, DeCherney AH, Corfman R, Coulam C, Robinson E, Haas G, Katz E, Vermesh M, Gleicher N**, Transcervical balloon tuboplasty: a multicenter trial, JAMA 264:2079, 1990.

78. **Quagliarello J, Arny M**, Inaccuracy of basal body temperature charts in predicting urinary luteinizing hormone surges, Fertil Steril 45:334, 1986.

79. **Luciano AA, Peluso J, Koch E, Maier D, Kuslis S, Davison E**, Temporal relationship and reliability of the clinical, hormonal, and ultrasonographic indices of ovulation in infertile women, Obstet Gynecol 75:412, 1990.

80. **Nulsen J, Wheeler C, Ausmanas M, Blasco L**, Cervical mucus changes in relationship to urinary luteinizing hormone, Fertil Steril 48:783, 1987.

81. **Corsan GH, Blotner MB, Bohrer MK, Sheldon R, Kemmann E**, The utility of a home urinary LH immunoassay in timing the postcoital test, Obstet Gynecol 81:736, 1993.

82. **Noyes RW, Hertig AT, Rock J**, Dating the endometrial biopsy, Fertil Steril 1:23, 1950.

83. **Wentz AC, Herbert CM III, Maxon WS, Hill GA, Pittaway DE**, Cycle of conception endometrial biopsy, Fertil Steril 46:196, 1986.

84. **Wathen NC, Perry L, Lilford RJ, Chard T**, Interpretation of single progesterone measurement in diagnosis of anovulation and defective luteal phase: observations on analysis of the normal range, Br Med J 288:7, 1984.

85. **Cooke ID, Morgan CA, Parry TE**, Correlation of endometrial biopsy and plasma progesterone levels in infertile women, J Obstet Gynaecol Br Comm 79:647, 1972.

86. **Shepard MK, Senturia YD**, Comparison of serum progesterone and endometrial biopsy for confirmation of ovulation and evaluation of luteal function, Fertil Steril 28:541, 1977.

87. **Rosenfeld DL, Chudow S, Bronson RA**, Diagnosis of luteal phase inadequacy, Obstet Gynecol 56:193, 1980.

88. **Cumming DC, Honore LH, Scott JZ, Williams KP**, The late luteal phase in infertile women: comparison of simultaneous endometrial biopsy and progesterone levels, Fertil Steril 43:715, 1985.

89. **Soules MR, McLachlan RI, Ek M, Dahl KD, Cohen, NL, Bremmer WJ,** Luteal phase deficiency: characterization of reproductive hormones over the menstrual cycle, J Clin Endocrinol Metab 69:804, 1989.

90. **Li T-C, Lenton EA, Dockery P, Rogers AW, Cooke ID,** The relation between daily salivary progesterone profile and endometrial development in the luteal phase of fertile and infertile women, Br J Obstet Gynaecol 96:445, 1989.

91. **Peters AJ, Lloyd RP, Coulam CP,** Prevalence of out-of-phase endometrial biopsy specimens, Am J Obstet Gynecol 166:1738, 1992.

92. **Jacobs MH, Balasch J, Gonzalez-Merlo JM, Vanrell JA, Wheeler C, Strauss JF III, Blasco L, Wheeler JE, Lyttle CR,** Endometrial cytosolic and nuclear progesterone receptors in the luteal phase defect, J Clin Endocrinol Metab 64:472, 1987.

93. **Shoupe D, Mishell DR Jr, Lacarra M, Lobo R, Horenstein J, d'Ablaing G, Moyer D,** Correlation of endometrial maturation with four methods of estimating day of ovulation, Obstet Gynecol 73:88, 1989.

94. **Batista MC, Cartledge TP, Merino MJ, Axiotis C, Platia MP, Merriam GR, Loriaux DL, Nieman LK,** Midluteal phase endometrial biopsy does not accurately predict luteal function, Fertil Steril 59:294, 1993.

95. **Li T-C, Dockery P, Rogers AW, Cooke ID,** How precise is histologic dating of endometrium using the standard dating criteria? Fertil Steril 51:759, 1989.

96. **Wentz AC, Kossoy L, Parker RA,** The impact of luteal phase inadequacy in an infertile population, Am J Obstet Gynecol 162:937, 1990.

97. **Balasch J, Fabreques F, Creus M, Vanrell JA,** The usefulness of endometrial biopsy for luteal phase evaluation in infertility, Hum Reprod 7:973, 1992.

98. **Navot D, Bergh PA, Williams M, Garrisi GJ, Guzman I, Sandler B, Fox J, Schreiner-Engel P, Hofmann GE, Grunfeld L,** An insight into early reproductive processes through the in vivo model of ovum donation, J Clin Endocrinol Metab 72:408, 1991.

99. **Downs KA, Gibson M,** Clomiphene citrate for luteal phase defect, Fertil Steril 39:34, 1983.

100. **Huang K-E,** The primary treatment of luteal phase inadequacy: progesterone versus clomiphene citrate, Am J Obstet Gynecol 155:824, 1986.

101. **Murray DL, Reich L, Adashi EY,** Oral clomiphene citrate and vaginal progesterone suppositories in the treatment of luteal phase dysfunction; a comparative study, Fertil Steril 51:35, 1989.

102. **DeVane GW, Guzick DS,** Bromocriptine therapy in normoprolactinemic women with unexplained infertility and galactorrhea, Fertil Steril 46:1026, 1986.

103. **Padilla SL, Person GK, McDonough PG, Reindollar RH,** The efficacy of bromocriptine in patients with ovulatory dysfunction and normoprolactinemic galactorrhea, Fertil Steril 44:695, 1985.

104. **Martinez AR, Bernardos RE, Voorhorst FJ, Vermeiden JPW, Schoemaker J,** Intrauterine insemination does and clomiphene citrate does not improve fecundity in couples with infertility due to male or idiopathic factors: a prospective, randomized, controlled study, Fertil Steril 53:847, 1990.

105. **Gnarpe H, Friberg J,** T-mycoplasmas as a possible cause for reproductive failure, Nature 242:120, 1973.

106. **de Louvois J, Blades M, Harrison RF, Hurley R, Stanley VC,** Frequency of mycoplasma in fertile and infertile couples, Lancet 1:1073, 1974.

107. **Harrison RF, de Louvois J, Blades M, Hurley R,** Doxycycline treatment and human infertility, Lancet 1:605, 1975.

108. **Toth A, Lesser ML, Brooks C, Labriola D,** Subsequent pregnancies among 161 couples treated for T-mycoplasma genital tract infection, New Engl J Med 308:505, 1983.

109. **Cassell GH, Younger JB, Brown MB, Blackwell RE, Davis JK, Marriott P, Stagno S,** Microbiologic study of infertile women at the time of diagnostic laparoscopy, New Engl J Med 308:502, 1983.

110. **Schlaff WD, Hassiakos DK, Damewood MD, Rock JA,** Neosalpingostomy for distal tubal obstruction: prognostic factors and impact of surgical technique, Fertil Steril 54:984, 1990.

111. **Crosignani PG, Collins J, Cooke ID, Duzfalusy E, Rubin B,** Unexplained infertility, Hum Reprod 8:977, 1993.

112. **Verkauf BS,** The incidence and outcome of single-factor, multifactorial and unexplained infertility, Am J Obstet Gynecol 147:175, 1983.

113. **Collins J, Rowe T,** Age of the female partner is a prognostic factor in prolonged unexplained infertility: a multicenter study, Fertil Steril 52:15, 1989.

114. **Kirby CA, Flaherty SP, Godfrey BM, Warnes GM, Matthews CD,** A prospective trial of intrauterine insemination of motile spermatozoa versus timed intercourse, Fertil Steril 56:102, 1991.

115. **Crosignani PG, Walters DS, Soliani A,** Addendum to the ESHRE multicentre trial: a summary of the abortion and birth statistics, Hum Reprod 7:286, 1992.

116. **Mackenna AI, Zegers-Hochschild F, Fernandez EO, Fabres CV, Huidobro CA, Prado JA, Roblero LS, Altieri EL, Guadarrama AR, Lopez TH,** Fertilization rate in couples with unexplained infertility, Hum Reprod 7:223, 1992.

117. **Simon A, Laufer N,** Unexplained infertility: a reappraisal, Assist Reprod Rev 3:26, 1993.

118. **Glazener CMA, Coulson C, Lambert PA, Watt EM, Hinton RA, Kelly NG, Hull MGR,** Clomiphene treatment for women with unexplained infertility: placebo-controlled study of hormonal responses and conception rates, Gynecol Endocrinol 4:75, 1990.

119. **Deaton JL, Gibson N, Blackmer KM, Nakajima ST, Badger GJ, Brumsted JR,** A randomized, controlled trial of clomiphene citrate and intrauterine insemination in couples with unexplained infertility, Fertil Steril 54:1083, 1990.

120. **Karlstrom P-O, Bergh T, Lundkvist O,** A prospective randomized trial of artificial insemination versus intercourse in cycles stimulated with human menopausal gonadotropin or clomiphene citrate, Fertil Steril 59:554, 1993.

121. **Dhont M, Serreyn R, Duvivier P, Vanluchene E, DeBoever J, Vandekerckhove D,** Ovulation stigma and concentration of progesterone and estradiol in peritoneal fluid: relation with fertility and endometriosis, Fertil Steril 41:872, 1984.

122. **Friedman R, Gradstein B,** *Surviving Pregnancy Loss*, Little, Brown and Co., Boston, 1992.

123. **Martin C,** *Beating the Adoption Game*. Harcourt Brace Jovanovich, New York, 1988.

124. **Lamb EJ, Leurgans S,** Does adoption affect subsequent fertility? Am J Obstet Gynecol 134:138, 1979.

125. **Taylor PJ, Graham G,** Is diagnostic curettage harmful in women with unexplained infertility? Br J Obstet Gynaecol 89:296, 1982.

27 Recurrent Early Pregnancy Losses

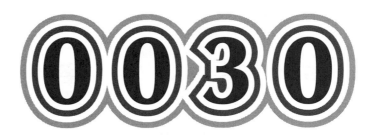

Early pregnancy loss (abortion) is defined as the termination of pregnancy before 20 weeks of gestation (dated from the last menstrual period) or below a fetal weight of 500 g. Approximately 15% of all pregnancies between 4–20 weeks of gestation will undergo clinically recognized spontaneous abortions. The true early pregnancy loss rate is closer to 50% because of the high rate of unrecognized abortions in the 2–4 weeks immediately following conception. The majority of these very early cases are caused by chromosomal abnormalities in the sperm or the egg.

"Habitual" abortion was classically defined as 3 or more consecutive abortions. In 1938, Malpas, using theoretical calculations, stated that a woman with a history of 3 consecutive abortions had a 73% chance of aborting in the next pregnancy.[1] In 1946, Eastman presented statistical calculations indicating that after 3 abortions the risk was 83.6%.[2] These early conclusions, based primarily upon intuition rather than clinical studies, established the notion that the chance for a subsequent abortion increases dramatically with each successive abortion; and that after 3 abortions the chances for a successful pregnancy are very low. Studies on the efficacy of many types of treatments used these pessimistic figures for comparison rather than containing their own controls. If treatment increased the salvage rate to 70% it was considered curative. However, clinical studies have indicated that the risk of pregnancy loss after 3 successive abortions is in fact 30–45%.[3-5] The chance of a successful live birth after 3 consecutive abortions without a live birth is 55–60%; with at least one previous normal pregnancy (live birth) in addition to the repetitive abortions, the chance is approximately 70%.[3,4]

The projections by Malpas and Eastman were theoretical exercises that were not confirmed when appropriate data were collected. Thus, it is not surprising that treatment with a wide range of approaches, including vitamins and psychotherapy, produced successful pregnancies in a reasonable percentage of women with recurrent abortions. These cures were not due to the therapy; the claims for success were based on a comparison with the discredited statistics of Malpas and Eastman.

The Risk of Recurrent Early Pregnancy Loss[3,4]

	Number of Prior Losses	% Risk of Loss in Next Pregnancy
Women who have had at least one liveborn infant:	0	12%
	1	24%
	2	26%
	3	32%
	4	26%
Women who have not had at least one liveborn infant:	2 or more	40–45%

The diagnostic and therapeutic response to a couple with pregnancy loss is not dictated by the number of abortions. The response is significantly influenced by the woman's age, the couple's level of anxiety, and factors readily identified in the family and medical history. The degree of response will range from an educational discussion to a full diagnostic evaluation with appropriate treatment. It is helpful to consider recurrent abortions according to the following influencing factors:

1. Normal statistics.
2. Genetic factors.
3. Environmental factors.
4. Endocrine factors.
5. Anatomic causes.
6. Infectious causes.
7. Immunologic problems.

Normal Statistics

The reproductive loss between conception and clinically recognizable pregnancy is significant; about 50% of fertilized ova do not progress to a viable pregnancy.[6,7] The use of sensitive assays for human chorionic gonadotropin (HCG) suggests that up to 30% of pregnancies are lost between implantation and the 6th week.[8] It is important for physicians and their patients to be aware of the high degree of reproductive loss, especially in older women due in part to the increasing frequency of trisomies with advancing age. However, the frequency of both euploid (normal) and aneuploid (abnormal) abortuses increases with maternal age.

Approximately 80% of spontaneous abortions occur in the first 12 weeks of pregnancy, and nearly 70% of these abortions in early pregnancy are due to chromosomal anomalies.[9] Clinically recognized abortion occurs in only 12% of women younger than age 20, but the incidence increases to 26% in women older than age 40. The overall abortion risk (recognized and unrecognized) in women over age 40 is approximately 75%! An appreciation for these statistics contributes significantly to a couple's ability to cope with a spontaneous abortion.

Once a live embryo is detected by ultrasonography in normal women or in women with infertility, the rate of fetal loss is 5%. However, in women with recurrent pregnancy loss, the rate of loss after detection of fetal cardiac activity is 4–5 times higher.[10]

Genetic Factors

Despite the knowledge that the spontaneous salvage rate is 55–70%, it is still worth trying to uncover causes for repetitive first trimester pregnancy losses. A recognized cause of the problem is a genetic abnormality, and karyotyping of couples will reveal that 3–8% have some abnormality, most frequently a balanced chromosomal rearrangement, a translocation.[11-16] Other abnormalities usually encountered include sex chromosome mosaicism, chromosome inversions, and ring chromosomes. Besides spontaneous abortions, these abnormalities are associated with a high risk of malformations and mental retardation. Karyotyping is especially vital if the couple has had a malformed infant or fetus in addition to abortions. It is important to emphasize that karyotyping uncovers only a percentage of those pregnancies lost due to genetic abnormalities. There may be single gene defects that are not manifested by chromosomal abnormalities, and it is very likely that a percentage of those patients now considered to have unexplained repetitive pregnancy loss have this type of genetic defect. In addition, karyotyping of blood cells misses abnormalities of meiosis, which can be found in sperm cell lines.

If the karyotype is abnormal, nothing can be done to lessen the chances for another abortion, however with most abnormalities there is a 50% chance the next pregnancy will be normal. Amniocentesis or chorionic villus biopsy should be encouraged in any pregnancy in couples with a previous abnormal karyotype because of the risk of an abnormal child. Today, couples with serious high risk abnormalities may elect to pursue a pregnancy by means of donor sperm or in vitro fertilization with donor oocytes (or both).

As noted, approximately 70% of early spontaneous abortions are associated with fetal chromsomal abnormalities.[17,18] In addition, 30% of second trimester abortions and 3% of stillbirths have abnormal chromosomes. In most cases, the couple is chromosomally normal and the fetal chromosomal abnormality is a random event. The abnormalities include maternal and paternal accidents in gametogenesis, as well as miscues after fertilization. The fetal chromsomal abnormalities in single spontaneous abortions are different than those in recurrent abortions. Autosomal trisomy is the most frequent anomaly (about 50% of early pregnancy abortions), due to nondisjunction or translocation.[19] Trisomies of chromosomes 13, 16, 18, 21, and 22 are the most common. The next most common anomaly (about 25%) is 45,X which is responsible for Turner syndrome when the fetus survives. Of the remaining anomalies, most are polyploidies.

Fetuses that abort later in gestation usually have normal chromosomes. Perhaps in this situation, the responsible factors are external to the fetus. Subtle chromosomal defects, however, may be revealed as our analytic techniques improve.

According to McDonough, treatment of endocrine factors yields a 90% normal child rate; correction of anatomic factors yields a 60–70% rate, but known genetic factors are associated with only a 32% expectation for a normal child.[20]

It is helpful to have a karyotype on a previous abortion to determine aneuploidy or euploidy. Once determined, there is an increased likelihood that subsequent abortions will be the same, although there is still a chance for women with recurrent pregnancy loss to have a normal pregnancy. If aneuploidy is documented, accurately timed inseminations could be considered based on animal studies relating aneuploidy to aging of ovum and sperm, otherwise the choice is between hoping for the best or donor insemination. Once pregnant, chorionic villus sampling should be considered. If euploidy has been documented, anatomic and endocrine factors should be corrected.

Karyotyping is expensive. A factor that can help in decision-making is a positive family history for recurrent abortions.[21] Translocations within families are usually associated with a mixed history: some normal pregnancies intermixed with recurrent abortions.

Karyotyping is indicated when family members can be identified with multiple sponta-neous abortions or the family has a malformed or mentally retarded child or a child with a known chromsomal abnormality. In any event, we recommend a karyotype when there is a history of 3 consecutive spontaneous early pregnancy losses and no previous normal liveborn.

Environmental Factors

Smoking, alcohol, and heavy coffee consumption are associated with an increased risk of recurrent abortions.[9,22] The increase in risk is proportional to the number of cigarettes smoked. In these cases, the fetal chromosomes are normal. Anesthetic gases and tetrachloroethylene (used in dry cleaning) have been implicated as causative agents of abortion, but exposure to video terminals does not appear to be a factor.[23] Exercise programs do not increase the risk of spontaneous abortion, and bed rest will not influence the risk of recurrent abortion. Isotretinoin (Accutane) is definitely associated with an increased incidence of spontaneous abortion.[24]

Endocrine Factors

Mild or subclinical endocrine diseases are not causes of recurrent abortion. Patients who have significant thyroid disease or uncontrolled diabetes mellitus may suffer spontane-ous abortions, but it is unlikely that laboratory assessments of thyroid function and carbohydrate metabolism are worthwhile in relatively healthy women.[25–27] Neverthe-less, the high frequency of hypothyroidism warrants screening with a measurement of thyrotropin-stimulating hormone (TSH).[15] No convincing evidence exists linking endo-metriosis with an increased risk of spontaneous abortion.[28]

An endocrine abnormality that may cause recurrent abortions is the inadequate luteal phase. Studies of the role of hormone deficiency as a cause of recurrent abortion have largely focused on deficiencies of progesterone or its metabolites. Attempts to implicate low progesterone or pregnanediol levels in early pregnancy as a cause for abortion, and, as a corollary, to treat with exogenous progesterone or progestins have been shown to be fruitless.[29]

A second approach has been to diagnose an inadequate luteal phase during the nonpreg-nant state and to initiate treatment with progesterone a few days after ovulation. Jones and Delfs[30] claimed that 30% of women with pregnancy wastage had an inadequate luteal phase, whereas more recent studies have found that 20–25% of women with recurrent abortions have an inadequate luteal phase.[11–16] Yet it is by no means certain that progestational treatment makes a difference. Indeed, a meta-analysis of randomized trials of pregnancies treated with progestational agents failed to find any evidence for a positive effect on the maintenance of pregnancy.[31] Nevertheless, clinicians continue to report, as we have noted, a significant incidence of luteal phase inadequacy in their series of patients with recurrent abortions.[15]

The uncertainty that plagues physicians in dealing with the inadequate luteal phase in infertility, therefore, is also apparent when considering recurrent abortion. If repetitive endometrial biopsies indicate a lag in histologic development of more than 2 days or if the basal body temperature chart shows a luteal phase of less than 11 days, it is reasonable to treat with clomiphene or progesterone vaginal suppositories (25 mg bid) and with a dopamine agonist if galactorrhea or an elevated prolactin is present. In the absence of galactorrhea or hyperprolactinemia, we prefer clomiphene because this avoids the situation of a prolonged luteal phase due to progesterone treatment, a false expectation of pregnancy, and a more difficult time for the couple in coping with the results of a negative pregnancy test.

Should clomiphene be offered empirically when no other cause for recurrent abortion can be identified? Placebo treatment may be useful in maintaining a physician/patient relationship in which the patient derives needed psychologic sustenance. Furthermore, there is no evidence of any major harmful consequences with clomiphene treatment (see Chapter 30). In view of the difficulty in establishing the diagnosis of an inadequate luteal phase and the uncertainties that surround this diagnosis, we believe there is a place for empirical treatment. It must be remembered, however, that there is a reasonable cure rate in unexplained recurrent abortion, even without treatment.

Anatomical Causes

Uterine abnormalities can result in impaired vascularization of a pregnancy and limited space for a fetus due to distortion of the uterine cavity. Approximately 12–15% of women with recurrent abortion have a uterine malformation, and this can be best diagnosed by vaginal ultrasonography, confirmed by magnetic resonance imaging. Hysterosalpingography is relatively inaccurate and decisions should not be based upon hysterosalpingography alone.[32] The various uterine anomalies, including leiomyomata and diethylstilbestrol (DES) exposure, are discussed in detail in Chapter 4. Surgical repair of these defects, often by hysteroscopy, is rewarded with delivery rates in the 70–80% range; however, this high rate of success must be tempered by the realization that it is not derived from randomized clinical trials. The septate uterus is the most frequent anatomic abnormality associated with recurrent early spontaneous abortions, and the results with hysteroscopic repair have been impressive.[33] Repeat procedures are occasionally necessary; the surgical result should be evaluated several weeks postoperatively by hysterosalpingography (which is sufficiently accurate for this purpose) or office hysteroscopy. Surgery is unlikely to make a difference in a patient who has successfully delivered a live born term infant. The prophylactic use of cervical cerclage has not been supported by results from randomized trials.[34] However, when there is nothing else to offer, cervical cerclage is worthwhile, e.g., in patients with late losses and müllerian anomalies such as a bicornuate or unicornuate uterus and in DES-exposed women with a hypoplastic cervix.

In addition to müllerian anomalies, another anatomic cause, although uncommon, of recurrent abortions is intrauterine synechiae (Asherman's syndrome). If an appropriate predisposing factor, such as uterine curettage or a severe uterine infection, can be identified, diagnostic hysterosalpingography or hysteroscopy should be performed.

Infectious Causes

Despite periodic reports that have implicated specific infectious agents as etiologic factors in recurrent spontaneous abortions, there currently is no hard evidence that bacterial or viral infections cause recurrent abortions. An impressive incidence of antichlamydial antibody has been reported in women with 3 or more spontaneous abortions, but it is not certain whether this an association with *Chlamydia trachomatis* or whether this is a marker of a different immune response in women with recurrent abortions.[35] Claims of effective antibiotic treatment have been derived without benefit of randomized studies. Perhaps an exception is infection with *Ureaplasma urealiticum*.[36] Other organisms that have been implicated, but not substantiated, include *Toxoplasma gondii, Listeria monocytogenes, Mycoplasma hominis,* herpes virus, and cytomegalovirus. It is more cost-effective and time efficient to prescribe couples a course of doxycycline (100 mg bid for 14 days) or erythromycin (250 mg qid for 14 days) than to pursue multiple and repeated cultures.

Immunologic Problems

Autoimmunity (Self Antigens)

In autoimmunity, a humoral or cellular response is directed against a specific component of the host. The lupus anticoagulant and anticardiolipin antibodies are antiphospholipid antibodies, which arise as the result of an autoimmune disease. The lupus anticoagulant is present in a variety of clinical conditions, not just with lupus erythematosus. The antiphospholipid antibodies are directed against platelets and the vascular endothelium and cause thrombosis, spontaneous abortion, and fetal wastage. These antibodies block prostacyclin formation, which results in unbalanced thromboxane activity, leading to vasoconstriction and thrombosis.[37] In several series, 10–16% of women with recurrent abortions have had antiphospholipid antibodies.[15,38] These antibodies are also associated with fetal growth retardation and fetal death in addition to recurrent abortion, and when present, there is a high rate of second trimester fetal deaths. The mechanism of pregnancy loss is probably decidual and placental insufficiency due to the thrombotic tendency.

Despite activating thrombosis, the antiphospholipid antibodies prolong the prothrombin time and the partial thromboplastin time. The activated partial thromboplastin time is a relatively sensitive screening test, but we also obtain a kaolin clotting time. The anticardiolipin antibody can be identified and titered by specific immunoassays. The antiphospholipid antibodies all produce the same clinical impact and have identical effects on clotting tests. Although the prevalence is uncertain, patients with recurrent abortions should be screened with the activated partial thromboplastin time, a kaolin clotting time, and the anticardiolipin antibody.[39–43]

In Europe, patients with recurrent abortions are studied with hysterosalpingography under pressure. It is claimed that an increase in pressure of injection correlates with a pattern in the uterine vasculature that could be secondary to vasospasm and thrombosis (and subsequent fibrosis). It remains to be seen whether this is an acceptable method to select patients for treatment of antiphospholipid antibodies.

Our preferred treatment for significant titers of antiphsopholipid antibodies consists of the combination of low dose aspirin and low dose heparin as soon as pregnancy is diagnosed.[44] Treatment is not always successful.[45] Others advocate the addition of a glucocorticoid in a dose sufficient to restore the clotting studies to normal.[46] The addition of glucocorticoids is not very effective in eliminating the anticardiolipin antibody. Many of these patients develop preeclampsia, often very severe, but approximately 75% of patients with antiphospholipid antibodies will deliver a viable infant in a treated pregnancy.

Alloimmunity (Foreign Antigens)

Alloimmunity includes all causes of recurrent abortion related to an abormal maternal immune response to antigens on placental or fetal tissues.[38] Normally, maintenance of pregnancy may require the formation of blocking factors (probably complexes of antibody and antigen) that prevent maternal rejection of fetal antigens. It has been argued that couples with repetitive abortion have an increased sharing of human leukocyte antigens (HLA), a condition that would not allow the mother to make blocking antibodies.

Immunotherapy to stimulate antibody formation has been offered to produce a favorable maternal immune response in order to protect the developing embryo. Women with recurrent abortions have been treated with infusions of their partner's lymphocytes. In one study, 77% of women receiving their husband's cells gave birth compared to 37% receiving their own cells.[47] Critics of this study have contended that success in the control group raises the question of the adequacy of matching in the selection of control patients. Others have claimed good results with transfusion of leukocyte-rich, erythrocyte-rich donor blood (3 transfusions every 4–8 weeks) or with intravenous immunoglobulin or seminal plasma vaginal suppositories.[48–50]

Women have been selected for immunotherapy by HLA typing, but its use is controversial. Many investigators have failed to confirm that sharing of HLA antigens is found in couples with recurrent abortions.[51,52] This agrees with experiments in animals where sharing of HLA antigens has not been found to affect reproduction. The sharing of genetic loci may be a broader problem that includes genetic loci critical for embryonic development, and the antigens available for measurement serve only as markers for a more fundamental genetic immunologic failure in pregnancy. There is also concern that immunization of mothers may affect placenta and fetus. There is no specific immunologic test which will predict the need for treatment.[53] Immunotherapy remains experimental with potential risks of adverse consequences on the immune systems of mother and child. The results of a world-wide prospective trial of immunotherapy, organized by the American Society of Reproductive Immunology, should be available in the mid 1990s. In the meantime, it is important to note that 3 randomized placebo-controlled studies have failed to demonstrate a beneficial effect of immunotherapy.[54–56]

Embryotoxic Factors
Women with a history of recurrent abortions produce soluble factors in response to sperm and trophoblast, which are toxic to mouse embryos and human trophoblastic cells. Hill has suggested that these embryotoxic factors can serve as a marker for an adverse outcome and can be used to select patients who may benefit from immunosuppressive therapy.[57] One therapeutic possibility is progesterone which has known immunosuppressive effects. Factors that are toxic for mouse embryos have also been obtained from fetal cord sera of women with endometriosis and unexplained infertility, as well as recurrent pregnancy losses. This wide range of clinical conditions raises questions regarding the specificity of this marker.

Summary of Immunologic Causes

Women whose recurrent abortions are more likely to have an immunologic cause have the following characteristics:[53]

1. Many previous spontaneous abortions.
2. No recent full term pregnancies.
3. Less than 35 years old.
4. Aborted conceptus with a normal karyotype.
5. Usually at least one loss after the first trimester.

| Summary of Laboratory Evaluation and Management for Repeated Early Pregnancy Losses | **Normal statistics:** Education and support; no specific laboratory tests. |
| | |

Normal statistics: Education and support; no specific laboratory tests.

Genetic factors: Karyotypes of both parents; counseling.

Environmental factors: No specific laboratory tests; counseling.

Endocrine factors: TSH screen for thyroid disease, evaluation of luteal phase including prolactin; empiric clomiphene.

Anatomic causes: Vaginal ultrasonography confirmed by MRI; surgery.

Infectious causes: No specific cultures unless clinically indicated; empiric doxycycline or erythromycin.

Immunologic problems: Activated partial thromboplastin time, kaolin clotting time, anticardiolipin antibody titer; aspirin and heparin.

Concluding Thoughts

The patient with early pregnancy losses usually presents as an anxious, frustrated individual on the verge of despair. Evaluation should be spaced over several visits, allowing the physician to establish communication and rapport with the patient. Frequent communication between the clinician and the patient during the first trimester of the next pregnancy is essential. The emotional support that the physician can bring to this interaction will be most useful and in some cases may be therapeutic.[13] It should be emphasized that continued attempts at conception are rewarded with success in the majority of women (70–75%) labeled as recurrent aborters and who have no identifiable cause. Except in the case of a second trimester loss which is associated with a poor prognosis in the subsequent pregnancy with increased risks for preterm delivery, stillbirth, and neonatal death, approximately 40–50% of women with histories of recurrent abortions have no identifiable abnormalities and do well in their next pregnancies.[12–16,58] All subsequent pregnancies should be closely monitored because there is a higher rate of ectopic pregnancies in women with recurrent abortions.[59]

References

1. **Malpas P,** A study of abortion sequence, J Obstet Gynaecol Br Emp 45:932, 1938.

2. **Eastman NJ,** Habitual abortion, in Meigs JV, Sturgis S, editors, *Progress in Gynecology,* Vol 1, Grune & Stratton, New York, 1946.

3. **Warburton D, Fraser FS,** Spontaneous abortion risks in man: data from reproductive histories collected in a medical genetics unit, Am J Hum Genet 16:1, 1964.

4. **Poland BJ, Miller JR, Jones DC, Trimble BK,** Reproductive counseling in patients who have had a spontaneous abortion, Am J Obstet Gynecol 127:685, 1977.

5. **Roman E,** Fetal loss rates and their relation to pregnancy order, J Epidemiol Community Health 38:29, 1984.

6. **Wramsby H, Fredga K, Liedholm P,** Chromosome analysis of human oocytes recovered from preovulatory follicles in stimulated cycles, New Engl J Med 316:121, 1987.

7. **Warburton D,** Reproductive loss: how much is preventable? New Engl J Med 316:158, 1987.

8. **Wilcox AJ, Weiberg CR, O'Connor JF, Baird DD, Schlatterer JP, Canfield RE, Armstrong EG, Nisula BC,** Incidence of early loss of pregnancy, New Engl J Med 319:189, 1988.

9. **Harlap S, Shiono PH,** Alcohol, smoking, and incidence of spontaneous abortions in the first and second trimester, Lancet 2:173, 1980.

10. **van Leeuwen I, Branch DW, Scott JR,** First trimester ultrasonography findings in women with a history of recurrent pregnancy loss, Am J Obstet Gynecol 168:111, 1993.

11. **Tho PT, Byrd Jr, McDonough PG,** Etiologies and subsequent reproductive performance of 100 couples with recurrent abortion, Fertil Steril 32:389, 1979.

12. **Harger JH, Archer DF, Marchese SG, Muracca-Clemens M, Garver KL,** Etiology of recurrent pregnancy losses and outcome of subsequent pregnancies, Obstet Gynecol 62:574, 1983.

13. **Stray-Pedersen B, Stray-Pedersen S,** Etiologic factors and subsequent reproductive performance in 195 couples with a prior history of habitual abortion, Am J Obstet Gynecol 148:140, 1984.

14. **Portnoi M-F, Joye N, van den Akker J, Morlier G, Taillemite JL,** Karyotypes of 1142 couples with recurrent abortion, Obstet Gynecol 72:31, 1988.

15. **Plouffe L Jr, White EW, Tho ST, Sweet CS, Layman LC, Whitman GF, McDonough PG,** Etiologic factors of recurrent abortion and subsequent reproductive performance of couples: have we made any progress in the past 10 years? Am J Obstet Gynecol 167:313, 1992.

16. **Tulppala M, Palosuo T, Ramsay T, Miettinen A, Salonen R, Ylikorkala O,** A prospective study of 63 couples with a history of recurrent spontaneous abortions: contributing factors and outcome of subsequent pregnancies, Hum Reprod 8:764, 1993.

17. **Boue J, Boue A, Lazar P,** Retrospective and prospective epidemiological studies of 1500 karyotyped spontaneous human abortions, Teratology 12:11, 1975.

18. **Guerneri S, Bettio D, Simoni G, Brambat B, Lanzani A, Fraccaro M,** Prevalence and distribution of chromosome abnormalities in a sample of first-trimester internal abortions, Hum Reprod 2:735, 1987.

19. **Carr DH,** Chromosome studies in selected spontaneous abortions and early pregnancy loss, Obstet Gynecol 37:570, 1971.

20. **McDonough PG,** Repeated first-trimester loss: evaluation and management, Am J Obstet Gynecol 153:1, 1985.

21. **Mowbray JF, Underwood J, Gill TJ III,** Familial recurrent spontaneous abortions, Am J Reprod Immunol 26:17, 1991.

22. **Armstrong BG, McDonald AD, Sloan M,** Cigarette, alcohol, and coffee consumption and spontaneous abortion, Am J Public Health 82:85, 1992.

23. **Schnorr TM, Grajewski BA, Hornung RW, Thun MJ, Egeland GM, Murray WE, Conover DL, Halperin WE,** Video display terminals and the risk of sponaneous abortion, New Engl J Med 324:727, 1991.

24. **Lammer EJ, Chen DT, Hoar RM, et al,** Retinoic acid embryopathy, New Engl J Med 313:837, 1985.

25. **Montoro M, Collea JV, Frasier D, Mestman J,** Successful outcome of pregnancy in women with hypothyroidism, Ann Intern Med 94:31, 1981.

26. **Sutherland HW, Pritchard CW,** Increased incidence of sponaneous abortion in pregnancies complicated by maternal diabetes mellitus, Am J Obstet Gynecol 155:135, 1986.

27. **Mills JE, Simpson JL, Driscoll SG,** Incidence of spontaneous abortion among normal women and insulin-dependent diabetic women whose pregnancies were identified within 21 days of conception, New Engl J Med 319:1617, 1988.

28. **Damewood MD,** The association of endometriosis and repetitive (early) spontaneous abortions, Seminars Reprod Endocrinol 7:155, 1989.

29. **Sherman RP, Garrett WJ,** Double blind study of effect of 17-hydroxyprogesterone caproate on abortion rate, Br Med J 1:292, 1963.

30. **Jones GES, Delfs E,** Endocrine patterns in term pregnancies following abortion, JAMA 146:1212, 1951.

31. **Goldstein P, Berrier J, Rosen S, Sacks HS, Chalmers TC,** A meta-analysis of randomized control trials of progestational agents in pregnancy, Br J Obstet Gynaecol 96:265, 1989.

32. **Pellerito JS, McCarthy SM, Doyle MB, Glickman MG, DeCherney AH,** Diagnosis of uterine anomalies: relative accuracy of MR imaging, endovaginal sonography, and hystero-salpingography, Genitourinary Radiol 183:795, 1992.

33. **Daly DC, Maier D, Soto-Alber RS,** Hysteroscopic metroplasty: 6 years' experience, Obstet Gynecol 73:201, 1989.

34. **Lazar P, Gueguen S, Dreyfus J, Renaud R, Pontonnier G, Papiernik E,** Multicentered controlled trial of cervical cerclage in women at moderate risk of preterm delivery, Br J Obstet Gynaecol 91:731, 1984.

35. **Witkin SS, Ledger WJ,** Antibodies to *Chlamydia trachomatis* in sera of women with recurrent spontaneous abortions, Am J Obstet Gynecol 167:135, 1992.

36. **Quinn PA, Shewchuk AB, Shuber J, Lie KI, Ryan E, Chipman ML, Nocilla DM,** Efficacy of antibiotic therapy in preventing spontaneous pregnancy loss among couples colonized with genital mycoplasmas, Am J Obstet Gynecol 145:239, 1983.

37. **Tulppala M, Viinikka L, Ylikorkala O,** Thromboxane dominence and prostacyclin deficiency in habitual abortion, Lancet 337:879, 1991.

38. **Scott JR, Rote NS, Branch DW,** Immunologic aspects of recurrent abortion and fetal death, Obstet Gynecol 70:645, 1987.

39. **Cowchock S, Smith JB, Gocial B,** Antibodies to phospholipids and nuclear antigens in patients with repeated abortions, Am J Obstet Gynecol 155:1002, 1986.

40. **Lockwood CJ, Romero R, Feinberg RF, Clyne LP, Coster B, Hobbins JC,** The prevalence and biologic significance of lupus anticoagulant and anticardiolipin antibodies in a general obstetric population, Am J Obstet Gynecol 161:369, 1989.

41. **Balasch J, Lopez-Soto A, Cervera R, Jove I, Casals FJ, Vanrell JA,** Antiphospholipid antibodies in unselected patients with repeated abortion, Hum Reprod 5:43, 1990.

42. **Parazzini F, Acaia B, Faden D, Lovotti M, Marelli G, Cortelozzo S,** Antiphospholipid antibodies in recurrent abortion, Obstet Gynecol 77:854, 1991.

43. **Infante-Rivard C, David M, Gauthier R, Rivard G-E,** Lupus anticoagulants, anticardiolipin antibodies, and fetal loss, New Engl J Med 325:1063, 1991.

44. **Cowchock FS, Reece EA, Balaban D, Branch DW, Plouffe L,** Repeated fetal losses associated with antiphospholipid antibodies: a collaborative randomized trial comparing prednisone with low-dose heparin treatment, Am J Obstet Gynecol 166:1318, 1992.

45. **Branch DW, Silver RM, Blackwell JL, Reading JC, Scott JR,** Outcome of treated pregnancies in women with antiphospholipid syndrome: an update of the Utah experience, Obstet Gynecol 80:614, 1992.

46. **Branch DW, Scott JR, Kochenour NK, Hershgold E,** Obstetric complications associated with the lupus anticoagulant, New Engl J Med 313:1322, 1985.

47. **Mowbray JF, Gibbings C, Liddell H, Reginald PW, Underwood JL, Beard RW,** Controlled trial of treatment of recurrent spontaneous abortion by immunization with paternal cells, Lancet 1:941, 1985.

48. **Unander AM, Lindholm A,** Transfusions of leukocyte-rich erythrocyte concentrates: a successful treatment in selected cases of habitual abortion, Am J Obstet Gynecol 154:516, 1986.

49. **Christiansen OB, Mathiesen O, Lauritsen JG, Grunnet N,** Intravenous imnmunoglobulin treatment of women with multiple miscarriages, Hum Reprod 7:718, 1992.

50. **Stern JJ, Coulam CB, Wagenknecht DR, Peters AJ, Faulk WP, McIntyre JA,** Seminal plasma treatment of recurrent spontaneous abortions, Am J Reprod Immunol 27:50, 1992.

51. **Adinolfi M,** Recurrent habitual abortion, HLA sharing and deliberate immunization with partner's cells: a controversial topic, Hum Reprod 1:45, 1986.

52. **Eroglu G, Betz G, Torregano C,** Impact of histocompatibility antigens on pregnancy outcome, Am J Obstet Gynecol 166:1364, 1992.

53. **Cowchuck S,** What's a mother to do? Analysis of trials evaluating new treatments for unexplained recurrent miscarriages and other complaints, Am J Reprod Immunol 26:156, 1991.

54. **Ho H-N, Gill TJ III, Hsieh H-J, Jian J-J, Hsieh C-Y,** Immunotherapy for recurrent spontaneous abortions in a Chinese population, Am J Reprod Immunol 25:10, 1991.

55. **Cauchi MN, Lim D, Young DE, Kloss M, Pepperell RJ,** Treatment of recurrent aborters by immunization with paternal cells: controlled trial, Am J Reprod Immunol 25:16, 1991.

56. **Christiansen OB, Christiansen BS, Husth M, Mathiesen O, Lauritsen JG, Grunnet N,** Prospective study of anticardiolipin antibodies in immunized and untreated women with recurrent spontaneous abortions, Fertil Steril 58:328, 1992.

57. **Ecker JL, Laufer MR, Hill JA,** Measurement of embryotoxic factors is predictive of pregnancy outcome in women with a history of recurrent abortions, Obstet Gynecol 81:84, 1993.

58. **Goldenberg RL, Mayberry SK, Copper RL, Dubard MB, Hauth JC,** Pregnancy outcome following a second-trimester loss, Obstet Gynecol 81:444, 1993.

59. **Fedele L, Acala B, Parazzine F, Ricciardiello, Cantiani GB,** Ectopic pregnancy and recurrent spontaneous abortion: two associated reproductive failures, Obstet Gynecol 73:206, 1989.

28   Endometriosis

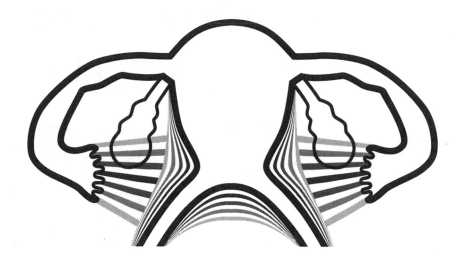

Endometriosis is a term indicating ectopic endometrial glands and stroma (outside the uterus), and in its clinical manifestations it is a progressive disease that is a vexing problem for both patient and clinician. However, clinical studies over the past decade have provided information for a better understanding of the disease and better decision-making regarding management options.[1,2] This chapter will review the more recent information regarding treatment as well as what is known concerning the etiology and pathogenesis of endometriosis.

Etiology of Endometriosis

Endometriosis was described in the medical literature in the 1800s, but it was not until this century that its common occurrence was appreciated. Based on clinical observation and examination of histopathologic specimens, John Sampson of Albany, New York, in 1921, suggested that peritoneal endometriosis in the pelvis arose from seedings from ovarian endometriosis. Subsequently, in 1927, he published his classic paper, "Peritoneal Endometriosis Due to Menstrual Dissemination of Endometrial Tissue Into the Peritoneal Cavity," which introduced the term "endometriosis" and established retrograde flow of endometrial tissue through the fallopian tubes and into the abdominal cavity as the probable cause of the disease.[3] The conclusions of Sampson have been validated by the following observations:

1. During laparoscopy, flow of blood from the fimbriated end of the tube has been observed in virtually all menstruating women.[4]

2. Endometriosis is most commonly found in dependent portions of the pelvis, most frequently on the ovaries, the anterior and posterior cul-de-sac, and the uterosacral ligaments, followed by the posterior uterus and posterior broad ligaments.[5,6]

3. Endometrial fragments from the menstrual flow can grow both in tissue culture and following injection beneath the abdominal skin, and can be retrieved from the peritoneal fluid of most menstruating women.[7]

4. Endometriosis developed when the cervices of monkeys were transposed so that menstruation occurred into the peritoneal cavity.[8]

5. A higher incidence of endometriosis is observed in women who have obstructions to the outward flow of the menstrual effluvium.[9]

6. The risk of endometriosis is increased in women with shorter menstrual cycles and longer flows, characteristics that give greater opportunity for ectopic endometrial implantation.[10]

Endometriosis at sites distant from the pelvis may be due to vascular or lymphatic transport of endometrial fragments. Even the common occurrence of endometriosis on the ovaries can be explained by lymphatic flow from the uterus to the ovary.[11]

Endometriosis can occur in almost every organ of the body.[12] For example, pulmonary endometriosis occurs and can be manifested by asymptomatic nodules or as pneumothrorax, hemothorax, or hemoptysis during menses.[13] Urologic endometriosis is of importance because of the possiblity for ureteral obstruction.

Extrapelvic endometriosis is occasionally encountered years after surgical removal of the uterus and the ovaries.[14] This endometriosis can be hormone-resistant, and we can only speculate as to why it grows. One possibility is transplantation of endometrial implants during the original surgery, or activation of residual disease. Another possibility is transformation by metaplasia of other tissue or activation of embryonic rest tissue. When the endometriosis is hormone-sensitive, a good possibility is that an ovarian remnant is left behind during the complicated surgery, and this allows continuing hormonal stimulation of residual endometriosis.

There are case reports of endometriosis in men who received treatment with estrogen, and therefore, another possible cause of endometriosis is the transformation of coelomic epithelium into endometrial-type glands as a result of unspecified stimuli. The following arguments can be used to defend the coelomic metaplasia theory:[15]

1. Endometriosis occurs in adolescent girls in the absence of müllerian anomalies, and it can be discovered a few years after menarche before many menstrual cycles have been experienced.[16]

2. Endometriosis has been reported in a prepubertal girl.[17]

3. Endometriosis has been encountered in women who never menstruated.[18]

4. Endometiosis in unusual sites such as thumb, thigh, or knee can be explained by the fact that mesenchymal limb buds develop adjacent to coelomic epithelium during early embryogenesis.

5. Although usually associated with high dose estrogen treatment, endometriosis does occur in men.[19,20]

Because many women have reflux seeding of menstrual debris into the peritoneal cavity, and not all develop endometriosis, there may be genetic or immunologic factors that influence the susceptibility of a woman to the disease. Simpson and coworkers reported 6.9% of first-degree relatives of patients with endometriosis had the disease, compared with 1.0% in a control group.[21] Dmowski and coworkers demonstrated that monkeys with endometriosis had decreased cellular immunity to endometrial tissue, suggesting that specific immunologic defects can render some individuals susceptible to endometriosis.[22] Others have found an increased prevalence of humoral antibodies directed against endometrial and ovarian tissue in the sera of women with endometriosis.[23] In addition, women with endometriosis demonstrate a decrease in various measurements of immune response.[24,25]

A consideration of the etiologic theories regarding endometriosis leads to the conclusion that all of these mechanisms may contribute to the clinical problem in an individual patient, and the degree of contribution for each probably varies from patient to patient. Endometrial cells can be spread by mechanical means, or perhaps can arise by metaplasia, and progression of the disease is influenced by the individual's immune mechanisms.

Prevalence of Endometriosis

Widely varying figures for the prevalence of endometriosis have been published, and a rough estimate is that 3–10% of women in the reproductive age group and 25–35% of infertile women have endometriosis.[2,26] About 4 per 1,000 women age 15–64 are hospitalized with endometriosis each year, slightly more than those admitted with breast cancer. The common perceptions that endometriosis only occurs in goal-oriented women over the age of 30 and is not found often in black women have now been discredited. Whereas endometriosis essentially does not occur before menarche, there are increasing reports of its occurrence in the teen years.[27] A number of these cases involve anatomic abnormalities that obstruct the outflow tract.[28] Endometriosis is not confined to nulliparous women, and physicians should be alert to the presence of endometriosis in cases of secondary infertility.

Diagnosis of Endometriosis

Endometriosis should be suspected in any woman complaining of infertility. Suspicion is heightened when there are also complaints of dysmenorrhea and dyspareunia.

Symptoms and Signs

Dysmenorrhea is even more suggestive of endometriosis if it begins after years of relatively pain-free menses. It should be recognized, however, that many women who have endometriosis are asymptomatic. A common observation is that some women with extensive endometriosis have little or no pain, whereas others with only minimal endometriosis complain of severe pain. Very severe pain, however, is associated with deeply infiltrating endometriosis.[29] Pain can be diffuse in the pelvis or it can be more localized, often in the area of the rectum. Symptoms also can arise from rectal, ureteral, or bladder involvement with endometriosis, and can be present throughout the month. Blockage of the ureter can occur, and urinary tract symptoms should be investigated with urologic and radiologic techniques. Low back pain, too, may be due to endometriosis. An association of endometriosis and premenstrual spotting has been suggested, but in most cases menstrual dysfunction is not increased with endometriosis. An association between galactorrhea and endometriosis has been claimed, but baseline elevations of prolactin are not higher in patients with endometriosis compared to normal women.

The CA-125 Assay

CA-125 is a cell surface antigen found on derivatives of the coelomic epithelium (which includes endometrium), and it is a useful marker in the monitoring of women with epithelial ovarian carcinoma. In addition, serum CA-125 levels are often elevated in patients with endometriosis and correlate with both the degree of disease and the response to treatment.[30,31] The sensitivity of this assay is too low to use it as a screening test, but it can be a marker of response to treatment and for recurrence; however, elevated levels which suppress during medical treatment often promptly return to pretreatment concentrations immediately after cessation of therapy, limiting its clinical usefulness.[32] Serum CA-125 determinations may be able to differentiate endometriotic from non-endometriotic benign adnexal cysts.[33] Note that CA-125 levels can be elevated by early pregnancy, acute pelvic inflammatory disease, leiomyomata, and menstruation.

Examination

The uterus is often in fixed retroversion and the ovaries may be enlarged. However, retroversion of the uterus is not an etiologic factor, and prophylactic uterine suspension is no longer recommended. Nodularity (which is usually tender) of the uterosacral ligaments and cul-de-sac can be found in one-third of patients with endometriosis. The diagnosis almost always should be confirmed by laparoscopy before treatment is initiated. Minimal findings such as slight beading and tenderness of the uterosacral ligaments in the young, asymptomatic patient can be treated, however, with combined, low dose oral contraceptives.

The classic chocolate cyst of the ovary is the result of a blood-filled cavity within an endometrioma. Ultrasonography and magnetic resonance imaging can be helpful in diagnosing endometriomas.[34,35] However, neither can diagnose small peritoneal implants or adhesions.

The appearance of endometriosis is quite varied. All too often the clinician fails to observe endometrial lesions because of a preconceived expectation limited to the classic blue or black powder burn appearance. Lesions can be red, black, blue, or white and nonpigmented.[36] Biopsies from visibly normal peritoneum can contain endometriosis in 6–13% of infertile women; however, the clinical significnce of this presence is uncertain (and, in our view, unlikely to be important).[37] Adhesions, peritoneal defects, and tan, creamy, fresh-appearing endometrium also can be observed. The dark pigmented lesions are later consequences of tissue bleeding responses to cyclic hormones. The ovary is the most common site for both implants and adhesions, followed by widespread distribution, anteriorly and posteriorly, over the broad ligament and cul-de-sac.

A Classification System

Because both treatment and prognosis are determined to some extent by the severity of the disease, it is desirable to have a uniform system of classification that takes into account both the extent and severity of the disease. A uniform classification is also crucial for comparing the results of different treatments. The American Fertility Society developed a classification system based on findings at laparoscopy or laparotomy, and forms are available from the Society.[38] However, there were weaknesses in the classification system, especially the fact that it was based upon the arbitrary impressions of the clinician. A second form was produced to standardize the documentation of findings in patients who have pelvic pain and endometriosis.[39] There can be a high intraobserver and interobserver variability in the evaluation of endometriosis using a classification system.[40] Therefore, efforts must continue to provide a useful method for staging.

Endometriosis and Infertility

When endometriosis involves the ovaries and causes adhesions that block tubal motility and pickup of the egg, there is no question of its role in causing mechanical interference with fertility. Less secure is the information on the role of peritoneal endometriosis on fertility. Many physicians believe that even minimal endometriosis can cause infertility. This argument has been weakened by a failure to find benefit from medical treatment of infertility associated with minimal to mild endometriosis.[41–44]

The absence of benefit from therapy, however, could represent a problem with the treatment rather than a lack of association between infertility and endometriosis.[45] Endometriosis diagnosed by laparoscopy is reported in a higher proportion of infertile women (38.5%) compared with fertile women (5.2%).[46] Moreover, fecundity rates in women with endometriosis tend to be lower than the normal fecundity rate.[2,47,48]

However, the long-term cumulative pregnancy rates are very high in women who have minimal to mild endometriosis but who are not treated.[49]

If minimal or mild endometriosis does affect fertility, what are the mechanisms? Certainly, dyspareunia secondary to endometriosis could play a role.

Another mediator could be prostaglandins produced by the implants, which could, in turn, affect tubal motility, or folliculogenesis and corpus luteum function. Patients with endometriosis have been reported to have an increase in both the volume of peritoneal fluid and the concentration of thromboxane B_2 and 6-keto-prostaglandin $F_{1\alpha}$ in the fluid.[50,51] Others, however, found neither an increase in peritoneal fluid nor an increase in concentration of peritoneal fluid prostaglandin E_2, prostaglandin $F_{2\alpha}$, 15-keto-13,14-dihydroprostaglandin $F_{2\alpha}$, and thromboxane B_2.[52,53]

Subsequent studies also have provided contradictory information. No elevation in peritoneal fluid prostanoid levels during the proliferative phase in women with endometriosis has been reported, and similarly no peritoneal fluid elevation in 6-keto prostaglandin $F_{1\alpha}$ levels has been observed in the luteal phase.[54,55] However, others have reported elevated concentrations of prostanoids in the peritoneal fluid of women with endometriosis.[56] These differences could be accounted for by differing levels of prostaglandin synthesis according to different morphologic characteristics of the lesions.[57] In summary, it has not been established that women with endometriosis have higher levels of prostanoids in peritoneal fluid compared to other infertile women. Even if higher levels were found consistently, their role in infertility still would be speculative. Nevertheless, interest in prostaglandins continues. A correlation can be demonstrated between the degree of dysmenorrhea experienced by women with endometriosis and the amount of prostaglandins produced by the endometriosis tissue.[58]

Peritoneal macrophages have been suggested as possible mediators of infertility, and increased activation of macrophages has been found in association with endometriosis.[59,60] Phagocytosis of sperm by macrophages could be one mechanism of action.[61] However, patients with and without endometriosis have the same number of motile sperm recoverable from the peritoneal cavity.[62] Peritoneal macrophages from women with endometriosis secrete interleukin-1 which is toxic to mouse embyros.[63] In addition, cytokines are elevated in the peritoneal fluid, which could recruit macrophages and lymphocytes and perpetuate the inflammatory reaction.

Endometriosis has been implicated as a factor in disordered follicle growth, ovulatory dysfunction, and failure of embryo development. Ultrasonography studies suggest that there is some retardation in growth of follicles in women with endometriosis.[64] Luteinized unruptured follicle syndrome (LUF) in which the oocyte is not released at the time of follicle rupture (or there is a failure of the follicle to rupture) has been suggested as a cause of both unexplained infertility and infertility secondary to endometriosis. Although an unruptured follicle can occur in women, there currently is no impressive evidence that this syndrome is secondary to endometriosis or is even a cause of infertility.[65]

The question of how minimal or mild endometriosis can affect fertility now has been superseded by the question of whether there is *any* effect of mild endometriosis on fertility. More importantly, should endometriosis be treated if the complaint is infertility and not pain? Many articles purporting to show that therapy overcomes endometriosis-associated infertility are flawed by lack of control groups and the failure to use life table analyses.[66] Moreover, expectant management of mild endometriosis is rewarded with reasonable pregnancy rates that are comparable to those obtained with treatment.[41–44,67–69] A cumulative pregnancy rate after 5 years of 90% has been reported in women not treated for minimal or mild endometriosis.[49]

Whereas the studies cited above strongly suggest that medical or surgical treatment of mild endometriosis may not be worthwhile, there are those who champion fulguration treatment under laparoscopic visualization.[70] Because of lack of proof of its efficacy, the occasional report of ureteral injury occurring during fulguration of endometrial implants on the uterosacral ligaments, and the suspicion of some clinicians that burned areas may become a nidus for adhesion formation, we would reserve laparoscopic fulguration of minimal or mild endometrial implants for those patients who have significant pelvic pain.[71] However, an argument can be made that active treatment of even mild endometriosis is warranted because endometriosis is often a progressive disease.

An aggressive method was used by Buttram and Betts who noted that of 56 women with mild endometriosis and an average duration of infertility of 37 months, 73.2% were pregnant within 15 months of conservative surgery by laparotomy.[72] Of those who conceived, 36.6% did so in 3 months and 55.7% within 6 months. Higher pregnancy rates with laparoscopic excision of mild and minimal endometrisois have been reported compared to results achieved with danazol (although the number of women in the danazol group was small).[73] *It should be emphasized, however, that based on monthly fecundity rates and life table analyses, no study has shown an advantage for conservative surgery as opposed to expectant management.*[74]

Surgical Treatment of Endometriosis

In contrast to the dispute over the proper treatment of mild endometriosis, there is little doubt that adhesive disease associated with endometriosis, or large (>2 cm) endometriomas, is best treated by surgery. The object of surgery should be to restore normal anatomical relationships and to excise or fulgurate as much of the endometriosis as possible. Removal of severely diseased adnexa when the other side is more normal produces better results than attempts to do major repairs. Presacral neurectomy does not enhance fertility, although many surgeons advocate it to alleviate dysmenorrhea. This may be less compelling now that prostaglandin inhibitors are available to accomplish the same purpose. A careful study of presacral neurectomy concluded that this procedure is only indicated in patients with pain limited to the midline area.[75] The text by Buttram and Reiter is recommended for a description of surgical techniques.[76]

The success of surgery in relieving infertility is directly related to the severity of endometriosis. Patients with moderate disease can expect a pregnancy success of approximately 60%, whereas the comparable figure is 35% in those with severe disease.[74] There is no convincing evidence that surgical treatment of early endometriosis enhances fertility.[77] There is support for selective use of danazol for 2–3 months following laparoscopy and prior to conservative surgery, especially in patients with pain due to major disease.[78] Similar favorable effects should result from the preoperative treatment with a progestin or a gonadotropin releasing hormone agonist. Preoperative treatment aids surgery by softening endometrial implants. Postoperative use of hormones has been the subject of greater controversy. The highest pregnancy rates following conservative surgery occur in the first year after surgery, and most physicians have been reluctant to use hormones that prevent pregnancy even for a few months. If pregnancy does not occur within 2 years of surgery for endometriosis, the chances are poor that pregnancy will occur. The recurrence rates reported for endometriosis after surgery are usually below 20%, but when it does recur, second surgeries to aid fertility have only a limited chance for success.

The type of surgery that we have been discussing is labeled "conservative" to indicate that reproductive function is maintained. When endometriomas are removed a vigorous attempt should be made to leave behind any normal ovarian tissue. Even one-tenth of an ovary can be enough to preserve function and fertility. Conservative surgery can be accomplished by laparoscopy which decreases costs and morbidity, yet provides results that are as efficacious in all stages of disease as laparotomy.

"Conservative" surgery is in contradistinction to "radical" surgery, which includes hysterectomy and usually bilateral salpingo-oophorectomy. When radical surgery is performed, an uninvolved ovary can be preserved in some cases if all of the nonovarian endometriosis is removed by fulguration or excision. This does provide a risk for recurrent disease, but the risk seems to be small.

Hormonal Treatment of Endometriosis

Although hormonal therapy of infertility associated with endometriosis is not of proven value, medical therapy for dysmenorrhea, dyspareunia, and pelvic pain associated with endometriosis is very successful (although relief may be short-term). The various agents used are comparable in terms of efficacy. Implants of endometriosis react to steroid hormones in a manner somewhat, but not exactly, similar to normally stimulated endometrium. However, endometriotic tissue displays histologic differences and biochemical differences, including enzyme activity and receptor levels which differ in concentration and response compared to normal endometrium. Nevertheless, estrogen stimulates growth of the implants. For this reason, endometriosis usually regresses following menopause and is usually not found prior to menarche unless there is a blockage of the outflow tract.

Hormone therapy is designed to interrupt the cycle of stimulation and bleeding. An early approach was the use of massive doses of diethylstilbestrol (DES), which, because of variable success, the risk of affecting the fetus, and side effects of severe bleeding and nausea, is now of only historical interest. Treatment with androgens (methyltestosterone linguets 5–10 mg/day) can provide only transient relief of the pain of endometriosis, and its effect on infertility appears to be negligible. In addition, ovulation can occur while on treatment, and there is a risk of exposure of the fetus to the androgen.

Until the late 1970s the most important alternative to conservative surgery was the use of combination oral contraceptives taken in a continuous fashion.[79] It seems to matter little which low dose monophasic product is used to accomplish the conversion of endometrial implants into decidualized cells associated with a few inactive endometrial glands. At this time the efficacy of the multiphasic formulations is unknown. The usual dose of the combined oral contraceptive is one pill per day continuously for 6–12 months. Estrogen (conjugated estrogens 1.25 mg or estradiol 2.0 mg daily for 1 week) is added if breakthrough bleeding occurs. The treatment with oral contraceptives was called pseudopregnancy because of the amenorrhea and the decidualization of the endometrial tissue induced by the estrogen-progestin combination. It also reflected the commonly held belief that pregnancy can improve endometriosis, a belief that has been disputed. The side effects of treatment are those associated with oral contraceptives (Chapter 22). Pregnancy rates after stopping medication are reported to be in the 40–50% range. Whereas published recurrence rates are not excessive, this therapy, as with all hormone treatment for endometriosis, must be viewed as suppressive rather than curative.

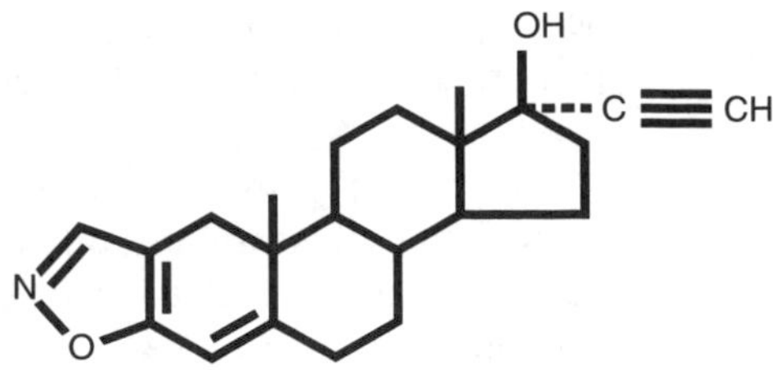

Danazol

Treatment with Danazol

The golden age for danazol has passed. Although its expense and side effects seemed a reasonable tradeoff for an effective treatment, it is now apparent that danazol is no more effective than the other medications used to treat endometriosis. In distinction to the pseudopregnancy induced by oral contraceptives, danazol produces what has been incorrectly termed as pseudomenopause. Danazol is an isoxazole derivative of the synthetic steroid 17α-ethinyltestosterone. It originally was thought to exert its effect solely by inhibition of pituitary gonadotropins. Although danazol can decrease follicle-stimulating hormone (FSH) and luteinizing hormone (LH) in castrated individuals, it does not alter basal gonadotropin concentrations in premenopausal women. It does, however, eliminate the midcycle surge of FSH and LH. Asch et al. demonstrated a shortening of the luteal phase in monkeys treated with danazol, an effect that was not reversed by injections of human chorionic gonadotropin (HCG), suggesting a direct effect on the ovary.[80] Similarly, danazol inhibits steroidogenesis in the human corpus luteum.[81] Danazol is metabolized to at least 60 different products, some of which may contribute to its many effects. The multiple actions of danazol include:[82]

1. Binding to androgen, progesterone, and glucocorticoid receptors, producing both agonistic and antagonistic actions.

2. No binding to intracellular estrogen receptors.

3. Binding to sex hormone binding globulin (displacing testosterone and thus increasing free testosterone) and to corticosteroid binding globulin (with a small increase in free cortisol).

4. Decrease in sex hormone binding globulin production by the liver as well as an increase in a host of other liver proteins.

5. Prevention of the midcyle surge of FSH and LH, but no significant suppression of basal FSH or LH (mainly an androgen agonistic action).

6. No effect on aromatization.

7. Inhibition of the following enzymes involved in steroidogenesis:
   cholesterol side chain cleavage enzyme (P450scc)
   3β-hydroxysteroid dehydrogenase
   17β-hydroxysteroid dehydrogenase
   17-hydroxylase, 17,20-lyase (P450 c17)
   11β-hydroxylase (P450c11)
   21-hydroxylase (P450c21)

The multiple effects of danazol produce a high androgen, low estrogen environment that does not support the growth of endometriosis, and the amenorrhea that is produced prevents new seeding from the uterus into the peritoneal cavity.

The side effects of danazol are related both to the hypoestrogenic environment it creates and to its androgenic properties. The most common side effects are weight gain, fluid retention, fatigue, decreased breast size, acne, oily skin, growth of facial hair, atrophic vaginitis, hot flushes, muscle cramps, and emotional lability. Some of these side effects occur in approximately 80% of women who are taking danazol, but less than 10% find the side effects sufficiently troublesome to warrant discontinuation of the drug. Because danazol has been associated with the development *in utero* of female pseudo-hermaphroditism, it should not be given if there is the possibility of pregnancy.[83] The androgenic action of danazol can irreversibly deepen the voice.[84,85] It is worth enquiring whether singing is an important part of your patient's life.

Danazol is metabolized largely in the liver, and in some patients it causes hepatocellular damage. Its use, therefore, is contraindicated in women with liver disease. Furthermore, liver enzymes should be monitored during treatment with danazol. The fluid retention that is often associated with danazol makes it dangerous to use when there is severe hypertension, congestive heart failure, or impaired renal function. It can produce increased cholesterol and low-density lipoprotein levels and decreased levels of high-density lipoprotein. It is unlikely that these short-term effects on lipids and lipoproteins are clinically important. The drug has been used to treat autoimmune disease, but it is not known if this action plays a role in its effects on endometriosis.

It should be noted again that treatment of mild endometriosis associated with infertility has been called into question because women with untreated mild endometriosis have pregnancy rates equal to women who have received treatment for the endometriosis. Thus, danazol treatment of infertility associated with mild endometriosis has no scientific support.

On the other hand, danazol is useful to relieve the pain of endometriosis and to prevent progression of the disease. Pain relief is obtained in 90% of patients. The usual dose is two 200 mg tablets twice a day (although some claim that spacing the drug at 6-hour intervals may be more effective) for 6 months. Dmowski and Cohen reviewed 99 women who completed danazol treatment for a period of 3–18 months (average 6 months) and who were reevaluated an average of 37 months later.[86] During the course of treatment all the patients had symptomatic improvement, and the majority (85%) were clinically improved. At the time of the reevaluation, however, approximately one-third were symptomatic and had clinical findings suggestive of recurrent endometriosis. In the majority of these patients, the symptoms recurred within the first year after discontinuation of the drug.

The success of danazol treatment is greatest in cases of peritoneal endometriosis or those with small lesions of the ovary. Endometriomas larger than 1.0 cm are less likely to respond to danazol, although quite surprising regression of endometriomas larger than 1.0 cm is sometimes seen.

Because of the significant side effects encountered with danazol, and its cost, there has been a trend toward the use of lower doses than the usual 800 mg daily. However, doses below 800 mg may be less effective.[87] The occurrence of amenorrhea appears to be correlated with improved outcome, and this is more consistently obtained at the 800 mg level. Others, however, do not believe that amenorrhea is an important consideration because many of the patients will bleed from an atrophic endometrium.

There is a general perception, but only limited experimental evidence, that danazol is more effective than oral contraceptives for the treatment of endometriosis.[88] Noble and Letchworth compared danazol with a high dose estrogen-progestin combination (Enovid).[89] The dose of both danazol and the oral contraceptive was increased until the patients became amenorrheic. One of 25 patients taking danazol could not complete 5 months of treatment, whereas 7 of 17 (41%) of the group taking oral contraceptives dropped out because of side effects. Danazol was more effective than estrogen-progestin in relieving symptoms, and laparoscopic assessment showed much better results with danazol. Seven of 12 danazol-treated patients became pregnant compared with 4 of the 10 women who had taken oral contraceptives. Unfortunately, the study size was too small to allow statistical analysis.

Treatment with a Progestational Agent

Both oral and injectable medroxyprogesterone acetate have been effective in treating endometriosis by causing decidualization and subsequent atrophy of endometrial tissue. Medroxyprogesterone acetate in an oral dose of 30 mg daily has been demonstrated to be as effective as danazol in treating endometriosis.[69] Similar results have been obtained with higher doses.[1] For this reason and because it is more cost-effective and there are fewer side effects, medroxyprogesterone acetate is often the first choice for medical treatment of endometriosis. High doses of medroxyprogesterone can adversely affect the lipoprotein profile; there is no reason to use a dose greater than 30 mg/day. Megestrol acetate has been administered in a dose of 40 mg daily with good results.[90]

Side effects include weight gain, fluid retention, and breakthrough bleeding. Breakthrough bleeding is a common occurrence, although it is usually cleared by short-term (7 days) administration of estrogen. Depression is a significant problem, and both patient and physician should be alert for its development. The usefulness of depo-medroxyprogesterone acetate (150 mg im every 3 months) in infertile patients is limited by the varying length of time it takes for ovulation to resume after discontinuation of therapy. This is not a problem with oral administration.

Medroxyprogesterone acetate, like danazol, can relieve the symptoms of endometriosis, but it is not effective in treating infertility. In a prospective, randomized clinical trial, there was no difference in pregnancy rates following treatment with medroxyprogesterone acetate (100 mg/day) or placebo.[91]

Treatment with GnRH Agonists

Gonadotropin releasing hormone has a short half-life because it is rapidly cleaved between amino acids 5–6, 6–7, and 9–10. Analogues of GnRH have been produced by altering the amino acids at these positions. Substitutions of amino acids at the 6 position and/or replacement of the C-terminal glycine-amide (inhibiting degradation) produce agonists. The GnRH agonists are administered intramuscularly, subcutaneously, or by intranasal absorption. After an initial agonistic action (the so-called flare response), down-regulation and desensitization of the pituitary produce a hypogonadotropic, hypogonad state. The depot formulation of leuprolide is administered intramuscularly and monthly. Goserelin consists of a small biodegradable cylinder which is inserted subcutaneously and monthly using a prepackaged syringe.

A long-acting GnRH agonist can create a pseudomenopause for the treatment of endometriosis.[92,93] At the end of 2–4 weeks of daily administration of the agonist, estrogen levels will decrease to those found in oophorectomized women. Dosage can be adjusted by monitoring serum estradiol levels; the best therapeutic effect is associated with a range of 20–40 pg/mL (75–150 pmol/L). Thus, the "medical oophorectomy" caused by the continuous use of a GnRH agonist has provided a new approach to the treatment of endometriosis. Excellent, large, well-designed studies (with advanced

Gonadotropin releasing
hormone

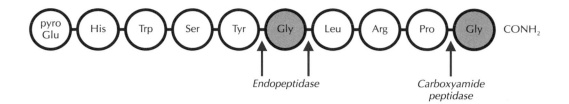

GnRH agonists

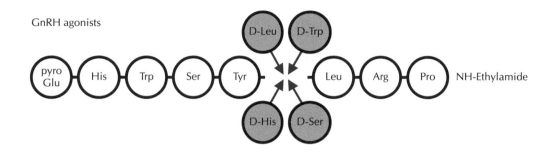

disease in nearly 50% of the patients) have compared GnRH agonist therapy (with various agents) with danazol.[94–98] The results in terms of reduction of disease (as demonstrated by post-treatment laparoscopies) and pregnancy rates have been the same with either treatment. However, GnRH agonist treatment does not have an adverse impact on serum lipids and lipoproteins compared to that observed with danazol.[99] An experimental comparison of agonist and progestin treatment in monkeys concluded that the progestin was just as effective as the agonist.[100]

An uneventful pregnancy delivering a normal infant has been reported despite GnRH agonist treatment (monthly treatment with a long-acting agonist was continued through the first two months of pregnancy).[101]

GnRH Agonists in Clinical Use

Position	1	2	3	4	5	6	7	8	9	10
Native GnRH	pGlu	His	Trp	Ser	Tyr	Gly	Leu	Arg	Pro	Gly-NH$_2$
Leuprolide						D-Leu				NH-Ethylamide
Buserelin						D-Ser (tertiary butanol)				NH-Ethylamide
Nafarelin						D-Naphthylalanine (2)				
Histrelin						D-His (tertiary benzyl)				NH-Ethylamide
Goserelin						D-Ser (tertiary butanol)				Aza-Gly
Deslorelin						D-Trp				NH-Ethylamide
Tryptorelin						D-Trp				

As with all other drug therapies of endometriosis, the GnRH agonist provides suppression rather than cure of the disease. The long-term consequences of the hypoestrogenic state on calcium metabolism and bone are of concern. Therefore, treatment is usually limited to 6 months to avoid bone loss, although even during this time period there can be a 6–8% decrease in trabecular bone density. This short-term bone loss is reversed after cessation of therapy; however, many patients as much as one year later have not regained the bone that was lost.[102,103] Long-term therapy, therefore, carries with it the concern over a lasting impact on the risk of osteoporosis. The addition of a progestational agent as add-back treatment can be effective in decreasing bone loss.[104,105] A postmenopausal estrogen-progestin program can be utilized (conjugated estrogens 0.625 mg daily and medroxyprogesterone acetate 2.5 mg daily). This combined add-back treatment is effective for endometriosis and prevents the hypoestrogenic symptoms (especially hot flushes and vaginal dryness) associated with GnRH agonist therapy, including loss of bone.[106] Endometriosis by itself is not a cause of accelerated bone loss.[107,108]

In well-designed trials, treatment with GnRH agonists has not increased pregnancy rates in women with infertility associated with minimal or mild endometriosis.[109]

Treatment with Gestrinone

Gestrinone, a 19-nortestosterone derivative, decreases the secretion of FSH and LH and has the advantage of requiring only twice a week administration. Used in Europe, it has been as effective as danazol in treating endometriosis.[110] The clinical side effects are also similar to those seen with danazol. As with other hormonal treatments, gestrinone has been ineffective for the infertility associated with endometriosis.[109]

Recurrence of Endometriosis

Endometriosis tends to recur unless definitive surgery is performed. The recurrence rate is approximately 5–20% per year (reaching a cumulative rate at 5 years as much as 40%). The recurrence rates 5 years after women were treated with various GnRH agonists were 37% for minimal disease and 74% for severe disease.[111] After 7 years, 56% of all treated women had a recurrence. In women treated for pelvic pain, the symptoms usually return rather quickly after cessation of therapy.[112] For a period of time after medical treatment, however, the intensity of symptoms is less severe.[95,113] The recurrence rates after treatment with GnRH agonists are similar to those after danazol, and both are greater than that obtained with surgical excision.

Speculation regarding the reason for recurrence focuses on endometriosis (perhaps microscopic) which escaped detection, incomplete treatment, or reestablishment of primary disease by whatever mechanism is responsible. The treatment choices and results are no different than when originally confronted.

Hormone Treatment after Surgery

Definitive surgery for severe endometriosis, which includes abdominal hysterectomy and bilateral salpingo-oophorectomy as well as resection of all endometriosis, is the only cure for the disease. If oophorectomy is performed, estrogen-progestin therapy at usual doses can be started immediately postoperatively with an essentially negligible risk of inciting growth of residual endometriosis. The addition of a progestational agent is strongly recommended because of reported cases of adenocarcinoma in endometriosis tissue in women treated with unopposed estrogen.[114,115]

Long-Term Hormonal Therapy

Long-term hormonal therapy without surgery is useful in patients with severe symptoms but with little in the way of palpable findings. Before undertaking prolonged therapy, diagnosis should be established by laparoscopy. Prolonged therapy also is indicated if symptoms recur after conservative surgery.

Prevention of Infertility

A common clinical problem is the incidental finding at surgery of mild endometriosis in a young woman who has no immediate interest in pregnancy. Cyclic combination oral contraceptives to prevent further seeding are appropriate for treatment of very mild disease, for example a few implants in the cul-de-sac. More advanced disease should be treated with 6 months of medroxyprogesterone acetate, a GnRH agonist, or danazol, followed by cyclic oral contraceptives to decrease the risks of progression of the disease. Although not well documented, clinical experience has suggested that continuous oral contraceptives are more effective as prophylaxis than the usual cyclic regimen. Indeed, we favor the continuous regimen without a break for this purpose.

As with all medical treatments, as time passes, endometriosis emerges. Although spontaneous regression occurs, endometriosis is usually progressive. The risk of endometriosis is reduced in women currently using oral contraceptives; however, effective prophylaxis requires long-term treatment.[116] Nevertheless, treatment of endometriosis does have a beneficial impact on the natural history of the disease.

Endometriosis and Spontaneous Abortion

Endometriosis has been purported to be associated with an increased risk of spontaneous abortion, a risk that is said to be substantially lessened by either hormonal or surgical treatment.[117] In appropriately controlled studies, however, the abortion rate was in the normal range in women with endometriosis who were not treated, and it is likely that previous studies were flawed by their choice of control abortion rates.[118,119]

Endometriosis and Ovulation

The frequency of anovulation and luteal phase defects is similar in women with and without endometriosis.[120,121] Thus, a woman need not be ovulating in order to have endometriosis. One report has suggested, however, that the success of ovulation induction in women with endometriosis is enhanced by prior treatment with danazol.[122]

Endometriosis and Assisted Reproduction

The use of superovulation with intrauterine insemination (Chapters 30 and 31) has been reported to increase fecundity rates in women with infertility associated with endometriosis.[123,124] However, although superovulation raised fecundity rates, it did not raise cumulative pregnancy rates.[125] This treatment may accelerate the occurrence of pregnancy without changing overall fertility.

Individuals with mild to moderate endometriosis do as well in in vitro fertilization programs as those with tubal disease. Although results with severe endometriosis have been poor in the past, more recent experience (perhaps reflecting improved technique and technology) has yielded good pregnancy rates (Chapter 31).

References

1. **Kauppila A,** Changing concepts of medical treatment of endometriosis, Acta Obstet Gynecol Scand 72:324, 1993.

2. **Olive DL, Schwartz LB,** Endometriosis, New Engl J Med 328:1759, 1993.

3. **Sampson JA,** Peritoneal endometriosis due to the menstrual dissemination of endometrial tissue into the peritoneal cavity, Am J Obstet Gynecol 14:422, 1927.

4. **Liu DTY, Hitchchock A,** Endometriosis: its association with retrograde menstruation, dysmenorrhea, and tubal pathology, Br J Obstet Gynaecol 93:859, 1986.

5. **Ishimaru T, Masuzaki H,** Peritoneal endometriosis: endometrial tissue implantation as its primary etiologic mechanism, Am J Obstet Gynecol 165:210, 1991.

6. **Jenkins S, Olive DL, Haney AF,** Endometriosis: pathogenetic implications of the anatomic distribution, Obstet Gynecol 67:335, 1986.

7. **Kruitwagen RFPM, Poels LG, Willemsen WNP, Jap PHK, Thomas CMG, Rolland R,** Endometrial epithelial cells in peritoneal fluid during the ealy follicular phase, Fertil Steril 55:297, 1991.

8. **Scott RB, TeLinde RW, Wharton LR Jr,** Further studies on experimental endometriosis, Am J Obstet Gynecol 66:1082, 1953.

9. **Olive DL, Henderson DY,** Endometriosis and müllerian anomalies, Obstet Gynecol 69:412, 1987.

10. **Cramer DW, Wilson E, Stillman RJ, Berger MJ, Belisle S, Schiff I, Albrecht B, Gibson M, Stadel BV,Schoenbaum SC,** The relation of endometriosis to menstrual characteristics, smoking and exercise, JAMA 355:1904, 1986.

11. **Ueki M,** Histologic study of endometriosis and examination of lymphatic drainage in and from the uterus, Am J Obstet Gynecol 165:201, 1991.

12. **Rock JA, Markham SM,** Extra pelvic endometriosis, in Wilson EA, editor, *Endometriosis,* Alan R. Liss, Inc., New York, 1987, pp 185–206.

13. **Foster DC, Stern JL, Buscema J, Rock JA, Woodruff JD,** Pleural and parenchymal pulmonary endometriosis, Obstet Gynecol 58:552, 1981.

14. **Metzger DA, Lessey BA, Soper JT, McCarty KS Jr, Haney AF,** Hormone-resistant endometriosis following total abdominal hysterectomy and bilateral salpingo-oophorectomy: correlation with histology and steroid receptor content, Obstet Gynecol 78:946, 1991.

15. **Suginami H,** A reappraisal of the coelomic metaplasia theory by reviewing endometriosis occurring in unusual sites and instances, Am J Obstet Gynecol 165:214, 1991.

16. **Schifrin BS, Erez S, Moore JG,** Teen-age endometriosis, Am J Obstet Gynecol 116:973, 1973.

17. **Clark AH,** Endometriosis in a young girl, JAMA 136:690, 1948.

18. **El-Mahgoub S, Yaseen S,** A positive proof for the theory of coelomic metaplasia, Am J Obstet Gynecol 137:137, 1980.

19. **Oliker AJ, Harris AE,** Endometriosis of the bladder in a male patient, J Urol 106:858, 1971.

20. **Schrodt GR, Alcorn MO, Ibanez J,** Endometriosis of the male urinary system: a case report, J Urol 124:722, 1980.

21. **Simpson JL, Elias J, Malinak LR, Buttram VC,** Heritable aspects of endometriosis. I. Genetic studies, Am J Obstet Gynecol 137:327, 1980.

22. **Dmowski WP, Steele RW, Baker GF,** Deficient cellular immunity in endometriosis, Am J Obstet Gynecol 141:377, 1981.

23. **Mathur S, Peress MR, Williamson HO, Youmans CD, Maney SA, Garvin AJ, Rust PF, Fudenberg HH,** Autoimmunity to endometrium and ovary in endometriosis, Clin Exp Immunol 50:259, 1982.

24. **Vigano P, Vercellini P, Di Blasio AM, Colombo A, Candiani GB, Vignali M,** Deficient antiendometrium lymphocyte-mediated cytotoxicity in patients with endometriosis, Fertil Steril 56:894, 1991.

25. **Oosterlynck DJ, Meuleman C, Waer M, Vandeputte M, Koninckx PR,** The natural killer activity of peritoneal fluid lymphocytes is decreased in women with endometriosis, Fertil Steril 58:292, 1992.

26. **Cramer DW,** Epidemiology of endometriosis, in Wilson EA, editor, *Endometriosis*, Alan R. Liss, Inc., New York, 1987, pp 5–22.

27. **Sanfillippo JS,** Endometriosis in adolescents, in Wilson EA, editor, *Endometriosis,* Alan R. Liss, Inc., New York, 1987, pp 161–172.

28. **Huffman JW,** Endometriosis in young teen-age girls, Pediatr Ann 10:501, 1981.

29. **Cornillie FJ, Oosterlynck D, Lauweryns JM, Konickx PR,** Deeply infiltrating pelvic endometriosis: histology and clinical significance, Fertil Steril 53:978, 1990.

30. **Barbieri RL, Niloff JM, Bast RC Jr, Schaetzl E, Kistner RW, Knapp RC,** Elevated serum concentrations of CA-125 in patients with advanced endometriosis, Fertil Steril 45:630, 1986.

31. **Pittaway DE,** The use of serial CA-125 concentrations to monitor endometriosis in infertile women, Am J Obstet Gynecol 163:1032, 1990.

32. **Franssen AMHW, van der Heijden PFM, Thomas CMG, Doesburg WH, Willemsen WNP, Rolland R,** On the origin and significance of serum CA-125 concentrations in 97 patients with endometriosis before, during, and after buserelin acetate, nafarelin, or danazol, Fertil Steril 57:974, 1992.

33. **Pittaway DE, Fayez JA,. Douglas JW,** Serum CA-125 in the evaluation of benign adnexal cysts, Am J Obstet Gynecol 157:1426, 1987.

34. **Friedman H, Vogelzang RL, Mendelson Eb, Neiman HL, Cohen M,** Endometriosis detection by US with laparoscopic correlation, Radiology 157.217, 1985.

35. **Arrivé L, Hricak H, Martin MC,** Pelvic endometriosis: MR imaging, Radiology 171:687, 1989.

36. **Jansen RPS, Russell P,** Nonpigmented endometriosis: clinical, laparoscopic and pathologic definition, Am J Obstet Gynecol 155:1154, 1986.

37. **Nisolle M, Paindaveine B, Bourdon A, Berlière M, Casanas-Roux F, Donnez J,** Histologic study of peritoneal endometriosis in infertile women, Fertil Steril 53:984, 1990.

38. **The American Fertility Society,** Revised American Fertility Society classification of endometriosis, Fertil Steril 43:351, 1985.

39. **The American Fertility Society,** Management of endometriosis in the presence of pelvic pain, Fertil Steril 60:952, 1993.

40. **Hornstein MD, Gleason RE, Orav J, Haas ST, Friedman AJ, Rein MS, Hill JA, Barbieri RL,** The reproducibility of the revised American Fertility Society classification of endometriosis, Fertil Steril 59:1015, 1993.

41. **Garcia CF, Davis SS,** Pelvic endometriosis: infertility and pelvic pain, Am J Obstet Gynecol 129:740, 1977.

42. **Schenken RS, Malinak LR,** Conservative surgery versus expectant management for the infertile patient with mild endometriosis, Fertil Steril 37:183, 1982.

43. **Seibel M, Berger MJ, Weinstein FG, Taymor ML,** The effectiveness of danazol on subsequent fertility in minimal endometriosis, Fertil Steril 38:534, 1982.

44. **Fedele L, Parazzini F, Radici E, Bocciolone L, Bianchi S, Bianci C, Candiani GB,** Buserelin acetate versus expectant management in the treatment of infertilty associated with minimal or mild endometriosis: a randomized clinical trial, Am J Obstet Gynecol 166:1345, 1992.

45. **Guzick DS,** Clinical epidemiology of endometriosis and infertility, Obstet Gynecol Clin North Am 16:43, 1989.

46. **Verkauf BS,** The incidence, symptoms and signs of endometriosis in fertile and infertile women, J Fla Med Assoc 74:671, 1987.

47. **Candiani GB, Vercellini P, Fedele L, Colombo A, Candiani M,** Mild endometriosis and infertility: a critical review of epidemiologic data, diagnostic pitfalls, and classification limits, Obstet Gynecol Survey 46:374, 1991.

48. **Toma SK, Stovall DW, Hammond MG,** The effect of laparoscopic ablation or Danocrine on pregnancy rates in patients with stage I or II endometriosis undergoing donor insemination, Obstet Gynecol 80:253, 1992.

49. **Badawy SZA, Elbakry MM, Samuel F, Dizer M,** Cumulative pregnancy rates in infertile women with endometriosis, J Reprod Med 33:757, 1988.

50. **Drake TS, Metz SA, Grunert GM, O'Brien WF,** Peritoneal fluid volume in endometriosis, Fertil Steril 34:280, 1980.

51. **Drake TS, O'Brien WF, Ramwell PW, Metz SA,** Peritoneal fluid thromboxane B_2 and 6-keto-prostaglandin $F_{1\alpha}$ in endometriosis, Am J Obstet Gynecol 140:401, 1981.

52. **Rock JA, Dubin NH, Ghodgaonkar RB, Berquist CA, Erozan YS, Kimball AW Jr,** Cul-de-sac fluid in women with endometriosis: fluid volume and prostanoid concentration during the proliferative phase of the cycle — days 8 to 12, Fertil Steril 37:747, 1982.

53. **Rezai N, Ghodgaonkar RB, Zacur HA, Rock JA, Dubin NH,** Cul-de-sac fluid in women with endometriosis: fluid volume, protein and prostanoid concentration during the periovulatory period — days 13 to 18, Fertil Steril 48:29, 1987.

54. **Sgarlatta CS, Hertelendy F, Mikhail G,** The prostanoid content in peritoneal fluid and plasma of women with endometriosis, Am J Obstet Gynecol 147:563, 1983.

55. **Mudge TJ, James MJ, Jones WR, Walsh JA,** Peritoneal fluid 6-keto-prostaglandin $F_{1\alpha}$ levels in women with endometriosis, Am J Obstet Gynecol 152:901, 1985.

56. **DeLeon FD, Vijayakumar R, Brown M, Rao CV, Yussman MA, Schultz G,** Peritoneal fluid volume, estrogen, progesterone, prostaglandin, and epidermal growth factor concentrations in patients with and without endometriosis, Obstet Gynecol 68:189, 1986.

57. **Vernon MW, Beard JS, Graves K, Wilson EA,** Classification of endometriotic implants by morphologic appearance and capacity to synthesize prostaglandin F, Fertil Steril 46:801, 1986.

58. **Koike H, Egawa H, Ohtsuka T, Yamaguchi M, Ikenoue T, Mori N,** Correlation between dysmenorrheic severity and prostaglandin production in women with endometriosis, Prostaglandins Leukot Essent Fatty Acids, 46:133, 1992.

59. **Halme J, Becker S, Wing R,** Accentuated cyclic activation of peritoneal macrophages in patients with endometriosis, Am J Obstet Gynecol 148:85, 1984.

60. **Chacho KJ, Chacho MS, Andresen PJ, Scommegna A,** Peritoneal fluid in patients with and without endometriosis: prostanoids and macrophages and their effect on the spermatozoa penetration assay, Am J Obstet Gynecol 154:1290, 1986.

61. **Muscato JJ, Haney AF, Weinberg JB,** Sperm phagocytosis by human peritoneal macrophages: a possible cause of infertility and endometriosis, Am J Obstet Gynecol 144:503, 1982.

62. **Stone SC, Himsl K,** Peritoneal recovery of motile and nonmotile sperm in the presence of endometriosis, Fertil Steril 46:338, 1986.

63. **Mori H, Sawairi M, Nakagawa M, Itoh N, Wada K, Tamaya T,** Expression of interleukin-1 (IL-1) beta messenger ribonucleic acid (mRNA) and IL-1 receptor antagonist mRNA in peritoneal macrophages from patients with endometriosis, Fertil Steril 57:535, 1992.

64. **Doody MC, Gibbons WE, Buttram VC Jr,** Linear regression analysis of ultrasound follicular growth series: evidence for an abnormality of follicular growth in endometriosis patients, Fertil Steril 49:47, 1988.

65. **Mahmood TA, Templeton A,** Folliculogenesis and ovulation in infertile women with mild endometriosis, Hum Reprod 6:227, 1991.

66. **Olive DL, Haney AF,** Endometriosis-associated infertility: a critical review of therapeutic approaches, Obstet Gynecol Survey 41:538, 1986.

67. **Portuondo JA, Echanojauregui AD, Herran C, Alijarte I,** Early conception in patients with untreated mild endometriosis, Fertil Steril 39:22, 1983.

68. **Olive DL, Stohs GF, Metzger DA, Franklin RR,** Expectant management and hydrotubations in the treatment of endometriosis-associated infertility, Fertil Steril 44:35, 1985.

69. **Hull ME, Moghissi KS, Magyar DF, Haves MF,** Comparison of different treatment modalities of endometriosis in infertile women, Fertil Steril 47:40, 1987.

70. **Tulandi T, Mouchawar M,** Treatment-dependent and treatment-independent pregnancy in women with minimal and mild endometriosis, Fertil Steril 56:790, 1991.

71. **Haney AF,** The risks/benefits of laparoscopic cautery for endometriosis, Fertil Steril 55:243, 1991.

72. **Buttram VC Jr, Betts JW,** Endometriosis, Curr Probl Obstet Gynecol 11:No. 11, 1979.

73. **Fayez JA, Collazo LM, Vernon C,** Comparison of different modalities of treatment for minimal and mild endometriosis, Am J Obstet Gynecol 159:927, 1988.

74. **Olive DL, Lee KL,** Analysis of sequential treatment protocols for endometriosis-associated infertility, Am J Obstet Gynecol 154:613, 1986.

75. **Candiani GB, Fedele L, Vercellini P, Bianchi S, Di Nola G,** Presacral neurectomy for the treatment of pelvic pain associated with endometriosis: a controlled study, Am J Obstet Gynecol 167:100, 1992.

76. **Buttram VC Jr, Reiter RC,** *Surgical Treatment of the Infertile Female,* Williams & Wilkins, Baltimore, 1985.

77. **Adamson GD, Hurd SJ, Pasta DJ, Rodriguez BD,** Laparoscopic endometriosis treatment: is it better? Fertil Steril 59:35, 1993.

78. **Donnez J, Lemaire-Rubbers M, Karaman Y, Nisolle-Pochet M, Casanas-Roux F,** Combined (hormonal and microsurgical) therapy in infertile women with endometriosis, Fertil Steril 48:239, 1987.

79. **Kistner RW,** Management of endometriosis in the infertile patient, Fertil Steril 26:1151, 1975.

80. **Asch RH, Fernandez EO, Siler-Khodr TM, Bartke A, Pauerstein CJ,** Mechanism of induction of luteal phase defects by danazol, Am J Obstet Gynecol 136:932, 1980.

81. **Barbieri RL, Osathanondh R, Ryan KJ,** Danazol inhibition of steroidogenesis in the human corpus luteum, Obstet Gynecol 57:722, 1981.

82. **Barbieri RL, Hornstein MD,** Medical therapy for endometriosis, in Wilson EA, editor, *Endometriosis,* Alan R. Liss, Inc., New York, 1987, pp 111–140.

83. **Quagliarello J, Alba Greco M,** Danazol and urogenital sinus formation in pregnancy, Fertil Steril 43:939, 1985.

84. **Wardle PG, Whitehead MI, Mills RP,** Nonreversible and wide ranging vocal changes after treatment with danazol, Br Med J 287:946, 1983.

85. **Mercaitis PA, Peaper RE, Schwartz PA,** Effect of danazol on vocal pitch: a case study, Obstet Gynecol 65:131, 1985.

86. **Dmowski WP, Cohen MR,** Antigonadotropin (danazol) in the treatment of endometriosis: evaluation of post-treatment fertility and three-year follow-up data, Am J Obstet Gynecol 130:41, 1978.

87. **Dmowski WP, Kapetanakis E, Scommegna A,** Variable effects of danazol on endometriosis at 4 low-dose levels, Obstet Gynecol 59:408, 1982.

88. **Barbieri RL, Evans S, Kistner RW,** Danazol in the treatment of endometriosis: analysis of 100 cases with a 4-year follow-up, Fertil Steril 37:737, 1982.

89. **Noble AD, Letchworth AT,** Medical treatment of endometriosis: a comparative trial, Postgrad Med J 55 (Suppl 5):37, 1979.

90. **Schlaff WD, Dugoff L, Damewood MD, Rock JA,** Megestrol acetate for treatment of endometriosis, Obstet Gynecol 75:646, 1990.

91. **Tellima S,** Danazol and medroxyprogesterone acetate inefficacious in the treatment of infertility in endometriosis, Fertil Steril 50:872, 1988.

92. **Meldrum DR,** Clinical management of endometriosis with luteinizing hormone-releasing hormone analogues, Seminars Reprod Endocrinol 3:371, 1985.

93. **Lemay A, Sandow J, Bureau M, Maheux R, Fontaine J-Y, Merat P,** Prevention of follicular maturation in endometriosis by subcutaneous infusion of luteinizing hormone-releasing hormone agonist started in the luteal phase, Fertil Steril 49:410, 1988.

94. **Henzl MR, Corson SL, Moghissi K, Buttram VC, Berqvist C, Jacobson J,** Administration of nasal nafarelin as compared with oral danazol for endometriosis, New Engl J Med 318:485, 1988.

95. **The Nafarelin European Endometriosis Trial Group,** Nafarelin for endometriosis: a large-scale, danazol-controlled trial of efficacy and safety, with 1-year follow-up, Fertil Steril 57:514, 1992.

96. **Wheeler JM, Knittle JD, Miller JD,** Depot leuprolide versus danazol in treatment of women with symptomatic endometriosis, Am J Obstet Gynecol 167:1367, 1992.

97. **Wheeler JM, Knittle JD, Miller JD, for the Lupron Endometriosis Study Group,** Depot leuprolide acetate versus danazol in the treatment of women with symptomatic endometriosis: a multicenter, double-blind randomized clinical trial. II. Assessment of safety, Am J Obstet Gynecol 169:26, 1993.

98. **Rock JA, Truglia JA, Caplan RJ, and the Zoladex Endometriosis Study Group,** Zoladex (goserelin acetate implant) in the treatment of endometriosis: a randomized comparison with danazol, Obstet Gynecol 82:198, 1993.

99. **Välimäki M, Nilsson G, Roine R, Ylikorkala O,** Comparison between the effects of nafarelin and danazol on serum lipids and lipoproteins in patients with endometriosis, J Clin Endocrinol Metab 69:1097, 1989.

100. **Mann DR, Collins DC, Smith MM, Kessler MJ, Gould KG,** Treatment of endometriosis in monkeys: effectiveness of continuous infusion of a gonadotropin-releasing hormone agonist compared to treatment with a progestational steroid, J Clin Endocrinol Metab 63:1277, 1986.

101. **Har-Toov J, Brenner SH, Jaffa A, Yavetz H, Peyser MR, Lessing JB,** Pregnancy during long-term gonadotropin-releasing hormone agonist therapy associated with clinical pseudomenopause, Fertil Steril 59:446, 1993.

102. **Henzl MR,** Gonadotropin-releasing analogs: update on new findings, Am J Obstet Gynecol 166:757, 1992.

103. **Dawood MY,** Impact of medical treatment of endometriosis on bone mass, Am J Obstet Gynecol 168:674, 1993.

104. **Cedars M, Lu JKH, Meldrum DR, Judd HL,** Treatment of endometriosis with a long acting gonadotropin-releasing hormone agonist plus medroxyprogesterone acetate, Obstet Gynecol 75:641, 1990.

105. **Surrey ES, Judd HL,** Reduction of vasomotor symtptoms and bone mineral density loss with combined norethindrone and long-acting gonadotropin-releasing hormone agonist therapy of symptomatic endometriosis: a prospective randomized trial, J Clin Endocrinol Metab 75:558, 1992.

106. **Friedman AJ, Hornstein MD,** Gonadotropin-releasing hormone agonist plus estrogen-progestin "add-back" therapy for endometriosis-related pelvic pain, Fertil Steril 60:236, 1993.

107. **Lane N, Baptista J, Snow-Harter C,** Bone mineral density of the lumbar spine in endometriosis subjects compared to an age-similar control population, J Clin Endocrinol Metab 72:510, 1991.

108. **Rico H, Revilla M, Arnanz F, Villa LF, Perera S, Arribas I,** Total and regional bone mass values and biochemical markers of bone remodeling in endometriosis, Obstet Gynecol 81:272, 1993.

109. **Hughes EG, Fedorkow DM, Collins JA,** A quantitative overview of controlled trials in endometriosis-associated infertility, Fertil Steril 59:963, 1993.

110. **Fedele L, Bianchi S, Viezzoli T, Arcaini L, Candiani GB,** Gestrinone versus danazol in the treatment of endometriosis, Fertil Steril 51:781, 1989.

111. **Waller KG, Shaw RW,** Gonadotropin-releasing hormone analogues for the treatment of endometriosis: long-term follow-up, Fertil Steril 59:511, 1993.

112. **Vercellini P, Trespidi L, Colombo A, Vendola N, Marchini M, Crosignani PG,** A gonadotropin-releasing hormone agonist versus a low-dose oral contraceptive for pelvic pain associated with endometriosis, Fertil Steril 60:75, 1993.

113. **Fedele L, Bianchi S, Bocciolone L, Di Nola G, Franchi D,** Buserelin acetate in the treatment of pelvic pain associated with minimal and mild endometriosis: a controlled study, Fertil Steril 59:516, 1993.

114. **Reimnitz C, Brand E, Nieberg RK, Hacker NF,** Malignancy arising in endometriosis associated with unopposed estrogen replacement, Obstet Gynecol 71:444, 1988.

115. **Heaps JM, Nieberg RK, Berek JS,** Malignant neoplasms arising in endometriosis, Obstet Gynecol 75:1023, 1990.

116. **Vessey MP, Villard-Mackintosh L, Painter R,** Epidemiology of endometriosis in women attending family-planning clinics, Br Med J 306:182, 1993.

117. **Groll M,** Endometriosis and spontaneous abortion, Fertil Steril 41:933, 1984.

118. **Metzger DA, Olive DL, Stohs GF, Franklin RR,** Association of endometriosis and spontaneous abortion: effect of control group selection, Fertil Steril 45:18, 1986.

119. **FitzSimmons J, Stahl R, Gocial B, Shapiro SS,** Spontaneous abortion and endometriosis, Fertil Steril 47:696, 1987.

120. **Pittaway DE, Maxson W, Daniell J, Herbert C, Wentz AC,** Luteal phase defects in infertility patients with endometriosis, Fertil Steril 39:712, 1983.

121. **Kusuhara K,** Luteal function in infertile patients with endometriosis, Am J Obstet Gynecol 167:274, 1992.

122. **Dmowski WP, Radwanska E, Binor Z, Rana N,** Mild endometriosis and ovulatory dysfunction: effect of danazol treatment on success of ovulation induction, Fertil Steril 46:784, 1986.

123. **Dodson WC, Whitesides DB, Hughes CL Jr, Easley HA III, Haney AF,** Superovulation with intrauterine insemination in the treatment of infertility: a possible alternative to gamete intrafallopian transfer and in vitro fertilization, Fertil Steril 48:441, 1987.

124. **Chaffkin LM, Nulsen JC, Luciano AA, Metzger DA,** A comparative analysis of the cycle fecundity rates associated with combined human menopausal gonadotropin (hMG) and intrauterine insemination (IUI) versus either hMG or IUI alone, Fertil Steril 55:252, 1991.

125. **Fedele L, Bianchi S, Marchini M, Villa L, Brioschi D, Parazzini F,** Superovulation with human menopausal gonadotropins in the treatment of infertility associated with minimal or mild endometriosis: a controlled randomized study, Fertil Steril 58:28, 1992.

29   Male Infertility

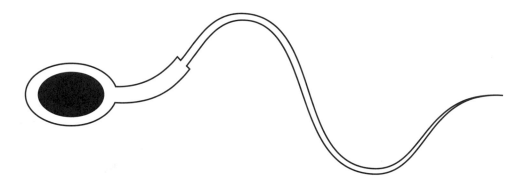

The perception of the degree of male involvement in infertility has undergone a number of revisions during the past 50 years. Initially, infertility was considered primarily a female problem. This notion gave way to the realization that 40% of infertility is wholly or in part due to a male factor. More recently, there have been attempts to redefine, in a downward direction, the lower limit of "normal" for a sperm count. Thus, many men who in the past would have been categorized as subfertile now are considered normal, and the focus has returned to their female partners.

Despite these changes, there is no doubt that a substantial percentage of infertility is due to deficiencies in the semen. For that reason it is important to be knowledgeable concerning male infertility. After initial evaluation, it is our responsibility to determine whether urologic consultation is required. This chapter will consider the analysis of semen and the newer functional tests, indicate factors responsible for abnormalities of the semen, and consider available treatment for problems of male infertility, including artificial insemination.

Regulation of the Testes

The testes have 2 distinct components, the seminiferous tubules (site of spermatogenesis) and the Leydig cells (source of testosterone). The function of these 2 components requires both pituitary gonadotropins, follicle-stimulating hormone (FSH) and luteinizing hormone (LH). The primary effect of LH is to stimulate the synthesis and secretion of testosterone by Leydig cells (about 5–10 mg per day), an effect that is enhanced by FSH, which also binds to Leydig cells and increases the number of LH receptors on the cells. Increasing levels of testosterone, in turn, inhibit LH secretion, acutely through the hypothalamus and chronically at the pituitary level. This negative feedback action does not require aromatization to estrogen. In men virtually all the estrone and estradiol present is derived from androstenedione and testosterone; there is essentially no direct secretion of estrogen.

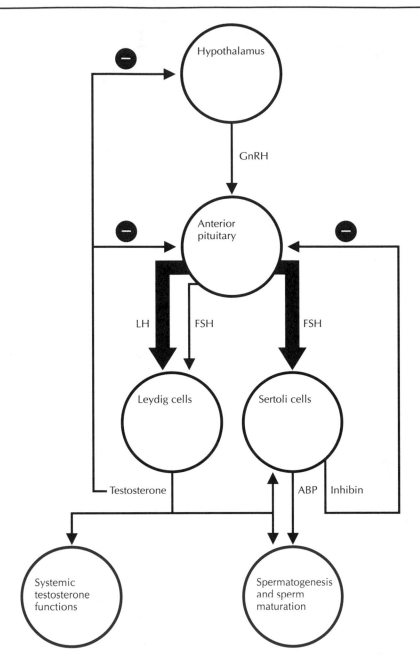

Leydig cells contain receptors for prolactin. Prolactin at normal levels stimulates testosterone secretion, whereas hypersecretion of prolactin leads to reduced testosterone secretion. Although studies suggest that prolactin synergises with LH and testosterone in the testes, a role for prolactin has not been established for normal testicular function.

FSH, in conjunction with testosterone, acts on the seminiferous tubules to stimulate spermatogenesis. This effect may be mediated by activation of Sertoli cell function. The Sertoli cells are controlled by 2 hormones, FSH and testosterone. FSH binds to Sertoli cells and stimulates the production of several proteins, chief of which is ABP, the androgen binding protein. Spermatogenesis requires a very high local concentration of testosterone and dihydrotestosterone, 50 times higher than that present in the circulation and greater than can be administered exogenously. The ABP is secreted into the tubule lumen and binds testosterone and dihydrotestosterone as they diffuse into the lumen, concentrating the androgens in the seminiferous epithelium for spermatogenesis and in the epididymis for sperm maturation.

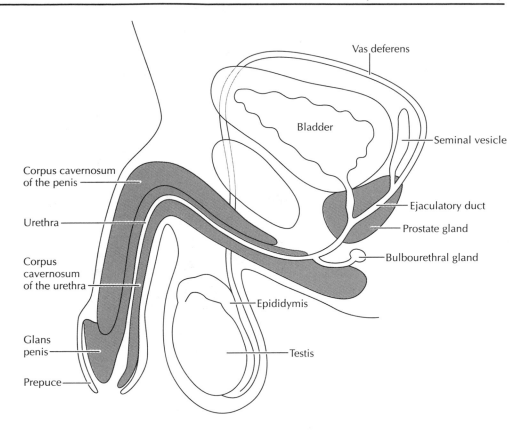

In contrast to the effects of testosterone on LH, steroid hormones at physiologic levels do not suppress FSH secretion. Orchiectomy is followed, however, by a rise in FSH levels. This phenomenon led to the discovery of inhibin. Inhibin is synthesized in the Sertoli cells in response to FSH and specifically inhibits FSH secretion in the pituitary.[1] Inhibin has been found in seminal fluid, spermatozoa, and Sertoli cells. The story is more complicated in that inhibin is also found in Leydig cells, and its secretion is further modulated by LH, human chorionic gonadotropin (HCG), and testosterone. Undoubtedly, autocrine/paracrine regulation by growth factors and local peptides is involved in a system analagous to the complex interaction in the ovarian follicle.

The seminiferous tubules and the intraluminal environment are controlled by the Sertoli cells. Tight junctions between the Sertoli cells effectively seal off the tubules, creating the blood-testis barrier. The seminiferous tubules, therefore, are essentially avascular, and regulatory substances must enter by diffusion. The blood-testis barrier protects the germ cells from antigens, antibodies, and environmental toxins. The Leydig cells are in the connective tissue between the seminiferous tubules.

Developing sperm are enveloped by Sertoli cells that influence the sequential process of spermatogenesis. Spermatogonia undergo mitotic division to form the primary spermatocytes, which in turn form the haploid (23 chromosomes) secondary spermatocytes by meiotic division. The secondary spermatocytes proceed through a maturation process to the spermatid stage, ultimately becoming the spermatozoa. In female somatic cells, one X chromosome is inactivated; however, in the oocyte both X chromosomes are genetically active. The opposite situation prevails in the male where the single X chromosome is genetically active in somatic cells but inactive in spermatogenesis. Normal spermatogenesis is directed by the genes on the Y chromosome, although many required regulating proteins are derived from autosomal chromosomes.[2]

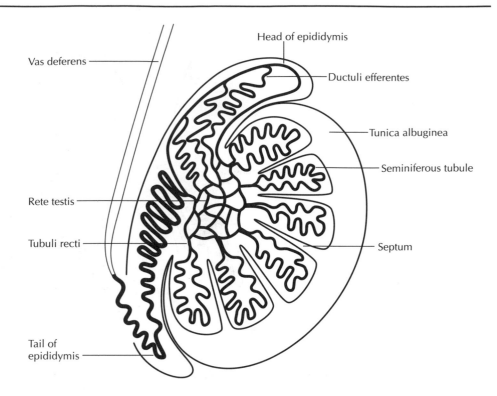

There is an age-related decline in spermatogenesis that results in some decline in male fertility. Precise estimates of the magnitude of this decline are not available because this issue has not been studied. There is no doubt, however, that many elderly men continue to have the ability to produce pregnancies.

Most of the testis is composed of the tightly coiled seminiferous tubule, which, if uncoiled, would reach a length of 70 cm. Approximately 74 days are required to produce spermatozoa, about 50 days of which are spent in the tubule. After leaving the testes, sperm take 12–21 days to travel the epididymis (which is 5–6 meters long) and appear in the ejaculate. The vas deferens is 30–35 cm in length, begins at the cauda epididymis and terminates in the ejaculatory duct near the prostate. Because of the long development and transit times the semen analysis can reflect events which occurred days or weeks earlier. The semen is composed of secretions contributed in a sequential fashion, first the prostatic fluid and contents of the distal vas deferens, followed by seminal vesicle secretions.

Semen Analysis

An abstinence period of 2–3 days prior to semen collection is adequate, although some urologists favor 5 days. Increasing the ejaculatory frequency reduces the volume and count but has no significant impact on quality (morphology and motility). The specimen should be collected directly into a clean container and not into a condom because the latter contains spermicidal agents. Sheathes are available that do not contain a spermicidal agent, and they can be used if the man cannot, or will not, obtain a specimen by masturbation. Collection of a specimen by withdrawal runs the risk of losing the first part of the specimen that contains the highest concentration of sperm. The specimen should be protected from the cold and delivered to the laboratory within 1 hour of collection. Semen liquefication, which occurs 20–30 minutes after ejaculation, is a necessary prerequisite for doing an accurate analysis. On occasion, a specimen does not undergo normal liquefication or is abnormally viscid, and, if this is associated with a poor postcoital test, it may be a factor in infertility. Techniques used to break up a viscid specimen in preparation for doing a sperm count or for artificial insemination include mechanically dispersing the gel by running the semen repeatedly through a number 19 needle, collecting the semen as a split ejaculate because the first part may be less viscid or treating the semen with proteolytic enzymes. If the postcoital test is normal, however, high viscosity probably is not an infertility factor.

There is reason to believe that sperm counts are decreasing.[3] In MacLeod's 1951 report, 5% of fertile men had counts below 20 million, while today 20–25% of fertile men have counts below 20 million.[4–7] The mean sperm count in Denmark in 1990 was 66 million/mL compared to 113 million/mL in 1940.[3] An argument can be made for an impact due to increased toxins in our environment. Despite suggestions that there is a decrease in sperm counts, the percent of American married couples who were infertile did not change significantly between 1962 and 1988. Thus, the apparent decrease in sperm count is not reflected in a parallel change in the rate of infertility.

Defining male infertility on the basis of sperm count or motility has become more complicated in the past decade. Whereas it is still true that very poor sperm counts (less than 5 million/mL) and very low motilities (less than 20%) indicate compromised fertility, values previously considered to be in the infertile range may, in fact, be compatible with normal fertility. Moreover, evaluation of sperm morphology, motion patterns, such as lateral head displacement, or sperm velocity may provide better prognostic information than count or motility. To add to the difficulties of diagnosing male infertility is the variability in count and motility that can be seen in successive semen specimens from the same individual. This leads to one truism: at least two or preferably three samples must be screened before an individual can be categorized as potentially fertile, subfertile, or infertile (azoospermia). Because it can take 2.5 months for the testes to recover from an insult, it is reasonable to space the specimens over a longer period of time.

There have been conflicting statements in textbooks and articles pertaining to the lower limit of normal for the sperm count. The most commonly cited figures are 60 million/mL, 40 million/mL, 20 million/mL, and 10 million/mL, with the 20 million/mL figure being the generally accepted standard.[4,7–9] Confidence in any figure is limited by the inaccuracies inherent in the methods used for counting sperm. When a group of technicians and pathologists used a counting chamber to do a semen analysis on the same pooled specimen, the mean sperm count was 46.7 million/mL with a range of values lying between 10 and 98 million/mL, giving a coefficient of variation of 37.8%.[10] These inconsistent results are not necessarily remedied even with computer-assisted semen analysis (CASA). Significant errors can still occur with CASA, especially with specimens containing low numbers where other cells can be miscounted as sperm.[11] Perhaps this is one reason it has been difficult to establish a prognostic value for the sperm count.[12] A similar, albeit somewhat lesser, uncertainty surrounds assessments of sperm motility.

The World Health Organization (WHO) suggests the following for normal values, but these should be viewed as rough guidelines only.[13]

Volume	**2.0 mL or more**
Sperm concentration	**20 million/mL or more**
Motility	**50% or more with forward progression, or 25% or more with rapid progression within 60 minutes of ejaculation**
Morphology	**30% or more normal forms**
White blood cells	**fewer than 1 million/mL**
Immunobead test	**fewer than 20% spermatozoa with adherent particles**
SpermMar test	**fewer than 10% spermatozoa with adherent particles**

In an attempt to increase the prognostic value of the routine semen analysis the results of the sperm count and the percentage of motility have been combined to give total motile sperm count (total sperm in the ejaculate x percent motility) or motile sperm per milliliter (sperm per mL x percent motility). The combining of count and motility allows determination of the number or concentration of active sperm and may provide a more informative way to present the data. Males with less than 24 months of infertility and a motile sperm count of greater than 10 million/mL have a higher pregnancy rate than those with 2–10 million/mL motile sperm.[14] Even with motile sperm counts less than 5.1 million/mL the pregnancy rate was 37.5%.[15] However, with counts between 60.1 and 100 million motile sperm/mL, the pregnancy rate rose to 78.6%. Whereas trends are evident, the overlapping results limit the prognostic power of combining sperm count and sperm motility.

Sperm Morphology

Until recently the clinician's trust in laboratory evaluations of sperm morphology was often misplaced. Interpretations of the normality of individual sperm varied widely among different observers. Even use of atlases of sperm morphology as guides was of only limited value. Then Katz and Overstreet introduced an overlay to use with video microscopy, which allowed a more standardized assessment of morphology.[16] With this method the coefficient of variation between observers was markedly reduced. Kruger and coworkers, in a series of articles, championed morphology as the best prognostic indicator for subsequent successful fertilization with in vitro fertilization.[17] They utilize "strict criteria" that shift many sperm out of the normal category by including as abnormal, sperm with even minor abnormalities as well as those with abnormalities of the acrosome (in addition to the usual head and tail abnormalities).

Using these strict criteria males with greater than 14% normal forms have normal rates of fertilization with in vitro fertilization, whereas those with less than 4% normal forms have fertilization rates of only 7–8%.[14] Values between 4% and 14% normal forms are associated with intermediate rates of fertilization. Technicians well trained in using strict criteria can provide highly reproducible results, but the standardization may not be possible on a more widespread scale. Interobserver differences in assessing sperm morphology could be eliminated if newly developed computer-assisted morphometric evaluations prove to be workable.[18]

Other Parameters

Whereas the count, motility, and morphology of the specimen constitute the major parameters on which the male's fertility is categorized, there are other characteristics of the semen that may impact on fertility potential. A volume of less than 1 mL may be too small to make contact with the cervix, and a volume greater than 7 mL may dilute the sperm concentration so that insufficient numbers are in close proximity to the cervix.

Round cells in the specimen can be either white cells or immature cells. The WHO standards manual states that a normal ejaculate should not contain more than 5 million round cells per mL (5 per high power field) while the number of leukocytes should not exceed 1 million per mL.[13] There are staining methods, biochemical tests, and immunologic techniques to differentiate immature cells from white cells, but these tests are not commonly performed.[19] In most laboratory reports all round cells are lumped together as white blood cells. It is reasonable to obtain a culture, perhaps by prostatic massage, when the report states that there are 5 or more white cells per high power field, even though some of these may be immature cells.

Repetitive agglutination of sperm (except when it is on pieces of debris) is suggestive of an immunologic effect or an infection. It may, however, be nonspecific and of no significance. Although it is common practice to evaluate the pH of semen because abnormalities may provide a clue to disorders of the accessory glands, in practice this measurement is of little value.

Tests of Sperm Function

In considering some of the other tests of sperm quality and function, it is of value to categorize them as being used commonly in clinical practice, those that are used occasionally in clinical practice, those that are probably not clinically useful, and those that are experimental.

A Test Used Commonly in Clinical Practice

Sperm penetration assay (SPA)

The zona pellucida of most mammalian species presents not only a block to polyspermia but also a barrier to fertilization of an egg by sperm of a different species. However, if the zona is removed by gentle enzyme digestion, foreign sperm can fuse with and penetrate an egg. In the sperm penetration assay, eggs are collected from superovulated golden hamsters; the zonae are removed by enzymes, and the denuded eggs are cultured for 2–3 hours with human sperm that have been washed and incubated overnight in culture media.[20] Presence of a swollen sperm head in the egg cytoplasm is evidence of successful penetration. Most laboratories report the percentage of eggs penetrated and compare this figure to the percent penetrated by a known fertile sperm specimen (some laboratories use the criterion of number of sperm penetrations per egg with 2 or more considered normal). Whereas the concept of the SPA as a measure of sperm fertilizing ability is an attractive one, the practical aspects of the test have hindered its standardization. For example, the source of the albumin used as the protein supplement in the media can influence the result as can use of resuspended compared to swimup sperm. Moreover, an individual's results in the SPA can vary over time. In addition, different laboratories utilize different cutoff points for the lower limit of normal penetration with the most common points being 0, 10, 14, and 20%.

Equally important has been a continuing controversy over the prognostic value of the test. A meta-analysis concluded that the test was not of value.[21] Other authors, however, have found correlations with eventual fertility. An SPA result of greater than 19% was associated with a pregnancy rate of 48%, whereas below 20% eggs penetrated was associated with a pregnancy rate of 20%.[22] However, even with an SPA of 0% the pregnancy rate in this series was 16%. This has been a common finding. Failure of the sperm to penetrate the hamster egg is not an absolute indication that the sperm cannot penetrate the human egg. Because of this limitation of the SPA, attempts have been made to optimize the test with a goal of eliminating these false negative results. Strategies to eliminate or to lower the number of false negative tests include treatment of sperm with follicular fluid, test yolk buffer, calcium ionophore, miniaturizing the test, and adjusting the concentration of albumin or the ions in the culture media.[23,24] With any of these maneuvers an SPA showing no or low penetration should be a more accurate harbinger of poor results in human in vitro fertilization (IVF). Although the tests are still not 100% accurate, if an optimized SPA has zero penetration, the couple should be given the option of considering use of donor sperm. In contrast to the problems with low SPAs, normal levels of sperm penetration correlate quite well, although not absolutely, with human fertilization in vivo and in vitro.

What is the value of the SPA in clinical practice? First, it may identify abnormalities of sperm not evident by studies of count, motility, or morphology. Thus, its major role is in screening couples with unexplained infertility. A second area is the screening of poor sperm specimens, but it is precisely in this important area that the accuracy of the SPA remains to be established. A third possible use of the SPA is as an endpoint for the study of sperm-enhancing procedures. For example, if treatment of sperm with follicular fluid increases penetration in the SPA, then this observation may provide a rationale for similar treatment in preparation for human IVF.

Tests Used Occasionally in Clinical Practice

Human Zona Binding Assay

Whereas the SPA tests the ability of sperm to penetrate or to be engulfed by the egg, it does not test the critical ability to pass through the zona pellucida. The zonae are, of course, removed in preparation for the SPA because they are, with rare exceptions, impervious to foreign sperm. Thus, to test zona penetrating or zona binding ability of human sperm requires the use of human zonae. One approach is to use zonae obtained from surgically removed ovarian tissue and slit them in half so that both patient sperm and donor sperm can be tested in parallel on different portions of the same zona.[25] The ratio of the number of sperm bound for the test subject to the number of sperm bound for fertile control sperm has been labeled the hemizona assay index (HZI). A breakpoint at an HZI value of 36 has provided a good correlation with results in human IVF.[26] Despite these good results the limited availability of zonae will restrict the overall utilization of this test. Moreover, variability in test results between laboratories can be anticipated, which means that each laboratory must establish its own range of normal values. In the future, development of materials that mimic the properties of the zona should allow widespread application of this attractive test.

On the basis of the available literature, currently the 2 best tests for assaying fertility potential for in vitro fertilization are the evaluation of sperm morphology by strict criteria and the human zona binding assay. However, both require standardization and some skills beyond the qualifications of most clinical laboratories, and thus they will not be universally applicable. The use of computer-driven assessments of sperm morphology may provide the information and universal availability needed to make this test a gold standard for evaluating the male. However, past experience suggests that no one test will ever be sufficient to test all the qualities of the sperm that are necessary for successful fertilization.

Thus the search continues for tests that provide information on any aspect of sperm function.

In Vitro Tests of Sperm Penetration into Mucus

A drop of sperm can be placed next to cervical mucus on a slide and progression of sperm into the mucus monitored under the microscope. To better standardize the test, tubes filled with bovine cervical mucus, available commercially, can be utilized and the length of mucus traversed by the sperm measured. The greatest usefulness of this assay is in individuals who have poor postcoital tests. If the sperm penetrate the bovine mucus but not human mucus, it suggests that the latter is the problem. One caveat is that antibody-affected sperm may not be handicapped in moving through bovine mucus while they generally would do poorly in human cervical mucus.

Because of the recent enthusiasm for empirically treating infertile couples with combinations of gonadotropin stimulation and intrauterine insemination (IUI), no matter what the sperm-mucus interaction, the sperm penetration test may no longer supply information that will influence clinical management.

Assessments of Sperm Motility

A sperm quality analyzer uses an electro-optical method to provide an assessment of the number of motile sperm in a specimen and, to some extent, the quality of the motility.[27] This may prove to be a useful instrument for assessing the functional capacity of sperm at a significantly lower expense than that of the computer-aided sperm analysis (CASA) systems.

Measurement of Sperm Velocity

In addition to the basic measurements, the CASA systems do provide information on sperm velocity that correlates with fertility, and measurements of lateral head displacement that has been championed as a good prognostic indicator. However, it is not yet established that these parameters provide unique information that cannot be obtained with less expensive instruments. Moreover, Davis and Katz have decried the lack of standardization of CASA instruments.[28] They warn that the resulting skepticism concerning accuracy may undermine the potential of CASA to become the standard tool for evaluation of semen.

Tests That Are Probably Not Clinically Useful

Hypo-osmotic Swelling Test

When sperm are placed in a hypo-osmotic solution of sodium citrate and fructose, a normal sperm tail will swell and coil as fluid is transported across the membrane. Conversely, if there is a functional disturbance of the tail membrane, the tail will appear unaffected. This test has been scrutinized by a number of investigators with the weight of opinion denying an important role for the hypo-osmotic test. Not all types of swelling are fully correlated with sperm parameters and the SPA. The best correlation has been with significant swelling at the tip of the tail.[29]

Measurement of Adenosine Triphosphate (ATP)

ATP is an important component of sperm metabolism. The levels of ATP in semen can be a strong discriminator between populations of fertile and infertile males.[30] A multi-center study sponsored by the World Health Organization concluded, however, that levels of semen ATP could not predict the occurrence of pregnancy when the female partner was normal and the male partner had a sperm concentration greater than 20 million/mL.[31]

Measurement of the Acrosome Reaction

The acrosome reaction (see Chapter 7) occurs on or near the zona pellucida. However, a low percentage of sperm will become reactive while in media or following treatment with a calcium ionophore that induces capacitation. Although the initiation of the acrosome reaction has been correlated with IVF results, the relatively small difference in acrosome-reactive sperm in the different groups leaves one hesitant to suggest that this approach is clinically important.[32]

Measurement of Acrosin

Acrosin is a proteolytic enzyme associated with the acrosome which may be important for aiding sperm to traverse the zona.[33] Low acrosin concentrations could be associated with infertility. Difficulties associated with accurately measuring acrosin have limited its clinical applicability; however, an assay kit is now available for clinical use.

Experimental Methods

There are a variety of surface ligands which have been identified as mediators of sperm attachment to the zona pellucida and to the egg membrane.[34,35] Theoretically, an absence or abnormality of these sites could interfere with fertilization and, in the future, these defects will be tested. A more severe abnormality, identified by electron microscopy, is the complete absence of the acrosome that gives the sperm a round-headed appearance and leaves them unable to achieve fertilization. A qualitative assessment of sperm activity can be obtained by a color change produced in the organic dye resazurin by metabolically active sperm.[36]

Sperm Antibodies

Whereas the previous assays measure sperm function or sperm numbers, sperm antibody tests determine reactions to sperm. It has been known for more than 100 years that animals, both male and female, can be rendered infertile by immunization with sperm.[37] Sperm are very antigenic and are normally isolated by the blood-testis barrier. Disruption of this anatomic and functional barrier in the seminiferous tubules can lead to antibody formation; hence antibodies can follow vasectomy, testicular torsion, infections, or trauma. In addition, there are women who have allergic reactions to semen manifested by reactions as diverse as irritation of the vagina and cardiovascular collapse following intercourse. The basic question for the infertility physician is whether more subtle immunologic reactions can occur that interfere with fertility.

Initial efforts to detect sperm antibodies involved incubating sperm in the sera of both males and females with agglutination being the endpoint. Despite the fact that substantial agglutination of sperm in semen on a repetitive basis is an indication of the presence of antibodies, agglutination in serum often is nonspecific. Thus, this test has been abandoned. Furthermore, it is now recognized that sperm antibodies in the circulation of men or women have no influence on fertility.[38]

The two tests now in clinical use both utilize immunologically mediated attachment of particles or beads to sperm that are assessed under a microscope.[39] The immunobead test has beads labeled with anti-IgG, anti-IgA, or anti-IgM and thus it provides identification of the class of antibodies on the sperm. The site on the sperm where the beads are adherent also can be noted. Anti-IgA localizes to the tail and anti-IgG to the head of the sperm. Antibody localized only to the tip of the tail usually is not significant, whereas antibody on the rest of the tail may interfere with sperm motility. Antibodies on the head of the sperm can cause failure of fusion with the egg. A second test, the mixed agglutination test (SpermMar), uses antiserum to IgG to bridge antibody-coated sperm and latex particles that have been conjugated with human IgG. The endpoint in this test is clumping, and the reactions against individual segments of the sperm cannot be identified. The SpermMar test can be used on unprepared semen, as opposed to the immunobead test where sperm washing is required, and thus SpermMar is suitable as an office laboratory screening test. If the SpermMar is positive, the immunobead test then can be used to determine which antibody is present and where it is localized.

For the SpermMar test the diagnosis of immunologic infertility is suggested when 10–39% of motile sperm are attached to latex particles, whereas immunologic infertility is very probable when 40% or more of the motile sperm are covered with beads. Using the immunobead test, if over 50% of sperm were antibody-bound, the subsequent pregnancy rate was 15.3%, whereas when the percentage of sperm positive for antibody was less than 50%, the pregnancy rate was 66.7%.[40] Others have used a cut off of 20%, and it is not clear at this time which is the more valid number.[13]

In testing the male the most accurate method is to incubate the individual's sperm with the immunobeads or to test with the SpermMar. To test the female for antibodies, sperm known to be free of antibody are mixed with the woman's serum. If the woman is positive, the sperm are presumably coated with antibody, and this shows up when the sperm are tested with the immunobead test or with the SpermMar. Male serum also can be tested in this way but it is less accurate than the direct test of the sperm surface. Levels of sperm antibodies in serum are similar in fertile and infertile individuals.[41] Similarly, the ability to conceive has not been influenced by serum antibodies to sperm.[38,42] Thus, testing of sera is of little value.

To add to the difficulty associated with sperm antibody testing there can be fluctuations in antibody levels even without therapy. In males receiving a placebo, 58% had a decrease in sperm-bound immunoglobulins.[43]

A high percentage of positive sperm antibody tests is associated with poor postcoital tests, and it would seem cost-effective to initially screen for antibodies only in individuals whose postcoital tests show no sperm, all dead sperm, a high percentage of shaking sperm, or less than 3 motile sperm per high power field. This latter number is somewhat arbitrary, and some may choose to use less than 5 or even less than 1 as the cut off value. On the other hand, there has been a movement toward screening all couples entering IVF programs for sperm antibodies. If the woman is positive, her serum is not used for the culture procedures. If the male is positive, his semen is collected in medium (see below). We also test for antibodies in men who have less than normal results with the sperm penetration assay.

Treatment of Sperm Antibodies	Use of condoms to avoid contact between sperm and the female with antibodies has been abandoned because of lack of efficacy. The current office treatments for sperm antibodies in the male are the use of steroids or ejaculation into media containing protein combined with intrauterine inseminations.[44,45] The latter may decrease adherence of seminal plasma antibodies to the sperm but will not remove antibodies bound to the sperm prior to ejaculation. In an alternative treatment the sperm are separated on Percoll gradients, and then incubated with antibody beads.[46] A population of sperm without antibody can be separated from the mix and utilized for insemination.

Moderate to high doses of corticosteroids have been used to treat sperm antibodies in the male. Reports of efficacy in reducing antibody levels and marginal increases in pregnancy rate have been balanced by sporadic reports of serious side effects such as aseptic necrosis of the femoral head and less severe side effects such as irritability. Hendry and coworkers[47] gave males with sperm antibodies prednisolone 20 mg bid from days 1 to 10 of their partners' cycles, followed by 5 mg on days 11 and 12. The dosage was increased if the antibody titer did not fall in 3 months. Nine of 29 who received prednisolone achieved pregnancy, whereas only 1 of 20 who received placebo was successful. An important point is that an advantage for prednisolone was not seen until after 5 months of treatment. Prior to that time pregnancy rates in the treated and the placebo groups were similar. Others have not seen success with steroid treatment although dosage may be a critical factor.[48] We have encountered antibody positive men with poor to zero performance on sperm penetration assays who have improved sperm penetration and achieved pregnancy with treatment consisting of prednisone, 5 mg tid for at least 3 months. Similar corticosteroid treatment in the female has not been aggressively investigated or used.

The most popular therapy involves intrauterine insemination of washed spermatozoa in conjunction with gonadotropin treatment of the female. Determination of the efficacy of this treatment has been hindered by difficulties in deciding what constitutes a positive sperm antibody test in the female and reports that lumped together patients who were antibody positive with others who may not have been afflicted with antibodies but who had poor postcoital tests.

Use of in vitro fertilization, with placement of sperm near the oocyte, is a reasonable final approach to the treatment of sperm antibodies in both the male and the female. If antibody is hampering sperm transport, IVF is a means of overcoming this problem. If the female is positive for antibodies, her serum is not used in the culture medium. If the male is positive for antibodies, he can ejaculate into medium containing protein as a preliminary to utilizing swimup or Percoll separation of the sperm. Even if many of the sperm continue to be hampered by antibody bound to their surface, there are almost always some sperm that are antibody-free. These sperm would gain a competitive advantage by being placed close to the egg in the IVF procedure. Success with in vitro fertilization is reduced in couples with sperm antibodies, but once fertilization occurs, the probability of pregnancy is not affected.[49] Micromanipulation (Chapter 31) should be considered when IVF fails.

Donor insemination is an alternative therapy for antibodies in the male and possibly in the female if she reacts only to her partner's sperm.

Investigation and Treatment of Male Infertility

If the semen analysis is abnormal, inquiry should be made concerning the presence of the following factors, any of which can produce abnormal sperm quality and quantity.

1. History of testicular injury, surgery, or mumps.

2. Heat. A small rise in scrotal temperature can adversely affect spermatogenesis and a febrile illness may produce striking changes in sperm count and motility. The effect of the illness can be seen in the sperm count and motility even 2–3 months later. This reflects the 74 days required for a spermatozoon to be generated from a primary germ cell. Environmental sources of heat, such as the use of jockey shorts instead of boxer shorts, excessively hot baths, hot tubs, or occupations that require long hours of sitting, e.g., long distance truck driving, may all decrease fertility potential; however, none of these factors has ever been substantiated by clinical study.

3. Severe allergic reactions.

4. Exposure to radiation or to industrial or environmental toxins. This area has received increasing attention, highlighted by studies suggesting a deterioration of semen quality over the past decades. One hypothesis is that industrial pollution may be responsible, and a study from Scandinavia did show lower sperm counts in males from an urban area compared to males in rural areas.[50] More direct evidence of a deleterious effect of environmental hazards is difficult to obtain because there is a reluctance of workers to produce the serial semen specimens that would be required for a thorough

industrial study. In any case, the physician should determine if a male with an abnormal semen specimen has had exposure to industrial or environmental toxins.

5. Heavy marijuana and alcohol use can depress sperm counts and testosterone levels, and there is evidence that cigarette smoking can depress sperm motility. Cocaine use within 2 years is associated with an increased risk of lower sperm counts. Certain drugs, including cimetidine, spironolactone, nitrofurans, sulfasalazine, erythromycin, tetracyclines, anabolic steroids, and chemotherapeutic agents, depress sperm quantity and quality. Cephalosporins, penicillins, quinolones, and the combination of sulfamethoxazole and trimethoprim are relatively safe to use when there is concern about effects on sperm.[51] Neurologic ejaculatory dysfunction can be caused by α-blockers, phentolamine, methyldopa, guanethidine, and reserpine.

6. Coital frequency. Counts at the lower levels of the normal range may be depressed to below normal levels by ejaculations occurring daily or more frequently. Conversely, abstinence for 10–14 days or more to save up sperm may be counterproductive because the gain in numbers can be offset by the lower motility produced by the increased proportion of older sperm. For most couples, coitus every 36 hours around the time of ovulation will give the optimal chance for pregnancy.

7. Exposure to diethylstilbestrol in utero has been suggested, but not proven, as a cause of male infertility.

Urologic Evaluation

In the presence of semen abnormalities referral is made to a urologist in order to look for an anatomic abnormality, an infection, an endocrine disorder, a varicocele, or an immunologic reaction to sperm.

Anatomic Abnormalities

Examination may reveal a physical impairment such as a marked hypospadias, which can cause sperm to be deposited outside the vagina. In rare cases of diabetes, with some neurologic diseases, or occasionally following prostatectomy, there can be retrograde ejaculation into the bladder. Pregnancies have been reported after insemination of sperm obtained from alkalinized urine or following treatment with a variety of drugs.[52] Retrograde ejaculation may be only partial, and some men with this condition have small amounts of ejaculate emitted from the urethra.

Obstruction or absence of the vas deferens is a relatively uncommon cause of male infertility; however more aggressive evaluation (including vasography) may detect obstructions that can be surgically corrected.[53] If the ducts are congenitally absent, fructose which is produced in the seminal vesicles will be absent from the semen. Testicular biopsy can differentiate between a block in the outflow tract or primary damage to the testes. In the latter case, if the biopsy reveals hyalinization and fibrosis of the seminiferous tubules, there is very little chance for fertility. Testicular damage or maldevelopment can be found following mumps orchitis, cryptorchidism, or in association with Klinefelter's syndrome. Males with the latter genetic abnormality (XXY) usually have small testes and azoospermia. With blockage of the vas, sperm can be aspirated from the epididymis and vasa efferentia. Successful fertilization in vitro can result in pregnancy.[54]

It is important that any infection in the genitourinary tract, including those caused by mycoplasma and chlamydia, be treated because white cells in the seminal plasma can significantly reduce sperm motility and egg penetration.

Endocrine Disorders

Although endocrine disorders are an uncommon cause for infertility, testing for thyroid, gonadotropins, prolactin, and testosterone may uncover unsuspected abnormalities. FSH levels are elevated with germ cell aplasia, and testosterone levels are decreased in men who are hypogonadotropic. Hyperprolactinemia is commonly associated with impotence, and in the absence of impotence, measuring a prolactin level is unlikely to aid in the diagnosis. Azoospermia has been reported in a man with a mutation that caused a substitution of arginine for glutamine in the beta-subunit of LH; this man presented with hypogonadism, a normal FSH level, and an elevated immunoactive (but biologically inactive) LH level.[55]

Infusion of gonadotropin releasing hormone (GnRH) can stimulate secretion of gonadotropins, and there have been occasional reports of the usefulness of this treatment in males who have an isolated gonadotropin deficiency. Although nonspecific therapy with thyroid, clomiphene citrate, and human chorionic gonadotropin has been used extensively, there is no compelling evidence that it is beneficial. Clomiphene citrate can elevate the sperm count, but an associated increase in fertility does not occur. Males with severe impairment of their semen have been treated with injections of pure FSH.[56] The dose was 150 IU three times a week for a minimum of 3 months. There was no improvement in sperm parameters but an increase in fertilization occurred with IVF. However, comparing current cycles with the patient's historical data may not be reasonable, and caution is needed in evaluating this study.

A fundamental problem in most studies of the efficacy of drug therapy in male fertility is the lack of a control group for comparison. Investigators make the erroneous assumption that the spontaneous cure rate of male infertility is zero and that any pregnancy that occurs during or following treatment is due solely to that treatment. A number of studies, however, have attested to the spontaneous cure rate of male infertility. In one study approximately one-third of males with counts below 10 million/mL who were not treated successfully impregnated their partners.[7] In summary, hormone treatment of infertile males who do not have an endocrine disorder is almost always unrewarding, and it does not improve fertility beyond what occurs by chance.

Varicocele

A varicocele is an abnormal tortuosity and dilatation of the veins of the pampiniform plexus within the spermatic cord. Approximately 25–30% of infertile males have a varicocele, usually on the left side because of the direct insertion of the spermatic vein into the renal vein. Varicoceles, in all likelihood, exert their effects by raising testicular temperature, an effect mediated by increased arterial blood flow.[57]

Approximately 10–15% of males in a general population have a varicocele on physical examination, but there is no evidence that males with normal semen characteristics need treatment even if a varicocele is present. They should be checked periodically, however, to be sure that there is no deterioration in their semen characteristics.

Ligation of varicoceles results in a 30–50% pregnancy rate. Although the beneficial effects of treatment of varicocele have been disputed by some investigators who found equal results without treatment, current clinical practice supports the utilization of varicocele ligation in those males who have infertility and an impaired semen specimen.[57] Nevertheless, there has not been a randomized study of varicocele repair. A group from Melbourne, Australia, tried but failed because of poor compliance.[58] Because the authors told their patients that varicocele repair might not make a difference, only 283 of 651 men chose to have it done. In those who had the repair, the only impact on the semen analysis was an improvement in motility from 33.5% to 39.3%, the classically reported finding. The same change, however, was noted in the nonoperated group, and the pregnancy rates in both the operated and nonoperated groups were the same! However, varicocele is more commonly found in men with abnormal semen, and there is evidence that a varicocele may exert an increasingly deleterious effect over time.[59]

Recent attention has focused on trying to identify those males with varicocele who have the best chance of benefiting from surgery. Decreased size of the left testicle may be an indication that the varicocele is exerting a pathologic effect and that surgery is the treatment of choice.

Some varicoceles only can be diagnosed by ultrasound examination, but it is questionable whether these small varicoceles have any clinical significance. Although surgical interruption of the internal spermatic vein is the usual treatment for clinically apparent varicoceles, there is also a nonsurgical approach that utilizes embolization to occlude the vein.[57]

Reactive Oxygen Species

Beyond these well-known problems is an increasing recognition that increased levels of reactive oxygen species can cause damage to the sperm membrane.[60] Although the exact contribution to infertility is uncertain, some protection can be gained by avoiding smoking and by ingestion of ascorbic acid.

Intrauterine Insemination of Washed Sperm (IUI)

Inseminations of whole semen have a limited role in infertility. They are useful when, either because of physical or psychologic factors, it is not possible to deposit sperm in the vagina by intercourse. In addition they are obviously useful in donor insemination. In the past small amounts of untreated semen were used for intrauterine insemination, but the potential for reactions to the proteins, prostaglandins, and bacteria in semen have made this approach an historic relic. In its place has emerged the use of washed sperm for intrauterine insemination (IUI).

The initial indications for IUI were failure of sperm to penetrate cervical mucus and male infertility. During the past decade the indications for IUI have been liberalized and now it is frequently employed, often in conjunction with the woman's use of clomiphene citrate or gonadotropins. Current controversies revolve around issues of techniques and those of efficacy.

There are a variety of methods that allow the separation of a more promising population of sperm. Most commonly used are washing and swimup or resuspension of sperm or separation of sperm on Percoll or other gradients. Other methods include allowing the sperm to swim into hyaluronidase or filtering the sperm on glass wool. All isolate a population of sperm with a higher percentage of motile forms and with a more uniform morphology than those found in untreated ejaculates. In the swimup techniques the semen is washed once or twice with one to three volumes of culture medium. A variety of media is available from commercial suppliers. After washing and centrifugation the supernatant is decanted and the pellet overlaid with 0.5 mL media. At this point the pellet can be agitated to resuspend the sperm and 0.3 or 0.4 mL of the preparation can be used for insemination. Because of the resuspension, the live sperm in the inseminate are accompanied by dead sperm and miscellaneous cellular elements. In the alternative swimup technique the unagitated pellet and overlying medium are placed in an incubator at 37° for 30–60 minutes. This provides lower numbers of sperm in the medium portion compared to the resuspension technique, but it achieves a cleaner specimen and for this reason it is the method we prefer. However, with severely oligospermic specimens it may be necessary to use resuspension to obtain sufficient sperm for insemination.

Percoll (silicone particles coated with polyvinyl pyrrolidone) provides a viscous medium for sperm to penetrate.[61] Sperm are layered over gradients of differing density. After centrifugation, the sperm in the densest fraction are retrieved by further washing and centrifugation, and the final product in a volume of 0.3–0.4 mL is inseminated. The percentage retrieval of motile sperm seems to be better with Percoll compared to the swimup method. Miniaturizing the process is necessary for severely impaired specimens.[62] Here the Percoll gradients consist of 0.3 mL each of 50%, 70%, and 90% Percoll. With this technique increased rates of fertilization can be achieved with IVF. An advantage for this method is that specimens separated by Percoll are less prone to damage by reactive oxygen species than are centrifuged swimup sperm.

Whereas all sperm separation methods produce specimens with better motility and more uniform morphology, this improvement may not necessarily translate into increased pregnancy rates. When equal numbers of motile sperm separated from good and from poor specimens were used in the sperm penetration assay, sperm separated from the good specimens were superior in achieving penetration.[63] Thus there may be intrinsic defects in sperm from poor specimens that may affect even the best sperm from that cohort.

At least 1 million motile sperm should be inseminated because lower numbers are seldom associated with success. When more than 15 million motile sperm were inseminated, there was no increase in the pregnancy rate; however, there was an increase in multiple births when the inseminate exceeded 20 million motile sperm.[64] Others have also reported increased pregnancy rates when higher numbers of donor sperm were inseminated.[65]

Empiric therapy consisting of clomiphene alone, gonadotropin alone, IUI, or IUI combined with clomiphene or gonadotropin in the female increasingly has been used for treatment of infertility of any origin. The greatest enthusiasm supports IUI combined with gonadotropin, which offers a number of possible advantages. It increases the number of oocytes that have the potential for fertilization. It raises the woman's hormone levels, eliminates seminal plasma, and markedly increases the number of sperm reaching the uterine cavity. The enthusiasm was fueled not only by these postulated advantages of gonadotropin-IUI but by a series of positive reports that appeared in the literature in the late 1980s and early 1990s. In a population selected for male factor infertility or poor postcoital tests, superovulation combined with IUI increased the monthly probability of pregnancy approximately four times compared to that following IUI timed by the LH surge.[66] The most striking advantage was seen in the subgroup of women who were treated with gonadotropin and HCG rather than clomiphene alone or clomiphene-gonadotropin/HCG combinations. Another study in couples with unexplained infertility demonstrated a pregnancy rate per cycle of 2.7% with IUI alone, 6.1% with gonadotropin alone, but 26.4% when gonadotropin/IUI was used.[67] Very similar experiences have been reported by others[68] (see Chapter 30).

Despite these outstanding results there are still questions concerning the combination of superovulation and IUI in cases of unexplained infertility. Although gonadotropin/IUI provided a 19% pregnancy rate per cycle compared to clomiphene/IUI where the pregnancy rate was 4%, the former result was not statistically different from that achieved with gonadotropin and timed intercourse (13%).[69] Moreover, the results with clomiphene and timed intercourse (17%) were better than those with clomiphene and IUI noted above. Another study found that timed intercourse was superior to IUI in GnRH down-regulated, gonadotropin stimulated cycles.[70] Dodson and Haney surveyed the literature and found that gonadotropin and IUI fecundity was 8.7% for male factor and 17% for unexplained infertility.[71] Their own experience, which was included in the survey figures, was 15% for each category.

Our current formulation concludes that IUI without associated superovulation is a useful treatment only for women with poor postcoital tests. Clomiphene, gonadotropin, or IUI alone are relatively ineffective treatments for male factor or unexplained infertility. Gonadotropin-IUI probably does not appreciably increase the pregnancy rate when there is a problem with the semen specimen, but it may be of some value for unexplained infertility. Its true effectiveness must be delineated by a multi-center randomized trial now in progress.

The timing of inseminations and the number of inseminations per cycle may influence the ultimate pregnancy rates. Most commonly IUI is timed for the day following the LH surge measured in the urine or at approximately 36 hours after an injection of human chorionic gonadotropin (HCG). Variations on these schedules can still be associated with reasonable pregnancy rates. Markedly increased pregnancy rates were obtained by doing two IUI's in a cycle at 18 hours and 42 hours after the ovulatory injection of HCG.[72] Because an earlier study found a similar increase in pregnancy rates with frozen donor sperm when two inseminations were used, this should provide an impetus to further assess the value of double inseminations combined with gonadotropin/IUI.

Prior down-regulation with GnRH agonist treatment does not seem to enhance results with gonadotropin/IUI.[73] Similarly, intraperitoneal or intratubal inseminations of sperm, although conceptually attractive, have no proven advantage over intrauterine insemination.[74] Moreover, intratubal transfer probably increases the risk of infection. Infection with IUI is rare, probably in the range of 1 in 500. Multiple pregnancies occur in approximately 20% of cases of gonadotropin/IUI, and the pregnancy loss rate is approximately 20%. Hyperstimulation can be minimized, but not eliminated, by monitoring of ovarian follicle numbers and growth by ultrasound, and by monitoring estrogen levels (reviewed in Chapter 30).

Treatment of sperm with methylxanthines such as caffeine and pentoxiphylline seems to enhance motility. The compounds inhibit cyclic AMP phosphodiesterase which results in an increase in cyclic AMP. Despite some earlier enthusiasm, pentoxiphylline offered no advantage in an IVF program, and a cautionary note was raised because the safety of the compound in early pregnancy has not been established.[75]

Therapeutic Donor Insemination

The combined problems of male infertility and decreased availability of adoptable babies have increased the interest and demand for therapeutic donor inseminations (TDI). Tens of thousands of babies are born each year as a result of TDI.[76]

The procedure raises emotional, ethical, and legal questions that must be considered and discussed. For obvious reasons the physician must never do inseminations without the consent of both partners. Increasingly, single women are seeking TDI. McGuire and Alexander[77] point out that children in single head of household families are as psychologically adjusted as those from two-parent households and that TDI should not be denied to single women solely on the basis of their lack of a male partner. Many states in the U.S. have specified the parental rights of the single woman and the donor, but most states have been silent on this issue.

Three points are worth emphasizing.

1. Donor inseminations do not guarantee pregnancy. The success rate with fresh semen is about 70% over 5–6 cycles. The use of frozen semen lowers the success rate.[78,79] The fecundibility (chance of getting pregnant per cycle) has been reported to be 18.9% with fresh semen and only 5.0% with frozen semen.[78] However, with exceptionally good frozen specimens suc-

cess can approach that achieved with fresh specimens. Over 80% of pregnancies that will occur do so within 6 months with fresh semen and within 12 months with frozen semen. In a summary of nearly 3,000 treatment cycles with frozen sperm, the cumulative pregnancy rates were 21% at 3 months, 40% at 6 months, and 62% at 12 months for women less than 30 years old.[80] For women over the age of 30, the pregnancy rates were 17%, 26%, and 44%, respectively. Because of the risk of acquired immunodeficiency syndrome (AIDS), use of frozen sperm that has been quarantined for 6 months is now accepted clinical practice. However, preparation of washed, swim-up sperm for intrauterine insemination appears to effectively remove human immunodeficiency virus (HIV)-infected cells and avoids HIV seroconversion, providing a safer method to achieve a healthy pregnancy and child for these couples.[81] Because of the importance and seriousness of this situation, these results require corroboration.

2. The couple needs to give some thought to their feelings should the child be born with a congenital anomaly. This will occur in perhaps 4–5% of all pregnancies, irrespective of whether they follow intercourse or therapeutic donor insemination.[82]

3. Both the man and the woman should sign a consent form. The procedure is covered by law in more than 20 states. It is worthwhile for the physician to know the legal status of TDI in his or her state so that correct information can be conveyed to patients.

As a rule the donor should be unknown to the couple. His health and fertility must be unimpeachable, and there should be no family history of genetic diseases. Screening for thalassemia in Mediterranean races, Tay-Sachs heterozygosity in Jews, and sickle cell disease in blacks is a wise precaution. Potential donors who are at high risk for AIDS (homosexuals, bisexuals, intravenous drug users) should be excluded as should individuals who have multiple sexual partners. Similar exclusions can include those individuals with histories of herpes, chronic hepatitis, and venereal warts. In addition, testing is recommended for human immunodeficiency virus (HIV), syphilis, serum hepatitis B antigen, gonorrhea, chlamydia, and cytomegalovirus. An initial screening test for HIV, if negative, should be repeated after 6 months. If both results are negative, the semen, which should be cryopreserved and quarantined for the 6 months, can be used.

The donor will not be a mirror image of the male partner, but an attempt should be made to match physical characteristics. TDI is usually a private matter between the physician and the couple. Discussions with friends or relatives should be discouraged. Use of friends or relatives as donors raises the potential for emotional problems in the future, although we have used a relative when it was requested by a stable, intelligent couple who understood the long-term implications. Requests to mix the partner's sperm with the donor's signifies that the couple may not have made the emotional adjustment to the thought of donor insemination. A partner's semen also may impair the donor's sperm, although this is in dispute.

Donor inseminations are useful in azoospermia, severe oligospermia, or asthenospermia refractory to treatment. They also are useful for the woman who has a history of fetal loss due to Rh sensitization. In that case an Rh-negative donor would be used. Genetic diseases may, on occasion, be an indication for donor insemination.

The basal body temperature (BBT) change, the woman's perception of vaginal wetness, and ovulatory pain, if present, are useful guides for timing of inseminations. More precise timing can be accomplished by ultrasound visualization of the preovulatory follicle and monitoring of the day of the LH surge either by measurements of LH in serum or by measurements of LH in urine with any of a number of commercially available kits. We prefer to time inseminations according to the measurement of the LH surge in urine. In our experience approximately 75% of women can successfully use the kits at home to identify their LH surge. Insemination is performed the day after the LH surge is identified. Alternative monitoring and treatment approaches utilize ultrasound to monitor preovulatory follicle growth and an injection of 5,000 or 10,000 IU human chorionic gonadotropin when the dominant follicle reaches 18 mm or greater in diameter. The insemination (if not IUI) is performed 24 hours after the HCG injection. Ultrasound, LH monitoring, or HCG injection also can be used to time partner inseminations.

If the BBT alone is used, an attempt is made to inseminate on the date just before or two days before the temperature rise with the timing based on reviewing 2 months of charts and/or the day of maximal vaginal wetness. Usually one to two donor inseminations are done each month.

Semen can be inseminated at the entrance to the cervical canal by means of a polyethylene catheter. The major portion of the semen overflows into the posterior fornix. The overflow collects on the posterior blade of the speculum, and the cervical os is allowed to dip into this pool while the woman rests for 10–15 minutes with her hips elevated. If pregnancy does not occur in the first two cycles, then intrauterine inseminations with washed, resuspended sperm are performed in subsequent cycles. Some, but not all, clinical studies indicate that the pregnancy rate per treatment cycle is greater with IUI.[83–85] With IUI of donor sperm it is preferable to have a 34–36-hour interval between HCG and IUI.

The children born after donor insemination have outcomes comparable to the general population.[82] Interestingly, approximately half of couples do and half do not tell their children of their origins. The divorce rate in families with children conceived with donor insemination is lower than the general rate.[82]

The Future

In the future more sophisticated investigative techniques may uncover causes of male infertility not diagnosable by current methods. Study of receptors on sperm may reveal abnormalities that preclude sperm-zona or sperm-oocyte interaction. Assessment of the role of ABP, the androgen binding protein, and the process of spermatogenesis and maturation may uncover specific disorders currently unknown. The genetic analysis of sperm may make it possible to be selective for "good" sperm. Finally, with micromanipulation it is now possible to place a single sperm within an egg. Pregnancies have been achieved by micromanipulation with men who have sperm counts less than 100,000/mL with zero motility and no normal forms (see Chapter 31).

References

1. **Plymate SR, Paulsen CA, McLachlan RI,** Relationship of serum inhibin levels to serum follicle stimulating hormone and sperm production in normal men and men with varicoceles, J Clin Endocrinol Metab 74:859, 1992.

2. **Burgoyne PS,** The role of the mammalian Y chromosome in spermatogenesis, Development 101(Suppl):133, 1987.

3. **Carlsen E, Giwercman A, Keidin N, Skakkebaek NE,** Evidence for decreasing quality of semen during past 50 years, Br Med J 305:609, 1992.

4. **MacLeod J, Gold RA,** The male factor in fertility and infertility. II. Spermatozoan counts in 1000 cases of known fertility and 1000 cases of infertile marriage, J Urol 66:436, 1951.

5. **Nelson CMK, Bunge RG,** Semen analysis: evidence for changing parameters of male fertility potential, Fertil Steril 25:503, 1974.

6. **Zukerman Z, Rodriguez-Rigau LJ, Smith KD, Steinberger E,** Frequency distribution of sperm counts in fertile and infertile males, Fertil Steril 28:1310, 1977.

7. **Smith KD, Rodriguez-Rigau LJ, Steinberger E,** Relationship between indices of semen analysis and pregnancy rate in infertile couples, Fertil Steril 28:1314, 1977.

8. **Bernstein GS, Siegel MS,** Male factor in infertility, in Mishell DR Jr, Davajan V, Lobo RA, editors, *Infertility, Contraception, and Reproductive Endocrinology,* Philadelphia, FA Davis Co., 1991, pp 612-641.

9. **Andrews WC,** Investigation of the infertile couple, in Gold JJ, Josimovich JB, editors, *Gynecologic Endocrinology,* Plenum Medical Book Co., New York, 1987, p 543.

10. **Jequier AM, Ukome EB,** Errors inherent in the performance of a routine semen analysis, Br J Urol 55:434, 1983.

11. **Neuwinger J, Behre HM, Nieschlag E,** External quality control in the andrology laboratory: an experimental multicenter trial, Fertil Steril 54:38, 1990.

12. **Polansky FF, Lamb EJ,** Do the results of semen analysis predict future fertility? A survival analysis study, Fertil Steril 49:1059, 1988.

13. **World Health Organization,** *Laboratory Manual for the Examination of Human Semen and Sperm — Cervical Mucus Interaction,* Cambridge University Press, Cambridge, 1992.

14. **Hargreave TB, Elton RA,** Fecundability rates from an infertile population, Br J Urol 58:194, 1986.

15. **Steinberger E, Rodriguez-Rigau LJ, Smith KD,** The interaction between the fertility potentials of the two members of an infertile couple, in Frajese G, Hafez ESE, Conti C, Fabbrini A, editors, *Oigospermia: Recent Progress in Andrology,* Raven Press, New York, 1981, p 9.

16. **Katz DF, Diel L, Overstreet JW,** Differences in the movement of morphologically normal and abnormal human seminal spermatozoa, Biol Reprod 26:66, 1982.

17. **Kruger TF, Acosta AA, Simmons KF, Swanson RJ, Matta JF, Oehninger S,** Predictive value of abnormal sperm morphology in in vitro fertilization, Fertil Steril 49:112, 1988.

18. **Kruger TF, Dutoit TC, Franken DR, Acosta AA, Oehninger SC, Menkveld R, Lombard CJ,** A new computerized method of reading sperm morphology (strict criteria) is as efficient as technician reading, Fertil Steril 59:202, 1993.

19. **Eggert-Krause W, Bellmann A, Rohr G, Tilgen W, Runnebaum B,** Differentiation of round cells in semen by means of monoclonal antibodies and relationship with male fertility, Fertil Steril 58:1046, 1992.

20. **Yanagimachi R,** Zona-free hamster eggs: their use in assessing fertilizing capacity and examining chromosomes of human spermatozoa, Gamete Res 10:187, 1984.

21. **Mao C, Grimes DA,** The sperm penetration assay: can it discriminate between fertile and infertile men? Am J Obstet Gynecol 159:279, 1988.

22. **Margalioth EJ, Feinmesser M, Navot D, Mordel N, Bronson RA,** The long-term predictive value of the zona-free hamster ova sperm penetration assay, Fertil Steril 52:490, 1989.

23. **McClure DR, Tom RA, Dandekar PV,** Optimizing the sperm penetration assay with human follicular fluid, Fertil Steril 53:546, 1990.

24. **Falk RM, Silverberg KM, Fetterolf PM, Kirschner FK, Rogers BJ,** Establishment of test-yolk buffer enhanced sperm penetration assay limits for fertile males, Fertil Steril 54:121, 1990.

25. **Burkman LJ, Coddington CC, Franken DR, Kruger TF, Rosenwaks Z, Hodgen GD,** The hemizona assay (HZA): development of a diagnostic test for the binding of human spermatozoa to the human hemizona pellucida to predict fertilization potential, Fertil Steril 49:688, 1988.

26. **Coddington CC III,** The hemizona assay (HZA) and considerations for its use in assisted reproductive technology, Seminars Reprod Endocrinol 10:1, 1992.

27. **Bartoov B, Ben-Barak J, Mayevsky A, Sneider M, Yogev L, Lightman A,** Sperm motility index: a new parameter for human sperm evaluation, Fertil Steril 56:108, 1991.

28. **Davis RO, Katz DF,** Computer-aided sperm analysis: technology at a crossroads, Fertil Steril 59:953, 1993.

29. **Mordel N, Dano I, Epstein-Eldan M, Shemesh A, Schenker JG, Laufer N,** Novel parameters of human sperm hypoosmotic swelling test and their correlation to standard spermatogram, total motile sperm fraction, and sperm penetration assay, Fertil Steril 59:1276, 1993.

30. **Comhaire FH, Vermeulen L, Schoonjans F,** Reassessment of the accuracy of traditional sperm characteristics and adenosine triphosphate (ATP) in estimating the fertilizing potential of human semen in vivo, Int J Androl 10:654, 1987.

31. **WHO Task Force on the Prevention and Management of Infertility,** Adenosine triphosphate in semen and other sperm characteristics: their relevance for fertility prediction in men with normal sperm concentration, Fertil Steril 57:877, 1992.

32. **Takahashi K, Wetzels AMM, Goverde HJM, Bastiaans BA, Janssen HJG, Rolland R,** The kinetics of the acrosome reaction of human spermatozoa and its correlation with in vitro fertilization, Fertil Steril 57:889, 1992.

33. **Liu DY, Baker HWG,** Inhibition of acrosin activity with a trypsin inhibitor blocks human sperm penetration of the zona pellucida, Biol Reprod 48:340, 1993.

34. **Blobel CP, Myles DG, Primakoff P, White JM,** Proteolytic processing of a protein involved in sperm-egg fusion correlates with acquisition of fertilization competence, J Cell Biol 111:69, 1990.

35. **Huszar G, Vigue L, Morshedi M,** Sperm creatine phosphokinase M-isoform ratios and fertilizing potential of men: a blinded study of 84 couples treated with in vitro fertilization, Fertil Steril 57:882, 1992.

36. **Glass, RH, Ericsson SA, Ericsson RJ, Drouin MT, Marcoux LJ, Sullivan H,** The resazurin reduction test provides an assessment of sperm activity, Fertil Steril 56:743, 1991.

37. **Adeghe J-HA,** Male subfertility due to sperm antibodies: a clinical overview, Obstet Gynecol Survey 48:1, 1992.

38. **Eggert-Kruse W, Christmann M, Gerhard I, Pohl S, Klinga K, Runnebaum B,** Circulating antisperm antibodies and fertility prognosis: a prospective study, Hum Reprod 4:513, 1989.

39. **Rajah SV, Parslow JM, Howell RJR, Hendry WF,** Comparison of mixed antiglobulin reaction and direct immunobead test for detection of sperm-bound antibodies in subfertile males, Fertil Steril 57:1300, 1992.

40. **Ayvaliotis B, Bronson R, Rosenfeld D, Cooper G,** Conception rates in couples where autoimmunity to sperm is detected, Fertil Steril 44:739, 1986.

41. **Critser JR, Villines PM, Coulam CB, Crister ES,** Evaluation of circulating antisperm antibodies in fertile and patient populations, Am J Reprod Immunol 21:137, 1989.

42. **Collins JA, Burrows EA, Yeo J, Younglai EV,** Frequency and predictive value of antisperm antibodies among infertile couples, Hum Reprod 8:592, 1993.

43. **Haas GG Jr, Manganiello P,** A double-blind placebo-controlled study of the use of methylprednisolone in infertile men with sperm-associated immunoglobins, Fertil Steril 47:295, 1987.

44. **Margalioth EJ, Sauter E, Bronson RA, Rosenfeld DL, Schou GM, Cooper GW,** Intrauterine insemination as treatment for antisperm antibodies in the female, Fertil Steril 50:441, 1988.

45. **Agarwal A,** Treatment of immunological infertility by sperm washing and intrauterine insemination, Arch Androl 29:207, 1992.

46. **Grundy CE, Robinson J, Gordon AG, Hay DM,** Selection of an antibody-free population of spermatozoa from semen samples of men suffering from immunological infertility, Hum Reprod 6:593, 1991.

47. **Hendry WF, Hughes L, Scammell G, Pryor JP, Hargreave TB,** Comparison of prednisolone and placebo in subfertile men with antibodies to spermatozoa, Lancet 335:85, 1990.

48. **Smarr SC, Wing R, Hammond MG,** Effect of therapy on infertile couples with antisperm antibodies, Am J Obstet Gynecol 158:969, 1988.

49. **Rajah SV, Parslow JM, Howell RJ, Hendry WF,** The effects on in-vitro fertilization of autoantibodies to spermatozoa in subfertile men, Hum Reprod 8:1079, 1993.

50. **Ledholm OP, Ranstam J,** Depressed semen quality: a study over two decades, Arch Androl 12:113, 1984.

51. **Schlegel PN, Chang TSK, Marshall FF,** Antibiotics: potential hazard to male fertility, Fertil Steril 55:235, 1991.

52. **Hershlag A, Schiff SF, DeCherney AH,** Retrograde ejaculation, Hum Reprod 6:255, 1991.

53. **Pryor JP, Hendry WF,** Ejaculatory duct obstruction in subfertile males: analysis of 87 patients, Fertil Steril 56:725, 1991.

54. **Silber SJ, Ord T, Balmaceda J, Patrizio P, Asch RH,** Congenital absence of the vas deferens: the fertilizing capacity of human epididymal sperm, New Engl J Med 323:1788, 1990.

55. **Weiss J, Axelrod L, Whitcomb RW, Harris PE, Crowley WF, Jameson JL,** Hypogonadism caused by a single amino acid substitution in the β subunit of luteinizing hormone, New Engl J Med 326:179, 1992.

56. **Acosta AA, Khalifa E, Oehninger S,** Pure human follicle stimulating hormone has a role in the treatment of severe male infertility by assisted reproduction: Norfolk's total experience, Hum Reprod 7:1067, 1992.

57. **Howards SS,** Varicocele, Infert Reprod Med Clin North Am 3:429, 1992.

58. **Baker HWG, Burger HG, de Kretser DM, Hudson B, Rennie GC, Straffon WGE,** Testicular vein ligation and fertility in men with varicoceles, Br Med J 291:1678, 1985.

59. **Gorelick JI, Goldstein M,** Loss of fertility in men with varicocele, Fertil Steril 59:613, 1993.

60. **Aitken RJ,** The role of free oxygen radicals and sperm function, Int J Androl 12:95, 1989.

61. **Berger T, Marrs RP, Moyer DL,** Comparison of techniques for selection of motile spermatozoa, Fertil Steril 43:268, 1985.

62. **Ord T, Patrizio P, Marello E, Balmaceda JP, Asch RH,** Mini-percoll: a new method of semen preparation for IVF in severe male factor infertility, Hum Reprod 5:987, 1990.

63. **Syms AJ, Johnson A, Lipshultz LI, Smith RG,** Reduced ability of motile human spermatozoa obtained from oligospermic males to penetrate zona-free hamster eggs, Fertil Steril 41:1055, 1984.

64. **Kerin J, Byrd W,** Supracervical placement of spermatozoa in Soules MR, editor, *Controversies in Reproductive Endocrinology and Infertility,* Elsevier, Amsterdam, 1989.

65. **Shapiro SS,** Strategies to improve efficiency of threapeutic donor insemination, Infertil Reprod Med Clin North Am 3:469, 1992.

66. **Kemmann E, Bohrer M, Shelden R, Fiasconaro G, Beardsley L,** Active ovulation management increases the monthly probability of pregnancy occurrence in ovulatory women who receive intrauterine insemination, Fertil Steril 48:916, 1987.

67. **Serhal PF, Katz M, Little V, Woronowski H,** Unexplained infertility — the value of pergonal superovulation combined with intrauterine insemination, Fertil Steril 49:602, 1988.

68. **Chaffkin LM, Nulsen JC, Luciano AA, Metzger DA,** A comparative analysis of the cycle fecundity rates associated with combined human menopausal gonadotropin (hMG) and intrauterine insemination (IUI) versus either hMG or IUI alone, Fertil Steril, 55:252, 1991.

69. **Karlstrom P-O, Bereh T, Lundkuist O,** A prospective randomized trial of artificial insemination versus intercourse in cycles stimulated with human menopausal gonadotropin or clomiphene citrate, Fertil Steril 59:554, 1993.

70. **Zikopoulos K, West CP, Thong PW, Kalser EM, Morrison J, Wu FCW,** Homologous intrauterine insemination has no advantage over timed natural intercourse when used in combination with ovulation induction for the treatment of unexplained infertility, Hum Reprod 8:563, 1993.

71. **Dodson WL, Haney AF,** Controlled ovarian hyperstimulation and intrauterine insemination for treatment of infertility, Fertil Steril 55:457, 1991.

72. **Silverberg, KM, Johnson JV, Olive DL, Burns WN, Schenken RS,** A prospective, randomized trial comparing two different intrauterine insemination regimens in controlled ovarian hyperstimulation cycles, Fertil Steril 57:357, 1992.

73. **Dodson WL, Walmer DK, Hughes CL Jr, Yancy SE, Haney AF,** Adjunctive leuprolide therapy does not improve cycle fecundity in controlled ovarian hyperstimulation and intrauterine insemination of subfertile women, Obstet Gynecol 78:187, 1991.

74. **Oei ML, Surrey ES, McCaleb B, Kerin JF,** A prospective, randomized study of pregnancy rates after transuterotubal and intrauterine insemination, Fertil Steril 58:167, 1992.

75. **Tournays H, Janssens R, Camus M, Staessen C, Devroey P, Van Steirteghem A,** Pentoxifylline is not useful in enhancing sperm function in cases with previous in vitro fertilization failure, Fertil Steril 59:210, 1993.

76. **Barratt CLR, Chauhan M, Cooke ID,** Donor insemination — a look to the future, Fertil Steril 54:375, 1990

77. **McGuire M, Alexander NJ,** Artificial insemination of single women, Fertil Steril 43:182, 1985.

78. **Richter MA, Haning RV Jr, Shapiro SS,** Artificial donor insemination: fresh versus frozen semen: the patient as her own control, Fertil Steril 41:277, 1984.

79. **Subak LL, Adamson GD, Boltz NL,** Therapeutic donor insemination: a prospective randomized trial of fresh versus frozen sperm, Am J Obstet Gynecol 166:1597, 1992.

80. **Shenfield F, Doyle P, Valentine A, Steele SJ, Tan S-L,** Effects of age, gravidity and male infertility status on cumulative conception rates following artificial insemination with cryopreserved donor semen: analysis of 2998 cycles of treatment in one centre over 10 years, Hum Reprod 8:60, 1993.

81. **Semprini AE, Levi-Setti P, Bozzo M, Ravizza M, Tagliorettie A, Sulpizio P, Albani E, Oneta M, Pardi G,** Insemination of HIV-negative women with processed semen of HIV-positive partners, Lancet 340:1317, 1992.

82. **Amuzu B, Laxova R, Shapiro SS,** Pregnancy outcome, health of children, and family adjustment after donor insemination, Obstet Gynecol 75:899, 1990.

83. **Byrd W, Edman C, Bradshaw K, Odom J, Carr B, Ackerman G,** A prospective randomized study of pregnancy rates following intrauterine and intracervical insemination using frozen donor sperm, Fertil Steril 53:521, 1990.

84. **Hurd WW, Menge AC, Randolph JF Jr, Ohl DA, Ansbacher R, Brown AN,** Comparison of intracervical, intrauterine, and intratubal techniques for donor insemination, Fertil Steril 59:339, 1993.

85. **Patton PE, Burry KA, Novy MJ, Wolf DP,** A comparative evaluation of intracervical and intrauterine routes in donor therapeutic insemination, Hum Reprod 5:263, 1990.

30   Induction of Ovulation

In previous editions of this book, we began this chapter with a statement in celebration of one of the greatest achievements of reproductive endocrinology, the ability to induce ovulation and attain pregnancy in women who in the past had little basis or hope for reversal of their ovulatory dysfunction. As we approach a half century of ovulation induction for infertility, this elation remains justified. A variety of logical strategies, often empirically defined, designed to respond to specific indications do yield excellent results. In many clinical circumstances accurate data confirm the theoretical expectation that treatment can result in pregnancy rates equivalent to those in the normal population.

As the field has matured, however, the initial exuberance has been tempered by the realities of objective review. Results of treatment, despite restriction to a single indication, are not uniform. Complications occur and unwanted consequences lead to reduced patient compliance or escalation to more costly and hazardous treatments. Perhaps most concerning is the vexingly persistent disparity between rates of successful ovulation (high) and pregnancy (relatively low). This paradox presents two challenges.

1. The informed consent dialogue with the infertile couple does not conclude with the initial outline of strategic options. Helping the couple deal with the frustration of repeated partial success but persistent ultimate failure requires special time, sensitivity, and compassion.

2. The disparity between ovulation and pregnancy rates is an emphatic reminder for the clinician of the imprecision of the diagnosis, "ovulatory dysfunction and/or failure," the inadequacy of the available tests to determine if induction of ovulation has actually occurred, and the existence of more basic inherent defects in the reproductive process not disclosed by our current thorough work-up or simply not discovered.

Nevertheless, as a somewhat perverse acknowledgment of these deficiencies, the field has seen the emergence of medical "superovulation" as a treatment, not solely for anovulation, but in the management of persistent, unexplained infertility.

These considerations are all the more reason for the clinician to understand thoroughly the various indications and the many options available for induction of ovulation. This chapter will review the principles which guide the use of clomiphene, human menopausal gonadotropins (HMG), purified follicle-stimulating hormone (FSH), bromocriptine, and gonadotropin releasing hormone (GnRH), and consider the results and complications of the medical induction of ovulation. In addition, laparoscopic ovarian multiple cystotomy (modified wedge resection) and the impact of GnRH agonist therapy will be reviewed.

Despite the specificity of the therapy and the promise of successful results, it is incumbent upon the practitioner to perform the appropriate medical evaluation to ensure that a contraindication to therapy is not overlooked. The reader is referred to Chapter 13 and Chapter 14 for a consideration of anovulation and hirsutism, and Chapter 12 for the evaluation of amenorrhea and galactorrhea.

For reference purposes, we provide the following definitions of ovulatory deficiencies according to the the World Health Organization.

1. **Group I: Hypothalamic-Pituitary Failure.** This classfication includes patients diagnosed as hypothalamic amenorrhea, and includes stress-related amenorrhea, anorexia nervosa and its variants, Kallmann's syndrome, and isolated gonadotropin deficiency. These patients display hypogonadotropic hypogonadism with low FSH and estrogen levels, normal prolactin concentrations, and a failure to bleed after the administration of a progestational agent (the progestational challenge).

2. **Group II: Hypothalamic-Pituitary Dysfunction.** This classification includes normogonadotropic, normoestrogenic, anovulatory, oligoamenorrheic women. The classic anovulatory polycystic ovary syndrome is in this category.

3. **Group III: Ovarian Failure.** Patients in this classification are hypergonadotropic hypogonadal individuals with low estrogen levels. All variants of ovarian failure and ovarian resistance are in this category.

For the purposes of this chapter, as well as the expression of our clinical philosophy, hyperprolactinemic ovulatory dysfunction is treated as a specific treatment entity.

Clomiphene Citrate

Clomiphene citrate was first synthesized in 1956, introduced for clinical trials in 1960, and approved for clinical use in the United States in 1967. Clomiphene citrate is an orally active nonsteroidal agent distantly related to diethylstilbestrol. Its chemical name is 2-[p-(2-chloro-1,2-diphenylvinyl)phenoxy] triethylamine dihydrogen citrate. Clomiphene is a racemic mixture of its 2 stereochemical isomers, originally described as the cis and trans isomers. This designation is now recognized to have been inaccurate, and the isomers have been relabeled as zuclomiphene and enclomiphene citrate.[1] Clomiphene is available in 50 mg tablets, under the trade names of Clomid and Serophene, which contain 38% of the active zuclomiphene form.

The similarity of clomiphene's structure to an estrogenic substance is the clue to its mechanism of action. Clomiphene exerts only a very weak biologic estrogenic effect. The structural similarity to estrogen is sufficient to achieve uptake and binding by estrogen receptors; however, there are several important different characteristics.[2,3] Perhaps most importantly, clomiphene occupies the nuclear receptor for long periods of time, for weeks rather than hours. Clomiphene modifies hypothalamic activity by

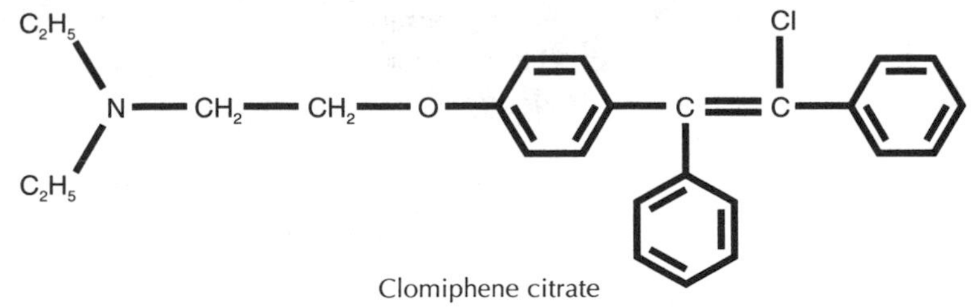

Clomiphene citrate

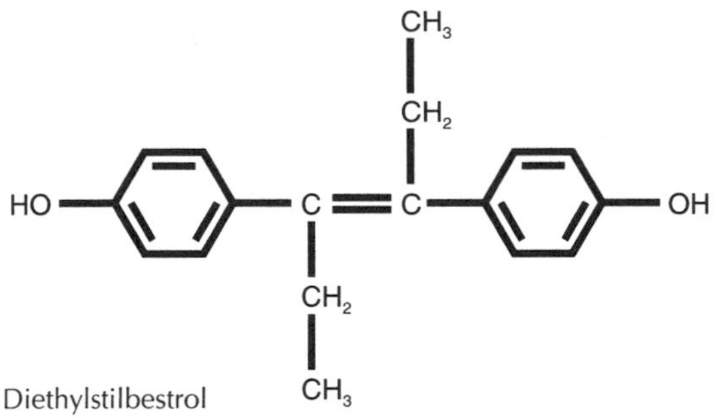

Diethylstilbestrol

affecting the concentration of the intracellular estrogen receptors. Specifically, the concentration of estrogen receptors is reduced by inhibition of the process of receptor replenishment.

When exposed to clomiphene, the hypothalamic-pituitary axis is blind to the endogenous estrogen level in the circulation. Because receptor capacity is reduced and the true estrogen signal falsely lowered, negative feedback is diminished and the neuroendocrine mechanism for GnRH secretion is activated. When clomiphene is administered to normally cycling women, FSH and luteinizing hormone (LH) pulse frequency (but not amplitude) is increased, suggesting an increase in GnRH pulse frequency.[4] Anovulatory women, however, respond in a different fashion. Clomiphene stimulates an increase in gonadotropin pulse amplitude, presumably because GnRH pulses are already operating at maximal frequency in anovulatory women with polycystic ovaries.[5] Nevertheless, the experimental data indicate that the primary site of action is the hypothalamus.

During clomiphene administration, circulating levels of FSH and LH rise. The subsequent ovulation that occurs after clomiphene therapy is a manifestation of the hormone and morphologic changes produced by the growing follicles. Clomiphene therapy does not directly stimulate ovulation, but it retrieves and magnifies the sequence of events that are the physiologic features of a normal cycle. The effectiveness of the drug, however, may not be restricted to its ability to cause an appropriate GnRH discharge.

In animal models, clomiphene exerts an estrogenic effect on the pituitary and directly stimulates gonadotropin release, independent of its action on GnRH.[3] In the presence of estrogen, clomiphene influences pituitary response to GnRH in women, preferentially promoting FSH secretion.[6] In addition, clomiphene exerts a direct ovarian effect. In the absence of estrogen, clomiphene is an estrogen agonist, directly enhancing FSH stimulation of LH receptors in granulosa cells.[7] In an important contrast, in the uterus, cervix, and vagina, clomiphene acts primarily as an antiestrogen. Thus vaginal cornification is attenuated, and the effect of estrogen on cervical mucus and endometrium is antagonized, potentially important actions affecting implantation, sperm transport, and early embryonic development.[8] However, no significant effects on luteal phase endometrial morphology could be detected when clomiphene was administered to normal women.[9] Nor could a detrimental impact on cervical mucus be documented in either anovulatory or normal women.[10] In addition, the administration of clomiphene failed to affect endometrial concentrations of estrogen and progesterone receptors in normal ovulatory women.[11] These latter observations suggest that the potential antiestrogenic, adverse effects of clomiphene do not appear when clomiphene is used clinically.

Clomiphene has no progestational, corticotropic, androgenic, or antiandrogenic effects. Clomiphene does not interfere with adrenal or thyroid function. Although the effect of the drug is brief, only 51% of the oral dose is excreted after 5 days, and radioactivity from labeled clomiphene appears in the feces up to 6 weeks after administration. Significant plasma concentrations of the active zu isomer can be detected up to 1 month after treatment with a single dose of 50 mg.[12]

This long half-life of clomiphene presents theoretical concern. Clomiphene has been detected both in the serum and in follicular fluid obtained from in vitro fertilization patients on the day of ovulation.[13] The presence of clomiphene at this time and during the luteal phase could have unwanted effects. In vitro, clomiphene inhibits progesterone production by luteal granulosa cells in a fashion that suggests that clomiphene in the presence of estrogen, by virtue of its antiestrogenic action, interferes with the induction of LH receptors.[14] Because this inhibition is reversed by human chorionic gonadotropin (HCG), pregnancy and the appearance of HCG may prevent this unwelcome effect.

In rats and rabbits, a dose-dependent increase in the incidence of fetal malformations is seen when clomiphene is given during the period of organogenesis. Clomiphene has been found to cause disruptions of the organization of the uterine mesenchyme and tubal epithelium in human fetal reproductive tissue transplanted to athymic nude mice.[15] Extremely high doses inhibit fetal development. In these experiments, exposure took place at later periods of gestation than those associated with clomiphene exposure when the drug is taken for the induction of ovulation. Although clomiphene therapy should be withheld if there is any possibility of pregnancy, there is no good evidence that clomiphene is teratogenic in humans.[16,17] Furthermore, infant survival and performance after delivery are normal.

Selection of Patients

Absent or infrequent ovulation is the chief indication for clomiphene therapy. It is the physician's responsibility to rule out disorders of pituitary, adrenal, and thyroid origin requiring specific treatment before initiating clomiphene therapy. A complete history and physical examination are mandatory, but only a minimum of laboratory procedures is necessary. Liver function evaluation should precede clomiphene therapy if history and physical examination findings suggest liver disease. The vast majority of patients are healthy women suffering only from infertility secondary to oligoovulation or anovulation.

If periods are infrequent, it is not absolutely necessary to document infrequent or absent ovulation by basal body temperature records and endometrial biopsy. An endometrial biopsy is a wise precaution in a patient who has been anovulatory for a long period of time because of the tendency for these patients to develop hyperplasia and even carcinoma of the endometrium. It is also wise to precede therapy with an evaluation of the semen, to avoid an unnecessary waste of time and effort in the presence of azoospermia. A dedicated effort must be made to detect galactorrhea, and the prolactin level must be measured. Galactorrhea or hyperprolactinemia dictate a different therapeutic approach: bromocriptine. The remainder of the infertility workup in a patient with no previous medical or surgical problems is deferred until after a trial of clomiphene therapy. Because approximately 75% of pregnancies occur during the first 3 treatment cycles, the infertility workup is pursued only after the patient has responded with 3 months of ovulatory cycles and has not become pregnant.[18] This is appropriate because clomiphene is simple, safe, and cost-effective.

Despite the antiestrogen action of clomiphene the incidence of poor cervical mucus on the postcoital test is only 15%.[19] In the past, estrogen (0.625 to 2.5 mg conjugated estrogens daily) was administered from day 10 to day 16 (for 1 week starting the day after the last day of clomiphene administration) in an effort to improve mucus production. Although high doses of estrogen do not interfere with the gonadotropin response, ovulation, or the pregnancy rate, there is reason to believe that estrogen treatment is ineffective.[20,21] Another alternative, the one we prefer, is to proceed with intrauterine inseminations of prepared sperm, bypassing the cervix.

Cases of ovarian failure are unresponsive to any form of ovulation induction. Therefore, the presence of ovarian tissue capable of responding to gonadotropins must be documented. This is only a problem in the patient with amenorrhea, since the presence of menstrual bleeding confirms the function (although perhaps limited) of the hypothalamic-pituitary-ovarian axis. The patient with amenorrhea who fails to produce a withdrawal bleed after a course of a progestational agent (medroxyprogesterone acetate, 10 mg daily for 5 days) must be further evaluated (Chapter 12). A case has been made by others for the usefulness of an ovarian biopsy, perhaps via the laparoscope, to establish the presence of competent ovarian tissue. It is our practice, however, to rely on the immunoassay of gonadotropin levels and the response to a progestin, thus avoiding unnecessary surgical and anesthetic risks, to accurately rule out hypergonadotropic hypogonadism (ovarian failure). Attempts at medical induction of ovulation in these patients would be a waste of time and money.

The patients most likely to respond to clomiphene display some evidence of pituitary-ovarian activity as expressed in the biologic presence of estrogen (spontaneous or withdrawal menstrual bleeding). These are anovulatory women who have gonadotropin and estrogen production, but do not cycle, or women with inadequate luteal phases.

If the mechanism of an inadequate corpus luteum is inadequate FSH stimulation during the follicular phase, it makes sense to treat this condition with clomiphene, and a good response has been observed by ourselves and others.[22] Two randomized trials comparing clomiphene to progesterone treatment for inadequate luteal phases demonstrated equal pregnancy rates with each treatment.[23,24] Clomiphene does not prolong the luteal phase (as progesterone supplementation does). This is an important advantage, avoiding the anxiety and heightened monthly emotional response of infertile couples.

The patient who is deficient in gonadotropin secretion and, as a result, is hypoestrogenic, cannot be expected to respond to further lowering of the estrogen signal and thus should not respond to clomiphene. However, this principle is not completely applicable to clinical practice. An occasional patient who is, by all criteria, hypoestrogenic will respond. Therefore, any otherwise medically uncomplicated patient with infertility secondary to lack of ovulation is a candidate for clomiphene therapy unless galactorrhea or hyperprolactinemia is present. Hypoestrogenic women respond so rarely, however, that it is appropriate to omit treatment with clomiphene and move to other more productive options.

In addition to anovulation, treatment with clomiphene is indicated to improve the timing and frequency of ovulation and to enhance the possibilities of conception in the patient who ovulates only occasionally. Clomiphene is also useful to regulate the timing of ovulation in women undergoing insemination.

There is one special group in whom clomiphene is indicated in women who ovulate regularly and spontaneously. Certain religious requirements, such as those in Orthodox Judaism, interfere with the normal reproductive process. In the devout Orthodox Jewish couple, intercourse is prohibited in the presence of menstrual flow and for 7 days following its conclusion. In some women menstrual flow is prolonged or the follicular phase is shortened, so that coitus cannot take place until after ovulation. In the usual mode of treatment, medication is begun on day 5 of the cycle. Ovulation can be delayed to a more appropriate time by starting clomiphene later, usually on day 7 or 8 of the cycle. Ovulation can be expected in the interval 5–10 days after the last day of medication. This manipulation has its limitations. Administration too late in the cycle, beyond day 9, may have no effect.

The question is often asked whether the indications for clomiphene therapy should be extended to include the initiation of cyclicity in the oligoamenorrheic patient who does not seek fertility. In our opinion, this is an inappropriate use of clomiphene for several reasons: 1) the effectiveness of clomiphene is restricted to the cycle in which it is used and it should not be expected to induce cyclicity following the conclusion of treatment, 2) the use of clomiphene may aggravate the clinical problems of acne and hirsutism during the treatment cycle by increasing LH stimulation of ovarian steroid production, and 3) the inability to induce cyclicity can be so discouraging to the patient that her acceptance of the drug will be impaired at some future date when it is legitimately offered as a fertility agent for the induction of ovulation.

Clomiphene and Unexplained Infertility

Clomiphene is used for the treatment of unexplained infertility, i.e., women who have prolonged (>3 years) infertility but who ovulate spontaneously and repeatedly by all available measures and do not have other abnormalities.[25] While the spontaneous pregnancy rate is high in these patients (cumulative rates approach 50%), patient pressure and physician enthusiasm have led to superovulation induction in these couples. The rationale is appealingly clear. With more than one ovulation, surely there is an increased probability of successful fertilization, and such therapy would reverse (if present) episodic, unpredictable, recurrent, occult ovulatory dysfunction. Despite the high spontaneous pregnancy rate, advocates believe clomiphene has value in the empiric treatment of unexplained infertility, particularly prior to undertaking the more expensive and more complicated assisted reproductive technologies. In well-designed studies, treatment with clomiphene was associated with a higher pregnancy rate, and in one study, combination with intrauterine insemination yielded a higher monthly fecundity rate than timed intercourse.[26,27]

How to Use Clomiphene

A program of clomiphene therapy is begun on the 5th day of a cycle following either spontaneous or induced bleeding. It has not been established that a progestin withdrawal bleed is necessary before starting clomiphene treatment; we often omit this step if we are certain that the patient is not pregnant. The initial dose is 50 mg daily for 5 days. There is no advantage to beginning with a higher dose for the following two reasons: 1) in a random distribution of our patients begun with initial doses of either 50 mg or 100 mg daily, the pregnancy rate was identical; and 2) the highest incidence of side effects in our experience occurs at the 50 mg dose; however, at 100 mg, patients may develop more serious reactions. About 50% of patients conceive at the 50 mg dose, and another 20% at 100 mg.[18,19] An occasional patient will be exceptionally sensitive to clomiphene and can achieve pregnancy at the reduced dose of 25 mg.

Beginning clomiphene on the 5th day is a method arrived at empirically; however, we can now offer a rational explanation based on current physiology. The clomiphene-induced increase in gonadotropins during days 5–9 occurs at a time when the dominant follicle is being selected. Beginning clomiphene earlier can be expected to stimulate multiple follicular maturation resulting in a greater incidence of multiple gestation. Indeed, clomiphene is administered earlier in in vitro fertilization programs in order to obtain more than one oocyte. However, in standard ovulation induction protocols, no

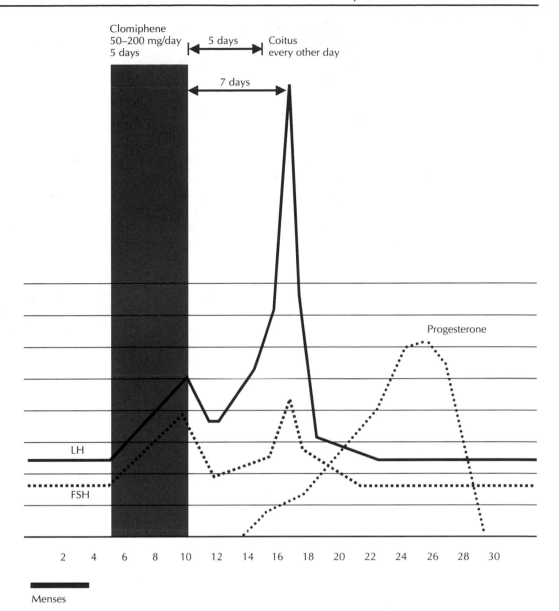

Clomiphene
50–200 mg/day
5 days

5 days

Coitus
every other day

7 days

Progesterone

LH

FSH

2   4   6   8   10   12   14   16   18   20   22   24   26   28   30

Menses

differences have been observed in the rates of ovulation, pregnancy, or spontaneous abortion whether clomiphene was started on day 2, 3, 4, or 5.[28]

If ovulation is not achieved in the very first cycle of treatment, dosage is increased to 100 mg. Thereafter, if ovulation and a normal luteal phase are not achieved in any cycle, dosage is increased in a staircase fashion by 50 mg increments to a maximum of 200–250 mg daily for 5 days. The highest dose is pursued for 3–4 months before considering the patient to be a clomiphene failure. The quantity of drug and the number of cycles go beyond those recommended by manufacturers. However, in our experience those recommendations are inappropriately limiting. We have achieved a 15% pregnancy rate at the 150 mg and 200 mg dose levels.[18]

There is a significant correlation between body weight and the dose of clomiphene required for ovulation.[29,30] One must adhere to the usual regimen, however, because the weight cannot be used to predict prospectively the correct ovulatory dose. In other words, some obese women ovulate at the same low dose which achieves ovulation in thin women. Clomiphene is not stored in adipose tissue, and the increased dose often necessary in obese women is more likely due to a more intense anovulatory state with higher androgen levels producing a more resistant hypothalamic-pituitary-ovarian axis. Increasing the dose of clomiphene will eventually achieve the same level of success in overweight women as can be attained in lean women.[31,32]

At the present time there is no clinical or laboratory parameter that can predict the dose of clomiphene necessary to achieve ovulation. Androgen and estrogen levels do not show any correlation with the dose of clomiphene that proves successful.[33]

Following the 5-day course of clomiphene, the ovulatory surge of gonadotropins can occur anywhere from 5 to 10 days after the last day of clomiphene administration. The patient is advised to have intercourse every other day for 1 week beginning 5 days after the last day of medication. In view of the role prostaglandins play in the physical expulsion of an oocyte, it is prudent to advise patients involved in programs of ovulation induction to avoid the use of agents that inhibit prostaglandin synthesis.

After the first treatment cycle the patient is evaluated for side effects, residual ovarian enlargement, and basal body temperature changes. We have found it unnecessary to perform a pelvic examination every month because significant ovarian enlargement is encountered infrequently, and it is usually symptomatic. It is more economical, for both patient and physician, to mail the temperature chart to the office and several days later plan by telephone for the following month. Cysts within a reasonable size range (3–5 cm) do not require a rest from treatment; they do not respond to further stimulation, and they do not impact upon subsequent response.

A basal body temperature record is necessary to follow the response. If an inadequate luteal phase is evident, (temperature elevation less than 11 days duration) the amount of clomiphene is increased to the next dose level. If the patient is already at the maximal level, consider the available options for dealing with clomiphene failure (detailed below). Biphasic changes are taken as an indication of ovulation and success. Maintenance of the temperature elevation beyond the expected time of menses is the earliest practical indication of pregnancy.

When the temperature chart is inconclusive or when the patient is not pregnant despite a period of apparently normal ovulations, an endometrial biopsy is indicated to document the adequacy of the luteal phase. One should also consider ultrasonographic monitoring for treatment failures, looking for follicles which do not reach mature size or the luteinized unruptured follicle syndrome (although it is by no means certain that luteinized unruptured follicles are a factor in infertility).

When inadequate luteal function is documented during clomiphene treatment, an increase in dosage is the logical solution. If this fails, consider the various methods for dealing with clomiphene failures. Keep in mind the effect of excess androgens (which may also be exerted at the endometrial level). When androgens are elevated, suppression with dexamethasone should be tried in combination with clomiphene treatment.

The additional use of HCG is limited to those cases in which there is a failure to ovulate at the maximal dose level or, when at that level, a short luteal phase is demonstrated. The rationale is to improve on the midcycle LH surge; therefore, 10,000 IU of HCG can be given as a single intramuscular dose on the 7th day after clomiphene when follicular maturation is at its peak. Because premature HCG administration may interfere with normal ovulation by down-regulating LH receptors, more accurate timing of HCG administration may be desirable. This requires either measurement of the blood estradiol level or estimation of follicular size (18–20 mm diameter) by sonography. When HCG is administered, intercourse is advised for that night and for the next 2 days. ***In our experience, the addition of HCG has not had a significant impact on the pregnancy rate.***

Care should be taken to review with the patient the pathophysiology of her condition, the principles of treatment, the prolonged course of therapy which may be necessary, and possible complications. Repeated failures accumulate frustration and despair in the couple, making each successive cycle of treatment more difficult. The anxiety and stress may hinder coital performance, and it is not uncommon for a couple to have difficulty performing scheduled intercourse.

Results

In properly selected patients, 80% can be expected to ovulate, and approximately 40% become pregnant. The percent of pregnancies per induced ovulatory cycle is about 20–25%. The multiple pregnancy rate is approximately 5%, almost entirely twins; there have been rare cases of quintuplet and sextuplet births. In our own experience, with standardization of therapy, the incidence of twins has decreased.

The abortion rate is not increased. Most importantly, the incidence of congenital malformations is not increased, and infant survival and performance after delivery are no different from normal.[17]

The discrepancy between ovulation rates and pregnancy rates is mainly due to 2 factors, the presence of other causes of infertility and a lack of persistence. ***In those patients with no other cause of infertility, the cumulative 6-month conception rate approaches a normal rate of 60–75%.***[19,33] The pregnancy rate per ovulatory cycle equals the normal rate. The pregnancy rate in 70 of our patients who received therapy sufficient to ovulate in at least 3 cycles was 55.7%, the same pregnancy rate after 3 months of exposure in the general population.[18] With additional treatment cycles, the pregnancy rate decreases, although the ovulatory rate remains high. Approximately 15% of patients treated with the higher doses of 150–250 mg will become pregnant.[18] Therefore there may be no need to attribute negative effects of clomiphene on oocyte, endometrium, the corpus luteum, and an early embryo.

If all factors are corrected, and conception has not occurred in 6 months, prognosis is poor. In one large series, only 7.8% of those who had one or more factors in addition to anovulation became pregnant.[19]

Complications

Side effects do not appear to be dose-related, occurring more frequently at the 50 mg dose. Patients requiring the high doses are probably less sensitive to the drug. The most common problems are vasomotor flushes (10%), abdominal distention, bloating, pain, or soreness (5.5%), breast discomfort (2%), nausea and vomiting (2.2%), visual symptoms (1.5%), headache (1.3%), and dryness or loss of hair (0.3%). Patients who are extremely sensitive to the side effects of clomiphene can be sucessfully treated with half a tablet (25 mg) daily for 5 days, and even with half a tablet daily for 3 days.

A common antiestrogenic effect is an increase in the basal body temperature during the 5-day period of clomiphene administration. Visual symptoms include blurring vision, scotoma (visual spots or flashes), or abnormal perception. The cause of these symptoms is unknown, but in every case studied thus far, the visual symptoms have disappeared upon discontinuation of the medication, and no permanent effects have been reported. Usually these symptoms disappear within a few days but may take 1 or 2 weeks.

Significant ovarian enlargement is associated with longer periods of treatment and is infrequent (5%) with the usual 5-day course. Maximal enlargement of the ovary usually occurs several days after discontinuing the clomiphene (in response to the increase in gonadotropins). If the patient is symptomatic, pelvic examination, intercourse, and undue physical exercise should be avoided because the enlarged ovaries are very fragile.

Ovarian enlargement dissipates rapidly and only rarely is a subsequent treatment cycle delayed.

What to Do with Clomiphene Failures

There are several options available for the 10–20% of women who fail to become pregnant with clomiphene up to the highest dose. Knowledge gained from experience with in vitro fertilization provides us with several explanations for failure to respond to clomiphene.[33] These include the effects of excessive LH in the follicular phase, the dysfunctional effects of an untimely LH surge, and excess local concentrations of androgens. These mechanisms may yield impaired folliculogenesis, increased atresia, poor oocyte quality, precocious or impaired oocyte maturation, low fertilization rates, variable implantation rates, and deficient corpus luteum function. Strategies have developed to mitigate or avoid many of these detrimental effects: the supplemental use of dexamethasone (to reduce androgen burden), GnRH agonists (to eliminate endogenous LH intrusion), pulsatile GnRH therapy (to preserve physiologic interactive feedback mechanisms), "pure" FSH (to diminish excessive LH in the follicular phase), and, finally, the use of human menopausal gonadotropins. We are also seeing the return of modified ovarian wedge resection by laparoscopic multiple ovarian tissue destruction by cautery or laser techniques.

First, make sure galactorrhea has not been overlooked and a prolactin level has been obtained. The good results with bromocriptine make it essential that this cause of anovulation be detected. After 6 months of clomiphene therapy, and in the absence of any other infertility factors, we proceed to one of the available options.

The Addition of Dexamethasone to Clomiphene

Patients with hirsutism and high circulating androgen concentrations are more resistant to clomiphene.[34–36] Dexamethasone, 0.5 mg at bedtime to blunt the nighttime peak of ACTH, is added to decrease the adrenal contribution to circulating androgens and thus diminish the androgen level in the microenvironment of the ovarian follicles. Higher ovulation and conception rates are achieved with this treatment when the circulating level of dehydroepiandrosterone sulfate (DHAS) is greater than the upper limit of normal. The dexamethasone is maintained daily until pregnancy is apparent. The dose of clomiphene is returned to the starting point of 50 mg and increased in incremental fashion as needed.

Extended Clomiphene Treatment

Two approaches have been reported for extending clomiphene treatment. We have very little experience with either. In the first, 250 mg of clomiphene are given for 8 days, followed by 10,000 IU HCG 6 days later. Three pregnancies were achieved out of 25 treatment cycles.[37] In another series, the clomiphene dose was increased every 5 days, with some patients receiving up to 25 days of consecutive treatment, the last 5 days at 250 mg daily.[38] Eight of 21 patients conceived and, in those patients who responded, measurement of gonadotropin revealed sustained elevations in FSH. This latter approach requires estrogen monitoring with discontinuation of the clomiphene when an increase in estrogen is detected. No patient ovulated after more than 21 days of treatment. A simple approach is to extend the duration of clomiphene treatment until a follicle of 18 mm diameter (on ultrasound) is obtained, then administer HCG. But extended clomiphene treatment is a lot of hassle for few results; couples might as well move on to HMG.

Pretreatment Suppression

The anovulatory state is a dysfunctional condition. It is reasonable to expect suppression of the contributing factors to be followed by a reassertion of the harmony operating in a normal menstrual cycle, at least for a short time. Clinicians have long advocated (without benefit of careful study) a period of suppression (at least 6 months) with an oral contraceptive, followed immediately by resumption of clomiphene administration. The same principle applies to the use of a GnRH agonist. Treatment with a GnRH agonist to the point of hypoestrogenism, followed by clomiphene administration when estradiol returned to a level greater than 40 pg/mL, has achieved ovulation and pregnancy in clomiphene failure patients.[39] This approach has an added attraction. There is reason to believe that women with elevated LH and testosterone levels not only have more difficulty achieving pregnancy, but also experience a higher spontaneous abortion rate.[40–42]

The Addition of Bromocriptine to Clomiphene

Although the use of bromocriptine to induce ovulation is clearly indicated in the presence of galactorrhea or hyperprolactinemia, its use in the clomiphene failure patient with a normal prolactin and no galactorrhea is controversial. Anovulatory patients with normal levels of prolactin do respond to bromocriptine, but the effectiveness of this treatment has not been established by controlled studies. Nevertheless, the clinical response is occasionally impressive.

Bromocriptine. Elevated prolactin levels interfere with the normal function of the menstrual cycle by suppressing the pulsatile secretion of GnRH. This is manifested clinically by a spectrum, ranging from a subtle inadequate luteal phase to total suppression and hypoestrogenic amenorrhea. Regardless of the prolactin level, we interpret the presence of galactorrhea to indicate excessive prolactin stimulation. We screen all patients with galactorrhea or any ovulatory disorder with an assessment of the prolactin level. After a consideration of the problems of amenorrhea, galactorrhea, and the pituitary adenoma (as discussed in Chapter 12), bromocriptine emerges as the drug of choice for the induction of ovulation in these patients.

Ovulatory dysfunction in the presence of galactorrhea responds well to bromocriptine, even if the prolactin level is normal.[43] Either biologic activity is not being detected by the immunoassay or a random blood sample fails to reveal subtle elevations in prolactin.

Bromocriptine is examined in detail in Chapter 12, but it would be helpful to review pertinent details here. Bromocriptine is a dopamine agonist that directly inhibits pituitary secretion of prolactin. Suppression of prolactin levels restores CNS-pituitary gonadotropin function and also appears to increase ovarian responsiveness. The increase in ovarian responsiveness is seen in patients with normal prolactin levels and no galactorrhea. This is the apparent mechanism for an increase in sensitivity to clomiphene when bromocriptine is added to the therapeutic regimen. In women with persistent anovulation and polycystic ovaries, LH secretion is decreased by bromocriptine treatment, thus providing a rationale for why it might enhance the ovulatory response in these patients.[44]

The gastrointestinal and cardiovascular systems react to the dopaminergic action of bromocriptine, and, therefore, the side effects are mainly nausea, diarrhea, dizziness, headache, and fatigue. Side effects can be minimized by slowly building tolerance toward the usual dose, 2.5 mg bid. We start treatment with an initial dose of 2.5 mg at bedtime. If intolerance occurs, the tablet can be cut in half, and a slower program, developed by the patient, can be followed to work up to the standard dose. Usually, the second dose is added after 1 week, at breakfast or at lunch. In some patients, elevated prolactin levels can be reduced to normal levels with very small doses of bromocriptine, as little as 0.625 or 1.25 mg.[45] Patients extremely sensitive to the side effects of bromocriptine can be treated by administering the drug intravaginally. Usually one tablet daily will be effective; if the prolactin level is elevated, the dose can be titrated to bring the prolactin level into the normal range.

The usual regimen is to administer bromocriptine daily until it is apparent the patient is pregnant, as usually determined by the basal body temperature chart. Although there has been no evidence of any harmful effects on the fetus, some patients and physicians prefer to avoid bromocriptine in the luteal phase and, therefore, during early pregnancy. The drug is stopped when a temperature rise occurs and resumed when menses begin.

Ovulatory menses and pregnancy are achieved in 80% of patients with galactorrhea and hyperprolactinemia. Response is rapid, and, therefore, if there is no indication of ovulation (a rise in the basal body temperature) within 2 months, clomiphene is added to the regimen. The starting dose of clomiphene is 50 mg daily for 5 days, given and increased in the usual fashion.

As discussed in Chapter 12, once pregnant, the majority of women with a pituitary-secreting adenoma remain asymptomatic. Women with both microadenomas and macroadenomas may undergo uneventful pregnancies. It is extremely rare for a patient to develop a problem that results in perinatal damage or serious maternal sequelae. Surveillance during pregnancy need only consist of an awareness for the development of symptoms, headaches and visual disturbances. Assessment of visual fields, prolactin assay, and sella turcica changes by imaging can await the onset of suspicious symptoms. Tumor expansion (and its symptoms) promptly regress with bromocriptine treatment. No adverse effects of bromocriptine on the pregnancy or the newborn have been reported.

Resolution of galactorrhea or hyperprolactinemia can occur spontaneously after a pregnancy. Perhaps a tumor can undergo infarction in response to the expansion and shrinkage during and after pregnancy, or the condition was associated with dysfunction of the hypothalamus, now corrected.

Bromocriptine for Euprolactinemic Women. Clinical experience suggests that successful induction of ovulation and achievement of pregnancy with bromocriptine can occur in the absence of galactorrhea and with a normal prolactin level in women who have failed to respond to clomiphene.[46] Some anovulatory women with normal prolactin levels who ovulated in response to bromocriptine have been found to have elevated nocturnal peaks of prolactin.[47] The mechanism of action may be an increase in follicular responsiveness either due to suppression of prolactin or suppression of LH (a known action of dopamine). A decrease in LH may alter local follicular steroidogenesis in such a way to create a more favorable microenvironment. The method of administration is the same as above. If, after 2 months of treatment, there is no response, clomiphene is reinitiated, working up again from the starting dose of 50 mg daily. A carefully designed study has demonstrated that bromocriptine has nothing to offer for ovulatory women with unexplained infertility.[48] On the other hand, bromocriptine or bromocriptine plus clomiphene treatment of ovulatory women with galactorrhea (and normal prolactin levels) yielded higher pregnancy rates when compared to a control group.[49] Once again the importance of detecting galactorrhea is emphasized.

Human Menopausal Gonadotropins (HMG)

Human menopausal gonadotropins consist of a purified preparation of gonadotropins extracted from the urine of postmenopausal women. The generic name is menotropins. The commercial preparation is available with either 75 units of FSH and 75 units of LH per ampule, or in an ampule with twice the amount, 150 units. The potency is expressed in terms of international units based on an international reference preparation. A significant factor in the use of HMG is its high cost. Treatment may cost from $1,000 to $1,500/cycle for the drug alone. HMG is inactive orally and, therefore, must be given by intramuscular injections.

Recombinant FSH has been produced through genetic engineering and successfully tested.[50] Recombinant FSH is homogeneous and free of contamination by proteins (characteristic of menopausal gonadotropins from urinary extracts); this allows simpler subcutaneous administration. Clinical studies should be forthcoming. Remember that while FSH will provide the necessary stimulus for follicular recruitment and growth, some LH is necessary for full ovarian steroidogenesis.

Selection of Patients

Not only because of its expense but because of its greater complication rate, patients should not receive HMG without a very careful evaluation. An absolute requirement is the demonstration of ovarian competence. Abnormally high serum gonadotropins with a failure to demonstrate withdrawal bleeding indicate ovarian failure and preclude induction of ovulation except in those special cases of ovarian failure discussed in Chapter 12. Successful induction of ovulation and pregnancy has been reported in women with apparent ovarian failure, treated with a combination of estrogen (to suppress FSH to normal levels) and HMG. Our own experience with this approach has been disappointing, and the chance of achieving pregnancy must be very low.

A thorough infertility investigation must be performed. In addition to the demonstration of ovarian competence, tubal and uterine pathology should be ruled out, anovulation documented, and semen analysis obtained. Nongynecologic endocrine problems must be treated. Hypogonadotropic function (low serum gonadotropins), including galactorrhea syndromes, requires evaluation for an intracranial lesion, with appropriate imaging and measurement of prolactin levels. It is imperative to take all steps necessary to exclude treatable pathology to which anovulation is secondary.

In our practice we sometimes, but not often, offer a course of clomiphene, not only because of the cost and complications associated with HMG, but also because some apparently hypogonadotropic patients will unpredictably respond to clomiphene. Because some patients cannot tolerate bromocriptine, it is important to know that hyperprolactinemia has no adverse effect on response to HMG.[51]

Superovulation and IUI for Unexplained Infertility

Because empiric superovulation (also called controlled ovarian hyperstimulation) combined with intrauterine inseminations (IUI) is associated with cycle fecundity rates (approximately 15%, which compares favorably to the spontaneous fertility rate of approximately 3% per month in these couples) similar to those of the more expensive and more invasive methods of the assisted reproductive technologies, a course of this treatment is often chosen by patients and clinicians.[52,53] The rationale is appealing: correction of occult defects in either the female or male. An improved pregnancy rate has been reported with two intrauterine inseminations, one before ovulation (18 hours after HCG) and one after (42 hours after HCG), compared to a single IUI 34 hours after HCG administration.[54] However, it is not certain whether the addition of IUI is critical for success. It is possible that the improved timing inherent in this procedure is important. On the other hand, the achievement of pregnancy may be entirely due to multiple ovulations, enhanced oocyte quality, and improved endometrium. Or, maybe both procedures make a contribution. Only randomized clinical trials can provide the answer. In two randomized trials, intrauterine insemination yielded no advantage over timed natural intercourse when combined with GnRH agonist and HMG treatments or when IUI alone was compared with HMG and IUI.[55,56] In another randomized trial of 148 couples, insemination again provided no increase in pregnancy rate compared to well-timed intercourse, although HMG yielded a higher pregnancy rate than clomiphene.[57] Nevertheless, the safety and reduced costs with clomiphene argue persuasively that several cycles of clomiphene-IUI should be completed prior to a regimen of HMG and IUI. With the accumulation of evidence from randomized trials, IUI may prove to be without benefit.

The incidence of multiple births and ovarian hyperstimulation is higher with this empiric treatment. Patients and clinicians undertaking empiric superovulation should have ready recourse to in vitro fertilization. *If HMG stimulation is excessive, several choices are available: avoiding HCG administration and cancelling the cycle, aspirating most of the ovarian follicles with ultrasound guidance, or proceeding with in vitro ferilization.*

How to Use HMG

Instruction and counseling of the couple are essential. A thorough understanding of the need for daily treatment and frequent observation is necessary prior to initiating therapy. As part of this instruction, the partner can be taught to administer injections. Daily recording of the basal body temperature and body weight is important for proper management. The couple should be told about the need for scheduled intercourse, the possibility that more than one course of treatment may be necessary, and the expense of the treatment. Above all, the patient must be prepared for the anguish that accompanies failure. Because this is a pressure-packed situation, unexpected impotence is occasionally encountered on the days of scheduled intercourse.

In the past there were 2 commonly used techniques of HMG administration, the variable and the fixed dosage methods. Pregnancy rates with the fixed dosage method are unacceptably low, and the variable dosage method should be used to achieve follicular growth and maturation. Follicle stimulation is achieved by 7–14 days of continuous HMG, beginning with 150 units daily. Response is judged by the degree of estrogen produced by the growing follicles. The patient is monitored periodically with the measurement of the circulating estradiol level and vaginal ultrasound assessment of the number and size of follicles. The patient is seen on the 7th day of treatment, and a decision is made to continue or increase the dose. After the 7th day, the patient is seen anywhere from daily to every 3rd day. Patients with polycystic ovaries are handled more gingerly because they are more responsive. These patients are usually started on 75 units daily, and monitoring begins on the 5th day of treatment.

HMG comes as a dry powder in a sealed glass ampule, along with a second ampule containing 2 mL of diluent. Based on clinical responses, there is no evidence that bioactivity varies among the different production lots of the standard commercial preparation.[58] One ampule of HMG requires 1 mL of diluent. When 2 ampules are to be administered, solution with 1 mL is accomplished in the first vial of HMG, and the solution is then deposited in the second vial. Thus, when giving 2 ampules of HMG the contents of 2 vials are dissolved in a total of 1 mL of diluent. When 4 ampules are given, a total of 2 mL of diluent are used. Should 6 ampules of HMG be required, 3 ampules are dissolved in 1.5 mL of diluent, and two injections are administered, each in the upper outer quadrant of each buttock. The HCG injection comes as a vial containing 10,000 units as a dry powder; one mL of the accompanying diluent is used for administration.

It cannot be emphasized too strongly that dosage administration and the judicious use of estrogen measurements depend upon the experience of the physician administering HMG. When estradiol and ultrasound monitoring indicate that the patient is ready to receive the ovulatory stimulus, 10,000 units of HCG are given as a single dose intramuscularly. Because of its structural and biologic similarity to LH, HCG, readily available from human pregnancy urine and placental tissue, is used to simulate the midcycle LH ovulatory surge. Neither manipulation of HCG dosage nor time of administration has been successful in changing the rates of multiple gestation and hyperstimulation.

The patient is advised to have intercourse the day of the HCG injection and for the next 2 days. In view of the fragility of hyperstimulated ovaries, further intercourse as well as strenuous physical exercise should be avoided.

Pregnancy is usually achieved with the administration of 150 units/day for 7–12 days. The best results are obtained when the treatment period covers 10–15 days; when less than 10 days, the spontaneous abortion rate is increased.[59] In general there is a direct relationship between dose and body weight; however, the same empiric approach is needed even in obese patients.[60] In some individuals, presumably with extremely hyposensitive ovaries, adequate follicular stimulation requires doses up to 4, 6, and more ampules/day. In this group of amenorrheic women massive doses of gonadotropins are necessary, and with proper monitoring, pregnancy can be achieved safely. The range between the dose that does not induce ovulation and the dose that results in hyperstimulation is narrow. The situation is made even more difficult because the ovaries may react differently to essentially similar doses from month to month. Close supervision and experience in the use of HMG are necessary to avoid difficulties. There is no reason to avoid consecutive cycles of ovarian stimulation; indeed, an increased cycle fecundity has been observed in consecutive treatment cycles when compared to alternating stimulation and nontreatment.[61,62]

Estrogen Monitoring

The use of estrogen measurements is necessary to choose the correct moment for administering the ovulatory dose of HCG in order to prevent hyperstimulation. On day 7 of the therapeutic cycle blood is assayed for estradiol. Depending on the findings, the dosage of HMG is individualized for the duration of the cycle. With experience, the physician can avoid daily estrogen measurements although sometimes this is necessary.

What should the blood estradiol level be? Because the blood estradiol is determined on a single sample of blood, the timing of the sampling with relationship to the previous injection of HMG becomes a significant variable. When HMG injections are given between 5 and 8 PM and blood samples are obtained first thing in the morning, an estradiol window of 1,000–1,500 pg/mL (3,700–5,500 pmol/L) is optimal.[63] The risk of hyperstimulation is significant from 1,500 to 2,000 pg/mL and, as a general rule, over 2,000 pg/mL (7,300 pmol/L), HCG should not be given, and the ovarian follicles should be allowed to regress. Careful correlation of estrogen levels with the ultrasonographic picture allows a more aggressive approach. Haning has calculated that an upper limit for estradiol of 3,800 pg/mL for anovulatory women (with polycystic ovaries) and 2,400 for women with hypothalamic amenorrhea gives a risk of severe hyperstimulation of 5% in pregnant cycles and 1% in nonconception cycles.[64]

Attempting to reproduce the normal midcycle levels of estradiol does not achieve a maximal pregnancy rate, and higher levels are required. The relative safety of this approach was seen in our series, where only 2 of 24 patients with estradiol levels over 1,000 pg/mL developed hyperstimulation and it was moderate in both cases.[63] When a patient nears ovulation, timing of the HCG administration can be predicted fairly accurately by plotting the estradiol values on semilogarithmic paper. The rate of increase in estradiol is the same in spontaneous and induced cycles, and does not differ in cycles that result in multiple gestation.[65] The level which is reached at the time of HCG administration is more critical than the slope of increase. Once a linear rise of estradiol is established, there is no need to increase the dose.

Ultrasound Monitoring

Ultrasound assessment of the growth and development of the ovarian follicle indicates the degree of follicular maturity and capability.[66] During normal cycles, the growing cohort of follicles can be first identified by ultrasonography on days 5 to 7 as small sonolucent cysts. The dominant follicle will become apparent by days 8–10. The maximal mean diameter, indicating ovum maturity, of the preovulatory dominant follicle varies from 20 to 24 mm (range 14–28 mm) in normal, spontaneous cycles. Individual women tend to produce the same maximal diameter on repeated cycles. Pregnancies have not been observed with follicles less than 17 mm diameter in normal cycles.[66] Subordinate follicles rarely exceed 14 mm in diameter. In 5–11% of cycles, two dominant follicles develop.

During the 5 days preceding ovum expulsion, the dominant follicle exhibits a linear growth pattern of approximately 2 to 3 mm per day, followed by rapid exponential growth during the last 24 hours prior to ovulation. *Ultrasonographic surveillance of ovaries reveals that mittelschmerz is associated not with follicular rupture but with the rapid expansion of the dominant follicle, thus the pain precedes follicular rupture.*

Ovulation is associated with complete emptying of the follicular contents in 1 to 45 minutes. Fluid can be detected frequently, but not always, in the cul-de-sac. The follicle either disappears or more commonly appears as a smaller, irregular cyst which diminishes in size over the next 4–5 days.

In response to clomiphene treatment, follicles pursue a linear but generally accelerated rate of growth compared to spontaneous cycles.[67] The maximal diameter of clomiphene-induced preovulatory follicles is similar to that seen with spontaneous cycles, 20–24 mm, but ovulation can be successfully induced with HCG administration when the diameter reaches 18–20 mm (by the time of ovulation, the follicle will have grown another 2–3 mm). With HMG, the maximal follicular diameter (15–18 mm) is smaller than that seen during spontaneous and clomiphene-induced cycles. When follicles reach this size, ovulation will occur approximately 36 hours after HCG is administered.

Ultrasound monitoring does not eliminate the risks of multiple gestation and hyperstimulation. It is claimed that a higher pregnancy rate can be achieved when ultrasound is combined with estrogen monitoring.[68] The guiding principle has been to administer HCG when mature follicles correlate with an estrogen level of 400 pg per follicle. The 400 pg principle only applies when there are several leading follicles, not when many intermediate (9–16 mm) and small (<9 mm) follicles are present. As a general rule, hyperstimulation is associated with the presence of more follicles. We believe that HCG should not be administered if there are more than 3–5 follicles 14 mm or greater in diameter (offering some protection against multiple gestation and hyperstimulation). Mild hyperstimulation has been associated with an increased number of intermediate size follicles, and severe hyperstimulation with an increase in small follicles.[69,70] A large number (11 or more) of smaller follicles also should preclude HCG administration.

Serial ultrasound observations of ovarian cycles has raised many questions. Alleged asynchronies have been identified involving the estradiol surge, the gonadotropin surge, deficient luteinization, and the growth and disappearance of follicles.[71] A new syndrome has emerged, the luteinized unruptured follicle syndrome. This condition, in which the follicle becomes luteinized without release of the ovum, cannot be diagnosed by the usual standard but indirect methods of ovulation assessment.[72] This phenomenon occurs in both fertile and infertile women, in perhaps as many as 5–10% of cycles. The actual relationship, if any, of these observations to infertility is uncertain.

Measurement of Endometrial Thickness. Ultrasonographic studies in cycles of in vitro fertilization have revealed that successful implantation is correlated with endometrial thickness on the day of HCG administration.[73] This same correlation has been observed in patients in non-IVF patients receiving HMG for ovulation induction.[74] Consistent with the antiestrogenic action of clomiphene, endometrial thickness is reduced in women treated with clomiphene (and reversed with estrogen). In a program utilizing clomiphene and timed administration of HCG for the purposes of intrauterine inseminations, no pregnancies occurred when the endometrial thickness measured less than 6 mm.[75] The chance of pregnancy is greatest, no matter what program of ovarian stimulation is being used, if endometrial thickness is 6–9 mm or more.[76]

The Effect of Persistent Ovarian Cysts. In contrast to results with IVF or GIFT, the presence of a baseline ovarian cyst greater than 10 mm in diameter is associated with decreased fecundity in ovulation induction with HMG.[77] With large cysts, treatment should be either delayed, or cyst suppression with a GnRH agonist or oral contaceptives should be considered, although it has never been proven that such treatment is effective. With this exception, there is no advantage in avoiding multiple successive treatment cycles (such as alternating treatment and nontreatment cycles).[61,62]

Clomiphene-HMG Combination

The combination of both clomiphene and HMG was explored in order to minimize the amount and the cost of HMG alone. As long as treatment is monitored with estrogen levels the side effects and complications should not be dissimilar to those with HMG alone. It has not been demonstrated that patients unresponsive to HMG alone would respond to the sequence method, and there is no logical reason to assume that this would be true.

The usual method of treatment is to administer clomiphene 100 mg for 5–7 days, then to immediately proceed with HMG beginning with 150 units per day. Estrogen levels are monitored as usual. This method may decrease the amount of HMG required by approximately 50%; however, the same risks of multiple pregnancy and hyperstimulation can be expected. This reduced requirement for HMG is found only in those patients who demonstrate a positive withdrawal bleeding following progestin medication or who have spontaneous menses.[78]

Pulsatile Administration of HMG

HMG can be administered in pulsatile fashion, either subcutaneously or intravenously, using an appropriate pump system.[79,80] The aim is to reproduce the pulsatile pattern of gonadotropin secretion during the normal menstrual cycle. The dose administered intravenously is 6–9 units per pulse every 90 minutes, with adjustments upward according to response. The usual monitoring with estradiol levels and ultrasonography is necessary. It is not certain whether this method is better beyond a decrease in dose and possibly a response in patients unresponsive to the traditional intramuscular regimen.

Results

The most significant aspect of this method of treatment is that it does achieve pregnancy in otherwise untreatable situations. A cumulative conception rate of 90% after 6 treatment cycles can be achieved in women with hypothalamic amenorrhea (this rate exceeds that observed in spontaneously ovulating women), with a 23% rate of spontaneous abortion.[81] Women with normogonadotropic anovulation achieve only a 40% cumulative conception rate with relatively higher rates of abortion (24–40%). A slightly higher rate of spontaneous abortion reflects the combination of better detection of early pregnancy loss, advanced maternal age, and the increased incidence of multiple pregnancies. As with clomiphene, there is a normal incidence of congenital malformations, and the children have a normal postnatal development.[17] *The risk of ectopic pregnancy is increased with ovulation induction, a consequence of multiple oocytes and high hormone levels.*[82] These patients should be closely monitored in the early weeks of their pregnancies.

Women with polycystic ovaries and moderate obesity require larger doses of HMG and ovulate at a lesser rate compared to leaner women with polycystic ovaries.[83] A comparable pregnancy rate (40%) is achieved. However, spontaneous abortion is more frequent which is consistent with the observation that spontaneous abortion is more frequent in obese women.

HCG disappears from the blood with an initial component having a half-life of about 6 hours and a second, slower, component with a half-life of about 24 hours. It is this relatively slow half-life that enables a single injection of 10,000 IU to maintain the corpus luteum until pregnancy takes over. The HCG concentration after the ovulation injection should be less than 50–100 IU/L by day 14 after the injection. A β-subunit assay of HCG at this time or one of the urine assays performed 2–4 weeks after the HCG injection are reliable tests for pregnancy. Additional HCG (during the luteal phase) does not improve pregnancy rates.[84] Luteal supplementation is required only with concurrent treatment with a GnRH agonist.

The likelihood of ovulation is dose related, and complications are likewise dose related. The rate of serious hyperstimulation has been 1–2%. Prior to the present era of more careful monitoring, the multiple pregnancy rate was reported as approximately 30% (triplets or more, 5%). Currently, the multiple pregnancy rate can be as low as 10% with careful monitoring and good medical judgment; however, rates as high as 40% are reported.[68] The multiple pregnancies are secondary to multiple ovulations, and therefore the siblings are not identical. The rate of spontaneous occurrence of twins is only about 1% and that of triplets 0.010–0.017% of the pregnant population. Dizygotic twinning varies among different populations and is inherited through the mother. The monozygotic twinning rate is about 0.3–0.4%, fairly constant, and uninfluenced by heredity. Surprisingly, induction of ovulation increases the frequency of monozygotic twinning 3-fold.[85] It is not known whether the multiple pregnancy rate with HMG is significantly affected by a maternal history of twinning.

Maternal complications and fetal loss caused by prematurity in the multiple pregnancies have been serious problems. In addition, the abortion rate with HMG is somewhat higher (25%) than normal, probably a combination of the effect of age, multiple pregnancies, and recognition of early abortions.[86]

After at least one HMG-induced pregnancy, the subsequent spontaneous pregnancy rate reaches 30% after 5 years.[87] Most of the pregnancies occur within 3 years of the HMG pregnancy, and the more endogenous hypothalamic-pituitary-ovarian function a patient has, the more likely a spontaneous pregnancy will occur.[88] This is consistent with a return to normal function in some women after suppression of a dysfunctional state. With time, it is logical to expect the original dysfunctional state to reestablish itself.

Multifetal Pregnancy Reduction

Therapeutic abortion in the case of triplets or more is an option, but it would be surprising if patient and physician would choose this solution. On the other hand, selective reduction of a number of embryos in multiple pregnancy can be accomplished.[89–92] Under ultrasound guidance, a gestational sac can be aspirated or a cardiotoxic drug (potassium chloride) can be injected into, or adjacent to, the fetal heart. The transvaginal procedure is best performed between the 8th and 9th weeks of gestation and the transabdominal procedure between the 11th and 12th weeks. A later procedure is worthwhile because there is an incidence of spontaneous disappearance of one or more gestational sacs in multiple gestations, approximately 5% after fetal heartbeats have been identified.[93] Selection of which gestational sac to be terminated is based solely on technical considerations, such as accessibility. The subsequent risk of losing one or more of the remaining fetuses is 4–9%, and of losing the pregnancy, 10% by experienced clinicians and higher with less experience. Reduction of a monochorionic pregnancy is not advisable because of shared vasculature and the high risk of losing all fetuses. The moral and ethical aspects of fetal reduction are significant, but in view of the potential problems associated with a multiple birth, it is a reasonable alternative for some.

Hyperstimulation Syndrome

Ovarian hyperstimulation can be life threatening. In mild cases the syndrome includes ovarian enlargement, abdominal distension, and weight gain. In severe cases, a critical condition develops with ascites, pleural effusion, electrolyte imbalance, and hypovolemia with hypotension and oliguria.[94–96] The ovaries are tremendously enlarged with multiple follicular cysts, stromal edema, and many corpora lutea. Because of this enlargement, torsion of the adnexa is a relatively common complication of this syndrome.[97]

The incidence of clinically important hyperstimulation is striking. Although it might be expected that the mild type would be relatively common, the moderate to severe form appears at an impressive rate (1–2%). Two-thirds of cases occur early in a conception cycle, the remainder in nonconception cycles. For purposes of one of the methods of assisted reproduction, the ovaries are stimulated at an even greater rate than for conventional ovulation induction; however, the incidence of hyperstimulation is no greater.[98] For this reason, it has been suggested that follicular aspiration offers partial protection against the hyperstimulation syndrome. Some reports have indicated a higher incidence of hyperstimulation in in vitro fertilization protocols using the combination of HMG and a GnRH agonist.[98] Because support during the luteal phase is required when GnRH agonist treatment is used, the additional HCG administered is responsible for greater stimulation. The use of progesterone for luteal support is probably safer, and therefore, when estradiol levels are high (>2,500 pg/mL [9,200 pmol/L]) and when the follicle number is greater than 15, intravaginal or intramuscular progesterone is recommended instead of HCG.

Anovulatory women with polycystic ovaries are at greatest risk for the hyperstimulation syndrome. The use of a GnRH agonist in combined therapy does not eliminate this risk. These patients should be treated slowly with careful titration of dose, and therapy should be started at a dose of 75 units per day.

The basic disturbance in hyperstimulation is a shift of fluid from the intravascular space into the abdominal cavity, creating a massive third space. The resulting hypovolemia leads to circulatory and excretory problems. The genesis of the ascites is unclear. The very high level of estrogen secretion by the ovaries may be the primary factor, inducing increased local capillary permeability and leakage of fluid from the peritoneal capillaries as well as the ovaries. Or the syndrome may result from overproduction of autocrine/paracrine factors which affect vascular permeability. The leakage of fluid is also critically related to the mass, volume, and surface area of the ovaries. Therefore, the larger the ovaries and the greater the steroid production, the more severe the condition. Experiments in animals have implicated a role for histamine and prostaglandins.

The loss of fluid and protein into the abdominal cavity accounts for the hypovolemia and hemoconcentration. This in turn results in low blood pressure and decreased central venous pressure. The major clinical complications are increased coagulability and decreased renal perfusion. Blood loss as the cause of the clinical picture can be easily ruled out since a hematocrit will reveal hemoconcentration. The decreased renal perfusion leads to increased salt and water reabsorption in the proximal tubule, producing oliguria and low urinary sodium excretion. With less sodium being presented to the distal tubule, there is a decrease in the exchange of hydrogen and potassium for sodium, resulting in hyperkalemic acidosis. A rise in the blood urea nitrogen (BUN) is due to decreased perfusion and increased urea reabsorption. Because it is only filtered, creatinine does not increase as much as the BUN. Thus, the patient is hypovolemic, azotemic, and hyperkalemic. In response to these changes, aldosterone, plasma renin activity, and antidiuretic hormone levels are all elevated.[99]

Treatment is conservative and empiric. When a patient displays excessive weight gain (usually 10 or more pounds), excessive pain, hemoconcentration (hematocrit over 50%, white blood count over 25,000), oliguria, dyspnea, or postural hypotension, she should be hospitalized. Pelvic and abdominal examinations are contraindicated in view of the extreme fragility of the enlarged ovaries. Ovarian rupture and hemorrhage are easily precipitated.

Upon admission, the patient is put on bed rest, with daily body weights, strict monitoring of intake and output, and frequent vital signs. Serial studies of the following are obtained: hematocrit, BUN, creatinine, electrolytes, total proteins with albumin:globulin ratio, coagulation studies, and urinary sodium and potassium. The electrocardiogram is utilized to follow and evaluate hyperkalemia. Fluid and salt restriction is controversial. It is argued that correction of the decreased circulating volume is not necessary as long as the BUN remains stable (an abnormally low urine output can be tolerated).[99] Others believe that plasma expanding agents and electrolyte supplements should be administered.[100] Human albumin (safe from viral contamination) is the volume expander of choice. Potassium exchange resins may be necessary. Diuretics are without effect and, indeed, may be disadvantageous. The fluid in the abdominal cavity is not responsive to diuretic treatment, and diuresis may further contract the intravascular volume and produce hypovolemic shock or thrombosis. Arterial and venous thromboses have been reported, and anticoagulant therapy should be considered in severely hemoconcentrated patients.[101,102] Although both antihistamines and indomethacin have been demonstrated to ameliorate the hyperstimulation in animal studies, their efficacy and safety in early human pregnancy are unknown. Inhibition of prostaglandin synthesis can worsen renal perfusion.

In severe cases, life-threatening adult respiratory distress syndrome can occur.[103] These patients require intensive care monitoring, including central venous and pulmonary wedge pressures. Adult respiratory distress syndrome is associated with a 50% mortality rate. Chlorpheniramine maleate, an H-1 receptor blocker, appears to maintain membrane stability, allowing the use of fluids and mannitol to retain intravascular volume.[104] With ultrasound guidance to avoid the enlarged ovaries, abdominal paracentesis can relieve severe pulmonary compromise. Aspiration of ascites can also be accomplished (and probably more easily) transvaginally (with ultrasound guidance).[105,106] With repeated aspirations, it is very important to replace the lost plasma proteins (autotransfusion of the ascitic fluid has been used in a small number of cases). On the average, repeat aspirations are necessary in 3 to 5 days.

In severe cases, transvaginal aspiration of follicular structures should be considered to interfere with the intraovarian mechanism responsible for the clinical picture; progesterone supplementation will be necessary to maintain an on-going pregnancy.[107]

The possibility of ovarian rupture should always be considered, and serial hematocrits may be the only clue to intraperitoneal hemorrhage. Of course, a falling hematocrit accompanied by diuresis is an indication of resolution, not hemorrhage. Laparotomy should be avoided in these precarious patients. If surgery is necessary, only hemostatic measures should be undertaken and the ovaries should be conserved if possible, since a return to normal size is inevitable. If torsion of the adnexa is encountered, unwinding the adnexa (and preserving the ovary in an infertile patient) is possible even when the adnexa are already ischemic.

The key point is that the hyperstimulation syndrome will undergo gradual resolution with time. In a patient who is not pregnant, the syndrome will cover a period of approximately 7 days. In a patient who is pregnant and in whom the ovaries are restimulated by the emerging endogenous HCG production, the syndrome will last 10–20 days.

The syndrome will not develop unless the ovulatory dose of HCG is given. Thus, the major emphasis in recent years has been to utilize monitoring to avoid hyperstimulation. The relationship between estrogen levels and hyperstimulation is not a perfect one. Hyperstimulation has been found with relatively low estrogen levels, and high estrogen is not necessarily followed by hyperstimulation. As a general rule, the more follicles present (on ultrasound examination) the greater the risk for hyperstimulation. But this too is not a perfect correlation. Nevertheless, monitoring is the major available deterrent to a potentially life-threatening situation.

What to Do with the HMG Failure?

At one time, management of the couple who had failed ovulation induction with HMG was difficult, but straightforward. Short of another costly round if funds and emotional reserves were sufficient, nothing was left to offer except adoption. Today a major option is now available in the assisted reproductive technologies (Chapter 31). Although even more costly and emotionally charged, these methods do offer significant additional opportunities for unsuccessful patients. Nevertheless, guidance to adoption services and emotional support continue to be part of the physician's obligation.

A very important question for patients is: when to stop? All clinicians have been confronted by the dismal and frustrating prospects of a woman who has squandered years in vain repetitive attempts at ovulation induction, only to arrive at age 40 for intervention with one of the methods of assisted reproductive technology. If a properly managed set of 6 HMG cycles is unsuccessful, the prudent counsel is to recommend a turn toward the methods of assisted reproductive technology.

An additional factor has intruded into the question of when to stop. An analysis of 3 case-control studies of ovarian cancer conducted in the U.S. from 1987–1989 concluded that the risk was increased among women who had used fertility drugs and among women who had been exposed to long periods of sexual activity without contraception.[108] However, this conclusion was limited by the small number of cases, and the exact drugs and dosage used by these cases were unknown. Nevertheless, the idea that superovulation can increase the risk of ovarian cancer is biologically plausible because there is a decreasing risk for invasive epithelial ovarian cancer associated with those conditions marked by a decrease in the number of ovulations: multiparity, increasing duration of breastfeeding, and the use of oral contraception.

It is worth noting that a long-term follow-up of 2,632 women in Israel who had received drugs for induction of ovulation did not record an increased incidence of ovarian cancer in the subsequent years.[109] Nevertheless, an anecdotal report of 12 cases of granulosa cell tumors developing during or after ovarian stimulation emphasizes the importance of careful monitoring of these patients.[110] A persistently enlarged ovary requires definitive evaluation and diagnosis.

Can Failure to Respond Be Predicted?

Women who present with "incipient" ovarian failure have elevated FSH levels and decreased levels of inhibin, but normal levels of estradiol.[111] This indicates that inhibin levels are regulated independently of estradiol, and that inhibin is a more sensitive marker of ovarian follicular competence. The changes in the later reproductive years reflect lesser follicular competence as the better primordial follicles respond early in life, leaving the lesser follicles for later. This is reflected in the decrease in fecundity that occurs with aging.

The rise in FSH during the later years is believed to represent declining inhibin production by the less competent ovarian follicles.[112,113] Inhibin levels are lower in the follicular phase in women 45–49 years old compared to younger women. This decline begins early, but accelerates after 40 years of age. The rise in FSH is usually not apparent until age 40, and there is no change in LH levels until menopause. The inability to suppress gonadotropins to a normal range during estrogen treatment of postmenopausal women reflects this loss of inhibin.

Elevated FSH levels on cycle day 3 (greater than 15, but especially greater than 20 IU/L) are associated with poor performance with in vitro fertilization.[114] Day 3 FSH levels increase with age. In normal women under age 40, a single day 3 FSH value less than 20 IU/L was highly predictive that day 3 values would stay under 20 the rest of the year.[115] However, in women over age 40, the levels were found to increase within a year's time. This is consistent with the wide swings in baseline FSH levels during the perimenopausal period. In repeated superovulation cycles, the use of day 3 FSH has little predictive value because of wide variation from cycle to cycle. A cycle day 3 FSH level that is 25 IU/L or more or an age of 44 years or more both independently are associated with a chance of pregnancy close to zero during ovulation induction or with assisted reproductive technology.[116] Women with one ovary have higher day 3 FSH levels which correlate with reduced outcomes in in vitro fertilization.[117] It is not certain whether this reflects the loss of the other ovary or the factors which were responsible for the unilateral oophorectomy. Keep in mind that there is no abrupt change at 40, and therefore these changes can apply to younger women.

The Clomiphene Challenge Test. Navot and colleagues developed the clomiphene challenge test as a bioassay of FSH response (which in turn probably reflects ovarian follicular inhibin capability).[118] Clomiphene is administered in a dose of 100 mg/day on days 5–9. The levels of FSH on days 9–11 are compared to the baseline levels on days 2–3. An exaggerated FSH response of 26 IU/L or more is 2 standard deviations above the control values, and this increase in FSH is associated with a significant prospect for failure to achieve pregnancy. There is a high incidence of abnormal responses in women over 35; 85% of women with increased FSH levels respond poorly to ovarian stimulation, and long-term pregnancy rates are drastically reduced.[119,120]

Regardless of age, women with elevated day 3 FSH levels and/or abnormal responses to the clomiphene challenge test should consider in vitro fertilization with young, donated oocytes.

GnRH Agonist Combination

Recognizing that women with significant estrogen, androgen, and gonadotropin levels do not respond well to induction of ovulation, attention was turned to a method that could turn off a woman's endogenous reproductive hormone production. The availability of GnRH agonists provided such a method. The thesis underlying the use of a GnRH agonist as an adjunctive therapy in ovulation induction is straightforward: convert normogonadotropic anovulators to a hypogonadotropic hypogonad state by the process of pituitary GnRH receptor down-regulation and desensitization.[121,122] Premature LH effects on the follicle and the burden of excess local androgen can be diminished and an improved therapeutic response achieved. There is reason to believe that women with anovulatory polycystic ovaries have a higher incidence of spontaneous abortion following induction of ovulation with HMG;[40–42] combining the GnRH agonist with HMG not only yields a greater pregnancy rate, but also reduces the abortion rate.[123] Furthermore, premature LH release is believed to contribute to the risk of ovarian hyperstimulation in women with polycystic ovaries.[124] Combining a GnRH agonist with HMG treatment could reduce (although not eliminate) the risk of this serious complication.

Leuprolide acetate (Lupron) is administered twice daily (0.5 mg subcutaneously) for 2 weeks.[122] Suppression of gonadotropin secretion is confirmed by measurement of the estradiol level; a concentration less than 25 pg/mL (90 pmol/L) should be achieved before treatment is initiated with gonadotropins. Lupron treatment is maintained throughout the HMG regimen until HCG is administered. It is not unusual to require higher doses of HMG. With this combination, no difference has been observed in the number of follicles recruited, the rate of rise and final estradiol level achieved, or the number of cycles canceled compared with HMG alone. Hyperstimulation is not avoided, but per cycle fecundity appears to be modestly increased. Buserelin and nafarelin can also be used for this purpose.

The administration of a GnRH agonist to a woman who has menstrual function will initially produce a stimulatory response, known as the "flare." The magnitude of the flare response depends upon when in the cycle the agonist is administered. During the follicular phase or in anovulatory women, the flare is greater, and enlarged follicular cysts can occur. This response can be minimized by beginning therapy during the midluteal phase or by administering a progestational agent (e.g., 10 mg medroxy-progesterone acetate daily for 10 days) and beginning GnRH agonist treatment after 3 days of progestin.

During the hypoestrogenic period of time, menopausal-like symptoms are common, especially hot flushes. Forewarning and reassurance are usually sufficient to help patients tolerate these short-lived reactions.

Utilization of a GnRH agonist suppresses endogenous LH levels to such a low level that, after ovulation, the corpus luteum requires additional exogenous support. One can administer HCG (2,000 IU) twice, 3 days, and 6 days after ovulation, or progesterone supplementation beginning 3 days after ovulation (4 days after the LH surge): intravaginal progesterone suppositories, 25 mg twice per day or intramuscular proges-terone, 50 mg per day. The pregnancy rates with either treatment are the same, but the use of HCG adds to the risk of hyperstimulation.[125,126]

Adding Growth Hormone

As discussed in Chapter 6, the primate ovarian follicular cycle is very dependent upon autocrine/paracrine factors. In view of the critical role played by insulin-like growth factor-I, it was quickly recognized that the addition of growth hormone (which stimu-lates insulin-like growth factor-I production), usually in a dose of 24 IU given intramuscularly every other day, might facilitate ovulation induction by gonadotropins, and especially, might convert poor responders to good responders. Initial results in poor responders were favorable, although this may be limited to patients with polycystic ovaries.[127,128] In women with normal responses, however, the addition of growth hormone did not improve results or reduce the total dose of HMG.[129] Thus, in normally responding women, the growth hormone and IGF-I system may be operating at maximal levels. In poorly responding women, concomitant treatment with growth hormone can reduce the amount of HMG necessary, shorten the duration of treatment, and increase the chance of pregnancy. However, not all poorly responding women respond favorably to growth hormone treatment.[130] The effective selection of patients, dosage, and treatment regimens remains to be standardized, and the extreme cost of growth hormone is a significant disadvantage. Another approach is to administer growth hormone-releasing hormone. In a small randomized trial (13 women), the addition of growth hormone-releasing hormone to HMG treatment was associated with a higher pregnancy rate.[131] However, others have administered 500 μg of growth hormone-releasing hormone twice daily to poor responders with little effect, although the dosage of HMG may be reduced.[132,133]

Purified FSH	Purified FSH is separated from LH by immunochromotography. One ampule contains 75 IU of FSH and less than 1 IU of LH. Recombinent gonadotropins (which, of course, would be completely pure) should eventually replace the HMG obtained from postmenopausal urine. Results with recombinent FSH should be the same as with purified FSH. However, relatively pure FSH has the benefit of self-administration by subcutaneous injection.

Daily low doses (1 ampule/day and increasing by 0.5–1.0 ampule every 7 days) of FSH can achieve pregnancy in women with polycystic ovaries.[134] Higher doses of FSH are associated with a risk of hyperstimulation despite only a modest rate of ovulatory response. Therefore, purified FSH must be administered with monitoring methods similar to those of HMG, and the problems and results are also similar.[135] With the exception of low dose treatment of women with polycystic ovaries, there is no reason to believe that results with purified FSH are superior to HMG. Even in women with polycystic ovaries, pregnancy rates with FSH and HMG are similar; however, the risks of hyperstimulation and multiple pregnancy appear to be reduced with the use of FSH.[136] On the other hand, others have reported that similar careful use of low doses of HMG can yield the same results.[137]

Gonadotropin Releasing Hormone (GnRH)

Numerous advantages can be cited in favor of pulsatile GnRH therapy for ovulation induction. GnRH methodology, once established, is simple to use, requires no extensive (or expensive) follicular monitoring, and, relative to its counterparts, is quite safe. Ovarian hyperstimulation and multiple gestations are rare because only "physiologic" levels of FSH should be generated. Because GnRH serves largely a permissive role, the internal feedback mechanisms between the ovary and pituitary should be operative, yielding follicular growth and development similar to a normal menstrual cycle in response to the "turning on" of the system by GnRH.

GnRH is administered constantly in a pulsatile fashion by a programmable portable minipump. Induction of ovulation with the GnRH pump is most effective in women with hypothalamic amenorrhea (absence of menstrual bleeding following a progestin challenge) where endogenous GnRH is dysfunctional or absent. Unfortunately, although it has been successful in some anovulatory women with polycystic ovaries, this success is far less than anticipated, and these patients are at greater risk for hyperstimulation and multiple pregnancy, therefore requiring a lower dose (2.5 μg per bolus).[138,139] Nevertheless, the GnRH pump is a safer, less expensive alternative for these patients than HMG. The GnRH pump is also effective in women with hyperprolactinemia, providing a good alternative if bromocriptine cannot be tolerated.

GnRH is available in crystalline form that when reconstituted in the aqueous diluent is stable for at least 3 weeks at room temperature. The pump must be worn constantly around the clock, requiring some ingenuity for bathing and sleeping. GnRH can be administered by either the intravenous or subcutaneous routes. The subcutaneous route requires a higher dose. Failure with subcutaneous administration is associated with a polycystic ovary-like picture, with high LH levels, anovulation, and even symptoms of androgen excess. This is not surprising in that subcutaneous administration results in an absorption curve with a broad base without a definite peak. For intravenous administration, heparin is added to the GnRH solution in a concentration of 1,000 U/mL. We favor starting with the intravenous route. The needle is left in place until there are signs of local reaction and then changed. Women at risk for bacterial endocarditis should be restricted to the subcutaneous route of administration.

Although some argue in favor of near-physiologic duplication of the pulse frequency, similar results can be obtained with empiric 90-minute cycles throughout treatment. The dose for subcutaneous administration is 20 μg per bolus, for intravenous administration, 5 μg per bolus. If the patient fails to respond (assessed by weekly measurement of estradiol), the dose should be increased by 5 μg increments.

After ovulation, the luteal phase is maintained by either continuing the pump or administering HCG (2,000 IU intramuscularly at the time of the temperature rise and then every 3 days for 3 doses). In our experience most patients would rather discontinue the pump.

One of the reasons that the GnRH pump is less expensive is that it reproduces physiologic hormonal events, and intensive monitoring is not necessary. The main problem is knowing with some accuracy when to have intercourse. Usually ovulation occurs by 14 days of treatment, but the range extends from 10 days to 22 days. Intercourse every other day during this period of time can be a formidable challenge. Ultrasonic monitoring of follicular development may be required, or more conveniently, the couple can use one of the urinary LH test kits to detect the LH surge and have intercourse for 2–3 days beginning the day of the color change.

Side effects with the GnRH pump are minimal, principally related to pump functioning and local reactions to the needle placement. The patient must be educated to pay close attention to proper function of the pump and maintenance of the GnRH reservoir. Hyperstimulation and multiple births have been encountered, but this is rare and associated with higher than recommended doses. The risk of dangerous hyperstimulation is essentially zero. Several cases of allergic response with the development of circulating antibodies have been reported.

The pregnancy rate in women with hypothalamic (hypogonadotropic) amenorrhea is 20–30% per treatment cycle which approximates the pregnancy rate of normal couples.[140] Persistence with repeated cycles is rewarded with high cumulative pregnancy rates, approximately 80% after 6 cycles and 93% after 12 cycles.[141] The abortion rate of 20% is typical of all methodologies. The incidence of multiple pregnancy is about twice normal (5%). The cumulative pregnancy rate in women with polycystic ovaries is approximately 30–40%. If this method is to be used for women with polycystic ovaries, it is recommended that down-regulation and desensitization of the pituitary with a GnRH agonist should precede treatment (and retreatment will be necessary with each cycle). This approach can yield a cumulative pregnancy rate of 60%.[142] Even then, obese patients are less likely to respond, and they have higher rates of spontaneous abortion.

The safety and simplicity of GnRH administration are powerful attractions. Despite the clear advantages, the GnRH pump has not received wide acceptance by patients. Many are irrationally fearful of the risk of needle displacement or equipment problems associated with the technology.

Ovarian Wedge Resection

Irving Stein and Michael Leventhal, in 1935, at the Michael Reese Hospital in Chicago, described 7 cases of the syndrome that bears their names.[143] They developed wedge resection of the ovaries when they observed that several of their amenorrheic (anovulatory) patients with polycystic ovaries menstruated after ovarian biopsies. In their original procedure, they removed 50 to 75% of each ovary. They concluded that the thickened surface of the ovary prevented follicles from reaching the surface. For years, the wedge resection was the only method available to induce ovulation in these patients, and it wasn't until 30–40 years later that an accurate understanding of the mechanism was achieved.

The purpose of wedge resection of the ovaries is to remove a significant amount of hormone-producing tissue. Documentation of hormone changes following wedge resection indicates that an important change is a sustained reduction in testosterone levels.[144,145] This suggests that the barrier to ovulation is the intraovarian, atresia-promoting effects of the high testosterone production. Removal of androgen-producing tissue effectively lowers this barrier, and ovulatory cycles can ensue. Another contributing factor is a reduction in circulating levels of inhibin which follows the loss of ovarian tissue.[146] A rise in FSH occurs in the days after wedge resection; successful ovulation reflects the combined effects of increased FSH and the removal of the local androgen obstruction to the emergence of a dominant follicle.

The response to ovarian wedge resection is variable. Some patients resume ovulation permanently. However, most patients return to their anovulatory state. Some patients fail to respond at all. Furthermore, the surgical procedure carries with it the potential problem of postoperative adhesion formation.

The operative risk, the variable response, and the possibility of postoperative adhesion formation are the liabilities of wedge resection. These must be weighed against the excellent results obtained with medical induction of ovulation (approximating the normal conception rate when anovulation is the only fertility problem present). It should truly be a rare patient in whom wedge resection of the ovaries is necessary.

Today, a new type of "wedge resection" is available. Using either cautery, diathermy, or laser vaporization by means of the laparoscope, destruction of ovarian tissue at multiple sites (15–20 per ovary) can achieve spontaneous ovulations or an increased sensitivity to clomiphene.[146–150] These procedures are associated with the same decrease in androgens and inhibin as observed with wedge resection. When clomiphene is reinstituted, 70–80% of patients will ovulate, and approximately 60% will achieve pregnancy. Adhesion formation remains a problem, but perhaps it is less profound than in the traditional surgery.[151] Second look laparoscopy with lysis of adhesions is indicated if pregnancy does not follow successful ovulations. This therapy can be performed at the time of a planned diagnostic laparoscopy in a patient with known anovulation and polycystic ovaries. These procedures are worth considering by patients who are reluctant to pursue the more expensive and difficult methods of the assisted reproductive technologies. These methods are the modern equivalent of the original ovarian wedge resection pioneered by Stein and Leventhal.

References

1. **Ernst S, Hite G, Cantrell JS, Richardson A Jr, Benson HD,** Stereochemistry of geometric isomers of clomiphene: a correction of the literature and a reexamination of structure-activity relationships, J Pharm Sci 65:148, 1976.

2. **Clark JH, Markaverich BM,** The agonistic-antagonistic properties of clomiphene: a review, Pharmacol Ther 15:467, 1982.

3. **Adashi EY,** Clomiphene citrate-initiated ovulation: a clinical update, Seminars Reprod Endocrinol 4:255, 1986.

4. **Kerin JF, Liu JH, Phillipou G, Yen SSC,** Evidence for a hypothalamic site of action of clomiphene citrate in women, J Clin Endocrinol Metab 61:265, 1985.

5. **Kettel LM, Roseff SJ, Berga SL, Mortola JF, Yen SSC,** Hypothalmic-pituitary-ovarian response to clomiphene citrate in women with polycystic ovarian syndrome, Fertil Steril 59:532, 1993.

6. **de Moura MD, Ferriani RA, de Sa MFS,** Effects of clomiphene citrate on pituitary luteinizing hormone and follicle-stimulating hormone release in women before and after treatment with ethinyl estradiol, Fertil Steril 58:504, 1992.

7. **Kessel B, Hsueh AJW,** Clomiphene citrate augments follicle-stimulating hormone-induced luteinizing hormone receptor content in cultured rat granulosa cells, Fertil Steril 46:334, 1987.

8. **Birkenfeld A, Beier HM, Schenker JG,** The effect of clomiphene citrate on early embryonic development, endometrium and implantation, Hum Reprod 1:387, 1986.

9. **Li TC, Warren MA, Murphy C, Sargeant S, Cooke ID,** A prospective, randomised, cross-over study comparing the effects of clomiphene citrate and cyclofenil on endometrial morphology in the luteal phase of normal, fertile women, Br J Obstet Gynaecol 99:1008, 1992.

10. **Thompson LA, Barratt CLR, Thornton SJ, Bolton AE, Cooke ID,** The effects of clomiphene citrate and cyclofenil on cervical mucus volume and receptivity over the periovulatory period, Fertil Steril 59:125, 1993.

11. **Fritz MA, Holmes RT, Keenan EJ,** Effect of clomiphene citrate treatment on endometrial estrogen and progesterone receptor induction in women, Am J Obstet Gynecol 165:177, 1991.

12. **Mikkelson TJ, Kroboth PD, Cameron WJ, Dittert LW, Chungi V, Manberg PJ,** Single-dose pharmacokinetics of clomiphene citrate in normal volunteers, Fertil Steril 46:392, 1986.

13. **Oelsner G, Barnea ER, Mullen MV, Mikkelson TJ, Tarlatzis BC, Naftolin F, DeCherney AH,** Simultaneous measurements of clomiphene citrate in plasma and follicular fluid in women undergoing IVF & ET, Program, American Fertility Society, Abstract 39, 1986.

14. **Lavy G, Diamond MP, Polan ML,** Reversal by human chorionic gonadotropin of the inhibitory effect of clomiphene on progesterone production by granulosa-luteal cells in culture, Int J Fertil 34:359, 1989.

15. **Cunha GR, Taguchi O, Namikawa R, Nishizuka Y, Robboy SJ,** Teratogenic effects of clomiphene, tamoxifen, and diethylstilbestrol on the developing human female genital tract, Human Pathol 18:1132, 1987.

16. **Mills JL, Simpson JL, Rhoads GG, Graubard BI, Hoffman H, Conley MR, Lassman M, Cunningham G,** Risk of neural tube defects in relation to maternal fertility and fertility drug use, Lancet 336:103, 1990.

17. **Shoham Z, Zosmer A, Insler V,** Early miscarriage and fetal malformations after induction of ovulation (by clomiphene citrate and/or human menotropins), in vitro fertilization, and gamete intrafallopian transfer, Fertil Steril 55:1, 1991.

18. **Gorlitsky GA, Kase NG, Speroff L,** Ovulation and pregnancy rates with clomiphene citrate, Obstet Gynecol 51:265, 1978.

19. **Gysler M, March CM, Mishell DR Jr, Bailey EJ,** A decade's experience with an individualized clomiphene treatment regimen including its effect on the postcoital test, Fertil Steril 37:161, 1982.

20. **Taubert H-D, Dericks-Tan, JE,** High doses of estrogens do not interfere with the ovulation-inducing effect of clomiphene citrate, Fertil Steril 27:375, 1976.

21. **Bateman BG, Nunley WC Jr, Kolp LA,** Exogenous estrogens therapy for treatment of clomiphene citrate-induced cervical mucus abnormalities: is it effective? Fertil Steril 54:577, 1990.

22. **Downs KA, Gibson M,** Clomiphene citrate therapy for luteal phase defect, Fertil Steril 39:34, 1983.

23. **Huang K-E,** The primary treatment of luteal phase inadequacy: progesterone versus clomiphene citrate, Am J Obstet Gynecol 155:824, 1986.

24. **Murray D, Reich L, Adashi EY,** Oral clomiphene citrate and vaginal progesterone suppositories in the treatment of luteal phase dysfunction: a comparative study, Fertil Steril 51:35, 1989.

25. **Collins JA,** Superovulation in the treatment of unexplained infertility, Seminars Reprod Endocrinol 8:165, 1990.

26. **Deaton JL, Gibson M, Blackmer KM, Nakajima ST, Badger GJ, Brumsted JR,** A randomized, controlled trial of clomiphene citrate and intrauterine insemination in couples with unexplained infertility or surgically corrected endometriosis, Fertil Steril 54:1083, 1990.

27. **Glazener CMA, Coulson C, Lambert PA, Watt EM, Hinton RA, Kelly NG, Hull MGR,** Clomiphene treatment for women with unexplained infertility: placebo-controlled study of hormonal responses and conception rates, Gynecol Endocrinol 4:75, 1990.

28. **Wu CH, Winkel CA,** The effect of therapy initiation day on clomiphene citrate therapy, Fertil Steril 52:564, 1989.

29. **Shepard MK, Balmaceda JP, Leija CG,** Relationship of weight to successful induction of ovulation with clomiphene citrate, Fertil Steril 32:641, 1979.

30. **Lobo RA, Gysler M, March CM, Goebelsmann U, Mishell DR Jr,** Clinical and laboratory predictors of clomiphene response, Fertil Steril 37:168, 1982.

31. **Hammond MG, Halme JK, Talbert LM,** Factors affecting the pregnancy rate in clomiphene citrate induction of ovulation, Obstet Gynecol 62:196, 1983.

32. **Tiitinen AE, Laatikainen TJ, Seppala MT,** Serum levels of insulin-like growth factor binding protein-1 and ovulatory responses to clomiphene citrate in women with polycystic ovarian disease, Fertil Steril 60:58, 1993.

33. **Lunenfeld B, Pariente C, Dor J, Menashe Y, Seppala M, Mortman H, Insler V,** Modern aspects of ovulation induction, Ann N Y Acad Sci 626:207, 1991.

34. **Lobo RA, Paul W, March CM, Granger L, Kletzky OA,** Clomiphene and dexamethasone in women unresponsive to clomiphene alone, Obstet Gynecol 60:497, 1982.

35. **Daly DC, Walters CA, Soto-Albers CE, Tohan N, Riddick DH,** A randomized study of dexamethasone in ovulation induction with clomiphene citrate, Fertil Steril 41:844, 1984.

36. **Hoffman D, Lobo RA,** Serum dehydroepiandrosterone sulfate and the use of clomiphene citrate in anovulatory women, Fertil Steril 43:196, 1985.

37. **Lobo RA, Granger LR, Davajan V, Mishell DR Jr,** An extended regimen of clomiphene citrate in women unresponsive to standard therapy, Fertil Steril 37:762, 1982.

38. **O'Herlihy C, Pepperell RJ, Brown JB, Smith MA, Sandri L, McBain JC,** Incremental clomiphene therapy: a new method for treating persistent anovulation, Obstet Gynecol 58:535, 1981.

39. **Cassidenti DL, Ary BA, Lobo RA,** Leuprolide acetate (LA) followed by clomiphene citrate (CC) induces ovulation in clomiphene resistant patients with polycystic ovary syndrome (PCO), Annual Meeting, American Fertility Society, 1992, Abstract 0-069.

40. **Homburg R, Armar NA, Eshel A, Adams J, Jacobs HS,** Influence of serum luteinising hormone concentrations on ovulation, conception, and early pregnancy loss in polycystic ovary syndrome, Br Med J 297:1024, 1988.

41. **Regan L, Owen EJ, Jacobs HS,** Hypersecretion of luteinising hormone, infertility and miscarriage, Lancet 336:1141, 1990.

42. **Watson H, Kiddy DS, Hamilton-Fairley D, Scanlon MJ, Barnard C, Collins WP, Bonney RC, Franks S,** Hypersecretion of luteinizing hormone and ovarian steroids in women with recurrent early miscarriage, Hum Reprod 8:829, 1993.

43. **Padilla SL, Person GK, McDonough PG, Reindollar RH,** The efficacy of bromocriptine in patients with ovulatory dysfunction and normoprolactinemic galactorrhea, Fertil Steril 44:695, 1985.

44. **Falaschi P, Rocco A, del Pozo E,** Inhibitory effect of bromocriptine treatment on luteinizing hormone secretion in polycystic ovary syndrome, J Clin Endocrinol Metab 62:348, 1986.

45. **Soto-Albers CE, Daly DC, Walters CA, Ying YK, Riddick DH,** Titrating the dose of bromocriptine when treating hyperprolactinemic women, Fertil Steril 43:485, 1985.

46. **Porcile A, Gallardo E, Venegas E,** Normoprolactinemic anovulation nonresponsive to clomiphene citrate: ovulation induction with bromocriptine, Fertil Steril 53:50, 1990.

47. **Suginami H, Hamada K, Yano K, Kuroda G, Matsuura S,** Ovulation induction with bromocriptine in normoprolactinemic anovulatory women, J Clin Endocrinol Metab 62:899, 1986.

48. **Weight CS, Steele SJ, Jacobs JS,** Value of bromocriptine in unexplained primary infertility: a double-blind controlled trial, Br Med J 1:1037, 1979.

49. **DeVane GW, Guzick DS,** Bromocriptine therapy in normoprolactinemic women with unexplained infertility and galactorrhea, Fertil Steril 46:1026, 1986.

50. **Germond M, Dessole S, Senn A, Loumaye E, Howles C, Beltrami V,** Successful in-vitro fertilisation and embryo transfer after treatment with recombinant FSH, Lancet 339:1170, 1992.

51. **Farine D, Dor J, Lupovici N, Lunenfeld B, Mashiach S,** Conception rate after gonadotropin therapy in hyperprolactinemia and normoprolactinemia, Obstet Gynecol 65:658, 1985.

52. **Dodson WC, Whitesides DB, Hughes CL Jr, Easley HA III, Haney AF,** Superovulation with intrauterine insemination in the treatment of infertility: a possible alternative to gamete intrafallopian transfer and in vitro fertilization, Fertil Steril 48:441, 1987

53. **Serhal PF, Katz M, Little V, Woronowski H,** Unexplained infertility — the value of Pergonal superovulation combined with intrauterine insemination, Fertil Steril 49:602, 1988.

54. **Silverberg KM, Johnson JV, Olive DL, Burns WN, Schenken RS,** A prospective, randomized trial comparing two different intrauterine insemination regimens in controlled ovarian hyperstimulation cycles, Fertil Steril 57:357, 1992.

55. **Zikopoulos K, West CP, Thong PW, Kacser EM, Morrison J, Wu FCW,** Homologous intrauterine insemination has no advantage over timed natural intercourse when used in combination with ovulation induction for the treatment of unexplained infertility, Hum Reprod 8:563, 1993.

56. **Nulsen JC, Walsh S, Dumez S, Metzger DA,** A randomized and longitudinal study of human menopausal gonadotropin with intrauterine insemination in the treatment of infertility, Obstet Gynecol 82:780, 1993.

57. **Karlstrom P-O, Bergh T, Lundkvist O,** A prospective randomized trial of artificial insemination versus intercourse in cycles stimulated with human menopausal gonadotropin or clomiphene citrate, Fertil Steril 59:554, 1993.

58. **Diamond MP, Polan ML, Blanchette M, Mazure CM, DeCherney AH, Lunenfeld B,** Comparison of ovarian response in the same women with the same or different lots of human menopausal gonadotropin, Gynecol Endocrinol 6:135, 1992.

59. **Gindoff PR, Jewelewicz R,** Use of gonadotropins in ovulation induction, N Y State J Med 85:580, 1985.

60. **Chong AP, Rafael RW, Forte CC,** Influence of weight in the induction of ovulation with human menopausal gonadotropin and human chorionic gonadotropin, Fertil Steril 46:599, 1986.

61. **Diamond MP, DeCherney AH, Baretto P, Lunenfeld B,** Multiple consecutive cycles of ovulation inductions with human menopausal gonadotropins, Gynecol Endocrinol 3:237, 1989.

62. **Silverberg KM, Klein NA, Burns WN, Schenken RS, Olive DL,** Consecutive versus alternating cycles of ovarian stimulation using human menopausal gonadotrophin, Hum Reprod 7:940, 1992.

63. **Haning RV Jr, Levin RM, Behrman HR, Kase NG, Speroff L,** Plasma estradiol window and urinary estriol glucuronide determination for monitoring menotropin induction of ovulation, Obstet Gynecol 54:442, 1979.

64. **Haning RV Jr, Boehnlein LM, Carlson IH, Kuzma DL, Zweibel WJ,** Diagnosis-specific serum 17β-estradiol (E_2) upper limits for treatment with menotropins using a ^{125}I direct E_2 assay, Fertil Steril 42:882, 1984.

65. **Wilson EA, Jawad MJ, Hayden TL,** Rates of exponential increase of serum estradiol concentrations in normal and human menopausal gonadotropin-induced cycles, Fertil Steril 37:46, 1982.

66. **Ritchie WGM,** Ultrasound in the evaluation of normal and induced ovulation, Fertil Steril 43:167, 1985.

67. **Leerentueld R, Van Gent I, Der Stoep M, Wladimiroff J,** Ultrasonographic assessment of Graffian follicle growth under monofollicular and multifollicular conditions in clomiphene citrate stimulated cycles, Fertil Steril 43:565, 1985.

68. **March CM,** Improved pregnancy rate with monitoring of gonadotropin therapy by three modalities, Am J Obstet Gynecol 156:1473, 1987.

69. **Tal J, Paz B, Samberg I, Lazarov N, Sharf M,** Ultrasonographic and clinical correlates of menotropin versus sequential clomiphene citrate: menotropin therapy for induction of ovulation, Fertil Steril 44:342, 1985.

70. **Blankstein J, Shalev J, Sasdon T, Kukia EE, Rabinovici J, Pariente C, Lunenfeld B, Serr DM, Mashiach S,** Ovarian hyperstimulation syndrome: prediction by number and size of preovulatory follicles, Fertil Steril 47:597, 1987.

71. **Elissa MK, Sawers RS, Docker MF, Lynch SES, Newton JR,** Characteristics and incidence of dysfunctional ovulation patterns detected by ultrasound, Fertil Steril 47:603, 1987.

72. **Hamilton C, Wetzels L, Evens J, Hoogland H, Mvijtjens A, DeHaan J,** Follicle growth curves and hormonal patterns in patients with the luteinized unruptured follicle syndrome, Fertil Steril 43:541, 1985.

73. **Ueno J, Ochninger S, Brzyski RG, Acosta AA, Philput B, Muasher SJ,** Ultrasonographic appearance of the endometrium in natural and stimulated in-vitro fertilization cycles and its correlation with outcome, Hum Reprod 6:901, 1991.

74. **Shoham Z, Di Carlo C, Patel A, Conway GS, Jacobs HS,** Is it possible to run a sucessful ovulation induction program based solely on ultrasound monitoring? The importance of endometrial measurements, Fertil Steril 56:836, 1991.

75. **Dickey RP, Olar TT, Taylor SN, Curole DN, Matulich EM,** Relationship of endometrial thickness and pattern to fecundity in ovulation induction cycles: effect of clomiphene citrate alone and with human menopausal gonadotropin, Fertil Steril 59:756, 1993.

76. **Shapiro H, Cowell C, Casper RF,** The use of vaginal ultrasound for monitoring endometrial preparation in a donor oocyte program, Fertil Steril 59:1055, 1993.

77. **Akin JW, Shepard MK,** The effects of baseline ovarian cysts on cycle fecundity in controlled ovarian hyperstimulation, Fertil Steril 59:453, 1993.

78. **March CM, Tredway DR, Mishell DR Jr,** Effect of clomiphene citrate upon amount and duration of human menopausal gonadotropin therapy, Am J Obstet Gynecol 125:699, 1976.

79. **Ho Yuen B, Pride SM, Burch-Callegari P, Leroux AM, Moon YS,** Clinical and endocrine response to pulsatile intravenous gonadotropins in refractory anovulation, Obstet Gynecol 74:763, 1989.

80. **Nakamura Y, Yoshimura Y, Yamada H, Ubukata Y, Yoshida K, Tamaoka Y, Suzuki M,** Clinical experience in the induction of ovulation and pregnancy with pulsatile subcutaneous administration of human menopausal gonadotropin: a low incidence of multiple pregnancy, Fertil Steril 51:423, 1989.

81. **Ho Yuen B, Pride S,** Induction of ovulation with exogenous gonadotropins in anovulatory infertile women, Seminars Reprod Endocrinol 8:1861, 1990.

82. **Fernandez H. Coste J, Job-Spira N,** Controlled ovarian hyperstimulation as a risk factor for ectopic pregnancy, Obstet Gynecol 78:656, 1991.

83. **Hamilton-Fairley D, Kiddy D, Watson H, Paterson C, Franks S,** Association of moderate obesity with a poor pregnancy outcome in women with polycystic ovary syndrome treated with low dose gonadotropin, Br J Obstet Gynaecol 99:128, 1992.

84. **Keenan JA, Moghissi KS,** Luteal phase support with hCG does not improve fecundity rate in human menopausal gonadotropin-stimulated cycles, Obstet Gynecol 79:983, 1992.

85. **Derom C, Derom R, Vlietink R, Van Den Berghe H, Thiery M,** Increased monozygotic twinning rate after ovulation induction, Lancet 1:1236, 1987.

86. **Bohrer M, Kemmann E,** Risk factors for spontaneous abortion in menotropin-treated women, Fertil Steril 48:571, 1987.

87. **Ben-Rafael Z, Mashiach S, Oelsner G, Farine D, Lunenfeld B, Serr DM,** Spontaneous pregnancy and its outcome after human menopausal gonadotropin/human chorionic gonadotropin-induced pregnancy, Fertil Steril 36:560, 1981.

88. **Aboulghar MA, Mansour RT, Serour GI, Rizk P, Riad R,** Improvement of spontaneous pregnancy rate after stopping gonadotropin therapy for anovulatory infertility, Fertil Steril 55:722, 1991.

89. **Evans MI, Fletcher JC, Zador IE, Newton BW, Quigg MH, Struyk CD,** Selective first-trimester termination in octuplet and quadruplet pregnancies: clinical and ethical issues, Obstet Gynecol 71:289, 1988.

90. **Lynch L, Berkowitz RL, Chitkara U, Alvarez M,** First-trimester transabdominal multifetal pregnancy reduction: a report of 85 cases, Obstet Gynecol 75:735, 1990.

91. **Evans MI, Dommergues M, Wapner RJ, Lynch, L, Dumez Y, Goldberg JD, Zador IE, Nicolaides KH, Johnson MP, Golbus MS, Boulot P, Berkowitz RL,** Efficacy of transabdominal multifetal pregnancy reduction: collaborative experience among the world's largest centers, Obstet Gynecol 82:61, 1993.

92. **Timor-Tritschd IE, Peisner DB, Monteagudo A, Lerner JP, Sharma S,** Multifetal pregnancy reduction by transvaginal puncture: evaluation of the technique used in 134 cases, Am J Obstet Gynecol 168:799, 1993.

93. **Kol S, Levron J, Lewit N, Drugan A, Itskovitz-Eldor J,** The natural history of multiple pregnancies after assisted reproduction: is spontaneous fetal demise a clinically significant phenomenon? Fertil Steril 60:127, 1993.

94. **Engel T, Jewelewicz R, Dyrenfurth I, Speroff L, Vande Wiele RL,** Ovarian hyperstimulation syndrome: report of a case with notes on pathogenesis and treatment, Am J Obstet Gynecol 112:1052, 1972.

95. **Navot D, Bergh PA, Laufer N,** Ovarian hyperstimulation syndrome in novel reproductive technologies: prevention and treatment, Fertil Steril 58:249, 1992.

96. **Schenker JG,** Prevention and treatment of ovarian hyperstimulation, Hum Reprod 8:653, 1993.

97. **Mashiach S, Bider D, Moran O, Goldenberg M, Ben-Rafael Z,** Adnexal torsion of hyperstimulated ovaries in pregnancies after gonadotropin therapy, Fertil Steril 53:76, 1990.

98. **Rizk B, Smitz J,** Ovarian hyperstimulation syndrome after superovulation using GnRH agonists for IVF and related procedures, Hum Reprod 7:320, 1992.

99. **Haning RV Jr, Strawn EY, Nolten WE,** Pathophysiology of the ovarian hyperstimulation syndrome, Obstet Gynecol 66:220, 1985.

100. **Rizk B, Aboulghar M,** Modern management of ovarian hyperstimulation syndrome, Hum Reprod 6:1082, 1991.

101. **Rizk B, Meagher S, Fisher AM,** Severe ovarian hyperstimulation syndrome and cerebrovascular accidents, Hum Reprod 5:697, 1990.

102. **Fournet N, Surrey E, Kerin J,** Internal jugular vein thrombosis after ovulation induction with gonadotropins, Fertil Steril 56:354, 1991.

103. **Zosmer A, Katz Z, Lancet M, Konichezky S, Schwartz-Shoham Z,** Adult respiratory distress syndrome complicating ovarian hyperstimulation syndrome, Fertil Steril 47:524, 1987.

104. **Kirshon B, Doody MC, Cotton DB, Gibbons W,** Management of ovarian hyperstimulation syndrome with chlorpheniramine maleate, mannitol, and invasive hemodynamic monitoring, Obstet Gynecol 71:485, 1988.

105. **Padilla SA, Zamaria S, Baramki TA, Garcia JE,** Abdominal paracentesis for the ovarian hyperstimulation syndrome with severe pulmonary compromise, Fertil Steril 53:365, 1990.

106. **Aboulghar MA, Mansour RT, Serour GI, Sattar MA, Amin YM, Elattar I,** Management of severe ovarian hyperstimulation syndrome by ascitic fluid aspiration and intensive intravenous fluid therapy, Obstet Gynecol 81:108, 1993.

107. **Fakih H, Bello S,** Ovarian cyst aspiration: a therapeutic approach to ovarian hyperstimulation syndrome, Fertil Steril 58:829, 1992.

108. **Whittemore AS, Harris R, Itnyre J, and the Collaborative Ovarian Cancer Group,** Characteristic relation to ovarian cancer risk: collaborative analysis of twelve US case-control studies. II. Invasive epithelial ovarian cancers in white women, Am J Epidemiol 136:1184, 1993.

109. **Ron E, Lunenfeld B, Menczer J, Blumstein T, Katz L, Oelsner G, Serr D,** Cancer incidence in a cohort of infertile women, Am J Epidemiol 125:780, 1987.

110. **Willemsen W, Kruitwagen R, Bastiaans B, Hanselaar T, Rolland R,** Ovarian stimulation and granulosa-cell tumour, Lancet 341:986, 1993.

111. **Buckler HM, Evans A, Mamlora H, Burger HG, Anderson DC,** Gonadotropin, steroid and inhibin levels in women with incipient ovarian failure duirng anovulatory and ovulatory 'rebound' cycles, J Clin Endocrinol Metab 72:116, 1991.

112. **Lenton EA, de Kretser DM, Woodward AJ, Robertson DM,** Inhibin concentrations throughout the menstrual cycles of normal, infertile, and older women compared with those during spontaneous conception cycles, J Clin Endocrinol Metab 73:1180, 1991.

113. **Hughes EG, Robertson DM, Handelsman DJ, Hayward S, Healey DL, de Kretser DM,** Inhibin and estradiol responses to ovarian hyperstimulation: effects of age and predictive value for in vitro fertilization outcome, J Clin Endocrinol Metab 70:358, 1990.

114. **Toner JP, Philput CB, Jones GS, Muasher SJ,** Basal follicle-stimulating hormone level is a better predictor of in vitro fertilization performance than age, Fertil Steril 55:784. 1991.

115. **Brown JR, Berkeley AS, Liu H, Sewitch KF,** Variability of day 3 FSH levels in normal women, Annual Meeting, American Fertility Society, 1992, abstract P-009.

116. **Pearlstone AC, Fournet N, Gambone JC, Pang SC, Buyalos RP,** Ovulation induction in women age 40 and older: the importance of basal follicle-stimulating hormone level and chronological age, Fertil Steril 58:674, 1992.

117. **Khalifa E, Toner JP, Muasher SJ, Acosta AA,** Significance of basal follicle-stimulating hormone levels in women with one ovary in a program of in vitro fertilization, Fertil Steril 57:835, 1992.

118. **Navot D, Rosenwaks Z, Margalioth EJ,** Prognostic assessment of female fecundity, Lancet 2:645, 1987.

119. **Tanbo T, Dale PO, Lunde O, Norman N, Abyholm T,** Prediction of response to controlled ovarian hyperstimulation: a comparison of basal and clomiphene citrate-stimulated follicle-stimulating hormone levels, Fertil Steril 57:819, 1992.

120. **Scott RT, Leonardi MR, Hofmann GE, Illions EH, Neal GS, Navot D,** A prospective evaluation of clomiphene citrate challenge test screening of the general infertility population, Obstet Gynecol 82:539, 1993.

121. **Dodson WC,** Gonadotropin releasing analogues as adjunctive therapy in ovulation induction, Seminars Reprod Endocrinol 8:198, 1990.

122. **Dodson WC, Hughes CL, Whitesides DB, Haney AF,** The effect of leuprolide acetate on ovulation induction with human menopausal gonadotropins in polycystic ovary syndrome, J Clin Endocrinol Metab 65:95, 1987.

123. **Homburg R, Levy T, Berkovitz D, Farchi J, Feldberg D, Ashkenazi J, Ben-Rafael Z,** Gonadotropin-releasing hormone agonist reduces the miscarriage rate for pregnancies achieved in women with polycystic ovarian syndrome, Fertil Steril 59:527, 1993.

124. **Mizunuma H, Andoh K, Yamada K, Takagi T, Kamijo T, Ibuki Y,** Prediction and prevention of ovarian hyperstimulation by monitoring endogenous luteinizing hormone release during purified follicle-stimulating hormone therapy, Fertil Steril 58:46, 1992.

125. **Smitz J, Devroey P, Camus M, Deschacht J, Khan I, Staessen C, Van Waesherghe L, Wisanto A, Van Steirteghem AC,** The luteal phase and early pregnancy after combined GnRH-agonist/hMG treatment for superovulation in IVF and GIFT, Hum Reprod 3:585, 1988.

126. **McClure N, Leya J, Radwanska E, Rawlins R, Haning RV Jr,** Luteal phase support and severe ovarian hyperstimulation syndrome, Hum Reprod 7:758, 1992.

127. **Ibrahim ZHZ, Lieberman BA, Matson PL, Buck P,** The use of biosynthetic growth hormone to augment ovulation induction with buserelin acetate/human menopausal gonadotrophin in women with a poor ovarian response, Fertil Steril 55:202, 1991.

128. **Owen EJ, Shoham Z, Mason BA, Ostergaard H, Jacobs HS,** Cotreatment with growth hormone, after pituitary suppression, for ovarian stimulation in in vitro fertilization: a randomized, double-blind, placebo-control trial, Fertil Steril 56:1104, 1991.

129. **Hughes SM, Huang ZH, Matson PL, Buck P, Lieberman BA, Morris ID,** Clinical and endocrinological changes in women following ovulation induction using buserelin acetate/human menopausal gonadotrophin augmented with biosynthetic human growth hormone, Hum Reprod 7:770, 1992.

130. **Levy T, Limor R, Villa Y, Eshel A, Eckstein N, Vagman I, Lidor A, Ayalon D,** Another look at co-treatment with growth hormone and human menopausal gonadotrophins in poor ovarian responders, Hum Reprod 8:834, 1993.

131. **Tulandi T, Galcone T, Guyda H, Hemmings R, Billiar R, Morris D,** Effects of synthetic growth hormone-releasing factor in women treated with gonadotrophin, Hum Reprod 8:525, 1993.

132. **Hugues JN, Torresani T, Herve F, Martin-Point B, Tamboise A, Santarelli J,** Interest of growth hormone-releasing hormone administration for improvement of ovarian repsonsiveness to gonadotropins in poor responder women, Fertil Steril 55:945, 1991.

133. **Volve A, Coukos G, Barreca A, Giordano G, Artini PG, Genazzani AR,** Clinical use of growth hormone-releasing factor for induction of superovulation, Hum Reprod 6:1228, 1991.

134. **Shoham Z, Patel A, Jacobs HS,** The polycystic ovarian syndrome: safety and effectiveness of stepwise and low-dose administration of purified follicle-stimulating hormone, Fertil Steril 55:1051, 1991.

135. **Claman P, Seibel MM,** Purified human follicle-stimulating hormone for ovulation induction: a critical review, Seminars Reprod Endocrinol 4:277, 1986.

136. **McFaul PB, Traub AI, Thompson W,** Treatment of clomiphene citrate-resistant polycystic ovarian syndrome with pure follicle-stimulating hormone or human menopausal gonadotropin, Fertil Steril 53:792, 1990.

137. **Sagle MA, Hamilton-Fairley D, Kiddy DS, Franks S,** A comparative, randomized study of low-dose human menopausal gonadotropin and follicle-stimulating hormone in women with polycystic ovarian syndrome, Fertil Steril 55:56, 1991.

138. **Bunger CW, Korsen TJM, Hompes PGA, Vankessel H, Schoemaker J,** Ovulation induction with pulsatile LHRH in women with clomiphene resistant polycystic ovary-like disease: clinical results, Fertil Steril 46:1045, 1986.

139. **Filicori M, Flamigni C, Meriggiola MC, Ferrari P, Michelacci L, Campaniello E, Valdiserri A, Cognigni G,** Endocrine response determines the clinical outcome of pulsatile gonadotropin-releasing hormone ovulation induction in different ovulatory disorders, J Clin Endocrinol Metab 72:965, 1991.

140. **Carr JS, Reid RL,** Ovulation induction with gonadotropin-releasing hormone (GnRH), Seminars Reprod Endocrinol 8:174, 1990.

141. **Braat DD, Schoemaker R, Schoemaker J,** Life table analysis of fecundity of intravenously gonadotropin-releasing hormone-treated patients with normogonadotropic and hypogonadotropic amenorrhea, Fertil Steril 55:266, 1991.

142. **Filicori M, Flamigni C, Campaniello E, Meriggiola MC, Michelacci L, Valdiserri A, Ferrari P,** Polycystic ovary syndrome: abnormalities and management with pulsatile gonadotropin-releasing hormone and gonadotropin-releasing hormone analogs, Am J Obstet Gynecol 163:1737, 1990.

143. **Stein IF, Leventhal ML,** Amenorrhea associated with bilateral polycystic ovaries, Am J Obstet Gynecol 29:181, 1935.

144. **Judd HL, Rigg LA, Anderson DC,** The effect of ovarian wedge resection on circulating gonadotropin and ovarian steroid levels in patients with polycystic ovaries, J Clin Endocrinol Metab 43:347, 1976.

145. **Katz M, Carr PJ, Cohen BM, Millar RP,** Hormonal effects of wedge resection of polycystic ovaries, Obstet Gynecol 51:437, 1978.

146. **Kovacs G, Buckler H, Gangah M, Burger H, Healy D, Baker G, Phillips S,** Treatment of anovulation due to polycystic ovarian syndrome by laparoscopic ovarian electrocautery, Br J Obstet Gyneacol 98:30, 1991.

147. **Daniell JF, Miller W,** Polycystic ovaries treated by laparoscopic laser vaporization, Fertil Steril 51:232, 1989.

148. **Gadir A, Mowafi RS, Alnaser HMI, Alrashid AH, Alonezi OM, Shaw RW,** Ovarian electro-cautery versus human menopausal gonadotrophins and pure follicle stimulating hormone therapy in the treatment of patients with polycystic ovarian disease, Clin Endocrinol 33:585, 1990.

149. **Naether OGJ, Fischer R, Weise HC, Geiger-Kotzler L, Delfs T, Rudolf K,** Laparoscopic electrocoagulation of the ovarian surface in infertile patients and polycystic ovarian disease, Fertil Steril 60:88, 1993.

150. **Armar NA, Lachelin GCL,** Laparoscopic ovarian diathermy: an effective treatment for anti-oestrogen resistant anovulatory infertility in women with polycystic ovarian syndrome, Br J Obstet Gynaecol 100:161, 1993.

151. **Naether OGJ, Fischer R,** Adhesion formation after laparoscopic electrocoagulation of the ovarian surface in polycystic ovary patients, Fertil Steril 60:95, 1993.

31   Assisted Reproduction

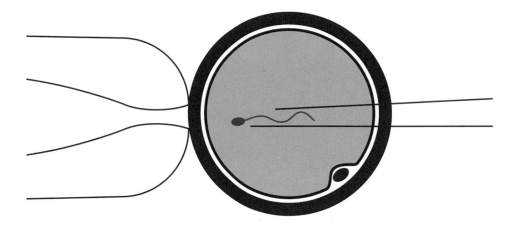

Assisted reproductive technology (ART) refers to all techniques involving direct retrieval of oocytes from the ovary. The first and still most common procedure is in vitro fertilization, but there is an ever increasing list of technologies.

IVF — In Vitro Fertilization: extraction of oocytes, fertilization in the laboratory, transcervical transfer of embryos into the uterus.

GIFT — Gamete Intrafallopian Transfer: the placement of oocytes and sperm into the fallopian tube.

ZIFT — Zygote Intrafallopian Transfer: the placement of fertilized oocytes into the fallopian tube.

TET — Tubal Embryo Transfer: the placement of cleaving embryos into the fallopian tube.

POST— Peritoneal Oocyte and Sperm Transfer: the placement of oocytes and sperm into the pelvic cavity.

SUZI — Subzonal insertion of sperm by microinjection.

ICZI — Intracytoplasmic sperm injection (of a single spermatozoon).

It has been almost two decades since the birth of the first child conceived by in vitro fertilization (IVF). During the intervening years the number of IVF programs has increased to over 200 in the United States alone, technology has evolved, the success rate has improved, and the number of indications for IVF has increased. Furthermore, procedures that utilize some, but not all, of the methodology of IVF have become a part of clinical practice.

Numerous volumes have been published which extensively cover all aspects of ART, and it is not our purpose to duplicate that effort. Rather, this chapter will focus on the evolving techniques and will review briefly the place of ART in the treatment of nontubal disease.

Patient Selection for IVF

The initial experience with in vitro fertilization involved women with tubal disease, but early in the 1980s, the treatment was extended to individuals with male factor infertility, unexplained infertility, endometriosis, and immunologic causes for infertility. In addition, successful pregnancies have occurred following the transfer of donor embryos developed from IVF to women with premature ovarian failure or decreased ovarian function. Women with severe pelvic adhesive disease who were denied IVF in the past because their ovaries could not be visualized by laparoscopy now can be treated by ultrasonically guided vaginal oocyte retrieval. Although it is reasonable to recommend tubal surgery in young women with mild distal tubal disease, IVF is the treatment of choice for patients with more severe distal disease, proximal obstruction (especially after 6 months have elapsed following cannulation or balloon tuboplasty), and for patients who have failed to achieve pregnancy within 2 years after tubal surgery or when tubal obstruction persists after surgery.

Whereas IVF can overcome a number of the barriers to fertility, it suffers the same limitation as does in vivo fertilization when it comes to age (discussed in Chapter 26). In successful IVF programs, where take-home baby rates can be in the 35% range for women 36 and younger, for women over 39 the figure is in the 10% range. Beyond the simple effect of age, there also may be a negative influence on IVF success from decreased ovarian responsiveness. This can be manifested by poor response to exogenous gonadotropin stimulation and by abnormal hormone profiles. The exact definition of a poor responder is uncertain but it encompasses those who respond to stimulation with the development of 4 or less follicles or with depressed estrogen levels. Pretreatment diagnosis of these individuals can be achieved by measuring basal FSH and estradiol levels. Elevated FSH levels, indicative of decreased ovarian reserve, result from a failure of aging ovaries to produce inhibin.

Three distinct populations have been identified on the basis of the cycle day three FSH.[1] With FSH values less than 15 IU/L, the pregnancy rate with IVF was 24%, whereas when the FSH values were 15 to 24.9 IU/L, the pregnancy rate was 13.6%. When the FSH was 25 IU/L or higher the pregnancy rate was 10.7%. However, the ongoing pregnancy rate in this latter group was only 3.6%. A common experience is that successful pregnancy is rare when the FSH is above 25 IU/L. Remember in all discussions pertaining to specific hormone levels that these may vary widely, even in the same sample, depending on which assay system is used. Thus, a figure cited as abnormal in one laboratory may not be abnormal in another.

In one series, if the day three estradiol was greater than 75 pg/mL (280 pmol/L) there were no pregnancies (or if the basal FSH were greater than 26 IU/L).[2] Another critical cut-off point for the day three estradiol was 45 pg/mL (170 pmol/L). There were no ongoing pregnancies if the estradiol was greater than 45 pg/mL and the FSH was greater than 17 IU/L. However, if either estradiol or FSH was below these levels, moderate elevations of the other did not depress pregnancy rates. The highest pregnancy rate (33.8%) occurred if both day three FSH and estradiol were low, less than 18 IU/L and less than 46 pg/mL, respectively. The poor prognosis associated with elevated basal estradiol levels could be on the basis of premature recruitment of a single dominant follicle. In addition to the prognostic value of the basal estradiol, it has another usefulness. High levels can artificially depress FSH, and thus an isolated FSH in the normal range can be misleading if the estradiol value is not measured.

Further attempts to gain prospective information on ovarian responsiveness has centered on provocative tests to stimulate FSH and estradiol. Navot and colleagues developed the clomiphene challenge test as a bioassay of FSH response.[3] Clomiphene is administered in a dose of 100 mg/day on days 5–9. The levels of FSH on days 9–11 are compared to the baseline levels on days 2–3. A poor response is characterized by elevated day 9–11 levels (FSH higher than 26 IU/L), reflecting failure of the stimulated follicles to produce sufficient amounts of inhibin. In the poor response group, 1 of 18 patients conceived compared to 14 of 32 who had normal tests. The clomiphene challenge test uncovered abnormalities not detected by the day three FSH. Combining the basal FSH with day 10 FSH (following a clomiphene challenge test) was the best predictor of future response to treatment with a gonadotropin releasing hormone agonist and human menopausal gonadotropins for IVF.[4] None of 10 women with abnormal values achieved a pregnancy. Scott and coworkers, not surprisingly, found older women had a higher incidence of abnormal clomiphene challenge tests, although, on occasion, they were found in women under age 35.[5] In a general infertility population, conception occurred in 92 of 213 (43%) women with normal results, but only 2 of 23 (9%) women with abnormal results. Of the 23 abnormal clomiphene challenge tests, 1 was abnormal because of an elevated day three FSH alone, 16 were abnormal because of elevated day 10 values alone (70%), and 6 (26%) had elevated levels on both day 3 and day 10. Thus, the clomiphene challenge test identified potential poor responders with greater sensitivity than the day three FSH measurement. Individuals with abnormal results are less likely to respond to stimulation, and they have decreased chances for conception.

Older women with infertility should seriously consider an early resort to hormonal stimulation for both multiple oocyte response and better support of the endometrium. Older couples should be provided the option of oocyte donation from young donors instead of standard assisted reproductive technologies.

Stimulation Protocol

The momentous work of Edwards and Steptoe was developed over more than 10 years. Success was achieved by utilizing a nonstimulated cycle with timing of oocyte retrieval based on measurements of luteinizing hormone (LH) at 3-hour intervals. Nonstimulated cycles are still used as a means of decreasing expenses, but the delivery rate per retrieval is approximately 6%.[6] The very low success rate associated with this approach led to the use of clomiphene citrate and human menopausal gonadotropins (HMG) to stimulate the development of multiple ovarian follicles. Injections of human chorionic gonadotropin (HCG), whose biologic activity mimics that of LH, were utilized to allow more certain timing of oocyte retrieval. It is still possible to reduce costs and the risks of multiple pregnancy by retrieval of a single oocyte from a natural menstrual cycle; however, it requires 3 natural cycles to achieve the pregnancy rate achieved in one stimulated cycle (eventually about one-half the cumulative pregnancy rate).[7]

In the late 1980s gonadotropin releasing hormone agonists (GnRH agonists) were introduced as a means of down-regulating the pituitary to prevent premature ovulation which in the past had necessitated canceling approximately 15% of IVF cycles. The down-regulating effects of GnRH agonists, as opposed to the stimulatory effects of GnRH, are related to the frequency of administration and the prolonged occupation of GnRH receptors by the agonists. Since their introduction, pregnancy rates have increased because of the opportunity to retrieve cycles that would have been lost to early ovulation and because of the increase in the number of oocytes obtained in GnRH agonist cycles.[8] However, use of an agonist increases the amount of gonadotropins needed to stimulate follicular growth, and thus, it also increases the expense. Despite this negative aspect, the combination of GnRH agonist and HMG controlled hyperstimulation of the ovary and substitution of exogenous HCG for the endogenous LH surge is now utilized by most IVF programs. This approach has another beneficial attribute; it allows more flexible scheduling of the necessary interventions.

In the early and mid 1980s questions were directed to the relative success of protocols using clomiphene, HMG, or combinations of the two. These questions have given way to comparisons of protocols utilizing luteal phase or follicular phase initiation of GnRH agonist treatment. Most commonly the GnRH agonist is started in the midluteal phase. Whereas leuprolide (Lupron) injected subcutaneously is the most commonly used GnRH agonist in the United States, a higher pregnancy rate has been achieved with the use of nafarelin (Synarel) which is administered as a nasal spray.[9] The menstrual period usually arrives on schedule after luteal phase initiation of GnRH agonist treatment, and the quiescent status of the ovaries and endometrium can be noted by ultrasonography. Confirmation, if desired, can be obtained by measuring an estrogen level (estradiol less than 40 pg/mL, 150 pmol/L). The GnRH agonist is continued during the stimulation with HMG, which can usually begin 10–21 days after GnRH agonist treatment is initiated. The dose of HMG is usually 225–300 IU/daily by intramuscular injection, except in young women or those with polycystic ovarian disease where a lower dose (150 IU/daily) is appropriate. The dose can be adjusted as cycle monitoring with ultrasonography and estradiol measurements proceeds. Use of a preparation which contains mostly FSH with only a small amount of LH does not seem to offer any striking advantages. It is thought to be of some value for ovulation induction in women with polycystic ovarian disease where endogenous baseline LH levels are elevated and when high doses (450–600 IU) of HMG are used. One of the goals in limiting the dose of LH is to decrease stimulation of the androgenic component of the ovarian response. A newer, purer preparation of FSH, which can be given subcutaneously, will replace the HMG and FSH preparations currently on the market. Eliminating the sometimes painful intramuscular injections will be a major benefit.

The use of a GnRH agonist, both in terms of dose and day initiated, can vary. In a "flare" protocol the drug is started, not in the luteal phase, but on day 2 of the cycle. HMG is started the next day or the day after to build on the initial agonist response to the GnRH agonist. We have used this protocol for poor responder patients with only limited success. Others have used GnRH agonist flare as their main protocol.[10] Most continue the agonist throughout the cycle while HMG is given, whereas others administer it for just a few days.

Whatever protocol is used there is a 10–30% cancellation rate because of inadequate follicular response. Measurements of basal FSH and estradiol and the clomiphene challenge test can provide information for discussing with patients the expectations for success. Ideally, a stimulation protocol could be tailored to boost the chances for an adequate response. However, it is evident that poor responders (and those with abnormal basal or provocative FSH and estradiol levels) only rarely can be converted to good responders. The 5 most common changes in protocol designed to accomplish that elusive goal are:

1. Increase the gonadotropin dose or change the mix of FSH-LH and FSH.

2. Use of the flare protocol.

3. Lower the dose of the GnRH agonist.

4. Omit the GnRH agonist and use HMG alone or a combination of clomiphene and HMG.

5. A less common approach limited by expense and availability of drugs is the use of growth hormone in conjunction with HMG.

No improvement in response was observed when the starting dose of FSH was increased from 4 to 6 ampules (300–450 IU) beginning on day 1 or 2 of the cycle.[11] Rosenwaks also reported similar discouraging results when increasing the dose with only 1 pregnancy in

20 transfers.[12] He did, however, find it useful to decrease the dose of the GnRH agonist. In our hands the flare protocols are only occasionally effective in poor responders. The alternative of omitting the GnRH agonist also has met with only limited success.

The expectation that administration of growth hormone with HMG might overcome the problem of poor response has not been totally realized to date (see Chapter 30). In poorly responding women, concomitant treatment with growth hormone can reduce the amount of HMG necessary, shorten the duration of treatment, and increase the chance of pregnancy.[13,14] However, not all poorly responding women respond favorably to growth hormone treatment.[15,16] The effective selection of patients, dosage, and treatment regimens remains to be standardized, and the extreme cost of growth hormone is a significant disadvantage.

Monitoring Ovarian Response

Most programs use both measurements of serum estradiol and ultrasound imaging of ovarian follicles to monitor the ovarian response to stimulation. The minimum goal of stimulation is to achieve the growth of a lead follicle to at least 17 mm diameter, and at least 3 or 4 other follicles with diameters of 14 mm or greater, combined with estradiol levels of approximately 200 pg/mL (740 pmol/L) per large (14 mm or greater) follicle. Once this rate of stimulation is achieved, a single injection of 5,000 or 10,000 IU of HCG is given to induce final follicular maturation. The time interval between HCG and retrieval is considered to be critical. Whereas 34–36 hours is standard, longer intervals (up to 39 hours) may allow for better maturation of the oocytes while only marginally increasing the risk for ovulation.[17] The values given for follicle size and estradiol levels on the day of decision for HCG injection are only rough guidelines because ultrasound measurements may differ among observers and machines. In addition, each program must establish, based on its own experience, its criteria for determining the adequacy of follicle size. Moreover, estradiol assays will differ from one laboratory to another, and comparisons therefore are difficult. Estradiol levels per follicle can vary widely and still be compatible with successful IVF. Some programs measure the estrogen level on the day following HCG, and if there is a marked drop in the value at that time, retrieval is canceled because that pattern is associated with a poor chance for pregnancy.

Cancellation and avoidance of HCG injections should also be considered if the ovaries are markedly hyperstimulated (greater than 25 follicles) or the total estradiol is greater than 5,000 pg/mL (18,500 pmol/L). (Hyperstimulation is discussed in Chapter 30.) Again, the specific values may not be valid with other assays, and each program must establish which estradiol level is its warning sign. Risks of hyperstimulation can be decreased by lowering the dose of HMG used to initiate the cycle. The use of FSH as opposed to HMG in women with polycystic ovaries is not protective; with all stimulation protocols, the key is careful use of appropriate doses. An important protection which can be accorded if the women proceed to retrieval is to use progesterone rather than HCG injections to support the luteal phase. Retrieval itself, with aspiration of follicular fluid and granulosa cells, is somewhat but not absolutely protective against hyperstimulation.[18]

When follicles are fully developed, the endometrium should be 8 mm wide or greater. If the endometrium is 6 mm or less, there is a reduced chance for pregnancy.[19] The suggestion that the endometrial pattern as seen by ultrasonography carries prognostic significance is in dispute, but a three-stripe lining is considered the best and a homogenous white-out pattern considered the worst.[19,20]

Oocyte Retrieval

Ultrasonically guided vaginal oocyte retrieval is performed approximately 34–36 hours after the HCG injection, but as late as 39 hours with the combined use of a GnRH agonist and HMG.[21] The HCG injection allows for confidence in this precise timing. Intravenous medication in the form of fentanyl and midazolam can be used for analgesia, and some programs use additional short acting anesthetics. A number 16 or number 17 needle is placed down a sterile needle guide that is attached to the upper side of the vaginal ultrasound transducer. A line on the monitor screen indicates the path the needle will traverse once it enters the abdominal cavity and the ovary. The ultrasound transducer is manipulated to position a follicle along this pathway. Usually only one puncture of each ovary is needed to allow sequential aspiration of the follicles. Accessibility of the ovaries is rarely a problem. Most women will experience only slight to moderate pain during the procedure, although an occasional woman will have a high level of pain despite analgesia. Rare complications of the procedure are intra-abdominal bleeding or introduction of infection into the ovary and pelvis. Recovery from transvaginal follicle aspiration is usually rapid without the side effects associated with general anesthesia.

Oocyte Culture

Skill is required to identify the oocytes under either a dissecting or an invert microscope. Often these can be seen easily in their cumulus masses but upon occasion they are obscured by cells and by blood. Critical is the minimizing of exposure of the oocytes to ambient temperature and room air.

One of the major breakthroughs in IVF was the discovery that sperm should not be added to the eggs immediately after retrieval; oocytes have a higher chance for fertilization if insemination follows retrieval by 4 to 6 hours.[22] Furthermore, if the oocytes are less mature or immature, much longer (12 to 30 hours) periods of incubation prior to insemination lead to better rates of fertilization. Maturity of the oocyte is determined by the morphology of the surrounding cumulus-corona cell complex or by the presence or absence of the germinal vesicle and the first polar body.[23]

Sperm are prepared by washing, centrifugation, overlaying the sperm pellet with fresh media and retrieval of the sperm that swim up into the media. Isolation of the most motile sperm also can be accomplished by separating the specimen on columns of liquid albumin or on Percoll gradients.

A variety of media has been used for embryo culture with Ham's F10 the most popular in the United States. The media for IVF are supplemented with a protein source, most commonly maternal serum or fetal cord serum. Less frequently, albumin is used. A higher pregnancy rate was achieved in Australia when fetal cord serum was the supplement compared to cases where maternal serum was used.[24] Maternal and fetal cord sera should be screened by testing their ability to support development of preimplantation mouse embryos as well as their freedom from HIV and hepatitis viruses. The complexity of the serum supplements, whether they are fetal or maternal, raises concern that they may contain factors that are deleterious to embryos. Protein-free media would obviate this problem, and pregnancies have been achieved with protein-free media.[25] Despite this success, most programs continue to use protein-supplemented Ham's F10.

Culture of oocytes and embryos on cell monolayers from a variety of sources has been advocated as a means of enhancing development.[26] Pregnancy rates were increased and blastomere fragmentation reduced when human embryos were cultured on outgrowths of bovine tissue.[27] The explanation for the beneficial effect could be the secretion of an "embryotrophic" factor by the somatic cells or their removal of detrimental components from the media. In a cautionary note, Bavister suggested that greater attention to culture media quality can yield the same gains as those seen with co-culture.[28] In addition, co-culture with granulosa cells did not help couples with previous fertilization failures.[29] The use of co-culture is an evolving story, and its promise needs to be validated by continuing study.

Fertilization

Approximately 50,000–100,000 motile sperm (and much higher for male factor cases) are added to each dish containing an oocyte. The day after insemination, cumulus cells that remain attached to the zona pellucida are removed, and the egg is examined for evidence of fertilization (the presence of 2 pronuclei). A failure to fertilize is viewed by clinicians as a "human egg test" for that specific couple. However, fertilization failure in one cycle is not an absolute indication of an insurmountable problem. Indeed, a high rate of fertilization has been reported in subsequent cycles after an initial fertilization failure, although the eventual pregnancy rate is a little lower than the usual rate in IVF programs.[30,31] To demonstrate a complete failure of fertilization, at least 3 IVF cycles are necessary.

Extra embryos can be cryopreserved at the 2 pronuclei stage. There is no known limit on duration of cryopreserved embryo storage. About two-thirds of embryos survive the process. The transfer of cryopreserved embryos adds significantly to success rates with IVF and lowers the cost. Increasing age is associated with a decrease in pregnancy rates because of a reduction in pre-embryo quality; cycle day 3 FSH levels greater than 15 IU/L are also associated with decreased pregnancy rates, in this case because of fewer embryos available for cryopreservation.[32] Neither age nor basal FSH levels, however, predict failure to survive cryopreservation and thawing.

Embryo Transfer

Embryos have been transferred successfully at any stage from the pronuclear to the blastocyst, although most commonly, they are transferred when development is between the 4 and 10 cell stage, approximately 48–80 hours after retrieval. Transfer of more than one embryo increases the chances for pregnancy, but in general no more than 4 or 5 embryos are transferred to limit the risks of multiple births. The multiple pregnancy rate with transfers of more than one embryo is approximately 30%. This risk decreases with advancing age. Thus, in women 40 or older it is reasonable to place higher numbers of embryos. The ability to use fetal reduction to limit the number of continuing fetuses has lessened slightly the concern over multiple births. In experienced hands the risk of losing the entire pregnancy from selective fetal reduction is less than 10%.[33] In some countries, strict guidelines or laws limit transfer to no more than 3 embryos in order to minimize the number of multiple pregnancies. Embryos that are not transferred can be cryopreserved and transferred in later cycles if the initial cycle is unsuccessful.

There does not seem to be any advantage to placing the patient in knee-chest compared to lithotomy position for transfer. Ancillary medications given around the time of transfer, such as prostaglandin inhibitors, tranquilizers, or antibiotics are of uncertain value. It is common practice to supplement the luteal phase with progesterone.[34] Progesterone vaginal suppositories, 25 mg bid, or progesterone in oil 25 mg im once or twice daily, are given for 12 days starting on the day of transfer. An alternative therapy is the use of HCG, 2,000 IU every 3 days for 4 doses; however, HCG supplementation increases the risk of ovarian hyperstimulation.. The value of luteal phase supplementation can be questioned, but there is no doubt that it provides some psychologic benefit for both patient and physician. An initial quantitative HCG measurement can be obtained 12 days after transfer. If the test is positive, a follow-up test is obtained 3 days later. This will establish the trend of the HCG and provide prognostic information.

Assisted hatching consists of making an opening in the zona pellucida to help the embryo emerge. Assisted hatching is associated with an increased implantation rate, especially in older women.

IVF Results

A certain skepticism has arisen concerning the pregnancy rates reported by IVF programs.[35] Competition for patients is seen as the motivation for some of the exaggerations and half-truths contained in public statements and letters to referring physicians. An associated problem is determining what constitutes a pregnancy. A slight unsustained rise in the HCG is properly termed a "chemical pregnancy," and it should not be counted as a success. To avoid confusion, only those pregnancies that contain identifiable products of conception, an amniotic sac, or a fetus with a heart beat on ultrasound examination should be considered a pregnancy for reporting purposes. The most important statistic, which is the number of live births per retrieval, should be the one used for comparison. Uniform reporting by clinics, monitored by the Society for Assisted Reproductive Technology, with results available to the public, has now been implemented.[36] Programs will be subject to audits of their work, and this should restore a measure of confidence in the reliability of published results. International results are also available.[37]

Many programs have now achieved delivery/retrieval pregnancy rates of more than 25%. Success rates are impacted by the ages of the women treated by the programs and the presence or absence of male factors. Surprisingly, 4–5% of pregnancies achieved through IVF are ectopic, emphasizing the need for close ultrasonographic and HCG titer surveillance. Pregnancies occurring simultaneously in different body sites (heterotropic pregnancies) are a rare condition, occurring in 1 of 30,000 spontaneous pregnancies. The incidence of combined pregnancy among patients who have undergone one of the assisted reproduction procedures is much higher, closer to 1 in 100 pregnancies.[38–40] A case-control study has concluded that the risk of ectopic pregnancy with assisted reproduction is due to the multiple ovulations and high hormone levels secondary to the stimulation protocols.[41]

Twenty percent of clinical pregnancies result in spontaneous abortions because that is close to the rate in infertility populations; there is no increase in the rate of congenital malformations.[42]

The multiple pregnancy rate is approximately 30% (25% twins and 5% triplets or more). The selective reduction of the number of embryos in a multiple pregnancy can be safely accomplished.[43,44] The subsequent risk of losing one or more of the remaining fetuses is 4–9%, and of losing the pregnancy, 10%, when the procedure is performed by experienced clinicians. This can be a difficult decision for some couples, but in view of the potential problems associated with a multiple pregnancy, it is an option deserving consideration.

A major factor influencing IVF results is the gross inefficiency of human reproduction in vivo. A number of studies have attested to the low fecundability of humans. Only 25% of normal women who attempt pregnancy in a given cycle are successful. There is a large loss of embryos prior to or around the time of implantation in vivo, and thus, many women have pregnancy losses without realizing that they have been pregnant because the menstrual period comes at the normal time. It can be concluded that many sperm and many oocytes, even from individuals who are fertile, do not have the ability to contribute to a normal pregnancy. This affects the success of both in vivo and in vitro fertilization.

Whereas the chance for success in successive IVF cycles does not change appreciably, women who commit themselves to 3 to 6 cycles of IVF will have a good chance of achieving pregnancy.

The cumulative pregnancy rates of the Norfolk Group for 1 to 6 cycles of treatment were as follows:[45]

1 cycle — 13.5%.
2 cycles — 25.3%.
3 cycles — 38.5%.
4 cycles — 47%.
5 cycles — 49.3%.
6 cycles — 57.8%.

These rates are similar to those achieved at the Hallam Medical Centre in London, where 45% of women under the age of 35 have a live birth within 5 cycles of treatment.[46] The figures exclude cases of male infertility. Subsequent transfers of cryopreserved embryos will add to the pregnancy rate that can be achieved from one retrieval. Most individuals will find the emotional, physical, and financial consequences of going beyond 3 to 6 cycles too difficult.

Male Infertility and IVF

The limited effectiveness of treatments for male infertility has provided a sizable number of individuals who desire IVF to overcome problems with sperm. Early experience with male factor infertility in IVF indicated that even placing sperm in the dish with the oocyte still left many sperm specimens with a handicap. Fertilization rates tended to be approximately one-half those achieved with normal sperm, and the pregnancy rates were correspondingly lower. On the other hand, it should be recognized that fertilization can at times occur with surprisingly few sperm. For example, sperm obtained from vas aspirations have been able to achieve fertilization, although their numbers may be so small that eggs need to be put together in one dish in order to meet a sufficient concentration of the sperm.

IVF provides the ability to visualize the results of sperm and egg interaction and thus to quickly determine if specific manipulations of the sperm can affect fertilization. A variety of sperm treatments have been attempted. One approach is to increase the number of sperm in the dish with the hope that even with abnormal specimens there will be a few normal sperm that can achieve fertilization. By increasing the numbers in each dish there will be more normal sperm per egg. A second approach is to isolate the best sperm from the specimen, not from the standard swim-up technique, but by using Percoll gradients. In some hands this has provided increased fertilization rates, but others have not found it to be a significant advantage. Similar contradictory results have been reported with drug treatment of the semen; the most popular such treatment has utilized pentoxifylline which acts by increasing cyclic AMP in cells.[47] The drug must be washed out from the sperm specimen before incubation with the egg because it may have adverse effects on the latter. Another treatment that has been used to enhance sperm is incubation in follicular fluid.[48] In men with sperm autoantibodies, in vitro fertilization is correlated with the extent the sperm are covered with antibodies, but if fertilization occurs, pregnancy follows at the usual rates.[49]

Micromanipulation

Many of these techniques now have been overshadowed by the use of sperm micromanipulation.[50] Initially, a microneedle was used to make a small puncture in the zona pellucida (partial zona dissection) with the presumption that sperm would be able to breach the opening and proceed on to the egg membrane. Limited success with this technique led to the development of subzonal insertion of sperm (SUZI) by microinjection. In this technique 5 to 10 sperm are injected into the perivitelline space. More than one sperm are injected because not all are physiologically prepared for membrane fusion. Injection of more than one sperm under the zona does increase somewhat the risk of forming triploid embryos.

939

The most startling of the microneedle approaches has been the direct injection of one sperm into the egg cytoplasm. Van Steirtenghen and his coworkers in Belgium pioneered the technique for intracytoplasmic sperm injection (ICSI) of a single spermatozoon and have reported it to be superior to subzonal insemination (SUZI).[51] Fifty-three percent of oocytes injected into the cytoplasm with a single sperm had two pronuclei compared to 17% with SUZI. The clinical pregnancy rate with ICSI was 26% per cycle. With ICSI, in vivo protective mechanisms against abnormal sperm are bypassed. However, it is reassuring that Van Steirtenghen reported that 151 normal karyotypes were obtained by prenatal diagnosis from his patients, and that follow-up of 119 children born following ICSI did not reveal an increase in major congenital anomalies. An alternative has been suggested, using "heavy insemination" (effective concentrations of 1 to 5 million sperm per mL in a microdroplet under oil) of individual oocytes.[52] These techniques have achieved pregnancies with sperm counts less than 100,000/mL and with zero motile spermatozoa and no normal forms.[52,53] Thus the andrologist and the embryologist now have a variety of techniques to call on to overcome that most difficult of problems — male infertility.

IVF for Endometriosis

Individuals with mild to moderate endometriosis do well in IVF programs, although one report suggested that this is true only if the endometriosis has been treated.[54] The results with severe endometriosis, on the other hand, have not been good. Decreased numbers of stimulated follicles have been the experience in women with severe endometriosis, and even when comparable numbers of embryos were transferred, the pregnancy rate was decreased. Only a 2% pregnancy rate was achieved in a group with the most severe endometriosis.[55] On the other hand, recent experience is more encouraging. The Cornell group has reported similar pregnancy rates in all stages of endometriosis.[56] Perhaps improved techniques now offer good success rates for patients with moderate to severe endometriosis.

Other Indications for IVF

The experience using IVF for immunologic infertility is limited. If the problem lies with the male, then semen is obtained by masturbation into media to dilute out the antigens carried by the seminal plasma. If sperm antibodies are in the woman's serum, it should not be used to culture the eggs and the sperm. With unexplained infertility the results may be as good as those obtained in cases of tubal disease.

Other Techniques

In addition to IVF, individuals with unexplained infertility have been offered a number of tactics to overcome hypothesized problems with gamete transport. For gamete intrafallopian transfer (GIFT), minilaparotomy or laparoscopy is used to aspirate oocytes following hyperstimulation of the ovary.[57] After the oocytes are identified in the laboratory, they are taken up into a transfer catheter which also contains 100,000 sperm separated by the swim-up technique. The transfer catheters are guided into the distal 1.5 to 2 cm of a fallopian tube and the contents gently discharged. Usually 2 oocytes are placed in each tube although placement in one tube is equally successful. Extra eggs obtained by aspiration can be utilized for IVF. Success with GIFT in the collected statistics from the United States and Canada (1991) was 26.5% deliveries per retrieval.[36] In the same year the success with IVF was 15.25% deliveries per retrieval (18% for women less than 40 and no male factor).[36] This difference is believed to be due largely to differences in patient selection. Ectopic pregnancy occurs in approximately 3% of GIFT pregnancies, somewhat less than the 5% reported with IVF. The multiple pregnancy rate with GIFT is similar to that of IVF, approximately 30%.

In a variation of GIFT, called ZIFT, oocytes are obtained by vaginal aspiration, fertilized in vitro, and then 1 day later at the pronuclear stage placed in the fallopian tubes by the GIFT technique. The 1991 figures for ZIFT were 19.7% pregnancies per retrieval.[36] Whereas there was an early impression that ZIFT was decidedly superior to IVF, this is not reflected in current statistics. Indeed, prospective comparisons within the same clinics demonstrate similar results with uterine (IVF) versus tubal transfers (GIFT, ZIFT).[58,59]

Other attempts to overcome problems of gamete transport include injections of washed sperm and oocytes into the peritoneal cavity (POST) and cannulation of the fallopian tube via the cervix, as a conduit for injecting sperm directly into the tube. Not all of these methods have been subjected to close scrutiny and appropriate studies, but currently they have only a minimal role to play. In a technique of limited applicability, because it risks pregnancy in a donor, a fertilized human ovum at the blastocyst stage can be removed by uterine lavage from a donor and placed transcervically in the uterus of an infertile recipient.[60]

A technique of proven value is ovum donation. The use of a young donor can lead to pregnancy rates of 40–50% when her embryos are transferred to the uterus of an older woman (a rate that is 1–2 times higher than that with standard IVF). The recipient's age can affect the success, but the lower success with older women can be reversed by a high dose of progesterone in the stimulation protocol.[61]

Choice of Methods

The choice of methods, IVF, GIFT, ZIFT, can be made on the basis of infertility factors, chance for success, cost, and risk. If the problem is male infertility then it is important to know if fertilization can occur, and therefore GIFT would not be an appropriate choice. If there is tubal damage, then GIFT or ZIFT would be unwise. In rare instances where there is scarring of the cervix one of the intratubal techniques would be preferable. The additional cost of GIFT or ZIFT because of the need for anesthesia and operating room time may be a deterrent for many individuals. Moreover, anesthesia entails an additional risk that is usually not associated with IVF. Also important in terms of choosing a technique is consideration of which one the program is most comfortable with, and with which it has achieved the best results. These individual results are more important than countrywide statistics. Both GIFT and ZIFT can be accomplished by transcervical cannulation of the fallopian tube with injection of gametes or embryos into the tube. Despite the attractiveness of these cannulation techniques because they do not require anesthesia, they have not provided an increase in pregnancy rates over that achieved with IVF.

Preimplantation Genetic Diagnosis

Diagnosing genetic disorders before implantation provides couples with the option of foregoing the attempt to establish a pregnancy. This avoids the difficult decision whether or not to continue an affected pregnancy when the diagnosis is made at amniocentesis or by chorionic villus biopsy. There are 3 possible approaches for preimplantation diagnosis.[62] The first is the removal of the first polar body. The polar body contains only one copy of the gene, but if the copy is found to be normal, it can be presumed that the oocyte contains the abnormal copy. However, this method is technically very difficult and subject to error if crossing-over occurs and both copies are present in the polar body. A second method is to biopsy cells which are destined to become placenta. This requires opening the zona pellucida in the 5–6 day embryo. The disadvantage is the lower pregnancy rate when the embryo is transferred at this later stage. The third method is the removal of a single cell from the 6–8 cell embryo (blastomere biopsy) for DNA amplification and analysis. The biopsy procedure does not affect development and implantation, and the diagnostic testing is rapid; the biopsy and DNA analysis are accomplished within 8 hours. This method has been used for preimplantation testing for cystic fibrosis.[63] In addition, preimplantation genetic diagnosis has successfully detected single gene defects in disorders such as Duchene's muscular dystrophy, sickle cell disease, hemophilia, Tay-Sachs disease, and Lesch-Nyhan syndrome. These methods

941

can also be used to predict the sex of embryos from couples who are at risk for transmitting X-linked disorders.

The utilization of molecular biology techniques for preimplantation genetic diagnosis is associated with some significant risks. Polymerase chain reaction amplification does not always succeed. An erroneous diagnosis can occur because of contamination by DNA from surrounding cells or from sperm which are attached to the zona pellucida. This less than 100% success rate must be coupled with the low pregnancy rate achieved by IVF per cycle as well as the high costs of these procedures.

Concluding Thoughts

The new reproductive techniques and the technology associated with in vitro fertilization have been presented in a somewhat mechanistic way in this chapter. This should not obscure the fact that this is an emotionally trying experience for almost everyone undertaking therapy. Psychological stresses are acute and anxiety is accentuated with each step of the process despite the fact that couples enter treatment knowing that there is a limited chance for success. However, they invariably harbor some optimism over their chances, and thus, failures at every stage are exceptionally difficult for both patients and physicians. Support groups such as those organized by RESOLVE are helpful for almost every couple going through an IVF or associated program.

References

1. **Scott RT, Toner JP, Muasher SJ, Oehninger S, Robinson S, Rosenwaks Z**, Follicle-stimulating hormone levels on cycle day 3 are predictive of in vitro fertilization outcome, Fertil Steril 51:651, 1989.

2. **Licciardi FL, Liu HC, Berkeley AS, Cholst I, Davis OK, Graf MJ, Grifo JA, Noyes NL, Rosenwaks Z**, Day 3 estradiol levels as prognosticators of pregnancy outcome in in vitro fertilization, both alone and in conjunction with day 3 FSH levels, Abstract 141, 38th Annual Meeting of the Society for Gynecologic Investigation, San Antonio, March 20–23, 1991.

3. **Navot D, Rosenwaks Z, Margalioth EJ**, Prognostic assessment of female fecundity, Lancet 2:645, 1987.

4. **Loumaye E, Billion J-M, Mine J-M, Psalti I, Pensis M, Thomas K**, Prediction of individual response to controlled ovarian hyperstimulation by means of a clomiphene citrate challenge test, Fertil Steril 53:295, 1990.

5. **Scott RT, Leonardi MR, Hofmann GE, Illions EM, Neals GS, Navot D**, A prospective evaluation of clomiphene citrate challenge test screening of the general infertility population, Obstet Gynecol 82:539, 1993.

6. **Claman P, Domingo M, Garner P, Leader A, Spence JEH**, Natural cycle in vitro fertilization — embryo transfer at the University of Ottawa: an inefficient therapy for tubal infertility, Fertil Steril 60:298, 1993.

7. **Paulson RJ, Sauer MV, Francis MM, Macaso TM, Lobo RA**, In vitro fertilization in unstimulated cycles; the University of Southern California experience, Fertil Steril 57:290, 1992.

8. **Hughes EG, Fedorkow DM, Daya S, Sagle MA, Van de Koppel P, Collins JA**, The routine use of gonadotropin-releasing hormone agonists prior to in vitro fertilization and gamete intra-fallopian transfer: a meta-analysis of randomized controlled trials, Fertil Steril 58:888, 1992.

9. **Martin M, Givens CR, Schriock ED, Glass RH, Dandekar PV**, The choice of GnRH analog influences outcome in in vitro fertilization treatment, Am J Obstet Gynecol, in press.

10. **Garcia JE, Padilla SL, Bayati J, Baramki TA**, Follicular phase gonadotropin-releasing hormone agonist and human gonadotropins: a better alternative for ovulation induction in in vitro fertilization, Fertil Steril 53:302, 1990.

11. **Karande VC, Jones GS, Veeck LL, Muasher SJ**, High-dose follicle-stimulatling hormone stimulation at the onset of the menstrual cycle does not improve the in vitro fertiization outcome in low-responder patients, Fertil Steril 53:486, 1990.

12. **Rosenwaks S**, Optimizing IVF success, 26th Annual Postgradute Course, American Fertility Society, Montreal, October 9–10, 1993.

13. **Ibrahim ZHZ, Matson PL, Buck P, Lieberman BA**, The use of biosynthetic growth hormone to augment ovulation induction with buserelin acetate/human menopausal gonadotropin in women with a poor ovarian response, Fertil Steril 55:202, 1991.

14. **Owen EJ, Shoham Z, Mason BA, Ostergaard H, Jacobs HS**, Cotreatment with growth hormone, after pituitary suppression, for ovarian stimulation in in vitro fertilization: a randomized, double-blind, placebo-control trial, Fertil Steril 56:1104, 1991.

15. **Shaker AG, Fleming R, Jamieson ME, Yates RWS, Coutts JRT**, Absence of effect of adjuvant growth horone therapy on follicular resonses to exogenous gonadotropins in women: normal and poor responders, Fertil Steril 58:919, 1992.

16. **Levy T, Limor R, Villa Y, Eshel A, Eckstein N, Vagman I, Lidor A, Ayalon D**, Another look at co-treatment with growth hormone and human menopausal gonadotrophins in poor ovarian responders, Hum Reprod 8:834, 1993.

17. **Jamieson ME, Fleming R, Kader S, Ross KS, Yates RWS, Coutts JRT**, In vivo and in vitro maturation of human oocytes: effects on embryo development and polyspermic fertilization, Fertil Steril 56:93, 1991.

18. **Aboulghar MA, Mansour RT, Serour GI, Elattar I, Amin Y**, Follicular aspiration does not protect against the development of ovarian hyperstimulation syndrome, J Assist Reprod Genetics 9:238, 1992.

19. **Gonen Y, Casper RF**, Prediction of implantation by the sonographic appearance of the endometrium during controlled ovarian stimulation for in vitro fertilization (IVF), J In Vitro Fertil Embryo Transfer 7:146, 1990.

20. **Sher G, Herbert C, Maassarani G, Jacob MH**, Assessment of the late proliferative phase endometrium by ultrasonography in patients undergoing in vitro fertilization and embryo transfer (IVF/ET), Hum Reprod 6:232, 1991.

21. **Tarlatzis BC,** Oocyte collection and quality, Assist Reprod Rev 2:16, 1992.

22. **Trounson AO, Mohr LR, WoodC, Leeton JF**, Effect of delayed insemination on in vitro fertilization, culture and transfer of human embryos, J Reprod Fertil 64:285, 1982.

23. **Veeck L**, Extracorporeal maturation: Norfolk, 1984, Ann NY Acad Sci 442:357, 1985.

24. **Leung PCS, Gronow MJ, Kellow GN, Lopata A, Speirs AL, McBain JC, duPlessis YP, Johnston I**, Serum supplement in human in vitro fertilization and embryo development, Fertil Steril 41:36, 1984.

25. **Caro CM, Trounson A**, Successful fertilization, embryo development, and pregnancy in human in vitro fertilization (IVF) using a chemically defined culture medium containing no protein, J In Vitro Fertil Embryo Transfer 3:215, 1986.

26. **Bongso A, Ng S-C, Sathanathan H, Ng PL, Rauff M, Ratnam S**, Improved quality of human embryos when co-cultured with human ampullary cells, Hum Reprod 4:706, 1989.

27. **Weimer KE, Hoffman DI, Maxson WS, Eager S, Muhlberger B, Fiore I, Cuervo M**, Embryonic morphology and rate of implantation of human embryos following co-culture on bovine oviductal epithelial cells, Hum Reprod 8:97, 1993.

28. **Bavister BD**, Co-culture for embryo development: Is it really necessary? Hum Reprod 7:1339, 1992.

29. **Plachot M, Mendelbaum J, Junca AM, Anatoine JM, Salat-Baroux J, Cohen J**, Co-culture with granulosa cells does not increase the fertilization rate in couples with previous fertilization failures, Hum Reprod 8:1455, 1993.

30. **Molloy D, Harrison K, Breen T, Hennessey J,** The predictive value of idiopathic failure to fertilize on the first in vitro fertilization attempt, Fertil Steril 56:285, 1991.

31. **Lipitz S, Rabinovici J, Ben-Shlomo I, Bider D, Ben-Rafael Z, Mashiach S, Dor J,** Complete failure of fertilization in couples with unexplained infertility: implications for subsequent in vitro fertilization cycles, Fertil Stcril 59:348, 1993.

32. **Toner JP, Veeck LL, Muasher SJ,** Basal follicle-stimulating hormone level and age affect the chance for and outcome of pre-embryo cryopreservation, Fertil Steril 59:664, 1993.

33. **Macones GA, Schemmer G, Pritts E, Weinblatt V, Wapner RJ**, Multifetal reduction of triplets to twins improves perinatal outcome, Am J Obstet Gynecol 169:982, 1993.

34. **Pados G, Devroey P,** Luteal phase support, Assist Reprod Rev 2:148, 1992.

35. **Soules MR**, The in vitro fertilization pregnancy rate: Let's be honest with one another, Fertil Steril 43:511, 1985.

36. **Society for Assisted Reproductive Technology, The American Fertility Society,** Assisted Reproductive Technology in the United States and Canada: 1991 results from the Society for Assisted Reproductive Technology generated from the American Fertiity Society Registry, Fertil Steril 59:956, 1993.

37. **Testart J, Plachot M, Mandelbaum J, Salat-Baroux J, Frydman R, Cohen J,** World collaborative report on IVF–ET and GIFT: 1989 results, Hum Reprod 7:362, 1992.

38. **Molloy D, Deambrosis W, Keeping D, Hynes J, Harrison K, Hennessey J,** Multiple-sited (heterotropoic) pregnancy after in vitro fertilization and gamete intrafallopian transfer, Fertil Steril 53:1068, 1990.

39. **Dor J, Seidman DS, Levran D, Ben-Rafael Z, Ben-Shlomo I, Mashiach S,** The incidence of combined intrauterine and extrauterine pregnancy after in vitro fertilization and embryo transfer, Fertil Steril 55:833, 1991.

40. **Savare J, Norup P, Thomsen SG, Hornes P, Maigaard S, Helm P, Petersen K, Andersen AN,** Heterotropic pregnancies after in-vitro fertilization and embryo transfer — a Danish survey, Hum Reprod 8:116, 1993.

41. **Fernandez H, Coste J, Job-Spira N,** Controlled ovarian hyperstimulation as a risk factor for ectopic pregnancy, Obstet Gynecol 78:656, 1991.

42. **Shoham Z, Zosmer A, Insler V,** Early miscarriage and fetal malformations after induction of ovulation (by clomiphene citrate and/or human menotropins), in vitro fertilization, and gamete intrafallopian transfer, Fertil Steril 55:1, 1991.

43. **Evans MI, Dommergues M, Wapner RJ, Lynch L, Dumez Y, Goldberg JD, Zador IE, Nicolaides KH, Johnson MP, Golbus MS, Boulot P, Berkowitz RL,** Efficacy of transabdominal multifetal pregnancy reduction: collaborative experience among the world's largest centers, Obstet Gynecol 82:61, 1993.

44. **Timor-Tritschd IE, Peisner DB, Monteagudo A, Lerner JP, Sharma S,** Multifetal pregnancy reduction by transvaginal puncture: evaluation of the technique used in 134 cases, Am J Obstet Gynecol 168:799, 1993.

45. **Guzick DS, Wilkes C, Jones HWJr,** Cumulative pregnancy rates for in vitro fertilization, Fertil Steril 46:663, 1986.

46. **Tan SL, Royston P, Campbell S, Jacobs HS, Betts J, Mason B, Edwards RG,** Cumulative conception and livebirth rates after in-vitro fertilisation, Lancet 339:1390, 1992.

47. **Yovich JL,** Pentoxifylline: actions and applications in assisted reproduction, Hum Reprod 8:1786, 1993.

48. **McClure RD, Tom RA, Dandekar PV,** Optimizing the sperm penetration assay with human follicular fluid, Fertil Steril 53:546, 1990.

49. **Rajah SW, Parslow JM, Howell RJ, Hendry WF,** The effects on in-vitro fertilization of autoantibodies to spermatozoa in subfertile men, Hum Reprod 8:1079, 1993.

50. **Cohen J, Adler A, Alikani M, Ferrara TA, Kissin E, Reing AM, Suzman M, Talansky BE, Rosenwaks Z,** Assisted fertilization and abnormal sperm function, Seminars Reprod Endocrinol 11:83, 1993.

51. **Van Steirteghem A, Liu J, Nagy Z, Joris H, Tournaye H, Liebaers I, Devroey P,** Use of assisted fertilization, Hum Reprod 8:1784, 1993.

52. **Tucker MJ, Wiker S, Massey J,** Rational approach to assisted fertilization, Hum Reprod 8:1778, 1993.

53. **Terriou P, Giorgetti C, Hans E, Spach J-L, Salzmann J, Carlon N, Navarro A, Roulier R,** Subzonal sperm insemination and total or extreme asthenozoospermia: an effective technique for an uncommon cause of male factor, Fertil Steril 60:1057, 1993.

54. **Wardle PG, Foster PA, Mitchell JD, McLaughlin EA, Sykes JAC, Corrigan E, Hull MGR, Ray BD, McDermott A,** Endometriosis and IVF: effects of prior therapy, Lancet 1:376, 1986.

55. **Mastson PL, Yovich JL,** The treatment of infertility associated with endometriosis by in vitro fertilization, Fertil Steril 46:432, 1986.

56. **Feldberg D, Davis O, Grifo J, Berkeley A, Graf M, Liu HC, Rosenwaks Z,** Severity of endometriosis does not impact on pregnancy success after in vitro fertilization, Abstract P-279, 7th World Congress on IVF and Assisted Procreations, Paris, June 28–30, 1991.

57. **Asch RH, Balmaceda JP, Ellsworth LR, Wong PC,** Preliminary experience with gamete intrafallopian transfer (GIFT), Fertil Steril 45:366, 1986.

58. **Tanbo T, Dale PO, Aabyholm T,** Assisted fertilization in infertile women with patent fallopian tubes. A comparison of in vitro fertilization, gamete intrafallopian transfer and tubal embryo stage transfer, Hum Reprod 5:266, 1990.

59. **Balmaceda JP, Alam V, Roszjtein D, Ord T, Snell K, Asch R,** Embryo implantation rates in oocyte donation: a prospective comparison of tubal versus uterine transfers, Fertil Steril 57:362, 1992.

60. **Sauer MV, Bustillo M, Gorrill MJ, Louw JA, Marshall JR, Buster JE,** An instrument for the recovery of preimplantation uterine ova, Obstet Gynecol 71:804, 1988.

61. **Meldrum DR,** Female reproductive aging — ovarian and uterine factors, Fertil Steril 59:1, 1993.

62. **Dubey AK, Layman LC,** Preimplantation genetic diagnosis, Assist Reprod Rev 3:224, 1993.

63. **Handyside AH, Lesko JG, Tarín JJ, Winston RML, Hughes MR,** Birth of a normal girl after in vitro fertilization and preimplantation diagnostic testing for cystic fibrosis, New Engl J Med 327:905, 1992.

32 Ectopic Pregnancy

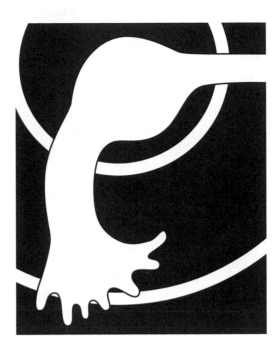

The modern management of ectopic pregnancy is one of medicine's greatest success stories. Ectopic pregnancy has been recognized for a very long time (it was first described in the 11th century), and for a long time, only as a universally fatal event. In medieval times, the ectopic pregnancy was believed to be located outside the uterus because of a violent emotion, usually fright or surprise, experienced by the woman during the coitus of conception.[1] Treatment was so unavailable that the only recourse was speculation.

The first documentation of an unruptured ectopic pregnancy was recorded in 1693 in the results of an autopsy performed on a woman prisoner condemned to death and executed. Previous infertility was linked to ectopic pregnancy in 1752 with the report of an extrauterine pregnancy in a prostitute with 20 years of sterility. In the mid 19th century, pathology reports began to stress pelvic inflammation as a cause of ectopic pregnancy. This knowledge was derived from women who died because of tubal rupture and hemorrhage. Although data were gradually accumulated from autopsies and the pathology was described, treatment remained unavailable.

Because the ectopic fetus was obviously responsible for the death of the mother, physicians recommended measures to kill the fetus. These measures included starvation, purging, bleeding, and even large doses of strychnine. Early attempts to surgically puncture ectopic sacs or to introduce electric current into the fetus were followed by sepsis and maternal death. Even into the early 1900s, a favored treatment was the introduction of electricity by means of the direct insertion of needles into the gestational sac. Another favored treatment was the injection of morphine into the ectopic pregnancy.

Around 1600, there were several isolated reports of abdominal surgical procedures in women with repeat ectopic pregnancies. Then for more than 100 years there was no mention of a surgical operation for this purpose. The first case in the 18th century was reported in France in 1714. The first American surgeon to operate abdominally and successfully (for the removal of a macerated fetus) was John Bard of New York City in 1759. The second successful American operation was performed in 1791 by William Baynham, a country physician in Virginia. In 30 abdominal operations in the first 80 years of the 1800s, only 5 women survived.[1] The survival rate in those not treated (one out of three) was better!

W.W. Harbert of Louisville was the first, in 1849, to suggest surgery early enough to stop fatal bleeding.[2] But the problem was that diagnosis was only certain when it was too late. In 1876, John S. Parry (of the Philadelphia Hospital) wrote:[3]

> ...when one is called to a case of this kind, it is his duty to look upon his unhappy patient as inevitably doomed to die, unless he can by some active measure wrest her from the grave already yawning before her.

Robert Lawson Tait in London, after experiencing the death of several women and at autopsy recognizing that appropriate dissection and ligation of bleeding vessels would be effective, for the first time in 1883, deliberately and successfully performed a laparotomy to ligate the broad ligament and a ruptured tube.[4] By 1885, Tait had accumulated a relatively large number of successful cases.

Asepsis, anesthesia, and antibiotics (and blood transfusions) combined to save the lives of many women. But diagnosis was still difficult, and surgical intervention was relatively late. Even in the first half of the 20th century, the maternal mortality rate in the United States ranged from 200 to 400 per 10,000 cases of ectopic pregnancies. As dramatic as the contribution of immediate salpingectomy coupled with simultaneous blood transfusion was, progress in the last 20 years has been even more impressive. Treatment has shifted from the saving of lives to the preservation of fertility.

The Centers for Disease Control first began to report the incidence of ectopic pregnancies in the U.S. in 1970. In 1970, there were 17,800 ectopic pregnancies, and by 1987, the number had increased to 88,000, a rate increase of 4.5 to 16.8 ectopic pregnancies per 1,000 pregnancies.[5] Since 1987, the number of ectopic pregnancies in the United States has stabilized.[6] *However, at the same time, the fatality rate decreased from 35.5 to 3.8 per 10,000 ectopic pregnancies, a decrease of 90%.*

The increase in ectopic pregnancies has not been paralleled by a similar increase in sexually transmitted diseases (STDs), and therefore, the increased incidence of ectopic pregnancies is not due to STDs alone.[5] Ectopic pregnancies do occur in totally normal tubes, suggesting that abnormalities of the conceptus or maternal hormonal changes can function as etiologic factors. The other important contributing factors are reconstructive tubal surgery, assisted reproductive technologies, and most importantly, earlier and more accurate diagnosis.

Today management intervention occurs prior to tubal rupture in more than 80% of cases.[7] This can be attributed directly to three diagnostic advances: a highly specific and sensitive immunoassay for human chorionic gonadotropin (HCG), ultrasonography, and the use of laparoscopy.

**Etiology and
Clinical Presentation**

Even though the risk of death from ectopic pregnancy has declined dramatically, ectopic pregnancy is the second leading cause of maternal mortality in the United States (12% of all maternal deaths in 1987).[8] This represents a combination of a lack of access to appropriate services and misdiagnosis.

Ectopic pregnancy is the great masquerader. The clinical presentation can vary from vaginal spotting to vasomotor shock with hematoperitoneum. The classic triad of delayed menses, irregular vaginal bleeding, and abdominal pain is most commonly ***not*** encountered. The exact frequency of clinical symptoms and signs is hard to assess. Standard descriptions in texts are based upon older reports and, thus, older methods of diagnosis. Suspicion of the diagnosis and rapid recourse to the methods of early diagnosis represent the best and most rewarding approach. Patients who present because of acute symptoms (frequently in emergency rooms) are usually at a more advanced gestational age compared to asymptomatic infertility patients being followed closely because of their increased risk for ectopic pregnancy.

Differential Diagnosis
- Normal intrauterine pregnancy.
- Ruptured ovarian cyst.
- Bleeding corpus luteum.
- Spontaneous abortion.
- Salpingitis.
- Appendicitis.
- Adnexal torsion.
- Endometriosis.

Relevant factors in a patient's medical history include previous pelvic inflammatory disease, prior tubal surgery, the use of assisted reproductive technology, exposure to diethylstilbestrol (DES), and the method of contraception. However, most patients presenting with an ectopic pregnancy do not have a recognized risk factor, suggesting dysfunctional problems in tubal transport or impaired implantation due to some abnormality in the conceptus. Nevertheless, pregnancies following tubal surgery or treatment with one of the methods of assisted reproduction should, ideally, be diagnosed immediately and followed closely with HCG titers and ultrasonography.

**Previous Pelvic
Inflammatory Disease**

In Westrom's classic report, women with a history of salpingitis (verified by laparoscopy) had a four-fold increased risk of ectopic pregnancy.[9] The one predisposing factor identified most often is previous pelvic inflammatory disease, either by history or histologic evidence in removed tubal tissue. Salpingitis damages the endosalpinx, resulting in agglutination of the mucosal folds and adhesion formation. The risk of an ectopic pregnancy increases with each inflammatory episode. Evidence of chlamydial infection (circulating antibodies) is associated with a greater than two-fold increased risk of ectopic pregnancy.[10] A similar increased risk is associated with douching, but the presence of infection may be the reason for the douching.

Prior Tubal Surgery

Women with tubal surgery have an increased risk of ectopic pregnancy. High risk surgery includes any infertility surgery on the tube, but not abdominal or pelvic surgery that avoids the tubes.[11] Women with an ectopic pregnancy treated by conservative surgery have a ten-fold increased risk of a subsequent ectopic. Ectopic pregnancies occur after tubal occlusion procedures for sterilization that are not performed immediately postpartum (interval sterilization); the risk with postpartum sterilization is very low, comparable to that observed in oral contraceptive users.[12] With interval sterilization, bipolar tubal coagulation is more likely to result in ectopic pregnancy than is mechanical occlusion. This is attributed to fistula formation that allows sperm passage, and this may explain the difference in ectopic pregnancy rates between interval and postpartum sterilization because postpartum procedures are mostly by the Pomeroy method. Ectopic pregnancies following tubal ligation usually occur two or more years after the sterilization, rather than immediately after. In the first year after sterilization, about 6% of sterilization failures will be ectopic pregnancies, but the majority of pregnancies that occur 2–3 years after occlusion will be ectopic.[13] Overall, the ectopic risk in women with interval sterilizations is 80% less than that in nonsterilized women; however, the relative risk is 3.7 times that of women using oral contraception and 2.8 times that with barrier methods of contraception.[12]

The Use of Assisted Reproductive Technology

Pregnancies occurring *simultaneously* in different body sites *(heterotopic pregnancies)* are a rare condition, occurring in 1 of 30,000 spontaneous pregnancies. The incidence of combined pregnancy among patients who have undergone one of the assisted reproduction procedures (in vitro fertilization, gamete intrafallopian transfer, and even superovulation) is much higher, closer to 1 in 100 pregnancies.[14–16] Close monitoring of pregnancies in these programs is important to prevent a deleterious delay in the treatment of an ectopic pregnancy. Is the increased risk with these treatment methods due to ovulation induction (with superovulation and elevated levels of hormone influence on the tubes) or due to previous tubal disease? A case-control study has concluded that the risk of ectopic pregnancy was increased four-fold with ovulation induction, but not further increased when ovulation induction was used for in vitro fertilization.[17] This would indicate that the multiple eggs and high hormone levels are the important factors.

Method of Contraception

The risk of ectopic pregnancy is reduced with all methods of contraception except the progesterone-containing intrauterine device.[6,18–20]

The IUD has been traditionally listed as a risk factor for ectopic pregnancy. It should be emphasized that the modern copper-bearing IUDs do **NOT** increase the risk of ectopic pregnancy and, in fact, offer considerable protection. The largest study, a World Health Organization multicenter study, concluded that IUD users were 50% less likely to have an ectopic pregnancy when compared to women using no contraception.[20] However, if an IUD user becomes pregnant, the pregnancy is more likely to be ectopic. About 3–4% of IUD pregnancies have been ectopic, making the actual occurrence a rare event. The protection against ectopic pregnancy provided by the copper and levonorgestrel IUDs makes these IUDs acceptable choices for contraception in women with previous ectopic pregnancies.

The risk of pelvic infection with the modern IUD is limited to contamination of the endometrial cavity at the time of insertion. With careful screening of patients to make sure they are at low risk for acquiring STDs and with good insertion technique, the risk of infection (and the risk of a subsequent ectopic pregnancy) is minimized and definitely not increased.

The risk of an ectopic pregnancy during use of Norplant is lower than the general rate. However, because of the impressive contraceptive efficacy of Norplant, when pregnancy does occur, ectopic pregnancy should be suspected. With the progestin-only minipill, ectopic pregnancy is not prevented as effectively as intrauterine pregnancy. Although the overall incidence is not increased, the situation is similar to that with Norplant. When pregnancy occurs, an ectopic gestation must be suspected.

Ectopic Pregnancy Rates per 1,000 Woman-Years[6,18–20]

All U.S. women	1.50
Noncontraceptive users	3.00
Copper T-380 IUD	0.20
Progesterone IUD	6.80
Levonorgestrel IUD	0.20
Norplant	0.28

Ectopic Sites

Almost all ectopic pregnancies are located in the tube. Although relatively uncommon, ectopic pregnancies in nontubal sites are very susceptible to complications, especially hemorrhage. For example, abdominal pregnancies are often misdiagnosed, and the mortality rate is 17 times greater compared to the overall ectopic rate.[21] Contrary to the experience with tubal pregnancy, recurrence in nontubal sites is rare.

Sites of Ectopic Implantation[22]

Fallopian tube:	
Ampullary segment	80 %
Isthmic segment	12 %
Fimbrial end	5 %
Cornual and interstitial	2 %
Abdominal	1.4%
Ovarian	0.2%
Cervical	0.2%

**The Methods of
Early Diagnosis**

Patients with normal intrauterine pregnancies can present with the same symptoms encountered in patients with unruptured ectopic pregnancies. The best way to diagnose ectopic pregnancy is to be highly suspicious and sensitive to its possibility, and to utilize the new tools of diagnosis: the quantitative measurement of HCG and ultrasonography. Laparoscopy is necessary only when the diagnosis is in doubt, or when laparoscopy is the technique selected for surgical treatment.

**The Quantitative
Measurement of HCG**

HCG is secreted by the syncytiotrophoblast and reaches a maximal level of 50,000–100,000 IU/L at 8–10 weeks of gestation. The maternal circulating HCG concentration is approximately 100 IU/L at the time of the expected but missed menses. Virtually 100% (but not absolutely all) of patients suspected of an ectopic pregnancy, but not pregnant, will have a negative blood HCG assay.[23] Contrast this present day sensitivity of the HCG assay with the urinary tests of the past. In the 1960s and early 1970s, the urinary pregnancy tests were positive in only 50% of patients with ectopic pregnancies.

In some laboratories, the lower limit of the assay is 10–15 IU/L, but even that level is almost never associated with a false negative. With a detection limit of less than 5 IU/L for the serum HCG assay, there should be no false negative results; however, this situation (very rarely) can be encountered.[24] When the clinical picture is confusing, a definitive diagnosis by laparoscopy is warranted.

A landmark observation was reported in 1981, documenting that HCG levels approximately double every 2 days in early, normal intrauterine pregnancies, and that a lesser increase is associated with ectopic pregnancies and spontaneous abortions.[25] In the first 6 weeks of normal pregnancy, the concentration of HCG in the maternal blood follows a well-recognized pattern.[26] The rate of increase is nonlinear, changing with advancing gestational age and increasing HCG concentrations.[27] However, during the time period when the diagnosis of ectopic pregnancy is most important, from 2 to 4 weeks after ovulation, the relationship between HCG titers and gestational age is linear, approximately doubling every 2 days until the titer is greater than 10,000.[28] Use of the HCG titer requires medical judgment. Some ectopic pregnancies will display a normal rise in titer (at least for awhile), and some normal pregnancies (about 10%) will have an abnormal doubling time.

The Clinical Usefulness of the Quantitative Measurement of HCG

1. **Assessment of pregnancy viability.** Most of the time, but not always, a normal rate of rise indicates a normal pregnancy. Clinical decisions require serial measurements of HCG.

2. **Correlation with ultrasonography.** When the titer exceeds 1,000–1,500 IU/L, vaginal ultrasonography should identify the presence of an intrauterine gestation. With multiple gestation, a gestational sac will not be apparent until the titer is a little higher.[29] In an asymptomatic patient, repeat ultrasonography 2–3 days later is warranted.

3. **Assessment of treatment results.** Declining levels are consistent with effective medical or surgical treatment. Persistent or rising levels indicate the presence of viable trophoblastic tissue.

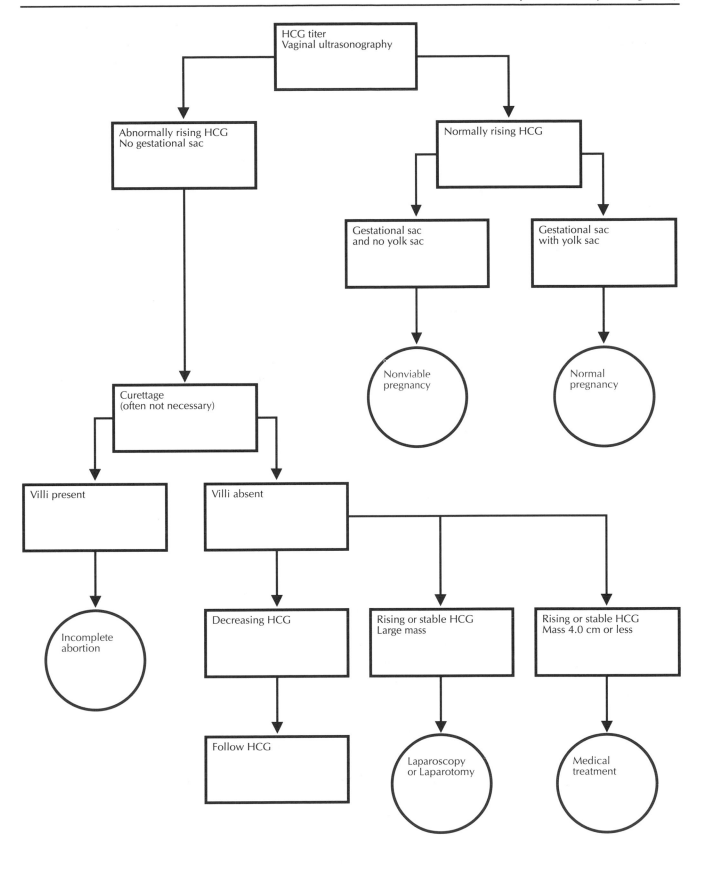

Vaginal Ultrasonography

The difficulty in diagnosis is establishing the cause of abnormal HCG levels: is it an ectopic pregnancy or a spontaneous abortion? The addition of ultrasonography has made an important contribution to this differential diagnosis.

The discriminatory zone is that HCG titer above which a gestational sac can be identified with ultrasonography. Previously, with abdominal ultrasonography, this level was approximately 6,000 IU/L. Transvaginal ultrasonography has now established the discriminatory zone at a level that varies from 1,000 to 1,500 IU/L (based on the International Reference Preparation). This level is achieved approximately one week after the time of expected menses. Institutions must establish their own exact discriminatory zone based on the sensitivity of their immunoassay and their equipment and the ability of their ultrasonographers. Keep in mind that in a multiple pregnancy, the discriminatory zone will be a little higher, requiring an extra 2–3 days for a gestational sac to become visible.

Demonstration of a viable intrauterine pregnancy does not absolutely exclude the possibility of an ectopic pregnancy. With the increase in incidence of ectopic pregnancy associated with superovulation, dizygotic twinning is more common, and thus a combined intrauterine pregnancy and extrauterine pregnancy (heterotopic pregnancy) is more frequent. *Heterotopic pregnancy should especially be considered when the pregnancy is the result of one of the methods of assisted reproductive technology.*

Color and pulsed Doppler increases the sensitivity of vaginal ultrasonography. This method adds physiologic information to the anatomic picture of regular ultrasonography. A small intrauterine gestational sac, without the double sac sign (decidua and membranes) or the presence of a yolk sac is hard to distinguish from the pseudosac of an ectopic pregnancy. A pseudogestational sac due to endometrial bleeding occurs in about 10% of ectopic pregnancies.[30] Local vascular changes associated with a true gestational sac differentiate an intrauterine pregnancy from the pseudosac of ectopic pregnancy. Vascular pulses increase with pregnancy and produce a "warm" appearance with color Doppler ultrasonography. In addition, high velocity arterial flow is detected even with very early pregnancies.

A failed intrauterine pregnancy can be associated with either elevated flow velocity around the trophoblast or very low velocities. Thus, a characteristic peritrophoblastic arterial flow correlates with gestational sac size and HCG levels.[31] Ectopic masses can also be distinguished by the surrounding abnormal color mapping. Doppler ultrasound, therefore, has greater sensitivity and is technically less challenging (and quicker). Although traditional ultrasonography can reveal an adnexal mass, Doppler flow imaging can indicate that the mass is an ectopic pregnancy by documenting abnormal vascular activity of the mass combined with the relatively cool uterine vasculature. This difference between Doppler and standard ultrasonography is greatest in early pregnancy, and thus this greater accuracy can allow earlier initiation of medical treatment.

Important Observations with Vaginal Ultrasonography

1. **Documentation of an intrauterine sac.** An experienced ultrasonographer should be able to identify a viable intrauterine pregnancy if the HCG titer is 1,000–1,500 IU/L or greater. An HCG titer of greater than 1,000–1,500 IU/L with no intrauterine sac is consistent with an ectopic pregnancy. Accurate assessment of ultrasonography is important, as well as correlation with the HCG titers.

2. **Adnexal masses.** An ectopic equal to or greater than 2 cm in diameter should be identified by ultrasonography. Vaginal ultrasonography should also establish large ectopics that require different consideration. Currently an ectopic pregnancy with a diameter of 4 cm or more is a relative contraindication to medical treatment, although this may change with increasing experience.

3. **Adnexal cardiac activity.** The presence of cardiac activity in an ectopic pregnancy, detectable when the HCG titer is approximately 15,000–20,000 IU/L, is a relative contraindication to medical treatment.

The Progesterone Level

Serum progesterone levels have a wide spectrum with considerable overlap between normal and ectopic pregnancies. This measurement must be viewed as an adjunct to HCG levels and ultrasonography. The concentration of the serum progesterone is usually lower in ectopic pregnancies. A value of 25 ng/mL (80 nmol/L) or more is 98% of the time associated with a normal intrauterine pregnancy, while a value of less than 5 ng/mL (16 nmol/L) identifies a nonviable pregnancy, regardless of location.[32] The value of the serum progesterone is to help make a decision regarding the viability of a possible intrauterine pregnancy prior to curettage. In most cases, however, this is a decision easily made by the combined results of the clinical presentation, the HCG titers, and ultrasonography. The great majority of patients will have a progesterone level between 10 and 20 ng/mL (30 and 60 nmol/L) at presentation, significantly limiting the clinical usefulness of progesterone measurement.[33] The value of 25 ng/mL as an indicator of a normal intrauterine pregnancy was established in women with spontaneous ovulations and pregnancies. The appropriate number for women receiving medication for the induction of ovulation is probably higher, and in these cases, the use of the progesterone level is even more limited.

Uterine Curettage

The purpose of uterine curettage is to determine the presence or absence of villi to rule out a nonviable intrauterine pregnancy. In most cases, this clinical situation will be associated with a serum progesterone less than 5 ng/mL (16 nmol/L). Curettage with examination of the curettings can be used to prevent unnecessary laparoscopies in patients undergoing spontaneous abortions. Floating the curettings in saline will usually identify villi if present, but not always. The saline flotation of curettings has been reported to be incorrect in 6.6% of patients with ectopic pregnancies and incorrect in 11.3% of patients with intrauterine pregnancies.[32] Because of this inaccuracy, permanent sections and follow-up HCG titers are necessary for confirmation.

Culdocentesis

Culdocentesis to seek the presence of unclotted blood was for a period of time a valuable technique to aid in the diagnosis of an ectopic pregnancy. We have progressed to the point where the relative accuracy of culdocentesis is no longer sufficient. Furthermore, the presence of blood in the cul-de-sac does not mean that an ectopic pregnancy has ruptured. Therefore, a positive culdocentesis is of no help in deciding whether to treat medically or surgically. Culdocentesis no longer has a place in the differential diagnosis of ectopic pregnancy.

The Treatment of Ectopic Pregnancy

Expectant Management

Part of the increased incidence of ectopic pregnancy is due to earlier diagnosis detecting ectopic pregnancies which previously resolved and remained clinically undiagnosed. Not all tubal pregnancies progress to clinical manifestations, and therefore expectant management of ectopic pregnancies diagnosed very early is an appropriate choice.[34] Expectant management includes the monitoring of clinical symptoms, HCG titers, and ultrasonography findings. Approximately one-fourth of women presenting with ectopic pregnancy can be managed expectantly, and 70% of this select group of patients will avoid surgery and experience successful outcomes.[35] The long-term outcome (subsequent intrauterine and ectopic pregnancies) is similar to that with active treatment interventions. The following criteria are reasonable requirements for expectant management:

Criteria for Expectant Management

1. Falling HCG titer.

2. Ectopic pregnancy definitely in the tube.

3. No significant bleeding.

4. No evidence of rupture.

5. Ectopic mass not larger than 4 cm in greatest diameter.

Medical Treatment

Medical treatment of unruptured ectopic pregnancies is appealing for several reasons: less tubal damage, less cost, and hopefully, enhanced potential for future fertility. Methotrexate, a folic acid antagonist that interferes with DNA synthesis, has a long history of effectiveness against trophoblastic tissue, derived from experience in the treatment of hydatiform moles and choriocarcinoma. Methotrexate was used in the 1960s to treat the difficult problem of trophoblastic tissue left in situ after removal of an abdominal pregnancy. Methotrexate was first used to treat an ectopic pregnancy in Japan in 1982.[36] The first U. S. experience was reported by Ory in 1986.[37] The guidelines for the safe and effective use of methotrexate were established by Stovall and his colleagues.[38,39]

Criteria for Patient Selection

1. The patient is healthy, hemodynamically stable, reliable, and compliant.

2. Ultrasonography should fail to find an intrauterine pregnancy, and uterine curettage should fail to obtain villi.

3. The ectopic pregnancy measures 4 cm or less in its greatest diameter.

4. There is no evidence of rupture of the ectopic pregnancy.

5. HCG titers greater than 10,000 IU/L and fetal cardiac activity are relative contraindications. However, even patients with fetal cardiac activity have been successfully treated.

Prior to Methotrexate Treatment

1. Administer Rhogam if patient is Rh negative and greater than 8 weeks gestation.

2. Obtain baseline liver and renal function tests, complete blood and platelet counts.

3. Consider uterine curettage.

Patient Instructions

The following are avoided until HCG titers are negative: alcohol use, sexual intercourse, and the use of folic acid-containing vitamins.

The Multiple Dose Method

The initial protocols for treatment utilized multiple doses of methotrexate together with citrovorum factor (folinic acid) to minimize side effects. Treatment with this method has been 95% successful. Failures have been more common with HCG levels greater than 5,000 IU/mL, and thus the presence of fetal cardiac activity is generally a contra-indication. Side effects (in 3–4% of patients) include mild stomatitis, gastritis, diarrhea, and transient elevations in liver enzymes. Significant reactions (bone marrow suppression, dermatitis, pleuritis) have been very rare. The incidence of nonresponders and/or tubal rupture is 3–4%.

In our own experience, the onset of abdominal cramping occurring 3–4 days after the initiation of methotrexate treatment produces some anxious moments. The concern, of course, is that the ectopic pregnancy is rupturing. Although this is always a possibility, the cramping is usually a side effect of the methotrexate and resolves in a day or two. Occasionally, hospitalization is necessary until hemodynamic stability is verified.

Multiple Dose Methotrexate Protocol

Treatment is discontinued when a decline is observed in two consecutive daily HCG titers, or after 4 doses of methotrexate.

Day 1:	Baseline studies.	
	Methotrexate	1.0 mg/kg im.
Day 2:	Citrovorum factor	0.1 mg/kg im.
Day 3:	Methotrexate	1.0 mg/kg im.
Day 4:	Citrovorum factor	0.1 mg/kg im.
	HCG titer.	
Day 5:	Methotrexate	1.0 mg/kg im.
	HCG titer.	
Day 6:	Citrovorum factor	0.1 mg/kg im.
	HCG titer.	
Day 7:	Methotrexate	1.0 mg/kg im.
	HCG titer.	

Day 8: Citrovorum factor   0.1 mg/kg im.
HCG titer.
Complete blood and platelet counts.
Renal and liver function tests.

Weekly: HCG titer until negative.

Approximately 20% of patients will require only one dose of methotrexate, and 20% will require 4 doses.[39–41] The side effects are encountered in those patients who require multiple doses. Changes in blood counts and liver enzymes are so infrequent and so mild, that daily monitoring is unnecessary.

In terms of subsequent fertility, methotrexate compares favorably with conservative laparoscopic surgery. In Stovall's experience, of those attempting pregnancy, 62.5% became pregnant with a recurrent ectopic rate of 10.8%.[41,42] The mean time to return of menses was 26 days (usually within the first month). These results match well with the 67% intrauterine pregnancy rate and 12% recurrent ectopic rate with laparoscopic surgery.[43]

The ultrasonographic picture of a mass persists after HCG titers become negative.[44] The time for resolution of the mass is variable, and often it takes several months. Thus, the persistence of a mass should not be interpreted as a treatment failure.

The Single Dose Method
Experience with the multiple dose method indicated that a significant number of patients responded promptly and did not require several doses. With lesser dosing, fewer side effects could be anticipated, and the use of citrovorum factor could be abandoned. The initial results with a single dose have been very encouraging, even with very high HCG titers and the presence of fetal cardiac activity.[40] The HCG titers usually keep rising for 3 days after treatment but by day 7 are declining. Full resolution requires 3 to as much as 6 weeks. Serious side effects are virtually absent. If there is less than a 15% decline on day 7 (the usual assay variation), the treatment protocol is repeated (necessary in approximately 3% of patients).[41] In a prospective series of 120 patients, 87.2% achieved a subsequent intrauterine gestation, whereas 12.8% experienced a subsequent ectopic pregnancy.[41]

Single Dose Methotrexate Protocol

Day 1: Baseline studies.
Methotrexate   50 mg/M^2 im.

Day 4: HCG titer.

Day 7: HCG titer
Complete blood and platelet count.
Liver and renal function tests.

Weekly: HCG titer until negative.

Oral Methotrexate
After baseline studies, methotrexate is administered orally in a dose of 0.3 mg/kg daily for 4 days. One week after beginning therapy, the HCG titer is measured and laboratory tests for side effect surveillance are obtained (complete blood and platelet count, liver and renal function tests). If the HCG titer is falling, weekly titers are followed until negative. If the HCG titer plateaus or rises, a second course of methotrexate can be

administered, or the ectopic pregnancy should be treated surgically. Experience with the oral method of treatment is still limited; assessment of efficacy may be available in the forthcoming medical literature.

Important Cautions

The medical treatment of ectopic pregnancy requires compulsive compliance. An ectopic pregnancy can exist in the absence of detectable HCG.[45] Although in this instance, the extrauterine pregnancy is usually degenerating and associated with an indolent clinical course, rupture can still occur. Clinicians should always be alert for the possibility of rupture (3–4% of medically treated cases). A satisfying decline in HCG titers does not guarantee against rupture.[46] The average time for HCG to return to nondetectable levels is about 4 weeks.

The risk of tubal rupture is about 10% when the HCG titer is less than 1,000 IU/L, and if the ectopic is isthmic, a risk of rupture is still present with a titer of 100 or less. Remember that a negative HCG assay means that HCG is not present in levels greater than the sensitivity of the assay; therefore, trophoblastic tissue can still be present, secreting minimal amounts of HCG (below the limits of the assay). Ectopic pregnancies will continue to adhere to their historical record; always expect behavior that is an exception to the general rule.

Although experience is limited with the medical treatment of relatively large masses (with a fetus present and high levels of HCG), case reports indicate a greater risk of bleeding and problems. Carefully selected cases with HCG titers greater than 10,000 IU/L might warrant medical treatment, but as a general rule these cases deserve surgical treatment.

Special Indications for Methotrexate

Treatment with methotrexate is especially useful when the pregnancy is located in a site (cervix, ovary, or cornua) where surgical treatment carries significant risk.[47,48] Methotrexate treatment is an attractive option when an ectopic pregnancy is in the interstitial portion of the tube, growing in the wall of the uterus (diagnosed by ultrasonography).[49]

Salpingocentesis

Salpingocentesis is the injection of a substance directly into the gestational sac within the tube, either at laparoscopy or under ultrasound guidance. Various substances have been used, including methotrexate, potassium chloride, prostaglandins, and hyperosmotic glucose. The efficacy, safety, and the long-term impact on fertility have not been established. Thus far local injections have been associated with inconsistent results; at least one clinical trial was discontinued because of poor results with tubal injection of methotrexate while another claimed excellent results, especially when the HCG level was under 5,000 IU/L.[50–52] Circulating levels of methotrexate are similar when gestational sac injection is compared to intramuscular injection.[53] Thus, local treatment with methotrexate offers no obvious advantage over systemic treatment. Hyperosmotic glucose (a 50% solution) appears to be safe and effective when the HCG titers are less than 2,500 IU/L.[54]

Surgical Treatment

With earlier diagnosis, conservative surgery to preserve fertility has replaced the life-saving procedure of salpingectomy. Linear salpingostomy along the antimesenteric border to remove the products of conception is the procedure of choice for ectopic pregnancies in the ampullary portion of the tube. Ectopic pregnancies in the ampulla are usually located between the lumen and the serosa, and thus these are ideal candidates for linear salpingostomy. Segmental excision with either simultaneous or delayed micro-surgical anastomosis is the preferred procedure for isthmic pregnancies. Although linear salpingostomy is possible for a small and unruptured gestation, isthmic pregnancies reflect a damaged endosalpinx, and these patients do poorly with linear salpingostomy (with a high rate of recurrent ectopic pregnancy).

Occasionally, an ampullary pregnancy can be expressed through the fimbrial end of the tube (milking the tube), but this procedure is associated with a higher incidence of persistent and recurrent ectopic pregnancy, undoubtedly due to invasion of the tube by the trophoblastic tissue. However, fimbrial expression of an ectopic pregnancy that is easily dislodged is acceptable. Interstitial pregnancy at the utero-tubal junction usually requires surgical excision, and even hysterectomy if bleeding cannot be controlled. The first unruptured ectopic pregnancy treated with methotrexate was an interstitial pregnancy, and this is now the treatment of choice if diagnosis is achieved early enough.

Patients with compromised fertility do better when the tube that contains the ectopic pregnancy is conserved (even when the opposite tube appears to be normal). However, in patients with a history positive for previous tubal disease, the risk of a recurrent ectopic pregnancy in the same tube is very much higher, and in this case, some argue in favor of salpingectomy. When performing a salpingectomy, a cornual wedge excision as prophylaxis against recannulation and a subsequent ectopic pregnancy is no longer considered to be necessary. An effort should be made to retain both ovaries when appropriate as a resource for the future use of in vitro fertilization.

Indications for Salpingectomy
Childbearing completed.
Second ectopic pregnancy in the same tube.
Uncontrolled bleeding.
Severely damaged tube.

These procedures can be accomplished either by laparotomy or laparoscopy. The choice of surgical method and specific procedure is determined by the patient's condition, desire for future fertility, the location, size, and state of the ectopic pregnancy, and the experience of the surgeon. The relative contraindications to laparoscopy include extensive pelvic adhesions, hematoperitoneum, and an ectopic pregnancy greater than 4 cm diameter. Hemodynamic instability is an absolute contraindication.

Linear salpingostomy through the laparoscope achieves results comparable with those obtained at laparotomy.[55,56] Hemostasis is the key and several methods are used, including the use of vasopressin, microcautery, and laser. The gains are notable: outpatient versus inpatient cost and a more rapid recovery. Almost all patients can now be successfully treated with conservative surgery. Comparisons of the different types of surgery (laparoscopic salpingostomy, laparotomy salpingostomy, and laparotomy salpingectomy) indicate that the surgical technique chosen is less important to the outcome than the causes of the ectopic pregnancy.[57]

Results with Laparoscopic Surgery

Successful	95%
Subsequent intrauterine pregnancy	70%
Subsequent tubal patency	84%
Subsequent ectopic pregnancy	12%
Persistent trophoblast	15%

Treatment of an Ectopic Pregnancy after Tubal Ligation

An ectopic pregnancy after a previous tubal ligation is usually located in the segment of tube containing the fimbria. The pregnancy occurs because of small channel recannulation through the ligation site, allowing sperm to migrate toward the oocyte. A prophylactic procedure should be highly considered. Removing both fimbrial segments and fulgurating the proximal segments (either by laparoscopy or laparotomy) will prevent the recurrence of another ectopic pregnancy.

Treatment of Persistent Trophoblastic Tissue

The risk of a persistent ectopic pregnancy with conservative surgery by laparotomy is 5%.[58] Laparoscopic salpingostomy is associated with a higher rate of persistent trophoblastic tissue; approximately 15% of patients will require further treatment.[59] Persistence of ectopic trophoblastic tissue can be associated with hemorrhage and tubal rupture (usually within 2 weeks); however, regression without clinical sequelae is the general rule. For this reason, *weekly HCG measurements are necessary following conservative surgery.* The incidence of persistent trophoblastic tissue is greater (not surprising) with higher HCG titers, and relatively rare with a titer less than 3,000 IU/L.[60] The risk of persistent trophoblastic tissue is very significant with a hematosalpinx greater than 6 cm in diameter, an HCG titer greater than 20,000 IU/L, and a hematoperitoneum greater than 2,000 mL.[61] Rupture is unlikely for an ampullary pregnancy with an HCG level of 100 or less, but not so for an isthmic pregnancy.

The average time for HCG levels to become undetectable is 4 weeks, but it can take 6 weeks. The need for treatment of persistent trophoblastic tissue can emerge in a few days or not until 1 month later. Although reoperation is always a treatment option, the use of methotrexate in one of the above protocols is preferable.[62] Even lower doses (15 mg im) have been successfully used.[63] Low and declining HCG levels warrant only close surveillance; only persistent or rising titers require treatment (a small minority of patients). Symptomatic patients, of course, usually demand surgical therapy.

The problem of persistent trophoblastic tissue after surgery makes earlier diagnosis of an ectopic pregnancy even more important. With sufficiently early diagnosis, medical treatment becomes the method of choice.

Rh Sensitization

Despite underutilization of Rhogam in Rh-negative women, no apparent increase in sensitization has been observed.[64,65] This indicates that ectopic pregnancies do not contain sufficiently large quantities of fetal red blood cells. The use of Rhogam should be considered only for ectopic pregnancies that are older than 8 weeks gestation.

References

1. **Graham H,** *Eternal Eve: The History of Gynaecology & Obstetrics,* Doubleday & Co., Inc., Garden City, NY, 1951, pp 503-508.

2. **Harbert WW,** A case of extra-uterine pregnancy, West J Med Surg 3:110, 1849.

3. **Parry JS,** *Extra-uterine Pregnancy: Its Causes, Species, Pathological Anatomy, Clinical History, Diagnosis, Prognosis, and Treatment,* H.C. Lea, Philadelphia, 1876, pp 211-212.

4. **Tait RL,** Five cases of extra-uterine pregnancy operated upon at the time of rupture, Br Med J 1:1250, 1884.

5. **Nederlof KP, Lawson HW, Saftlas AF, Atrash HK, Finch EL,** Ectopic pregnancy surveillance, United States, 1970-1987, MMWR 39:9, 1990.

6. **Centers for Disease Control,** Ectopic pregnancy — United States, 1988–1989, MMWR 41:591, 1992.

7. **Pansky M, Golan A, Bukovsky I, Caspi E,** Nonsurgical management of tubal pregnancy: necessity in view of the changing clincal appearance, Am J Obstet Gynecol 164:888, 1991.

8. **Atrash HK, Friede A, Hogue CJ,** Ectopic pregnancy mortality in the United States, 1970-1983, Obstet Gynecol 70:817, 1987.

9. **Westrom L, Joesoef R, Reynolds G, Hagdu A, Thompson SE,** Pelvic inflammatory disease and fertility, Sex Trans Dis 19:185, 1992.

10. **Chow JM, Yonekura L, Richwald GA, Greenland S, Sweet RL, Schachter J,** The association between Chlamydia trachomatis and ectopic pregnancy: a matched-pair, case-control study, JAMA 263:3164, 1990.

11. **Ni H, Daling J, Chu J, Stergachis A, Voigt L, Weiss N,** Previous abdominal surgery and tubal pregnancy, Obstet Gynecol 75:919, 1990.

12. **Holt VL, Chu J, Daling JR, Stergachis AS, Weiss NS,** Tubal sterilization and subsequent ectopic pregnancy, JAMA 266:242, 1991.

13. **Chi IC, Laufe LE, Atwed R,** Ectopic pregnancy following female sterilization procedures, Adv Plann Parenthood 16:52, 1981.

14. **Molloy D, Deambrosis W, Keeping D, Hynes J, Harrison K, Hennessey J,** Multiple-sited (heterotopic) pregnancy after in vitro fertilization and gamete intrafallopian transfer, Fertil Steril 53:1068, 1990.

15. **Dor J, Seidman DS, Levran D, Ben-Rafael Z, Ben-Shlomo I, Mashiach S,** The incidence of combined intrauterine and extrauterine pregnancy after in vitro fertilization and embryo transfer, Fertil Steril 55:833, 1991.

16. **Savare J, Norup P, Thomsen SG, Hornes P, Maigaard S, Helm P, Petersen K, Andersen AN,** Heterotropic pregnancies after in-vitro fertilization and embryo transfer — a Danish survey, Hum Reprod 8:116, 1993.

17. **Fernandez H. Coste J, Job-Spira N,** Controlled ovarian hyperstimulation as a risk factor for ectopic pregnancy, Obstet Gynecol 78:656, 1991.

18. **Franks AL, Beral V, Cates W Jr, Hogue CJ,** Contraception and ectopic pregnancy risk, Am J Obstet Gynecol 163:1120, 1990.

19. **Sivin I,** Dose- and age-dependent ectopic pregnancy risks with intrauterine contraception, Obstet Gynecol 78:291, 1991.

20. **WHO Special Programme of Research, Development and Research Training in Human Reproduction, Task Force on Intrauterine Devices for Fertility Regulation,** A multinational case-control study of ectopic pregnancy, Clin Reprod Fertil 3:131, 1985.

21. **Atrash HK, Friede A, Hogue CJ,** Abdominal pregnancy in the United States: frequency and maternal mortality, Obstet Gynecol 69:333, 1987.

22. **Breen JL,** A 21 year survey of 654 ectopic pregnancies, Am J Obstet Gynecol 106:1004, 1970.

23. **Schwartz RO, DiPietro DL,** β-HCG as a diagnostic aid for suspected ectopic pregnancy, Obstet Gynecol 56:197, 1980.

24. **Maccato ML, Estrada R, Faro S,** Ectopic pregnancy with undetectable serum and urine β-hCG levels and detection of β-hCG in the ectopic trophoblast by immunocytochemical evaluation, Obstet Gynecol 81:878, 1993.

25. **Kadar N, Caldwell BV, Romero R,** A method of screening for ectopic pregnancy and its indications, Obstet Gynecol 58:162, 1981.

26. **Kadar N, Romero R,** Observations on the long human chorionic gonadotropin-time relationship in early pregnancy and its practical implications, Am J Obstet Gynecol 157:73, 1987.

27. **Fritz, MA, Guo S,** Doubling time of human chorionic gonadotropin (hCG) in early normal pregnancy: relationship to hCG concentration and gestational age, Fertil Steril 47:584, 1987.

28. **Kadar N, Freedman M, Zacher M,** Further observations on the doubling time of human chorionic gonadotropin in early asymptomatic pregnancies, Fertil Steril 54:783, 1990.

29. **Keith SC, London SN, Weitzman GA, O'Brien TJ, Miller MJ,** Serial transvaginal ultrasound scans and β-human chorionic gonadotropin levels in early singleton and multiple pregnancies, Fertil Steril 59:1007, 1993.

30. **Chambers S, Muir B, Haddad N,** Ultrasound evaluation of ectopic pregnancy including correlation with human chorionic gonadotropin levels, Br J Radiol 63:246, 1990.

31. **Emerson DS, Cartier MS, Altier LA, Felker RE, Smith WC, Stovall TG, Gray LA,** Diagnostic efficacy of endovaginal color Doppler flow imaging in an ectopic pregnancy screening program, Radiology 183:413, 1992.

32. **Stovall TG, Ling FW, Carson SA, Buster JE,** Serum progesterone and uterine curettage in differential diagnosis of ectopic pregnancy, Fertil Steril 57:456, 1992.

33. **Gelder MS, Boots LR, Younger JB,** Use of a single random serum progesterone value as a diagnostic aid for ectopic pregnancy, Fertil Steril 55:497, 1991.

34. **Garcia AJ, Aubert JM, Sama J, Josimovich JB,** Expectant management of presumed ectopic pregnancies, Fertil Steril 48:395, 1987.

35. **Ylostalo P, Cacciatore B, Sjoberg J, Kaariainen M, Tenhunen A, Stenman U-H,** Expectant management of ectopic pregnancy, Obstet Gynecol 80:345, 1992.

36. **Tanaka T, Hayashi H, Kutsuzawa T, Ichinoe K,** Treatment of interstitial ectopic pregnancy with methotrexate: report of a successful case, Fertil Steril 37:851, 1982.

37. **Ory SJ, Villanueva AL, Sand PK, Tamura RK,** Conservative treatment of ectopic pregnancy with methotrexate, Am J Obstet Gynecol 154:1299, 1986.

38. **Stovall TG, Ling RW, Buster JE,** Outpatient chemotherapy of unruptured ectopic pregnancy, Fertil Steril 51:435, 1989.

39. **Stovall TG, Ling FW, Gray LA, Carson SA, Buster JE,** Methotrexate treatment of unruptured ectopic pregnancy: a report of 100 cases, Obstet Gynecol 77:749, 1991.

40. **Stovall TG, Ling FW, Gray LA,** Single-dose methotrexate for treatment of ectopic pregnancy, Obstet Gynecol 77:754, 1991.

41. **Stovall TG, Ling FW,** Single-dose methotrexate: an expanded clinical trial, in press.

42. **Stovall TG, Ling FW, Buster JE,** Reproductive performance after methotrexate treatment of ectopic pregnancy, Am J Obstet Gynecol 162:1620, 1990.

43. **Pouly JL, Chapron C, Manhes H, Canis M, Wattiez A, Bruhat MA,** Multifactorial analysis of fertility after conservative laparoscopic treatment of ectopic pregnancy in a series of 223 patients, Fertil Steril 56:453, 1991.

44. **Brown DL, Felker RE, Stovall TG, Emerson DS, Ling FW,** Serial endovaginal sonography of ectopic pregnancies treated with methotrexate, Obstet Gynecol 77:406, 1991.

45. **Hochner-Celnikier D, Ron M, Goshen R, Azcut D, Amir G, Yagel S,** Rupture of ectopic pregnancy following disappearance of serum beta subunit of HCG, Obstet Gynecol 79:826, 1992.

46. **Tulandi T, Hemmings R, Khalifa F,** Rupture of ectopic pregnancy in women with low and declining serum β-chorionic gonadotropin concentration, Fertil Steril 56:786, 1991.

47. **Yankowitz J, Leake J, Huggins G, Gazaway P, Gates E,** Cervical ectopic pregnancy: review of the literature and report of a case treated by single-dose methotrexate therapy, Obstet Gynecol Survey 45:405, 1990.

48. **Timor-Tritsch IE, Monteagudo A, Matera C, Veit CR,** Sonographic evolution of cornual pregnancies treated without surgery, Obstet Gynecol 79:1044, 1992.

49. **Karsdorp VHM, Van der Veen F, Schats R, Boer-Meisel ME, Kenemans P,** Successful treatment with methotrexate of five vital interstitial pregnancies, Hum Reprod 7:1164, 1992.

50. **Menard A, Crequat J, Mandelbrot L, Hauuy JP, Madelenat P,** Treatment of unruptured tubal pregnancy by local injection of methotrexate under transvaginal sonographic control, Fertil Steril 54:47, 1990.

51. **Mottla GL, Rulin MC. Guzick DS,** Lack of resolution of ectopic pregnancy by intratubal injection of methotrexate, Fertil Steril 57:685, 1992.

52. **Fernandez H, Benifla J-L, Lelaidier C, Baton C, Frydman R,** Methotrexate treatment of ectopic pregnancy: 100 cases treated by primary transvaginal injection under sonographic control, Fertil Steril 59:773, 1993.

53. **Schiff E, Shalev E, Bustan M, Tsafari A, Mashiach S, Winer E,** Pharmacokinetics of methotrexate after local tubal injection for conservative treatment of ectopic pregnancy, Fertil Steril 57:688, 1992.

54. **Lang PF, Tamussino K, Honigl W, Ralph G,** Treatment of unruptured tubal pregnancy by laparoscopic instillation of hyperosmolar glucose solution, Am J Obstet Gynecol 166:1378, 1992.

55. **Vermesh M, Presser SC,** Reproductive outcome after linear salpingostomy for ectopic gestation: a prospective 3-year follow-up, Fertil Steril 57:682, 1992.

56. **Lundorff P, Thorburn J, Lindblom B,** Fertility outcome after conservative surgical treatment of ectopic pregnancy evaluated in a randomized trial, Fertil Steril 57:998, 1992.

57. **Sultana CJ, Easley K, Collins RL,** Outcome of laparoscopic versus traditional surgery for ectopic pregnancies, Fertil Steril 57:285, 1992.

58. **DiMarchi JM, Kosasa TS, Kobara TY, Hale RW,** Persistent ectopic pregnancy, Obstet Gynecol 70:555, 1987.

59. **Seifer DB, Gutman JN, Grant WD, Kamps CA, DeCherney AH,** Comparison of persistent ectopic pregnancy after laparoscopic salpingostomy versus salpingostomy at·laparotomy for ectopic pregnancy, Obstet Gynecol 81:378, 1993.

60. **Lundorff P, Hahlin M, Sjoblom P, Lindblom B,** Persistent trophoblast after conservative treatment of tubal pregnancy: prediction and detection, Obstet Gynecol 77:129, 1991.

61. **Pouly JL, Chapron C, Mage G, Manhes H, Wattiez A, Canis M, Gaillard G, Bruhat MA,** The drop in the levels of hCG after conservative laparoscopic treatment of ectopic pregnancy, J Gynecol Surg 4:211, 1991.

62. **Rose PG, Cohen SM,** Methotrexate therapy for persistent ectopic pregnancy after conservative laparoscopic management, Obstet Gynecol 76:947, 1990

63. **Bengtsson G, Bryman I, Thorburn J, Lindblom B,** Low-dose methotrexate as a second-line therapy for persistent trophoblast after conservative treatment of ectopic pregnancy, Obstet Gynecol 79:589, 1992.

64. **Grimes D, Geary F, Harcher R,** Rh immunoglobulin utilization after ectopic pregnancy, Am J Obstet Gynecol 140:246, 1981.

65. **Grant J, Hyslop M,** Underutilization of Rh prophylaxis in the emergency department: A retrospective survey, Ann Emer Med 21:181, 1992.

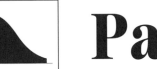

Part V

Clinical Assays

33 Clinical Assays

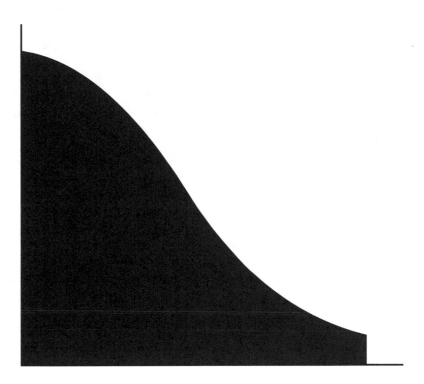

The purpose of this chapter is to review the laboratory assays that are commonly used in clinical gynecologic endocrinology. With this information, the clinician will have confidence in the selection of specific laboratory tests, and will be secure in the personal interpretation of the data.

Classically, hormones were measured in blood by bioassays, i.e., dose-response measurements based upon organ responses in animals. Some of the principles fundamental to endocrinology were established by such methods. However, bioassay methods, although adequate for qualitative statements, were relatively imprecise, nonspecific, time-consuming, expensive, and required too large an amount of the biologic sample in order to meet the quantitative requirements of modern research and clinical practice.

The International System of Units

The International System of Units (SI units — Systeme International) has been adopted throughout the world in all areas of science and industry. In medicine, the major change is the expression of concentration as amount per volume (moles per liter) instead of mass per volume (milligrams per deciliter). Because we are in the midst of this change, the table provides ranges for the most relevant laboratory values in reproductive endocrinology, in conventional and SI units. Because the conversion from conventional units to SI units is based on the molecular weight of the analyte, a conversion factor can be derived and utilized; to convert from conventional to SI units, multiply by the conversion factor; to convert from SI to conventional units, divide by the conversion factor.

Laboratory Values for Selected Measurements in Urine

Substance	Conventional Units	Conversion Factor	SI Units
Cortisol, free	10–90 µg/24 hr	2.759	28–250 nmol/24 hr
Estrogens, total	5–25 µg/24 hr	3.67	18–92 nmol/24 hr
17-Hydroxycorticosteroids	2–6 mg/24 hr	2.759	5.5–15.5 µmol/24 hr
17-Ketosteroids	6.0–15 mEq/24 hr	3.467	21–52.5 µmol/24 hr

SI Prefixes and Their Symbols

10^9	giga	G
10^6	mega	M
10^3	kilo	k
10^2	hecto	h
10^1	deka	da
10^{-1}	deci	d
10^{-2}	centi	c
10^{-3}	milli	m
10^{-6}	micro	µ
10^{-9}	nano	n
10^{-12}	pico	p
10^{-15}	femto	f
10^{-18}	alto	a

Laboratory Values for Selected Measurements in Blood, Plasma, and Serum

Substance	Conventional Units	Conversion Factor	SI Units
ACTH, adrenocorticotropin hormone			
6:00 AM	10–80 pg/mL	0.2202	2.2–17.6 pmol/L
6:00 PM	<50 pg/mL	0.2202	<11 pmol/L
Androstenedione	60–300 ng/dL	0.0349	2.1–10.5 nmol/L
Calcium, total	8.5–10.5 mg/dL	0.25	2.1–2.6 mmol/L
Cholesterol	<200 mg/dL	0.0259	<5.2 mmol/L
LDL-cholesterol	60–130 mg/dL	0.0259	1.6–3.4 mmol/L
HDL-cholesterol	30–70 mg/dL	0.0259	0.8–1.8 mmol/L
Cortisol			
8:00 AM	5–25 µg/dL	27.9	140–700 nmol/L
4:00 PM	3–12 µg/dL	27.9	80–330 nmol/L
10:00 PM	<50% of AM value	27.9	<50% of AM value
DHAS, Dehydroepiandrosterone sulfate	80–350 µg/dL	0.0027	2.2–9.5 µmol/L
11-Deoxycortisol	0.05–0.25 µg/dL	28.86	1.5–7.3 nmol/L
11-Deoxycorticosterone	2–10 ng/dL	30.3	60–300 pmol/L
Estradiol	20–400 pg/mL	3.67	70–1500 pmol/L
Estrone	30–200 pg/mL	3.7	110–740 pmol/L
FSH, reproductive years	5–30 mIU/mL	1.0	5–30 IU/L
Glucose, fasting	70–110 mg/dL	0.0556	4.0–6.0 mmol/L
Growth hormone	<10 ng/mL	1.0	<10 µg/L
17-Hydroxyprogesterone	100–300 ng/dL	0.03	3–9 nmol/L
Insulin, fasting	5–25 µU/mL	7.175	35–180 pmol/L
Insulin-like growth factor-I	0.3–2.2 U/mL	1000	300–2200 U/L
LH, reproductive years	5–20 mIU/mL	1.0	5–20 IU/L
Progesterone			
Follicular phase	<3 ng/mL	3.18	<9.5 nmol/L
Secretory phase	5–30 ng/mL	3.18	16–95 nmol/L
Prolactin	1–20 ng/mL	44.4	44.4–888 pmol/L
Testosterone, total	20–80 ng/dL	0.0347	0.7–2.8 nmol/L
Testosterone, free	100–200 pg/dL	0.0347	35–700 pmol/L
TSH, thyroid stimulating hormone	0.35–6.7 µU/mL	1.0	0.35–6.7 mU/L
Thyroxine, free T_4	0.8–2.3 ng/dL	1.29	10–30 nmol/L
Triglycerides	40–250 mg/dL	0.0113	0.5–2.8 mmol/L
Triidothyronine, T_3, total	80–220 ng/dL	0.0154	1.2–3.4 nmol/L
Triidothyronine, T_3, free	0.13–0.55 ng/dL	15.4	2.0–8.5 pmol/L
Triidothyronine, reverse	8–35 ng/dL	15.4	120–540 pmol/L

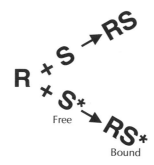

Saturation Analysis (Immunoassay, Competitive Protein Binding)

Basic Principles

The methods of saturation analysis yield greater simplicity, sensitivity, and precision. Reactions in saturation analysis follow the law of mass action. A protein or antibody (R) is mixed with a substance (S) for which it has specific binding sites, forming a complex, RS. The radioactive form of the substance (S*) also forms a complex, RS*. Since the number of binding sites on the protein or antibody are limited, the labeled and unlabeled compound, S and S*, will compete for binding sites in proportion to their concentrations. Since the binding reagent, R (protein or antibody), is kept constant, increasing the unlabeled compound, S, will displace more and more labeled tracer, S*. Plotting the change in either bound or unbound (free) tracer, S*, against the amount of unlabeled compound, S, added will produce a standard curve. The amount of radioactivity bound or free in the presence of an unknown level of compound will reveal the concentration of the compound when compared to the standard curve. The requirements for saturation analysis are, therefore, either a suitable binding protein, or an antibody, and a labeled pure form of the compound to be measured. The need for radioisotopes can be eliminated by the use bioluminescence, chemiluminescence, fluoroimmunoassays, and enzyme-linked assays.

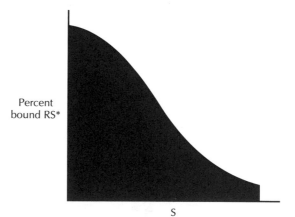

Methodology

A purified, labeled amount of the substance to be measured is added to the biologic sample (e.g., plasma) to be assayed. The radioactive tracer equilibrates with the unlabeled and unknown amount of compound in the sample. The sample is now mixed with an appropriate solvent to extract the desired compound and tracer. The extraction process usually removes several compounds that may interfere with the assay, and separation (purification) of the desired substance is frequently necessary. A chromatographic separation utilizing thin layer chromatography or column chromatography was used for most steroid assays, but solid phase systems and even magnetic separation of bound and free fractions are currently utilized. Direct assays on untreated serum are less accurate.

The next step is to mix the extracted compound with a specific reagent. In the case of immunoassay, this reagent is an antiserum, and in the case of competitive protein binding, this reagent is a protein that has affinity for the compound to be measured. The combination of the compound with this reagent (antiserum or specific protein) is called binding. Since the compound is in equilibrium with a small amount of labeled compound, the labeled compound will bind to the reagent in proportion to the amount of unlabeled compound present. This is the fundamental principle: the distribution of bound and unbound radioactivity (or the color/light provoking agent) is dependent upon the total concentration of the compound in the system. Measurement of the radioactivity, color, or light, therefore, can be utilized to calculate the unknown amount of compound in the system.

Since steroid compounds are not antigenic, the production of a specific antiserum depends upon the linkage of a steroid to a large protein molecule. The protein molecule is antigenic in itself, but when combined with a steroid, the steroid-protein complex (hapten) stimulates a variety of antibodies, some of which recognize and are specific for the steroid. Thus, when the steroid-protein complex is injected into an animal the antiserum formed may be utilized as a reagent (R) for measurement of the steroid (S) in the technique of saturation analysis.

Immunoradiometric Assays

In immunoradiometric assays (IRMAs), the antibody is labeled instead of the hormone. The advantage is the greater stability in iodinated immunoglobulins compared to iodinated hormones.

Monoclonal Antibodies

Antibodies are produced by the B lymphocytes present in the bone marrow, spleen, lymph nodes, and other lymphoid glands. Monoclonal antibodies are homogeneous, eliminating the heterogeneity and variability associated with antiserum obtained by the regular immunization process (polyclonal antibodies). An animal is first immunized against an antigen (anti-X in the illustration). The antibody can be derived from specific cells in the spleen or elsewhere, or from the B lymphocytes. Production of monoclonal antibodies depends upon the development of a hybridoma cell line. Usually a tumor cell is fused with the cell from the animal, e.g., a combination of a myeloma and lymphocytes. The tumor cell can be maintained in culture essentially forever. The medium is manipulated so that only the fused hybridoma cells grow. For example in the illustration, the tumor B lymphocytes have a defective secondary pathway for the synthesis of nucleic acids. Therefore only those cells fused to normal lymphocytes will continue to grow in the medium that contains an inhibitor of the main biosynthetic pathway for nucleic acids. The normal lymphocytes die after only a few days in culture.

The supernatant in each well is tested for the presence of the antibody. Ultimately a well will contain only a single cell line producing homogeneous, identical, monoclonal antibodies.

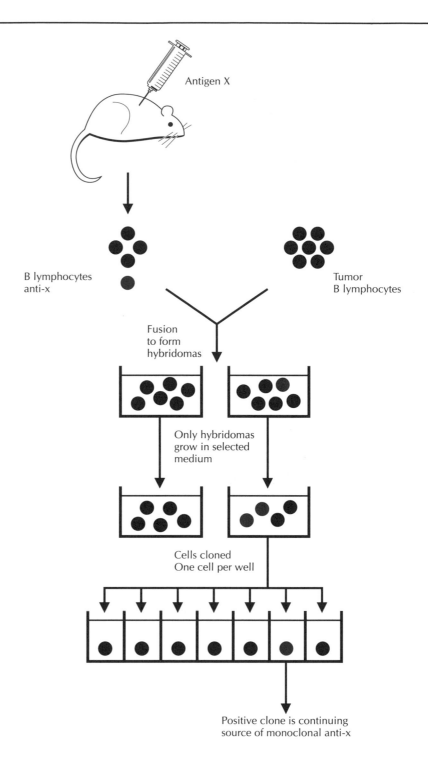

The ELISA technique

ELISA stands for enzyme-linked immunosorbent assay, also known as the sandwiched technique. This method does not require a radioactive tracer. A monoclonal antibody is coupled to an enzyme, e.g., horseradish peroxidase, that provides a color endpoint which can be measured by spectrophotometry. For the measurement of the glycopeptides (HCG, LH, TSH), this technique uses two monoclonal antibodies, one against the alpha-subunit and coupled to a bead or a plastic tube, and the other antibody against the beta-subunit is coupled to the enzyme. The antibody to the alpha-subunit binds the intact glycoprotein molecule; the beta-subunit antibody and the enzyme then sandwich the intact molecule by binding to the exposed beta-subunit. The result is obtained by comparing the enzyme reading on the spectrophotometer to a standard curve. Antibodies

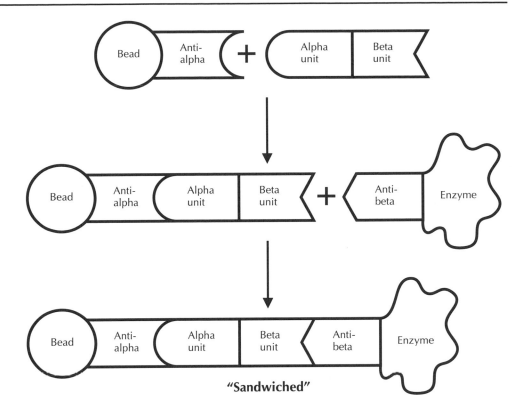

"Sandwiched"

can be attached to other active substances that produce luminescence. ELISA technology is utilized for most over-the-counter LH tests and pregnancy tests.

Problems

These methods are not without problems. Utmost precision and care in technique are necessary. An unknown variation in technique may completely disrupt an assay. The periodic appearance of the well known laboratory "gremlin" may be traced to a simple thing like the water supply or a change in glassware-washing routine. The accuracy of the results depends upon the following:

1. Specificity of the antibody or protein for the hormone to be measured, and therefore, the degree of interference or cross-reaction with other substances.

2. Purity and specificity of the radiolabeled tracer.

3. Purity and availability of the standard reference hormone.

4. *Sensitivity* (the smallest amount that can be measured) of the assay.

5. *Precision*, the variation observed when multiple measurements are obtained with the same sample, expressed as the coefficient of variation for intraassay precision and interassay precision.

If cross-reaction of the binding protein exists for other hormones, these cross-reacting substances must be removed. The radiolabeled tracer must have a high specific radioactivity, and purity is essential to ensure that it behaves identically as the substance being measured. Experimental error between assays as well as within an assay is an important determinant of assay reliability. A coefficient of variation of less than 15% for each is considered acceptable.

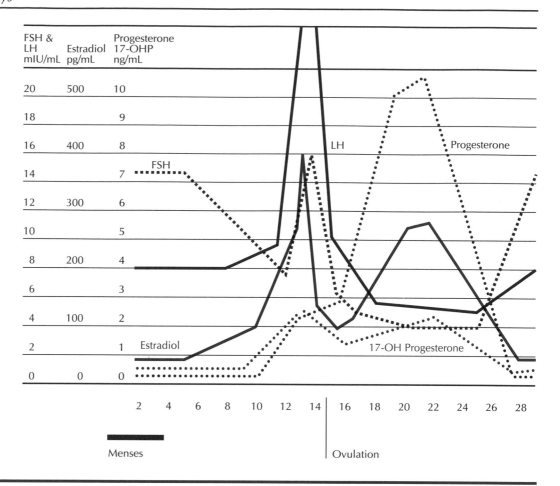

FSH & LH mIU/mL	Estradiol pg/mL	Progesterone 17-OHP ng/mL
20	500	10
18		9
16	400	8
14		7
12	300	6
10		5
8	200	4
6		3
4	100	2
2		1
0	0	0

Measurement of Pituitary Gonadotropins

In the case of polypeptide hormones (gonadotropins), immunoassay techniques are based upon the use of antibodies prepared by injecting the protein hormone of one species into another. The protein hormones vary in their physicochemical characteristics and amino acid composition from species to species, and, therefore, antibodies for use in immunoassay are formed when protein hormones are administered cross-species. A highly specific monoclonal antibody can be produced to be utilized as the binding reagent. This specificity makes chromatographic separation that ordinarily follows extraction unnecessary.

Over-the-counter LH kits are readily available to detect the LH midcycle surge in urine, utilizing enzyme immunoassays with monoclonal antibodies. The enzymes linked to the antibodies produce a color change in tubes, strips, or absorbent pads. The tests will detect the presence of LH in the urine 24–40 hours before ovulation, and thus provide a means to time conception. Intercourse or insemination is recommended the day after a positive test. Clinicians should keep in mind that this is not a test for ovulation. A midcycle surge in LH does not guarantee that ovulation and a normal luteal phase will follow.

Normal serum levels for pituitary gonadotropins during the normal menstrual cycle are illustrated above.

For clinical purposes, the following ranges are useful:

Clinical State	Serum FSH	Serum LH
Normal adult female	5–30 IU/L, with the ovulatory midcycle peak about 2 times the base level	5–20 IU/L, with the ovulatory midcycle peak about 3 times the base level
Hypogonadotropic state: Prepubertal, hypothalamic and pituitary dysfunction	Less than 5 IU/L	Less than 5 IU/L
Hypergonadotropic state: Postmenopausal, castrate and ovarian failure	Greater than 30 IU/L	Greater than 40 IU/L

Measurement of Blood Steroids

The normal levels for estradiol and progesterone during the normal menstrual cycle have been illustrated. Variation is seen from individual to individual, however, and the following ranges in gonadal steroids are normally reported:

	Estradiol	Progesterone	Testosterone
Follicular phase	25–75 pg/mL	Less than 1 ng/mL	20–80 ng/dL
Midcycle peak	200–600 pg/mL		20–80 ng/dL
Luteal phase	100–300 pg/mL	5–20 ng/mL	20–80 ng/dL
Pregnancy: 1st trimester	1–5 ng/mL	20–30 ng/mL	
Pregnancy: 2nd trimester	5–15 ng/mL	50–100 ng/mL	
Pregnancy: 3rd trimester	10–40 ng/mL	100–400 ng/mL	
Postmenopause	5–25 pg/mL	Less than 1 ng/mL	10–40 ng/dL

The immunoassay of 17-hydroxyprogesterone has replaced measurement of the urinary pregnanetriol level for the diagnosis of adrenal enzyme deficiency. Dramatic differences exist between normal individuals and patients with adrenal hyperplasia. Levels from 5 to 2,000 times greater than normal have been observed.

17-Hydroxyprogesterone	
Children	3–90 ng/dL
Adult females Follicular phase Luteal phase	15–70 ng/dL 35–290 ng/dL

The immunoassay of dehydroepiandrosterone sulfate (DHAS) has replaced the measurement of urinary 17-ketosteroids for the routine evaluation of adrenal androgen production. A random sample is sufficient, needing no corrections for body weight, creatinine excretion, or random variation. Variations are minimized because of its high circulating concentration and its long half-life. It is a direct measure of adrenal androgen activity correlating clinically with the urinary 17-ketosteroids. As with urinary 17-ketosteroids, aging is associated with a decrease in DHAS, accelerating after menopause with DHAS becoming almost undetectable after age 70.

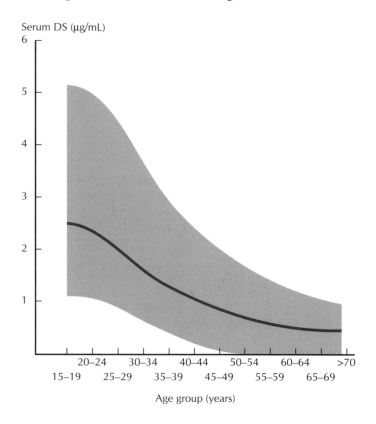

Urinary Steroid Assays

The measurement of estrogen in a 24-hour urine collection in the past was utilized during administration of human menopausal gonadotropins. Currently, there are no significant clinical uses for the measurement of estrogen in urine.

Total Urinary Estrogen	
Prepubertal	0–5 µg/24 hr
Follicular phase	10–25 µg/24 hr
Midcycle peak	35–100 µg/24 hr
Luteal phase	25–75 µg/24 hr
Postmenopausal	5–15 µg/24 hr

Pregnanediol is the main urinary metabolite of progesterone, although it accounts for only 7–20% of total progesterone production. Measurement of pregnanediol in a 24-hour urine sample has been used in the past to document pregnancy and especially the well-being of an early pregnancy. However, with the advent of the measurement of plasma progesterone, the use of urinary pregnanediol has waned.

Urinary Pregnanediol	
Follicular phase	Less than 1 mg/24 hr
Luteal phase	2–5 mg/24 hr
Pregnancy: 20 weeks	40 mg/24 hr
Pregnancy: 30 weeks	80 mg/24 hr
Pregnancy: 40 weeks	100 mg/24 hr

Pregnanetriol is the urinary metabolite of 17-hydroxyprogesterone and was used for the diagnosis of adrenal hyperplasia (the adrenogenital syndrome). Very little pregnanetriol is found in the urine of normal adults, but with the increased production of 17-hydroxyprogesterone due to an enzyme deficiency in the adrenal gland, increased urinary excretion of pregnanetriol will occur.

Urinary Pregnanetriol	
Children	Less than 0.5 mg/24 hr
Adults	0.2 to 2–4 mg/24 hr, the upper limit varying among laboratories

Measurement of Human Chorionic Gonadotropin

Secretion of human chorionic gonadotropin (HCG) by the syncytiotrophoblast cells of the placenta is predominantly into the maternal circulation. The assay of HCG in maternal urine has been the basis of pregnancy tests for many years. Aschheim and Zondek originated the bioassay pregnancy test in immature mice (the A-Z test) in 1922.

The biologic tests for HCG depended upon the response of ovaries or testes in immature animals (rabbits, rats, mice, frogs, and toads). This response was due to the gonadotropic properties of HCG and was measured either in terms of increased gonadal weight or hyperemia, or the secondary response in sex organs due to the increased gonadal steroidogenesis induced by the HCG. The expulsion of ova or sperm in amphibia was widely utilized as an end point for HCG. These biologic assays have now been succeeded by immunoassays for HCG in urine and blood.

HCG is similar to LH in its structure, and thus antibodies to the whole molecules cross-react with each other. The sensitivity of most commercial assays in the past had to be limited in order to avoid false positive tests due to cross-reactivity with LH. Modern assays utilizing highly specific monoclonal antibodies against the beta-subunit of HCG have a greater sensitivity and specificity. These antibodies are usually not directed to the unique C-terminal sequence of HCG, but to other sites on the molecule.

Most of HCG in the circulation is in the form of the intact hormone, and this is what is measured by immunoassays with beta-subunit antibodies. Small amounts of free alpha- and beta-subunits are also present. In the urine, a large fraction of HCG material is a metabolic fragment known as the "beta core" which consists of two polypeptide chains derived from the beta-subunit, joined by disulfide bridges. Fortunately, this fragment also reacts with the beta-subunit antibodies in immunoassays.

The most widely used current standard is the First International Reference Preparation provided by the World Health Organization. The 1st IRP succeeded the Second International Standard; 2 units of the 1st IRP are approximately equivalent to 1 unit of the 2nd IS. A third standard is appearing, the 3rd International Standard. Care must be taken in comparing values obtained in different assays with different standards.

An excellent assay can measure levels of HCG in nonpregnant premenopausal women in the range of 0.02–0.8 IU/L. HCG can be detected in the blood 7–9 days after the LH peak, 6–8 days after ovulation. A concentration of 100 IU/L is reached about the date of expected menses. Most clinical immunoassays for the β-subunit of HCG have a lower sensitivity of 2–5 IU/L. In general a titer less than 5 IU/L is assuredly a negative result, and a titer greater than 25 IU/L is a positive result. Values between 5 and 25 IU/L can be false positives and require verification.

Peak levels of HCG (mean values of 50,000 to 100,000 IU/L and a range of 20,000 to 200,000 IU/L) occur at 8–10 weeks of gestation, declining and remaining at approximately 10,000–20,000 IU/L by 12–14 weeks. Evaluation of a patient following a spontaneous or therapeutic abortion is occasionally a difficult problem. The urinary pregnancy test will be negative 3 weeks after abortion.

All current pregnancy tests measure HCG by an immunoassay of one type or another. The sensitivity of the rapid slide and dipstick tests is usually between 20 and 50 IU/L. Tests in this range of sensitivity can yield positive results even before the time of expected menses. Around the time of the expected period, these tests should be positive almost 100% of the time. This is quite a contrast to the situation in the 1960s when the most sensitive bioassay, the rabbit test, achieved a 75% rate of positive results not until the first week after the expected menses.

About the only cause of a false positive test is the modest increase in pituitary secretion of HCG after menopause. Modern tests are not affected by any interfering agents.

There are two clinical conditions in which blood HCG titers are very helpful, trophoblastic disease and ectopic pregnancies. Following molar pregnancies, in patients without persistent disease, the HCG titer should fall to a nondetectable level after 16 weeks. Patients with trophoblastic disease show an abnormal curve (a titer greater than 500 IU/L) frequently by 3 weeks and usually by 6 weeks.

Virtually 100% of patients suspected of an ectopic pregnancy, but not having the condition, will have a negative blood HCG assay. A positive test can also be utilized in diagnosis. The HCG level increases at different rates in normal and ectopic pregnancies. In a normal pregnancy the HCG should approximately double every 2 days in the 2–4 weeks after ovulation. When the HCG titer exceeds 1,000–1,500 IU/L, vaginal ultrasonograpy will identify the presence of an intrauterine gestation. When the HCG titer is below 1,500 IU/L and ultrasound examination fails to identify an intrauterine pregnancy, a patient may be managed expectantly if the HCG titer doubles in 2 days. If the titer does not double, an ectopic pregnancy must be suspected.

In clinical practice, these guidelines are not always so clear and definitive. The rate of HCG increase changes with advancing gestational age and increasing HCG concentrations. While the HCG level approximately doubles every 2 days below a level of 1,200 IU/L, from 1,200–6,000 IU/L, it takes nearly 3 days to double, and above 6,000 IU/L, about 4 days. In addition the zone at which a gestational sac is seen by ultrasound varies for different assays and different reference preparations. One should be sure that the discriminatory zone of 1,000–1,500 IU/mL applies to your local assay.

Measurement of 17-Ketosteroids, 17-Ketogenic Steroids, and 17-Hydroxy-corticoidsteroids

These assays provide essential clinical information, yet misunderstanding of their meaning and limitations is common. A basic appreciation for the methods and what they measure is necessary for the proper interpretation of these urinary assays.

A 24-hour urine specimen is required to avoid the variations in steroid excretion which occur throughout a day. Refrigeration is essential to avoid degradation of metabolites. It is wise to obtain a urinary creatinine as a check of the validity of the 24-hour collection. Urinary creatinine excretion is a reflection of body muscle mass and remains relatively constant, approximately 1,000 mg/24 hours.

The name "17-ketosteroids" (17-KS) is descriptive, designating compounds with a ketone group at the 17 position (C-17). The 17-KS are composed of the major urinary androgenic metabolites, but testosterone itself is not a 17-KS, and significant levels of testosterone may be associated with normal levels of 17-KS.

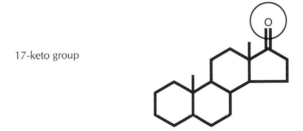

17-keto group

The commonly measured 17-ketosteroids are also known as the neutral 17-KS. Other compounds have a ketone group in the 17 position, but are not "neutral," for example, estrone. Estrone, due to its phenolic structure in ring A, is acidic, and therefore is removed from the urinary extract when washed with alkali in the procedure.

The 17-KS are divided into two groups: the major part being 11-deoxy-17-KS, produced by the gonads and adrenal cortex, and the 11-oxy-17-KS, produced *only* by the adrenal cortex.

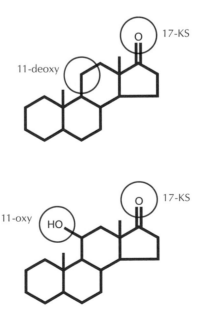

17-KS

11-deoxy

17-KS

11-oxy

The three major urinary 11-deoxy-17-KS and, therefore, the three major urinary metabolites of androgens are dehydroepiandrosterone (DHA), etiocholanolone, and androsterone. Note that the only difference between etiocholanolone and androsterone is the stereochemistry at the 5 position: alpha (α) in androsterone and beta (β) in etiocholanolone.

Dehydroepiandrosterone (DHA)

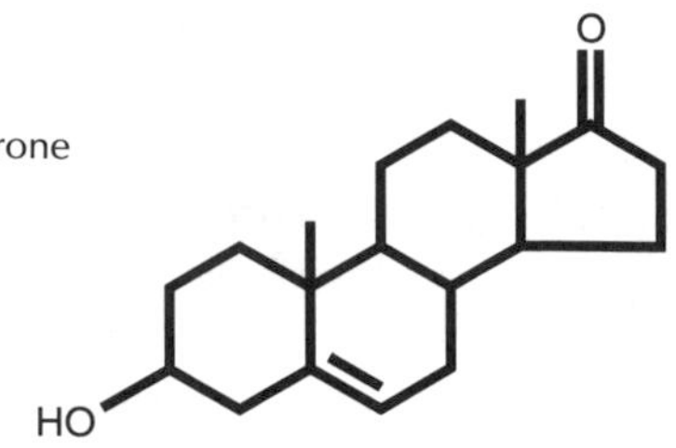

Etiocholanolone

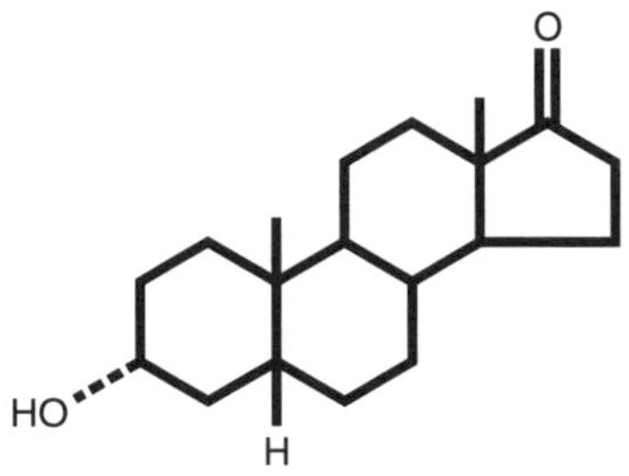

Androsterone

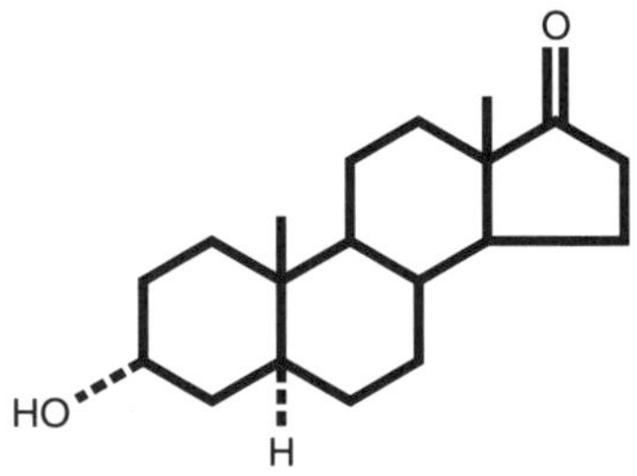

The major 11-oxy-17-KS are of adrenal origin: 11-hydroxyetiocholanolone and 11-ketoetiocholanolone (metabolites of corticosteroids) and 11β-hydroxyandrosterone (metabolite of 11β-hydroxyandrostenedione).

11β-Hydroxyandrosterone

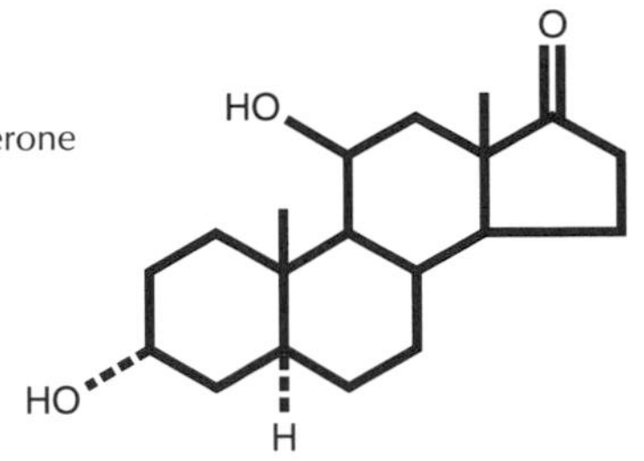

11-Hydroxyetiocholanolone

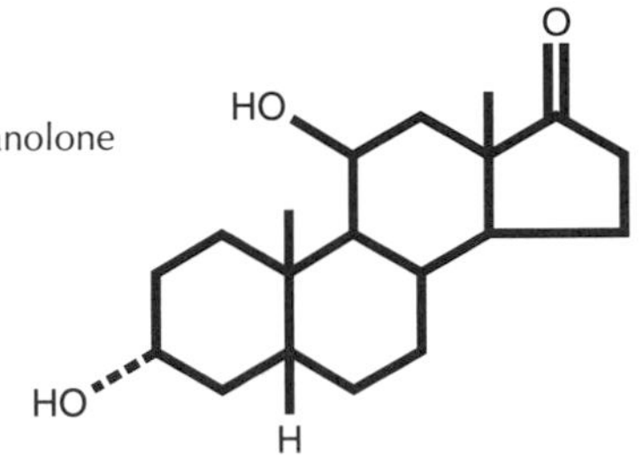

11-Ketoetiocholanolone

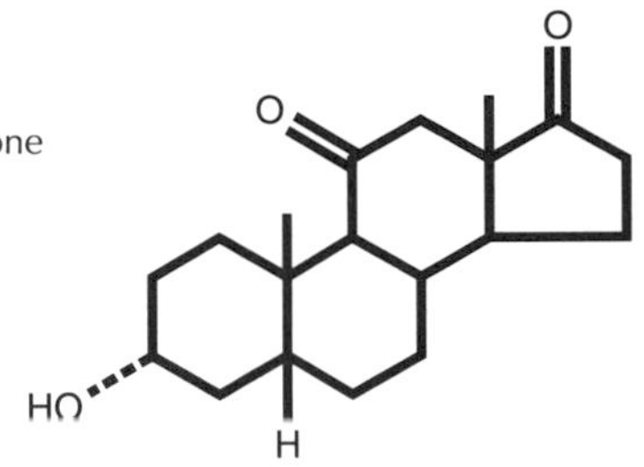

The majority of methods in clinical use for the assay of 17-KS include five major steps:

1. Hydrolysis of the 17-KS conjugates by acid to liberate the free steroids for extraction.

2. Extraction with organic solvents.

3. Removal of acidic material by washing with alkali.

4. Development of color, usually by the Zimmermann reaction (17-KS will give a purple color when treated with dinitrobenzene in the presence of alkali).

5. Measurement by colorimetric methods.

Normal 17-KS

The normal level of 17-ketosteroid excretion in a female is 10 ± 3 mg/24 hours. It should be kept in mind that excretion of 17-KS in the urine changes with age. This can be especially important in the evaluation of an elderly woman.

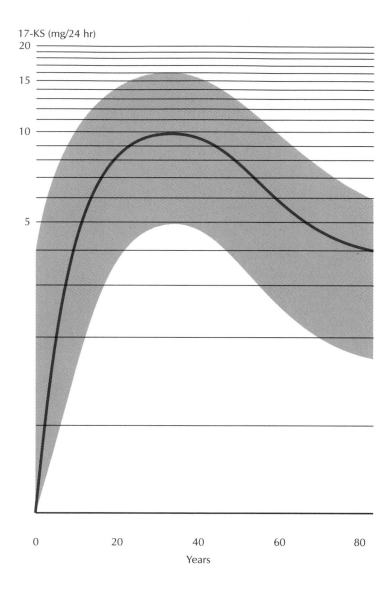

As stated above, the urinary 17-KS arise from precursors secreted by the adrenal cortex and the ovaries. In addition, a certain minimum of nonspecific pigments is present in every urine sample. The composition of normal 17-KS excretion is illustrated.

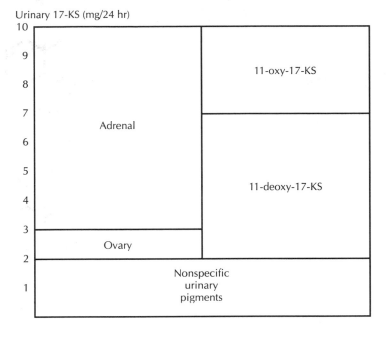

17-Ketogenic Steroids and 17-Hydroxycorticosteroids

17-Ketogenic steroid (17-KG) and 17-hydroxycorticosteroid (17-OHC) determinations measure urinary metabolites of glucocorticoids. There are significant differences in the two tests because more metabolites are measured by the 17-KG test.

The 17-KG and 17-OHC assays require the presence of a 17α-hydroxyl group. The mineralocorticoids (deoxycorticosterone (DOC), corticosterone (Compound B), and aldosterone) do not have a 17-hydroxyl group, and therefore are not measured in 17-KG and 17-OHC assays.

17-hydroxyl group

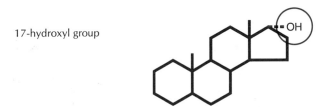

Deoxycorticosterone
(DOC)

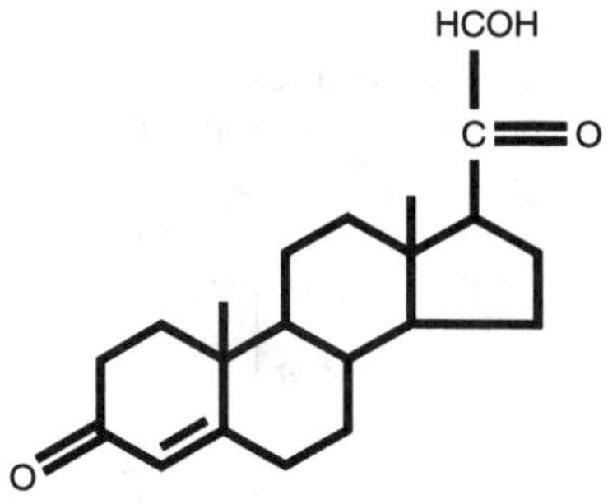

Corticosterone
(B)

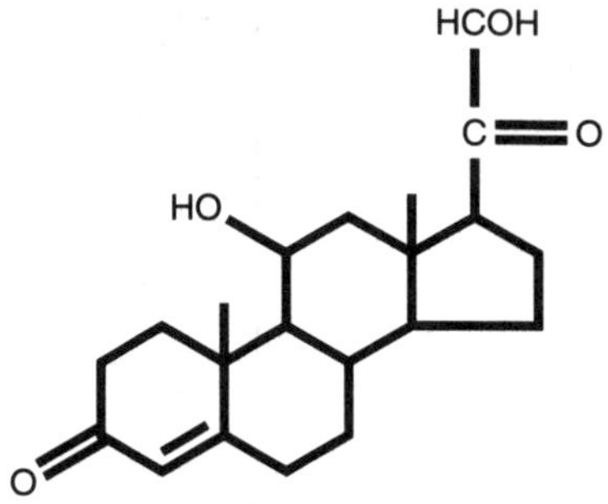

Aldosterone

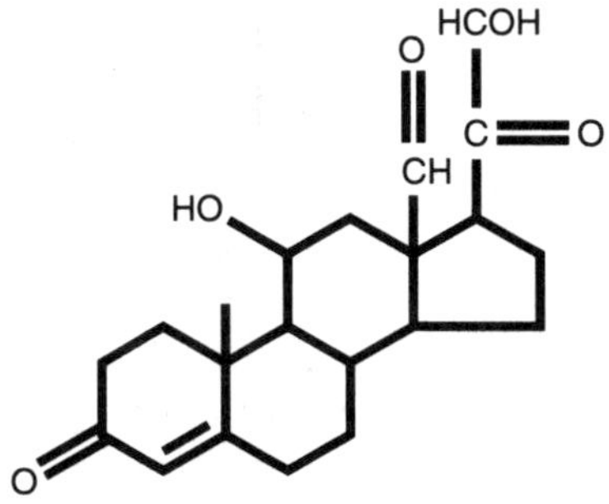

The principal glucocorticoid in the human is cortisol (hydrocortisone, Compound F). Cortisone (Compound E) is a metabolite of cortisol in the human.

Cortisol

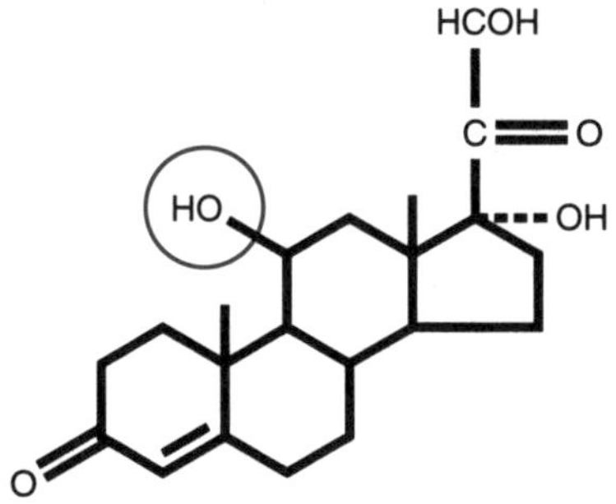

Cortisone

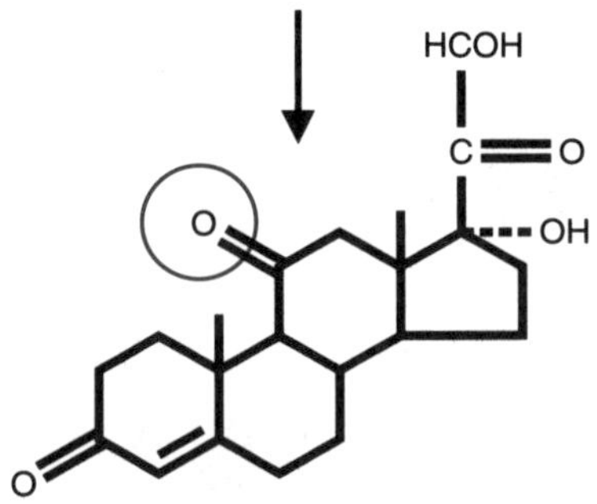

Enzymatic reductions produce the principal urinary metabolite of cortisol: tetra-hydrocortisol.

Cortisol

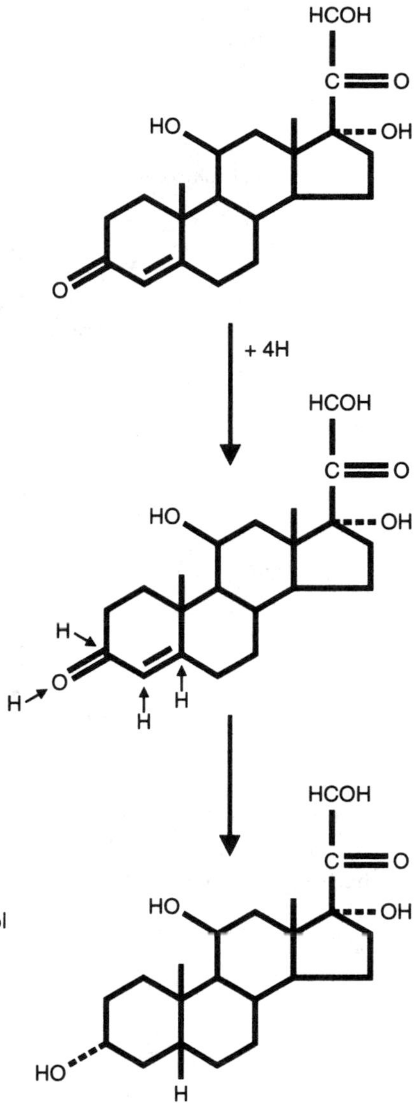

+ 4H

Tetrahydrocortisol

A similar reduction sequence applies to cortisone, yielding tetrahydrocortisone. Further reduction of tetrahydrocortisol and tetrahydrocortisone involves the ketone at the carbon-20 position, yielding cortol and cortolone.

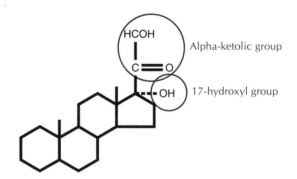

Tetrahydrocortisol

+ 2H

Cortol

The Porter-Silber reaction produces a color with phenylhydrazine and sulfuric acid. The reaction requires an alpha-ketolic group plus the 17-hydroxyl group. Therefore, a hydroxyl group must be at C-21 and C-17, and a ketone must be present at C-20. This reaction measures the 17-hydroxycorticosteroids, abbreviated as 17-OHC.

Alpha-ketolic group

17-hydroxyl group

The 17-OHC assay, therefore, cannot measure cortol and cortolone, the further reduction products of tetrahydrocortisol and tetrahydrocortisone, because the C-20 group is reduced and is not a ketone. Nor can the 17-OHC assay measure pregnanetriol since the α-ketolic group is not present.

Pregnanetriol

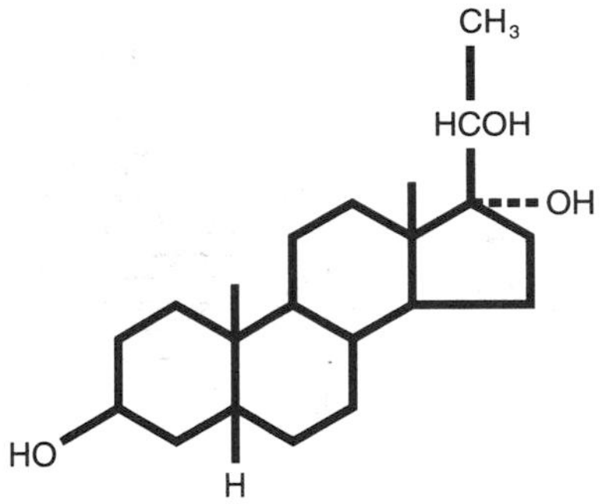

Normal 17-OHC

The normal urinary content of 17-hydroxycorticosteroids is 7 ± 3 mg/24 hours.

The 17-ketogenic (17-KG) steroids are compounds which, when oxidized with sodium bismuthate ($NaBiO_3$), give rise to 17-ketosteroids (17-KS), which can then be measured by the Zimmermann reaction. The initial measurement of 17-KS is subtracted, and the difference represents the 17-KG steroids. The requirement is a 17-hydroxyl group and a second hydroxyl group on either the C-20 or the C-21 position.

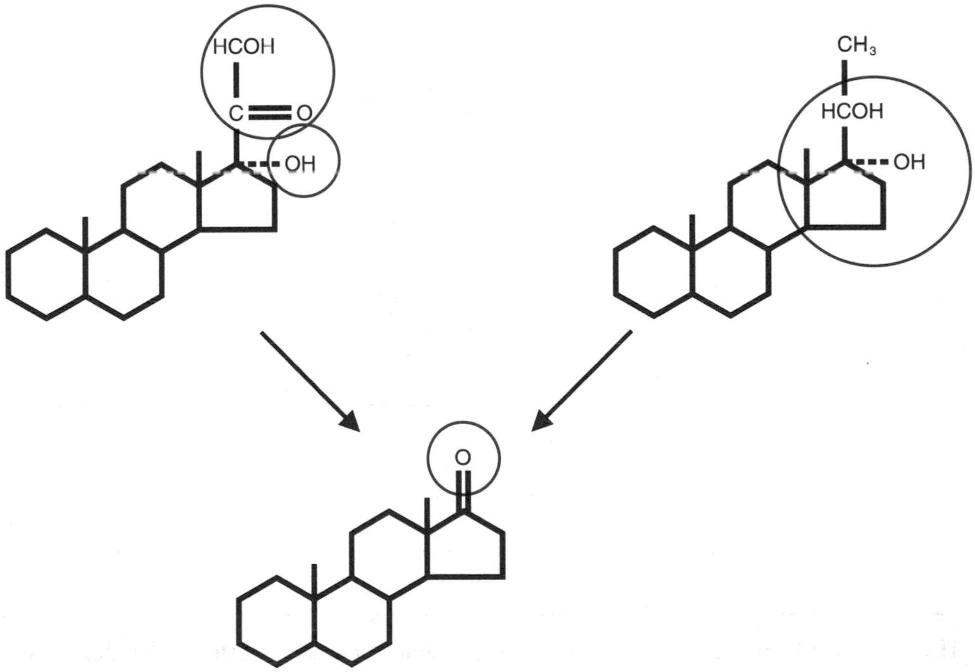

Therefore, the following compounds are measured: tetrahydrocortisol, tetrahydrocortisone, cortol, cortolone, and pregnanetriol (the latter three compounds are not measured in the 17-OHC assay). The compounds missing a 17-hydroxyl group, mainly mineralocorticoids (DOC, corticosterone, and aldosterone), will not be measured by either 17-OHC or 17-KG procedures.

Normal 17-KG

The normal urinary content of 17-KG is 10 ± 3 mg/24 hours. The measurement of additional steroids, when compared to the 17-OHC assay, may be troublesome in the adrenogenital syndrome where pregnanetriol excretion is elevated. Therefore, the 17-KG in the adrenogenital syndrome may be high, while the 17-OHC will be normal.

One should also keep in mind that values change with age.

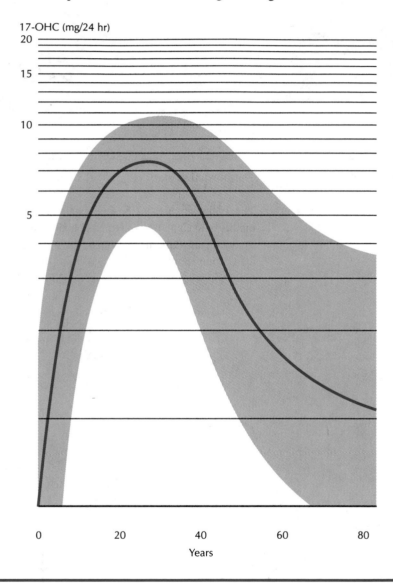

Adrenal Tests

The 24-Hour Urinary Free Cortisol

This measurement accurately reflects the daily production rate and the amount of cortisol which is free and active in the circulation. The normal value ranges from 20 to 90 µg/24 hours.

The Blood Cortisol Level

ACTH is secreted in a pulsatile fashion with the pulses being more frequent and of greater magnitude in the early morning hours, shortly before waking. A nadir in secretion is reached in the evening. Blood levels of ACTH and cortisol are highest in the early morning and lowest in the evening. When the sleep-awake cycle is altered, the diurnal rhythm shifts over about a week's time to resume the same sleep-awake pattern. A 8 AM, the normal plasma cortisol concentration ranges from 10 to 25 µg/dL. At 8 PM, the level is about half the morning concentration, and at 10 PM the level is usually less than 12 µg/dL.

The ACTH Stimulation Test

This is a test for adrenal reserve. Adrenal glands not exposed to ACTH over a long period of time will not have a normal response. Synthetic ACTH is injected in a bolus of 0.25 mg. The plasma cortisol should increase 2–3 times over baseline at 30 and 60 minutes.

The Metyrapone Test

This is a test for hypothalamic-pituitary-adrenal function (a test of ACTH reserve). Metyrapone blocks 11β-hydroxylase enzyme activity in the adrenal gland, thus interfering with cortisol production. After a baseline 24-hour urinary 17-hydroxycorticosteroid or plasma 11-deoxycortisol is obtained, metyrapone is given orally, 250 mg every 4 hours for 6 doses. The 17-OHC should at least double during the 24 hours of metyrapone administration or the next day. A plasma 11-deoxycortisol at 8 AM, 4 hours after the last dose of metyrapone, should exceed 7 µg/dL.

Index

Page numbers in **bold** denote figures or tables.

D

Dalkon Shield 778
Danazol
  endometriosis and 860–862
    recurrence 861
    success rates 861
  liver and 861
  mastalgia and 561
  multiple actions of 860
  side effects of 861
  structure of **860**
  treatment of infertility 861
  usual dose 861
De Graaf, Reinier 94
Decidua 125–126
Decidualization 118
Dehydroepiandrosterone **980**
  origin of 486
Dehydroepiandrosterone sulfate 255, 336, 976
  aging and 493
  hirsutism and 493–494
  hyperprolactinemia and 494
  marker for abnormal adrenal function 494
  origin of 486
Dehydrogenase
  17β-hydroxysteroid 42
  3β-hydroxysteroid 41
Dehydrogenase reactions 39
Delayed puberty 382–386
  history and physical examination 382
  laboratory assessments of 383–385
  relative frequency of abnormalities **384**
  treatment of 385–386
Demographics
  female **693**
Depletion
  of estrogen receptors 55
Depo Provera. *See* Medroxyprogesterone acetate
Depot-bromocriptine 429
Depression
  medroxyprogesterone acetate and 771
  menopause and 596
  oral contraception and 727, 744
Desensitization
  of adenylate cyclase 83
Deslorelin **160**
20-22-desmolase deficiency 334
Desmolase reaction 39
Desmopressin
  dysfunctional uterine bleeding and 540
Desogestrel **720**, 721
Development
  of anterior pituitary 172
  of kidney 325
  of müllerian system 110–111, 325
  of ovary 95
  of testes 97
  of urogenital sinus 98
  of urogenital tubercle 98
  of wolffian duct structures 98, 325
Dexamethasone 336
  clomiphene citrate and 906
  hirsutism and 506
  overnight test 492
DHA. *See* Dehydroepiandrosterone
DHAS. *See* Dehydroepiandrosterone sulfate
DHT. *See* Dihydrotestosterone

Diabetes
  gestational 273
Diabetes insipidus 164
  postoperative 428
Diabetes mellitus
  estrogen and 630
  hyperandrogenism and 475
  intrauterine device and 787
  noninsulin dependent 468
    estrogen and 608
  oral contraception and 726, 737, 743
  recurrent early pregnancy loss and 844
Diaphragm 797–799
  care of 799
  efficacy of 797
  failure rates 797
  fitting of 798
  gonorrhea and 798
  human immunodeficiency virus and 798
  pelvic inflammatory disease and 798
  side effects of 797–798
  timing of use 798–801
  toxic shock syndrome and 798
  tubal infertility and 798
  types of 798
  urinary tract infections and 797
  vaginal irritation and 797
Diazepam
  oral contraception and 742
Diethylstilbestrol
  breast cancer and 568
Diethylstilbestrol-associated anomaly 130
Differentiation
  of central nervous system 328
  of external genitalia 326–328
  of gonads 322–325
  of internal genitalia 330
  of müllerian system 325
  of Sertoli cell 97
  of testes, timing of 97, 324
  of wolffian system 98, 325
  stage of 96–98
Dihydrotestosterone 50, 327
  blood level of 51
  hair and 488
  mediation of androgen events 326–329
Dilantin
  oral contraception and 742
Dilatation and evacuation 710
Diplotene 5
Disappearing testis syndrome 345
Discriminatory zone 954
Dissociation rate
  of hormone-receptor complex 53
Diurnal rhythm
  of FSH and LH secretion 193
Djerassi, Carl 716
DNA
  base pair 7
  cloning 22–23
  complementary 13, 17
  double helix 7
  histone 8
  homeobox 9
  library 22
  molecule 6
  mutations of 15
  nucleosome 8